ENDOCRINE SURGERY

edited by

ARTHUR E. SCHWARTZ, M.D., F.A.C.S.
Clinical Professor of Surgery
Mount Sinai School of Medicine, New York University
New York, New York, U.S.A.

DEMETRIUS PERTSEMLIDIS, M.D., F.A.C.S.
Clinical Professor of Surgery
Mount Sinai School of Medicine, New York University
New York, New York, U.S.A.

MICHEL GAGNER, M.D., F.A.C.S.
Professor of Surgery
Chief, Division of Laparoscopic Surgery
Mount Sinai School of Medicine, New York University
New York, New York, U.S.A.

MARCEL DEKKER, INC. NEW YORK • BASEL

Library of Congress Cataloging-in-Publication Data
A catalog record for this book is available from the Library of Congress.

ISBN: 0-8247-4297-4

This book is printed on acid-free paper.

Headquarters
Marcel Dekker, Inc.
270 Madison Avenue, New York, NY 10016, U.S.A.
tel: 212-696-9000; fax: 212-685-4540

Distribution and Customer Service
Marcel Dekker, Inc.
Cimarron Road, Monticello, New York 12701, U.S.A.
tel: 800-228-1160; fax: 845-796-1772

Eastern Hemisphere Distribution
Marcel Dekker AG
Hutgasse 4, Postfach 812, CH-4001 Basel, Switzerland
tel: 41-61-260-6300; fax: 41-61-260-6333

World Wide Web
http://www.dekker.com

The publisher offers discounts on this book when ordered in bulk quantities. For more information, write to Special Sales/Professional Marketing at the headquarters address above.

Current printing (last digit):

10 9 8 7 6 5 4 3 2 1

PRINTED IN CANADA

To
Those who learn
Those who teach
Those who hope
Those who help

For Joan, who is always there, Nancy, Susan, and Emily. *Arthur E. Schwartz*

For my wife Lois and my sons Alexander and David. *Demetrius Pertsemlidis*

For my wife France Lapointe, my three sons, Xavier, Guillaume, and Maxime, with love. My father, Raymond Gagner, M.D., F.R.C.S.C., F.A.C.O.G., who inspired me to pursue a career in medicine and surgery. My mother Louise Duchaine and my three brothers, Francois, Richard, and Sebastien, for their support during all those years of studying and training. *Michel Gagner*

The encouragement, advice, and expertise of Mr. Robert Siegel, Dr. Alan Freedman, and Ms. Fran Shaller are gratefully acknowledged.

Foreword

Drs. Demetrius Pertsemlidis, Arthur E. Schwartz and Michel Gagner have assembled a distinguished faculty from the Mount Sinai School of Medicine in New York and an international cadre of "who's who" in endocrinology, to contribute to this comprehensive text.

This is much more than a book on endocrine surgery, focused as it is on covering all aspects of endocrinology. The text includes molecular endocrinology, pituitary, thyroid, parathyroid, adrenal, pancreatic and GI tract endocrine neoplasms, and concludes with an integrated review of multiple endocrine neoplasia. The presentation deals with each organ system, with a sequential concentration on pathology, imaging, individual syndromes, and surgical management in a very comprehensive manner. New approaches to imaging are succinctly summarized. Minimally invasive surgery and video-assisted surgery are counter-balanced by aggressive approaches to advanced disease, including organ transplantation and tumor debulking.

There should be something here for everyone interested in endocrine tumors, from diagnosis and localization to surgical approaches and nonsurgical management.

While heavily weighted to the Mount Sinai faculty, readers will find the contributions exciting, with some of the true international leaders featured within their own discipline. This provides a strong flavor of both standardized and alternative approaches to a series of complex diseases. For me, it was a pleasure to revisit areas of my own personal interest and I am sure other readers will similarly enjoy the vast array of information contained within this most attractive text.

In this age of increasing demands for clinical care, it is most encouraging to see clinicians committed to such a comprehensive and educational text.

Murray F. Brennan, M.D.
Chairman, Department of Surgery
Memorial Sloan-Kettering Cancer Center
New York, New York, U.S.A.

Preface

We offer an exposition of the current status of surgical care in the management of endocrine disorders. *Endocrine Surgery* includes a summary of present and evolving approaches to surgery of the pituitary, thyroid, parathyroid, adrenal, and pancreas. The text is comprehensive but not exhaustive, emphasizing practical approaches. Contributors with great experience have been encouraged to present logical differences in viewpoint, as well as controversies and alternative approaches to the management of problems. New diagnostic and therapeutic methods are brought to the attention of the reader. Operative techniques are presented and illustrated in detail.

The expanded understanding of endocrine disease, the increasing availability of sophisticated diagnostic methods, and the development of innovative surgical techniques, have changed the landscape of the management of endocrine disorders, profoundly influencing the practice of surgical endocrinology. Diagnostic capability expands at an exponential rate. The body is becoming virtually transparent as new x-ray imaging methods, radioisotope scanning, and ultrasound evolve rapidly. These techniques are presented, discussed, and illustrated.

New developments in surgery are stunning. Intraoperative hormone assays make it possible to confirm success while the patient is still on the operating table. Robotic surgery, made feasible by advanced computer capabilities and instant communication techniques, offers operative expertise at a great distance, and also constitutes a huge resource for surgical training. Small endoscopic instruments with intrinsic cameras can visualize almost any part of the body, giving surgeons access to nearly every organ, and in addition, to virtual spaces such as the hands, neck, retroperitoneal area, subcutaneous and intramuscular planes. The surgery can be executed through minimally invasive portals while the procedure is monitored on a television screen in real time.

Endocrine Surgery brings together the expertise of many authorities in their fields. It provides a perspective on present treatment and new developments. A practical summary of diagnostic methods, choices of management, and surgical techniques is offered that we hope will be helpful to those involved in the management of endocrine disorders.

Arthur E. Schwartz
Demetrius Persemlidis
Michel Gagner

Introduction: Science, Surgery, and the Endocrine Patient

Our generation learned little about RNA and DNA in medical school, considering it mostly irrelevant and arcane. How this attitude has changed! As young doctors we were overwhelmed by the seminal concept of immunoassay, pioneered by Berson and Yalow, that made it possible to determine the concentration of virtually any biological material with exquisite accuracy. The watershed development of monoclonal antibodies by Milstein enabled the fusion of myeloma cells, possessing an infinite ability to multiply, to B cells that secrete a specific antibody. This created a hybrid cell that continually produces a chosen, identifiable, monoclonal antibody. Unbelievable applications of such concepts were just beginning.

It was not until the beginning of the 1980s that molecular biology loomed large in our minds., and not until the 1990s that physicians realized that its relevance to clinical practice was enormous. It was then that seminars were organized to learn the new biology, making it possible for physicians to read and understand the many articles discussing the use of these new techniques.

At first blush it may seem that the rapid advances in molecular medicine have been so spectacular that by comparison the art and science of surgery have not moved an inch. But how wrong that is! If it had been suggested that a microscope would be useful at surgery or that large openings were not necessary for good views, surgeons, residents, and medical students at the time of our training would have laughed. Microsurgery of every organ is now possible. The introduction of endoscopic surgical approaches has been nothing but spectacular. Endoscopes as small as 2.7 mm in diameter offer great magnification and easy visualization in pituitary surgery. Every body cavity is accessible to this approach. Identification of small nerves and blood vessels is easy. Chest-splitting incisions can be avoided by a thoracoscopic approach to mediastinal parathyroid adenomas. Even virtual spaces, subcutaneous and intermuscular planes such as the neck, retroperitneum, and hand, can be explored endoscopically. No surgical subspecialty has been more affected by this enormous change than endocrine surgery.

1 MOLECULAR ENDOCRINOLOGY

Molecular endocrinology, the decoding and sequencing of the human genome, the development of our ability to manipulate genes, genetic engineering, and modern clinical technology will profoundly change our way of life. Our molecular understanding of endocrine diseases will continue to extend our therapeutic horizons. The study of intact organisms and cellular models is being supplanted by molecular genetics and new technology.

Development of a large biotechnology industry, combined with a new understanding of disease mechanisms, has resulted in successful treatments for a wide variety of diseases and holds even greater promise for others. The use of recombinant interferon in the treatment of hepatitis C and the stimulation of hematopoiesis by recombinant erythropoiesis in chronic renal failure are recent examples of the biotechnological approach. Within classical endocrinology, the development of human growth hormone and insulin comes to mind. The clinical use of recombinant thyrotropin

(TSH) in the search for thyroid-cancer metastases, monitoring the level of thyroglobulin to identify the presence and extent of recurrent disease, as well as the treatment of osteoporosis with recombinant parathyroid hormone augur an exciting and expanding horizon. The relationship of gene abnormalities, and the possibility of manipulating and altering them, offer promise in conditions such as hemophilia, cystic fibrosis, sickle cell anemia, Niemann-Pick disease, and others. At our own institution, a recent example involves Fabry disease, a painful and ultimately fatal metabolic disorder in which fatty deposits gradually clog the blood vessels of the heart, brain, and kidneys. The cause is a deficiency of the enzyme alpha-calactosidase A. The normal gene for this enzyme was isolated and a method developed to produce large quantities of the recombinant human enzyme. Clinical trials have demonstrated the enzyme replacement to be safe and effective.

There is evidence that schizophrenia and bipolar disease as well as many other conditions are a function of gene abnormalities. These deviations are certainly complex, but the aberrant mechanisms will ultimately be identified and ingenious methods devised for their treatment or prevention.

2 THE MALIGNANT CELL

The discovery of genes able to drive a cell into a cancerous state (oncogenes) and the concept that a normal cell may need multiple hits to activate a number of oncogenes before becoming malignant (multiple-hit hypothesis) have had an enormous impact on our understanding of cancer biology. But our understanding is far from complete and has still not yet translated in a large way into the clinical arena. The future holds great promise as drugs are developed to intercept oncogene signals and attempt to reverse the mutations a cell may develop. The preventive screening potential of these observation is huge (e.g., BRCA 1 and 2 breast cancer genes). The ability to predict diseases such as breast cancer, medullary thyroid carcinoma in multiple endocrine neoplasia (MEN) patients, and other forms of malignancy, in addition to noncancerous conditions such as Huntington's chorea, diabetes, and the glycogen storage diseases, engenders controversy concerning the ethics of knowing the risk profile of patients, but offers hope in their treatment and possible prevention.

The identification of cancer-screening proteins such as hCG, thyroglobulin, prostrate specific antigen, and the ovarian cancer antigens, combined with improved scanning procedures, has resulted in a more aggressive surgical approach to the control of cancer and its metastases. We can anticipate that future developments will enable the treatment of many more conditions at an early or even incipient stage. Witness the successful prevention of medullary carcinoma by thyroidectomy in MEN patients with C cell hyperplasia as early as 6 years of age, made possible by the widespread application of calcitonin immunoassays. Other conditions will surely follow.

3 THERAPEUTIC DRUGS

The development of ingenious and potent drugs by a robust pharmaceutical industry is changing the panorama of modern medicine. The prevention of gastric acid secretion, control of prostatic hypertrophy, more powerful anti-inflammatory drugs, new classes of drugs for diabetes, monoclonal antibodies to prevent myocardial thrombosis and inflammation, and more powerful immunosuppressants and chemotherapeutic agents are examples of recent success; all have reduced the number of patients needing surgery.

In addition, large-scale epidemiological studies of medical and surgical therapies are demonstrating that applications that appear to be sensible at first sight may in the end prove to have adverse effects, to wit, the downside of female hormone replacement therapy and the ineffectiveness of arthroscopic surgery for osteoarthritis of the knee It has taken years to discover that drugs such as cortisone, thalidomide, nicotine, and cocaine have their risks as well as benefits. Bloodletting was employed for generations until it was shown to do more harm than good. The concept of long-term, controlled, double-blind studies has emerged as an invaluable research tool to develop evidence-based approaches.

Problems such as an effective diet for weight control (e.g., the relative importance of fat and carbohydrates) remain to be evaluated. Intestinal bypasses and banding procedures for morbid obesity can now be performed endoscopically through minimal incisions and offer good treatment when indicated. But obesity itself is certainly a metabolic dysfunction that will eventually be managed by physiological means. The recognition that the hormone PPY, originating in the small intestine, switches off the urge to eat is the forerunner of others. An understanding of the metabolic causes of obesity will lead to the therapy of the future.

4 ANESTHESIA

Anesthesia has progressed to a point that extensive operation can be undertaken with ever-decreasing risk.

Local anesthesia has had a resurgence, particularly for minimally invasive procedures. Adjuncts such as propofol, midazolam, and fentanyl make local anesthesia much more comfortable for the patient as well as the surgeon. Regional nerve block can also be used effectively, particularly in neck surgery. In addition, many new and effective agents, as well as technical developments such as the pulse oximeter for the continuous monitoring of oxygen saturation, have made anesthesia much safer.

5 ORGAN TRANSPLANTATION

Transplantation of tissues and organs is developing at an exciting pace: the replacement of pancreas, heart and lungs (sometimes together), bowel, and liver and kidney (at times combined) are becoming routine. The pioneers of transplantation are all in debt to the development of powerful immunosuppressants and the sophisticated knowledge of how to use such drugs, as well as the advances in surgical techniques of anastamoses, prostheses, and the use of cadaveric tissues. The concept of delivering transplanted infused cells to treat disease is anticipated with excitement (e.g., islet cells for diabetes and the return of cells to the patient after gene transfer).

In addition to the technical aspects of transplantation, large organizational networks are required to procure tissues and distribute them effectively and equitably. These are being developed to an ever-greater extent, and we marvel at the progress.

6 STEM CELLS AND ARTIFICIAL ORGANS

Despite the political, religious, and ethical aspects of stem cells, there can be no doubt that the potential for their therapeutic use is enormous. In endocrinology, the replacement of hormone-secreting cells would be seminal. Such possibilities are on the horizon. Whether cells are engineered or grown from stem cells is unlikely to matter, as long as they work long term and are not subject to immune attack. The indentification of insulin-secreting stem cells and dopamine-secreting stem cells are obvious areas of hope in the management of diabetes and Parkinson's disease. More technological development is needed, but the future is inevitable. The success of cloning in a variety of mammals is now well established. If we can clone a whole animal it is likely that we can clone individual cell supplies and organs for each future patient. What a different world it will be when we can grow whatever organ we each need and replace the damage rendered by disease and age.

7 SERUM AND CELL MARKERS OF DISEASE

The identification and sensitive measurement of a wide variety of molecular and metabolic markers have been other emblems of modern medicine. With increasing frequency, the diagnosis or suspicion of disease is based on the chemistry of a patient rather than the physical examination. The success of parathyroid surgery can now be confirmed intraoperatively by very rapid assays of parathormone, taking advantage of its 3-minute half–life. Intraoperative adrenocorticotropic hormone confers the same advantage in surgery for Cushing's disease. The identification of disease markers offers powerful future possibilities. Serum calcitonin in medullary thyroid cancer, thyroglobulin in thyroid cancer, and prostate specific antigen have been noted earlier. More are needed.

8 IMAGING

The development of CT and MRI scanning is taken for granted because we use them every day, but these have been amazing advances over classical radiology. Even the coronary arteries can now be examined by such techniques. This approach, as well as other new noninvasive methods, will certainly be extended to a variety of additional sites and organs.

Isotopic scintigraphic methods that permit the identification of the anatomical site and function of primary tumors and metastatic disease are becoming increasingly useful in distinguishing benign from malignant tumors. Molecular serum and cellular markers with high-resolution noninvasive or invasive imaging make it possible to diagnose and localize endocrine tumors and nonneoplastic hypersecretory states of the adrenals and pancreas.

Ultrasound is invaluable in the preoperative diagnosis of pancreatic and adrenal lesions. The intraoperative use of ultrasound can effectively guide the surgical excision of adrenal tumors. In addition, laparoscopic ultrasound can successfully identify lesions deep within the parenchyma of the pancreas, such as islet cell adenomas. Intraoperative use of ultrasound for localization of tumors in the adrenal, pancreas, and liver during celiotomy or laparoscopy has virtually eliminated preoperative angiography and transportal selective venous sampling with their inherent risks.

The use of scintigraphy for the imaging and locating of parathyroid tumors has become the standard of care. PET and octreotide scans are becoming routine in the management of a variety of malignancies.

Indeed, the accuracy of imaging (CT, MRI, and ultrasound) has advanced to the point that masses are revealed that do not have clinical significance ("incidentalomas"), with the accompanying danger of unnecessary surgical procedures. Does every nonpalpable thyroid nodule require intervention? At what point should incidental nodules in the adrenal or kidney be removed? The parameters to decide when intervention is required are still being developed.

Real-time imaging using sonography and scintigraphy has made a great impact on everyday medicine. Equipment has been miniaturized and the images greatly improved. These modalities make more accurate needle biopsies possible. They have dramatically influenced the information available to the surgeon, many of whom perform the imaging themselves in their offices or at the operating table, for example, as an aid in exploration for parathyroid adenomas or pancreatic lesions.

9 NEEDLE BIOPSIES

Surgeons and physicians have become more aggressive at obtaining needle aspirates from diverse sites, including the thyroid, adrenal, breast, pancreas, lung, liver, and even parathyroids. Nevertheless, most of these samples continue to rely on crude morphological descriptions of the cell types obtained. While sometimes the diagnosis can be confirmed by immunoassay of the aspirate or immunohistochemical assessment (e.g., validation of a parathyroid adenoma by the presence of PTH), such an approach in the absence of specific cancer antigens has been limited. We badly need a technological revolution in the examination of cell aspirates that will utilize the molecular techniques that are becoming available. Needle aspiration biopsies can allow the amplifications of all the genomic and expressed genes present in the sample. Specific amplification of DNA and RNA by the polymerase chain reaction (PCR) now permits the amplification of known genes (DNA) and/or the expressed genes (RNA) present in the samples. This approach should provide a more scientific assessment of many biopsies. T-cell receptors and many other genes have been amplified in this way from tissue aspirates, but the diagnostic applications of these initial attempts have yet to be exploited.

10 BIOINFORMATICS AND IMAGE TRANSFER

Transmission of images on the Internet and robotic surgery loom large in the foreseeable future as methods of enormous capability. All our information is now on the computer. We no longer have x-ray films; we just consult the screen. Laboratory results are available instantly. You can look up the last 500 patients with hypercalcemia at the push of a button. Information is available in vast quantities and with ease. What is more, you can see all this in your home office or on your laptop while traveling. Such changes have engendered new ways of investigating and managing many diseases and have raised patient's expectations. The information can be made useful at remote locations. Long-distance consultations are readily available. The performance of surgery by robotic methods makes it possible for the operating surgeon to be a continent away.

11 NEW SURGICAL TECHNIQUES

There have been many improvements in surgical techniques, but there is little doubt that the horizon has expanded with the miniaturization of instrumentation, the availability of large screen displays to view surgery as it is performed, and the expanding use of endoscopic methods with video cameras that provide great magnification. Whether it means operating on the pituitary gland with miniature instruments under magnification via an endoscope 3 mm or less in diameter, using endoscopic techniques to remove a thyroid nodule, or performing and intestinal bypass for obesity, the sophistication of these approaches is astounding. And there is more to come. We have certainly not reached the limits of miniaturization, and the promises of in situ scanning and in situ malignant cell identification remain to be exploited.

The endocrine glands, often small in size, are especially suited to the use of endoscopic techniques. These glands secrete hormones that sustain our metabolism; derangements can have devastating effects. Tumors of the pituitary and parathyroid glands as small as several millimeters can be responsible for severe illness.

The modest size of many endocrine tumors facilitates removal by endoscopic approaches. Many are benign and therefore suitable for removal by enucleation or resection. Frequently no reconstruction is required. Endoscopes a few millimeters in diameter are available for these procedures and can be combined with an operating microscope. The magnification that these instruments offer makes the surgery easier and safer. It is possible to employ innovative anatomical approaches such as a nasal approach to the pituitary through the sphenoid bone or a retroperitoneal endoscopic approach to the adrenal tumors. Minimally invasive surgery has become the standard of care for benign adrenal tumors and nonmalignant tumors of the distal pancreas.

12 THE FUTURE

In early years an exploration for hyperparathyroidism was a trying and difficult affair requiring a long and extensive search for enlarged parathyroid glands that might, or might not, be in their normal location. It was not unusual for the diagnosis to be wrong because it was made based on clinical features that frequently overlapped other conditions. No biochemical confirmatory test was available. There were many disheartening outcomes to the surgery.

Compare that to what is at hand today. The diagnosis is easily established with precise accuracy by immunoassay of PTH. The location of the diseased gland is now frequently known preoperatively, using scintigraphy, ultrasound, MRI with gadolinium, CT scanning, or selective venous sampling for reexplorations—a range of choices previously unknown. The surgery is performed through minimal incisions or even via an endoscope. It can be performed under local anesthesia, if desired. When an abnormal gland is excised, a rapid parathormone assay can establish cure while the patient is still on the operating table.

Fear of surgery has diminished; expectations of patients and their physicians have increased. It appears that surgeons have mostly delivered. Progress in surgical techniques is likely to continue. Benign prostatic hypertrophy is now being treated with microwaves, often removing the need for surgery. Hormone replacement by tissue preservation and stem cell transplantation will eventually become a reality.

The development of robotic techniques and advanced intraoperative imaging, together with continuing progress in miniaturization, are all in play at this time without even considering the likely advances in transplantation. Robotic surgery is in its infancy offering a huge potential to make quality precision surgery available throughout the world. New computer-enhanced surgical systems, which use sensitive remote-controlled surgical instruments, guided by a surgeon who may be miles away at a computer keyboard, are rapidly evolving in the field of cardiac and abdominal surgery. Adrenalectomies and partial resections of the pancreas have already been performed using these devices. These systems also permit the availability of expertise, by remote control, to use virtual reality in the teaching of operative procedural techniques and preparing new surgeons for rare situations and challenges.

The future is bright!

Terry F. Davies, M.D., F.R.C.P.
Arthur E. Schwartz, M.D., F.A.C.S.
Demetrius Pertsemlidis, M.D., F.A.C.S.
Michel Gagner, M.D., F.A.C.S., F.R.C.S.C.

Contents

Contributors

Håkan Ahlman, M.D., Ph.D. Professor, Department of Surgery, Sahlgrenska University Hospital, Göteborg, Sweden

David C. Aron, M.D., M.S. Professor, Medicine and Epidemiology and Biostatistics, Division of Clinical and Molecular Endocrinology, Department of Medicine, Case Western Reserve University School of Medicine, and Center for Quality Improvement Research, Louis Stokes Department of Veterans Affairs Medical Center, Cleveland, Ohio, U.S.A.

Ahmad Assalia, M.D. Division of Minimally Invasive Surgery, Department of Surgery, Mount Sinai School of Medicine, New York University, New York, New York, U.S.A.

Maha T. Barakat, M.B.B.Chir., M.A., Ph.D., M.R.C.P. Clinical Lecturer, Division of Investigative Science, Department of Metabolic Medicine, Imperial College London, London, England

Angela R. Berning, M.D. Fellow in Body MRI, Department of Radiology, Mount Sinai School of Medicine, New York University, New York, New York, U.S.A.

Piero Berti, M.D. Department of Surgery, University of Pisa, Pisa, Italy

Laurent Biertho, M.D. Department of Abdominal Surgery, Les Cliniques Saint Joseph, Liege, Belgium

John P. Bilezikian, M.D. Professor of Medicine and Pharmacology and Chief, Division of Endocrinology, College of Physicians and Surgeons, Columbia University, New York, New York, U.S.A.

Stephen R. Bloom, M.A., M.D., D.Sc., F.R.C.Path., F.R.C.P, F.Med.Sci. Professor of Medicine, Division of Investigative Science, Department of Metabolic Medicine, Imperial College London, London, England

H. Jaap Bonjer, M.D., Ph.D. Professor, Department of Surgery, Erasmus Medical Center, Rotterdam, The Netherlands

Margaret Brandwein-Gensler, M.D. Associate Professor, Department of Pathology, Mount Sinai School of Medicine, New York University, New York, New York, U.S.A.

Christine A. Chu, M.D. Bay Area Surgical Associates, Inc., and John Muir/Mount Diablo Health System, Walnut Creek, California, U.S.A.

Terry F. Davies, M.D., F.R.C.P. Florence and Theodore Baumritter Professor and Director, Division of Endocrinology, Diabetes and Bone Diseases, Department of Medicine, Mount Sinai School of Medicine, New York University, New York, New York, U.S.A.

Stephen E. Dolgin, M.D. Professor and Chief, Pediatric Surgery, Department of Surgery, Mount Sinai School of Medicine, New York University, New York, New York, U.S.A.

Laura Bertani Dziedzic, Ph.D. Clinical Assistant Professor, Department of Medicine, Mount Sinai School of Medicine, New York University, New York, New York, U.S.A.

Stanley Walter Dziedzic, M.D., Ph.D. Clinical Assistant Professor, Department of Medicine, Mount Sinai School of Medicine, New York University, New York, New York, U.S.A.

Guido Eibl, M.D. Associate Researcher, Division of General Surgery, David Geffen School of Medicine at UCLA, Los Angeles, California, U.S.A.

Stephen G. Farrell, M.B.B.S., F.R.A.C.S. Visiting Medical Officer, Department of Surgery, University of Melbourne, and Endocrine Surgery Unit, St. Vincent's Hospital, Melbourne, Australia

Sander S. Florman, M.D. Assistant Professor, Department of Surgery, Recanati/Miller Transplantation Institute, Mount Sinai School of Medicine, New York University, New York, New York, U.S.A.

J. Lester Gabrilove, M.D. Florence and Theodore Baumritter Professor of Medicine Emeritus, Division of Endocrinology, Diabetes and Bone Diseases, Department of Endocrinology, Mount Sinai School of Medicine, New York University, New York, New York, U.S.A.

Michel Gagner, M.D., F.A.C.S., F.R.C.S.C. Franz W. Sichel Professor of Surgery, Chief, Division of Laparoscopic Surgery, Director, Minimally Invasive Surgery Center, Mount Sinai School of Medicine, New York University, New York, New York, U.S.A.

Jeffrey P. Goldman, M.D. Assistant Professor, Department of Radiology, Mount Sinai School of Medicine, New York University, New York, New York, U.S.A.

John R. Gosney, D.Sc., M.D., F.R.C.Path. Consultant Thoracic Pathologist, Honorary Reader in Thoracic Pathology, Department of Pathology, Royal Liverpool University Hospital, Liverpool, England

Loukas Gourgiotis, M.D. Clinical Endocrinology Branch, National Institute of Diabetes and Digestive and Kidney Diseases, National Institute of Health, Bethesda, Maryland, U.S.A.

Sydney S. Guo, M.D. Resident, Department of Surgery, West Los Angeles Veterans Administration Hospital and David Geffen School of Medicine at UCLA, Los Angeles, California,U.S.A.

Richard S. Haber, M.D. Associate Professor of Medicine, Division of Endocrinology, Diabetes and Bone Diseases, Department of Medicine, Mount Sinai School of Medicine, New York University, New York, New York, U.S.A.

Per Hellman, M.D., Ph.D. Associate Professor, Department of Surgery, University Hospital, Uppsala, Sweden

Jean-François Henry, M.D. Professor, Division of General and Endocrine Surgery, Hôpital de la Timone, Marseille, France

Oscar J. Hines, M.D. Associate Professor, Division of General Surgery, David Geffen School of Medicine at UCLA, Los Angeles, California, U.S.A.

William B. Inabnet, M.D., F.A.C.S. Assistant Professor, Division of Laparoscopic Surgery, Minimally Invasive Surgery Center, Mount Sinai School of Medicine, New York University, New York, New York, U.S.A.

Brian P. Jacob, M.D. Division of Laparoscopic Surgery, Minimally Invasive Surgery Center, Mount Sinai School of Medicine, New York University, New York, New York, U.S.A.

Mark Kidd, Ph.D. Post-Doctoral Fellow, Department of Surgery, Yale University School of Medicine, New Haven, Connecticut, U.S.A.

Job Kievit, M.D., Ph.D. Associate Professor of Surgery and Professor and Head of the Medical Decision Making Unit Section, Endocrine/Head and Neck Surgery, Departments of Surgery and Medical Decision Making, Leiden University Medical Center, Leiden, The Netherlands

Chun Ki Kim, M.D. Associate Professor of Radiology, Division of Nuclear Medicine, Mount Sinai School of Medicine, New York University, New York, New York. U.S.A.

Wesley A. King, M.D. Associate Professor, Department of Neurosurgery, Mount Sinai School of Medicine, New York University, New York, New York, U.S.A.

Borys R. Krynyckyi, M.D. Assistant Professor of Radiology, Division of Nuclear Medicine, Department of Radiology, Mount Sinai School of Medicine, New York University, New York, New York, U.S.A.

Kevin Lye, M.D. Resident, Department of Surgery, Yale University School of Medicine, New Haven, Connecticut, U.S.A.

John A. Lynn, M.S., F.R.C.S. Consultant Endocrine Surgeon and Honorary Senior Lecturer, Department of Surgery, Imperial College London, London, England

Josef Machac, M.D. Professor, Division of Nuclear Medicine, Department of Radiology, Mount Sinai School of Medicine, New York University, New York, New York, U.S.A.

Gabriele Materazzi, M.D. Department of Surgery, University of Pisa, Pisa, Italy

Ernest L. Mazzaferri, M.D., M.A.C.P. Emeritus Professor and Chairman of Medicine, Department of Medicine, Ohio State University, Columbus, Ohio, and Adjunct Professor of Medicine, Department of Medicine, University of Florida, Gainesville, Florida, U.S.A.

Jeffrey I. Mechanick, M.D., F.A.C.P., F.A.C.E., F.A.C.N. Associate Clinical Professor of Medicine, Division of Endocrinology, Diabetes and Bone Diseases, Department of Medicine, Mount Sinai School of Medicine, New York University, New York, New York, U.S.A.

David S. Mendelson, M.D. Associate Professor, Department of Radiology, Mount Sinai School of Medicine, New York University, New York, New York, U.S.A.

Paolo Miccoli, M.D. Professor, Clinical Chair, Department of Surgery, University of Pisa, Pisa, Italy

Harold A. Mitty, M.D. Professor, Department of Radiology, Mount Sinai School of Medicine, New York University, New York, New York, U.S.A.

Irvin M. Modlin, M.D., Ph.D., F.A.C.S., F.R.C.S. Proofessor, Department of Surgery, Yale University School of Medicine, New Haven, Connecticut, U.S.A.

Kjell Öberg, M.D., Ph.D. Professor, Department of Endocrine Oncology, Uppsala University Hospital, Uppsala, Sweden

Michael Olausson, M.D., Ph.D. Professor, Department of Surgery, Sahlgrenska University Hospital, Göteborg, Sweden

John A. Olson, Jr., M.D., Ph.D. Assistant Professor, Department of Surgery, Duke University Medical Center, Durham, North Carolina, U.S.A.

Neeta Pandit-Taskar, M.D. Department of Radiology, Memorial Sloan-Kettering Cancer Institute, New York, New York, U.S.A.

Aman B. Patel, M.D. Assistant Professor, Departments of Neurosurgery and Radiology, Mount Sinai School of Medicine, New York University, New York, New York, U.S.A.

David S. Pertsemlidis, M.D. Assistant Clinical Professor, Department of Surgery, Mount Sinai School of Medicine, New York University, New York, New York, U.S.A.

Demetrius Pertsemlidis, M.D., F.A.C.S. Clinical Professor, Department of Surgery, Mount Sinai School of Medicine, New York University, New York, New York, U.S.A.

Kalmon D. Post, M.D. Professor and Chairman, Department of Neurosurgery, Mount Sinai School of Medicine, New York University, New York, New York, U.S.A.

Charles A. G. Proye, M.D., F.R.C.S. Ed. (Hon.) Professor of Surgery, Department of Medicine, University of Lille II, and Department of Endocrine Surgery, Hôpital Claude Huriez, Lille, France

Daniel F. Roses, M.D. Jules Leonard Whitehill Professor of Surgery and Co-Director, Division of Oncology, Department of Surgery, New York University School of Medicine and Attending Surgeon, Tisch Hospital, New York University Medical Center, New York, New York, U.S.A.

Francesco Rubino, M.D. IRCAD-European Institute of Telesurgery, Strasbourg, France

Nicholas J. Sarlis, M.D., Ph.D., F.A.C.E., F.A.C.P. Division of Intramural Research, National Institutes of Diabetes, Digestive and Kidney Diseases, National Institute of Health, Bethesda, Maryland, U.S.A.

Mark P. Sawicki, M.D. Associate Professor, Department of Surgery, West Los Angeles Veterans Administration Hospital and David Geffen School of Medicine at UCLA, Los Angeles, California, U.S.A.

Arthur E. Schwartz, M.D., F.A.C.S. Clinical Professor of Surgery, Mount Sinai School of Medicine, New York University, New York, New York, U.S.A.

Myron E. Schwartz, M.D. Professor, Department of Surgery, Recanati/Miller Transplantation Institute, Mount Sinai School of Medicine, New York University, New York, New York, U.S.A.

Frédéric Sebag, M.D. Division of General and Endocrine Surgery, Hôpital de la Timone, Marseille, France

Bruno Sgromo, M.D. Department of Surgery, Erasmus Medical Center, Rotterdam, The Netherlands

Ashok Shaha, M.D. F.A.C.S. Professor, Department of Surgery, Cornell Medical School, and Attending Surgeon, Memorial Sloan-Kettering Cancer Institute, New York, New York, U.S.A.

Raj K. Shrivastava, M.D. Department of Neurosurgery, Mount Sinai School of Medicine, New York University, New York, New York, U.S.A.

Shonni J. Silverberg, M.D. Clinical Professor of Medicine, Division of Endocrinology, College of Physicians and Surgeons, Columbia University, New York, New York, U.S.A.

William L. Simpson, Jr., M.D. Assistant Professor, Department of Radiology, Mount Sinai School of Medicine, New York University, New York, New York, U.S.A.

Sotirios G. Stergiopoulos, M.D. Research Associate, Unit on Genetics and Endocrinology, Developmental Endocrinology Branch, National Institutes of Child Health and Human Development and National Institute of Health, Bethesda, Maryland, U.S.A.

Constantine A. Stratakis, M.D., D.Sc. Section of Endocrinology and Genetics, Developmental Endocrinology Branch, National Institute of Child Health and Human Development, National Institute of Health, Bethesda, Maryland, U.S.A.

Lars-Erik Tisell, M.D., Ph.D. Retired Chief of Endocrine Surgery, Department of Surgery, Sahlgrenska University Hospital, Göteborg, Sweden

David J. Torpy, M.D., M.B.B.S., Ph.D., F.R.A.C.P. Associate Professor, Unit of Genetics and Endocrinology, Developmental Endocrinology Branch, National Institutes of Child Health and Human Development, National Institute of Health, Bethesda, Maryland, U.S.A.

Pamela Unger, M.D. Associate Professor, Department of Pathology, Mount Sinai School of Medicine, New York University, New York, New York, U.S.A.

Moritz N. Wente, M.D. Resident, Department of General Surgery, University of Heidelberg, Heidelberg, Germany

Hsu-Chong Yeh, M.D. Department of Radiology, Mount Sinai School of Medicine, New York University, New York, New York, U.S.A.

Samuel D. J. Yeh, M.D. Professor, Department of Radiology, Memorial Sloan-Kettering Cancer Institute, and Associate Professor, Weill School of Medicine, Cornell Medical School, New York, New York, U.S.A.

1

Molecular Endocrinology

Nicholas J. Sarlis* and Loukas Gourgiotis

National Institute of Health, Bethesda, Maryland, U.S.A.

1 INTRODUCTION

Molecular endocrinology is the domain of biomedical science focused on the study of mechanisms underlying (1) hormone synthesis and secretion, (2) hormone action, (3) the ontogenesis of the endocrine system, and (4) the pathogenesis of various endocrine disorders at the cellular, molecular, and genetic levels. Hormones are defined as molecules synthesized and secreted by specialized cells within the endocrine organs, diffuse cellular groups with endocrine function (e.g., the neuropeptide-producing cells within the gastrointestinal tract and the bronchial tree), or—in selected cases—other nonendocrine organs [e.g., erythropoietin (EPO) secretion from the renal cortex and atrial natriuretic peptide from cardiac myocytes] (1). Hormones exert their action (1) at a distance from their site of origin after their release into the circulation and eventual access to target cells (*endocrine* action), (2) upon adjacent cells (*paraacrine* action; e.g., the effects of cortisol on catecholamine production by the adrenal medulla), or (3) upon cells that themselves have produced the relevant hormone (*autocrine* action; e.g., the inhibitory effect of β-endorphin upon secretion of proopiomelanocortin cleavage products by the anterior pituitary corticotrophs) (1,2). The traditional concept of hormones as intercellular signaling molecules has been expanded to include substances produced in the nervous and immune systems. Indeed, neurons secrete molecules acting as local hormones, while several hormones act as neurotransmitters or neuromodulators. In a similar fashion the immune system shares molecules with the endocrine system, whereas an ever-increasing number of immune peptides is shown to influence endocrine function (3).

At the crux of the endocrine system control lie the concepts of positive and negative feedback (4). Negative feedback denotes that a specific consequence of hormone action is the inhibition or attenuation of further hormone secretion [e.g., the negative effect of cortisol on hypothalamic corticotropin-releasing hormone (CRH) and pituitary adrenocorticotropin (ACTH) secretion]. The much rarer positive feedback denotes that the consequence of hormone action is the enhancement of further hormone secretion (e.g., cervical dilatation during labor strongly and continuously stimulates oxytocin secretion from the posterior pituitary). Both above apparently "simple" mechanisms of endocrine regulation in the context of the whole organism are mediated at the cellular level by a complex network of interconnecting signals from hormones, their receptors, and "downstream" effector pathways.

The relationship between endocrine surgery and molecular endocrinology is founded upon several prin-

* Current affiliation: Dept. of Endocrine Neoplasia and Hormonal Disorders, The University of Texas–M.D. Anderson Cancer Center, Houston, Texas, U.S.A.

ciples. Indeed, surgical intervention is frequently indicated for disorders, the manifestations of which stem from specific defects at the molecular or cellular level. Selected examples include (1) removal of hypercellular parathyroid glands, pituitary and pancreatic tumors in patients with multiple endocrine neoplasia type 1 (MEN1), caused by mutations in the *menin* gene, (2) total thyroidectomy or adrenalectomy in patients with MEN2 at risk for medullary thyroid cancer and pheochromocytoma due to *RET* proto-oncogene activation, and (3) extirpation of toxic thyroid adenomas. Additionally, the acquisition of an adequate knowledge basis in molecular endocrinology is of cardinal importance for the surgeon-researcher, as it can help considerably in the design of rational basic and clinical studies. This is exemplified by the surgical research efforts in the domain of gene therapy for endocrine malignancies (5) and the development of techniques for xenotransplantation of pancreatic islet β-cells for the treatment of type 1 diabetes mellitus (T1DM) (6).

In this chapter, we will describe the fundamental concepts of hormone action via their cognate receptors, with emphasis on the processes leading from a specific molecular defect to a human disease phenotype.

2 MECHANISMS OF HORMONE ACTION

Hormones exert their actions by binding to specific receptors, which show high specificity and affinity for their cognate ligands. A hormone can be either an agonist—when its binding to the cognate receptor activates "downstream" cellular effector mechanisms—or an antagonist—when hormone binding to the receptor site prevents activation of the aforementioned mechanisms. Of note, partial agonists also exist, i.e., a hormone can act as an agonist at its specific receptor site only in the absence of a more potent ligand, while it acts as an antagonist in the presence of such a ligand (1).

As a general principle, the magnitude of target tissue responses to a specific hormone signal depends on (1) the concentration of the hormone, (2) the number of target cells exhibiting functional receptors, and (3) the inherent sensitivity of the target cells to hormonal stimulation. The latter, in turn, depends mainly on the number of functional receptors expressed, the affinity of these receptors for the cognate ligand, and the specific post–receptor effector mechanisms that are responsible for transduction of the hormonal signal (7). The most commonly used parameter to reflect the sensitivity of a target tissue to a given hormone is the concentration of that hormone needed to achieve half-maximal response. Similarly, the affinity of the receptor for a given hormone is defined as the concentration of that hormone needed to occupy 50% of its cognate receptors within the tissue/cell under consideration (8). Importantly, hormones are capable of achieving maximal physiological responses in target tissues, even when only a small percentage of receptors are occupied therein, e.g., the muscle uptake of glucose stimulated by insulin becomes maximal when only 2% of insulin receptors are occupied. The above example denotes the principle of "spare receptors." Because of the presence of the latter in various tissues, the concentration of a given hormone needed to produce half-maximal responses is less than that needed to saturate half of its cognate receptors (9). The above phenomenology usually leads in sigmoid type curves for the graphic description of the relationship between hormone concentration and physiological effect; however, the exact position and shape of these curves are modified by several factors, depending on the particular hormone action system or target tissue under study (Fig. 1).

The mechanisms of hormone action can be classified into two major categories those mediated by plasma membrane receptors, which have a predilection for hydrophilic hormones, and those mediated by intra-

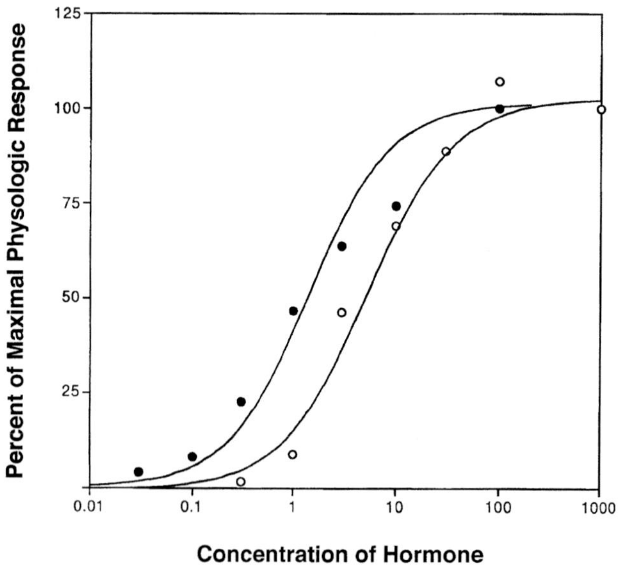

Figure 1 Percent of maximal biological response as a function of hormone concentration in a representative receptor-dependent cell system. Various factors can modulate the level of hormonal response and move the sigmoid dose-effect curve to the left or the right. The % receptor occupancy as a function of hormone concentration for a given total number of hormone receptors per cell can also be depicted by a similar graph.

cellular receptors, which have a predilection for lipophilic hormones. Although the vast majority of hormone receptors are peptidic in nature, some plasma membrane receptors are glycolipids (10). Many receptor proteins can undergo posttranslational modifications (glycosylation, phosphorylation, myristoylation, etc.) that are occasionally extensive (11).

Mutations of specific hormone receptors have been shown to be responsible for a variety of endocrine diseases. Generally, there are two types of mutations (1):

1. Gain-of-function (activating) mutations, whereby the receptor becomes constitutively active and leads to unregulated stimulation of post–receptor effector mechanisms in a ligand-independent fashion
2. Loss-of-function (inactivating) mutations, whereby the receptor is unable to perform its usual function because it may be absent, unable to bind to its ligand, or unable to activate post–receptor effector mechanisms

Specific examples of diseases caused by receptor-activating or -inactivating mutations will be provided in the following sections.

2.1 Plasma Membrane Receptors

Hydrophilic (mainly peptidic) as well as a few lipophilic hormones (e.g., melatonin and eicosanoids) exert their action by binding to plasma membrane receptors. These receptors share a general common structure: they have an extracellular domain that binds to the hormone, one or several transmembrane domains (TMDs) (usually an α-helix comprised of hydrophobic amino acid residues), and an intracellular domain that is responsible for the transduction of the hormonal signal to "downstream" effector mechanisms upon ligand binding. There are three main classes of plasma membrane receptors: G-protein–coupled (GPCRs), enzyme coupled, and ion channel coupled (1). The features of these classes are summarized in Table 1.

2.1.1 G-Protein–Coupled Receptors

G-protein–coupled receptors represent the largest family of plasma membrane receptors. They are activated by a variety of ligands of both peptidic and nonpeptidic nature, including "classical" hormones, neurotransmitters, growth factors, odorant molecules, and light. More than 1% of the human genome encodes approximately 1500 different GPCRs. These receptors constitute the target of more than 50% of the therapeutic agents currently in clinical use (12).

GPCRs share a common structure, as they all are single polypeptide chains with seven α-helical TMDs (Fig. 2) (13). Their name stems from the fact that they interact with heterotrimeric, guanosine triphosphate (GTP)–binding regulatory proteins, which relay signals from the cell surface to "downstream" intracellular effector mechanisms. Each G-protein consists of an α-subunit and a $\beta\gamma$-subunit dimer. Mammalian α-subunits can be categorized into four distinct classes, depending on their amino acid sequence and presumed evolutionary distance: (1) α_s and α_{olf}, (2) α_{t1}, α_{t2}, α_{gust},

Table 1 The Main Classes of Plasma Membrane Hormone Receptors

Receptor class	Receptor conformation	Receptor subtypes	Examples
G-protein–coupled	7-transmembrane domain	Numerous; depending on subtype of Gα protein	ACTHR; FSHR; LHR; TSHR; GHRHR; TRHR; adrenergic Rc's (α_1, α_2, β); glucagon Rcs; Ca^{2+}-sensing Rcs; V2-vasopressin Rcs
Enzyme coupled	Single TMD	Receptor tyrosine kinases	Insulin rc; Rcs for various growth factors
		TK-associated receptors	Cytokine Rcs; GHR; PRLR; leptin rc
		Serine threonine kinases	Rcs for the TGFβ superfamily[a]
Ion channel–coupled	Ligand-gated ion channel complex (usually pentameric)	N/A	Numerous; mainly relevant to neurotransmission/neuromodulation; SUR1 of endocrine interest[a]

ACTH: adrenocorticotropin; FSH: follitropin; GH: growth hormone; GHRH: growth hormone–releasing hormone; GPCR: G-protein–coupled receptor; LH: luteinizing hormone; N/A: not applicable; PRL: prolactin; Rc: receptor; RTK: receptor tyrosine kinase; STK: serine/threonine kinase; SUR1: sulfonylurea receptor type-1; TGFβ: transforming growth factor-β; TMD: transmembrane domain; TRH: thyrotropin-releasing hormone; TSH: thyrotropin.

[a] For details, please refer to text.

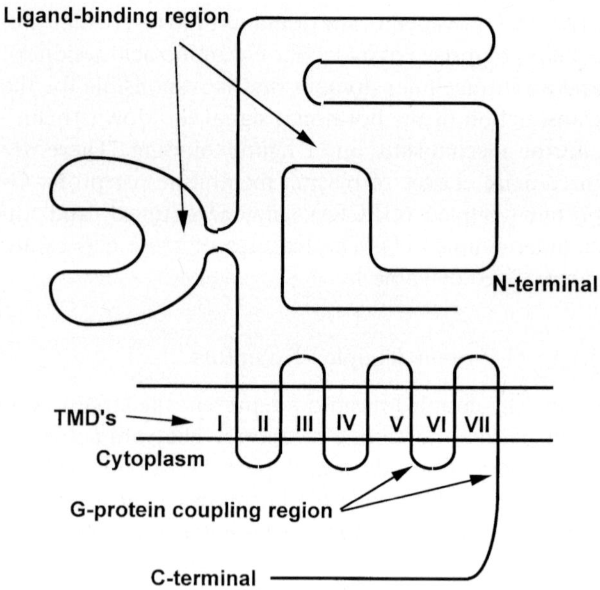

Figure 2 Schematic structure of the TSH receptor as a prototype of the G–protein–coupled heptahelical transmembrane domain (TMD) receptors. TMDs are designated in Latin numbers.

α_{i1}, α_{i2}, α_{i3}, α_0, and α_z, (3) α_q, α_{11}, α_{14}, and $\alpha_{15/16}$, and (4) α_{12} and α_{13}. Tissue expression varies vastly among the above types, with some being ubiquitously expressed (α_s, α_{i2}, α_q, α_{11}, α_{12}, and α_{13}) and others exhibiting specific tissue expression (14). Similar diversity is observed for the β- and γ-subunits: there are at least four distinct transcript variants for the β-subunit gene and at least as many for the γ-subunit (15). The type of α-subunit defines the role of the G-protein by activating a different effector mechanism. In the resting state, G-proteins bind guanosine diphospate (GDP) via their α-subunit, while the three subunits (α-, β-, and γ-) are tightly bound in a trimer configuration. Upon binding of the ligand, GDP is dissociated from the α-subunit and replaced by GTP, thus leading to dissociation of the α-subunit from the β- and γ-subunits, and the formation of an active α-subunit. The latter binds to "downstream" effectors and modulates their action. The α-subunit possesses intrinsic GTPase activity, hydrolyzing the bound GTP to GDP, and thus rendering itself inactive. In that state, the α-subunit is able to reassociate with the β- and γ-subunits, rendering the conformation of the αβγ complex to its inactive state and terminating the action of the ligand (16).

The above system has been recently shown to be significantly more complicated, as it involves (1) RGS proteins (regulators of G-protein signaling), which accelerate the hydrolysis of GTP to GDP leading to termination of the hormone signal (17), (2) receptor phosphorylation, which rapidly attenuates early signal transduction by receptor desensitization (18), and (3) receptor downregulation, i.e., the reduction in the number of receptors after long-term exposure to agonistic ligands, which occurs via decreased synthesis or increased degradation of these receptors (18).

Both germline and somatic mutations of G-proteins or GPCRs have been described in a variety of human diseases (19), and their role has also been implicated in carcinogenesis and cardiovascular disease. Examples include:

1. Gain-of-function mutations (with resultant defective termination of signal): pituitary, thyroid (20), adrenal and ovarian adenomas (21,22), McCune-Albright syndrome (23), familial male precocious puberty (24), autosomal dominant hypoparathyroidism (25), and essential hypertension (16)
2. Loss-of-function mutations (resulting in absent or inactive Gα protein): pseudohypoparathyroidism type-Ia, pseudo-pseudohypoparathyroidism (26), night blindness, retinitis pigmentosa (22,27), familial hypercalcemic hypocalciuria, and severe neonatal hyperparathyroidism (28)

2.1.2 Enzyme-Coupled Receptors

Receptors belonging to this group either have intrinsic enzymatic activity or are directly bound to an enzyme, though importantly without the intervention of a submembrane G-protein system. They are usually single TMD proteins and often form dimers with each other, either upon ligand binding or spontaneously.

Receptor Tyrosine Kinases. The ligands for these receptors include insulin and various growth factors (GFs) (1). They have intrinsic tyrosine kinase (TK) activity and phosphorylate tyrosine residues. These receptors can also undergo autophosphorylation. The latter modification provides docking sides for other proteins, which become bound to the receptor and thus activate themselves (29). Examples include the various insulin receptor substrates (IRSs), phospholipase C-γ (PLC-γ), phosphatidylinositol 3-kinase (PI3K), and the GTPase-activating proteins (GAPs) (30–33). These molecules constitute the first step of complex intracellular pathways via which ligands exert their actions.

The relevance of this type of receptors and their cognate "downstream" intracellular signaling molecules for human disease cannot be overemphasized.

Indeed, mutations in the insulin receptor can affect differentially its synthesis, transport to plasma membrane, capacity for insulin binding, transmembrane signaling or its degradation, thus resulting in type A insulin resistance. It is estimated that approximately 1% of patients with type 2 diabetes mellitus (T2DM) may carry germline mutations of the insulin receptor gene (14).

TK-Associated Receptors. The ligands for the receptors in this group include growth hormone (GH), prolactin (PRL), leptin, various interleukins (ILs), EPO, granulocyte-macrophage colony-stimulating factor(GM-CSF), and granulocyte colony-stimulating factor (type I TK-receptor subclass), as well as interferons (IFNs)-α, -β, and -γ (type II receptor subclass) (34). The structure of TK-associated receptors is similar to that of the previous group (RTKs), with the exception that they lack the intrinsic TK activity within their intracellular domain. Instead, in this case, ligand binding leads to activation of "downstream" intracellular TKs. The main signaling pathway activated by this class of receptors is known as the "Jak-STAT pathway," which includes phosphorylation and activation of Janus kinases (Jak). The latter subsequently phosphorylate and activate one of the signal transducer and activator of transcription (STAT) proteins, eventually resulting in the regulation of transcription of specific genes (35,36).

The clinical relevance of these receptors in endocrinology becomes apparent by the following: mutations in the leptin receptor are a well-recognized, albeit rare, cause of human obesity (37), and loss-of-function mutations in the GH receptor gene result in Laron dwarfism (38).

Serine/Threonine Kinase Receptors. The ligands for this group of receptors are members of the transforming growth factor-β (TGF-β) superfamily, which play a significant role during embryonic development and adult tissue homeostasis. Representative members of this superfamily of ligands include TGF-β, activin, bone morphogenetic proteins, several growth and differentiation factors, and anti-Mullerian hormone (39). Serine/threonine kinase (STK) receptors consist of a single TMD with STK activity within their intracellular part, which is activated upon receptor dimerization. Two types (I and II) of STK receptors have been described, the only known function of type II receptors being the activation of type I receptors via phosphorylation (40). The "downstream" signal transduction cascade includes activation (via phosphorylation) of cytoplasmic SMAD (−1 to−8) proteins, which then translocate to the cell nucleus and regulate specific gene transcription. The acronym SMAD is derived from the initially described members of this protein family, i.e., the *C. elegans* protein SMA ("small body size") and the *Drosophila* protein MAD ("mothers against decapentaplegic") (41). The STK receptor-dependent signaling system is under tight control by multiple other intracellular regulators, as this pathway is not only relevant to transduction of selected hormonal signals, but has been also been closely implicated in the initiation and promotion of tumorigenesis. Indeed, loss of the cell growth inhibition induced by TGF-β leads to tumor formation in several in vitro models (42), while SMAD-3 inactivation in the mouse has been shown to promote the development of metastatic colonic carcinoma (43).

2.1.3 Ion Channel–Coupled Receptors

Ion channels control the flux of specific ions across the plasma membrane. These channels can be either voltage-gated (i.e., ionic flux through them is regulated by charge gradients across the cell membrane) or ligand-gated (i.e., the flux is regulated by the binding of specific ligands to the channel itself or proteins associated with it). Members of the latter group include the nicotinic cholinergic, γ-aminobutyric acid (GABA), glutamate, glycine, and kainic acid receptors (1).

Ion channel–coupled receptors share a common general structure as they consist of a five-subunit complex (two α and one β, γ, and δ). Each subunit resembles the GPCRs, in that it consists of an extracellular, four transmembrane, and one short intracellular domains. Interestingly, some of the ligand-gated ion channel–coupled receptors utilize G-proteins for further signal transduction (1). No bona fide endocrine disorder has yet been associated with defects in a ion channel-coupled hormone receptor; however, mutations in sulfonylurea receptor-1 (SUR1), which in association with the Kir6.2 complex constitutes the functional ATP-sensitive potassium channel of the pancreatic β-cell, have been recently linked to persistent hyperinsulinemic hypoglycemia of infancy (44).

2.2 Intracellular Receptors

Intracellular receptors are not bound to the plasma cell membrane; instead, they reside either in the cytoplasm (cytoplasmic receptors, e.g., the receptors for mineralocorticoid and glucocorticoid hormones) or in the cell nucleus (nuclear receptors, e.g., the receptors for progesterone and estrogens) (45). Intracellular receptors bind ligands that easily penetrate the cell membrane. The most important members of this group are the receptors for the steroid-thyroid hormone superfamily, which also includes compounds such as retinoids, eicosanoids, and the long-chain fatty acids (LCFAs) (1). The features of the members of the above superfamily are summarized in Table 2. All above ligands have a profound effect on homeostasis, growth, reproduction, and organism behavior. The effects of hormones that bind to intracellular receptors are mediated by the interaction of these receptors (in their liganded form) with DNA and a wide variety of other nuclear proteins, e.g., the trascription pro-initiation complex, leading to regulation of transcription of specific target genes (46).

Intracellular receptors have been found to share a common structure, shown schematically in Figure 3A. Further, certain receptor regions are highly evolutionarily conserved among different receptor types and subtypes. As a rule, each intracellular receptor consists of four parts: (1) an N-terminal region that serves as a transactivation domain [transactivation function (TAF)-1] and controls gene transcription, (2) a central, highly conserved, DNA-binding domain (DBD), (3) a short "hinge" region, and (4) a C-terminal ligand-binding domain (LBD), which also contains amino acid sequences mediating receptor dimerization, nuclear localization, and subsequent transactivation (TAF-2) (47).

Inactive [unbound to ligand (or unliganded)] cytoplasmic intracellular receptors exist in molecular complexes with other proteins, such as heat shock proteins (hsps) and immunophilin/p59 (48,49). Ligand binding causes a conformational change in the receptor, its disassociation from the above proteins, receptor homo- or hetero-dimerization, and entrance into the nucleus. Once inside the nucleus, the ligand-receptor complex binds to specific DNA areas, called hormone response elements (HREs), which are located in the promoter regions of hormone-responsive genes, and modulates their transcription via a complex interaction with intranuclear transcription factors (Fig. 3B) (50).

It is worth emphasizing the following points:

1. Intracellular receptors can be activated independently of their ligands (possibly through receptor phosphorylation) (51).
2. Cross-talk exists between "downstream" effector systems transducing signals derived from plasma membrane receptors and intracellular receptors (52).
3. Steroid and thyroid hormones can also exert nongenomic (usually rapid-onset) actions (53).

Table 2 The Main Classes of Intracellular Hormone Receptors

Receptor classification	Receptor	Ligands	hsp association
Steroid/thyroid hormone superfamily			
Type-I Rc families	Glucocorticoid Rc (GR) -α, -β types	cortisol, corticosterone, aldosterone, progesterone, DOC	Yes
	Mineralocorticoid Rc (MR)	aldosterone, DOC, cortisol	Yes
	Progesterone Rc (PR) A- and B-types	progesterone	Yes
	Androgen Rc (AR)	dihydrotestosterone, testosterone, androstenedione, DHEA	Yes
Type II Rc families	Estrogen Rc (ER) -α, -β types	estradiol, estrone, estriol	Yes
	Vitamin D Rc (VDR)	1,25 $(OH)_2$-vitD_3	No
	Thyroid hormone rcs (TRs) -α, -β subfamilies	T3, T4	No
	Retinoid rcs (RAR, RXR) -α, -β, -γ subfamilies	9-*cis*-retinoic acid, all-*trans*-retinoic acid	No
RevErb/ROR superfamily			
PPAR family	PPARs -α, -γ, -δ subfamilies	15Δ-PGJ2, PGI2, DHEA-S, LCFAs	No

DHEA (-S): dihydroepiandrosterone (sulfate); DOC: deoxycorticosterone; Hsp: heat shock protein; LCFAs: long-chain fatty acids; PPAR: peroxisome proliferator-activated receptor; PG: prostaglandin; RAR: retinoic acid receptor; RXR: retonoid-X receptor; rc: receptor; T3: triiodothyronine; T4: thyroxine.

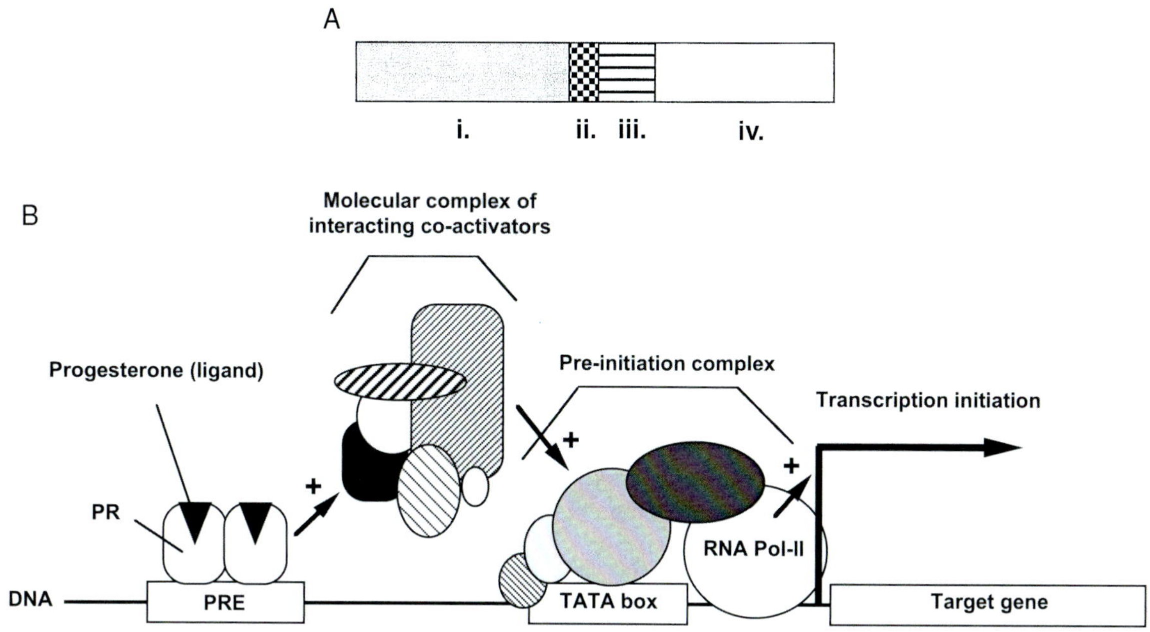

Figure 3 (A) Schematic representation of the structure of intracellular receptors. The following domains are identified: N-terminal/immunogenic (containing the TAF-1 region); DNA-binding (DBD); hinge; and ligand-binding (LBD; containing the TAF-2 region). (B) A model of transcriptional effects from the activation of the progesterone receptor (PR) as a prototype of intracellular receptors. Ligand binding leads to PR dimerization and attachment of the resulting complex upon a hormone-response element (in this case, PRE). This element is located within the nuclear DNA at the promoter region of a target gene. The PR dimer–PRE complex, via a specific molecular conformation, attracts transcription factors called co-activators, leading to the assembly and activation of basal RNA polymerase-II (RNA Pol-II) preinitiation complexes and eventually to gene transcription. The example given pertains to a target gene promoter that contains a defined TATA box; the mechanisms at play are somewhat different for genes with TATA-less promoters. The (+) symbol denotes activation of a molecular complex or action.

We will offer a brief discussion of one of the subclasses of the intracellular receptor superfamily, the peroxisome proliferator-activated receptors (PPARs), primarily because of their impact in the pharmacological treatment of T2DM. PPARs (-α, -γ, and -δ) were initially discovered as "orphan" receptors, i.e., receptors with no known ligand at that time. Subsequently, a variety of LCFAs and eicosanoids were found to be endogenous ligands for this type of receptors (54). Among them, PPAR-γ is the most extensively studied. PPAR-γs are abundant in adipose tissue and skeletal muscle and have been shown to promote adipogenesis. The synthetic PPAR-γ ligands thiazolidinediones (TZDs) increase insulin sensitivity and glucose uptake in diabetic individuals, although the specific target tissues of TZDs and the mechanism of decrease in insulin resistance remain unknown (55). Finally, PPAR-γs have been implicated in tumorigenesis: a recent study suggested that PPAR-γs have a tumor suppression function in human colon (56), whereas favorable responses have been observed in men with metastatic prostatic cancer treated with TZDs (57).

Notably, mutations of steroid hormone receptors are responsible for a variety of human diseases. Loss-of-function mutations in the androgen receptor are the basis for testicular feminization or androgen insensitivity syndromes (58). Similarly, inactivating mutations of the vitamin D receptor and thyroid receptor-β cause vitamin D–resistant rickets type II (59) and the syndrome of resistance to thyroid hormone (60), respectively. Qualitative and/or quantitative defects in the glucocorticoid receptor are associated with primary sporadic or familial glucocorticoid resistance (61).

3 CONCLUSION

Molecular endocrinology is a continuously evolving field. In this chapter, we have described the schemes of hormone action and signaling in a general fashion. It is evident that complex intricacies exist within each step of the pathways of expression and action of hormones, including the regulation of their secretion, modification(s) of their molecular structure, interactions with their cognate receptors, activation of assorted "downstream" (postreceptor) pathways of signal transduction, and, finally, the convergence of such pathways in the nucleus for the generation of an appropriate homeostatic genomic response.

Moreover, hormone signaling via different receptor types should be envisaged as a complex lattice or network, where different "downstream" signals, generated after hormone receptor activation, interact synchronously or metachronously with each other. This cross-signaling property of this network of effectors is far from being fully understood at this time.

Finally, the Human Genome Project has wide implications for molecular endocrinology, as it not only provides potential for the identification of the genetic basis of endocrine diseases, but will most probably allow a more comprehensive approach to the molecular basis of hormone synthesis and action. It is only through such an approach that future advances in the management of endocrine disorders will be optimally spearheaded, which of course applies to surgical treatment thereof.

ACKNOWLEDGMENTS

We wish to thank Drs. Paul M. Yen and Derek LeRoith, both of NIDDK, NIH, for their thorough review of the manuscript, as well as constructive comments and suggestions.

REFERENCES

1. Kacsoh B. Endocrine Physiology. Philadelphia: McGraw-Hill. 2000.
2. Taylor T, Dluhy RG, Williams GH. Beta-endorphin suppresses adrenocorticotropin and cortisol levels in normal human subjects. J Clin Endocrinol Metab 1983; 57:592–596.
3. Knight R, Sarlis N, Stephanou A. Interleukins and neurohormones: a common language. Postgrad Med J 1992; 68:603–605.
4. Yates FE, Brennan RD, Urquhart J. Application of control systems theory to physiology. Adrenal glucocorticoid control system. Fed Proc 1969; 28:71–83.
5. Castro MG, Southgate T, Lowenstein PR. Molecular therapy in a model neuroendocrine disease: developing clinical gene therapy for pituitary tumours. Trends Endocrinol Metab 2001; 12:58–64.
6. Weber CJ, Hagler M, Konieczny B, Chryssochoos J, Rajotte R, Lakkis F, Lowry R. Encapsulated islet iso-, allo-, and xenografts in diabetic NOD mice. Transplant Proc 1995; 27:3308–3311.
7. Simons SS, Oshima H, Szapary D. Higher levels of control: modulation of steroid hormone-regulated gene transcription. Mol Endocrinol 1992; 6:995–1002.
8. Steinberg RA, Levinson BB, Tomkins GM. Kinetics of steroid induction and deinduction of tyrosine aminotransferase synthesis in cultured hepatoma cells. Proc Natl Acad Sci USA 1975; 72:2007–2011.
9. Svec F. The relationship between glucocorticoid biopotency and receptor binding in the AtT-20 cell. Endocrinology 1984; 114:1250–1258.
10. Ohanian J, Ohanian V. Sphingolipids in mammalian cell signalling. Cell Mol Life Sci 2001; 58:2053–2068.
11. Chen CA, Manning DR. Regulation of G-proteins by covalent modification. Oncogene 2001; 20:1643–1652.
12. Marinissen MJ, Gutkind JS. G-protein-coupled receptors and signaling networks: emerging paradigms. Trends Pharmacol Sci 2001; 22:368–376.
13. Wess J. G-protein-coupled receptors: molecular mechanisms involved in receptor activation and selectivity of G-protein recognition. FASEB J 1997; 11:346–354.
14. Weintraub BD. Molecular Endocrinology: Basic Concepts and Clinical Correlations. New York: Raven Press, 1995.
15. Gautam N, Northup J, Tamir H, Simon MI. G protein diversity is increased by associations with a variety of gamma subunits. Proc Natl Acad Sci USA 1990; 87:7973–7977.
16. Farfel Z, Bourne HR, Iiri T. The expanding spectrum of G protein diseases. N Engl J Med 1999; 340:1012–1020.
17. Hepler JR. Emerging roles for RGS proteins in cell signalling. Trends Pharmacol Sci 1999; 20:376–382.
18. Bohm SK, Grady EF, Bunnett NW. Regulatory mechanisms that modulate signalling by G-protein-coupled receptors. Biochem J 1997; 322:1–18.
19. Spiegel AM. G protein defects in signal transduction. Horm Res 2000; 53:17–22.
20. Duprez L, Parma J, Van Sande J, Rodien P, Sabine C, Abramowicz M, Dumont JE, Vassart G. Pathology of the TSH receptor. J Pediatr Endocrinol Metab 1999; 12:(suppl 1):295–302.
21. Lania A, Mantovani G, Spada A. G protein mutations in endocrine diseases. Eur J Endocrinol 2001; 145:543–559.
22. Coughlin SR. Expanding horizons for receptors coupled to G proteins: diversity and disease. Curr Opin Cell Biol 1994; 6:191–197.
23. Shenker A, Weinstein LS, Moran A, Pescovitz OH, Charest NJ, Boney CM, Van Wyk JJ, Merino MJ, Feuillan PP, Spiegel AM. Severe endocrine and non-endocrine manifestations of the McCune-Albright syndrome associated with activating mutations of stimulatory G protein GS. J Pediatr 1993; 123:509–518.
24. Shenker A, Laue L, Kosugi S, Merendino JJ, Minegishi

T, Cutler GB, Jr. A constitutively activating mutation of the luteinizing hormone receptor in familial male precocious puberty. Nature 1993; 365:652–654.
25. Hirai H, Nakajima S, Miyauchi A, Nishimura K, Shimizu N, Shima M, Michigami T, Ozono K, Okada S. A novel activating mutation (C129S) in the calcium-sensing receptor gene in a Japanese family with autosomal dominant hypocalcemia. J Hum Genet 2001; 46:41–44.
26. Weinstein LS, Yu S, Warner DR, Liu J. Endocrine manifestations of stimulatory G protein alpha-subunit mutations and the role of genomic imprinting. Endocr Rev 2001; 22:675–705.
27. Robinson PR, Cohen GB, Zhukovsky EA, Oprian DD. Constitutively active mutants of rhodopsin. Neuron 1992; 9:719–725.
28. Brown EM, Pollak M, Hebert SC. The extracellular calcium-sensing receptor: its role in health and disease. Annu Rev Med 1998; 49:15–29.
29. van der Geer P, Hunter T, Lindberg RA. Receptor protein-tyrosine kinases and their signal transduction pathways. Annu Rev Cell Biol 1994; 10:251–337.
30. Nystrom FH, Quon MJ. Insulin signalling: metabolic pathways and mechanisms for specificity. Cell Signal 1999; 11:563–574.
31. Schlessinger J. Cellular signaling by receptor tyrosine kinases. Harvey Lect 1993; 89:105–123.
32. Songyang Z, Shoelson SE, Chaudhuri M, Gish G, Pawson T, Haser WG, King F, Roberts T, Ratnofsky S, Lechleider RJ. SH2 domains recognize specific phosphopeptide sequences. Cell 1993; 72:767–778.
33. Sun XJ, Wang LM, Zhang Y, Yenush L, Myers MG, Jr., Glasheen E, Lane WS, Pierce JH, White MF. Role of IRS-2 in insulin and cytokine signalling. Nature 1995; 377:173–177.
34. Gadina M, Hilton D, Johnston JA, Morinobu A, Lighvani A, Zhou YJ, Visconti R, O'Shea JJ. Signaling by type I and II cytokine receptors: ten years after. Curr Opin Immunol 2001; 13:363 373.
35. Kotenko SV, Pestka S. Jak-Stat signal transduction pathway through the eyes of cytokine class II receptor complexes. Oncogene 2000; 19:2557–2565.
36. Yeh TC, Pellegrini S. The Janus kinase family of protein tyrosine kinases and their role in signaling. Cell Mol Life Sci 1999; 55:1523–1534.
37. Friedman JM. Leptin and the regulation of body weight. Harvey Lect. 1999–2000; 95:107–136.
38. Laron Z. Prismatic cases: Laron syndrome (primary growth hormone resistance) from patient to laboratory to patient. J Clin Endocrinol Metab 1995; 80:1526–1531.
39. Massagué J, Wotton D. Transcriptional control by the TGF-beta/Smad signaling system. EMBO J 2000; 19:1745–1754.
40. Massagué J. TGF-beta signal transduction. Annu Rev Biochem 1998; 67:753–791.
41. Raftery LA, Sutherland DJ. TGF-beta family signal transduction in *Drosophila* development: from Mad to Smads. Dev Biol 1999; 210:251–268.
42. Datto MB, Frederick JP, Pan L, Borton AJ, Zhuang Y, Wang XF. Targeted disruption of Smad3 reveals an essential role in transforming growth factor beta-mediated signal transduction. Mol Cell Biol 1999; 19:2495–2504.
43. Zhu Y, Richardson JA, Parada LF, Graff JM. Smad3 mutant mice develop metastatic colorectal cancer. Cell 1998; 94:703–714.
44. Partridge CJ, Beech DJ, Sivaprasadarao A. Identification and pharmacological correction of a membrane trafficking defect associated with a mutation in the sulfonylurea receptor causing familial hyperinsulinism. J Biol Chem 2001; 276:35947–35952.
45. Bagchi M. Molecular mechanisms of nuclear receptor-mediated transcriptional activation and basal repression. Freedman LP, ed. Molecular Biology of Steroid and Nuclear Hormone Receptors. Boston: Birkhauser, 1998: 159–189.
46. Beato M, Chavez S, Truss M. Transcriptional regulation by steroid hormones. Steroids 1996; 61:240–251.
47. Simons SS, Jr. Function/activity of specific amino acids in glucocorticoid receptors. Vitam Horm 1994; 49:49–130.
48. Rehberger P, Rexin M, Gehring U. Heterotetrameric structure of the human progesterone receptor. Proc Natl Acad Sci USA 1992; 89:8001–8005.
49. Rexin M, Busch W, Segnitz B, Gehring U. Structure of the glucocorticoid receptor in intact cells in the absence of hormone. J Biol Chem 1992; 267:9619–9621.
50. Truss M, Beato M. Steroid hormone receptors: interaction with deoxyribonucleic acid and transcription factors. Endocr Rev 1993; 14:459–479.
51. Power RF, Mani SK, Codina J, Conneely OM, O'Malley BW. Dopaminergic and ligand-independent activation of steroid hormone receptors. Science 1991; 254:1636–1639.
52. Bjørnstrom L, Kilic E, Norman M, Parker MG, Sjøberg M. Cross-talk between Stat5b and estrogen receptor-alpha and -beta in mammary epithelial cells. J Mol Endocrinol 2001; 27:93–106.
53. Falkenstein E, Tillmann HC, Christ M, Feuring M, Wehling M. Multiple actions of steroid hormones—a focus on rapid, nongenomic effects. Pharmacol Rev 2000; 52:513–556.
54. Rosen ED, Spiegelman BM. PPAR-gamma: a nuclear regulator of metabolism, differentiation, and cell growth. J Biol Chem 2001; 276:37731–37734.
55. Kletzien RF, Clarke SD, Ulrich RG. Enhancement of adipocyte differentiation by an insulin-sensitizing agent. Mol Pharmacol 1992; 41:393–398.
56. Saez E, Tontoñoz P, Nelson MC, Alvarez JG, Ming UT, Baird SM, Thomazy VA, Evans RM. Activators of

the nuclear receptor PPAR-gamma enhance colon polyp formation. Nat Med 1998; 4:1058–1061.
57. Mueller E, Smith M, Sarraf P, Kroll T, Aiyer A, Kaufman DS, Oh W, Demetri G, Figg WD, Zhou XP, Eng C, Spiegelman BM, Kantoff PW. Effects of ligand activation of peroxisome proliferator-activated receptor gamma in human prostate cancer. Proc Natl Acad Sci USA 2000; 97:10990–10995.
58. Brinkmann AO. Molecular basis of androgen insensitivity. Mol Cell Endocrinol 2001; 179:105–109.
59. Malloy PJ, Feldman D. Vitamin D resistance. Am J Med 1999; 106:355–370.
60. Weiss RE, Refetoff S. Resistance to thyroid hormone. Rev Endocr Metab Disord 2000; 1:97–108.
61. Arai K, Chrousos GP. Syndromes of glucocorticoid and mineralocorticoid resistance. Steroids 1995; 60:173–179.

2

Robotic Endocrine Surgery

Brian P. Jacob and Michel Gagner

Mount Sinai School of Medicine, New York University, New York, New York, U.S.A.

1 INTRODUCTION

Robots have been in the operating room for approximately 10 years now, but their use in assisting laparoscopic endocrine surgery is very new. This chapter begins with a review of the history of endocrine surgery to show how it has evolved to include the use of surgical robots. Next we will describe the different types of surgical robots, and finally we will review the published data on robot-assisted laparoscopic adrenalectomies.

2 HISTORY OF ENDOCRINE SURGERY—FROM OPEN CASES TO ROBOTICS

The field of endocrine surgery encompasses a wide number of operations for diseases of the thyroid, parathyroid, pituitary, pancreas, adrenal, as well as breast, and gonadal glands. The history of endocrine surgery actually began with the social and religious practice of castration around 380 B.C., but it wasn't until the nineteenth century that the therapeutic removal of the ovaries and testes was performed (1).

The early 1900s marked many of the firsts in endocrine surgery. In 1905, Ernest Starling proposed the term "hormone" from the Greek word meaning "to excite," which marked the beginning of the science of endocrinology. From this point forward, the different surgical treatments for the various endocrine diseases would be described. Although the excision of thyroid goiter was described in the twelfth century, it wasn't until the early twentieth century that masters like Emil Theodor Kocher (1841–1917) of Bern refined the technique and the traditional open thyroidectomy became popular. Parathyroid surgery began in 1925 with the work of Felix Mandl (1892–1957) in Vienna, and in 1926 the first two adrenalectomies were performed by Cesar Roux (1857–1934) in Lausanne and Charles Mayo (1865–1939) in Rochester, Minnesota. In 1929 Roscoe Graham (1890–1948) from Toledo successfully removed a pancreatic insulinoma. Soon after, numerous surgeons began performing endocrine gland excisions around the world. Around this time, Oliver Cope (1902–1994) of Boston became one of the first surgeons to treat a large number of patients specifically diagnosed with endocrine-related diseases, thus marking the beginning of the modern-day era of endocrine surgery (1).

Research and development in endocrine surgery from the late 1950s through the present time was focused on refining surgical technique, limiting morbidity and mortality, and increasing postsurgical successful outcomes. Today, the main endocrine glands operated on by general surgeons who specialize in endocrine surgery include the thyroid/parathyroid, the endocrine pancreas, and the adrenal glands, leaving most of the pituitary and gonad operations for other specialists (1–3).

Traditional surgical endocrinology is performed through large incisions, and most of the original surgical incisions for the various endocrine glands are still used today. The thyroid and parathyroid glands are removed traditionally through a small curvilinear incision approximately 3 cm above the sternal notch. The adrenals were originally approached through an abdominal midline incision, and later through a lateral and then posterior approach. Pancreatic endocrine tumors once required a large midline incision as well. While these original incisions allow for optimal exposure and successful removal of the diseased organ, they tend to subject the patients to lengthy hospital stays, significant postoperative pain, and in some cases, cosmetically undesirable results.

By the end of the twentieth century, laparoscopy was already accepted worldwide for a large number of operations in general surgery. By minimizing the size of the skin incisions while still permitting superior visualization of the operative field, laparoscopy was proven for certain operations to lessen postoperative pain, improve cosmesis, and shorten postoperative hospital stays. It is therefore no surprise that endocrine surgeons soon adopted laparoscopic and endoscopic surgical procedures for the treatment of endocrine disease (4).

Endoscopic endocrine gland surgery has been evolving for over a decade now, but the specialty first appeared in the literature in 1992 when Gagner and colleagues published their work with laparoscopic adrenalectomies on humans (5). Numerous masters of laparoscopy have improved and refined the technique, and it is now the recommended gold standard for the treatment of benign adrenal lesions (4,6,7). The feasibility and safety of laparoscopic distal pancreatectomy was first reported by Soper and colleagues in a study on a porcine model in 1994, but the first reported human cases of a laparoscopically resected pancreatic endocrine tumor were by Gagner et al. and Sussman et al., both in 1996 (9–11). Laparoscopic pancreatic surgery now has several applications including roles in staging, palliation, resection, and drainage procedures (8). Later that same year, Gagner and colleagues also published the first few cases of an endoscopic parathyroidectomy in humans, marking the beginning of endoscopic neck surgery for endocrine pathology (12).

As minimally invasive surgery became more popular, surgeons realized some true limitations. Sensory information is limited due to lack of tactile feedback and restriction to a two-dimensional (2D) image. In addition, compared to the human hand in an open case, laparoscopic instruments have restricted degrees of freedom mainly due to the lack of a wrist-like joint in the instrument tip and the lack of maneuverability due to a fixed axis point at the trocar (13). Finally, others have reported inferior ergonomics, increased surgeon fatigue, and increased surgeon physical stress compared to routine open surgery (4). Improvements in laparoscopic endocrine surgery techniques (specifically thyroid/parathyroid and adrenal) are a current topic of debate but are beyond the scope of this chapter. However, in trying to improve minimally invasive techniques, many authors have suggested the need for laparoscopic instruments that could reproduce the movements of the hand as well as imaging devices that could reproduce the three dimensions with laparoscopy (13–17). It is this demand for more improvements in laparoscopic visualization and instrumentation that has led to the development of robotics.

The advent of robot-assisted laparoscopic surgery seems to deal with many of the recognized limitations of hand-held laparoscopic surgery and will be discussed later in the chapter. In general, robots reduce the natural tremor of the human hand, reestablish comfortable ergonomics, reducing stress and surgeon fatigue, and, in certain cases, reestablish the three-dimensional (3D) view of the surgical field. In addition, surgical robots have the potential to be more precise and permit greater accuracy when it comes to suturing tasks and careful perivascular dissections.

Since robotic surgery is still in its infancy, it is no surprise that at this time there has been no published work on robotics with the thyroid gland, the parathyroid gland, or pancreatic endocrine tumors. On the other hand, an increasing amount of work is being done with robotics and adrenal surgery (16,18–22), and for this reason the remainder of this chapter will focus on that topic.

3 HISTORY OF ROBOTICS AND SURGERY

The blending of robotics and surgery is approximately 10 years in evolution. In general, the surgical robot is necessary to reduce patient risks attributed to inappropriate endoscope movements and surgeon tremor that could increase the difficulty of delicate dissections. At one point, laparoscopy was performed with the chief surgeon holding and viewing images directly through a monocular scope. However, when technology permitted the images to be transmitted to an overhead monitor, a second operator was needed to hold the laparoscope. Now the surgeon would rely on an assistant to manipulate the camera, which has the potential to prolong the duration of cases, create unnecessary

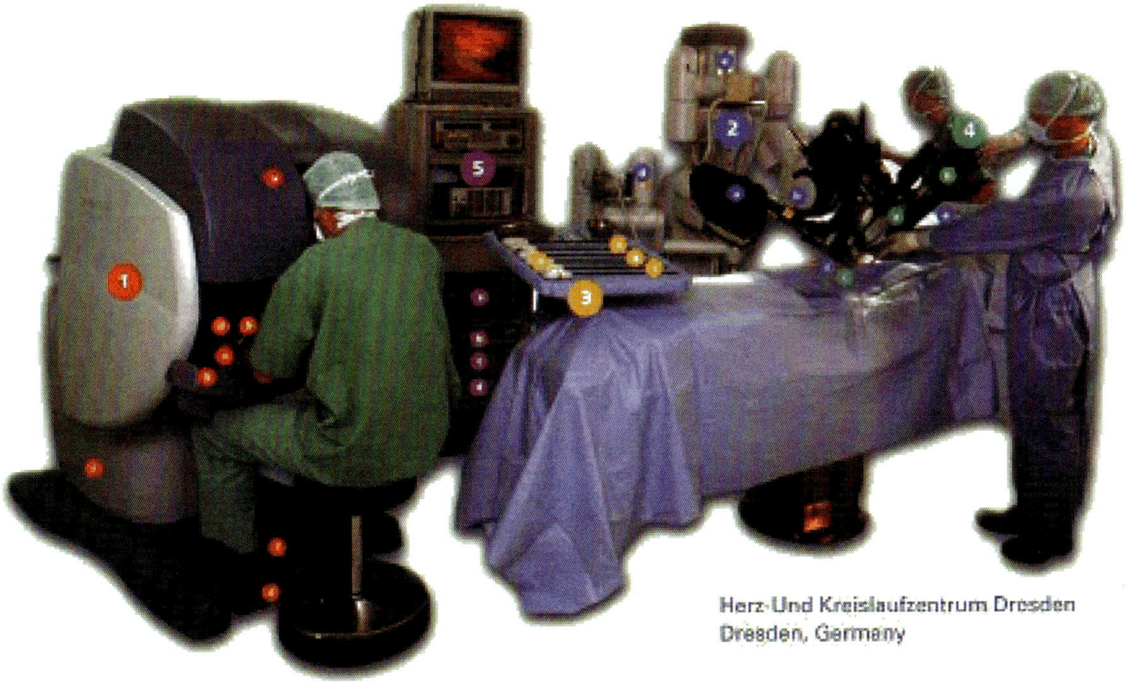

Figure 1 Da Vinci Robot System, including the InSite Vision System with 3D visualization.

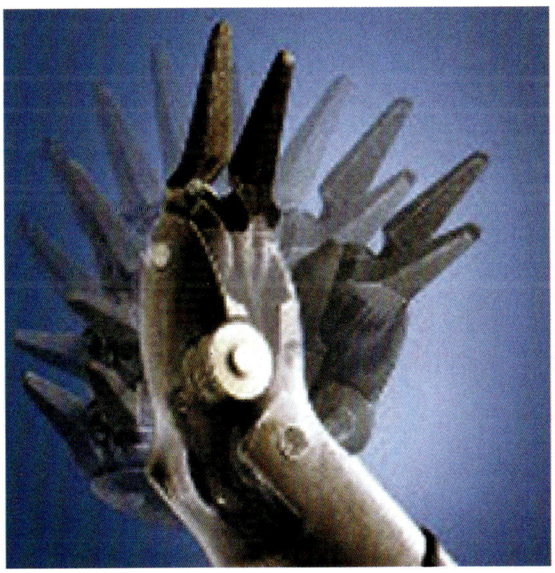

Figure 2 Closer view of the endowrist systems at the tip of Da Vinci, these instruments have 7 degrees of freedom and replicate the exact movement of the surgeon's hand. (Courtesy of Intuitive Surgical.)

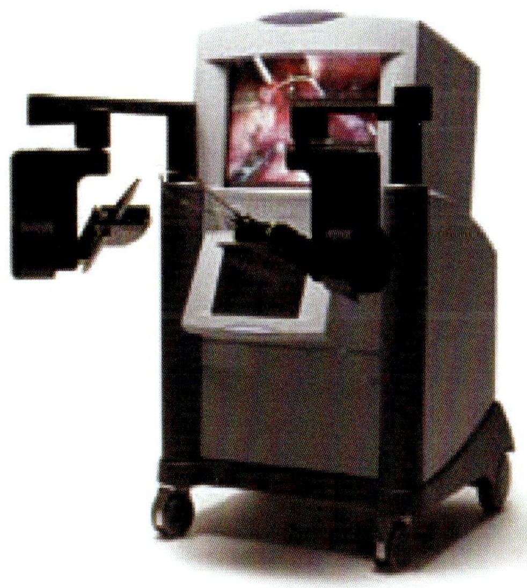

Figure 3 The Zeus Robot System, recently approved by the FDA, has a computer that filters hand tremor, permits scaling of human motion, and adds dexterity precision. (Courtesy of Computer Motion.)

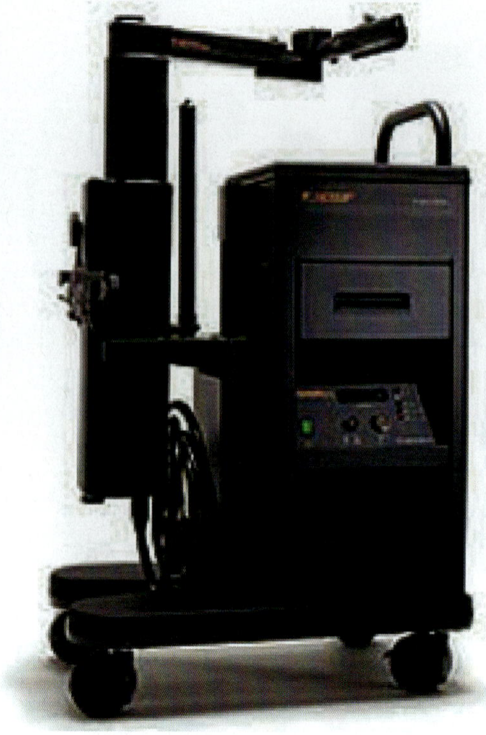

Figure 4 AESOP, the endoscope holder for advanced laparoscopic procedures and also part of Zeus. (Courtesy of Computer Motion.)

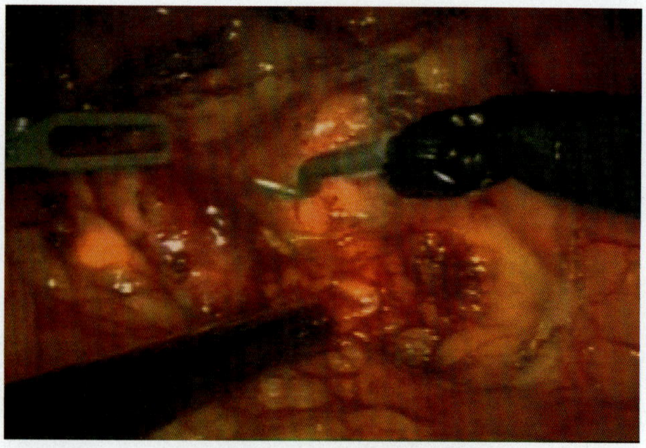

Figure 5 Laparoscopic robotic-assisted adrenalectomy using the Da Vinci system (Courtesy of Dr. S. Horgan, University of Illinois, Chicago, IL).

unsteadiness, and possibly increase patient risk during surgery (15). As early as 1992, reports of robots in the operating room showed that the use of mechanical retractors and robotic camera holders could be beneficial (13,14, 23,24). In a study by Kavoussi and colleagues (25), robotic controlled laparoscopic camera positioning was significantly steadier ($p < 0.005$) with fewer unnecessary movements than a hand-held camera. By limiting surgeon-dependent tremors that vary from case to case, robots may help standardize surgical outcomes.

In 1996, the invention of a "master-slave" manipulator system called ARTEMIS in Germany became the first surgical robot equipped with a surgeon end (the master) and a patient-end (robotic instruments or the slave end) (14). The master-slave manipulator allows the surgeon to electronically control the laparoscopic instruments while remaining seated at a distance from the patient. These original robotic telemanipulators sparked the development of future robotic surgical systems (discussed in a later section) that would soon allow for complete robot-assisted laparoscopic surgeries.

The first reported robot-assisted procedures in a human were by Cadiere and colleagues in Belgium in March 1997 (26). With the creation of advanced computer interfaces that could electronically control special instruments equipped with tips that allowed for intra-abdominal articulations, surgeons could now regain the dexterity of their hands inside the abdomen without making a large incision.

Surgical robots are currently in use for a variety of procedures in the areas of urology, cardiovascular surgery, neurosurgery, and general surgery. However, the use of robotics in endocrine surgery is still limited, and there are only a handful of case reports on robot-assisted laparoscopic adrenalectomies at this time (19–22,27) (and no reported cases of robot-assisted thyroid, parathyroid, or pancreatic tumor cases.) The limited practice of robotic-assisted endocrine surgery at this time is probably due to a number of reasons, including the novelty of the procedure, the cost of surgical robots ($750,000–$1,000,000), the limited number of surgeons trained in the procedure, and, most importantly, the lack of prospective studies showing a significant advantage for their use. Robotics seems to answer some of the limitations of standard laparoscopy, though at the current time it still lacks the ability to replace the lost tactile sensation. As technology evolves, more innovative devices will be created that will continue to expand the ability of the surgeon to treat disease while minimizing patient trauma and improving post-operative outcomes.

4 SURGICAL ROBOTS

There are currently two surgical telemanipulating robots with U.S. Food and Drug Administration regulatory clearance being used to assist minimally invasive procedures for general surgery: the Da Vinci Robotic Surgical System (Intuitive Surgical, Mountain View, CA) and the Zeus Robotic Surgical System (Computer Motion, Goleta, CA) (18,27,28).

The Da Vinci Surgical System consists of a "surgeon console" and a "surgical arm cart." An overview of the system can be seen in Figure 1. The surgical arm cart holds the robotic instruments and the endoscopic camera. The endoscope for the Da Vinci system is a specially designed 12 mm dual-camera endoscope that is capable of sending a 3D image to a specialized viewing screen in the console called the InSite Vision System. By looking into this 3D-image system, which eliminates all extraperipheral images other than those on the screen, the surgeon immerses himself in the operative field. The camera and instruments are both controlled by maneuvering the joysticks on the console. To alternate the digital handle's control back and forth between control of the camera and control of the instruments, the surgeon taps a foot pedal at the base of the console. At the current time there are 18 different robotic instruments in the Da Vinci system, which are appropriately called "endowrist instruments." The unique design of the instrument tip literally recreates the flexible movements of a human wrist (see Fig. 2). This wrist movement allows the laparoscopic surgeon to have the same 7 degrees of freedom mobility as the human hand at the tip of the laparoscopic instrument. This is in contrast to the traditional laparoscopic instrument, which is limited by a fixed pivot point and only 5 degrees of freedom (1—in and out; 2—left and right; 3—up and down; and 4—rotational; 5—grip).

Once immersed in the Da Vinci's virtual field, the surgeon inserts his fingers into the handles, sits in an ergonomically correct position, and then maneuvers the endowrist instruments with up to 7 degrees freedom: yaw (side-to-side), pitch (up/down), insertion (in and out), grip, and three additional degrees of freedom provided by the second joint in the instrument tip. In effect, maneuvering the Da Vinci instruments is like miniaturizing your hands and wrists and placing them into cavities they normally could never fit into, thus permitting the performance of delicate, precise dissection and suturing in the smallest cavity—all through small skin incisions.

The Zeus Robotic Surgical System also has two components: the surgeon console (Fig. 3) and the robotic instrument arms connected by a computer interface that can filter tremor and adjust the movement and rotational scale of the instruments. Unlike the Da Vinci system, the Zeus robotic arms are not on a cart, but instead can be attached directly to the operating room table. A second difference between the Zeus and the Da Vinci is that the Zeus uses a voice-activated camera control system called the AESOP Robotic Endoscope Positioner (Fig. 4). Instead of requiring a special 12 mm endoscope as with the Da Vinci, the Zeus allows the use of routine 5 or 10 mm endoscopes with the AESOP arm. With this system the surgeon can continuously maneuver the camera's position with simple voice commands like "camera in, camera out." The third difference between the two robotic surgery systems is that currently the Zeus system uses robotic laparoscopic instruments that mimic the hand-held laparoscopic instruments, thus lacking the additional degrees of freedom that you would get with an "endorist" instrument tip designed to mimic the human hand. Like standard laparoscopic instruments, these current Zeus instruments have only 5 degrees of freedom.

As the robotic technology is advancing rapidly, the Zeus is already in its third phase of design and is now available with instruments called "Microwrist technology." These new instruments, like the Da Vinci, have tips that offer a second joint mimicking the movements of the human wrist. Because this technology has just become available, there are no studies or published results demonstrating their efficiency, but the ability to perform wrist-like articulations inside the abdomen through small skin incisions is obviously promising.

The advantages and disadvantages of robotic-assisted surgery are currently being evaluated in various specialties including urology, cardiovascular surgery, neurosurgery, and general surgery. Each robotic system has been used for a large number of different surgical procedures, and there are now many published case reports and small series describing their feasibility. However, the only published paper to date that compares the performance of the two surgical robots in animals is by Gill et al. from Cleveland (18). They concluded that the Da Vinci and Zeus surgical systems were comparable in reducing surgeon tremor and fatigue, but that the Da Vinci and its endowrist instruments allowed for significantly shorter operating time and more "intuitive executions of surgical maneuvers" compared to the Zeus. Although this is the first time the two robots have been compared in a study on live subjects, this paper failed to compare these new robotic systems to the current standard of hand-held laparoscopy.

Dakin et al. compared the use of the two different surgical robots to the routine hand-held laparoscope and evaluated speed and precision in performing basic laparoscopic tasks (29). For basic laparoscopic tasks and speed, although the Da Vinci was significantly faster than the Zeus, standard instruments were significantly faster than either of the robotic systems. For fine (7–0) suturing and speed, the Da Vinci and standard instruments were similar, yet both were significantly faster than the Zeus. Finally, for fine suturing and precision, the robotic systems were similar but significantly more precise than standard instruments. In conclusion, for fine motor tasks, neither robot was faster than the standard instruments. For precision, robotics may have an advantage over standard instruments. Most subjects in this study had no prior experience with the robotic systems and limited experience with standard laparoscopy, therefore the results are limited as they reflect the times for first-time users and not for experienced robotic surgeons. Randomized, prospective comparison data are still scarce, and at this time it is premature to draw solid conclusions as to which is a better system for various procedures.

5 ROBOTIC-ASSISTED LAPAROSCOPIC ADRENALECTOMY

In general, robot-assisted laparoscopic surgery is another minimally invasive technique that well-trained robotic surgeons can add to their armamentarium for adrenal operations. Minimally invasive adrenalectomies began when the laparoscopic adrenalectomy was first described in 1992, and since then it has become the gold standard for the removal of benign adrenal tumors (4–6). The main advantages of laparoscopic adrenalectomy over routine open adrenalectomy include shorter operative times for unilateral adrenalectomies and less postoperative pain, fewer perioperative and postoperative complications, and quicker recovery times and return to work for patients receiving either unilateral or bilateral adrenalectomies (4). On the other hand, as is true for routine laparoscopic surgery, the lap adrenalectomy lacks 3D visualization, limits tactile feedback, restricts the degrees of freedom of movements, and has the potential for inaccuracy during the delicate dissection of the adrenal parenchyma, veins, and arteries. Both surgical robotic systems on the market seem to address the limitations of routine laparoscopy including recreating a 3D image, increasing precision and freedom of movement, eliminating tremor, reducing surgeon fatigue, and increasing natural ergonomics.

The published data on robotic adrenalectomy are extremely scarce at this time, but it is the most studied robotic-assisted endocrine procedure to date. The first published robotic assisted adrenalectomy was by Piazza and colleagues in Italy in 1999, when they successfully used the AESOP to assist a laparoscopic right adrenalectomy for Conn's syndrome (21). They reported an operating time of 180 minutes and no complications. In addition, that same year Hubens et al. from Belgium also used AESOP to successfully assist a laparoscopic adrenalectomy (22). Since then, numerous surgeons have begun to perform robotic-assisted adrenalectomies; at this time the Da Vinci Surgical System seems to be more widely used for this procedure. (Fig. 5). Gill and Sung from Cleveland compared the two surgical robotic systems with robotic-assisted laparoscopic adrenals in pigs and concluded that the Da Vinci system permitted shorter operating times (12.2 vs. 26.0 mins; $p = 0.006$) than did the Zeus system (18). Of note, the Zeus system used in their experiment was not equipped with the Microwrist technology, which would likely produce similar results. Their reported complications included adrenal parenchymal tears on both the right and the left and an IVC tear that was repairable with a robotic primary closure. These surgical systems have yet to be compared in humans.

Horgan and Vanuno from Chicago reported the use of the Da Vinci in a bilateral adrenalectomy (19). They concluded that the Da Vinci system provided superior articulation that greatly improved the precision and efficiency of the lateral and posterior dissection of the adrenal gland (Fig. 5). They agreed that the total operative time is longer than with conventional laparoscopy, but with proper training and experience for both the surgeon and the nursing staff, the operating times should eventually be comparable to routine laparoscopy.

Surgeons around the country are beginning to use the Da Vinci for unilateral and bilateral adrenalectomies, although many of these cases are not yet reported. We interviewed some of these surgeons and most of them agree that there is a steep learning curve. Approximately 5–10 cases are needed before the operating times are comparable to standard laparoscopic adrenalectomy. The 3D vision provided by the Insite vision system and the intraabdominal articulations of the "endowrist" instruments allow for precise dissections that facilitate the difficult operation while leaving only small scars and minimal postoperative pain.

6 CONCLUSIONS

Robotics and surgery are in its infancy, yet the advantages of increased precision, magnified 3D vision, and increased intraabdominal dexterity have already proven the robots as assets to a laparoscopist's armamentarium. While maintaining the advantages of tiny incisions, decreased postoperative pain, and shorter hospital stays, robot-assisted laparoscopy when applied to endocrine surgery offers patients a safe procedure with minimal postoperative trauma. As the price of the surgical robots decrease and training improves their use across the nation will grow. Eventually, hand-held laparoscopic instruments with intraabdominal articulating capabilities will replace the expensive and bulky surgical robots of today, and will continue to revolutionize laparoscopy as we know it. Until then, robot-assisted laparoscopic endocrine surgery seems appropriate for selected patients.

REFERENCES

1. Welbourn RB. Highlighs from endocrine surgical history. World J Surg 1996; 20(5):603–612.
2. Van Heerden JA. Endocrine surgery. J Am Coll Surg 1998; 186(2):142–148.
3. Roe SM. What's new in endocrine surgery. J Am Coll Surg 2001; 193(2):202–205.
4. Hansen P, Bax T, Swanstrom L. Laparoscopic adrenalectomy: history, indications, and current techniques for a minimally invasive approach to adrenal pathology. Endoscopy 1997; 29:309–314.
5. Gagner M, Lacroix A, Bolte E. Laparoscopic adrenalectomy in Cushings's syndrome and pheochromocytoma. N Engl J Med 1992; 327:1033.
6. Smith CD, Weber CJ, Amerson JR. Laparoscopic adrenalectomy: new gold standard. World J Surg 1999; 23:389–396.
7. Raeburn CD, McIntyre RC. Laparoscopic approach to adrenal and endocrine pancreatic tumors. Surg Clin North Am 2000; 80(5):1427–1441.
8. Park A, Schwartz R, Tandan V, et al. Laparoscopic pancreatic surgery. Am J Surg 1999; 177:158–163.
9. Soper NJ, Brunt LM, Dunnegan DL, Meininger TA. Laparoscopic distal pancreatectomy in the porcine model. Surg Endosc 1994; 8(1):57–60.
10. Sussman LA, Christie R, Whittle DE. Laparoscopic

excision of distal pancreas including insulinoma. Aust NZ J Surg 1996; 66:414–416.
11. Gagner M, Pomp A, Herrera MF. Early experience with laparoscopic resections of islet cell tumors. Surgery 1996; 120(6):1051–1054.
12. Gagner M. Endoscopic subtotal parathyroidectomy in patients with primary hyperparathyroidism [letter]. Br J Surg 1996; 83:875.
13. Begin E, Gagner M, Hurteau R, Santis S, Pomp A. A robotic camera for laparoscopic surgery: conception and experimental results. Surg Laparosc Endosc 1995; 5(1): 6–11.
14. Melzer A, Schurr MO, Kunert W, Buers G, Voges U, Meyer JU. Intelligent surgical instrument system (ISIS). Concept and preliminary experimental application of components and prototypes. Endosc Surg 1993; 1:166–170.
15. Sackier JM, Wang Y. Robotically assisted laparoscopic surgery. From concept to development. Surg Endosc 1994; 8(1):63–66.
16. Gill IS, Sung GT, Hsu TH, Meraney AM. Robotic remote laparoscopic nephrectomy and adrenalectomy: the initial experience. J Urol 2000; 164:2082–2085.
17. Mack MJ. Minimally invasive and robotic surgery. JAMA 2001; 285(5):568–572.
18. Sung GT, Gill IS. Robotic laparoscopic surgery: a comparison of the Da Vinci and Zeus systems. Urology 2001; 58(6):893–898.
19. Horgan S, Vanuno D. Robots in laparoscopic surgery. J Laparoendosc Adv Surg Tech A 2001; 11(6):415–419.
20. Pautler SE, McWilliams GW, Harrington FS, Walther MM. An articulating retractor holder to facilitate laparoscopic adrenalectomy and nephrectomy. J Urol 2001; 166: 198–199.
21. Piazza L, Caragliano P, Scardilli M, Sgroi AV, Marino G, Giannone G. Laparoscopic robot-assisted right adrenalectomy and left ovariectomy (case reports). Chir Ital 1999; 51(6):465–466.
22. Hubens G. Laparoscopic adrenalectomy with the aid of the AESOP 2000 robot. Acta Chir Belg 1999; 99(3):125–127.
23. Rhinisland HH. Basics of robotics and manipulator in endoscopic surgery. Endosc Surg 1993; 1:154–159.
24. Greenstein RJ. Mechanical retraction in laparoscopic surgery: cholecystectomy. J Laparoendosc Surg 1992; 2: 332–336.
25. Kavoussi LR, Moore RG, Adams JB, Partin AW. Comparison of robotic versus human laparoscopic camera control. J Urol 1995; 154:2134–2136.
26. Cadiere GB, Himpens J, Germay O, Izizaw R, Degueldre M, Vandromme J, Capelluto E, Bruyns J. Feasibility of robotic laparoscopic surgery: 146 cases. World J Surg 2001; 25(11):1467–1477.
27. www.intuitivesurgical.com
28. www.computermotion.com
29. Dakin GF, Gagner M. Comparison of laparoscopic skills performance between standard instruments and two robotic systems. Surg Endosc 2003. In press.

3

Selective Venous Sampling for Pituitary Tumors

Aman B. Patel

Mount Sinai School of Medicine, New York University, New York, New York, U.S.A.

1 INTRODUCTION AND RATIONALE

The primary reason for venous sampling in the head and neck region has been the evaluation of the secretory nature of a possible pituitary microadenoma, most commonly to distinguish between pituitary and other causes of Cushing's syndrome (CS). Pituitary-dependent hypercortisolism accounts for over 70% of cases of CS (1,2). The differentiation between pituitary and ectopic adrenocorticotropin (ACTH) secretion requires the integrated evaluation of biochemical tests and imaging techniques, none of which has a 100% diagnostic accuracy (3). Inferior petrosal sinus (IPS) sampling was devised in an attempt to improve the diagnostic work-up of CS (4,5). The rationale for IPS sampling is that a large proportion of the venous drainage of the pituitary glands is via the IPSs, allowing for analysis of samples uncontaminated from other sources. Therefore, in Cushing's disease (CD), the concentration of ACTH is expected to be higher in the IPS draining the hemi-hypophysis bearing the tumor than in the contralateral IPS or in the peripheral vessels (4,5).

A ratio between IPS and peripheral basal ACTH concentrations (IPS:P ratio) of 2:1 or greater is classically considered to be indicative of CD (4). After administration of corticotropin-releasing hormone (CRH) to stimulate ACTH secretion during IPS sampling, an IPS:P ratio of 3:1 or greater is classically considered to be indicative of CD (4). Finally, in patients with true CD, a ratio of greater than 1.4 in the detected ACTH concentration from one sinus to the other indicates that the adenoma is located on the corresponding side (6) (Table 1).

Early studies showed that IPS sampling had an extremely high sensitivity and specificity, up to 100%, in differentiating pituitary from ectopic ACTH hypersecretion (4). In addition, this technique was demonstrated to be a safe procedure, with the only frequent untoward effect being transient ear discomfort (4). Due to these results, it was suggested that IPS sampling should be performed in all cases of suspected CD without radiological evidence of a pituitary tumor. However, later studies have shown that IPS sampling is less reliable than formerly believed in the differential diagnosis of CS (3,7–14). Despite these results, IPS sampling continues to be an extremely reliable technique in the differentiation of pituitary from ectopic CS with sensitivity and specificity levels of greater than 90% (7,15–18). With CRH stimulation, the ability of sampling to correctly differentiate pituitary from ectopic CS increases.

The ability of IPS sampling to localize the side of an adenoma is less reliable than the ability to differentiate the source of CS. Studies have shown that IPS sampling correctly predicted the intra-pituitary tumor side with an average 78% diagnostic accuracy (3,6,15,19,20). An explanation for this could be the mixing of blood from the two sides of the pituitary gland (21). Another possibility is discordant sizes between the two IPSs,

Table 1 Inferior Petrosal Sinus Sampling ACTH Levels, Normal Anatomy

	Right IPS	Left IPS	Peripheral	IPS:P ratio	R: L ratio
Baseline	691	477	59	11.7:1	1.4:1
2 min Post-CRH	2245	1509	55	40.8:1	1.5:1
5 min Post-CRH	1740	528	89	19.5:1	3.3:1
10 min Post-CRH	1264	529	92	13.7:1	2.4:1
15 min Post-CRH	1060	299	94	11.3:1	3.5:1

Results of petrosal sinus sampling demonstrate petrosal to peripheral ACTH gradient before and after CRH stimulation, confirming Cushing's disease (see Fig. 1). In addition, a gradient between right and left IPSs was found, suggesting an adenoma within the right hemi-hyphosis. Transsphenoidal surgery confirmed an ACTH-secreting microadenoma within the right side of the pituitary gland.

resulting in a greater drainage via one sinus. Cavernous sinus sampling has been reported to be a better predictor of intra-pituitary tumor location and to have the same accuracy as IPS sampling in differentiating between pituitary and ectopic ACTH secretion (22,23). However, due to its higher costs and greater risks of adverse events, cavernous sinus sampling is not recommended at present (24).

In conclusion, IPS sampling has an important role in the work-up of CS in the carefully chosen patient. Sampling has a high specificity in the diagnosis of CD; thus, no patient with extra-pituitary CS risks being submitted to transsphenoidal surgery, although one must remember there is a percentage of false-negative results. In addition, the lateralizing gradient can guide the surgeon to the correct side of the pituitary gland affected by the tumor, taking into consideration that the localization is mistaken in 25–30% of cases. Therefore, IPS sampling is useful to distinguish CD from ectopic ACTH secretion, but it should be restricted to cases with conflicting hormonal and radiological findings.

2 SAMPLING TECHNIQUE

The venous drainage of the pituitary gland is via the cavernous sinus. The cavernous sinus then usually drains into the inferior petrosal sinuses, superior petrosal sinuses, and the basilar venous plexus. These all have a variable drainage course into the internal jugular vein and paraspinal venous plexus. Venous sampling must be obtained from a source that represents the venous drainage of the pituitary gland. In addition, bilateral simultaneous sampling is required to evaluate the side of a possible pituitary microadenoma. The IPSs are usually the best sites to obtain venous samples from, since they usually capture a large portion of the cavernous sinus drainage from their respective side.

2.1 Anticoagulation

Venous thrombosis of the IPS, cavernous sinuses, or jugular veins is an undesired event. Therefore, systemic anticoagulation is maintained during the procedure (4) with a bolus of 5000 U of intravenous heparin followed by a 1000 U bolus intravenously every hour thereafter. At the minimum the catheters will be in place for 30 minutes, and in cases of difficult catheterization it is not unusual to have a catheter in place for several hours.

2.2 Jugular Vein Catheterization

Bilateral venous access is established by the standard transfemoral venous approach (4). On one side a 6 French sheath is placed so that concomitant peripheral venous sampling can be obtained during the procedure. A 4 Fr. sheath is placed into the contralateral femoral vein. The jugular veins and, subsequently, the IPSs, are catheterized with 4 Fr. catheters (4). The catheter used should have an angled tip with an angle of 20–30 degrees, followed by a 2 cm straight segment. Occasionally, a different angle or shape may be necessary depending upon the specific anatomy. Each access site should be used to access the respective IPS because when the sampling is being performed, it is easier to keep track of which catheter goes where if the sampling catheters match the side they are sampling.

On the left, the junction of the innominate vein and superior vena cava is relatively large. Once the catheter is aimed in the right direction, a hydrophilic-coated guidewire should allow easy passage from the superior vena cava to the left subclavian vein. Catheterization of the left internal jugular vein can be challenging, usually because of a valve located at the thoracic inlet. Getting the wire to enter the internal jugular vein is usually a matter of luck and repetitive prodding during various phases of respiration. A forceful contrast injection into the subclavian vein will often show the location of various inflow veins as stumps, due to the venous valve system, which can then be used as guides.

Accessing the right jugular vein is usually more straightforward than the left, as the course is relatively straight. There can be variations that make the catheterization more difficult, but access can usually be achieved with a small amount of searching. The valve is usually not as much of a problem as on the left.

2.3 Inferior Petrosal Sinus Catheterization

The venous drainage at the skull base is variable, making the entry of the IPSs into the jugular system more difficult to find. In fact, advancing the catheter into the IPS is often the most challenging aspect of the procedure. Usually the IPS enters the internal jugular vein at the junction between the vein and the sigmoid sinus. The most common site of IPS entrance is at the apex of this jugular/sigmoid sinus curve and is typically located anterior and medial. Careful probing with a hydrophilic guidewire aimed in the appropriate direction will allow one to find the IPS. Occasionally a contrast injection will be needed to identify the location of the IPS. Once the guidewire is positioned into the IPS the 4 French catheter can be passed into the distal aspect of the IPS. Once the catheter is within the IPS, AP and lateral venograms are performed to confirm position and to assess the venous drainage. With good positioning, retrograde filling of both cavernous sinuses, inferior petrosal sinuses, and the basilar venous plexus is commonly seen (Fig. 1; Table 1).

Anomalous venous anatomy can make catheterization of the IPS difficult for even the most skilled practitioners. If difficulty is encountered, suspect a duplicated jugular vein or anomalous drainage of the IPS. In these circumstances, venography of the other IPS would invariably fill across the midline, clearly demonstrating the contralateral IPS. It is then possible to locate the exact entry point of the IPS into the opposite internal jugular vein. In the most difficult cases it is necessary to catheterize the arterial system, select the internal carotid artery, and perform a standard angiogram to locate the cavernous sinuses and visualize its drainage.

2.4 Venous Sampling Procedure

After the catheters are in position bilaterally, baseline samples are taken from each IPS catheter and the peripheral 6 Fr. sheath simultaneously. One must take care to place the samples into the appropriate specimen

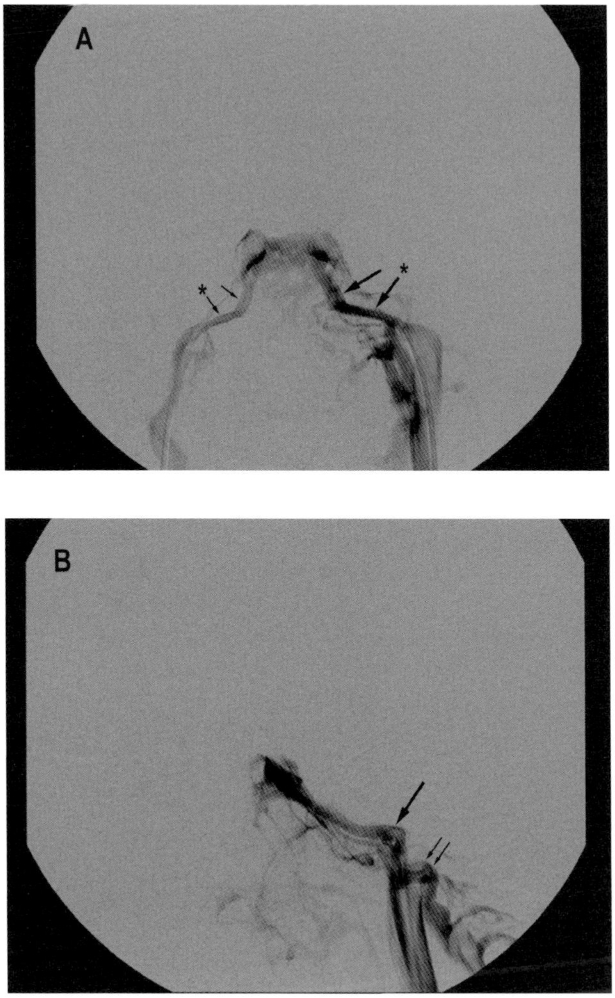

Figure 1 Normal symmetrical inferior petrosal sinuses (IPSs). (A) AP venogram obtained via injection of the left IPS (large arrows). Note filling of bilateral IPSs and cavernous sinuses. In addition, normal size of IPSs results in drainage into bilateral internal jugular veins. Arrows with label (*) indicate correct site of sampling catheter. (B) Lateral venograms via injection of left IPS. Drainage into bilateral internal jugular veins is noted (arrows). See Table 1 for sampling results.

tubes. For ACTH, samples are usually placed in the same tubes used for complete blood counts and kept on ice. Prolactin and growth hormone samples are placed in serum-chemistry tubes. These are guidelines, and for each institution prior contact with the appropriate laboratory should be made for confirmation of these instructions and coordination of handling.

After the baseline samples are collected, challenge or stimulation testing can be performed. This is most

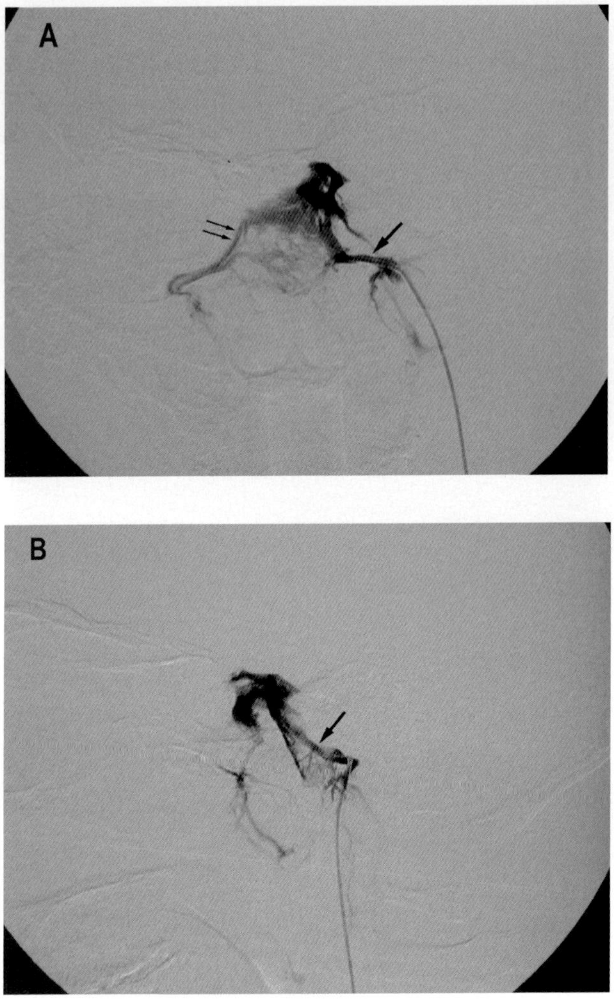

Figure 2 Hypoplastic IPSs. (A) AP venograms obtained via injection of the left IPS (large arrow). A hypoplastic right IPS (small arrows) with no drainage into the right internal jugular vein is seen. In addition, the left IPS (large arrow) is also smaller than normal, as indicated by the lack of drainage into the left internal jugular vein. (B) Lateral venogram via injection of left IPS (large arrow) also demonstrates lack of drainage into either internal jugular vein. See Table 2 for sampling results.

commonly performed for the work-up of CS. For ACTH testing, corticotropin-releasing hormone or Acthrel (ovine corticotropin-releasing hormone) is administered in a 1 μg/kg (up to a maximum of 100 μg) intravenous bolus peripherally. After administration of CRH, 2-, 5-, 10-, and 15-minute samples are obtained simultaneously from the IPSs and the peripheral vein. These samples are then placed in the appropriate tubes, labeled, placed on ice, and then sent to the laboratory for the appropriate analysis.

After the samples have been obtained, the IPS catheters are removed, heparin is reversed using protamine, and the sheaths are withdrawn. Pressure is applied to the femoral veins until hemostasis is obtained. The patient is observed for 2 hours post-procedure and then discharged.

3 FALSE-NEGATIVE RESULTS: REASONS

Doppman et al. (25), reviewing retrograde IPS venograms of 501 patients with surgically proven CD and negative pituitary imaging, reported that all patients with false-negative results had a hypoplastic or plexiform IPS ipsilateral to the adenoma (Figs. 2 and 3;

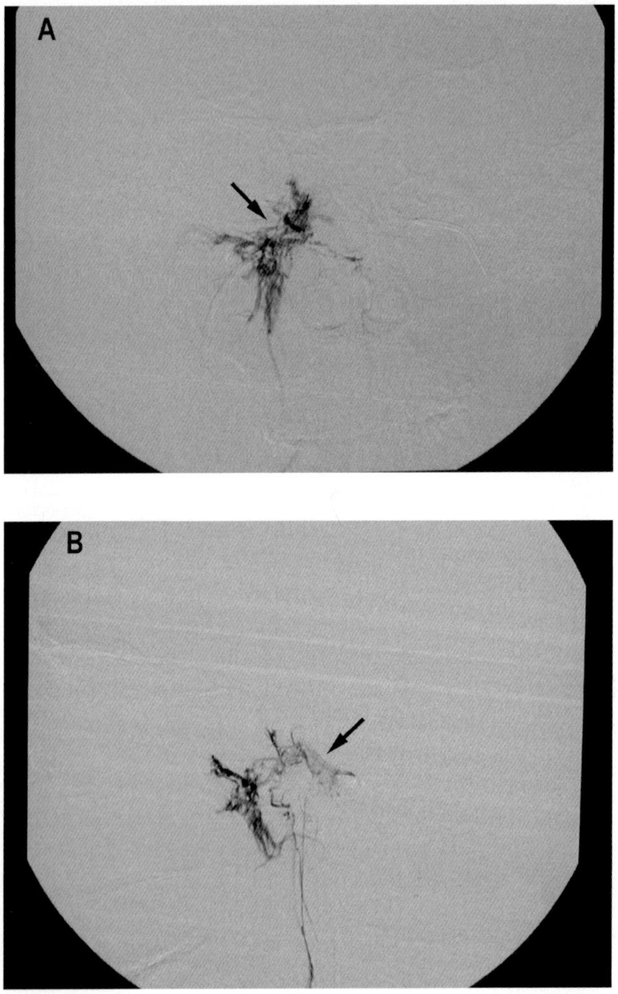

Figure 3 Right plexiform IPS (arrows) prevented catheter positioning. Petrosal sampling results were inconclusive and resulted in a false-negative test result. Transsphenoidal surgery revealed a microadenoma: (A) AP; (B) lateral.

Table 2 Inferior Petrosal Sinus Sampling ACTH Levels, Hypoplastic Sinuses

	Right IPS	Left IPS	Peripheral	IPS:P ratio	R: L ratio
Baseline	52	53	0	1:1	1:1
2 min Post-CRH	88	83	60	1.5:1	1:1
5 min Post-CRH	178	183	140	1.3:1	1:1
10 min Post-CRH	237	265	201	1.3:1	1.1:1
15 min Post-CRH	338	356	263	1.4:1	1.1:1

Results of petrosal sinus sampling demonstrate no petrosal to peripheral ACTH gradient before and after CRH stimulation in a patient with hypoplastic IPSs (see Fig. 2). This patient subsequently had a surgically proven ACTH-secreting pituitary microadenoma.

Table 2). Another explanation for a false-negative result is a potential additional drainage through the portal sinuses, ascending through the pituitary stalk into the hypothalamus (26). Sampling errors may also occur due to dilution of pituitary blood from nonpituitary sources secondary to extensive anastomosis between the IPS and the basilar venous plexus, retrograde drainage of superior petrosal sinuses, or misplaced catheters (21). Presampling visualization of anatomical variants may give an indication of the possibility of a false-negative result. However, even when venograms show correct positioning of the catheter, there is no definitive proof of correct sampling of pituitary blood from both IPSs.

4 COMPLICATIONS

IPS sampling is a safe and reliable procedure; however, it is an invasive test and should be used with caution. Although extremely rare, brain-stem vascular damage and transient or permanent neurological deficit can occur (incidence ~0.2%) (27,28). However, in most cases, IPS sampling causes only minor complications such as hematomas, vasovagal reaction (29); or transient ear discomfort. Due to vascular fragility and hypercoagulability of hypercortisolemic patients, heparin should be given to prevent thrombotic events. Injury to the vascular wall with subsequent thrombosis is the presumed caused of venous thromboembolism after IPS sampling (30,31). Therefore, since severe adverse reactions can occur during the procedure, although rare, IPS sampling should be performed only in specialized referral centers, where the safety of this procedure is greatly elevated.

REFERENCES

1. Aron DC, Findling JW, Tyrrell JB. Cushing's disease. Endocrinol Metab Clin North Am 1987; 16:705–730.
2. Orth DN. Cushing's syndrome. N Engl J Med 1995; 332:791–803.
3. Newell-Price J, Trainer P, Besser M, Grossman A. The diagnosis and differential diagnosis of Cushing's syndrome and pseudo-Cushing's states. Endocr Rev 1998; 19:647–672.
4. Oldfield EH, Doppman JL, Nieman LK, Chrousos GP, Miller DL, Katz DA, Cutler GBJr., Loriaux DL. Petrosal sinus sampling with and without corticotropin-releasing hormone for the differential diagnosis of Cushing's syndrome. N Engl J Med 1991; 325:897–905.
5. Corrigan DF, Schaaf M, Whaley RA, Czerwinski CL, Earll JM. Selective venous sampling to differentiate ectopic ACTH secretion from pituitary Cushing's sundrome. N Engl J Med 1977; 296:861–862.
6. Oldfield EH, Chrousos GP, Schulte HM, Schaaf M, McKeeven PE, Krudy AG. Preoperative lateralization of ACTH-secreting pituitary microadenomas by bilateral and simultaneous inferior petrosal sinus sampling. N Engl J Med 1985; 312:100–103.
7. Boscaro M, Rampazzo A, Paoletta A, Roseano P, Pagotto U, Fallo F, Sonino N. Selective venous sampling in the differential diagnosis of ACTH-dependent Cushing's syndrome. Neuroendocrinology 1992; 55:264–268.
8. Colao A, Merola B, Tripodi F.S, Di Sarno A, Esposito V, Marzullo P, La Tessa G, Spaziante R, Lombardi G. Simultaneous and bilateral inferior petrosal sinus sampling for the diagnosis of Cushing's syndrome: comparison of multihormonal assay, baseline multiple sampling and ACTH-releasing hormone test. Horm Res 1993; 40:209–216.
9. de Herder WW, Uitterlinden P, Pieterman H, Tanghe HL, Kwekkeboom DJ, Pols HA, Singh R, van de Berge JH, Lamberts SW. Pituitary tumour localization in patients with Cushing's disease by magnetic resonance imaging. Is there a place for petrosal sinus sampling? Clin Endocrinol (Oxf) 1994; 40:87–92.
10. Zarrilli L, Colao A, Merola B, La Tessa G, Spaziante R, Tripodi FS, Di Sarno A, Marzano LA, Lombardi G. Corticotropin-releasing hormone test: improvement of the diagnostic accuracy of simultaneous and bilateral inferior petrosal sinus sampling in patients

with Cushing syndrome. World J Surg 1995; 19:150–153.

11. Yamamoto Y, Davis DH, Nippoldt TB, Young WF Jr., Huston J3rd, Parisi JE. False-positive inferior petrosal sinus sampling in the diagnosis of Cushing's disease. Report of two cases. J Neurosurg 1995; 83:1087–1091.
12. Lopez J, Barcelo B, Lucas T, Salame F, Alameda C, Boronat M, Salto L, Estrada J. Petrosal sinus sampling for diagnosis of Cushing's disease: evidence of false negative results. Clin Endocrinol (Oxf) 1996; 45:147–156.
13. Heppner C, Becker K, Saeger W, Gunther RW, Allolio B, Krone W, Winkelmann W. Occult eutopic Cushing's syndrome—failure of simultaneous bilateral petrosal sinus sampling to diagnose pituitary-dependent Cushing's syndrome. Eur J Endocrinol 1997; 137:74–78.
14. Young J, Deneux C, Grino M, Oliver C, Chanson P, Schaison G. Pitfall of petrosal sinus sampling in a Cushing's syndrome secondary to ectopic adrenocorticotropin-corticotropin releasing hormone (ACTH-CRH) secretion. J Clin Endocrinol Metab 1998; 83:305–308.
15. Colao A, Faggiano A, Pivonello R, Giraldi FP, Cavagnini F, Lombardi G. Inferior petrosal sinus sampling in the differential diagnosis of Cushing's syndrome: results of an Italian multicenter study. Eur J Endocrinol 2001; 144:499–507.
16. Kaltsas GA, Giannulis MG, Newell-Price JD, Dacie JE, Thakkar C, Afshar F, Monson JP, Grossman AB, Besser GM, Trainer PJ. A critical analysis of the value of simultaneous inferior petrosal sinus sampling in Cushing's disease and the occult ectopic adrenocorticotropin syndrome. J Clin Endocrinol Metab 1999; 84:487–492.
17. Wiggam MI, Heaney AP, McIlrath EM, McCance DR, Sheridan B, Hadden DR, Atkinson AB. Bilateral inferior petrosal sinus sampling in the differential diagnosis of adrenocorticotropin-dependent Cushing's syndrome: a comparison with other diagnostic tests. J Clin Endocrinol Metab 2000; 85:1525–1532.
18. Bonelli FS, Huston J 3rd, Carpenter PC, Erickson D, Young WFJr., Meyer FB. Adrenocorticotropic hormone-dependent Cushing's syndrome: sensitivity and specificity of inferior petrosal sinus sampling. Am J Neuroradiol 2000; 21:690–696.
19. Booth GL, Redelmeier DA, Grosman H, Kovacs K, Smyth HS, Ezzat S. Improved diagnostic accuracy of inferior petrosal sinus sampling over imaging for localizing pituitary pathology in patients with Cushing's disease. J Clin Endocrinol Metab 1998; 83:2291–2295.
20. Frank SJ, Gesundheit N, Doppman JL, Miller DL, Merriam GR, Oldfield EH, Weintraub BD. Preoperative lateralization of pituitary microadenomas by petrosal sinus sampling: utility in two patients with non-ACTH-secreting tumors. Am J Med 1989; 87:679–682.
21. Doppman JL, Krudy AG, Girton ME, Oldfield EH. Basilar venous plexus of the posterior fossa: a potential source of error in petrosal sinus sampling. Radiology 1985; 155:375–378.
22. Graham KE, Samuels MH, Nesbit GM, Cook DM, O'Neill OR, Barnwell SL, Loriaux DL. Cavernous sinus sampling is highly accurate in distinguishing Cushing's disease from the ectopic adrenocorticotropin syndrome and in predicting intrapituitary tumor location. J Clin Endocrinol Metab 1999; 84:1602–1610.
23. Teramoto A, Yoshida Y, Sanno N, Nemoto S. Cavernous sinus sampling in patients with adrenocorticotrophic hormone-dependent Cushing's syndrome with emphasis on inter- and intracavernous adrenocorticotrophic hormone gradients. J Neurosurg 1998; 89:762–768.
24. Doppman JL, Nieman LK, Chang R, Yanovski JA, Cutler GBJr., Chrousos G. Selective venous sampling from the cavernous sinuses is not a more reliable technique than sampling from the inferior petrosal sinuses in Cushing's syndrome. J Clin Endocrinol Metab 1995; 80:2485–2489.
25. Doppman JL, Chang R, Oldfield EH, Chrousos G, Stratakis CA, Nieman LK. The hypoplastic inferior petrosal sinus: a potential source of false-negative results in petrosal sampling for Cushing's disease. J Clin Endocrinol Metab 1999; 84:533–540.
26. Bergland RM, Page RB. Can the pituitary secrete directly to the brain? (affirmative anatomical evidence). Endocrinology 1978; 102:1325–1338.
27. Lefournier V, Gatta B, Martinie M, Vasdev A, Tabarin A, Bessou P, Berge J, Bachelot I, Chabre O. One transient neurological complication (sixth nerve palsy) in 166 consecutive inferior petrosal sinus samplings for the etiological diagnosis of Cushing's syndrome. J Clin Endocrinol Metab 1999; 84:3401–3402.
28. Bonelli FS, Huston J3rd, Meyer FB, Carpenter PC. Venous subarachnoid hemorrhage after inferior petrosal sinus sampling for adrenocorticotropic hormone. Am J Neuroradiol 1999; 20:306–307.
29. Sturrock ND, Jeffcoate WJ. A neurological complication of inferior petrosal sinus sampling during investigation for Cushing's disease: a case report. J Neurol Neurosurg Psychiatry 1997; 62:527–528.
30. Diez JJ, Iglesias P. Complications of inferior petrosal sinus sampling for the etiological diagnosis of Cushing's syndrome. J Endocrinol Invest 2002; 25:195–196.
31. Obuobie K, Davies JS, Ogunko A, Scanlon MF. Venous thrombo-embolism following inferior petrosal sinus sampling in Cushing's disease. J Endocrinol Invest 2000; 23:542–544.

4

Pituitary Tumors

Raj K. Shrivastava, Wesley A. King, and Kalmon D. Post

Mount Sinai School of Medicine, New York University, New York City, New York, U.S.A.

1 THE HYPOTHALAMIC-PITUITARY UNIT

The anterior pituitary gland is under predominantly stimulatory control by the hypothalamus. Function of the normal pituitary gland depends on the integrity of the hypothalamus, the portal circulation, and the pituitary stalk. Portal vessels originate in a capillary bed in the median eminence and extend through long portal vessels into the pituitary stalk and to the adenohypophysis. The pituitary hormones adrenocorticotropic hormone (ACTH), growth hormone (GH), prolactin (PRL), thyroid-stimulating hormone (TSH), luteinizing hormone (LH), and follicle-stimulating hormone (FSH) are controlled by the hypothalamic hormones corticotropin-releasing factor (CRF), dopamine [or prolactin inhibitory factor (PIF)], growth hormon–ereleasing factor (GRF), thyroid-releasing hormone (TRH), and gonadotropin-releasing hormone (Gn-RH), respectively. This is efficiently accomplished via a portal vascular system connecting the hypothalamus with the anterior pituitary gland. These hypothalamic releasing factors are then under negative feedback control from the end-organ products (adrenal gland products, thyroid hormone, etc.), thereby completing the axis loop (1). The predominant net hypothalamic regulatory influence is stimulatory for all pituitary hormones except prolactin, which is under dominant inhibitory control (2). Any interruption or compression of the network of portal vessels as a result of pressure or invasion by any perisellar mass can alter the delivery of these hypothalamic factors to the anterior pituitary and cause impairment in its function.

The anterior pituitary gland is responsible for the secretion and regulation of a variety of peptide hormones and regulating factors. Tumors originating in the anterior pituitary gland may therefore produce excess quantities of a particular peptide hormone. Pituitary adenomas are benign monoclonal tumors that arise from the cells comprising the anterior pituitary gland. They account for approximately 15% of all intracranial tumors. The alterations in hormone secretion seen in patients with pituitary adenomas are often caused directly by the tumor itself or as a complication of its expansion and compression of surrounding structures, as is often seen in patients with partial or complete hypopituitarism. When this occurs, the resulting adenoma is classified as a functioning or secretory adenoma. Tumors without hormonal activity are logically classified as nonfunctioning or nonsecretory adenomas. In this chapter we will briefly review the different types of functioning pituitary tumors. To this end we will first review the hypothalamic-pituitary organ axis to help understand the diagnosis and treatment of patients with functioning pituitary tumors.

Anterior pituitary gland adenomas are identified pathologically both by their in vivo endocrine activity and by their in vitro immunohistochemical staining characteristics. The advent of immunohistochemical staining for the various peptide hormones has revealed the fact that many adenomas once thought to be nonsecretory actually secrete endocrinologically inactive peptides (3).

Adenomas maybe further subdivided into micro- or macroadenomas based upon size (4). Tumors less than 1 cm in diameter are considered microadenomas and are predictably located solely within the sella turcica. They characteristically do not invade neighboring structures such as the sphenoid and cavernous sinuses. Macroadenomas, by definition greater than 1 cm, typically enlarge the sella turcica and frequently invade neighboring structures. Microadenomas usually are discovered because of an endocrinopathy, whereas macroadenomas present with compressive effects of the tumor, i.e., bitemporal hemianopsia, as well as endocrinopathy. The endocrinopathy may be one of either oversecretion of undersecretion.

The evaluation of a patient with a suspected functioning pituitary tumor will be discussed in relation to each tumor type; however, because of the protean and often subtle manifestations of these endocrinopathies, a detailed history and physical examination are mandatory in guiding the rest of the work-up. Subtle changes in hair growth, skin texture or color, and body mass may be the only heralds of early endocrine dysfunction. Magnetic resonance imaging (MRI) technology has dramatically changed the radiographic evaluation of pituitary adenomas. MRI with and without gadolinium enhancement is now considered the study of choice in evaluating patients with suspected pituitary abnormalities (5–8). The normal pituitary gland will enhance within 5 minutes of contrast administration, leaving the adenoma hypointense compared to the surrounding pituitary. Findings on high-resolution MRI studies are highly sensitive, with a 60–70% sensitivity on unenhanced studies and increasing by 10% on postcontrast studies. Computed tomography (CT) scans are helpful in evaluating bony changes in the sella and surrounding structures but are much less sensitive than MRI in detecting small adenomas (9–12). All patients with pituitary adenomas must undergo detailed visual field testing, which is most important in those patients with macroadenomas.

2 PITUITARY TUMORS AND NEUROSURGERY

2.1 Prolactin-Secreting Adenomas

Prolactin-secreting pituitary adenomas are the most common form of pituitary tumor and represent the most common cause of hyperprolactinemia. Prolactin is classified as a somatomammotropic hormone along with growth hormone and chorionic somatomammotropin (13). It is a 198-amino-acids peptide chain necessary for the normal lactation in postpartum women. Prolactin levels begin to rise shortly after conception and reach levels of 150–200 ng/mL at term, but it is not until the postpartum decline in estrogen is complete that lactation may occur. Stimulation of tactile receptors on the nipple and areola of the breast leads to prolactin secretion that in the postpartum estrogen-primed breast results in lactation. Hyperprolactinemia disrupts normal reproductive function by altering the pulsatile gonadotropin secretion, interfering with sex steroid feedback at the level of the hypothalamus, and inhibiting gonadal steroidogenesis. TRH and vasoactive intestinal peptide (VIP) both appear to have minor prolactin-releasing activity, although their significance is presently unclear. Although the above stimuli lead to increases in prolactin secretion, the overwhelming control of prolactin release is inhibitory in nature, via dopamine. Dopamine, also known as prolactin-inhibiting factor, is released by the hypothalamus and leads to a decrease in prolactin secretion. As mentioned earlier, this inhibitory control becomes vitally important in the medical management of prolactinomas (14,15). Normal prolactin levels are less than 15 ng/mL in men and less than 20 ng/mL in nonpregnant women. Causes of hyperprolactinemia other than a pituitary adenoma include pregnancy, stress, hypoglycemia, renal failure, hypothyroidism, and phenothiazine-like medications. These, as well as several other etiologies, must be considered prior to a detailed investigation of a patient's pituitary gland (16).

2.2 Signs and Symptoms

Prolactin-secreting tumors represent 40% of all pituitary adenomas and are typically more symptomatic in women. Hyperprolactinemia in women leads to amenorrhea, galactorrhea, and osteoporosis, while in men it may result in diminished sexual drive and impotence or it may be asymptomatic. Menstrual disturbances are present in 93% of premenopausal women with prolactinomas. Because of this difference, men are not usually diagnosed until the tumor has reached a size sufficient to cause compressive effects on neighboring structures (17).

2.3 Diagnosis

Random measurement of serum prolactin levels are reliable to establish the diagnosis of hyperprolactinemia. This should begin with MRI with contrast, which often discloses a pituitary macroadenoma. Hyperprolactinemia in the presence of a macroadenoma does not mean a priori that the tumor is a prolactinoma. The degree of prolactin elevation is believed to be directly related to the functionality of the tumor. Serum prolactin levels greater than 150 ng/mL correlate well with the presence of a prolactinoma; however, milder elevations may be due to stalk compression leading to interference with the inhibitory effects of dopamine.

2.4 Treatment

The dopamine agonist bromocriptine has fundamentally changed the treatment of symptomatic prolactinomas (18–32). Other than selected indications, bromocriptine therapy has virtually replaced transsphenoidal resection as the therapy of choice. Bromocriptine is a dopamine agonist that directly stimulates the dopamine receptors located on lactotrophs (prolactin-secreting cells). Dosages of 2.5–7.5 mg/day are usually sufficient to treat most patients. The response to medical therapy can be dramatic. Prolactin levels begin to decrease in a matter of hours following the first dose, and tumor size often diminishes within a few days. Patients with visual field deficits may begin to improve after a few days of treatment. Other than pregnancy or a rapidly deteriorating visual/neurological function, there are virtually no contraindications to an initial trial of bromocriptine therapy. Follow-up with periodic serum prolactin measurements and imaging studies of the sella is necessary to ensure that therapy is effective. In approximately 66% of patients, tumor size will be reduced by as much as 75%, with the best response seen in patients with large tumors (21). Endocrine functions often return to normal with establishment of cyclic menses in women and return of libido in men. Many previously infertile women have, in fact, been able to conceive while on bromocriptine therapy.

Since bromocriptine is not tumoricidal, tumor reexpansion will occur when therapy is stopped (33). There is, however, a subset of patients in which neither discontinuation of therapy nor microdosage leads to a return of symptoms (20,34). Since there is no way of knowing which patients will have a response to medical therapy, it is prudent to stop therapy every few years and determine if there is continued need for treatment (35). There now exist newer nonergot dopamine agonists, such as CV 502-205, which has shown promise in a once-daily administration.

The side effects of bromocriptine usually consist of nausea and vomiting. Women with tumors larger than 12 mm who wish to conceive are often referred for surgery prior to pregnancy to avoid the pregnancy-induced enlargement of the tumor and its secondary neurological symptoms. For women with tumors less than 12 mm there is a 1% risk of neurological dysfunction (36).

The indication for surgery in patients with prolactinomas is for those who are either completely intolerant or show minimal response to medical therapy, as well as for patients with a severe or worsening visual field deficit. Surgery is also recommended for those patients who do not improve after 2 months of medical therapy (37).

The role of radiation therapy in prolactinomas is limited. Primary radiation therapy is reserved for elderly or debilitated patients who have large tumors and who are not helped by medical therapy. Radiation therapy is mostly used as adjunctive to surgery in those patients with residual tumor who are unresponsive to medical therapy.

Pretreatment with bromocriptine prior to surgery to "shrink" the tumor has been suggested to increase the cure rate (38,39). Since long-term treatment with bromocriptine has been associated with tumor fibrosis, if surgery is indicated it is best performed within a year of therapy (40,41).

There exists a subset of patients with so-called asymptomatic microprolactinomas whose tumor size and serum prolactin levels remain unchanged or even decrease over many years in follow-up. For this population, regular surveillance without treatment may be sufficient (42,43). It still remains to be determined whether there are any beneficial effects to normalizing prolactin levels in this population (44,45).

3 GROWTH HORMONE SECRETING ADENOMAS (ACROMEGALY)

Acromegaly or gigantism results from the hypersecretion of growth hormone. The term acromegaly, derived from the Greek *akron* (extremity) and *megale* (large), describes only one aspect of the clinical features through which the disease process presents. Harvey Cushing is credited with relating the overproduction of growth hormone to a pituitary source (46). GH is a polypeptide, 191 amino acids long, normally produced and released by the somatotropic cells found in the anterior pituitary in response to hypothalamic GRF (47). Somatostatin is a 14-amino-acid cyclic peptide-releasing factor that inhibits GH release (48). Three or four bursts of GH secretions occur per day, punctuating a basal state of minimal activity (49). Sleep, physical exertion or stress, hyper- and hypoglycemia, and a variety of pharmacological agents can also precipitate GH release. Circulating GH results in the secretion from the liver of a family of peptides called somatomedins. Somatomedin-C (insulin-like growth factor I) is the most familiar somatomedin measured. These secondary hormones, in turn, produce a variety of anabolic effects throughout the body and mediate the effects of GH at the end-organ level. Unlike GH, the somatomedins do not exhibit significant diurnal variation in serun levels and therefore may be a better means of evaluating patients (50).

Hypersecretion of GH can result from a number of conditions. The most common, and the focus of this section, is a pituitary adenoma. GH may also be produced by ectopic adenomas derived from remnants of the embryonic pituitary diverticulum or from tumors of the breast, lung, or ovary (51). Acromegaly may rarely be caused be excessive production of GRF by a hypothalamic tumor or from peripheral sources, such as carcinoid tumors of the abdomen (52).

3.1 Signs and Symptoms

Acromegaly affects males and females equally in the fifth decade (53). The effects of chronically elevated growth hormone are gradual and will result in gigantism in a child whose epiphyseal plates have not yet closed or in classic acromegalic features in an adult. Typically there is an insidious coarsening of the facial features and an increase in the soft tissues. The somatic changes may be so insidious as to go unnoticed until old photographs are used for comparison. Classically, patients first note an increase in shoe size or inability to wear rings that previously fit well. Later in the disease process, patients may develop visceromegaly, arthralgias, nerve entrapment syndromes, hyperhidrosis, prognathism, and acrochordon (skin tags). It has been noted in several studies that as many as 46% of patients will have colonic polyps, of which more than 50% are adenomatous (54). Some studies have also shown that the incidence of true colon carcinoma in acromegalics may be higher than in the general population. Because of this relationship, it has been recommended that acromegalic patients older than 50 years, patients with a more than 10-year history of acromegaly, or patients with more than three skin tags should have careful screening for colonic disease (55).

3.2 Diagnosis

The laboratory diagnosis of acromegaly is hampered by the normally wide daily variations in serum GH levels. In fact, the daily burst of secretion is maintained even in the presence of oversecretion of GH from an adenoma. Unlike the other secretory adenomas, static measurements of serum GH are, therefore, unreliable in establishing the diagnosis of acromegaly. Normal basal GH levels are generally below 1 ng/mL, with several secretory bursts seen throughout the day (56). In acromegaly the basal level is often elevated to levels above 5 ng/mL, although some patients may have normal basal levels with elevations only during the daily secretory burst.

Fortunately, somatomedin-C levels are not only even throughout the day, but are consistently elevated in acromegaly. Static measurements of somatomedin-C are an effective and reliable method for confirming the diagnosis of acromegaly (57,58). Alternatively, a glucose tolerance test can be performed. Normally, GH is suppressed to levels below 2 ng/mL after an oral glucose load (100 g). Failure of this normal suppression is consistent with hypersecretion of GH. In addition, infusions of either GRF or TRH will lead to increased GH in affected individuals but not in normal subjects.

Once a patient is confirmed as having a hypersecretory state, the goal is to discover the source. The overwhelming majority of patients will have an anterior pituitary adenoma, and therefore, the radiographic work-up should begin with a contrast MRI. Only in the few cases where no pituitary mass is demonstrated should a search be made for ectopic sources of GH.

3.3 Treatment

The effects of untreated acromegaly are eventually fatal. Patients will develop cardiac failure, diabetes, disfigurement, and possibly blindness, leading to a markedly shortened life expectancy (59). The goal of treatment, therefore, is the safe and rapid reduction of GH levels, elimination of any mass effect, and preservation of normal hormonal balance. The type of treatment must be judged by its ability to normalize GH levels and thereby to eliminate the development of the various metabolic derangements associated with hypersecretory states. The criteria for successful treatment of acromegaly are controversial. The accepted postoperative levels of GH that are indicative of a cure have declined in recent years. The current standard for cure is clinical remission associated with a postoperative GH level of <5 ng/mL with a normal somatomedin-C level (60). Growth hormone levels may return to normal in hours or days, but it has been our experience that somatomedin-C levels may take weeks or months to normalize.

Postoperative adjuvant therapy should be reserved for patients that do not meet these criteria.

Transsphenoidal resection remains the primary treatment modality for acromegaly. Successful resection results in a rapid reduction in GH levels and can be achieved with very low morbidity and mortality, even in older patients (4,61–66). In addition, the preservation of pituitary function has been reported to be as high as 95%, avoiding the need for lifelong hormone replacement. For larger tumors not amenable to curative resection, surgery still plays a significant role in reducing tumor load prior to any adjuvant therapy.

While transsphenoidal resection of pituitary adenomas is a safe and well-tolerated procedure, there are still many patients who are not surgical candidates. In those cases medical therapy and radiotherapy have therapeutic importance. The medical treatment of acromegalics has undergone considerable change in the past 10–15 years. Medical therapy that included estrogens, chlorpromazine, and antiserotoninergic agents had met with only limited success. Bromocriptine therapy, when used for its dopaminergic effects, was able to reduce GH levels to 5–10 ng/mL in more than 20% of patients (67–71). Most patients did achieve some relief of their somatic symptomatology, with reduced soft tissue swelling and decreased perspiration, even though GH levels were still elevated. The dosages necessary to achieve these effects are much higher than the dosages needed to control a prolactinoma, and the consequent incidence of side effects and drug intolerance is much higher.

Somatostatin naturally suppresses GH production, but it has a short half-life (2 min). A recently developed somatostatin analogue, octreotide, has a longer half-life and has been shown to be very effective (72–80). It must be administered three times each day as a subcutaneous injection or as a continuous subcutaneous infusion. The most common side effects reported include diarrhea and cholelithiasis (81), and the incidence of these side effects increases the longer the drug is administered. Some recent studies have shown dramatic reductions in GH levels and moderate tumor shrinkage. The perioperative period may be significantly improved by using octreotide for 3–4 months preoperatively. The soft tissue changes above the tongue and throat may lessen the risks of anesthesia.

The only other treatment option for patients is radiation therapy. Not only is this treatment fraught with difficulties such as hypopituitarism (in up to 25%) and radiation necrosis, but it has not been shown to be uniformly effective (82). Many patients will have persistently elevated GH levels for years following radiation therapy and may never reach normal levels, resulting in delayed or incomplete remission (83).

4 GLYCOPROTEIN-SECRETING ADENOMAS: TSH, FSH, LH

The glycoprotein hormones produced in the mammalian pituitary gland are TSH, LH, and FSH. Although these hormones are clearly related structurally, their roles are markedly different. TSH, as its name implies, regulates the metabolic rate via thyroid hormones, while the gonadotropic hormones LH, and FSH are responsible for sexual maturation and play pivotal roles in reproduction. Structurally, all three are composed of a common α subunit bonded to a β subunit that is unique to each hormone.

A number of laboratory advances have changed our understanding of glycoprotein-secreting adenomas. Two in particular were the development of specific immunohistochemical techniques for looking at tumor specimens and the improved techniques of measuring hormone and subunit levels in vivo. It has always been taught that glycoprotein-secreting adenomas represent a very small percentage of all pituitary tumors (approximately 1%). These improved techniques are revealing that many so-called "nonfunctioning" adenomas have evidence of glycoprotein production by immunohistochemical staining and serum radioimmunoassay techniques (3).

4.1 Signs and Symptoms

Except for TSH-secreting tumors, which may present as hyperthyroidism, the glycoprotein-secreting adenomas do not produce any specific clinical syndrome. Consequently, these adenomas are not diagnosed until they produce compressive effects. This unfortunately means that many of these tumors will grow to a size and extent that precludes any curative resection.

Hyperthyroidism caused by a TSH adenoma differs significantly from Graves' disease, for which it is often mistaken (84,85). The typical features of Graves' disease, including opthalmopathy, pretibial edema, female preponderance, and serum thyroid-stimulating immunoglobin, are lacking in hyperthyroidism of pituitary origin. Of note is a rare inherited disorder (autosomal dominant) designated as "selective pituitary resistance to thyroid hormone," in which the normal feedback effect of thyroid hormone upon TSH secretion is defective. This leads to TSH hypersecretion and continued production of active thyroid hormone, resulting in clinical hyperthyroidism. The TSH levels increase with TRH simulation, and this disorder is often associated with deaf-mutism, stippled epiphyses, and goiter, distinguishing it from a pituitary adenoma.

4.2 Diagnosis

As mentioned above, these tumors do not typically present with symptoms of hormone hypersecretion. As a result the determination that a pituitary tumor is secreting one of the glycoproteins is usually made after the tumor itself is discovered. Each of the hormones is composed of an α and a β subunit. Although the α subunit is the same for all three hormones, the β subunit is specific to each type. We are currently only able to assay intact hormone levels (α + β), or α subunit levels alone. The measurement of β subunit levels is possible, but is only available in some research laboratories. We have learned that not all patients will have an elevated intact hormone level, and some may in fact have low intact hormone levels with evidence of hormone production seen on pathological examinations (86). Fortunately, α subunit levels are elevated consistently in these tumors, decrease after successful treatment, and rise with tumor recurrence, although 22% of truly nonfunctional adenomas will have an associated α subunit association (87,88).

As with all other pituitary adenomas, MRI with contrast has replaced all other imaging modalities for evaluation of tumor anatomy. Specific to glycoprotein-secreting adenomas is the tendency to be larger and involve adjacent structures more often (89). Aside from this there is no way to distinguish these adenomas from any other pituitary adenoma based on radiographic studies alone.

4.3 Treatment

The treatment of patients with glycoprotein-secreting adeomas is often difficult. Because of the delay in clinical presentation, these tumors usually have suprasellar extension and involvement of the cavernous sinuses, lowering the chances for a surgical cure. Transsphenoidal resection is necessary for tissue diagnosis as well as decompression of the optic chiasma. Most patients have adequate symptomatic relief postoperatively; however, surgery is very often combined with radiotherapy or adjuvant medical therapy. Since the response of the tumor to radiation has not been impressive, the indications for it remain controversial (90). Trials with a somatostatin analogue and bromocriptine in the treatment of these tumors have met with some success, but not as much as in the treatment of acromegaly and prolactinomas, respectively (91). At our institution, these patients are managed with transsphenoidal adenomectomy followed by radiation therapy if residual tumor is seen on postoperative scans. If the postoperative studies suggest a "cure," they are repeated every 6 months.

5 ACTH-SECRETING ADENOMAS: CUSHING'S DISEASE

Cushing's syndrome, was first described by Harvey Cushing in 1912. Cushing's syndrome is a condition of hypercortisolemia from any source, while the term Cushing's disease refers exclusively to an ACTH-secreting pituitary adenoma. Cushing's disease, more than any other pituitary tumor, remains the most diagnostically and therapeutically challenging. Hypercortisolemia can cause a myriad of clinically significant problems. In general, patients tend to feel poorly and have diffused muscle weakness and pain, emotional lability, and profound fatigue. The presence of cortisol-induced or accelerated atherosclerosis, hypertension, diabetes, osteoporosis, obesity, susceptibility to infections, and perhaps peptic ulcer disease and thrombosis provide compelling evidence to identify the diagnosis (92).

The usefulness of standard radiological imaging in Cushing's disease has been either negative or nonspecifically (thereby misleadingly) positive (9,93–100). More recent advances in MRI imaging with contrast may change this (101,102).

Most cases of hypercortisolemia seen in the adult population are caused by microadenomas of the anterior pituitary gland (103). Other sources that are less common include ectopic overproduction of ACTH (104,105) and/or CRH (106,107), benign or malignant adrenal tumors, iatrogenic or exogenous hypercortisolemia, and alcoholic or depressive "pseudo-Cushing's" states. The presence of neural tissue within a distinct adenoma, or diffuse or nodular hyperplasia, may support the concept that pituitary Cushing's disease is actually a heterogeneous disorder (99,109).

The implications of this pathological finding is important in the clinical management. Primary pituitary Cushing's (with a single adenoma) might be curable by selective adenomectomy. Hyperplasia (perhaps from central overstimulation of the pituitary) might best be treated by complete hypophysectomy or medication aimed at modulating that stimulation (110). Intermediate-lobe Cushing's, on the other hand, may be responsive to bromocriptine, a medication that normally has no effect in other types of Cushing's (111).

5.1 Signs and Symptoms

There is a female preponderance with a median age of approximately 40 years. All patients present clinically with varying hypercortisolemia. Typically patients will have truncal obesity, hypertension, easy bruisability, abdominal striae, and plethoric or moon facies. Because of this impressive clinical picture, patients generally present early in terms of tumor growth, making detection and identification of a source challenging.

5.2 Diagnosis

The diagnosis of Cushing's disease is linked to the complex endocrine pathway involved with ACTH action. ACTH, stimulated by CRH, increases the production and secretion of cortisol from the adrenal cortex. There is a normal diurnal pattern to cortisol release, with the highest level seen in the morning and lowest seen in the evening. Cortisol negatively feeds back to reduce ACTH secretion. ACTH is difficult to measure clinically: therefore, circulating levels of cortisol and/or its urinary metabolites are used for diagnosis.

While Cushing's syndrome is easy to recognize clinically, its etiology is difficult to determine. Various diagnostic protocols have been developed, but no main paradigm has emerged (103,104,108,112–124). Measurements of plasma and urinary cortisol and its derivatives, basally and in response to dexamethasone or metryapone, as well as determination of plasma ACTH, may suggest either a primary adrenal, pituitary, or ectopic neoplastic source of disease (119,125). If these data are equivocal, CRH measurements (106,107,115,126) and CRH stimulation testing with measurement of ACTH and or cortisol (102,112,113,117,118,123), peripherally or in the bilateral venous effluent from the petrosal sinuses (116,120,122,124), are now frequently employed to provide additional biochemical evidence for the diagnosis of Cushing's disease.

Once it has been determined that a patient has a pituitary source of ACTH hypersecretion (Cushing's disease), it can be extremely difficult to identify the pituitary source. Since most ACTH-producing adenomas are small, their radiographic detection is difficult at best. Improvements in MRI, with contrast have identified many microadenomas that would be radiographically invisible. Because many cases have no evidence of tumor on MRI, the technique of petrosal sinus sampling has been developed to confirm the diagnosis and guide the surgical resection. The rationale behind this techique, described in detail elsewhere, is straightforward (122). Patients with Cushing's disease should have high (or inappropriately high) levels of ACTH production coming directly from the pituitary gland (116), and the levels should lateralize (122–124) to the side containing the adenoma. Those with ectopic ACTH secretion whose pituitary glands are suppressed should have neither an elevated pituitary-to-peripheral gradient nor a difference between sides. Patients without a discrete pituitary tumor (i.e., with hyperplasia of the corticotrophs) may have an increased central level of ACTH that is equal in blood from both sides of the gland. Some have advocated petrosal sinus sampling in all patients with ACTH-dependent disease, either to supplement or to supplant the conventional methods for establishing the etiology of the hypercortisolism (112,120,125). Published series indicate that the usefulness and reliability of this technique may be variable.

In Mampalam et al.'s series, (98), 39 of 116 subjects (34%) had selective venous sampling of ACTH. An inferior petrosal sinus to peripheral gradient was seen in 36. Of these 36, 31 (86%) where found to have adenomas. In three patients without a significant gradient, two had adenomas. Nine percent had false localization as to the site of the adenoma. In Ludecke's series (121), 6 of 19 (31%) had incorrect lateralization of the adenoma by inferior petrosal sinus sampling. Ludecke recommended intraoperative measurement of ACTH in the pituitary blood as a means of lateralizing the adenoma. In our institution we use the technique in the following situations:

1. Patients with equivocal lab data, if doubt exists as to the source of ACTH overproduction, and radiographic studies are not helpful.
2. Patients with laboratory data clearly pointing to the pituitary gland but with normal radiographic studies. A petrosal-sinus-directed hemihypophysectomy is done if an adenoma is not seen at surgery.
3. Young patients, especially women, for whom preservation of fertility is an important consideration and whose radiological studies are not grossly abnormal. Even when the lab studies clearly indicate pituitary-dependent disease, we routinely study these patients to lateralize the tumor. If nothing is found at the time of surgery hemihypophysectomy on the side with the higher CRH-stimulated ACTH levels would then be done.

4. Patients not cured following transsphenoidal surgery. In these patients the question to be answered is whether the diagnosis of Cushing's disease was truly correct.

In the most skilled hands, this sampling of venous effluent from the petrosal sinuses appears to be reliable and safe.

5.3 Treatment

The treatment of Cushing's disease has advanced by the development of microsurgical transsphenoidal surgery. Successful surgery can cause reversal of hypercortisolism and eventual return of normal pituitary corticotropic function.

Most cases of Cushing's disease are caused by isolated adenomas of the anterior gland. Basophilic hyperplasia occurs in less than 10% of patients. The treatment of choice for Cushing's disease is transsphenoidal surgery with either selective adenomectomy or partial or hemihypophysectomy (95–99,127,128). For those patients with very large tumors, surgery followed by conventional radiation therapy would be indicated and, very rarely, adrenalectomy. The surgical treatment paradigm remains controversial. The cure rate for this illness in all series remains under 90%. The surgical options for initial intervention include visual exploration of the gland, with removal of abnormal tissue (98), petrosal-sinus–directed hemihypophysectomy (97), to total hypophysectomy (129). Recurrence rates from 3.7 to 9.3% have been reported (95,97–99,128,130). Many of these patients have been reexplored. According to Nakane et al. (99), verification of all pituitary adenomas was done by reoperation, during which time no corticotroph cell hyperplasia was found. It was concluded that late recurrence of Cushing's disease may follow adenomectomy due to regrowth of adenoma cells not removed from peritumoral tissue during the original surgery. The alternative explanation is that the primary etiology was not an isolated pituitary tumor but rather overstimulation; thus, as remaining pituitary tissue continues to be overstimulated, relapse is inevitable. In Friedman et al.'s study (131) of the efficacy of repeat surgery for recurrent Cushing's disease, the incidence of remission of hypercortisolism was highest if an adenoma was identified at surgery and the patient received selective adenomectomy.

Patients who are not cured by selective resection fall into several groups: (1) those with invasive adenomas, (2) those with unidentified microadenomas, (3) those with corticotropic hyperplasia without a discrete adenoma, and (4) those with ectopic secretion of ACTH or CRH. Those with lateral invasive extension will not be cured by any surgical procedure, and therefore, hypophysectomy is not a consideration. Patients with microadenomas that are unidentified preoperatively are often cured by partial or total hypophysectomy; the microadenomas may be discovered within the excised tissue. If surgery has completely removed the tumor, the patient will be hypocorticsolemic for 3–6 months. Patients who are eucortisolemic immediately postoperatively have a high incidence of recurrence (132,133).

While transsphenoidal resection remains the primary procedure of choice, it does not attain a 100% success rate. There are other treatment modalities available for use as adjuvants for those cases in which initial or repeat surgical therapy has failed.

Stereotactic radiation has been used alone or incombination with surgery for the treatment of Cushing's disease (134,135); reports on its efficacy vary from 50 to 100%. Because of the length of time needed to effect a cure and because of the high incidence of hypopituitarism, we currently suggest that radiation therapy be used only when pituitary surgery has failed.

The medical therapies for Cushing's disease currently only address the symptomatic effects of the disease process rather than treat the underlying tumor pathology. These therapies primarily block ACTH or cortisol production at its end stage rather than treat the release process. Ketoconazole, a potent antifungal agent, inhibits adrenal steroidogenesis by blocking the 11-β-hydroxylase (and other enzymes involved in both cortisol and testosterone production). It is generally well tolerated, although sedation is a potential side effect. It is difficult to titrate the dose to achieve eucortisolemia. Often the aim is to achieve complete adrenal suppression, at which time supplemental steroid treatment is begun (136). Because several steps in steroid production are halted, effects on cholesterol, vitamin D, mineralocorticoid, and estrogen and androgen production need to be evaluated more closely before using ketoconazole on a long-term basis can be recommended. We often use this drug if there is to be a delay between diagnosis and treatment or if precise etiological diagnosis is in doubt (depression vs. mild Cushing's) as well as some interim treatment, if desirable.

6 ENDOSCOPIC PITUITARY SURGERY

The endoscopic or "minimally invasive" approaches to the pituitary have only recently been employed (Figs. 1–7). Transsphenoidal surgery is unique in neuro-

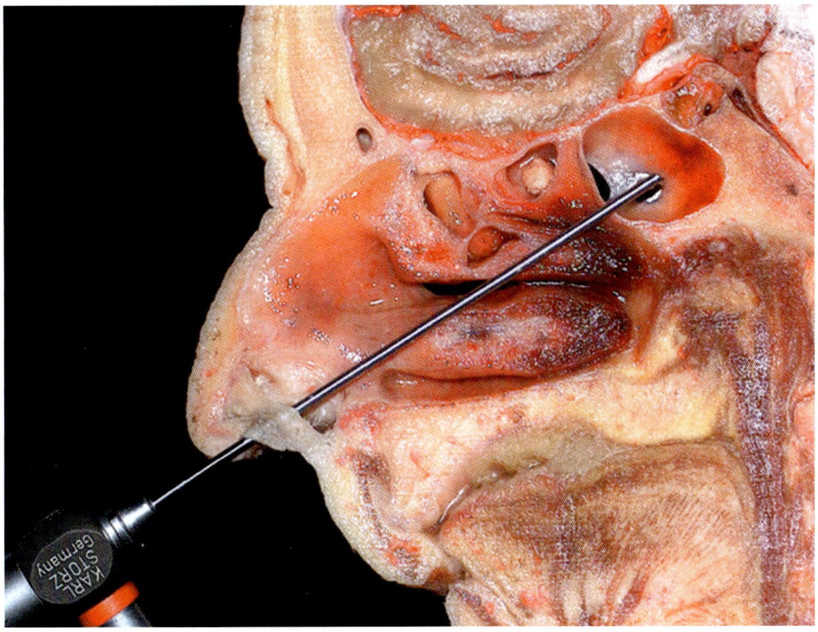

Figure 1 Endoscopic endonasal transsphenoidal approach on cadaveric specimen. (Image courtesy of Karl Storz Inc.)

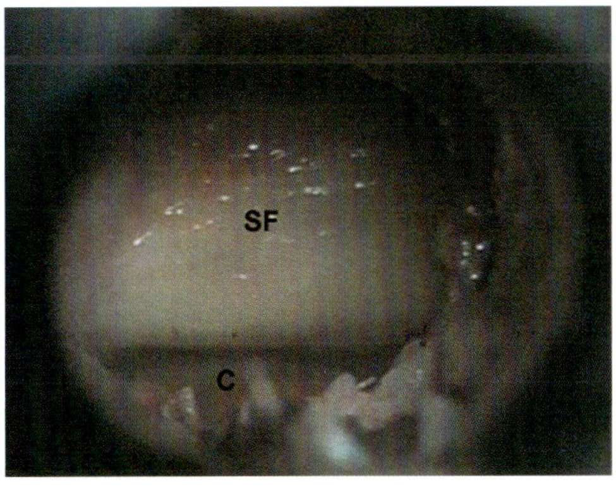

Figure 2 Microscopic image of the sellar floor (SF) and the clivus (C) from conventional transsphenoidal microsurgical approach. (Image courtesy of Karl Storz Inc.)

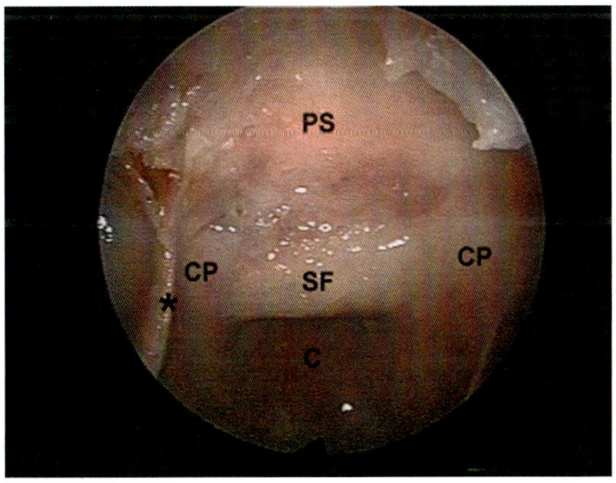

Figure 3 Endoscopic view of the same case as in Figure #2. The endoscopic view allows visualization of the clivus (C), carotid prominences (CP), planum sphenoidale (PS), sellar floor (SF) and the sphenoid septum (*) through movement of the scope forward into the sphenoid cavity. Enlargement of the sphenoid ostium provides an enlarged working angle in all three spatial directions. (Image courtesy of Karl Storz Inc.)

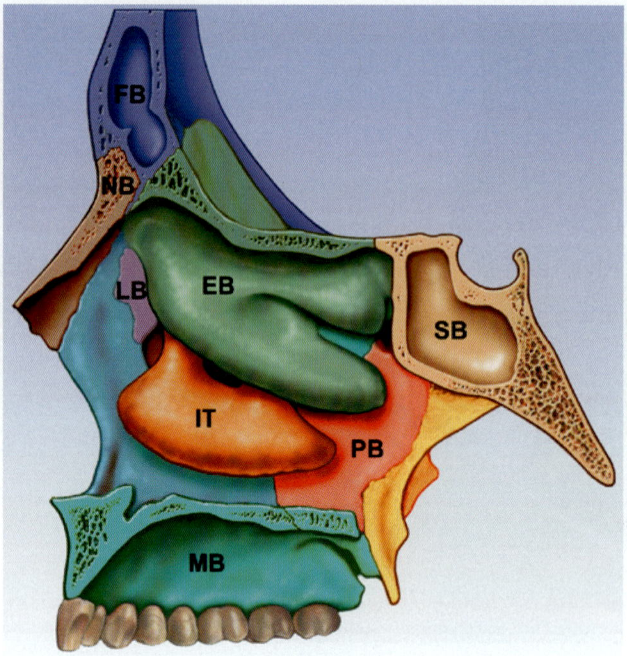

Figure 4 Schematic anatomical color-coded Figure of the lateral wall of the nasal cavity. From the Figure, the six bones that make up the lateral wall are identified. The ethmoid bone (EB), frontal bone (FB), inferior turbinate (IT), lacrimal bone (LB), maxillary bone (MB), nasal bone (NB), palatine bone (PB), and sphenoid bone (SB) can all be visualized. (Image courtesy of Karl Storz Inc.)

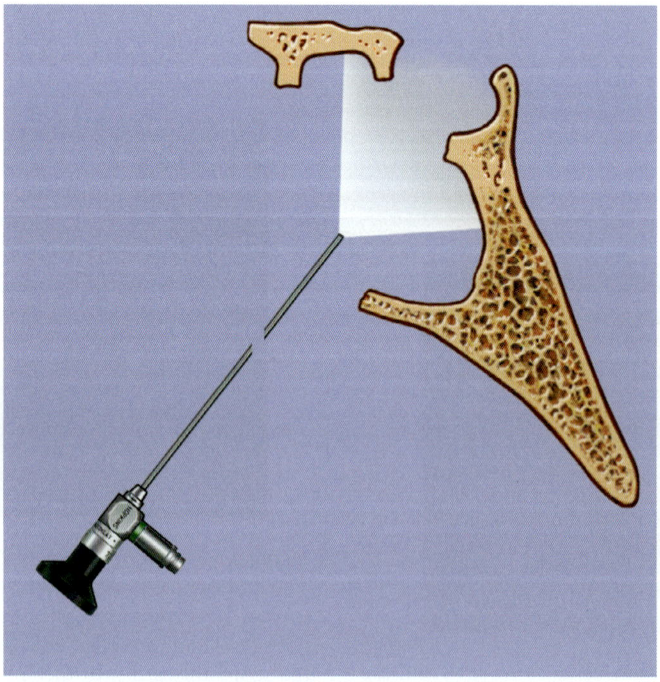

Figure 5 Schematic Figure of the view afforded through a 0 degree endoscope into the sella. The surgery is performed with the 0 degree scope, while exploration of the lesion is performed with the 30 degree or 45 degree scope after the lesion has been removed. (Image courtesy of Karl Storz Inc.)

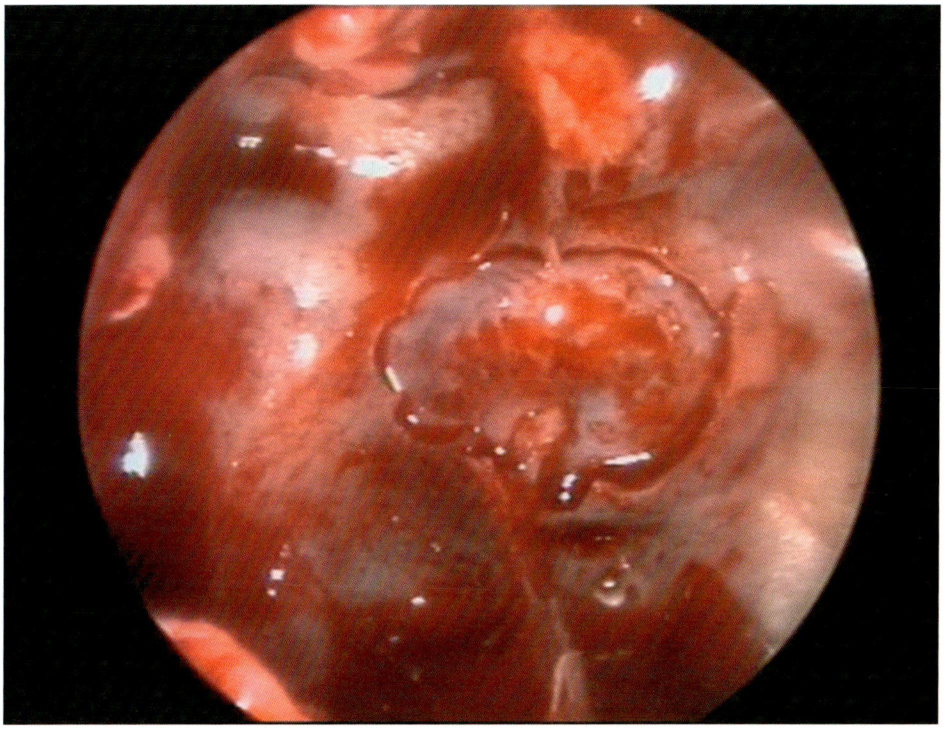

Figure 6 Intraoperative view of the sellar floor with the endoscope demonstrating a broad opening and an underlying macroadenoma. (Image courtesy of Karl Storz Inc.)

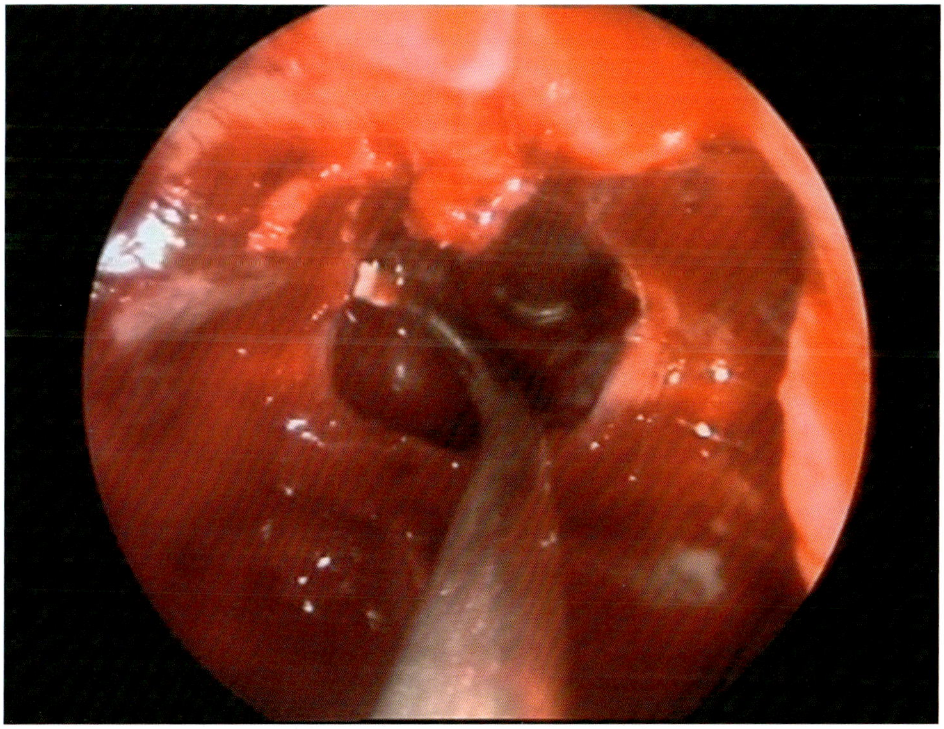

Figure 7 Intraoperative view of the resection of the intrasellar lesion. The angled curette is shown during the resection of the right lateral portion of the sellar lesion. Different size and angled direction curettes are used for the resection. (Image courtesy of Karl Storz Inc.)

surgery in that the operating surgical corridor is narrow, limiting the surgeon's view. In addition, during tumor removal only a fraction of the tumor can be visualized, which makes the confirmation of complete tumor removal often difficult. The indications for the use of endoscopic transsphenoidal surgery are essentially the same as for the standard approach. Endoscopic surgery through use of the short focal length offers the advantages of enhanced illumination and a wider angle of viewing than the microscope. The tumor morphology often dictates the approach in each case. Tumors with extensive suprasellar extension may require a craniotomy rather than a transsphenoidal resection. In addition to a detailed history, physical, and endocrinological work-up, the use of high-resolution MRI with and without contrast is imperative before surgery. Special coronal sella windows help delineate the sella anatomy, especially the location of the carotids and the optic chiasma. The extent of sphenoid sinus pneumatization is also important when planning the appropriate surgical approach. Many endoscopic surgeons also favor high-resolution computed tomography of the sphenoid and sella to better assess the bony anatomy of the sphenoid.

The operative technique employed in endoscopic transphenoidal surgery varies with the instrumentation used. While a variety of techniques have been described, almost all approaches utilize either the 3.7 mm 0-degree, 30-degree, or 70-degree endoscope. The angled endoscopes provide oblique views into the sinuses and lateral walls of the sphenoid and sella. A smaller 2.7 mm endoscope is also available for use in children or in patients with small nares. As in all endoscopes, the smaller size reduces the optical resolution and illumination. Optional self-retaining retractors hold the endoscope in place and allow the surgeon to operate with both hands. While specialized instruments for the endoscope are being designed, the same microsurgical instruments used in standard transsphenoidal surgery are currently employed. The instruments used in endoscopic sinus surgery are also useful in approaches to the pituitary.

There are only a few reports in the literature comparing endoscopic versus standard transphenoidal surgery. Sheehan et al. (138) retrospectively reviewed 26 patients who underwent endoscopic transnasal macroadenoma resection versus 44 matched control patients in the standard approach. Their conclusion was that surgical resection, anterior pituitary function, visual fields, and complications were not significantly different between the two groups. While their study cited a reduced surgical time, our personal results have not yet shown that to be the case. Koren et al. (139) retrospectively compared 20 patients undergoing an endoscopic approach to the sella with 20 patients undergoing a sublabial approach. The endoscopic approach was associated in their series with a shorter operative time, shorter hospitalization time, and lower incidence of septal perforation.

Endoscopic transsphenoidal surgery, though rapidly developing in its techniques and instrumentation, remains in its infancy in terms of its utilization potential. The limitations of endoscopic transsphenoidal surgery are a lack of stereoscopic depth perception and limited visualization when bleeding is encountered. Incomplete pneumatization of the sphenoid sinus makes an endoscopic approach very difficult anatomically. In these scenarios a conversion to the standard microsurgical technique is often necessary. We currently favor the endoscope as a proven adjunct to microsurgical resection that allows for direct angled inspection of residual tumor as well as the anatomical borders of the resection area (i.e., the carotid arteries). There is a need for continued refinement of the technique in order to display its advantage over the known low morbidity and high efficacy of standard transsphenoidal surgery.

7 CONCLUSION

Patients with functioning pituitary adenomas pose very different management problems and decisions than do patients with nonfunctioning adenomas. The unique pathology of each tumor requires careful history and physical examinations coupled with a detailed endocrinological work-up. The therapy employed should include not only surgery but also the current best-indicated medical therapy that is specific to the presentation of the individual patient. The recent advances in endoscopic and minimally invasive transsphenoidal surgery will continue to reduce the already low morbidity and enhance the high efficacy achieved through microsurgical resection. Meticulous follow-up is crucial in maintaining tumor control and treating possible tumor recurrence.

REFERENCES

1. Reichlin S. Anatomical and physiological basis of hypothalamic-pituitary regulation. In: Post KD, Jackson IMD, Reichlin S, eds. The Pituitary Adenoma. New York: Plenum, 1980:3–28.

2. Klibanski A. Nonsecreting pituitary tumors Endocrinol Metab Clin North Am 1987; 16:793–804.
3. Hardy J. Transsphenoidal microsurgery of the normal and pathological pituitary. Clin Neurosurg 1969; 16: 185–217.
4. Hardy J, Somma M. Acromegaly: surgical treatment by transsphenoidal microsurgical removal of the pituitary adenoma. In: Tindall GT, Collins WF, eds. Clinical Management of Pituitary Disorders. New York: Raven Press, 1979:209–217.
5. Litt AW, Kricheff II. Magnetic resonance imaging of pituitary tumors. In: Cooper PR, ed. Contemporary Diagnosis and Management of Pituitary Adenomas. Chicago, IL: Am Association of Neurologic Surgeons, 1991:1–19.
6. Macpherson P, Hadley DM, Teasdale E, et al. Pituitary microadenomas: does gadolinium enhance their demonstration? Neuroradiology 1989; 31:293–298.
7. Kulkarni MV, Lee KF, McArdle CB, et al. 1.5T MR imaging of pituitary microadenomas: technical considerations and CT correlation AJNR 1988; 9:5–11.
8. Doppman JL, Frank JA, Dwyer AJ, et al. Gadolinium DTPA enhanced MR imaging of ACTH-secreting microadenomas of the pituitary gland. J Comput Assist Tomogr 1988; 12:728–735.
9. Marcovitz S, Wee R, Chan J, et al. The diagnostic accuracy of preoperative CT scanning in the evaluation of pituitary ACTH-secreting adenomas. AJR 1987; 149:803–806.
10. Marcovitz S, Wee R, Chan J, et al. Diagnostic accuracy of preoperative CT scanning of pituitary prolactinomas AJNR 1988; 9:13–17.
11. Marcovitz S, Wee R, Chan J, et al. Diagnostic accuracy of preoperative CT scanning of pituitary somatotroph adenomas AJNR 1988; 9:19–22.
12. Davis PC, Hoffman JC Jr, tindall GT, et al. Prolactin-secreting pituitary microadenomas: inaccuracy of high-resolution Ct imaging. AJR. 1985;144;1541–156.
13. Frantz AG. Prolactin. N Engl J Med 1978; 298:201–207.
14. Jaquet P, Guibout M, Lucioni J, et al. Hypothalamo-pituitary regulation of prolactin in hypersecreting prolactinoma. In: Robyn C, Harter M, eds. Progress in Prolactin, Physiology and Pathology. New York: Elsevier-North Holland Biochemical Press, 1978:371–382.
15. Boyd AE, Reichlin S. Neural control of prolactin secretion in man Psychoneuroendocrinology 1978; 3: 113–130.
16. Kleinberg DL, Noel GL, Frantz AG. Galactorrhea: a study of 235 cases including 48 with pituitary tumors. N Engl J Med 1977; 296:589–600.
17. Goodman RH, Molitch MD, Post KD, Jackson IMD. Prolactin secreting adenomas in the male. In: Post KD, Jackson IMD, Reichlin S, eds. The Pituitary Adenoma. New York: Plenum Press, 1980:91–108.
18. Thorner MO, McNeilly AS, Hagan C, Besser GM. Long-term treatment of galactorrhea and hypogonadism with bromocriptine. Br Med J 1974; 2:419–422.
19. Vance ML, Evans WS, Thorner MO. Bromocriptine. Ann Intern Med 1984; 100:78–91.
20. Zarate A, Canales ES, Cano C, Pilonieta CJ. Follow-up of patients with prolactinomas after discontinuation of long-term therapy with bromocriptine. Acta Endocrinol (Copenh) 1983; 104:139–142.
21. Molitch ME, Elton RL, Blackwell RE, et al. Bromocriptine as primary therapy for prolactin-secreting macroadenomas: results of a prospective multicenter study. J Clin Endocrinol Metab 1985; 60:698–705.
22. Thorner MO, Martin WH, Rogol AD, et al. Rapid regression of pituitary prolactinomas during bromocriptine treatment. J Clin Endocrinol Metab 1980; 51:438–445.
23. Tindall GT, Kovacs K, Horvath E, et al. Human prolactin-producing adenomas and bromocriptine: a histological, immunocytochemical, ultrastructural, and morphometric study. J Clin Endocrinol Metab 1982; 55:1178–1183.
24. Barrow DL, Tindall GT, Kovacs K, et al. Clinical and pathological effects of bromocriptine on prolactin-secreting and other pituitary tumors. J Neurosurg 1984; 60:1–7.
25. Barrow DL, Mizuno J, Tindall GT. Management of prolactinomas associated with very high serum prolactin levels. J Neurosurg 1988; 68:554–558.
26. Molitch ME, Reichlin S. Hyperprolactinemic disorders. Dis Mon. June 1982;281–58.
27. Reichlin S. The prolactinoma problem. N Engl J Med 1979; 300:313–315.
28. Thorner MO, Schran HF, Evans WS, et al. A broad spectrum of prolactin suppression by bromocriptine in hyperprolactinemic women: a study of serum prolactin and bromocriptine levels after acute and chronic administration of bromocriptine. J Clin Endocrinol Metab 1980; 50:1026–1033.
29. Thorner MO, Edwards CRW, Charlesworth M, et al. Pregnancy in patients presenting with hyperprolactinemia. Br Med J 1979; 2:771–774.
30. Tindall GT, Barrow DL, Tindall SC. Current management of pituitary tumors, II. Contemp Neurosurg 1988; 10:1–6.
31. Vance ML, Cragun JR, Reimnitz C, et al. CV 205-502 treatment of hyperprolactinemia. J Clin Endocrinol Metab 1989; 68:336–339.
32. Wang C, Lam KSL, Ma JTC, et al. Long-term treatment of hyperprolactinemia with bromocriptine: effect of drug withdrawal. Clin Endocrinol (Oxf) 1987; 27:363–371.
33. Thorner MO, Perryman RL, Rogol AD, et al. Rapid changes of prolactinoma volume after withdrawal and reinstitution of bromocriptine. J Clin Endocrinol Metab 1981; 53:480–483.

34. Liuzzi A, Dallabonzana D, Oppizzi G, et al. Low doses of dopamine agonists in the long-term treatment of macroprolactinomas. N Engl J Med 1985; 313:656–659.
35. Kleinberg DL, Boyd AE, Wardlaw S, et al. Pergolide for the treatment of pituitary tumors secreting prolactin or growth hormone. N Engl J Med 1983; 309:704–709.
36. Molitch ME. Pregnancy and the hyperprolactinemic woman. N Engl Med 1985; 312:1364–1370.
37. Post KD. Surgical approaches to the treatment of prolactinomas. In: Olefsky JM, Robbins RJ, eds. Prolactinomas: Practical Diagnosis and Management. New York: Churchill Livingstone, 1986:159–194.
38. Fahlbusch R, Buchfelder M, Schrell U. Short-term preoperative treatment of macroprolactinomas by dopamine agonists. J Neurosurg 1987; 67:807–815.
39. Hubbard JL, Scheithauer BW, Abboud CF, Laws ER Jr. Prolactin-secreting adenomas: the preoperative response to bromocriptine treatment and surgical outcome. J Neurosurg 1987; 67:816–821.
40. Landolt AM, Osterwalder V. Perivascular fibrosis in prolactinomas: is it increased by bromocriptine? J Clin Endocrinol Metab 1984; 58:1179–1183.
41. Landolt AM, Keller PJ, Froesch ER, et al. Bromocriptine: does it jeopardize the result of later surgery for prolactinomas? Lancet 1982; 2:657.
42. Weiss MH, Teal J, Gott P, et al. Natural history of microprolactinomas: six-year follow-up. Neurosurgery 1983; 12:180–183.
43. Sisam DA, Sheehan JP, Sheeler LR. The natural history of untreated microprolactinoma. Fertil Steril 1987; 48:67–71.
44. Klibanski A, Greenspan SL. Increase in bone mass after treatment of hyperprolactinemic amenorrhea. N Engl J Med 1986; 315:542–546.
45. Klibanski A, Biller BMK, Rosenthal DI, Schoenfeld DA, Saxe V. Effects of prolactin and estrogen deficiency in amenorrheic bone loss. J Clin Endocrinol Metab 1988; 67:124–130.
46. Cushing H. Partial hypophysectomy for acromegaly with remarks on the function of the hypophysis. Ann Surg 1909; 50:1002–1017.
47. Lewis UJ, Singh RN, Tutwiler GF, Sigel MB, Vanderlaan EF, Vanderlaan WP. Human growth hormone: a complex of proteins. Recent Prog Horm Res 1980; 36:477–508.
48. Reichlin S. Somatostatin. N Engl J Med 1983; 309:1495–1501.
49. Vance ML, Kaiser DL, Evans WS, et al. Pulsatile growth hormone secretion in normal man during a continous infusion of human growth hormone releasing factor (1-40): evidence for intermittent somatostatin secretion. J Clin Invest 1985; 75: 1584–1590.
50. Van Wyk JJ. The somatomedins: biological actions and physiologic control mechanisms. In: Li CH, ed. Growth Factors. New York: Academic Press, 198:81–125.
51. Frohman La, Szabo M, Berelowitz, Stachura ME. Partial purification and acharacterization of a peptide with growth hormone-releasing activity from extrapituitary tumors in patients with acromegaly. J Clin Invest 1980; 65:43–54.
52. Melmed S, Ziel FH, Braunstein GD, Downs T, Frohman LA. Medical management of acromegaly due to ectopic production of growth hormone-releasing hormone by a carcinoid tumor. J Clin Endocrinol Metab 1988; 67:395–399.
53. Melmed S. Acromegaly. N Engl J Med 1990; 322:966–977.
54. Klein I, Parveen G, VanThiel DH. Colonic Polyps in patients with acromegaly. Ann Intern Med 1982; 97: 27–30.
55. Leavitt J, Klein I, Kendricks F, Gavaler J, VanThiel DH. Skin tags: a cutaneous marker for colonic polyps. Ann Intern Med 1983; 98:928–930.
56. Thorner MO, Vance ML. Growth hormone, 1988. J Clin Invest 1988; 82:745–747.
57. Clemmons DR, Van Wyk JJ, Ridqway EC, Kliman B, Kjellberg RN, Underwood LE. Evaluation of acromegaly by radioimmunoassay of somato medin-C. N Engl J Med 1979; 301:1138–1142.
58. Barkan AI, Beitins IZ, Kelch RP. Plasma insulin-like growth factor-1/somatomedin-C in acromegaly: correlation with the degree of growth hormone hypersecretion. J Clin Endocrinol Metab 1988; 67: 69–73.
59. Wright AD, Hill DM, Lowy C, Fraser TR. Mortality in acromegaly. QJ Med 1970; 39:1–16.
60. Baumann G. Acromegaly. Endocrinol Metab Clin North Am 1987; 16:685–703.
61. Ross DA, Wilson CB. Results of transsphenoidal microsurgery for growth hormone-secreting pituitary adenomas in a series of 214 patients. J Neurosurg 1988; 68:854 867.
62. Grisoli F, Leclercq T, Jaquet P, et al. Transsphenoidal surgery for acromegaly—long-term results in 100 patients. Surg Neurol 1986; 25:513–519.
63. Serri O, Somma M, Comtois R, et al. Acromegaly: biochemical assessment of cure after long-term follow-up of transsphenoidal selective adenomectomy. J Clin Endocrinol Metab 1985; 61:1185–1189.
64. Roelfsema F, van Dulken H, Frolich M. Long-term results of transsphenoidal pituitary microsurgery in 60 acromegalic patients. Clin Endocrinol (Oxf) 1985; 23: 555–565.
65. Ludecke DK, Saeger W, William T. Effectiveness of microsurgery in acromegaly: study of 210 cases. Period Biol 1983; 85:59–66.
66. Laws ER Jr, Randall RV, Abboud CF. Surgical treatment of acromegaly: results in 140 patients. In: Givens J, ed. Hormone-Secreting Pituitary Tumors.

Chicago, IL: Year Book Medical Publishers, 1982: 225–228.
67. Liuzzi A, Chiodini PG, Botalla A, Cremascoli G, Muller EE, Silvestrini F. Decreased plasma growth hormone (GH) levels in acromegalics following CB 154 (2-Br-alpha-ergocriptine) administration. J Clin Endocrinol Metab 1974; 38:910–912.
68. Lindholm J, Riishede J, Verstergaard S, Hummer L, Faber O, Hagen C. No effect of bromocriptine in acromegaly: a controlled trial. N Engl J Med 1981; 304: 1450–1454.
69. Wass JAH, Thorner MO, Morris DV, et al. Long-term treatment of acromegaly with bromocriptine. Br Med J 1977; 1:875–878.
70. Bell P, Atkinson AB, Hadden DR, et al. Bromocriptine reduces growth hormone in acromegaly. Arch Intern Med 1986; 146:1145–1149.
71. Besser GM, Wass JAH, Thorner MO. Acromegaly-results of long-term treatment with bromocriptine. Acta Endocrinol Suppl (Copenh) 1978; 88(suppl 216):187–198.
72. Lamberts SWJ, Zweens M, Verschoor L, del Pozo E. A comparison among the growth hormone-lowering effects in acromegaly of the somatostatin analolg SMS 201-995, bromocriptine, and the combination of both drugs. J Clin Endocrinol Metab 1986; 63:16–19.
73. Halse J, Harris AG, Kvistborg A, et al. A randomized study of SMS 201-995 versus bromocriptine treatment in acromegaly: clinical and biochemical effects. J Clin Endocrinol Metab 1990; 70:1254–1261.
74. Chiodini PG, Cozi R, Dallabonzana D, et al. Medical treatment of acromegaly with SMS 201-995, a somatostatin analog: a comparison with bromocriptine. J Clin Endocrinol Metab 1987; 64:447–453.
75. Lamberts SW. The role of somatostatin in the regulation of anterior pituitary hormone secretion and the use of its analogs in the treatment of human pituitary tumors. Endoc Rev 1988; 9:417–436.
76. Kohler PO. Treatment of pituitary adenomas. N Engl J Med 1987; 317:45–46.
77. Lamberts SWJ, Uitterlinden P, Verschoor L, van Dongen KJ, del Pozo E. Long-term treatment of acromegaly with the somatostatin analogue SMS 201-995. N Engl J Med 1985; 313:1576–1580.
78. Comi RJ, Gorden P. The response of serum growth hormone levels to the long-acting somatostatin analog SMS 201-995 in acromegaly. J Clin Endocrinol Metab 1987; 64:37–42.
79. Barnard LB, Grantham WG, Lambewrton P, O'Dorsio TM, Jackson IMD. Treatment of resistant acromegaly with long-acting somatostatin analogue (SMS 201-995). Ann Intern Med 1986; 105:856–861.
80. Harris AG, Prestele H, Herold K, et al. Long-term efficacy of Sandostatin (SMS 201-995, octreotide) in 178 acromegalic patients: results from the International Multicentre Acromegaly Study Group. Lamberts SWJ, ed. Sandostatin in the Treatment of Acromegaly. New York: Springer-Verlag, 1988: 117–125.
81. Ho KY, Weissberger AJ, Marbach P, Lazarus L. Therapeutic efficacy of the somatostatin analog SMS 201-995 (octreotide) in acromegaly: effects of dose and frequency and long-term safety. Ann Intern Med 1990; 112:173–181.
82. Snyder PJ, Fowble BF, Schatz NJ, Savino PJ, Gennarelli TA. Hypopituitarism following radiation therapy of pituitary adenomas. Am J Med 1986; 81:457–462.
83. Eastman RC, Gorden P, Roth J. Conventional supervoltage irradiation is an effective treatment for acromegaly. J Clin Endocrinol Metab 1979; 48:931–940.
84. Smallridge RC. Thyrotropin-secreting pituitary tumors. Endocrinol Metab Clin North Am 1987; 16: 765–792.
85. Smallridge RC, Smith CE. Hyperthyroidism due to thyrotropin-secreting pituitary tumors: diagnostic and therapeutic consideration. Arch Intern Med 1983; 143: 503–507.
86. Snyder PJ, Johnson J, Muzyka R. Abnormal secretion of glycoprotein alpha-subunit and follicle stimulating hormone (FSH) beta-subunit in men with pituitary adenomas and FSH hypersecretion. J Clin Endocrinol Metab 1980; 51:579–584.
87. Oppenheim DS, Kana AR, Sangha JS, Klibanski A. prevalence of alpha-subunit hypersecretion in patients with pituitary tumors: clinically nonfunctioning and somatotroph adenomas. J Clin Endocrinol Metab 1990; 70:859–864.
88. Kourides IA, Weintraub BD, Rosen SW, Ridgway EC, Kilman B, Maloof. Secretion of alpha subunit of glycoprotein hormones by pituitary adenomas. J Clin Endocrinol Metab 1976; 43:97–106.
89. Snyder PJ. Gonadotroph cell adenomas of the pituitary. Endocr Rev 1985; 6:552–563.
90. Ebersold MJ, Quast LM, Laws ER Jr, Scheithauer B, Randall RV. Long-term results in transsphenoidal removal of nonfunctioning pituitary adenomas. J Neurosurg 1986; 64:713–719.
91. Comi RJ, Gesundheit N, Murray L, Gorden P, Weintraub BD. Response of thyrotropin-secreting pituitary adenomas to a long-acting somatostatin analogue. N Engl J Med 1987; 317:12–17.
92. Burch W. Cushing's disease, a review. Arch Intern Med 1985; 145:1106–1111.
93. Burrow GN, Wortzman G, Rewcastle NB, et al. Microadenomas of the pituitary and abnormal sellar tomograms in an unselected autopsy seris. N Engl J Med 1981; 304:156–158.
94. Chandler WF, Schteingart DE, Lloyd RV, et al. Surgical treatment of Cushing's disease. J Neurosurg 1987; 66:204–212.

95. Fahlbusch R, Buchfelder M, Muller OA. Transsphenoidal surgery for Cushing's disease. J R Soc Med 1986; 79:262–269.
96. Guilhaume B, Bertagna X, Thomsen Me, et al. Transsphenoidal pituitary surgery for the treatment of Cushing's disease: results in 64 patients and long term follow-up studies. J Clin Endocrinol Metab 1988; 66:1056–1064.
97. Hardy J. Cushing's disease: 50 years later. Can J Neurol Sci 1982; 2:375–380.
98. Mampalam TJ, Tyrell JB, Wilson CB. Transsphenoidal microsurgery for Cushing's disease. Ann Intern Med 1988; 109:487–493.
99. Nakane R, Kuwayama A, Watanabe M, et al. Long-term results of transsphenoidal adenomectomy in patients with Cushing's disease. Neurosurgery 1987; 21:218–222.
100. Dwyer AJ, Frank JA, Doppman JL, et al. Pituitary adenomas in patients with Cushing's disease: initial experience with Gd-DTPA-enhanced MR imaging. Neuroradiology 1987; 163:421–426.
101. Newton DR, Dillon WP, Normal D, et al. Gd-DTPA-enhanced MR imaging of pituitary adenomas. AJNR 1989; 10:949–954.
102. Saris SC, Patronas NJ, Doppman JL, et al. Cushing's syndrome: pituitary CT scanning. Radiology 1987; 162:775–777.
103. Orth DN. The old and new in Cushing's syndrome. N Engl J Med 1984; 310:649–651.
104. Case records of MGH. Case 53-1981. N Engl J Med 1981; 305:1637–1643.
105. Suda T, Kondo M, Totani R, et al. Ectopic adrenocorticotropin syndrome caused by lung cancer that responded to corticotropin-releasing hormone. J Clin Endocrinol Metab 1986; 63:1047–1051.
106. Case Records of the MGH. Case 52-1987. N Engl J Med 1987; 317:1648–1658.
107. Schteingart DE, Lloyd RV, Akil H, et al. Cushing's syndrome secondary to ectopic corticotropin-releasing hormone-adrenocorticotropin secretion. J Clin Endocrinol Metab 1986; 63:770–775.
108. Nieman LK, Chrousos GP, Oldfield EH, et al. The ovine corticotropin-releasing hormone stimulation test and the dexamethasone suppression test in the differential diagnosis of Cushing's syndrome. Ann Intern Med 1986; 105:862–867.
109. Lloyd RV, Chandler WF, McKeever PE, Schteingart DE. The spectrum of ACTH-producing pituitary lesions. Am J Surg Pathol 1986; 10:618–626.
110. Post KD, Habas JE. Cushing's disease. In: Samii M, ed. Surgery of the Sellar Region and Paranasal Sinuses Berlin: Springer-Verlag, 1991:294–301.
111. Reith P, Monnot EA, Bathija PJ. Prolonged suppression of a corticotropin-producing bronchial carcinoid by oral bromocriptine. Ann Intern Med 1987; 147: 989–991.
112. Chrousos GP, Sculte HM, Oldfield EH, et al. The corticotropin-releasing factor stimulation test. N Engl J Med 1984; 310:622–626.
113. Chrousos GP, Schuermeyer TH, Doppman JL, et al. Clinical applications of corticotropin-releasing factor. Ann Intern Med 1985; 102:344–358.
114. Crapo L. Cushing's syndrome: a review of diagnostic tests. Metabolism 1979; 28:955–977.
115. Cunnah D, Jessop DS, Besser GM, Rees LH. Measurement of circulating-releasing factor in man. J Endocrinol 1987; 113:1123–1131.
116. Findling JW, Aron DC, Tyrell JB, et al. Selective venous sampling for ACTH in Cushing's syndrome. Ann Intern Med 1981; 94:641–652.
117. Fukata J, Nakai Y, Imura H, et al. Human corticotropin-releasing hormone test in normal subjects and patients with hypothalamic, pituitary or adrenocortical disorders. Endocrinol Jpn 1988; 35:491–502.
118. Hermus AR, Pieters GF, Pesman GJ, et al. The corticotropin-releasing hormone test versus the high dose dexamethasone test in the differential diagnosis of Cushing's syndrome. Lancet 1986; 2: 540–543.
119. Howlett TA, Drury PL, Perry L, et al. Diagnosis and management of ACTH-dependent Cushing's syndrome: comparison of the features in ectopic and pituitary ACTh production. Clin Endocrinol (Oxf) 1986; 24:699–713.
120. Landolt AM, Valvanis A, Girard J, Eberle AN. Corticotropin-releasing factor test used with bilateral, simultaneous inferior petrosal sinus blood-sampling for the diagnosis of pituitary-dependent Cushing's disease. Clin Endocrinol (Oxf) 1986; 25:687–696.
121. Ludecke DK. Intraoperative measurement of adrenocorticotrophic hormone in peripituitary blood in Cushing's disease. Neurosurgery 1989; 24:201–205.
122. Oldfield EH, Chrousos GP, Schulte HM, et al. Preoperative lateralization of ACTH-secreting pituitary microadenomas by bilateral and simultaneous inferior petrosal venous sinus sampling. N Engl J Med 1985; 312:98–103.
123. Schrell U, Fahlbusch R, Buchfelder M, et al. Corticotropin-releasing hormone stimulation test before and after transsphenoidal selective microadenomectomy in 30 patients with Cushing's disease. J Clin Endocrinol Metab 1987; 64:1150–1159.
124. Zovickian J, Oldfield EH, Doppman JL, et al. Usefulness of inferior petrosal sinus venous endocrine markers in Cushing's disease. J Neurosurg 1988; 68:205–210.
125. Findling JW, Tyrell JB. Occult ectopic secretion of corticotropin. Am J Med 1986; 146:929–933.
126. Carey RM, Varma SK, Drake CR, et al. Ectopic secretion of corticotropin-releasing factor as a cause of Cushing's syndrome. N Engl J Med 1984; 311: 13–20.
127. Boggan JE, Tyrell JB, Wilson CB. Transsphenoidal

microsurgical management of Cushing's disease: a report of 100 cases. J Neurosurg 1983; 59:195–200.

128. Tindall GT, Herring CJ, Clark RV, et al. Cushing's disease: results of transsphenoidal microsurgery with emphasis on surgical failures. J Neurosurg 1990; 72: 363–369.
129. Krieger DT. Physiopathology of Cushing's disease. Endocr Rev 1983; 4:22–43.
130. Salassa RM, Laws ER, Carpenter PC. Cushing's disease—50 years later. Trans Am Clin Climatol Assoc 1982; 94:122–129.
131. Friedman RB, Oldfield EH, Nieman LK, et al. Repeat transsphenoidal surgery for Cushing's disease. J Neurosurg 1989; 71:520–527.
132. Fitzgerald PA, Aron DC, Findling JW, et al. Cushing's disease: transient secondary adrenal insufficiency after selective removal of pituitary microadenomas; evidence for a pituitary origin. J Clin Endocrinol Metab 1982; 54:413–422.
133. Derome PJ, Delalande O, Visot A, Jedynac CP, Dupuy M. In: Landolt AM, ed. Progress in Pituitary Adenoma Research. London: Pergamon Press, 1988 375–379.
134. Degerblad M, Rahn T, Bergstrand G, Thoren M. Long-term results of stereotactic radiosurgery to the pituitary gland in Cushing's disease. Acta Endocrinol (Copenh) 1986; 112:310–314.
135. Sandler LM, Richards NT, Carr DH, et al. Long term follow-up of patients with Cushing's disease treated by interstitial irradiation. J Clin Endocrinol Metab 1987; 65:441–447.
136. Loli P, Berselli ME, Tagliaferri M. Use of ketoconazole in the treatment of Cushing's syndrome. J Clin Endocrinol Metab 1986; 63:1365–1371.
137. Sonino NThe use of ketoconazole as an inhibitor of steroid production. N Engl J Med 1987; 317: 812–818.
138. Sheehan MT, Atkinson JL, Kasperbauer JL, et al. Preliminary comparison of the endoscopic transnasal vs. the sublabial transseptal approach for clinically nonfunctioning pituitary macroadenomas. Mayo Clin Proc 1999; 74:661–670.
139. Koren I, Hadar T, Rappaport ZH, et al. Endoscopic transnasal transsphenoidal microsurgery versus the sublabial approach for the treatment of pituitary tumors: endonasal complications. Laryngoscope 1999; 109:1838–1840.

5

The Neuroendocrine Lung

John R. Gosney

Royal Liverpool University Hospital, Liverpool, England

1 INTRODUCTION

In 1938, an Austrian pathologist, Friedrich Feyrter, published a monograph (1) in which he described a system of regulatory cells, a "diffuse endocrine epithelial organ," distributed throughout the various organs and exerting an influence upon them by local release of chemical messengers, a mode of secretion he called "paracrine." This was not a fundamentally new idea (2,3), but Feyrter was the first to suggest that such cells were ubiquitous throughout the tissues, constituting a unified system of local endocrine control. This concept was consolidated largely by the work of Pearse and colleagues in the late 1960s (4–7), and the existence of what is now generally known as the diffuse neuroendocrine system (DNS), the cells of which are characterized by the secretion of amine, protein, and peptide hormones that are stored in cytoplasmic dense core (neurosecretory) vesicles (DCVs) (Fig. 1), has became universally accepted. It is with the pulmonary component of this system, its structure and function in healthy lungs, and the changes it undergoes in pulmonary disease that the first two sections of this chapter are concerned.

A unique feature of the respiratory epithelium is the frequency with which it gives rise to tumors characterized by neuroendocrine differentiation (8). Why this should happen so frequently is unclear. Admittedly, the more benign of the pulmonary neuroendocrine tumors (PNTs), the typical and atypical carcinoids, are rare, but small cell carcinoma accounts for about a fifth of all malignant pulmonary neoplasms. If those morphologically nonneuroendocrine pulmonary tumors that display immunochemical or ultrastructural features of this line of differentiation (see below) are added to those that display it overtly, some degree of neuroendocrine differentiation in neoplasms of the lung can be seen to be commonplace. It is the pathology of PNTs and the lesions that may precede them that the third part of this chapter will review.

The functional essence of neuroendocrine differentiation is the secretion of hormones, so it is only to be expected that pulmonary neoplasms following this line of differentiation would recapitulate this normal biological function. This is indeed the case, but the range of substances produced by such tumors is far in excess of that secreted by their normal cellular counterparts. This functional manifestation of neoplasia actually outstrips in its diversity the structural changes that more obviously characterize the process. Strenuous attempts have been made over the years to exploit the propensity of PNTs to secrete so-called serum markers of their presence as an aid to their diagnosis and management, albeit it with generally disappointing results (8). This functional aspect of the biology of PNTs is reviewed in the fourth section of this chapter.

Finally, an enduringly fascinating aspect of pulmonary oncology and endocrinology is the tendency of pulmonary tumors to produce clinical paraneoplastic effects (9). This is, in large part, a further consequence of

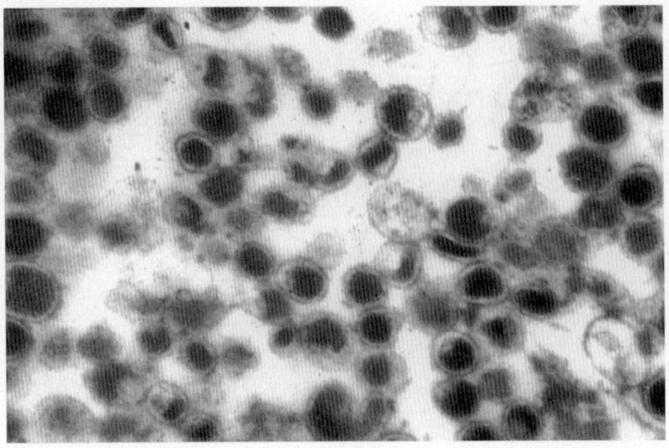

Figure 1 The dense core (neurosecretory) vesicles that are the ultrastructural hallmark of cells of the diffuse neuroendocrine system and of neuroendocrine tumors.

the neuroendocrine differentiation that so often characterizes them; the substances they secrete interfere with normal physiological functions and the unique antigens they display provoke abnormal immunological reactions. It is the often peculiar clinical effects that these processes can induce that the final part of this chapter will describe.

2 THE NORMAL PULMONARY NEUROENDOCRINE CELL SYSTEM

Over 10 years after Feyrter wrote his monograph, the first comprehensive study of the neuroendocrine cells of normal mammalian lungs was made by Fröhlich (10). He wrote a detailed account of their characteristics in a variety of species, including three condemned prisoners from the local jail on whom necropsies were performed shortly after execution. Since then, knowledge of the morphology, number, distribution, content, and putative functions of these pulmonary neuroendocrine cells (PNCs) has increased steadily, although many questions remain (8,11–15).

In early studies of the DNS, capricious histochemical techniques were all that were available to reveal its various components, but the advent of more specific and reliable immunochemical markers of neuroendocrine differentiation made their identification easier and greatly aided their study. Of these general markers of neuroendocrine differentiation, neuron-specific enolase (NSE), protein gene product (PGP) 9.5, and chromogranin have been most widely employed in the identification of PNCs (8). In healthy adult human lungs, PNCs are found at all levels from the larynx to alveoli but are most numerous in bronchi and bronchioles; in the airways, there is about one PNC for every 2500 epithelial cells (16). The vast majority of PNCs in humans are solitary (Fig. 2), only a very small number forming the highly organized, innervated clusters known as neuroepithelial bodies (NEBs) (Fig. 3) (17) that are so frequent in lower species (13). In human lungs, in common with other species, PNCs are most numerous in the late fetal and early neonatal periods, gradually falling in number as the lungs mature, to reach a steady state that persists into old age (18).

A variety of secretory products has been described in human PNCs (19), but those established as such by repeated demonstration in normal lungs are gastrin-releasing peptide (GRP), the mammalian analogue of amphibean bombesin (20), calcitonin (CT) (21), calcitonin gene–related peptide (CGRP) (22), and the amine serotonin (5-hydroxytryptamine; 5-HT) (23). In healthy human lungs, about 65% of PNCs contain GRP and the vast majority of the rest CT (16).

The functions of the pulmonary component of the DNS are a matter of continuing debate. Evidence for PNCs having a chemoreceptive role in lower animals grows ever stronger (15). In the 1970s, Lauweryns and colleagues (24–27) showed how rabbit PNCs organized into NEBs degranulate in response to hypoxia, generating activity in the afferent nerves supplying them, at least some of which relay in the vagus, as well as releasing their products locally. More recently, it has been shown that the membranes of these cells contain an

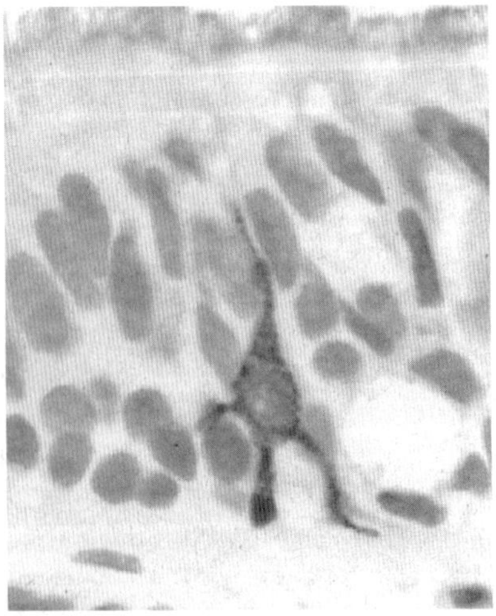

Figure 2 A solitary human pulmonary neuroendocrine cell labeled with neuron-specific enolase. The basal concentration of its secretory granules, and its cytoplasmic extension to the lumen of the airway are characteristic.

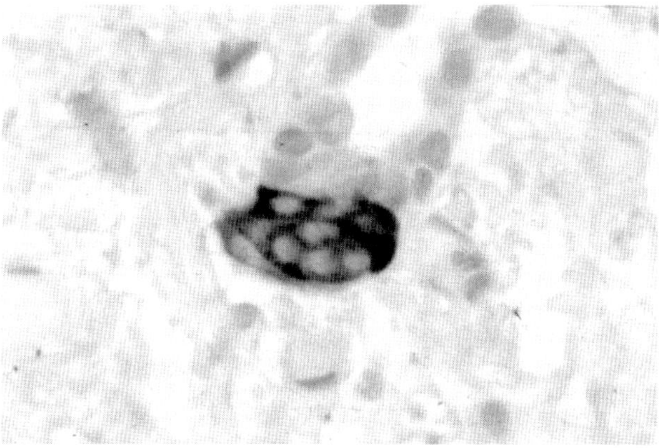

Figure 3 An innervated cluster of pulmonary neuroendocrine cells constituting a neureopithelial body, labeled with neuron-specific enolase, in the lung of a rabbit. These highly organized structures have a chemoreceptive role.

oxygen-sensing protein (28). The sparsity of PNCs in healthy adult human lungs, however, compounded by continuing doubt as to their function, has led some to believe that they are of little significance in humans, perhaps just vestigial elements that have lost any role they might have possessed in lower species as evolution advanced. However, more recent studies of PNCs during fetal pulmonary development and in human lungs affected by naturally occurring pulmonary disease have shown that this system of cells almost certainly plays a crucial role in regulating the development, regeneration, and repair of human pulmonary tissues (29–31).

Three pieces of evidence in particular point strongly to a role for PNCs in human fetal pulmonary growth and development. First, GRP, the predominant peptide in these cells in health, is powerfully trophic to human bronchial epithelial cells in vitro (32). Second, numbers of GRP-containing PNCs as well as levels of GRP, its mRNA, and its receptor, are markedly but transiently elevated during the canalicular period of human pulmonary development (33–35). And third, GRP stimulates fetal lung growth and maturation, including stimulation of branching morphogenesis, in vivo and in organ culture, in the murine and rhesus monkey fetus (36–38).

3 THE PULMONARY NEUROENDOCRINE CELL SYSTEM IN DISEASED LUNGS

The only other situation in which human PNCs are ever again so active as in fetal lungs is when they proliferate in diseased lungs (8,29,31). Most conditions in which they have been studied have involved inflammatory injury or, less often, some other form of pulmonary damage (Table 1).

Their pattern of proliferation follows a fairly predictable sequence (Fig. 4). The earliest change involves a linear proliferation of PNCs along the epithelial basement membrane to produce interrupted rows (Fig. 4b). If damage is persistent, recurrent, or particularly severe, a more disorderly proliferation occurs in which the cells pile up within the epithelium forming nodular aggregates (Fig. 4c). If injury proceeds to chronicity, it is likely that the process eventually and exceptionally gives rise to tumorlets (39), the small (2–3 mm) aggregates of PNCs that grow across the basement membrane into the parenchyma immediately adjacent to the airway, developing their own conspicuously fibrous stroma (Fig. 4d).

As proliferation progresses, the gradually increasing morphological disorder is accompanied by changes in the secretory content of the cells. In the earlier stages, when interrupted rows form, CT comes to predominate over GRP in a reversal of the normal situation (8,29,31). This may well be the morphological basis of the hypercalcitoninemia and hypercalcitoninuria demonstrable in patients with inflammatory pulmonary disease (see below). If nodular aggregates develop, and even more so if tumorlets form, aberrant peptides such as adrenocorticotropin hormone (ACTH), growth hormone, vasoactive intestinal polypeptide, and human chorionic gonadotropin (hCG) may appear (8,29,31,40–43).

It is likely that this proliferation is a fundamentally physiological response to injury involved with the control of repair and regeneration of damaged pulmonary tissues. This might be indirect, via the actions of its secretory products (30), or even direct, with PNCs acting as a reservoir of progenitor epithelial cells (44). What-

Table 1 Conditions in Which Increased Numbers of Pulmonary Neuroendocrine Cells have been Described

Asthma	Bronchopulmonary dysplasia
Pneumonia	Wilson-Mikity syndrome
Pulmonary fibrosis	Brainstem injury due to birth asphyxia
Bronchiectasis	Sudden infant death syndrome
Cystic fibrosis	
Chronic bronchitis and emphysema	
In pulmonary tissue around tumors	
Eosinophilic granuloma	
Plexogenic pulmonary arteriopathy	
Mechanical ventilation with oxygen	

Source: Ref. 8.

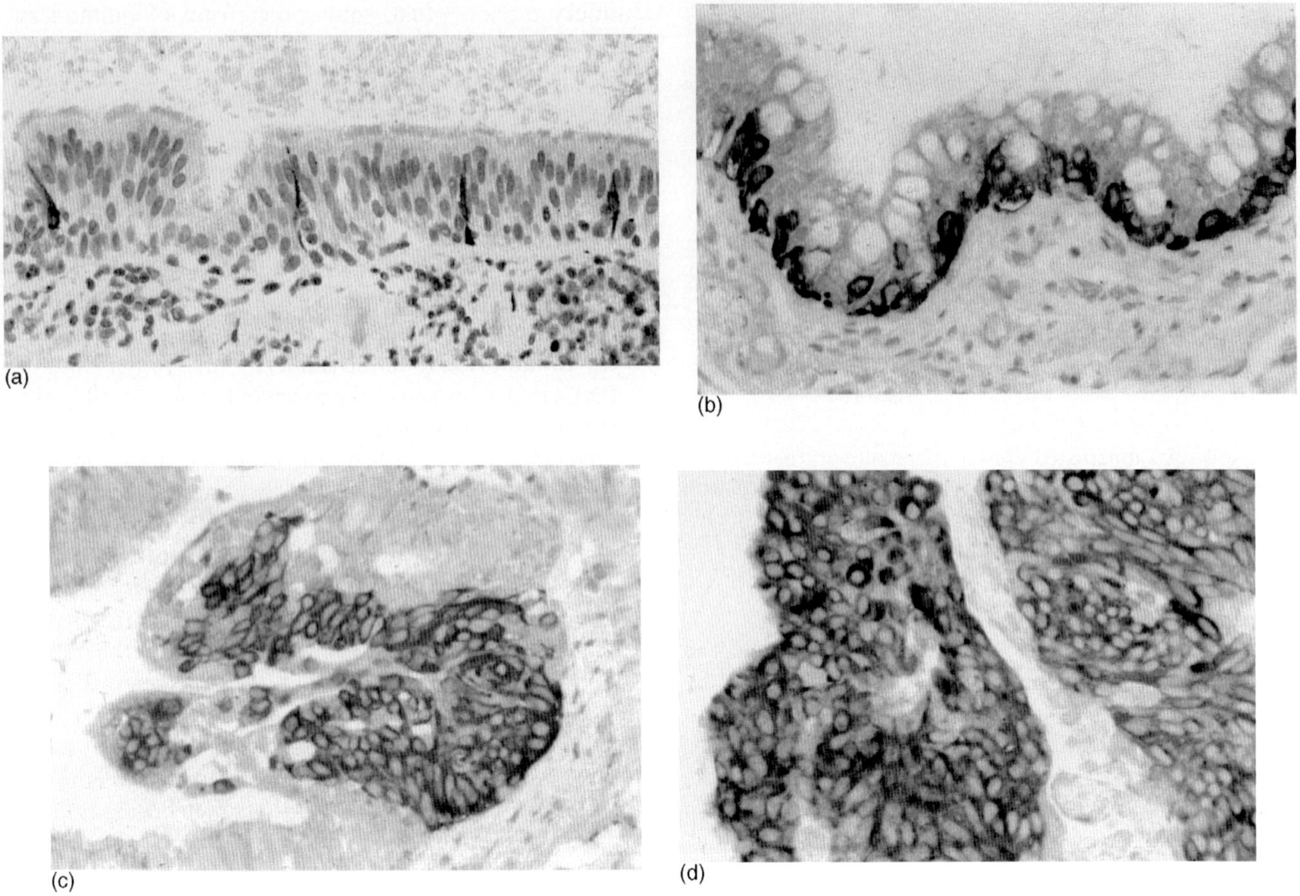

Figure 4 The pattern of proliferation of neuroendocrine cells, labeled with neuron-specific enolase, in injured human pulmonary epithelium. Replacement of their normal, sparse, regular distribution (a) by interrupted rows (b) is the earliest change. With persistent or repeated injury, larger, less orderly nodular aggregates appear (c). Exceptionally, proliferation extends across the basement membrane (d), giving rise to the locally infiltrative lesions known as tumorlets.

ever the case, the process would clearly be analogous to that controlling development of the lungs in utero. Its tendency as described to become morphologically and functionally disordered, however, is notable and raises the question of whether what is a basically reactive proliferation might ever become neoplastic. This intriguing possibility is addressed later in this chapter.

4 PULMONARY NEUROENDOCRINE TUMORS

4.1 Introduction

The fact that the lungs contain a dynamic system of neuroendocrine cells as described above makes it unsurprising that they generate neoplasms showing neuroendocrine features. The frequency with which they display this line of differentiation, however, is uniquely high and, at present, unexplained. It contrasts with the situation in other epithelial tissues, such as those lining the gastrointestinal and urinary tracts, in which neuroendocrine cells are also present, but neuroendocrine tumours are uncommon. Despite the prevalence of neuroendocrine differentiation in pulmonary tumours, their recognition as such has been a slow process. Although reports of so-called "ectopic" secretion by malignant pulmonary tumors had begun to appear by the early 1960s (see below) and DCVs had been described in both pulmonary carcinoids and small cell carcinoma by the end of the decade (45–47), these two tumors continued to be seen as separate and distinct, even in the 1982 World Health Organization (WHO) classification of pulmonary tumors (48) that was current until so recently (49). In the intervening years, however, the idea that pulmonary carcinoids and small cell carcinomas (SCCs) are related by their neuroendocrine phenotype and that tumors intermediate in their characteristics could be defined became established by morphological and immunochemical studies (50–53) and has been further supported by investigation of their molecular biology (54–57).

4.2 Classification

That part of the recently revised 1999 WHO classification of lung and pleural tumors that deals with pulmonary neuroendocrine tumours (49) is shown in Table 2. Overtly neuroendocrine pulmonary tumors are defined by their neuroendocrine morphology on light microscopy and are considered to comprise a spectrum in which four reasonably well-defined entities can be recognized. These share not only morphological, but also immunochemical and molecular pathological characteristics that vary quantitatively rather than qualitatively across this neuroendocrine spectrum, but they vary markedly in their behavior. The best differentiated PNTs, the typical carcinoids (TCs), occupy the benign extreme of the spectrum, with the most poorly differentiated, the small cell carcinomas, being the opposite, most malignant, extreme. In between are the atypical carcinoids (ACs), resembling TCs in many of their features but behaving with more aggression, and the large cell neuroendocrine carcinomas (LCNECs), which are more aggressive still and closer to SCCs in biology and behavior. These tumors are discussed in detail below.

Table 2 Neuroendocrine Proliferations and Neoplasms

NE cell hyperplasia and tumorlets
NE cell hyperplasia
NE cell hyperplasia associated with fibrosis and/or inflammation
NE cell hyperplasia adjacent to carcinoid tumors
Diffuse idiopathic NE cell hyperplasia with or without airway fibrosis/obstruction
Tumorlets
Tumors with NE morphology
Typical carcinoid
Atypical carcinoid
Large cell neuroendocrine carcinoma
Small cell carcinoma
Non–small cell carcinomas with NE differentiation
Other tumors with NE properties
Pulmonary blastoma
Primitive neuroectodermal tumor
Desmoplastic round cell tumor
Carcinomas with rhabdoid phenotype
Paraganglioma

Source: Ref. 49.

Pulmonary neoplasms with elements of neuroendocrine differentiation inapparent from their appearance also exist. These do not have the neuroendocrine morphology that characterizes the tumors in the neuroendocrine spectrum described above, but are often typical squamous or adenocarcinomas that display their concealed neuroendocrine phenotype either ultrastructurally, in the form of cytoplasmic DCVs, or immunochemically, by expressing one or more of the neuroendocrine markers described below (58,59). These non–small cell carcinomas with neuroendocrine differentiation are now explicitly recognized in the current WHO 1999 classification (Table 2) and will be considered in more detail later.

Also included in the classification (Table 2) is a group of very rare neoplasms that fit into neither of the above categories, but display features of neuroendocrine differentiation as part of their biology. These comprise the pulmonary blastoma, the primitive neuroectodermal tumor (PNET), the desmoplastic round cell tumor, carcinomas with rhabdoid phenotype, and paraganglioma. They are rare and will not be discussed further here.

Finally, there is now included in the new classification a group of PNC proliferations under suspicion of being possible precursors of the overtly neuroendocrine tumors described above, particularly the pulmonary carcinoids. This category of neuroendocrine cell hyperplasia and tumorlets (Table 2) includes those proliferations generally still considered reactive, discussed earlier in this chapter, as well as the recently recognized condition of diffuse idiopathic pulmonary neuroendocrine cell hyperplasia (DIPNECH). This is an interesting entity that poses intriguing questions about the relationship between PNC proliferation and bona fide neoplasia and will be discussed in more detail below.

4.3 Pathology

4.3.1 Typical Carcinoids

Typical pulmonary carcinoids (8,49,50,53,60–63) occupy the benign end of the spectrum of pulmonary neuroendocrine tumours. Although indolent, with a low rate of recurrence and metastasis after resection, they should always be considered potentially malignant. Their incidence is stable, peaking in the fifth decade, earlier in life than other PNTs, and their cause is unknown; they are not related to cigarette smoking.

Typical carcinoids most often arise in proximal airways as well-defined, yellow to red-brown masses,

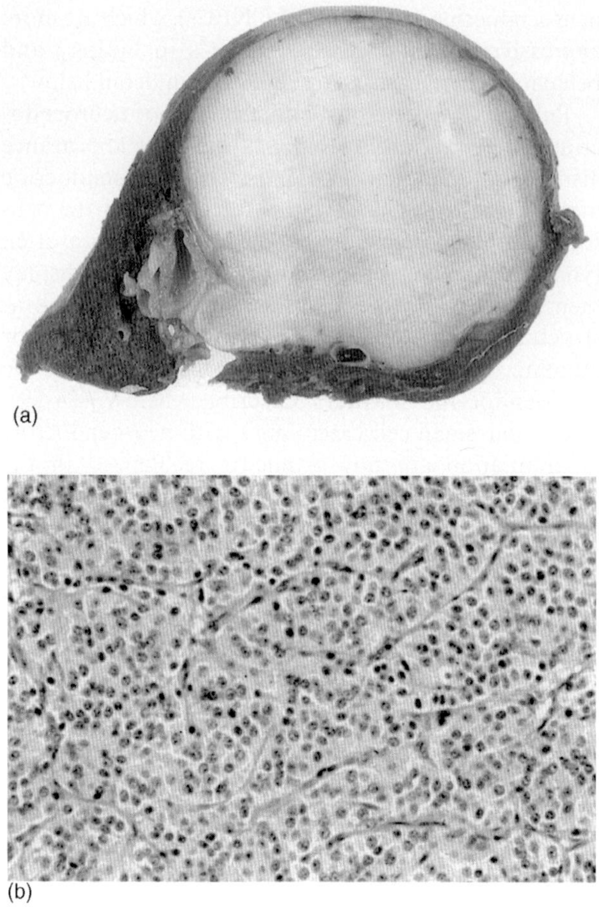

Figure 5 Characteristic gross (a) and microscopic (b) features of a typical pulmonary carcinoid tumor. These indolent lesions are well circumscribed and homogeneous (a) and characterized histologically by bland, monomorphic cells with a highly organized pattern of growth (b). There is no necrosis, and mitoses are rare.

usually 2–5 cm in diameter at diagnosis, and are characterized histologically by their highly organized "carcinoid" architecture and the bland uniformity of their cells (Fig. 5). These cells have copious cytoplasm, centrally placed nuclei, and are arranged within a delicate stroma in a well-ordered nodular, trabecular, acinar, or papillary pattern. Mitoses are rare (less than two per 2 mm^2), and there is no necrosis. The cytoplasm of their cells contains numerous DCVs and they strongly express a range of neuroendocrine markers (see below).

4.3.2 Atypical Carcinoids

Atypical pulmonary carcinoids (8,49,50,53,60–63) present, on average, a decade later in life than TCs and are usually larger and more obviously invasive at diagnosis. They are also more often peripheral within the lung. Like TCs, however, their incidence appears stable and they are not related to cigarette smoking. They are more aggressive tumors, with local recurrence common and eventual mestastasis in about three quarters of cases, often leading to death some years from diagnosis.

Atypical carcinoids are grossly and histologically similar to TCs (Fig. 6) but have a less well-organized architecture with some pleomorphism of their cells, a greater degree of mitotic activity (up to 10 mitoses per

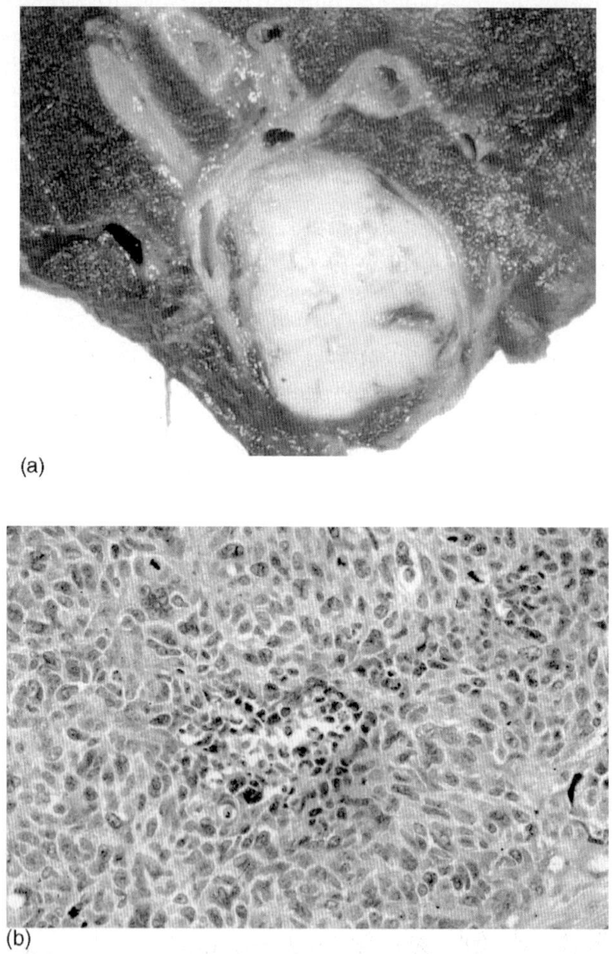

Figure 6 Characteristic features of an atypical carcinoid tumor. Often larger than typical carcinoids at diagnosis (a), foci of softening and hemorrhage are sometimes apparent, but they are usually well-defined tumors. Histologically (b), there is a lesser degree of organization than with typical carcinoids, occasional mitoses are seen, and punctate necrosis is characteristic.

mm^2), and show focal "punctate" necrosis. Their cells are often crowded and sometimes fusiform. Stromal fibrosis is not uncommon. Their cytoplasm contains smaller numbers of DCVs than that in the cells of TCs, and expression of neuroendocrine markers, although still prevalent, is less strong.

4.3.3 Large Cell Neuroendocrine Carcinoma

These neoplasms (49,52,60–65) are the most recently defined of the four entities within the spectrum of pulmonary neuroendocrine tumors, and their histopathological variability is greater than that of the other tumors within it, making the accurate diagnosis of LCNEC more difficult. Because of this, data with regard to their behavior is less reliable than for the other tumors within the spectrum, but they appear to be more closely related to SCCs than to ACs in their biology, generally behaving aggressively with early dissemination, and there is a growing tendency to refer to both LCNECs and SCCs together as "poorly differentiated neuroendocrine carcinomas." Their age incidence, appropriately, overlaps that of ACs and SCCs, and they are probably smoking-related.

Grossly, LCNECs are usually frankly malignant grey-white masses, often with obvious necrosis (Fig. 7a), although the better differentiated examples may be well circumscribed and homogeneous. Histologically, as already mentioned, the range of features they display is wider than that of other PNTs. Those examples most closely related to ACs have a well-developed neuroendocrine growth pattern, differing from ACs largely by displaying greater mitotic activity (more than 10 mitoses per 2 mm^2) and confluent necrosis. Those closer to SCC have lost much of their neuroendocrine morphology and appear frankly malignant cytologically and histologically, but they always retain some degree of it, usually in the form of a vague palisading or trabeculation (Fig. 7b). Electron microscopy reveals few DCVs, and neuroendocrine markers are often only weakly expressed.

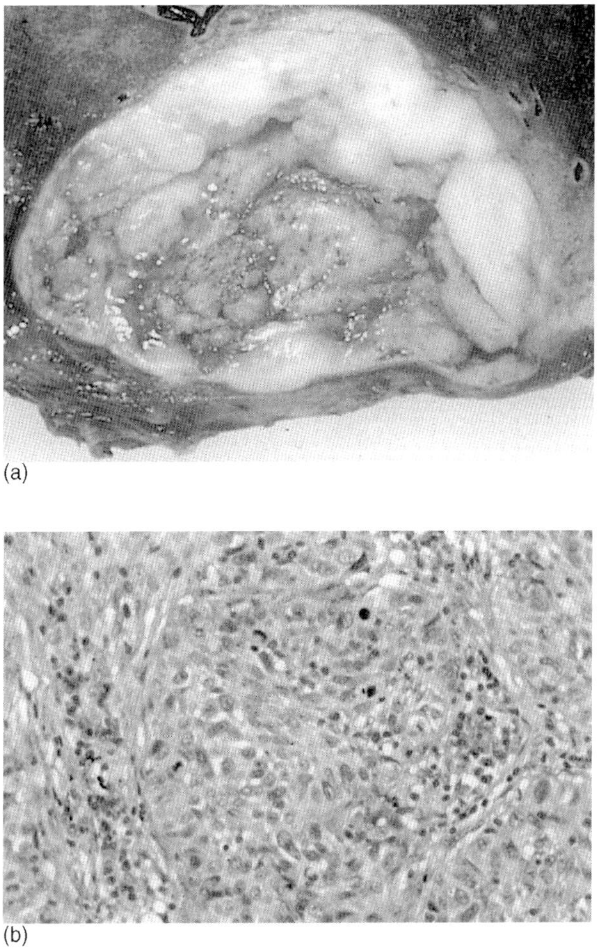

Figure 7 Characteristic features of a large cell neuroendocrine carcinoma. Usually obviously malignant on gross (a) and microscopic (b) examination, they nevertheless retain some degree of a neuroendocrine growth pattern. Cells are large with copious cytoplasm, necrosis is often confluent, and mitoses are numerous.

4.3.4 Small Cell Carcinoma

Small cell carcinoma (8,49,60–63) is the most common of the PNTs and the most aggressive, often spreading beyond the thorax by the time of diagnosis. They are closely related to cigarette smoking and arise predominantly in the seventh and eighth decades of life. They usually arise in major bronchi as frankly malignant, partly necrotic, grey-white masses. Most present with local effects, a smaller number because of metastases, and about one in 10 with paraneoplastic manifestations (see below), which are more common in SCC than in the other types of PNT.

Their histopathology is characteristic (Fig. 8); almost devoid of stroma, they comprise densely packed masses of small cells with large nuclei occupying much of their cytoplasm. These cells compress and distort each other. Mitoses are numerous, necrosis widespread, and connective tissue and blood vessels become impregnated with extruded nucleic acid. Dense core vesicles may be impossible to find on electron microscopy and expression of neuroendocrine markers may be weak or even absent.

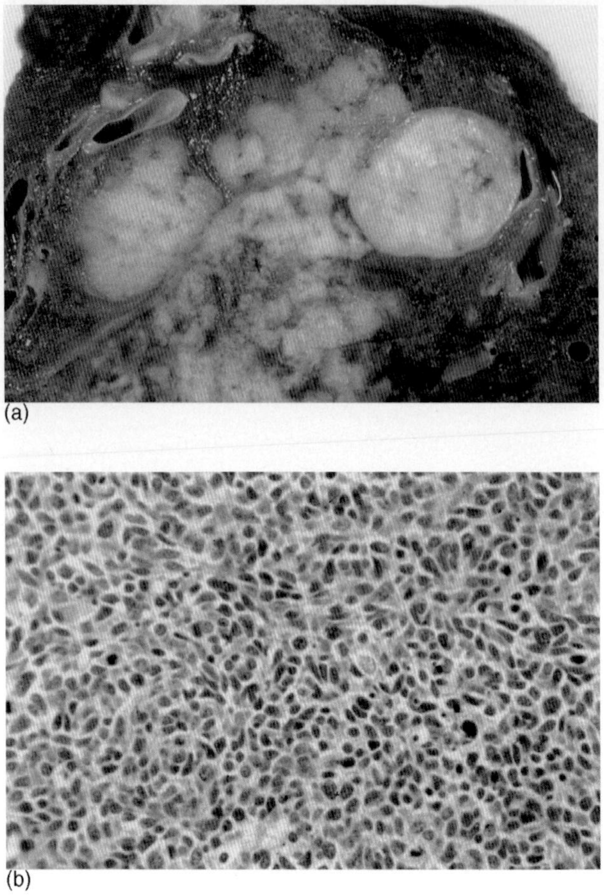

Figure 8 Characteristic features of small cell carcinoma. Clearly malignant on gross examination (a) and often disseminated at diagnosis, they are characterized histologically by small, densely packed cells, with large nuclei and minimal cytoplasm (b). Stroma is minimal, necrosis widespread, and mitoses numerous. Connective tissue is often impregnated with extruded nucleic acid.

4.3.5 Neuroendocrine Markers in Diagnosis

A wide range of immunochemical markers of neuroendocrine differentiation has become available over the years to asssist in the histological differential diagnosis of PNTs, but their sensitivity and specificity is variable and their practical utility is actually quite limited (8,63). They include cytoplasmic antigens such as NSE (66) and PGP 9.5 (67), components of secretory vesicles like chromogranin (68) and synaptophysin (69), and the membrane-based neural cell adhesion molecule (NCAM) (70), which is probably the most sensitive and specific of those markers currently available.

Although these markers are expressed more strongly by the better differentiated PNTs (TCs and ACs) than by the more malignant one (LCNECs and SCCs), the difference between tumor types is inconsistent and cannot be used to distinguish between individual tumors in the neuroendocrine spectrum. Nor are they able to distinguish neuroendocrine tumors arising in the lungs from those metastasizing into the thorax from elsewhere; medullary carcinoma of the thyroid and malignant carcinoids metastasizing from the gatrointestinal tract or pancreas are obvious examples. Where they are of use, however, is in distinguishing PNTs from nonneuroendocrine tumors arising within or metastasizing into the lungs, to which they may be histologically similar. For example, pulmonary metastases of adenocarcinomas of the thyroid or kidney may mimic pulmonary carcinoids. Similarly, poorly differentiated carcinomas arising either within the lungs or metastasizing to them from extrathoracic sites may be difficult to distinguish from LCNEC and SCC, especially with small bronchoscopic or needle biopsies, and the distinction between SCC and lymphoma can be particularly difficult on histological grounds alone. In situations like these, judicious use of a panel of markers, including not only neuroendocrine markers but those able to distinguish the possible diagnostic alternatives, can be extremely useful.

4.4 Possible Preneoplastic Neuroendocrine Proliferations

The proliferative response of normal PNCs to pulmonary injury and its occasional tendency to become disordered with the secretion of aberrant products and the formation of the locally infiltrative lesions known as tumorlets were described earlier in this chapter. It has generally been accepted that this proliferation, even to the extent of the development of tumorlets, is a reactive process with no propensity for neoplasia, a belief supported by recent description of the contrasting molecular pathology of pulmonary tumorlets and carcinoids (71). In the early 1990s, however, a disorder characterized by diffuse proliferation of PNCs, including linear rows, nodular aggregates, and tumorlets, in intimate association with small, peripheral carcinoid tumors, was repeatedly described (72–74). This condition, now generally known as diffuse idiopathic pulmonary neuroendocrine cell hyperplasia (DIPNECH), has resurrected intriguing questions about the relationship between presumed-reactive proliferation of PNCs and bona fide neuroendocrine neoplasia (Fig. 9).

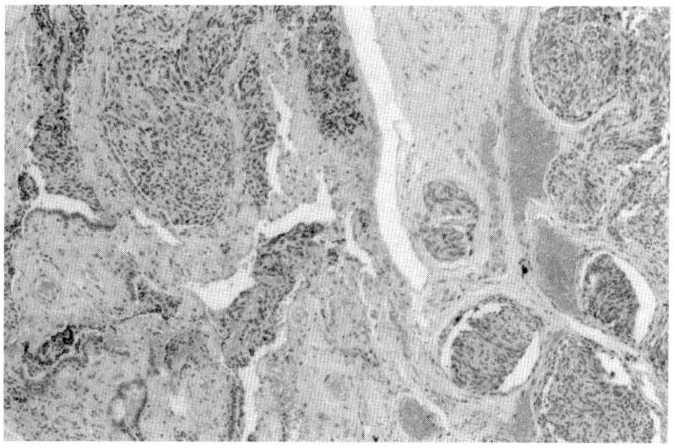

Figure 9 Proliferating neuroendocrine cells in a case of diffuse idiopathic pulmonary neuroendocrine cell hyperplasia (DIPNECH). Intraluminal and extraluminal proliferation, a tumorlet, and the edge of a small carcinoid tumor all are evident in this microscopic field.

Diffuse idiopathic pulmonary neuroendocrine cell hyperplasia arises in young to middle age and is perhaps more common in women. The history is one of a very slowly worsening dry cough and breathlessness, often over many years, often diagnosed as asthma or bronchitis. Radiographs show a diffuse reticulonodular pulmonary infiltrate, and respiratory function tests reveal a mixed obstructive-restrictive pattern of impairment with reduced diffusing capacity. Histopathological examination of tissue removed for diagnosis reveals variable proliferation of PNCs, with intraluminal and extraluminal aggregates, interrupted rows, nodular aggregates, and tumorlets together with, in many but not all cases, typical peripheral carcinoid tumors of variable size, most of them very small (Fig. 8). Often, there is intra- and extramural fibrosis of small airways. Some have considered this the cause of the proliferation, but the wider belief is that it is a consequence of the release of fibrogenic products from the proliferating cells.

It is still not certain that DIPNECH arises spontaneously. It might, for example, result from previous pulmonary injury no longer apparent—possibly an inhaled toxin. It is also not uncommon to see foci of PNC proliferation, including tumorlets, around pulmonary tumors of all types, not just carcinoids, in which situation it is often attributable to collapse and consolidation of the parenchyma in the vicinity of the tumour (75). Nevertheless, it is difficult to avoid the conclusion that, in at least some of these cases, PNC proliferation has developed without obvious cause, in normal lungs, and not only caused damage by injuring small airways, but also proceeded to the formation of true neuroendocrine neoplasms.

5 SERUM MARKERS OF PULMONARY NEUROENDOCRINE TUMORS

Serum markers of PNTs fall into three groups (Table 3): general tumor markers, endocrine markers, and actual secretory products.

5.1 General Tumour Markers

Like all neoplasms, PNTs can cause elevation of serum levels of a range of unrelated substances. These general tumor markers are numerous (Table 3) and not specific to their neuroendocrine phenotype. They include oncofetal antigens such as carcinoembryonic antigen (76), placental glycoproteins like hCG (77), enzymes such as

Table 3 Serum Markers of Pulmonary Neuroendocrine Tumors

General Markers	Endocrine markers
Oncofetal antigens	Neuron-specific enolase
Carcinoembryonic antigen	Brain isoenzyme of creatine kinase
Alpha-fetoprotein	Chromogranins and related proteins
Pancreatic oncofetal antigen	Diamine oxidase
Placental glycoproteins	Secretory products
Human chorionic gonadotropin	Adrenocorticotropin and related peptides
Human chorionic somatomammotropin	Calcitonin and calcitonin gene–related peptide
Enzymes	Arginine vasopressin and related peptides
Alkaline phosphatase	Bombesin-like peptides
Aspartate aminotransferase	Growth hormone and related peptides
Gamma aminotranspeptidase	Serotonin
Lactate dehydrogenase	Pituitary gonadotropins
Thymidine kinase	Prolactin
Phosphohexose isomerase	Thyroid-stimulating hormone
Fucosyl transferase	Vasoactive intestinal polypeptide
Sialyl transferase	Somatostatin
Others	Insulin
β_2-Microglobulin	Gastrin
α_1-Acid glycoprotein	Parathyroid hormone
Glucagon	Renin
Ferritin	
Prostaglandins	
Tissue polypeptide antigen	
Carbohydrate antigens	

Source: Ref. 8.

lactate dehydrogenase (78), and a miscellany of other substances including β_2-microglobulin (79), ferritin (80), and various carbohydrate antigens (81).

5.2 Neuroendocrine Markers

A second group of serum markers comprises substances released from PETs that reflect their neuroendocrine phenotype. To some extent these neuroendocrine markers are common to all tumors following the line of differentiation of the DNS, but in the case of PNTs their study has been confined almost entirely to SCC. They include three enzymes—NSE, the brain isoenzyme of creatine kinase (CK-BB), and diamine oxidase (DAO; histaminase)—and the group of proteins known as the chromogranins (Table 3).

The best documented of the enzymes is NSE. Since its presence in cultures of SCC and in the serum of patients with the tumor were first described (82,83), its efficacy as a marker of the presence and extent of the disease has been widely researched (8). Although there is reasonable correlation between serum levels of the enzyme and tumor burden, NSE has not proven either specific or sensitive enough to be of real practical utility in the management of patients with PNTs. Serum levels of CK-BB are elevated in about half of patients with SCC (84) and, like NSE, correlate with tumor burden (85). Levels of DAO have been reported to be elevated in about one third of patients with SCC (86), but it has been relatively little studied as a serum marker of the disease.

The chromogranins have been widely used as tissue markers of tumors following the line of differentiation of the DNS, including those arising in the lung, but they are also demonstrable in the serum of patients with these neoplasms (87). Employing antisera recognizing more than one of the chromogranins increases their sensitivity as serum markers (88), but, like the other markers in this group, they appear to be of little practical utility in the management of patients with PNTs.

5.3 Secretory Products

A third group of serum markers of PNTs comprises their actual secretory products (Table 3). Some of these are found in normal PNCs, others in PNCs only in diseased lungs, and a further group seems to be unique to PNTs. Since these tumors are characterized by neuroendocrine differentiation, it is unsurprising that they produce amine, peptide, and protein hormones; the fact that they recapitulate the line of differentiation of the pulmonary component of the DNS means that synthesis and release of substances found in normal PNCs or even in PNCs in diseased lungs are only to be expected. Many secretory products of PNTs, however, especially of those tumors towards the malignant end of the spectrum, do not fall into these categories, having not been demonstrated in PNCs under any circumstances. These substances and the processes of their synthesis and secretion are generally referred to as "inappropriate."

This concept of inappropriate secretion originally developed from the observation that even neoplasms arising in nonendocrine tissues occasionally produced hormones, the alternative but now less used term "ectopic secretion" having been originally introduced by Liddle et al. (89) to describe the release of ACTH from nonpituitary tumors. Such inappropriate products include peptide, protein, and glycoprotein hormones with their precursors and fragments, amines, prostaglandins, growth factors, and enzymes. Various theories have been proposed to explain the phenomenon (8,90) and will not be debated here, but it clearly is a functional equivalent of the morphological disorganization that characterizes malignant neoplastic populations.

The range of secretory products, appropriate and inappropriate, that has been demonstrated in the serum of subjects with PNTs is remarkable (Table 3), but only three of these have been studied extensively and will be discussed further here. The first, CT, is a product of PNCs in healthy lungs, the second, ACTH, an occasional product of these cells in diseased lungs, and the third, arginine vasopressin (AVP; antidiuretic hormone) does not appear to have been described in PNCs under any circumstances. Thus, whereas secretion of CT by these tumors is clearly appropriate, that of ACTH may or may not be depending upon whether its secretion by PNCs in diseased lungs is considered physiological or pathological, and that of AVP is clearly inappropriate.

5.3.1 Calcitonin

Since the first report of elevated levels of CT in the serum of a patient with bronchial carcinoma (91), the relationship between hypercalcitoninemia and pulmonary tumors has been extensively investigated (8). Numerous investigations describe its elevation in patients with SCC ranging in prevalence from about one fourth (92) to more than three fourths (93) of those with the disease, and it is present in a smaller proportion of subjects with non-neuroendocrine pulmonary tumors (94). Although its origin from the tumor has been clearly demonstrated on a number of occasions (95–97), the possibility that it sometimes has an alternative source, either from the thyroid gland (98) or from the proliferating PECs in the surrounding lung (75), has been raised. Such a possibility is supported by the observations that CT is the predominant peptide in proliferating PNCs in inflamed lungs (see above) and that hypercalcitoninemia and hypercalcitoninuria are not uncommon in patients with inflammatory pulmonary diseases like pneumonia, tuberculosis, cystic fibrosis, and chronic obstructive pulmonary disease (8,99). Indeed, sequential measurements of CT in patients with pneumonia showed a return of levels to normal as the infection resolved (99). A potential role for CT as a marker of disease in subjects with SCC has been investigated in a number of studies, but findings have been inconsistent (8).

5.3.2 Adrenocorticotrophin

Elevated levels of ACTH, its precursors and fragments, have been repeatedly demonstrated in the serum of patients with PNTs, carcinoid tumors, as well as those at the malignant end of the spectrum (100,101), when other peptides derived from the proopiocortin precursor are though often to accompany it (102,103). As with CT, elevated serum levels of ACTH have been described in subjects with nonneuroendocrine pulmonary tumors (104) and in those with inflammatory pulmonary disease (105,106). Nonsuppressible elevation of ACTH has also been described in a patient with a pulmonary abscess in whom it not only fell to normal after the abscess was resected, but was demonstrable within it by immunolabelling (107). Origin of the peptide from proliferating PNCs in diseased lung accompanying the tumor is again an alternative explanation for its elevation in the serum of some patients with pulmonary neoplasms (75). Like CT, the correlation between levels of ACTH and presence and extent of disease in patients with SCC has been extensively studied, but it appears neither particularly specific nor sensitive in this regard (8).

5.3.3 Arginine Vasopressin

Arginine vasopressin is responsible for the most common endocrine manifestation of SCC, namely the syndrome of inappropriate ADH secretion (SIADH). Since the earliest reports of the association (108,109), many authors have described levels of AVP inappropriate to plasma osmolality in the serum or urine of subjects with pulmonary tumors (8), and it has been demonstrated in tissue from SCCs by extraction and assay (96). Although AVP has not been demonstrated in PNCs, SIADH complicating pulmonary tuberculosis was described many years ago (110) and the peptide has been demonstrated in tuberculous pulmonary tissue (111). It appears to have no utility as a marker of presence and extent of disease in patients with PNTs (112).

6 PARANEOPLASTIC EFFECTS OF PULMONARY NEUROENDOCRINE TUMORS

The most obvious effects of pulmonary tumors, including those showing neuroendocrine differentiation, are a direct physical consequence of their growth. Many present locally by obstructing an airway, provoking collapse and consolidation, or by invading the wall of the chest or the structures of the mediastinum. Physical effects of metastases are also common; pathological fracture, raised intracranial pressure, or adrenocortical failure are obvious examples of ways in which a disseminated tumor might present. In addition, and as might be inferred from the preceding discussion, PNTs recapitulate the features of PNCs and, like other neuroendocrine tumors, have a capacity for secreting peptides and amines. Of the products produced by PNCs in healthy lungs, however, secretion of only serotonin by a PNT is likely to have any clinical effect, theoretically contributing to the carcinoid syndrome (see below). Such secretion and its consequences, if any, are a result of appropriate secretion and are predictable and explicable.

These are not the only ways in which PNTs present, however. Sometimes clinical manifestations of any tumor occur that are clearly a consequence of it, but attributable to neither its physical presence nor the secretion of substances appropriate to it. These effects are conventionally known as paraneoplastic phenomena (9) and are especially likely to arise in patients with pulmonary tumors, particularly those that show neuroendocrine differentiation.

6.1 Mechanisms of Paraneoplasia

It is likely that all paraneoplastic phenomena are due to the expression or release by neoplastic cells of substances that differ qualitatively or quantitatively from those expressed or released by their normal counterparts. These substances then exert their effects in one of two ways.

The first mechanism involves interference with normal physiological processes either because the substances are themselves biologically active or because they interfere with the function of their normal counterparts. In these cases the substances responsible often result from the process of inappropriate secretion described above. It is this mechanism that underlies many of the nonneurological paraneoplastic phenomena.

The second mechanism involves the provocation of an immune response by substances produced by the tumor that are unique or normally concealed. This results in either formation of immune complexes, a hypersensitivity reaction, or cross-reaction of the resulting antibodies with normal tissue components which happen to share antigenic sites with the substance expressed by the neoplastic cells. It is this mechanism that underlies many of the neurological paraneoplastic phenomena.

Many paraneoplastic manifestations of neoplasia are not associated particularly with PNTs, being seen in patients with a range of neoplasms (9). These include pyrexia, cachexia, coagulopathy, amyloidosis, and a variety of cutaneous and rheumatological abnormalities. Some paraneoplastic effects, however, are closely associated with PNTs and may be unique to them, whereas others are associated with pulmonary tumors in general but likely to be mediated by a peptide or protein hormone and probably reflect an element within the tumor of neuroendocrine differentiation.

6.2 Paraneoplastic Phenomena Associated with Pulmonary Neuroendocrine Tumors

The most practical classification of paraneoplastic phenomena is according to the anatomical or physiological system they disturb, in which scheme they are divisible into four broad groups (Table 4). Paraneoplastic endocrine disturbances are more often due to PNTs than to any other tumor and to some extent correlate with tumor type, the carcinoid syndrome, for example, being largely confined to TCs and ACs, whereas SIADH is almost exclusive to SCC. Cushing's syndrome arising in a patient with a PNT is the classical and most often cited example of inappropriate hormone secretion. A peculiar variety of cutaneous changes are among the more mysterious of the paraneoplastic effects of PNTs and largely unexplained, as are digital clubbing and hypertrophic osteoarthropathy, two paraneoplastic osteoarticular effects that have fascinated physicians throughout medical history. Finally, there is a large group of paraneoplastic neurological phenomena, most if not all immune mediated, that can affect any level of the nervous system from the cerebral cortex to the myoneural junction.

Table 4 Paraneoplastic Phenomena Occurring in Patients with Pulmonary Carcinoma That have an Established or Suspected Pulmonary Association with Neuroendocrine Differentiation in the Tumor

- Endocrine
  - The carcinoid syndrome
  - Cushing's syndrome and variants
  - The syndrome of inappropiate secretion of antidiuretic hormone (SIADH)
  - Gynecomastia
- Cutaneous
  - Epithelial proliferations (acanthosis nigricans, tripe palms, Bazex's syndrome, the sign of Leser-Trélat)
  - Erythema gyratum repens
  - Hypertrichosis lanuginosa
  - Dermatomyositis
- Osteoarticular
  - Digital clubbing
  - Hypertrophic osteoarthropathy
- Neurological
  - Effects on the cerebrum
    - Encephalomyelitis
    - Angioendotheliosis
  - Effects on the cerebellum
    - Cerebellar degeneration
  - Effects on the eye
    - Visual paraneoplastic syndrome
  - Other effects on the brain and cranial nerves
    - Optic neuritis
    - Extrapyramidal disorders of movement
    - Opsoclonus
  - Effects on the spinal cord
    - Subacute necrotic myelopathy
    - Amyotrophic lateral sclerosis
  - Effects on peripheral nerves
    - Sensory, motor, and mixed neuropathies
  - Autonomic effects
    - Orthostatic hypotension
    - Alimentary dysfunction
  - Effects on the myoneural junction
    - Eaton-Lambert myasthenic syndrome

Source: Ref. 8.

6.2.1 Endocrine Disturbances

The Carcinoid Syndrome. The carcinoid syndrome is probably caused to some extent by serotonin, a product of normal PNCs, and in this regard is not strictly paraneoplastic, but continuing doubt as to its pathogenesis and the likely involvement of other substances not normally found in these cells justifies its discussion here.

The syndrome is most often seen in patients with extensive hepatic metastases from carcinoids arising in the gut and is a rare manifestation of PNTs. This is because it is largely confined to tumors at the benign end of the spectrum of PNTs, being very rarely associated with SCC, and requires a large bulk of tumor tissue (113), whereas pulmonary carcinoids rarely metastasize to produce large secondary deposits. Its prevalence in patients with pulmonary carcinoids is probably about 5% (8).

The carcinoid syndrome has four main clinical components. These are, with their approximate prevalences, flushing, especially of the head and neck, often causing hyperpigmentation (75%), diarrhea, often of distressing frequency and associated with colic (75%), carcinoid heart disease, which takes the form of a plaque-like subendocardial fibrosis and affects predominantly the valves on that side of the heart through which blood draining the bulk of the tumor first passes (40%), and wheezing, due to bronchoconstriction (20%) (114). Ever since serotonin was first described in a carcinoid tumor (115), it has been considered an important mediator of the carcinoid syndrome, but it cannot explain all its components (114). Histamine, 5-hydroxytryptophan, kinins, tachykinins, and prostaglandins have all been implicated, but none has been confirmed as a consistent mediator of it.

Cushing's Syndrome and Variants. What is generally considered to be the first report of Cushing's syndrome due to secretion of ACTH by a PNT (116) actually predated description of the syndrome itself (117). Although the full-blown syndrome appears in only 2–3% of patients with SCC, elevated serum levels of ACTH are demonstrable in 10 times as many and impaired suppression of adrenal corticosteroid secretion in about half (8).

The syndrome that develops in patients with SCC differs from that due to pituitary hypersecretion in that hypokalemia is almost always a feature, but truncal obesity, striae, and pigmentation are less often present (9). The adrenal glands postmortem are markedly hyperplastic; there is expansion of the zona reticularis, obliterating the lipid-rich zona fasciculata (Fig. 10a), and a single gland may way 20 g. In the 15% of patients with Cushing's syndrome in whom a PNT is the cause, three features suggest such a tumor to be responsible: markedly increased levels of ACTH, markedly increased levels of urinary cortisol, and an inability to suppress plasma levels of cortisol with dexamethasone.

Inappropriate Secretion of Antidiuretic Hormone. Hyponatremia and high urinary sodium excretion in patients with tuberculosis and pulmonary carcinoma was first reported in 1938 (118), but it was some time before inappropriate secretion of AVP was suggested to be responsible (119) and the classical description of SIADH did not appear for another 10 years (120). The strict criteria for its diagnosis are hypo-osmolar plasma in the presence of hyperosmolar urine inappropriate to plasma osmolality and a persistent natriuresis with no evidence of volume depletion and providing there is normal cardiac, renal, and adrenal function and the changes cannot be attributed to drugs inhibiting water secretion (121). The syndrome according to these criteria occurs in 10–15% of patients with SCC, although abnormalities of water secretion and/or elevated serum levels of AVP are demonstrable in as many as 30–40% (8,9,122).

Gynecomastia. Considering the frequency with which elevated levels of the subunits of hCG are demonstrable in patients with pulmonary tumors (see above), gynecomastia is surprisingly rare, developing in only about one in 100 male patients (123). This may be because their synthesis is unbalanced and production of the complete, biologically active molecule is uncommon.

6.2.2 Cutaneous Changes

Althouth rare, developing in no more than 1% of patients with pulmonary carcinoma (8,9,124), paraneoplastic cutaneous manifestations are important because they often develop well before the tumor becomes apparent. They are not as closely associated with PNTs as most of the other paraneoplastic phenomena described here, however, and some are actually more often associated with neoplasms growing outside the lungs (9).

A variety of proliferative cutaneous processes are the most common of these. They include acanthosis nigricans, a symmetrical, velvety hyperkeratosis of the flexural and intertriginous areas, tripe palms, which is a similar process occurring on the palms, paraneoplastic acrokeratosis (Bazex's syndrome) in which erythematous or violaceous scaly lesions develop on the extrem-

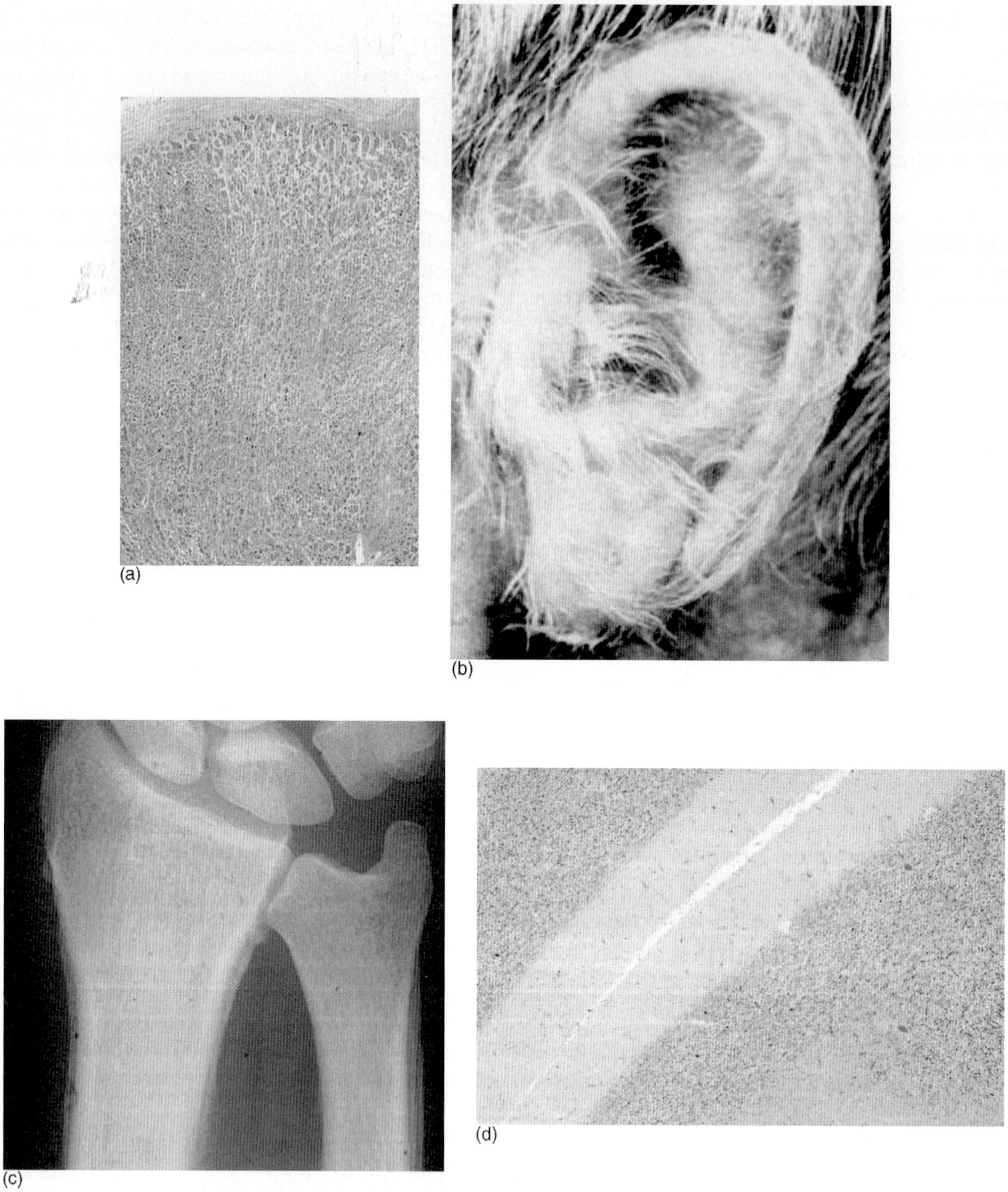

Figure 10 Four examples of paraneoplastic effects of pulmonary carcinoma. (a) The markedly hyperplastic adrenal cortices of a patient dying of disseminated adrenocorticotropin-producing small cell carcinoma. The normal lipid-rich cells of the zona fasciculata have disappeared as the cortex has expanded. (b) Growth of soft, silky hair characteristic of hypertrichosis lanuginosa on the ear of a patient with disseminated pulmonary carcinoma. (Courtesy of *CMA Journal* and Dr. M. A. Knowling.) (c) The wrist of a patient with a large cell neuroendocrine carcinoma and painful hypertrophic pulmonary osteoarthropathy that partly resolved after the tumor was resected. Subperiosteal new bone is evident. (d) Absence of Purkinje cells from the cerebellum of a patient dying of small cell carcinoma. Severe ataxia and hypotonia were present during life.

ities, and rapid, widespread growth of seborrheic warts, known as the sign of Leser-Trélat.

Several erythematous and blistering lesions are associated with malignant tumors in general (9), and, excluding the flushing of the carcinoid syndrome and the facial pigmentation this may produce, the only one to show a particular association with pulmonary carcinoma is a peculiar migratory circinate and serpiginous eruption known as erythema gyratum repens (125). Demonstration of IgG and C3 at the dermoepidermal junction suggests that erythema gyratum repens has an immunological basis (126).

Hypertrichosis lanuginosa (malignant down) is a remarkable manifestation of malignancy characterized by rapid growth of long, fine, silky hair, especially on the face and ears (127) (Fig. 10b). Like the erythematous and blistering lesions, it is not specific for PNTs, but pulmonary tumors are a frequent underlying cause.

Finally, mention should be made of dermatomyositis, an immune-mediated inflammatory disorder of the skin and skeletal muscles with a well-established association with malignant tumors of many types (128). The most common underlying tumor is probably pulmonary carcinoma (129), although there is no particularly close association with neuroendocrine differentiation.

6.2.3 Osteoarticular Effects

Two closely related conditions strongly associated with pulmonary carcinoma, digital clubbing and hypertrophic pulmonary osteoarthropathy [HPOA; Marie-Bamberger syndrome (130)], have been of abiding interest for many years, not least because of their uncertain pathogenesis; digital clubbing was described in the time of Hippocrates, but its cause, and that of HPOA, remain a matter of debate (8).

Clubbing is due to expansion of the soft tissues around the terminal phalanges, but whether new bone is laid down is uncertain (131). Osteogenesis is certainly a factor in HPOA, however, and characteristically forms beneath the periosteum, the changes characteristically affecting the ankles and wrists (Fig. 10c). Increased local blood flow due to vasodilatation is probably the crucial event in the development of both conditions and a variety of possible vasodilators has been proposed (132–134). Hypertrophic osteoarthropathy tends to resolve with removal of the tumor (135), but clubbing is more persistent. The fact that vagotomy often relieves the pain of HPOA and may also result in its resolution suggests that neural mechanisms are a factor in its causation, but this effect is not seen with clubbing and its basis is obscure (136).

6.2.4 Neurological Phenomena

Nonmetastatic neurological disturbances are pareneoplastic phenomena particularly closely associated with SCC. This is almost certainly because the tumor commonly expresses neural-type antigens that provoke an immune reaction damaging whichever part of the nervous system that happens to share them (137–139), and damage can occur at all levels.

Encephalomyelitis and cerebellar degeneration damage the cerebral and cerebellar cortices, respectively. The former characteristically presents with progressive dementia, although it is often complicated by accompanying injury at lower levels, particularly the dorsal root ganglia (140,141). The latter is characterized by loss of Purkinje cells (142) (Fig. 10d) and manifests clinically with progressive symmetrical ataxia, hypotonia, and pendular reflexes, although nystagmus is often absent. Loss of vision may occur due to destruction of photoreceptors (143). A clinical triad of photosensitivity, ring scotomas, and attenuated caliber of retinal arterioles characterizes this form of progressive blindness (144). Various other abnormalities due to damage above the level of the spinal cord have been described. These include optic neuritis (145), extrapyramidal disorders of movement (146), and opsoclonus (147), an involuntary saccadic movement of the eyes attributable to injury to a group of neurons in the brain stem.

Effects on the spinal cord and peripheral nerves include the two reasonably well-defined entities of subacute necrotic myelopathy and amyotrophic lateral sclerosis, and peripheral neuropathy may also occur. Subacute necrotic myelopathy is due to focal cavitation of the spinal cord, especially its thoracic segment, producing flaccid paraplegia with incontinence and sensory loss (148). Amyotrophic lateral sclerosis is the form of motor neuron disease involving loss of anterior horn cells and is occasionally associated with pulmonary carcinoma (149). Sensory, motor, and mixed sensorimotor neuropathies may also develop in association with pulmonary tumors (150), the purely sensory form being particularly closely associated with SCC (151).

Autonomic dysfunction is increasingly recognized as a paraneoplastic effect of PNTs (8). It usually presents as either orthostatic hypotension (152) or altered alimentary function in the shape of intestinal pseudo-obstruction (153). The histopathology comprises inflammatory destruction of the appropriate autonomic nerves (154).

Finally, SCC is closely associated with a neurological syndrome characterized by weakness and fatigueability of muscles, especially those of the pelvic girdle, accompanied by increased sensitivity to muscle relaxants. This myasthenic syndrome, which resembles mya sthenia gravis but differs in certain important aspects, was first reported in full by Eaton and Lambert in 1957 (155) and usually bears their names. In contrast to myasthenia gravis, it affects older subjects, involves different muscles, shows a transient muscle strengthening rather than a weakening in response to exercise, responds poorly to anticholinesterases, and is not associated with thymic pathology. Characteristic electromyographic features of increasing muscle action potentials on repeated stimulation of motor nerves are generally considered diagnostic but are probably not always evident, even when the syndrome is clearly related to SCC (156). The essence of the pathology is reduced quantal release of acetylcholine from presynaptic motor nerve terminals as a result of immune damage to voltage-gated calcium channels (157–160).

REFERENCES

1. Feyrter F. Über diffuse endokrine epitheliale Organe. Leipzig: JA Barth, 1938.
2. Masson P. La glande endocrine de l'intestin chez l'homme. CR Acad Sci (Paris) 1914; 158:59–61.
3. Hamperl H. Was sind argentaffine Zellen? Virchows Arch Pathol Anat 1932; 286:811–833.
4. Pearse AGE. The cytochemistry of the thyroid C cells and their relationship to calcitonin. Proc R Soc Lond Ser B Biol Sci 1966; 164:478–487.
5. Pearse AGE. Common cytochemical properties of cells producing polypeptide hormones with particular reference to calcitonin and the thyroid C cells. Vet Rec 1966; 79:587–590.
6. Pearse AGE. Common cytochemical and ultrastructural characteristics of cells producing polypeptide hormones (the APUD series) and their relevance to thyroid and ultimobranchial C cells and calcitonin. Proc R Soc Lond Ser B Biol Sci 1968; 170:71–80.
7. Pearse AGE. The cytochemistry and ultrastructure of polypeptide hormone-producing cells of the APUD series and the embryologic, physiologic and pathologic implications of the concept. J Histochem Cytochem 1969; 17:303–313.
8. Gosney JR. Pulmonary Endocrine Pathology: Endocrine Cells and Endocrine Tumours of the Lung. Oxford: Butterworth-Heinemann, 1992.
9. Arnold SM, Patchell R, Lowy AM, Foon KA. Paraneoplastic syndromes. In: DeVita VT, Hellman S, Rosenberg SA, eds. Cancer: Principles and Practice of Oncology. 6th ed. Philadelphia: Lippincott Williams & Wilkins, 2001;2511–2536.
10. Fröhlich F. Die helle Zelle der Bronchialschleimhaut und ihre Beziehungen zum Problem der Chemoreceptoren. Frank Z Pathol 1949; 60:517–559.
11. Hage E. Endocrine-like cells of the pulmonary epithelium. In: Coupland RE, Fujita T, eds. Chromaffin, Enterochromaffin and Related Cells.New York: Elsevier, 1976;317–332.
12. Scheuermann DW. Morphology and cytochemistry of the endocrine epithelial system in the lung. Int Rev Cytol 1987; 106:35–88.
13. Sorokin SP, Hoyt RF. Neuroepithelial bodies and solitary small granule cells. In: Massaro D, ed. Lung Cell Biology. New York: Marcel Dekker, 1989;191–344.
14. Sunday ME. Pulmonary neuroendocrine cells and lung development. Endocrine Pathol 1996; 7:173–201.
15. Van Lommel A, Bolle T, Fannes W, Lauweryns JM. The pulmonary neuroendocrine system: the past decade. Arch Histol Cytol 62:1999; 1–16.
16. Gosney JR, Sissons MCJ, Allibone RO. Neuroendocrine cell populations in normal human lungs: a quantitative study. Thorax 1988; 43:878–882.
17. Lauweryns JM, Peuskens JC. Neuroepithelial bodies (neuroreceptor or secretory organs?) in human infant bronchial epithelium. Anat Rec 1972; 172:471–482.
18. Gosney JR. Neuroendocrine cell populations in postnatal human lungs: minimal variation from childhood to old age. Anat Rec 1993; 236:177–180.
19. Polak J, Becker KL, Becker E, Cutz E, Gail DB, Goniakowska-Witalinska L, Gosney JR, Lauweryns JM, Linnoila I, McDowell EM, Miller YE, Scheuermann DW, Springall DR, Sunday ME, Zaccone G. Lung endocrine cell markers, peptides and amines. Anat Rec 1993; 236:169–171.
20. Wharton J, Polak JM, Bloom SR, Ghatei MA, Solcia E, Brown MR, Pearse AG. Bombesin-like immunoreactivity in the lung. Nature 1978; 273:769–770.
21. Becker KL, Monaghan KG, Silva OL. Immunocytochemical localization of calcitonin in Kulchitsky cells of human lung. Arch Pathol Lab Med 1980; 104:196–198.
22. Johnson DE, Wobken JD. Calcitonin gene-related peptide immunoreactivity in airway epithelial cells of the human fetus and infant. Cell Tissue Res 1987; 250:579–583.
23. Lauweryns JM, de Bock V, Verhofstad AAJ, Steinbusch HWM. Immunohisto-chemical localization of serotonin in intrapulmonary neuroepithelial bodies. Cell Tissue Res 1982; 226:215–223.
24. Lauweryns JM, Cokelaere M. Hypoxia-sensitive neuroepithelial bodies. Intrapulmonary secretory neuroreceptors, modulated by the CNS. Z Zellforsch Mikroskop Anat 1973; 145:521–540.
25. Lauweryns JM, Cokelaere M. Intrapulmonary neuroepithelial bodies: hypoxia-sensitive neuro-(chemo)receptors. Experientia 1973; 29:1384–1386.
26. Lauweryns JM, Cokelaere M, Deleersnyder M,

Liebens M. Intrapulmonary neuro-epithelial bodies in newborn rabbits. Influence of hypoxia, hyperoxia, hypercapnia, nicotine, reserpine, L-dopa and 5-HTP. Cell Tissue Res 1977; 182:425–440.

27. Lauweryns JM, Cokelaere M, Lerut T, Theunynck P. Cross-circulation studies on the influence of hypoxia and hypoxaemia on the neuroepithelial bodies in young rabbits. Cell Tissue Res 1978; 193:373–386.
28. Youngsen C, Nurse C, Yeger H, Cornutte JT, Vollmer C, Wong V, Cutz E. Immunocytochemical localization of O_2 sensing protein (NADPH oxidase) in chemoreceptor cells. Microsc Res Tech 1997; 37:101–106.
29. Gosney JR. Endocrine pathology of the lung. In: Anthony PP, MacSween RNM, eds. Recent Advances in Histopathology Vol. 16. Edinburgh: Churchill Livingstone, 1994;147–165.
30. Cutz E, Gillan JE, Perrin DG. Pulmonary neuroendocrine cell system: an overview of cell biology and pathology with emphasis on pediatric lung disease. Perspect Pediatr Pathol 1995; 18:32–70.
31. Gosney JR. Pulmonary neuroendocrine cell system in pediatric and adult lung disease. Microsc Res Tech 1997; 37:107–113.
32. Siegfried JM, Guentert PJ, Gaither AL. Effects of bombesin and gastrin-releasing peptide on human bronchial epithelial cells from a series of donors: individual variation and modulation by bombesin analogs. Anat Rec 1993; 236:241–247.
33. Spindel ER, Sunday ME, Hofler H, Wolfe HJ, Habener JF, Chin WW. Transient elevation of mRNAs encoding gastrin-releasing peptide (GRP), a putative pulmonary growth factor, in human fetal lung. J Clin Invest 1987; 80:1172–1179.
34. Sunday ME, Hua J, Dai HB, Nusrat A, Torday JS. Bombesin increases fetal lung growth and maturation in utero and in organ culture. Am J Respir Cell Mol Biol 1990; 3:199–205.
35. Wang D, Yeger H, Cutz E. Expression of gastrin-releasing peptide receptor gene in developing lung. Am J Respir Cell Mol Biol 1996; 14:409–416.
36. Sunday ME, Hua J, Reyes B, Masui H, Torday JS. Anti-bombesin moloclonal antibodies modulate fetal mouse lung growth and maturation in utero and in organ cultures. Anat Rec 1993; 236:25–32.
37. Aguayo SM, Schuyler WE, Murtagh JJ, Roman J. Regulation of lung branching morphogenesis by bombesin-like peptides and neutral endopeptidase. Am J Respir Cell Mol Biol 1994; 19:635–642.
38. Li K, Nagalla SR, Spindel ER. A rhesus monkey model to characterize the role of gastrin-releasing peptide (GRP) in lung development. J Clin Invest 1994; 94:1605–1615.
39. Whitwell F. Tumourlets of the lung. J Pathol Bacteriol 1955; 70:529–541.
40. Tsutsumi Y, Osamura RY, Watanabe K, Yanaihara N. Simultaneous histochemical localization of gastrin-releasing peptide (GRP) and calcitonin (CT) in human bronchial endocrine-type cells. Virchows Arch A Pathol Anat Histol 1983; 400:163–171.
41. Tsutsumi Y. Expression of the alpha subunit of human chorionic gonadotropin in normal and neoplastic neuroendocrine cells. An immunohistochemical study. Acta Pathol Jpn 1989; 39:413–419.
42. Fukayama M, Hayashi Y, Shiozawa Y, Furukawa E, Funata N, Koike M. Human chorionic gonadotropin alpha subunit in endocrine cells of fibrotic and neoplastic lung. Lab Invest 1990; 62:444–451.
43. Gosney J, Green ART, Taylor W. Appropriate and inappropriate neuroendocrine products in pulmonary tumourlets. Thorax 1990; 45:679–683.
44. Reynolds SD, Giangreco A, Power JH, Stripp BR. Neuroepithelial bodies of pulmonary airways serve as a reservoir of progenitor cells capable of epithelial regeneration. Am J Pathol 2000; 156:269–278.
45. Bensch KG, Gordon GB, Miller LR. Electron microscopic and biochemical studies on the bronchial carcinoid tumour. Cancer 1965; 18:592–602.
46. Bensch KG, Corrin B, Pariente R, Spencer H. Oat cell carcinoma of the lung: its origin and relationship to bronchial carcinoid. Cancer 1968; 22:1163–1172.
47. Hattori S, Matsuda M, Tateishi R, Tatsumi N, Terazawa T. Oat-cell carcinoma of the lung containing serotonin granules. Jpn J Cancer Res 1968; 59:123–129.
48. World Health Organization. The World Health Organization histological typing of lung tumours. 2nd ed.. Am J Clin Pathol 1982; 77:123–136.
49. Travis WT, Colby TV, Corrin B, Shimosato Y, Brambilla E. Histological Typing of Lung and Pleural Tumours. Geneva: Springer Verlag, 1999.
50. Gould VE, Linnoila RI, Memoli VA, Warren WH. Neuroendocrine components of the bronchopulmonary tract: hyperplasias, dysplasias and neoplasms. Lab Invest 1983; 49:519–537.
51. Warren WH, Faber LP, Gould VE. Neuroendocrine neoplasms of the lung: a clinico-pathologic update. J Thorac Cardiovasc Surg 1989; 98:321–332.
52. Travis WD, Linnoila RI, Tsokos MG, Hitchcock CL, Cutler GB, Nieman L, Chrousos G, Pass H, Doppman J. Neuroendocrine tumours of the lung with proposed criteria for large-cell neuroendocrine carcinoma. An ultrastructural, immunohistochemical, and flow cytometric study of 35 cases. Am J Surg Pathol 1991; 15:529–553.
53. Travis WD, Rush W, Flieder DB, Falk R, Fleming MV, Gal AA, Koss MN. Survival analysis of 200 pulmonary neuroendocrine tumors with clarification of criteria for atypical carcinoid and its separation from typical carcinoid. Am J Surg Pathol 1998; 22:934–944.
54. Brambilla E, Negoescu A, Gazzeri S, Lantuejoul S,

Moro D, Brambilla C, Coll JL. Apoptosis-related factors p53, Bcl2, and Bax in neuroendocrine lung tumors. Am J Pathol 1996; 149:1941–1952.

55. Przygodzki RM, Finkelstein SD, Langer JC, Swalsky PA, Fishback N, Bakker A, Guinee DG, Koss M, Travis WD. Analysis of p53, K-ras-2 and C-raf-1 in pulmonary neuroendocrine tumors. Correlation with histological subtype and clinical outcome. Am J Pathol 1996; 148:1531–1541.
56. Onuki N, Wistuba II, Travis WD, Virmani AK, Yashima K, Brambilla E, Hasleton P, Gazdar AF. Genetic changes in the spectrum of neuroendocrine lung tumors. Cancer 1999; 85:600–607.
57. Gugger M, Burckhardt E, Kappeler A, Hirsiger H, Laissue JA, Mazzucchelli L. Quantitative expression of structural genomic alterations in the spectrum of neuroendocrine lung carcinomas. J Pathol 2002; 196:408–415.
58. Graziano SL, Mazid R, Newman N, Tatum A, Oler A, Mortimer JA, Gullo JJ, DeFino SM, Scalzo AJ. The use of neuroendocrine immunoperoxidase markers to predict chemotherapy response in patients with non-small cell lung cancer. J Clin Oncol 1989; 7:1298–1406.
59. Schleusener JT, Tazelaar HD, Jung SH, Cha SS, Cera PJ, Myers JL, Creagan ET, Goldberg RM, Marschke RF Jr. Neuroendocrine differentiation is an independent prognostic factor in chemotherapy treated non-small cell lung carcinoma. Cancer 1996; 77:1284–1291.
60. Colby TV, Koss MN, Travis WD. Tumors of the Lower Respiratory Tract. Atlas of Tumor Pathology 3rd ed. Washington, DC: Armed Forces Institute of Pathology, 1995.
61. Marchevsky AM. Neuroendocrine tumors of the lung. Pathology 1996; 4:103–123.
62. Vuitch F, Sekido Y, Fong K, Mackay B, Minna JD, Gazdar AF. Neuroendocrine tumors of the lung. Pathology and molecular biology. Chest Surg Clin North Am 1997; 7:21–47.
63. Gosney JR. Neuroendocrine tumours of the lung. Curr Diag Pathol 2000; 6:64–70.
64. Wick MR, Berg LC, Hertz MI. Large cell carcinoma of the lung with neuroendocrine differentiation. A comparison with large cell 'undifferentiated' pulmonary tumors. Am J Clin Pathol 1992; 97:796–805.
65. Dressler CM, Ritter JH, Patterson GA, Ross E, Bailey WS, Wick MR. Clinico-pathologic analysis of 40 patients with large cell neuroendocrine carcinoma of the lung. Ann Thorac Surg 1997; 63:180–185.
66. Sheppard MN, Corrin B, Bennett MH, Marangos PJ, Bloom SR, Polak JM. Immunocytochemical localization of neuron specific enolase in small cell carcinomas and carcinoid tumours of the lung. Histopathology 1984; 8:171–181.
67. Rode J, Dhillon AP, Doran JF, Jackson P, Thompson RJ. PGP 9.5 a new marker for human neuroendocrine tumuors. Histopathology 1985; 9:147–158.
68. Wiedenmann B, Huttner WB. Synaptophysin and chromogranins/secretogranins—widespread constituents of distinct types of neuroendocrine vesicles and new tools in tumour diagnosis. Virchows Arch B (Cell Pathol) 1989; 58:95–121.
69. Gould VE. Synaptophysin: a new and promising pan-neuroendocrine marker. Arch Pathol Lab Med 1987; 111:791–794.
70. Lantuejoul S, Moro D, Michalides RJAM, Brambilla C, Brambilla E. Neural cell adhesion molecules (NCAM) and NCAM-PSA expression in neuroendocrine lung tumors. Am J Surg Pathol 1998; 22:1267–1276.
71. Finkelstein SD, Hasegawa T, Colby T, Yousem SA. 11q13 allelic imbalance discriminates pulmonary carcinoids from tumorlets. Am J Pathol 1999; 155: 633–640.
72. Aguayo SM, Miller YE, Waldron JA, et al. Brief report: idiopathic diffuse hyperplasia of pulmonary neuroendocrine cells and airways disease. N Engl J Med 1992; 327:1285–1288.
73. Armas OA, White DA, Erlandson RA, Rosai J. Diffuse idiopathic neuroendocrine cell proliferation presenting as interstitial lung disease. Am J Surg Pathol 1995; 19:963–970.
74. Miller RR, Muller NL. Neuroendocrine cell hyperplasia and obliterative bronchiolitis in patients with peripheral carcinoid tumors. Am J Surg Pathol 1995; 19:653–658.
75. Sheard JDH, Gosney JR. Endocrine cells in tumour-bearing lungs. Thorax 1996; 51:721–726.
76. Goslin RH, O'Brien MJ, Skarin AT, Zamcheck N. Immunocytochemical staining for CEA in small cell carcinoma of lung predicts clinical usefulness of the plasma assay. Cancer 1983; 52:301–306.
77. Francini G, Inaudi P, Gotti G, Gonnelli S, Lucani B, Perrone AF, Gennari C. Circulating levels of immunoreactive peptides and steroid hormones in bronchogenic carcinoma. Int J Biol Markers 1986; 1:93–100.
78. Lehtinen M, Wigren T, Lehtinen T, Kallioniemi O-P, Aine R, Aaran R-K, Ojala A. Correlation between serum tumor marker levels and tumor proliferation in small cell lung cancer. Tumor Biol 1988; 9:287–292.
79. Nissen MH, Plesner T, Roth M. Modification of beta-2-microglobulin in serum from patients with small cell bronchial carcinoma of the lung. Correlation with clinical course. Clin Chim Acta 1980; 141:41–50.
80. Lombardi C, Tassi GF, Pizzocolo G, Donata F. Clinical significance of a multiple biomarker assay in patients with lung cancer. A study with logistic regression analysis. Chest 1990; 897:639–644.
81. Glaubit D, Cordoni-Voutsas M. Tumor markers in serum with particular reference to CA 125 and CA 19.9 in patients with non small cell lung cancer. In: Gretin H, Klapdor R, eds. New Tumour Associated Antigens. Stuttgart: Georg Thieme Verlag, 1986;204–209.

82. Marangos PJ, Gazdar AF, Carney DN. Neuron specific enolase in human small cell carcinoma cultures. Cancer Lett 1982; 15:67–71.
83. Carney DN, Marangos PJ, Ihde DC, Bunn PA, Cohen MH, Minna JD, Gazdar AF. Serum neuron-specific enolase: a marker for disease extent and response to therapy of small-cell lung cancer. Lancet 1982; 1:583–585.
84. Jaques G, Bepler G, Holle R, Wolf M, Hannich T, Gropp C, Havemann K. Prognostic value of carcinoembryonic antigen, neuron-specific enolase, and creatine kinase-BB levels in sera of patients with small lung cancer. Cancer 1988; 62:125–134.
85. Carney DN, Zweig MH, Ihde DC, Cohen MH, Makuch RW, Gazdar AF. Elevated serum creatine kinase BB levels in patients with small cell lung cancer. Cancer Res 1984; 44:5399–5403.
86. Baylin SB, Abeloff MD, Wieman KC, Tomford JW, Ettinger DS. Elevated histaminase (diamine oxidase) activity in small-cell carcinoma of the lung. N Engl J Med 1975; 293:1286–1290.
87. O'Connor DT, Deftos LJ. Secretion of chromogranin A by peptide-producing endocrine neoplasms. N Engl J Med 1986; 314:1145–1151.
88. Eriksson B, Arnberg H, Oberg K, Hallman U, Lundqvist G, Warnstedt C, Wilander E. A polyclonal antiserum against chromogranin A and B—a new sensitive marker for neuroendocrine tumours. Acta Endocrinol 1990; 122:145–155.
89. Liddle GW, Island DP, Ney RL, Nicholson WE, Shimuzu N. Nonpituitary neoplasms and Cushing's syndrome. Arch Intern Med 1963; 111:471–475.
90. Baylin SB, Mendelsohn G. Ectopic (inappropriate) hormone production by tumors: mechanisms involved and the biological and clinical implications. Endocr Rev 1980; 1:45–77.
91. Silva OL, Becker KL, Primack A, Doppman JL, Snider RH. Ectopic production of calcitonin. Lancet 1973; 1:317.
92. Roos BA, Lindall AW, Baylin SB, O'Neil J, Frelinger AL, Birnbaum RS, Lambert PW. Plasma immunoreactive calcitonin in lung cancer. Endocr Res Commun 1979; 6:169–190.
93. Wallach SR, Royston I, Taetle R, Wohl H, Deftos LJ. Plasma calcitonin as a marker of disease activity in patients with small cell carcinoma of the lung. J Clin Endocrinol Metab 1981; 53:602–606.
94. Becker KL, Silva OL, Gazdar AF, Snider RH, Moore CF. Calcitonin and small cell cancer of the lung. In: Becker KL, Gazdar AF, eds. The Endocrine Lung in Health and Disease. Philadelphia: Saunders, 1984; 528–548.
95. Silva OL, Becker KL, Primack A, Doppman JL, Snider RH. Ectopic secretion of calcitonin by oat cell carcinoma. N Engl J Med 1974; 290:1122–1124.
96. Yamaguchi K, Abe K, Adachi I, Kimura S, Suzuki M, Shimada A, Kodama T, Kameya T, Shimosato Y. Peptide hormone production in primary lung tumors. Rec Res Cancer Res 1985; 99:107–116.
97. Sano T, Saito H, Yamasaki R, Hamaguchi K, Ooiwa K, Shimoda T, Hosoi E, Saito S, Hizawa K. Immunoreactive somatostatin and calcitonin in pulmonary neuroendocrine tumour. Cancer 1986; 57:64–68.
98. Silva OL, Broder LE, Doppmann JL, Snider RH, Moore CF, Cohen MH, Becker KL. Calcitonin as a marker for bronchogenic cancer. Cancer 1979; 44:680–684.
99. Becker KL, Silva OL, Snider RH, Moore CF, Geelhoed GW, Nash D. The pathophysiology of pulmonary calcitonin. In: Becker KL, Gazdar AF, eds. The Endocrine Lung in Health and Disease. Philadelphia: Saunders, 1984;277–299.
100. Coates PJ, Doniach I, Howlett TA, Rees LH, Besser GM. Immunocytochemical study of 18 tumours causing ectopic Cushing's syndrome. J Clin Pathol 1986; 39:955–960.
101. Del Gaudio A. Ectopic ACTH syndrome. Int Surg 1988; 73:44–49.
102. Ratcliffe JG. ACTH and related peptides in lung cancer. Rec Res Cancer Res 1985; 99:46–55.
103. White A, Clark AJ, Stewart MF. The synthesis of ACTH and related peptides by tumours. Clin Endocrinol Metab 1990; 4:1–27.
104. Southgate HJ, Archibold GPR, El-Sayed ME, Wright J, Marks V. Ectopic release of GHRH and ACTH from an adenoid cystic carcinoma resulting in acromegaly and complicated by pituitary infarction. Postgrad Med J 1988; 64:145–148.
105. Gewirtz G, Yalow RS. Ectopic ACTH production in carcinoma of the lung. J Clin Invest 1974; 53:1022–1032.
106. Ayvazian LF, Schneider B, Gewirtz G, Yalow RS. Ectopic production of big ACTH in carcinoma of the lung: its clinical usefulness as a biologic marker. Am Rev Respir Dis 1975; 111.279–287.
107. Dupont AG, Somers G, VanSteirteghem AC, Watson F, Vanhaelst L. Ectopic adrenocorticotropin production: disappearance after removal of inflammatory tissue. J Clin Endocrinol Metab 1984; 58:654–658.
108. Thorne NA, Transbol I. Hyponatraemia and bronchogenic carcinoma associated with renal excretion of large amounts of antidiuretic material. Am J Med 1963; 35:257–268.
109. Bower BF, Mason DM, Forsham PH. Bronchogenic carcinoma with inappropriate antidiuretic activity in plasma and tumour. N Engl J Med 1964; 271:934–938.
110. Müller P, Quincke H. Untersuchungen über den Stoffwechsel bei Tuberkulose. Tuberkulose und Chlorstoffwechsel II. Dtsch Arch Klin Med 1928; 160:24–39.
111. Vorherr H, Massry SG, Fallet R, Kaplan L, Kleeman CR. Antidiuretic principal in tuberculous lung tissue

of a patient with pulmonary tuberculosis and hyponatraemia. Ann Int Med 1970; 72:383–387.
112. Hansen M, Hammer M, Hummer L. ACTH, ADH and calcitonin concentrations as markers of response and relapse in small cell carcinoma of the lung. Cancer 1980; 46:2062–2067.
113. Moertel CG. An odyssey in the land of small tumors. J Clin Oncol 1987; 5:1503–1522.
114. Feldmen JM. Carcinoid tumors and syndrome. Semin Oncol 1987; 14:237–246.
115. Lembeck F. 5-Hydroxytryptamine in a carcinoid tumour. Nature 1953; 172:910–911.
116. Brown WH. A case of pluriglandular syndrome: diabetes of bearded women. Lancet 1928; 2:1022–1023.
117. Cushing H. The basophil adenomas of the pituitary body and their clinical manifestations (pituitary basophilism). Bull Johns Hopkins Hosp 1932; 50:137–195.
118. Winkler WA, Crankshaw OF. Chloride depletion in conditions other than Addison's disease. J Clin Invest 1938; 17:1–6.
119. Schwartz WB, Bennett W, Curelop S, Bartter FC. A syndrome of renal sodium loss and hyponatremia probably resulting from inappropriate secretion of antidiuretic hormone. Am J Med 1957; 23:529–542.
120. Bartter FC, Schwartz WB. The syndrome of inappropriate secretion of antidiuretic hormone. Am J Med 1967; 42:790–806.
121. Bayliss PH. Syndrome of inappropriate antidiuretic hormone secretion. In: Sheaves R, Jenkins PJ, Wass JAH, eds. Clinical Endocrine Oncology. Oxford: Blackwell Science, 1997;479–483.
122. Greco FA, Hainsworth J, Sismani A, Richardson RL, Hande JR, Oldham RK. Hormone production and paraneoplastic syndromes. In: Greco FA, Oldham RK, Bunn PA, eds. Small Cell Lung Cancer. New York: Grune and Stratton, 1981;177–223.
123. Rassam JW, Anderson G. Incidence of paramalignant disorders in bronchogenic carcinoma. Thorax 1975; 30:86–90.
124. Anderson G. Paramalignant syndromes in lung cancer. London: Heinemann, 1973.
125. Gammell JA. Erythema gyratum repens. Arch Dermatol 1952; 66:494–505.
126. Holt PJA, Davies MG. Erythema gyratum repens, an immunologically-mediated dermatosis. Br J Dermatol 1977; 96:343–347.
127. Fretzin DF. Malignant down. Arch Dermatol 1967; 95:294–297.
128. Barnes BE. Dermatomyositis and malignancy. A review of the literature. Ann Intern Med 1976; 84:68–76.
129. Cox NH, Lawrence CM, Langtry JAA, Ive FA. Dermatomyositis: disease associations and an evaluation of screening investigations for malignancy. Arch Dermatol 1990; 126:61–65.
130. Pankow W, Neumann K, V-Wichert P. Bronchial carcinoma associated with pulmonary osteoarthropathy (Marie-Bamberger disease). Pneumologie 1990; 44:1306–1311.
131. Pineda CJ, Guerra J, Weisman MH, Resnick D, Martinez-Lavin M. The skeletal manifestations of clubbing: a study in patients with cyanotic congenital heart disease and hypertrophic osteoarthropathy. Semin Arthritis Rheum 1985; 14:263–273.
132. Shneerson JM. Digital clubbing and hypertrophic osteoarthropathy: the underlying mechanisms. Br J Dis Chest 1981; 75:113–131.
133. Dickinson CJ, Martin JF. Megakaryocytes and platelet clumps as the cause of finger clubbing. Lancet 1987; 2:1434–1435.
134. Braegger CP, Corrigan CJ, MacDonald TT. Finger clubbing and tumour necrosis factor alpha. Lancet 1990; 336:759–760.
135. El-Salhy M, Simonsson M, Stenling R, Grimelius L. Recovery from Marie-Bamberger's syndrome and diabetes insipidus after removal of a lung adenocarcinoma with neuroendocrine features. J Int Med 1998; 243:171–175.
136. Huckstep RL, Bodkin PE. Vagotomy in hypertrophic pulmonary osteoarthropathy associated with bronchial carcinoma. Lancet 1958; 2:343–345.
137. Anderson NE, Rosenblum MK, Graus F, Wiley RG, Posner JB. Autoantibodies in paraneoplastic syndromes associated with small-cell lung cancer. Neurology 1988; 38:1391–1398.
138. Dalmau J, Furneaux HM, Gralla RJ, Kris MG, Posner JB. Detection of the anti-Hu antibody in the serum of patients with small cell lung cancer. A quantitative Western blot analysis. Ann Neurol 1990; 27:544–552.
139. Furneaux HF, Reich L, Posner JB. Autoantibody synthesis in the central nervous system of patients with paraneoplastic syndromes. Neurology 1990; 40:1085–1091.
140. Graus F, Elkon KB, Lloberes P, Ribalta T, Torres A, Ussetti P, Valls J, Obach J, Agusti-Vidal A. Neuronal antinuclear antibody (anti-Hu) in paraneoplastic encephalomyelitis simulating acute polyneuritis. Acta Neurol Scand 1987; 75:249–252.
141. Veilleux M, Bernier JP, Lamarche JB. Paraneoplastic encephalomyelitis and subacute dysautonomia due to an occult ayptical carcinoid tumour of the lung. Can J Neurol Sci 1990; 17:324–328.
142. Henson RA, Urich H. Cancer and the Nervous System: The Neurological Manifestations of Systemic Malignant Disease. Oxford: Blackwell, 1982.
143. Sawyer RA, Selhorst JB, Zimmerman LE, Hoyt WF. Blindness caused by photoreceptor degeneration as a remote effect of cancer. Am J Ophthalmol 1976; 81: 606–613.
144. Jacobson DM, Thirkill CE, Tipping SJ. A clinical triad to diagnose paraneoplastic retinopathy. Ann Neurol 1990; 28:162–167.
145. Boghen D, Sebag M, Michaud J. Paraneoplastic optic

neuritis and encephalo-myelitis. Report of a case. Arch Neurol 1988; 45:353–356.
146. Albin RL, Bromberg MB, Penney JB, Knapp R. Chorea and dystonia: a remote effect of carcinoma. Move Disord 1988; 3:162–169.
147. Giordana MT, Soffietti R, Schiffer D. Paraneoplastic opsoclonus: a neuropathologic study of two cases. Clin Neuropathol 1989; 8:295–300.
148. Handforth A, Nag S, Sharp D, Robertson DM. Paraneoplastic subacute necrotic myelopathy. Can J Neurol Sci 1983; 10:204–207.
149. Brain WR, Croft PB, Wilkinson M. Motor neurone disease as a manifestation of neoplasm. Brain 1965; 88:478–500.
150. Croft PB, Urich H, Wilkinson M. Peripheral neuropathy of sensorimotor type associated with malignant disease. Brain 1967; 90:3–66.
151. Graus F, Elkon KB, Cordon-Cardo C, Posner JB. Sensory neuronopathy and small cell lung cancer: antineuronal antibody that also reacts with the tumor. Am J Med 1986; 80:45–52.
152. Park DM, Johnson RH, Crean GP, Robinson JF. Orthostatic hypotension in bronchial carcinoma. Br Med J 1972; 3:510–511.
153. Schuffler MD, Baird HW, Fleming CR, Bell CE, Bouldin TW, Malagelada JR, McGill DB, LeBauer SM, Abrams M, Love J. Intestinal pseudo-obstruction as the presenting manifestation of small cell carcinoma of the lung. Ann Intern Med 1983; 98:129–134.
154. Chinn JS, Schuffler MD. Paraneoplastic visceral neuropathy as a cause of severe gastrointestinal motor dysfunction. Gastroenterology 1988; 95:1279–1286.
155. Eaton LM, Lambert EH. Electromyography and electric stimulation of nerves in diseases of motor unit. Observations on myasthenic syndrome associated with malignant tumors. J Am Med Ass 1957; 163: 1117–1124.
156. Ferroir JP, Milleron B, Ropert A, Billy C, Nahum L, Tcherakian S, Carette MF. Atypical paraneoplastic myasthenic syndrome: Lambert-Eaton syndrome or myasthenia? Rev Pneumol Clin 1999; 55: 168–170.
157. Fukunaga H, Engel AG, Lang B, Newsom-Davis J, Vincent A. Passive transfer of Lambert-Eaton myasthenic syndrome with IgG from man to mouse depletes the presynaptic membrane active zones. Proc Natl Acad Sci USA 1983; 80:7636–7640.
158. Fukunaga H, Engel AG, Osame M, Lambert EH. Paucity and disorganization of presynaptic membrane active zones in the Lambert-Eaton myasthenic syndrome. Muscle Nerve 1982; 5:686–697.
159. Chester KA, Lang B, Gill J, Vincent A, Newsom-Davis J. Lambert-Eaton syndrome antibodies: reaction with membranes from a small cell lung cancer xenograft. J Neuroimmunol 1988; 18:97–104.
160. Sher E, Pandiella A, Clementi F. Voltage-operated calcium channels in small cell lung carcinoma cell lines: pharmacological, functional, and immunological properties. Cancer Res 1990; 50:3892–3896.

6

Surgery for Differentiated Thyroid Cancer

Ashok Shaha

Memorial Sloan–Kettering Cancer Institute and Cornell Medical School, New York, New York, U.S.A.

Arthur E. Schwartz

Mount Sinai School of Medicine, New York University, New York, New York, U.S.A.

1 INTRODUCTION

Thyroid cancer is fascinating in many ways. The wide spectrum of aggressiveness is extraordinary, ranging from differentiated malignancies in which most patients live out close to their normal lifespan, to anaplastic varieties that are almost universally lethal.

Among many unique features of differentiated thyroid cancer, two require special mention. Age is the most important prognostic factor. It is interesting to note that the mortality in patients with thyroid cancer in the younger age group is extremely low, while the mortality in elderly patients is quite high. There is no other human cancer that parallels this biological behavior. This is the only cancer where age is included in the staging system. There is no Stage III and IV cancer in patients below the age of 45 (1–4).

Another unique feature is that the presence of nodal metastasis has almost no prognostic bearing. This clinical behavior is not seen in any other malignancy. In the majority of cancers, the presence of nodal metastasis decreases the survival by almost 50%: in well-differentiated thyroid cancer, there is no apparent effect on outcome (5).

Thyroid cancer is one of the most common endocrine neoplasms. Most deaths are the result of medullary or anaplastic thyroid tumors, rather than differentiated types. There appears to be a steadily increasing incidence in the United States, as well as an increased proportion of the disease in women; in the 1970s approximately 8000 new patients with thyroid cancer were seen, but the mortality remained steady at 1000 per year over the past two decades. In 2002 there were 20,700 new cases of thyroid cancer (15,800 women and 4900 men). During the same year there were 1300 deaths from thyroid malignancy (800 women and 500 men), suggesting that the prognosis is worse in men (6).

The mortality of differentiated thyroid cancer remains low; most deaths are directly related to the high-risk group, generally elderly patients with poorly differentiated histology or locally aggressive tumors. There is considerable debate and controversy about the management of the disease. Although most patients with well-differentiated thyroid cancer do well, there is contention related to the extent of thyroidectomy and postoperative management. There are vigorous proponents of routine total thyroidectomy, whereas other authors recommend less than total thyroidectomy, depending on the prognostic factors and risk groups. Approximately 2000 new peer-reviewed papers are published every year on the subject of thyroid cancer, reporting a large worldwide experience. Most of these studies are retrospective, with a substantial institu-

Table 1 Incidence and Survival of Histological Types of Thyroid Carcinoma

Histological type	Incidence, (1985–1990) (%)	10-Year overall survival (%)
Papillary	77.9	93
Follicular	14.2	85
Hürthle cell[a]	2.7	76
Medullary	3.7	75
Undifferentiated/ anaplastic[b]	1.6	14

[a] Although the survival of patients with Hürthle cell carcinoma closely matched that of patients with follicular carcinoma at 5 years, survival at 10 years was 9% lower, suggesting a marginally worse prognosis.
[b] In this report, the 14% survival of anaplastic and undifferentiated carcinoma does not discriminate between the two types. Classic anaplastic carcinoma (giant and spindle cell tumors) has a survival that is much worse than undifferentiated types.
Source: Ref. 2.

tional bias reflected in the conclusions. Prospective randomized studies, though strongly recommended by the American College of Surgeons Oncology Group, are difficult to undertake. The relatively benign course of the disease requires a large number of patients and a long duration of follow-up for a prospective randomized study. Hundahl et al. (2) recently reviewed the data from the National Cancer Data Base describing the demographics of 53,856 patients seen over a period of 10 years from 1985 to 1995. Their review reports that during that period the incidence of papillary cancer was 78% while the incidence of follicular, medullary, and anaplastic thyroid malignancy is 13, 4, and 2%, respectively (Table 1).

Our understanding of thyroid cancer has improved considerably in the last two decades with various reports describing the prognostic factors and analysis of risk groups. Hay (7,8) from the Mayo Clinic and Cady (9–11) from the Lahey Clinic have divided patients into low and high-risk groups. The mortality in the low-risk group was less than 2%, while the mortality in the high-risk group was approximately 46%. Shaha et al. from Memorial Sloan-Kettering Cancer Center divided the patients into low, intermediate, and high-risk groups with mortalities of 1, 13, and 43%, respectively (1).

2 APPROACH TO THYROID NODULES

It is almost always preferable to remove the entire thyroid lobe and isthmus than to perform an incisional biopsy or to remove a nodule; this is because of the difficulty of establishing a definitive diagnosis on frozen section (see Chapter xx). It is disheartening to receive a final diagnosis of malignancy several days after a frozen section has been reported to be benign—not an unusual occurrence. The surgeon who has initially performed only an incisional biopsy or partial lobectomy then faces the arduous task of excising the remainder of the lobe, with increased danger to the recurrent nerve and the parathyroid glands, as well as a higher incidence of local recurrence (12,13).

It is far better to remove the entire lobe and isthmus at the initial procedure, eliminating the need to go back to a previously dissected area. If the opposite lobe later requires removal, the surgeon has a virgin field to explore and the best opportunity to preserve the parathyroid glands and the recurrent nerve.

3 SPREAD OF THYROID CANCER NODAL AND DISTANT METASTASIS

The spread of thyroid cancer can be divided into local extension, cervical and mediastinal lymph node involvement, and distant metastasis (14,15). It is interesting to note that even with a small or occult primary tumor, particularly in the adolescent to 30-year age group, there may be bulky neck node metastases, whereas in elderly patients it is not unusual to find a large primary tumor without palpable neck disease. Distant metastases, however, are more likely to be seen in advanced local disease or with massive nodal metastasis. The incidence of nodal metastases ranges from 50 to 60%, while distant metastases are noted at the time of initial presentation in only 5% of patients. Most of the distant metastases, especially in papillary carcinoma, occur in the lungs. Follicular tumors may also present with disseminated metastases, especially to the bones of the pelvis and vertebral column (16,17). The incidence of clinically apparent neck node metastases in papillary thyroid cancer ranges from 15 to 50% (18).

There is a rich lymphatic drainage from the thyroid gland with an extensive network of intraglandular lymphatics. Generally they follow the venous channels, with the first echelon nodes appearing in the tracheoesophageal groove. Subsequently, patients often develop enlarged lymph nodes in the jugular chain or in the superior mediastinum. In addition, differentiated thyroid cancer is known to spread to contralateral jugular lymph nodes in approximately 10% of cases. The lower jugular or Level IV nodes (see Fig. 6) are commonly involved in patients with well-differentiated thyroid cancer; the majority of lymph node metastases are seen in the paratracheal and jugular chains. Superior mediastinal nodes are also frequently involved. Level I lymph nodes (in the submandibular and submental area), however, are rarely affected in differentiated thyroid cancer, with an incidence of less than 3% (19–24).

4 EVALUATING RISK GROUPS IN DIFFERENTIATED THYROID CANCER

Before making any decisions regarding the extent of thyroidectomy, it is valuable to understand the prognostic factors and risk groups in thyroid cancer. The European Organization for Research on Treatment of Cancer (EORTC) initially defined variables such as age, sex, histological type, extrathyroidal extension, and distant metastasis in their report in 1979. A complicated scoring system was addressed in this review (25).

Many prognostic systems are available, but essentially they all relate to the above features. Understanding the components of these indicators is important in the overall management of differentiated thyroid cancer. Other prognostic factors such as DNA ploidy, p53 mutation, EGF receptor, and adenylate cyclase activity are reported, but these molecular prognostic factors are not useful in clinical practice at this time.

Hay et al. from the Mayo Clinic defined the prognostic factors as AGES—age, grade of tumor, extrathyroidal extension, and size of tumor (2,26). The grade of the tumor was difficult to interpret at many other institutions; Cady et al. from the Lahey Clinic defined the prognostic factors as AMES—age, distant metastasis, extrathyroidal extension, and size of the tumor (9–11). The Mayo Clinic revisited the prognostic factors and defined the new system as MACIS—metastasis, age, completeness of resection, local invasion, and size of the tumor (27). Completeness of resection is a critical prognostic factor; the goal of any surgical procedure should be to remove all gross tumor. Based on these prognostic factors, the Mayo Clinic and the Lahey Clinic divided the patients into low- and high-risk groups.

The reviewers from Memorial Sloan-Kettering Cancer Center formulated prognostic factors based on patient-related and tumor-related factors, dividing their patients into low, intermediate, and high-risk groups. The low-risk group included patients under the age of 45 with low-risk tumors, while the high-risk group included patients above the age of 45 with high-risk tumor. The intermediate-risk group was divided into two categories: young patients with aggressive tumors or older patients with less aggressive tumors. Long-term survival in the low, intermediate, and high-risk groups was reported to be 99, 87, and 57%, respectively. Interestingly, when these data were reviewed for the patients in the low risk-group who died, it was found that all four had had aggressive histolological features that were not initially reported (28–30).

These prognostic scoring systems are critical to surgeons who selectively employ lobectomy or total thyroidectomy for the management of differentiated cancer. For others who routinely perform total or near-total thyroidectomy without regard to risk group criteria, they offer a valuable prognostic indicator and the opportunity to evaluate the results of treatment.

5 PAPILLARY CARCINOMA

Papillary, papillary-follicular carcinoma, and papillary variant of follicular carcinoma comprise about 85% of differentiated thyroid cancer and share the same prognosis (31–33). The realization that the follicular variant of papillary carcinoma is a form of papillary carcinoma rather than a follicular cancer, which has a less favorable outlook, explains the erroneously better cure rates for follicular cancer in the older literature. Other rarer types of papillary carcinoma such as tall cell, insular, diffusely sclerotic, and columnar cell are more aggressive and usually present at a higher stage.

Papillary cancers characteristically spread to neck nodes and at times to the lungs. Neck node metastases generally do not affect survival. The most critical prognostic feature is the age of the patient; those who are over 45 have a much poorer outlook than those who are younger.

Small papillary carcinomas (≤ 1 cm), sometimes referred to as "occult" or microcarcinoma, have an excellent prognosis, but the outcome becomes worse as the size of the primary tumor increases; those >4 cm. in diameter have a distinctly decreased survival (34, 35).

Extension of the tumor beyond the capsule of the thyroid, invasion of adjacent tissues, or distant metastases are adverse factors in the overall cure rates (36–38).

6 FOLLICULAR CARCINOMA

These tumors are less frequent than the papillary type, comprising approximately 15% of thyroid cancers, and have a less favorable prognosis (39–41). The incidence increases in iodine-deficient areas. There is no evidence that benign follicular adenomas develop into cancer. The overwhelming proportion are nonfunctional and appear cold on radioactive scan.

Follicular cancers are less likely to spread to regional lymph nodes and have a higher incidence of distant metastases than papillary cancer. Metastases presenting at the time of diagnosis portend a poor outlook; bone and lungs are the most frequent sites.

The Hürthle cell variant has been of special interest, with some authorities finding that they are more likely to metastasize, exhibit a more aggressive behavior, and have a decreased survival. This has been challenged by others who state that stage for stage they have the same outlook as other follicular cancers. In a recent study it was noted that, unlike other differentiated thyroid cancers, nodal metastases augur a worse outcome (42–47).

7 EXTENT OF SURGERY FOR DIFFERENTIATED THYROID CANCER

Microscopic cancer that does not influence the outcome of the disease is an important factor in the management of differentiated thyroid cancer. The issue is whether or not it should be surgically removed. After years of contention it is now almost universally accepted that neck dissection is not indicated in patients with clinically negative nodes—even though a high percentage are positive on microscopic evaluation. Controversy remains in regard to the extent of thyroidectomy required for differentiated thyroid cancer in relation to its frequent microscopic presence in the opposite lobe (30–50%).

The major indications for total thyroidectomy include high-risk patients with high-risk tumors, young patients with bulky nodal metastasis, patients with gross disease in both lobes of the thyroid, major extrathyroidal extension, or a preoperative diagnosis of poorly differentiated thyroid cancer (48). A thyroid malignancy in a patient with a history of radiation to the neck is also an indication for total thyroidectomy because of the risk of developing disease in the opposite lobe. Patients who present initially with distant metastasis are advised to undergo total thyroidectomy to facilitate radioactive iodine ablation.

Authors who advocate routine use of total thyroidectomy point to the following (49):

1. The high incidence of microscopic disease in the opposite lobe (40–70%). Although clinical recurrence is 5% or less, it can be reduced by total thyroidectomy.
2. Total thyroidectomy permits ablation of all thyroid tissue, increasing the sensitivity of early detection of pulmonary metastasis or other metastatic disease by radioactive iodine and monitoring with serum thyroglobulin levels. The location of metastatic disease and its treatment by RAI ablation becomes easier.
3. It removes the minimal possibility that anaplastic or poorly differentiated thyroid cancer could develop in the thyroid remnant.
4. Although many authors advocate a decision on whether to perform total thyroidectomy or lobectomy by the use of staging systems that define- high and low-risk categories, these classifications are postoperative evaluations. Factors such as aggressive tumor pathology or the extent of local tissue invasion are not available preoperatively. Distant metastases may not be apparent until postoperative radioactive iodine studies or thyroglobulin levels reveal them (50).

Wong (51) states that when patients are treated by total or near-total thyroidectomy with postoperative radioiodine, the "benefit of improved survival is similar to that obtained by not smoking, or surgery for three-vessel coronary artery disease." In a report on optimal treatment strategy in patients with papillary thyroid cancer, Esnaola et al. from the M.D. Anderson Cancer Center report that total thyroidectomy maximizes life expectancy in low as well as high-risk patients (31). Mazzaferri et al. advise that all patients with follicular carcinoma should have total thyroidectomy to facilitate postoperative radioiodine therapy, noting that most deaths are due to distant metastases (39).

Others disagree, finding survival rates in low-risk patients with differentiated thyroid carcinoma essentially the same, whether treated by lobectomy or total thyroidectomy. There is general agreement, however, that high-risk patients or those who present with distant metastases should have total thyroidectomy and radioiodine ablation.

The proponents of less than total thyroidectomy appreciate these logical points, but they base their treatment philosophy on the risk group analysis. The long-term results in the low-risk group are a survival of 99%; routine total thyroidectomy in this group does not appear to be warranted. The major argument for total thyroidectomy is the presence of microscopic disease in the opposite lobe, but the clinical appearance of recurrent disease in the opposite lobe is less than 5%. Multicentric microscopic disease is considered a "laboratory cancer" with no significant prognostic implication. Authors who favor hemithyroidectomy for low-risk cancer state that a minority of patients will require postoperative radioactive iodine. This would represent patients in the high-risk group, those with locally aggressive tumors, or poorly differentiated histology. These authors feel that for a patient presenting with a solitary thyroid nodule less than 1–1.5 cm in diameter and no other adverse features, lobectomy and isthmusectomy is effective treatment and usually the maximum surgical procedure necessary. Routine application of total thyroidectomy in every patient presenting with solitary thyroid nodule is probably unnecessary (1,48).

8 TECHNIQUE OF THYROIDECTOMY

The complications of thyroid surgery are directly related to the extent of surgery and inversely proportional to the experience of the operating surgeon. Total thyroidectomy would be the treatment of choice for all primary thyroid malignancy if it were not for the risk of hypoparathyroidism and recurrent nerve injury. It offers the advantage of removing the primary lesion and all foci of malignant tissue within the thyroid gland. The elimination of the total thyroid parenchyma (which might require radioactive iodine ablation of any remnant) would enable the physician to monitor the patient for recurrence with radioactive iodine scanning and serum thyroglobulin levels.

In practice, the benefits of total thyroidectomy must be weighed against a risk of permanent hypoparathyroidism ranging up to 4–5% and the hazard of recurrent nerve injury of 1–3%. The usual extended course and good prognosis of well-differentiated thyroid carcinoma makes it difficult to select those patients who warrant the risk of total thyroidectomy.

The initial approach for the surgery of differentiated thyroid carcinoma is total lobectomy on the side of the lesion with resection of the isthmus and pyramidal lobe. We emphasize visualization of the recurrent nerve and parathyroid glands. With experience it becomes possible to identify them and preserve their blood supply. Careful hemostasis is needed so that the distinctive appearance of the parathyroid glands will not be altered. The normal parathyroid is bean shaped, 3–6 mm. This is in marked contrast to the globular, oval or rounded appearance of a lymph node. The color is a dark yellow, tan, or brownish hue, different from the lighter yellow color of fat, or the darker gray, pink, or varying flesh tones of lymph nodes. It is usually cradled in a fat pad creating a distinctive combination. As the gland is manipulated, its color becomes darker because of vascular impairment, a feature not found with fat or lymph nodes.

The thyroid incision is placed transversely across the neck below the cricoid and at least two fingerbreadths above the sternal notch (Fig. 1). Many surgeons outline the incision by placing a suture across a crease line in the neck, creating pressure, and then making the incision in the depressed line. We prefer to carefully mark the midline and draw a line across the neck at a level that is measured and marked by a pen. A slightly upward curve is desirable. This has proved more predictable for us than the string method. The use of a natural crease line in the neck is attractive if the line is horizontal, but if the natural line is oblique, such an incision becomes unsightly. A higher location in the neck produces a more pleasing appearance; an incision close to the sternum tends to spread. A position closer to the cricoid cartilage makes dissection of the upper portion of the recurrent laryngeal nerve easier than a lower one because of better exposure in the area where the nerve ascends below the cricothyroid muscle. A more superiorly placed incision also facilitates a cosmetic extension of the wound laterally and upward, should a neck dissection be required.

Recently we have used the "harmonic scalpel," an ultrasonic knife that seals as it cuts, as an adjunct in the performance of thyroidectomy. This instrument makes it possible to divide tissue without the need for ligatures. It is useful in dividing the superior pole vessels, transecting the ima vessels, and dividing the

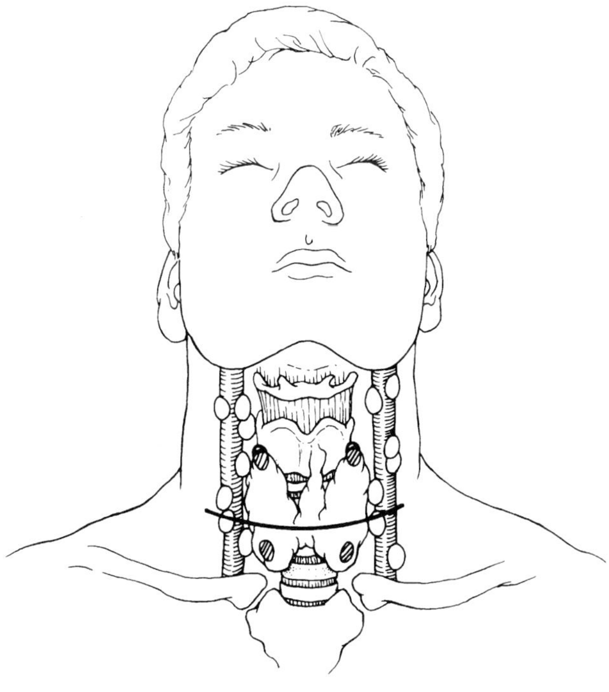

Figure 1 Placement of thyroid incision.

thyroid isthmus as the gland is separated from the trachea. Other portions of the operation are performed with traditional instruments.

A key to facile and elegant neck and thyroid surgery is to take advantage of tissue planes of the deep cervical fascia. Elevating the superior and inferior flaps is almost bloodless if the layer just beneath the platysma is followed and dissected. The strap muscles, which are enclosed by the cervical fascia, can be cleanly separated from the thyroid by identifying this investing layer. The larynx, thyroid, trachea, pharynx, and esophagus are contained within separate compartments. A fascial layer also encloses the thyroid gland, facilitating its mobilization. The parathyroid glands have their own separately derived capsules that ease their separation from the thyroid.

Good exposure is obtained by separating the strap muscles in the midline and retracting them laterally. Transverse division of the medial portion of the sternohyoid muscle near its insertion provides marked additional increase in access. Since the muscles form an "A" shape, the additional incision at the narrowed space between their upper portions offers a geometric increase in visibility. The sternothyroid muscle is routinely divided completely for better visibility (Fig. 2).

If the tumor is large or inaccessible, there should be no hesitation to completely divide the strap muscles transversely at their lower third. At the end of the procedure sternohyoid muscles are repaired. We have found it unnecessary to reapproximate the sternothyroids. If the strap muscles are adherent to the thyroid gland, especially to the tumor, they are resected with the gland. It is not unusual for malignant disease of the thyroid to penetrate the musculature.

After the thyroid gland is exposed, the middle thyroid vein is divided. This vessel drains directly into the jugular vein; failure to ligate it securely may risk hemorrhage that would make it more difficult to identify the parathyroid glands and recurrent nerve. It is then possible to mobilize the thyroid lobe—often by blunt dissection. The next goal is the division of the upper pole vessels. The thyroid lobe is first retracted downward and laterally to expose the superior pole vessels. Visualizing the cricothyroid muscle is the key to safe dissection of the upper pole. It is often helpful to divide the cricothyroid branch of the superior thyroid artery to gain access to the space between the cricothyroid muscle and upper pole vessels (Fig. 2). By clearing this space and placing a curved clamp from medial to lateral beneath the upper pole vessels, it is possible to avoid injury to the cricothyroid muscle's close companions: the superior and recurrent laryngeal nerves. The superior laryngeal nerve, which may be close to the vessels or even accompany them, is best preserved by awareness of its presence, isolating and dividing the superior pole vessels individually close to the upper pole of the thyroid. Sometimes the nerve can be seen as it descends with the vessels and on to the cricoid muscle, but usually it is not visualized (Fig. 3). A recent study showed that identification and dissection of the superior laryngeal nerve offered no better protection from damage than simply transecting the superior vessels close to the thyroid (52). We prefer to divide the superior pole vessels initially because it increases the mobility of the thyroid lobe, facilitating exposure of the parathyroid glands and recurrent nerve. Rotating the thyroid lobe medially and pulling it upward stretches the nerve, aiding in its identification and dissection. It also makes it easier to look for a superior parathyroid gland or a suggestive fat pad posterior and lateral to the upper pole (Fig. 3). When not present in its classic position, it is often located lower, close to the main trunk of the superior thyroid artery, or a centimeter or so above the inferior thyroid

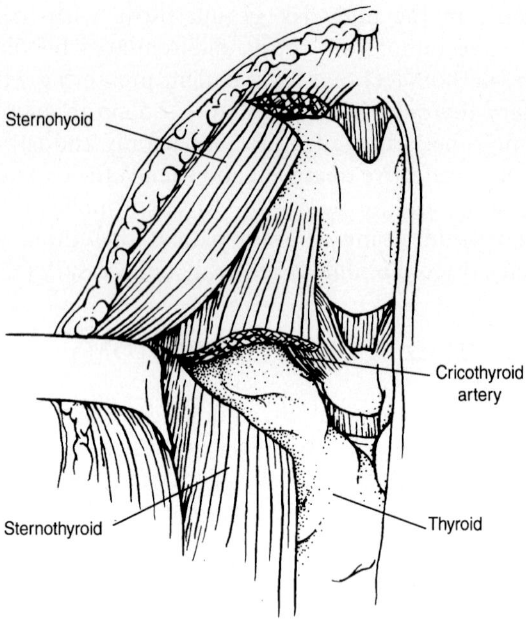

Figure 2 Exposure of the thyroid gland. The medial third of the sternohyoid muscle has been divided to provide greater access to the thyroid gland, particularly the upper pole. Transection of the sternothyroid muscle, as diagrammed, will offer direct and easy access of the thyroid lobe and the superior pole vessels. Division of the cricoid branch of the superior thyroid artery offers increased exposure to the space between the cricothyroideus and the superior pole of the thyroid. (From Ref. 13.)

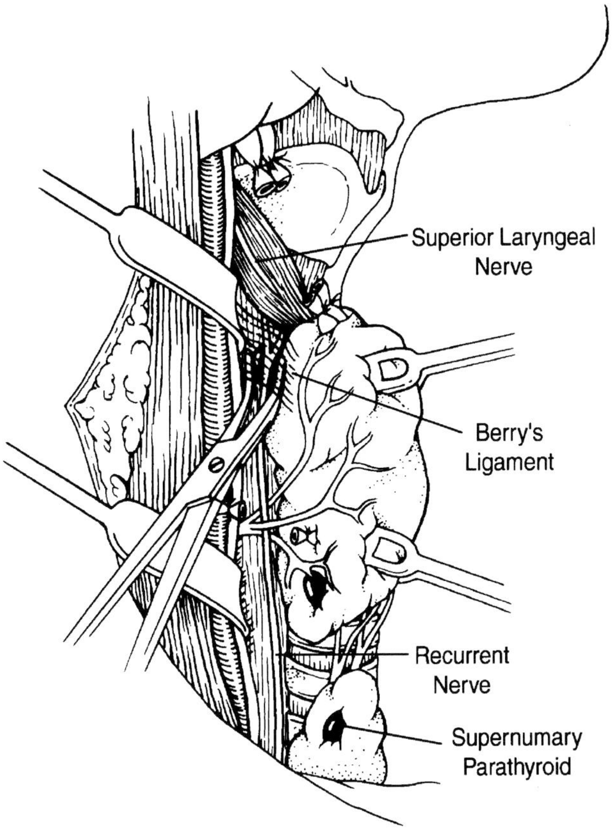

Figure 3 The middle thyroid vein and the superior pole vessels have been divided and ligated. The thyroid is retracted medially, visualizing the recurrent nerve coursing between branches of the inferior thyroid artery and continuing upward to split just as it travels beneath the cricothyroideus. The superior laryngeal nerve is seen as it enters the cricothyroideus. A curved hemostat elevates Berry's ligament as it is divided, displaying the superior parathyroid just posterior to the recurrent nerve. A supernumary parathyroid is present in the thymus.

artery. If visualized, the gland is not mobilized at this time. Dissection of the upper pole is discontinued. Berry's ligament is not blindly transected. This avoids injury to the parathyroid gland or its blood supply, which if not already located, may be present in the areolar and fatty tissue posterior to the superior pole vessels. It also avoids damage to the recurrent nerve, which may traverse the ligament (13) (Fig. 3).

Once the superior vessels are divided, attention is directed to searching for the recurrent laryngeal nerve and inferior parathyroid gland; the inferior thyroid artery is the key to both. The common carotid artery is a good landmark; the inferior thyroid artery is found at a right angle to the carotid artery entering the midportion of a normal thyroid lobe. In order to locate the midpoint of the lobe, the surgeon must mentally discount the distortions produced by tumors or other abnormal enlargements in varying portions of the lobe and visualize its original size and shape.

The recurrent nerve courses under the inferior thyroid artery in 80% of patients, forming the hypotenuse of a triangle with the carotid artery as the third limb (Fig. 3). In 20% of patients it travels above the inferior thyroid artery. The right recurrent nerve follows an upward course obliquely cephelad from lateral to medial as it recurs around the subclavian artery. The left nerve ascends directly upward in the tracheoesophageal groove after it recurs around the arch of the aorta. The nerves can frequently be palpated before they are seen by running a finger transversely across the trachea below the level of the inferior thyroid artery; they feel like a taught cord. In rare situations the right

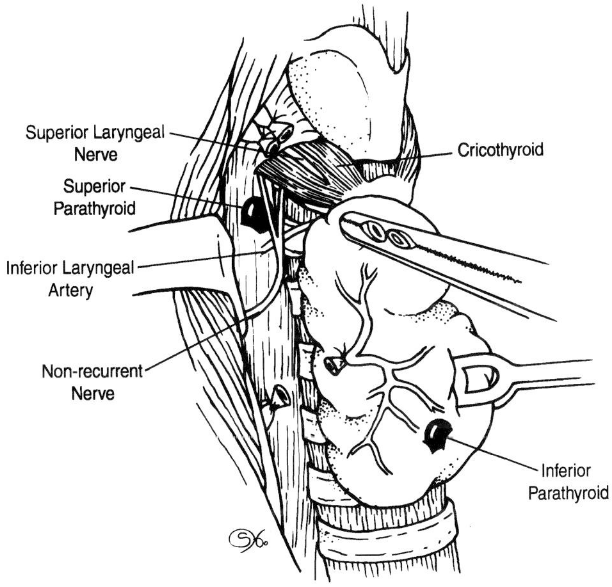

Figure 4 The upper pole has been divided, the inferior thyroid artery transected, and the recurrent nerve had been dissected. In this patient the nerve is "nonrecurrent," coming directly from the vagus. The superior parathyroid gland has been mobilized, displaced posteriorly, and preserved. The inferior laryngeal artery will be divided as close as possible to the thyroid lobe to avoid bleeding in this critical area and injury to the recurrent nerve. The inferior parathyroid gland is located too far from a branch of the inferior artery to be preserved with its blood supply. It will be necessary to remove the gland and implant its fragments into the sternomastoid muscle in order to preserve its function. (From Ref. 13.)

recurrent laryngeal nerve enters directly from the vagus and is "nonrecurrent" (Fig. 4). If the surgeon has difficulty finding the nerve in the lower area of the neck, an excellent alternative approach is to search for it at the inferior margin of the cricothyroid muscle, at the junction of the anterior third and the posterior two thirds. It often splits just below this point. This is a reliable location for finding the nerve, and it can then be traced downward along the trachea. A small area of thyroid parenchyma, the tuberculum Zuckerkandl, overlies the superior portion of the recurrent nerve. This tissue is dissected carefully to avoid injury to the underlying nerve.

Exploration of the distal branches of the inferior thyroid artery may lead to the lower parathyroid, which is nourished by a terminal branch. This branch or loop must be carefully sought and preserved; meticulous dissection is required to accomplish this. Great care must be taken to divide the inferior thyroid artery distal to the parathyroid branch (Fig. 5). It is good judgment to preserve as much of the inferior thyroid artery and its branches as possible, since it supplies the blood to the upper as well as the lower parathyroid glands. The location of the inferior parathyroid is less constant than that of the superior gland. Often it may be at some distance from the thyroid, and at times it may not be found. The practice of dividing the inferior thyroid artery as far distally as possible often preserves the blood supply to such a gland. Sometimes, however, the parathyroid gland may be found so far anteriorly on the thyroid lobe that it cannot be preserved with its blood supply. In these instances it should be removed, minced into 1–2 mm fragments, and implanted into the sternomastoid muscle (see Chapter 19). Placing the gland in a bath of iced saline until it is ready for use makes it firmer and easier to handle.

After the recurrent nerve has been identified, the thyroidea ima vessels can be safely divided inferiorly. The thyroid lobe is retracted upward, and by placing a scissors on the top of the recurrent nerve and spreading the blades, a plane is developed superior to the nerve that can be followed cephelad. The nerve is dissected by separating the tissues that are superior to it. The undersurface is not disturbed to avoid damaging its blood supply. It is followed upward to the point where it enters the larynx just below the cricothyroideus muscle. In more that half of patients the nerve splits, sometimes into more than two strands. All branches must be preserved. Berry's ligament, which anchors the posterior portion of the upper pole to the trachea and pharynx, is encountered near this point. The ligament is now divided under direct vision as the nerve is kept in

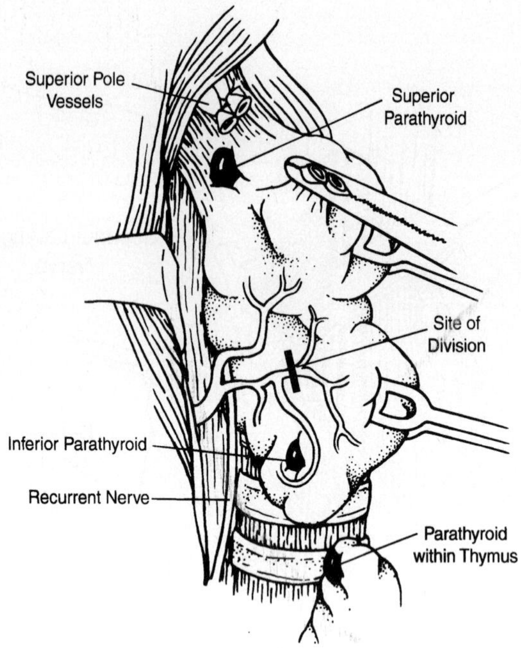

Figure 5 The superior parathyroid gland is not found in its classic position, but in the areolar tissue adjacent to Berry's ligament, which has not yet been divided. The gland is located only after division of the upper pole vessels and rotating the thyroid gland medially. A long segment of the inferior thyroid artery must be preserved to maintain the arterial loop, which returns backward to nourish the inferior parathyroid gland. The preferred site for division of the vessel is shown. An additional parathyroid gland present in the thymus will be preserved. (From Ref. 13.)

sight, and the superior parathyroid gland is mobilized posteriorly to avoid damage to these structures. It is important to note a constant branch of the inferior thyroid artery, the inferior laryngeal artery, emerging medially from beneath the recurrent laryngeal nerve just before the nerve enters beneath the cricothyroid muscle (Fig. 4). Careful clamping, division, and ligation of this vessel before the thyroid is resected from the trachea avoids hemorrhage at a site where the nerve would be at considerable risk. Sudden bleeding is best handled by sponge gauze compression so that, being constantly aware of the presence of the nerve, and with the aid of suction if necessary, the bleeding source can be methodically and carefully identified and clamped in a controlled and safe fashion. It is then a simple matter to remove the thyroid lobe by sharp dissection from the fascia overlying the trachea. Care must be taken to trace the pyramidal lobe upwards and remove it as completely as possible. It is often overlooked and later appears as residual uptake in postoperative scans. The isthmus is also routinely removed as part of a thyroid lobectomy to eliminate the later possibility of a mass in the anterior neck.

In some instances the recurrent nerve may not be in its usual position; it may be stretched and displaced anteriorly or posteriorly by a large goiter or nodule; the nerve must be carefully sought and separated to avoid injury. Delivery of substernal extensions of goiters without confirming the location of the nerve is hazardous; awareness of the site of the nerve is critical before removal of the tumor.

If a parathyroid gland appears nonviable at the end of the operation and is sufficiently removed from the tumor, it should be removed, minced, and transplanted into the sternomastoid muscle. We find it valuable to inspect the postlobectomy specimen for a gland that may have been inadvertently removed. If so, it can be transplanted.

We make the decision of whether to embark on total thyroidectomy by evaluating the postlobectomy status of the parathyroid glands on the side of the dominant lesion. If the parathyroid glands on the initial side are problematic, we prefer to preserve a posterior shell of normal thyroid on the uninvolved side to protect the glands and the recurrent laryngeal nerve ("near total thyroidectomy") (see Chapter 9). There is almost always grossly normal parenchyma that can be saved posteriorly. The patient will be far better off with a bit of residual thyroid tissue than with permanent hypoparathyroidism.

In most cases drainage is not required. When it does seem necessary, we prefer the use of a large (#10) Jackson Pratt drain connected to suction. It is important to note that the presence of a drain does not necessarily remove the risk of compression in the closed space of the neck. Clots within the neck and in the drain can render it nonfunctional. We prefer a simple light dressing so that the neck can be observed readily and the wound can be opened quickly if necessary.

9 COMPLETION THYROIDECTOMY

The subject of completion thyroidectomy is complex; it essentially mirrors the preference of the surgeon or endocrinologist in the management of thyroid carcinoma. Although there is general agreement that small, differentiated thyroid cancers are well treated by lobectomy, the situation becomes more involved when the tumor is larger, the extent of the disease is greater, and differing histological types are considered.

The usual situation is a change in the diagnosis from benign follicular tumor on frozen section to malignant on final examination. If the lesion is large, has adverse features such as major extension beyond the thyroid capsule, or vascular invasion, completion thyroidectomy is recommended; it removes all thyroid parenchyma that might contain additional disease and permits effective radioiodine identification and treatment of metastatic tumor. It also makes it possible to follow the patient with thyroglobulin levels. Adverse histological features found on final section (e.g., tall or columnar cell carcinoma, diffuse sclerosing variant, extension beyond the thyroid capsule, or areas of undifferentiated carcinoma) militate towards completion thyroidectomy. Unsuspected medullary carcinoma requires total thyroidectomy.

Some authors feel that Hürthle cell carcinoma is more aggressive and warrants completion thyroidectomy. However, the most important prognostic factor in Hürthle cell tumor is the extent of capsular invasion. Minimal capsular invasion indicates excellent prognosis, while patients with widely invasive Hürthle cell tumors do poorly (53).

In experienced hands there should be no increased risk in completion thyroidectomy. We prefer a lateral approach to avoid midline scarring, exposing the thyroid between the sternomastoid and strap muscles. The lobe will not have been scarred by previous dissection and resection should be no more difficult than a primary lobectomy.

There are no studies demonstrating the effect of completion thyroidectomy on survival. Although microscopic disease is present in the opposite lobe in 25–60% of patients with differentiated thyroid cancer, it does not correlate with a clinical recurrence rate of 5% in the contralateral thyroid lobe.

10 SURGICAL MANAGEMENT OF NECK NODES

Reports in the literature have concluded that the prognosis in papillary cancer of the thyroid is usually not affected by the presence or absence of lymph node metastasis. However, in patients above the age of 45, it does represent an adverse prognostic factor, especially as related to recurrent neck disease or distant metastasis.

The incidence of nodal metastasis is much higher in young individuals, but most of these patients will do extremely well, probably related to their age. The cumulative incidence of cervical lymph node metastasis in papillary, follicular, and Hürthle cell tumors is reported by Shaha et al. to be 61, 30, and 21%, respectively (54). Hughes et al. (5) studied the impact of lymph node metastasis in differentiated thyroid cancer by matched-pair analysis. They selected 100 patients with N0 and N1 disease. Overall, there was no survival difference in these two groups. However, their analysis demonstrated a higher incidence of recurrence in N1 patients above the age of 45. The long-term survival in patients with nodal metastasis above the age of 45 was slightly lower. Below the age of 45, there was no survival difference. They concluded that nodal metastases in older patients increase the risk of neck recurrence.

An important issue in the management of cervical node metastasis in differentiated thyroid cancer is the role of elective neck dissection. The incidence of nodal metastasis in the paratracheal area and central compartment is quite high; a central compartment clearance is recommended if there are obvious clinically enlarged lymph nodes at the time of surgery. However, elective neck dissection in the absence of grossly enlarged lymph nodes is generally not advocated. The usual practice during the intraoperative management is to evaluate the central compartment, the paratracheal nodes, the nodes in the tracheoesophageal groove, and the superior mediastinal nodes. If there are suspicious nodes in the tracheoesophageal groove, central compartment clearance is generally advocated, with removal of the lymph nodes at Level VI. Along with this, the superior mediastinum should be evaluated; if there are any obvious enlarged lymph nodes, they should be removed as well. Whether routine central compartment neck dissection should be performed in papillary thyroid cancer remains controversial. Generally, if the lymph nodes are clinically not suspicious or not enlarged, routine central compartment neck dissection is not advocated because of the high likelihood of permanent hypoparathyroidism.

The surgical procedure of selective node dissection, or "berry picking," is not recommended because of the high incidence of recurrent disease in the neck. If clinically positive nodes are apparent, a modified neck dissection is advocated. In individuals with bulky nodal metastasis, routine total thyroidectomy should be performed to remove disease and to facilitate the use of radioactive iodine ablation and follow-up. These patients may already have pulmonary metastases that can be documented only after radioactive iodine ablation.

10.1 Neck Dissection

Lymph nodes in the neck are classified by location (Fig. 6). The standard radical neck dissection popular-

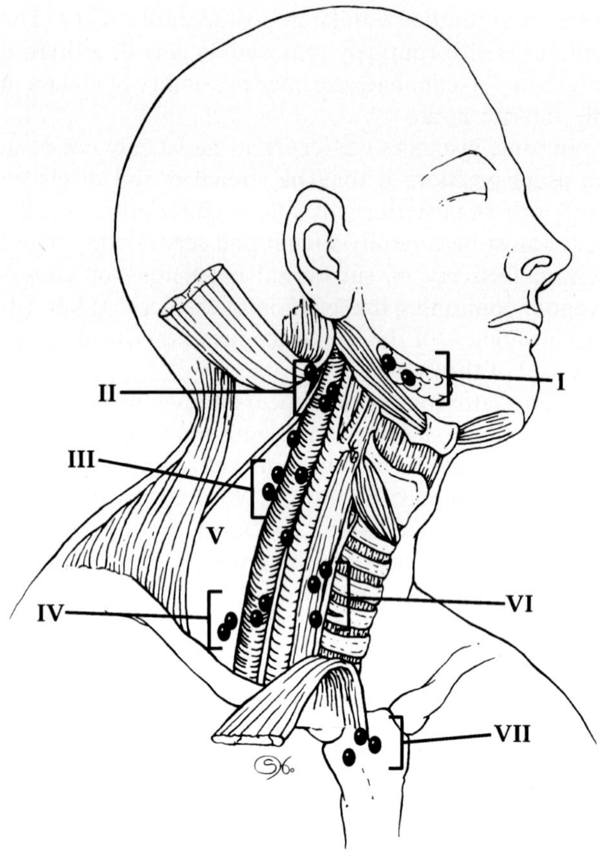

Figure 6 Lymph nodes leFvels in the neck. Level I: submandibular triangle; Levels II, III, IV: nodes accompanying the jugular vein; (high, mid, and low, respectively); Level V: posterior triangle and supraclavicular fossa; Level VI: paratracheal; Level VII: superior mediastinal.

ized by George Crile in 1906 includes removal of lymph nodes in the neck along with three important structures: sternomastoid muscle, internal jugular vein, and the accessory nerve. Considering the low biological aggressiveness of thyroid cancer, the standard classical neck dissection is rarely indicated for patients with differentiated thyroid cancer. Generally, these three significant structures can be preserved. Occasionally the sternomastoid muscle or the jugular vein may have to be sacrificed due to extensive metastatic disease or if the muscle is directly invaded by tumor. The jugular vein should be resected if it is invaded by nodal or gross disease or if is intimately adherent to tumor. There is minimal adverse effect on the patient from the loss of one jugular vein. Every effort, however, should be made to preserve the accessory nerve, which is important for shoulder function. Since the involvement of submaxillary nodes is rare in thyroid cancer, routine dissection of this area is usually not undertaken.

10.2 Central Compartment Dissection

The central compartment extends from the jugular vein to that on the opposite side. The superior boundary is the hyoid bone, and the inferior is the suprasternal notch. The lymph nodes included in this area are the pretracheal (Delphian) nodes, paratracheal nodes, and lymph nodes in the tracheoesophageal groove. Central compartment clearance is undertaken in locally aggressive thyroid cancers, poorly differentiated thyroid cancers, or those with adverse histological features—or if clinically positive enlarged lymph nodes are present. The jugular area is also evaluated; if no enlarged lymph nodes are present along the jugular vein, central compartment neck dissection is usually not performed.

Special attention to the parathyroids is required since they are at great risk in central compartment clearance. If a parathyroid becomes devascularized, it should be implanted into the sternomastoid muscle.

11 MANAGEMENT OF LOCALLY AGGRESSIVE THYROID CANCER

The philosophy of management of locally aggressive thyroid cancer is different from that of low-risk disease. A critical prognostic factor in differentiated thyroid cancer is the presence of extrathyroidal extension. The overall outcome in patients presenting with locally aggressive thyroid cancer or that invading the surrounding structures is poor. The presence of extrathyroidal invasion is associated with an increased frequency of local recurrence, metastatic nodal disease, and distant metastasis. In addition, patients presenting with extrathyroidal extension of disease have a high incidence of local recurrence, with a subsequent mortality of almost 50%. Involvement of the trachea or larynx may lead to airway obstruction and acute hemorrhage. The majority of deaths in differentiated thyroid cancer are directly related to central compartment recurrence.

Locally aggressive disease usually involves anatomical extension from thyroid into the surrounding structures in the midline of the neck. It may also be related to the histological grade of the tumor such as poorly differentiated thyroid cancer, tall cell, insular, trabecular, or columnar cell variants. In addition it may be a reflection of molecular characteristics that still need to be studied in detail. In the future, interest in molecular markers such as EGF receptor, p53, ploidy, CGH, and DNA array may shed more light on the aggressiveness of locally advanced thyroid cancer.

The location of the thyroid gland adjacent to the upper aerodigestive tract facilitates direct invasion of the tumor into the thyroid cartilage, trachea, recurrent laryngeal nerve, and esophageal musculature. The most common sites of locally aggressive thyroid cancer include the strap muscles, followed by tracheal wall, recurrent laryngeal nerve, or esophageal musculature.

Laryngeal structures are infrequently involved. Invasion of the larynx may be from direct extension of disease through the thyroid cartilage or spread behind the thyroid cartilage into the paraglottic space. When there is extension to the trachea, it can occur between the tracheal rings, or tumor may directly penetrate the cartilaginous structures. The recurrent laryngeal nerve may be invaded by the tumor at the cricothyroid area near the ligament of Berry, or it may be involved by the nodal metastasis in the paratracheal region. Preoperative evaluation of vocal cord mobility is critical to determine the extrathyroidal spread of the disease. Once there is intraluminal extension, the prognosis is poor, with a high incidence of local recurrence. Andersen et al. (55) from Memorial Sloan-Kettering Cancer Center recently noted that in patients below the age of 45, complete excision of tumors with extrathyroidal extension resulted in improved survival. Complete excision of tumor in patients over 45, however, did not. This is most likely due to the increased aggressiveness of the disease in older patients. Still, complete resection should always be the goal in order to improve survival and avoid local recurrence.

11.1 Evaluation of Locally Aggressive Thyroid Cancer

The most important clinical findings include fixed central compartment neck mass, fixed thyroid gland, hoarseness, dysphagia, difficulty in breathing, and hemoptysis. The presence of hemoptysis with a thyroid mass and a paralyzed vocal cord essentially indicates intraluminal extension of disease. Indirect or fiberoptic laryngoscopy should be a routine part of the preoperative evaluation in thyroid surgery. Patients may also have a paralyzed vocal cord without a change in their voice. Imaging studies are helpful to evaluate the extent of the disease and location of the extrathyroidal spread. If a CT scan is performed, it is preferable not to use contrast, which would delay postoperative radioactive iodine ablation. Preoperative endoscopy is crucial if it suspected that extensive surgery may be required; laryngoscopy, tracheoscopy, and bronchoscopy will define the intraluminal disease.

11.2 Surgical Management of Locally Advanced Thyroid Cancer

The anterior extension of the disease may infiltrate the strap muscles. This finding does not appear to result in poor outcome; all gross tumor can usually be removed without difficulty at the time of surgery (36,38). If the strap muscles are involved by extrathyroidal extension of the disease, they should be sacrificed from the thyroid cartilage to the sternum. It is easy to resect anterior extension of extrathyroidal disease en bloc with the strap muscles.

The decision regarding the management of recurrent laryngeal nerve is complex. If the nerve is paralyzed preoperatively, it is wise to sacrifice it along with resection of the surrounding soft tissues for better oncological clearance. However, if the nerve is functioning preoperatively, every attempt should be made to preserve it in continuity. In the event that the nerve appears to be involved by tumor, it should be resected. The tumor may occasionally encircle the nerve, at which time one has to make a critical decision regarding sacrifice of the nerve. The nodal disease can also be split in front of the nerve and resected in toto. However, it is crucial not to leave any gross tumor behind near the recurrent laryngeal nerve. If tumor invades the esophageal musculature, a local resection may be possible. Sometimes it may be feasible to remove disease without entry into the mucosa of the esophagus. It is important to avoid injury to the esophageal mucosa and a resulting mediastinal fistula. If small opening of the mucosa is noted, it should be sutured securely with an esophageal bougie in place to avoid esophageal stenosis.

When the tumor invades the trachea, the management decisions are complex. It is extremely important to evaluate the extent of the disease on the tracheal wall and to note whether there is intraluminal tumor or peritracheal disease adherent to the tracheal rings. Grillo and Zannini (37) described four types of tracheal involvement extending from the tumor adherent to the tracheal wall and cartilage to the intraluminal extension of the disease. If the tumor does not directly invade the trachea and can be removed by sharp dissection, the procedure is satisfactory and preserves vital functions. However, if the tumor invades the lumen of the trachea, appropriate excision is required. If the tumor invades intraluminally, it will usually necessitate a sleeve resection with end-to-end anastomosis. In rare circumstances, if the involvement is minimal, a tracheal window can be removed and reconstruction accomplished by using surrounding musculature or a sternomastoid periosteal flap from the sternomastoid and periosteum of the clavicle. A variety of techniques are described in the literature for reconstruction of the partial tracheal defect, including the insertion of the tracheostomy tube. However, it is important to remove all gross tumor—even though this may require resection of the tracheal segment. Involvement of the laryngeal cartilage may necessitate either resection of the laryngeal cartilage with its perichondrium or partial laryngectomy. If the entire larynx is destroyed or there is major intraluminal disease, total laryngectomy is undertaken. However, the necessity of primary total laryngectomy in well-differentiated thyroid cancer is extremely rare. If the tumor invades the cricoid cartilage, the surgical resection is quite complex and may require total laryngectomy. If the tumor invades the trachea and the esophagus, a total laryngopharyngectomy with reconstruction of the hypopharynx can be performed with jejunal free flap.

12 COMPLICATIONS OF THYROIDECTOMY

A variety of complications are well recognized as being specific to thyroid surgery. These can be distressing, especially those related to postoperative hemorrhage, airway distress, recurrent laryngeal nerve injury, permanent hypoparathyroidism, and chyle leakage.

12.1 Postoperative Hemorrhage

The thyroid is an extremely vascular organ; postoperative hemorrhage can occur due to continuous bleeding from the cut surface of the thyroid gland, slipping of a ligature, or increased cervical pressure due to coughing or bucking, especially during extubation. Drains have little impact on bleeding or postoperative hematoma; their most valuable feature is that they call attention to the bleeding. Suction drains can control limited bleeding as well as giving notice of the problem, but when there is a combination of continued hemorrhage and hematomas, they invariably cease to function. Bleeding usually occurs within 8–24 hours of the surgery; the patient may complain of tightness of the neck, increasing difficulty in breathing, and obvious swelling in the neck. It is important not to cover the thyroid incision with extensive dressings that may mask postoperative bleeding and hematoma. If the hemorrhage continues, it can produce life-threatening airway compression related to decreased venous return and laryngeal edema. The wound should be opened immediately at the bedside to relieve the pressure. If the airway is compromised, emergency intubation may be required. If there is difficulty in intubation because of laryngeal edema, tracheostomy or cricothyrotomy must be performed promptly, through the wound. The patient can then be brought safely to the operating room for appropriate control of the problem. Even if the wound is opened at the bedside and the hematoma, bleeding, and pressure are relieved, it is frequently necessary to bring the patient to the operating room for wound irrigation, removal of remaining clots, and to search for the bleeding vessels. Not infrequently the bleeding point cannot be found at reexploration. At other times bleeding may originate in the region of the recurrent laryngeal nerve, adjacent to Berry's ligament. Great care is necessary in reexploration to avoid injury to the recurrent laryngeal nerve.

Although it is popular to perform thyroidectomy as an outpatient procedure, sending the patient home a few hours later, postoperative hemorrhage in a situation where it cannot be controlled can be lethal. The authors feel that an overnight stay is safer. In a decision analysis with historical outcome data, Schwartz et al. predicted that for every 100,000 thyroidectomies performed, 94 deaths secondary to postoperative bleeding could be prevented by a 24-hour hospitalization compared to a 6-hour observation (12).

12.2 Recurrent Laryngeal Nerve Injury

The incidence of permanent recurrent laryngeal nerve injury in thyroidectomy is 0.5–3%. Common sites of recurrent laryngeal nerve injury are at the paratracheal area where the nerve crosses the inferior thyroid artery, or in the region of Berry's ligament where it enters the cricoid cartilage. Frequently the injury is related to attempts to control venous bleeding around the recurrent laryngeal nerve. In addition, small arterial branches such as the inferior laryngeal and cricothyroid artery are a risk in the area just below the cricothyroideus; they must be carefully divided and ligated. Bilateral recurrent laryngeal nerve injury is rare, but it can lead to respiratory difficulty and glottic narrowing. If the patient has suffered previous unilateral recurrent laryngeal nerve injury, contralateral thyroid lobectomy can be hazardous. Careful dissection in the tracheoesophageal groove and the use of magnifying loops and micro-clamps (along with bipolar cautery) reduce the incidence of recurrent laryngeal nerve injury and facilitate surgical exploration. Postoperative follow-up should include fiberoptic laryngoscopy. If the nerve injury is identified at the time of surgery, nerve repair with microsurgical instruments should be considered. Whether this will restore the function or not remains undefined at this time. Recurrent laryngeal nerve injury leads to breathiness in the voice and obvious hoarseness. If the superior laryngeal nerve is also injured, the patient may develop aspiration. The vocal cord may resume median or paramedian position at which time the voice may improve over months. Voice therapy during this time may be helpful. If there is considerable difficulty in voice projection or vocal incompetence, laryngoplasty or medialization procedures may be considered. Teflon injection in the vocal cord may give immediate relief from these distressing symptoms. A Gortex graft can be inserted in the cricothyroid area by a surgical procedure. Bilateral vocal paralysis, though rare, may lead to acute airway distress necessitating reintubation and subsequently a tracheostomy. A variety of endolaryngeal procedures such as arytenoid abduction or laser arytenoidectomy may be performed. The airway may also be opened with cordotomy.

12.3 Superior Laryngeal Nerve Injury

The external branch of the superior laryngeal nerve is critical in thyroid surgery; it runs along the medial border of the superior thyroid pedicle and superior thyroid vessels. The superior laryngeal nerve may be identified during surgery in approximately two thirds of patients; however, in large goiters or high riding superior poles, the nerve is more likely to be injured than recognized. Every effort should be made to ligate the superior thyroid pedicle very close to the thyroid substance to avoid injury to the superior laryngeal nerve. The exact incidence of superior laryngeal nerve injury is difficult to appreciate since the manifestations of this nerve injury may be quite subtle. Fiberoptic laryngoscopy may not document the superior laryngeal nerve injury, although the patient may not be able to raise the tone and pitch of the voice. This is especially disabling to singers or professional speakers. There is no effective therapy at this time.

12.4 Hypoparathyroidism

One of the most disabling complications of total thyroidectomy is permanent hypoparathyroidism. Temporary hypocalcemia is reported to range between 5 and 25%, while the incidence of permanent hypoparathyroidism is reported to vary from 0.5 to 5%, depending upon the extent of the surgical procedure and paratracheal nodal clearance. The frequency of permanent hypoparathyroidism has diminished in recent years as surgical expertise has increased. In a series of 183 total thyroidectomies, 152 of whom had extensive carcinoma, Schwartz and Friedman reported an incidence of 0.55% permanent recurrent nerve injury and a 3.3% rate of permanent hypoparathyroidism (13). Others report an even lower incidence.

The best way to avoid hypoparathyroidism is to recognize and preserve the parathyroid glands. If a gland is devascularized during the operation, it should be transplanted into the sternomastoid muscle. There is no need to autotransplant parathyroid glands into the forearm. These are normal glands in contrast to those of hyperplasia; they do not become hyperfunctional, and the easy access of forearm transplant is not required. It may take anywhere from 6 to 12 weeks for the autotransplanted parathyroid to function, and during this time the patient may require continued calcium and vitamin D supplementation. The goal is to maintain normocalcemia in the postoperative period, although symptoms are unlikely to appear unless the serum calcium drops to less than 8 mg/dL. Ionized calcium may offer a more accurate way to track serum calcium since it is not influenced by serum albumen levels. Patients should be observed for symptoms of tingling, numbness, and circumoral paresthesia. Tetany can be life threatening. Postoperative serum calcium levels should be checked within 4–8 hours and followed twice daily if the patient is symptomatic; intravenous calcium gluconate, 10–20 cc on an urgent basis, may be necessary. The active form of vitamin D (Rocaltrol) is a valuable adjunct, making it possible to reduce the amount of calcium required (0.25–0.5 μg 1–4 times a day). As the condition stabilizes the patient should be switched to oral calcium supplements as soon as possible. In most cases, the patient will improve in 12–24 hours. However, some may require calcium supplementation for 2–3 weeks ranging from 2 to 8 g/day.

Transient or permanent hypocalcemia is very unlikely after hemithyroidectomy, since the opposite lobe is not disturbed. Although the incidence of permanent hypoparathyroidism is low, it is one of the most distressing complications—one that can considerably change the patient's quality of life.

12.5 Chyle Leak

One of the most distressing complications of neck dissection is a chyle leak (or chyle fistula), which is more common in patients with extensive dissection in the supraclavicular fossa, or bulky nodal metastasis where the lymphatic channels are blocked and markedly enlarged. The easiest way to avoid this complication is to be aware of it at the time of surgery and to continue meticulous dissection, identifying small lymphatic ducts and ligating them with nonabsorbable suture material. There may occasionally be a chyle leak near the jugular vein, which can be quite distressing in the operating room. Figure of eight suture ligature in this area can be helpful. During surgery it is important to make certain that all chyle leakage is controlled. The wound should be dry on closure. Regardless of the surgeon's attention, there may occasionally be a delayed leak in the postoperative period. Generally, most of these patients can be treated conservatively with repeated aspirations. The wound may occasionally require opening if there is excessive drainage, although it is preferable to avoid this. The chylous leak on rare occasions may be voluminous, ranging from 1.0 to 3.0 L per 24 hours. In such a situation, maintenance of nutrition always becomes a problem; these patients require a low-fat diet and possible total parenteral nutrition. If the problem continues for an extended period of time, one may consider reexploration and ligation of the chyle leak. However, during the reexploration, there is invariably considerable inflamed tissue; locating the site of leakage may be quite difficult. The most satisfactory approach is to be especially conscious of the risk and to avoid injury to the fragile and easily damaged thoracic duct during the surgery, especially if the neck dissection is performed on the left side where the duct is vulnerable.

REFERENCES

1. Shaha AR. Controversies in the management of thyroid nodule. Laryngoscope 1999; 110(2 part 1):183–193.
2. Hundahl SA, Fleming ID, Fremgen AM, et al. A National Cancer Data Base report on 53,856 cases of thyroid carcinoma treated in the US, 1985–1995. Cancer 1998; (83):2638–2648.
3. Gilliland FD, Hunt WC, Morris DM, et al. Prognostic factors for thyroid carcinoma: a population-based study of 15,698 cases from the Surveillance, Epidemiology and End Results (SEER) program, 1973–1991. Cancer 1997; (79):564–573.
4. Fleming ID, Cooper JS, Henson DE, et al, eds. AJCC Cancer Staging Manual. 5th Ed. American Joint Committee on Cancer. 5th ed. Philadelphia: Lippencott-Raven, 1997.
5. Hughes CJ, Shaha AR, Shah JP, Loree TR. Impact of

lymph node metastasis in differentiated carcinoma of the thyroid—a matched pair analysis. Head Neck 1996; 18:127–132.
6. Jemal A, Thomas T, Murray M. Cancer statistics. CA 2002; 52(1):23–47.
7. Hay ID, Grant CS, Taylor WF, et al. Ipsilateral lobectomy versus bilateral lobar resection in papillary thyroid carcinoma: a retrospective analysis of surgical outcome using a novel prognostic scoring system. Surgery 1987; (102):1088–1095.
8. Hay ID, Bergstralh EJ, Goellner JR, et al. Predicting outcome in papillary thyroid carcinoma: development of a reliable prognostic scoring system in a cohort of 1779 patients surgically treated at one institution during 1940 through 1989. Surgery 1993; (104):947–953.
9. Cady B. Staging in thyroid carcinoma. Cancer 1998; (83):844–847.
10. Cady B. Hayes Martin Lecture. Our AMES is true: how an old concept still hits the mark, or risk group assignment points the arrow to rational therapy selection in differentiated thyroid cancer. Am J Surg 1997; (174): 462–468.
11. Cady B, Rossi R. An expanded view of risk-group definition in differentiated thyroid carcinoma. Surgery 1988; (104):947–953.
12. Schwartz AE, Clark OH, Ituarte P, Lo Gerfo P. Therapeutic controversy, thyroid surgery—the choice. J Clin Endocrinol Metab 1998; 83:1097–1105.
13. Schwartz AE, Friedman EW. Preservation of the parathyroid glands in total thyroidectomy. Surg Gynecol Obstet 1987; 165:327–332.
14. Noguchi M, Mizukami Y, Mizukami Y, Michigishi T, et al. Multivariate study of prognostic factors of differentiated thyroid carcinoma: The significance of histologic subtype. Int Surg 1993; (78):10–15.
15. Shah JP, Loree TR, Dharker D, et al. Prognostic factors in differentiated carcinoma of the thyroid gland. Am J Surg 1992; (164):658–661.
16. Simpson WJ, McKinney SE, Carruthers JS, et al. Papillary and follicular thyroid cancer: prognostic factors in 1578 patients. Am J Med 1987; (83):479–488.
17. Massin JP, Savoie JC, Garnier H, et al. Pulmonary metastases in differentiated thyroid carcinoma. Study of 58 cases with implications for the primary tumor treatment. Cancer 1984; 53:982–992.
18. Attie JN, Khafif RA, Steckler RM. Elective neck dissection in papillary carcinoma of the thyroid. Am J Surg 1971; 122:464–471.
19. Noguchi S, Murakami N. The value of lymph-node dissection in patients with differentiated thyroid cancer. Surg Clin North Am 1987; 67:251–261.
20. Scheumann GF, Gimm O, Wegener G, et al. Prognostic significance and surgical management of locoregional lymph node metastases in papillary thyroid cancer. World J Surg 1994; 18:359–367.
21. Noguchi S, Noguchi A, Murakami N. Papillary carcinoma of the thyroid gland: developing patterns of metastases. Cancer 1970; 26:1053–1060.
22. Hamming JF, Roukema JA. Management of regional lymph nodes in papillary, follicular, and medullary thyroid carcinoma. In: Clark OH, Duh QY, eds. Textbook of Endocrine Surgery. Philadelphia: WB Saunders, 1997:155.
23. McGregor GI, Luoma A, Jackson SM. Lymph node metastases from well-differentiated thyroid cancer: a clinical review. Am J Surg 1985; 149:610–612.
24. McHenry CR, Rosen IB, Walfish PG. Prospective management of nodal metastases in differentiated thyroid cancer. Am J Surg 1991; 162:353–356.
25. Byar DP, Green SB, Dor P, et al. A prognostic index for thyroid carcinoma: a study of the EORTC Thyroid Cancer Cooperative Group. Eur J Cancer 1979; (15): 1033–1041.
26. Hay ID, Grant CS, Bergstralh EJ, et al. Unilateral total lobectomy: is it sufficient surgical treatment for patients with AMES low-risk papillary thyroid carcinoma? Surgery 1998; (124):958–966.
27. Hay ID, Bergstralh EJ, Goellner JR, et al. Predicting outcome in papillary thyroid carcinoma: development of a reliable prognostic scoring system in a cohort of 1779 patients surgically treated at one institution during 1940 through 1989. Surgery 1993; (114):1050–1058.
28. Shaha AR, Shah JP, Loree T. Patterns of nodal and distant metastasis based on histologic varieties in differentiated carcinoma of the thyroid. Am J Surg 1996; 172(6):692–694.
29. Shaha AR, Clark OH, Goepfert H, Kaplan EL, Loree TR, Udelsman EL. Symposium—Part 2: therapy. Current concepts in the management of thyroid cancer. Contemp Surg 2000; 56(2):105–118.
30. Shaha AR, Shah JP, Loree TR. Low-risk differentiated thyroid cancer: the need for selective treatment. Ann Surg Oncol 1997; 4(4):328–333.
31. Esnaola NF, Cantor SB, Sherman SI, et al. Optimal treatment strategy in patients with papillary thyroid cancer. Surgery 2001; 130(6):923–930.
32. Mazzaferri EL. Review. Papillary thyroid carcinoma: factors influencing prognosis and current therapy. Semin Oncol 1987; (14):315–332.
33. Mazzaferri EL, Jhiang SM. Long-term impact of initial surgical and medical therapy on papillary and follicular thyroid cancer. Am J Med 1994; (97):418–428.
34. Cunningham MP, Duda RB, Recant W, et al. Survival discriminants for differentiated thyroid cancer. Am J Surg 1990; 160(4):344–347.
35. Hay ID, Grant CS, van Heerden JA, et al. Papillary thyroid microcarcinoma: a study of 535 cases observed in a 50-year period. Surgery 1992; (112):1139–1147.
36. Czaja JM, McCaffrey TV. The surgical management of laryngotracheal invasion by well-differentiated papillary thyroid carcinoma. Arch Otolaryngol Head Neck Surg 1997; (123):484–490.

37. Grillo HC, Zannini P. Resectional management of airway invasion by thyroid carcinoma. Ann Thorac Surg 1986; (42):287–298.
38. McCaffrey TV, Bergstralh EJ, Hay ID. Locally invasive papillary thyroid carcinoma: 1940–1990. Head Neck 1994; (16):165–172.
39. Young RL, Mazzaferri EL, Rahe AJ, Dorfman SG. Pure follicular thyroid carcinoma: impact of therapy in 214 patients. J Nucl Med 1980; (21):733–737.
40. Shaha AR, Loree TR, Shah JP. Prognostic factors and risk group analysis in follicular carcinoma of the thyroid. Surgery 1995; (118):1131–1138.
41. van Heerden JA, Hay ID, Goellner JR, et al. Follicular thyroid carcinoma with capsular invasion alone: a non-threatening malignancy. Surgery 1992; (112):1130–1136.
42. Stojadinvic A, Ghossein RA, Hoos A, et al. Hurthle cell carcinoma: a critical histopathid appraisal. J Clin Oncol 2001; 19(10):2616–2625.
43. Rosai J, Carcangiu ML, DeLellis RA. Tumors of the Thyroid Gland. Atlas of Tumor Pathology. Third Series, Vol 5, Fascicle 5. Washington, DC: Armed Forces Institute of Pathology, 1992.
44. Thompson NW, Dunn EL, Batsakis JG, et al. Hürthle cell lesions of the thyroid gland. Surg Gynecol Obstet 1974; 139:555–560.
45. McLeod MK, Thompson NW. Hürthle cell neoplasms of the thyroid. Otolaryngol Clin North Am 1990; 23: 441–452.
46. Carcangiu ML, Bianchi S, Savino D, et al. Follicular Hürthle cell tumors of the thyroid. Cancer 1991; 68: 1944–1953.
47. Grant CS, Barr D, Goellner JR, et al. Benign Hürthle cell tumors of the thyroid: a diagnosis to be trusted? World J Surg 1988; 12:488–495.
48. Shaha AR. Thyroid cancer: extent of thyroidectomy. Cancer Control 2000; 7(3):240–245.
49. Clark OH. Total thyroidectomy: the treatment of choice for patients with differentiated thyroid cancer. Ann Surg 1982; (196):361–370.
50. Sherman SI, Brierley JD, Sperling M, et al. Prospective multicenter study of thyroid carcinoma treatment: initial analysis of staging and outcome. National Thyroid Cancer Treatment Cooperative Study Registry Group. Cancer 1998; (83):1012–1021.
51. Wong JB, Kaplan MN, Meyer KB, Pauker SG. Ablative radioactive iodine therapy for apparently localized thyroid carcinoma: a decision analytic perspective. Endocrinol Metab Clin North Am 1990; 19(3):741–760.
52. Bellantone R, Boscherini M, Lombardi CP, et al. Is the identification of the external branch of the superior laryngeal nerve mandatory in thyroid operation? Results of a prospective randomized study. Surgery 2001; 130(6):1055–1059.
53. Chen H, Udelsman R. Hürthle cell adenoma and carcinoma. In: Clark OH, Duh QY, eds. Textbook of Endocrine Surgery. Philadelphia: WB Saunders, 1997: 101–106.
54. Shaha AR, Shah JP, Loree T. Patterns of failure in differentiated carcinoma of the thyroid based on risk groups. Head Neck 1998; 20(1):26–30.
55. Andersen PE, Cambronero E, Shaha AR, Shah JP. The extent of neck disease after regional failure during observation of the N0 neck. Am J Surg 1996; 172(6): 689–691.

7

A Guide to the Physiology and Testing of Thyroid Function

Terry F. Davies

Mount Sinai School of Medicine, New York University, New York, New York, U.S.A.

1 INTRODUCTION

The safe patient for surgery is the euthyroid patient. Though urgent surgery on unstable thyroid patients can produce good results, it is everyone's experience that the risk of surgery is increased in those who are dysthyroid. It is critical to the surgeon that the patient about to undergo surgery has normal thyroid function. Hence, an understanding of thyroid physiology and thyroid function tests is a great asset to every surgeon and especially an endocrine surgeon.

The normal thyroid gland is under the control of the pituitary (Fig. 1). Understanding this relationship is the key to understanding thyroid physiology. The pituitary gland controls the output of thyroid hormones via thyroid-stimulating hormone (TSH). The thyroid hormones then feed back, via a classical loop at the level of the hypothalamus and pituitary, to suppress the release of TSH-releasing hormone (TRH) and TSH. Hence, the level of easily measured serum TSH is often the only "comfort information" a surgeon will find necessary for reassurance.

2 THYROID HORMONE SYNTHESIS

Thyroid hormones are necessary for the essential metabolism of almost all cells; their excessive or diminished levels has a marked influence on cell function. Thyroid hormone synthesis is localized to the thyroid follicular cells; thyroxine (T4) and a small amount of triiodothyronine (T3) are released from the basal side of these cells into the circulation. However, most T3 is obtained from T4 by 5′-deiodinase enzymes, found in peripheral tissues, that contain the rare element selenium (1). This process of deiodination is essential since T4 is biologically inactive; T3 is the true thyroid hormone that binds to a thyroid hormone receptor. Any interruption in the hypothalamic-pituitary-thyroid axis, or deficiency (e.g., in the availability of iodide (or selenium)), will cause problems with thyroid hormone availability.

3 THE ROLE OF IODIDE

Iodide is essential for the production of thyroid hormones; it has been estimated that 100–150 μg of iodine a day are required. This mostly comes from the diet, especially with the introduction of iodination of salt, bread, and milk, giving total intakes of approximately 300–700 μg/day. Inorganic iodide is transported into the thyroid cells by an iodide transporter, which acts like a pump exchanging iodide for sodium (the sodium iodide symporter, or NIS). This transporter is under the control of TSH. However, NIS is not confined to the thyroid gland being also present in salivary glands, gastric mucosa, and mammary glands (2). These sites are often seen on high-dose whole-body radioiodine scans used in the investigation of thyroid cancer. The

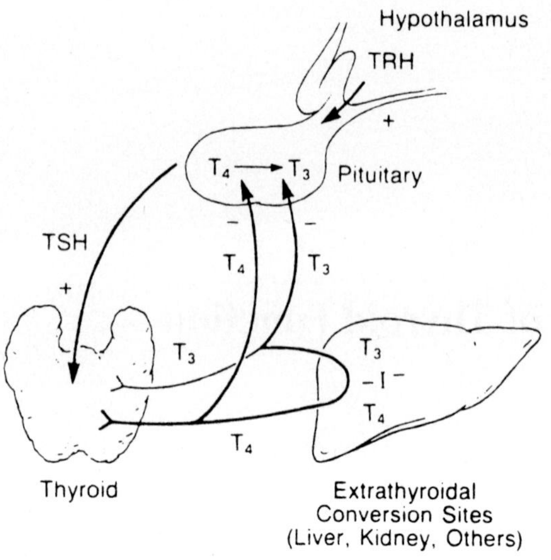

Figure 1 The hypothalamo-pituitary-thyroid axis. The regulation of TSH secretion by the anterior pituitary. Positive effects of TRH from the hypothalamus and the negative effects of circulating T3 and also T3 from intra-pituitary conversion of T4. (From Ref. 28.)

physiological role of these extrathyroidal iodide pumps remains unclear.

Decreasing total intake of iodine in the United States has been well documented in recent years (3), something of particular concern for pregnant women because of the increased turnover of iodide in pregnancy. However, up to the current time, iodine deficiency remains a major health problem only in those parts of the world where the diet is poor in iodine and where there has been no iodization of salt (4). Severe iodine deficiency may lead to reduced thyroid hormone synthesis and thus to chronic hypothyroidism. This reduces the negative feedback at the pituitary and hypothalamus, resulting in a rise in TSH output. With continuing failure of thyroid hormone feedback, there will be a persistently increased TSH level, which will lead to the TSH induction and development of thyroid nodules causing multinodular goiters seen so commonly in the developing world. The World Health Organization (WHO) and others have exerted considerable effort to combat iodine deficiency with its consequences to the children of hypothyroid mothers. The effects include not only overt cretinism caused by lack of maternal thyroid hormone during critical periods of brain formation, but also markedly reduced intelligence in large numbers of the population where maternal iodine deficiency is less severe (5). Similar outcomes have been seen in women with thyroid failure and inadequate thyroid hormone replacement (6). This has been and continues to be a major public health problem in the United States. In addition, the effective use of iodine has been suggested to be an important evolutionary step in human development, perhaps by providing more thyroid hormone during brain development (7).

4 THYROGLOBULIN

With a molecular weight of 660,000 kDa, thyroglobulin is the second largest gene in the human genome (8). It is the major secretion of the thyroid follicular cell and is exported through the apical membrane to be stored as colloid in the center of the follicle. Prior to storage and at the apical membrane, iodination of thyroglobulin occurs forming the thyroid hormones. Under TSH stimulation, thyroglobulin loaded with thyroid hormones is withdrawn from the colloid and taken into the thyroid cell by endocytosis, forming colloid droplets within the cell cytoplasm. These droplets fuse with lysosomes leading to degradation of Tg and release of thyroid hormones (Fig. 2) (9). The complex is then transported to the basal membrane, where thyroid hormones and thyroglobulin are released into the circulation, once again under the influence of TSH. Any released iodide is largely recycled within the cell.

5 THYROID HORMONE CONSTRUCTION

Thyroid hormones are synthesized from iodide, under the control of TSH, in reactions that occur on the backbone of thyroglobulin (Tg) using a highly effective and immunogenic enzyme called thyroid peroxidase (TPO). Synthesis takes place at specific iodination sites on thyroglobulin and consists of binding of iodide to specific tyrosyl residues to form iodotyrosyls, which are then coupled to form iodothyronines (10). T4 results from the combination of two diiodotyrosines (DIT, or T2), and T3 results from the union of one monoiodotyrosine (MIT or T1) and one DIT (Fig. 3). Only in states of iodine deficiency is more T3 made than T4. As described earlier, the thyroid hormone–loaded Tg is then stored in the colloid of the thyroid follicle (Fig. 2). TSH causes the synthesis of thyroid hormones and also Tg. Colloidal Tg is taken back into the thyroid cell and exported at its base into the blood stream. It is easy to see that, in addition to disease of the thyroid itself, interruption in the pituitary control of the thyroid or a

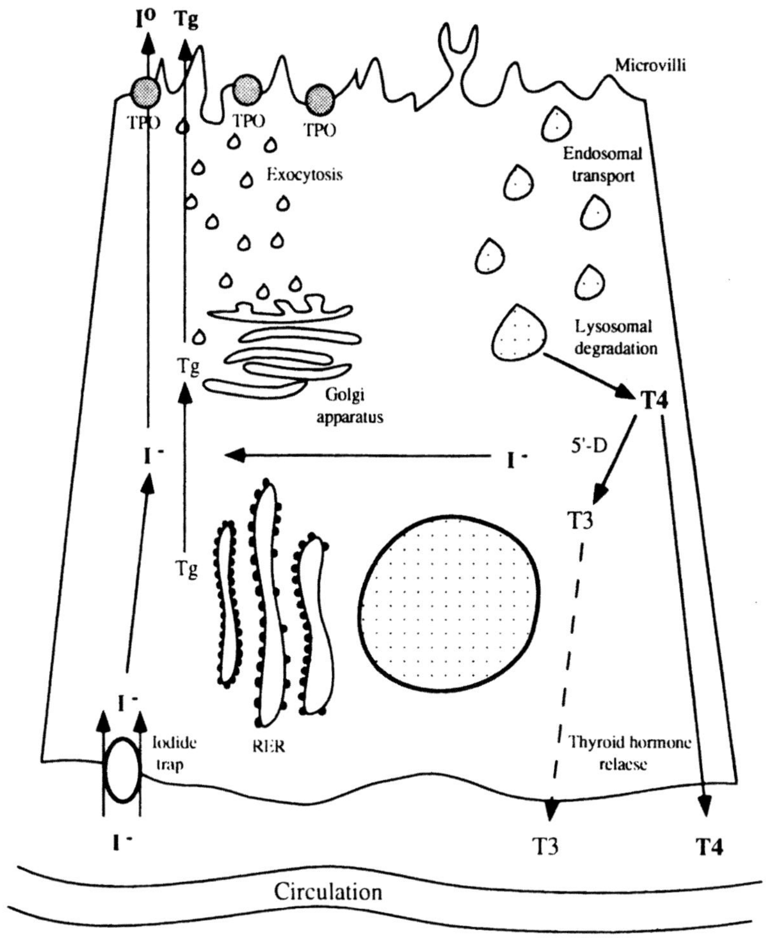

Figure 2 The thyroglobulin cycle. Steps in the synthesis and secretion of the thyroid hormones. Note the basal-apical-basal nature of this process. Iodide is trapped at the basal surface of the cell and moves quickly to the apical surface. Thyroglobulin (Tg) is initially synthesized in the endoplasmic reticulum (RER), and synthesis is completed in the Golgi apparatus. Tg is transported to the apical surface by exocytosis. Iodination of the Tg is catalyzed by thyroid peroxidase (TPO) at the apical portion of the cell. After reuptake into the cell as colloid droplets, the Tg moves to the basal surface by endosomal transport. T4 and T3 are released from the Tg via lysosomal degradation. The T4 and T3 are then secreted into the circulation at the basal membrane. TSH regulates all these steps of thyroid hormone synthesis and release. (From Ref. 29.)

shortage of iodide may compromise the synthetic ability of the thyroid cell. In fact the intake of iodide has been shown to influence the T2:T1 ratio in thyroglobulin (11).

6 RELEASE AND METABOLISM OF THYROID HORMONES

As described previously, pituitary TSH induces the resorption of stored iodinated thyroglobulin from the colloid and its transportation from the apical to the basal surface of the thyroid follicular cell. During this transport, T4 and a smaller amount of T3 are released from the thyroglobulin molecule and then into the circulation. Hence, thyroid hormone levels are a balance between the amount released by the thyroid gland and the amount entering the tissues, especially the liver and kidney. Most thyroid hormone released is T4, and this undergoes peripheral deiodination to T3 (1). Peripheral deiodination of T4 is best understood by considering T4 as a prohormone and T3 as the active hormone. T4 is converted to T3 by a widely available family of enzymes called the 5′-deiodinases (D) (Table 1). T3, therefore, is mainly produced from T4 in the tissues, where it is then available

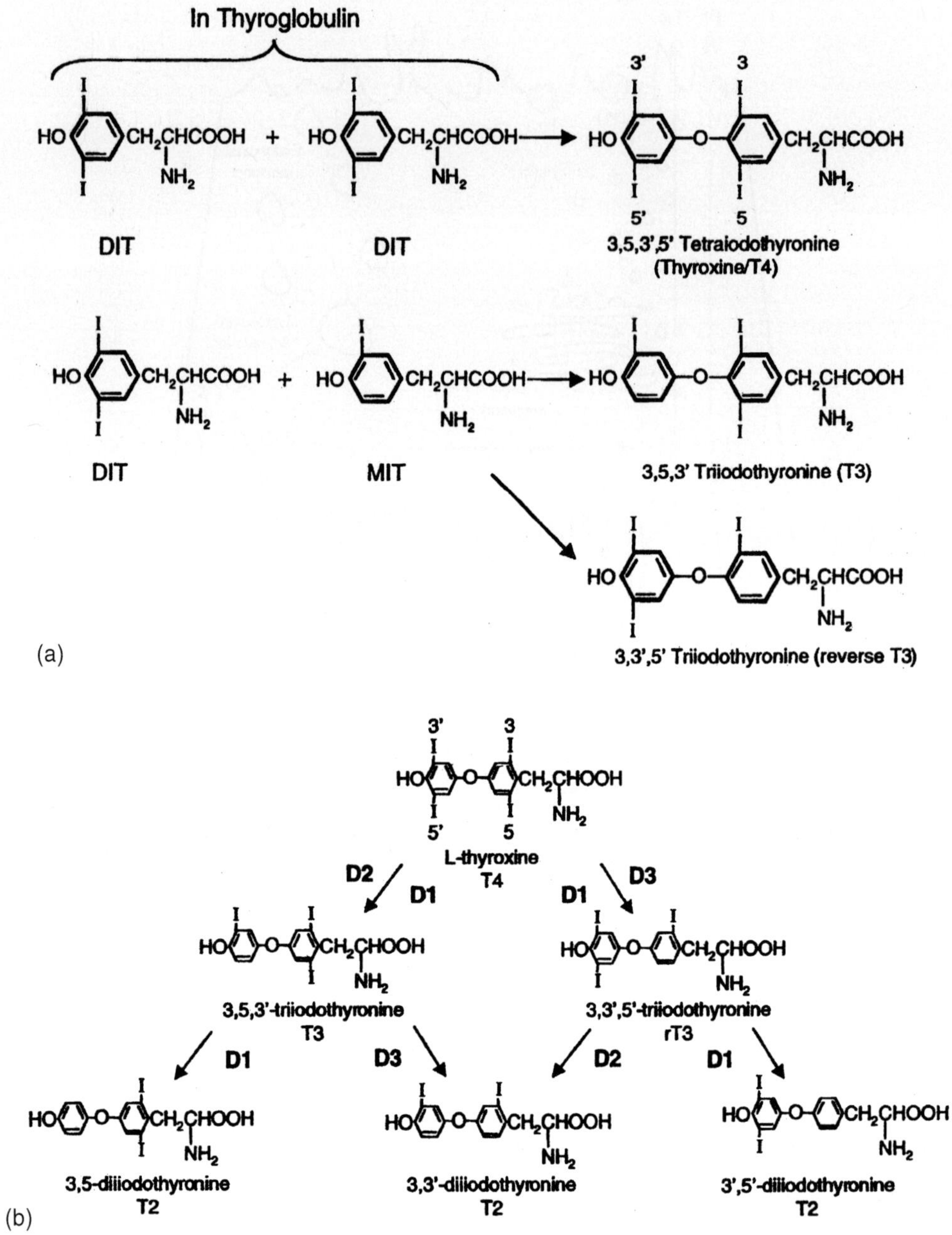

Figure 3 Thyroid hormone synthesis and degradation. (a) Synthetic pathway for T4, T3, and reverse T3. (b) Degradation pathway for T4 showing the different deiodinase enzymes (D1,D2, and D3) involved.

Table 1 The Deiodinase Enzymes

	Type I	Type II	Type III
Location	Liver, kidney Thyroid	CNS, pituitary Placenta, brown	Placenta, CNS Skin
Substrate	$rT_3 >$ sulfated thyronines $> T_4 > T_3$	$T_4 > rT_3 > T_3$	$T_4 \geq rT_3$
PTU	Inhibits	No effect	No effect
Selenium	Present	Absent	Absent
Km for T_4	High	Low	Low

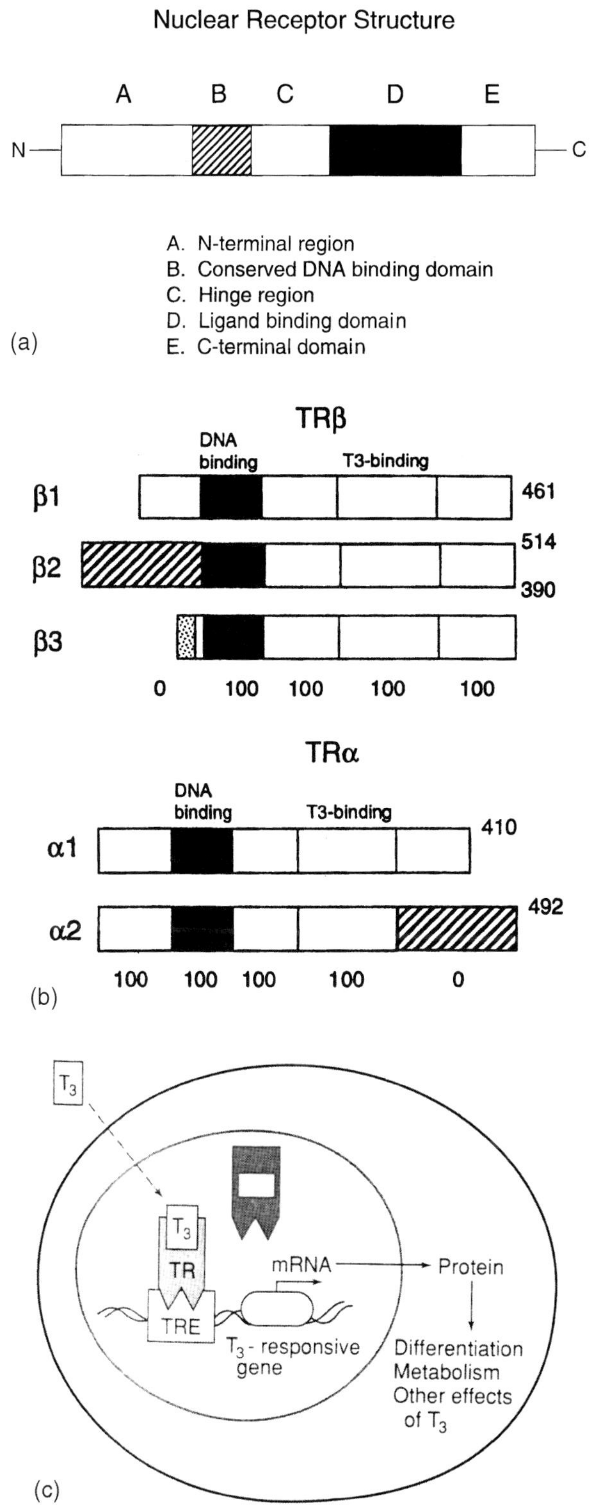

Table 2 Some Influences on Thyroxine Binding Globulin (TBG) Levels That Also Influence Total Serum T4 Levels

TBG is increased in:
Pregnancy
Estrogen therapy
Early hepatitis
Hypothyroidism
TBG is decreased in:
Androgen therapy
Hyperthyroidism
Liver failure
Renal failure

for action (Fig. 4). Recent data indicate that an intrathyroidal deiodinase enzyme can also influence this ratio of T4 to T3. In addition, T3 may be inactivated by further deiodination and the formation of sulfate conjugates or by the generation of acetic acid analogs. Similarly, the production of inactive reverse T3 also helps regulate circulating T3 levels.

7 MECHANISM OF ACTION OF THYROID HORMONES

Unbound, free T3 crosses the cell membrane to bind to intracellular T3 receptors, which are located in the cell nucleus and act as transcription factors in a complex network of influences on the genes that regulate cell growth, differentiation, and energy release among other actions (12). Four T3 nuclear receptors have been well characterized (Table 2) and designated α1, α2, β1, and β2 isoforms. The β2 receptors are unique to the pituitary gland and central to the phenomenon of TSH suppression by thyroid hormone

Figure 4 Thyroid hormone action. (a) Generic nuclear receptor structure; (b) thyroid hormone receptor structures; (c) T3 action via thyroid hormone receptors. T3 enters the cell or is derived from intracellular deiodination of T4. Nuclear interaction between a T3-bound thyroid hormone receptor (TR) and a thyroid hormone response element (TRE) results in increased or decreased activity of RNA polymerase on a T3-responsive gene. The TRE has two half-sites and may bind as a dimer. In the absence of T3, the TRE-bound TR may repress basal transcription. Many other transcriptional modulators are present, which may influence the binding of Trs and activation of T3-responsive genes.

feedback (Fig. 1). The other isoforms are widely distributed, and their varying proportions help explain the different influences of thyroid hormone on multiple tissues. Knocking out these receptors in the mouse has provided important new information on thyroid hormone action (13). For example, the α1 receptor is now thought to be important in the influence of thyroid hormone on the heart (14). In addition, mutations in the thyroid hormone β receptors have helped explain the rare syndrome of thyroid hormone resistance, which may vary from mildly abnormal thyroid function tests to reduced growth and mental retardation as well as hypothyroidism (15).

8 SERUM BINDING OF THYROID HORMONES

It is critically important to understand that thyroid hormones circulate in the blood in two forms—bound and free. Thyroid hormones are bound primarily to serum thyroxine-binding globulin (TBG) but also to other circulating liver proteins such as transthyretin (TTR), lipoproteins, and albumin. This binding is noncovalent and reversible, but only 0.03% of T4 and 0.3% of T3 is unbound and available as free thyroid hormones (free T4 and free T3). These free levels are reached by equilibration following changes in the levels of thyroid hormone or binding proteins. All measurements of thyroid hormone must, therefore, be identified as measurements of serum total or free hormone. Lastly, because much more of T4 than T3 binds to serum protein, the half-life of T4 is much longer (7 days) than that of T3 (1 day) and so serum T3 levels are subject to much more rapid changes than those of T4.

Many factors influence the concentration of TBG, to which 80% of T4 is bound. For example, estrogen increases TBG levels by enhancing synthesis and altering TBG glycosylation in such a way that the half-life of TBG is prolonged. Recent data remind us that even oral contraceptive pills may result in an increase in TBG significant enough that normal free T4 levels are not maintained and T4 supplementation may need to be increased in hypothyroid patients (16). Because there are many influences on the level of thyroid-binding proteins, the measurement of total T4 and total T3 levels must be corrected for the level of serum-binding protein. This results in the expression of T4:TBG ratios in varying forms. Hence the increasing preference by physicians for direct or indirect measurements of free T3 and free T4 (17).

9 THYROID FUNCTION TESTING

9.1 The Pituitary-Thyroid Axis and the Response of Serum TSH to Changes in Thyroid Hormone Levels

From the explanations provided so far, we can deduce that serum TSH levels will respond to changes in serum thyroid hormone levels. An increased T4 level will lead to increased T3 levels within the TSH-secreting cells of the anterior pituitary after 5′-deiodination by Type 2 DI. The T3 will then bind to an α2 intracellular thyroid hormone receptor (TR), which acts as a transcription factor, and the complex will then bind to a thyroid response element (TRE) in the 5′ region of the TSH-β gene. This binding acts in a negative manner, suppressing activation of the TSH-β gene and leading to decreased TSH synthesis and release. A similar phenomenon is employed to control TRH release in the hypothalamus. At the opposite extreme, a lack of T4 will mean less T3 available to bind to its receptor and fewer complexes binding to the TREs. Hence, less negative regulation will lead to increased TSH synthesis and release. This feedback control has allowed the measurement of serum TSH levels to be developed as the most sensitive and useful thyroid function test, with suppressed TSH levels indicating hyperthyroidism and raised TSH levels as evidence of hypothyroidism (18). Nevertheless, any changes in serum TSH should always be confirmed, if possible, with thyroid hormone measurements (Fig. 5).

9.2 The Measurement of Serum TSH

The wide availability of rapid and highly sensitive immunoassays for the measurement of serum TSH has transformed thyroid function testing into a logical area of understanding and greatly reduced the need for additional T4 and T3 testing in the majority of patients with normal TSH results. TSH assays are often referred to as belonging to a particular developmental generation dependent on their sensitivity (18). These days there is no need to use anything but a third-generation assay with a sensitivity of <0.01 μU/mL. These TSH assays allow the clear diagnosis of even mild thyroid dysfunction. In the absence of obvious pituitary disease, the serum TSH will increase in thyroid failure (>4.0 μU/mL) and be markedly decreased in the presence of an overactive thyroid gland (>0.1 μU/mL). The former may be confirmed with a free T4 assay and the latter with both free T4 and T3 assays. However, mild thyroid disease may present with only changes in TSH while

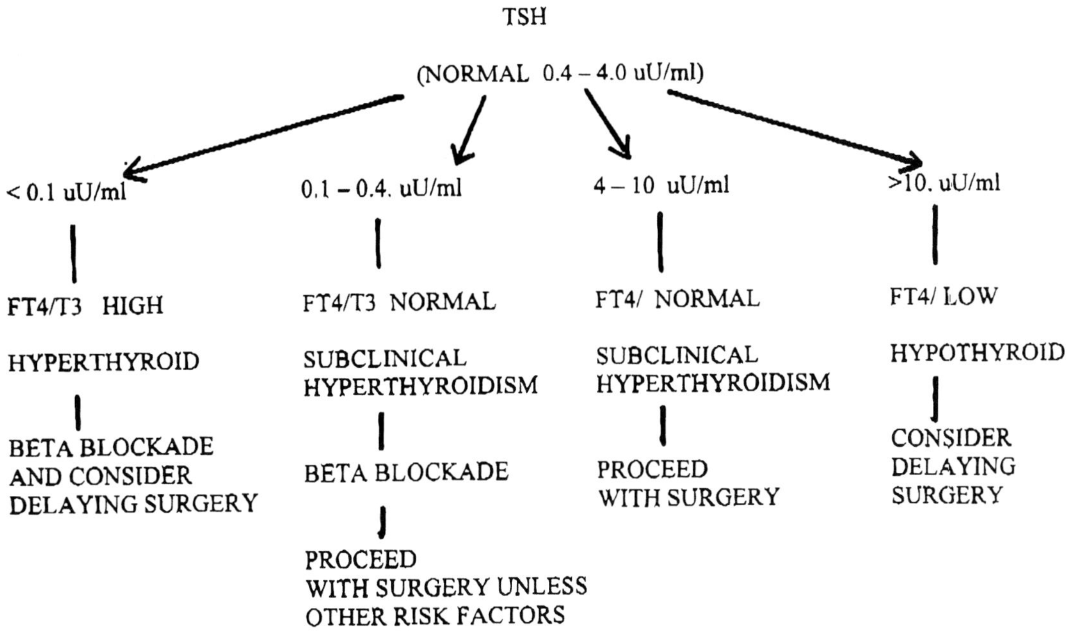

Figure 5 Thyroid function testing in surgical practice.

thyroid hormone levels remain within the normal range (so-called subclinical disease).

9.3 Total and Free T4

The measurement of total T4 remains the easiest thyroid function test to perform and is an important part of our investigative armamentarium. It is essential to try to confirm a high TSH with a measurement indicating a low T4 level since this allows the distinction between mild (normal T4) and significant (low T4) thyroid failure. However, the disadvantage of total T4 measurement is that a correction must be applied for the level of serum-binding proteins. This can be made using a resin uptake test (Fig. 6) or a direct measurement of TBG. Alternatively, a free T4 measurement may be derived directly from increasingly popular binding tests now available on many automatic analyzers or by the classical dialysis method. The latter, however, is an expensive technique and should be reserved for very extreme situations when TBG is very high or very low, causing the derived methods of estimating free T4 to be unreliable (19).

9.4 Total T3 and Free T3

After serum TSH measurement, serum T3 levels are the best confirmation of an overactive thyroid gland. Less T3 is bound to the serum-binding proteins than T4, and therefore the measurement of Total T3 is not as affected by changes in protein binding as is total T4. However, it remains helpful to know that there are no major binding protein changes when the total T3 level is abnormal, although in practice free T3 levels are not often needed (19).

9.5 Radioiodine Scanning Versus Sonography

The scanning of the thyroid gland using radioiodine (either I^{131} or I^{123}, which causes less radiation exposure) has been largely superceded by real-time sonography. When the serum TSH is suppressed, a thyroid nodule or multinodular gland must have active nodular tissue ("hot") secreting thyroid hormone causing the TSH suppression. When the TSH is normal, the gland is most likely to harbor predominantly underactive nodules ("cold"), with the euthyroid state maintained by the remaining normal tissue. However, sonography gives much more reliable identification and sizing of thyroid nodules than any scanning procedure. The major use of radioiodine scanning today, therefore, is to detect small residual thyroid cancer metastases after total thyroidectomy (20). In contrast, 24-hour radioiodine uptake measurements remain frequently used to differentiate chemical hyperthyroidism secondary to thyroiditis (no uptake due to cellular

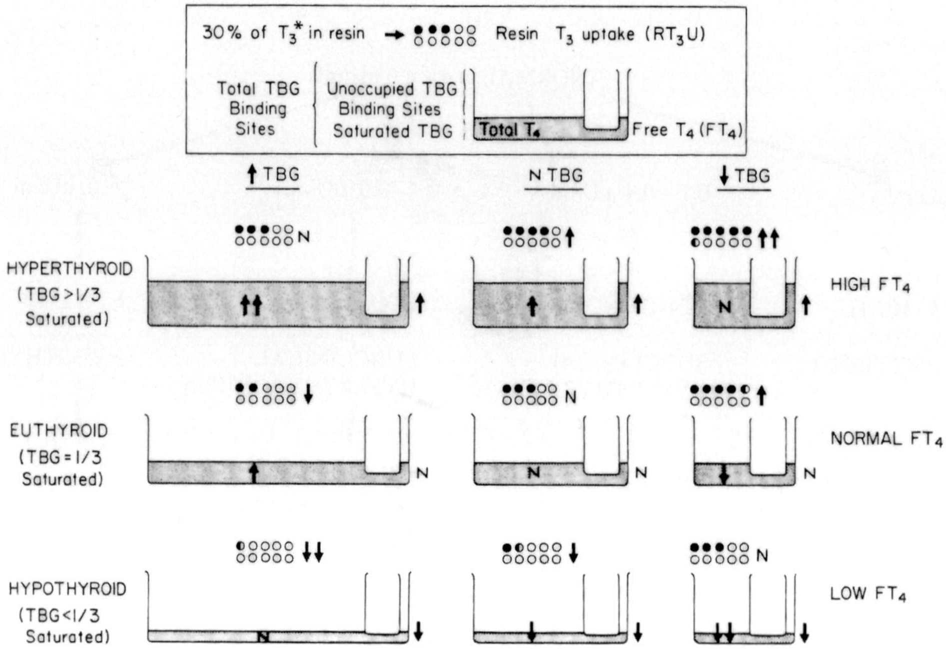

Figure 6 The T3 resin uptake test. Graphic representation of the relationship between the serum TT4 concentration, the RT3U test, and the FT4 concentration in various metabolic conditions and in association with changes in TBG. The principle of communicating vessels is used as an illustration. The height of the fluid in the small vessel represents the level of FT4; the total amount of fluid in the large vessel, the TT4; and the total volume of the large vessel, the TBG capacity. The RT3U test result (black dots) is inversely proportional to the unfilled capacity of the large vessel (unoccupied TBG). (From Ref. 30.)

destruction) from hyperthyroidism caused by Graves' disease (normal or increased uptake induced by thyroid-stimulating antibodies).

9.6 The Serum Thyroglobulin Assay

Most thyroid disease causes an increase in serum Tg levels, making this determination an unreliable measurement in thyroid dysfunction. However, the thyroid gland is the major source of serum Tg, and therefore the measurement of serum Tg has become a clinically useful test for the presence of residual thyroid tissue (21). This is particularly valuable in the follow-up of patients with thyroid cancer who have been treated by total thyroidectomy followed by radioiodine ablation to remove the presence of all residual thyroid tissue. Under such circumstances, the persistence or development of serum Tg indicates the persistence of residual thyroid tissue. Furthermore, if the serum Tg rises while the patient is receiving thyroid hormone replacement (maintaining a low TSH level), then this is very suggestive of metastatic disease. Recently, it has been shown that significant residual metastatic disease can be stimulated to secrete Tg in thyroid cancer patients using recombinant human TSH (22). This can be performed while the patient remains on thyroid hormone suppression, avoiding the unpleasant prolonged withdrawal of thyroid hormone in order to raise endogenous TSH.

9.7 Thyroid Autoantibody Testing

Thyroid antibody testing does not help the assessment of thyroid function. Such tests are used only in the diagnosis and prediction of autoimmune thyroid disease (Graves' disease and Hashimoto's thyroiditis) and are complicated by the presence of such antibodies in up to 20% of the normal population (23). The most commonly measured thyroid antibodies are those to the enzyme thyroid peroxidase (anti-TPO) and to thyroglobulin (anti-Tg) that are easily measured by enzyme-linked immunoabsorbent assay or competitive binding assays (24). These antibodies are usually present in all patients with autoimmune thyroid disease and in very high titers in patients with Hashimoto's thyroiditis. Another commonly measured antibody is found in Graves' disease. The cause of hyperthyroid Graves' disease is the development of thyroid-stimulating antibodies that bind to and stimulate the TSH receptor. These unique antibodies are usually measured clinically as antibodies to the TSH receptor by using competition with radiolabeled TSH for binding to soluble TSH receptors. Only rarely, such as in pregnancy, are biological assays for thyroid-stimulating activity needed. These assays can be performed using thyroid cells or model cells transfected with the TSH receptor (24–26). Some 15% of patients with Hashimoto's thyroiditis have TSH receptor antibodies, which block the TSH receptor rather than stimulate it.

10 THE SICK EUTHYROID SYNDROME

Despite "normal" thyroid function, total T3 and T4 levels are decreased in the presence of severe and chronic illness leading to the concept of the sick euthyroid syndrome (27). There are many reasons for the fall in T3 and T4 levels in this situation, which often first presents with a low T3 and only later with a fall in T4. The half-life of T3 is much shorter than that of T4, and it is bound to binding proteins with much lower affinity than T4, explaining why serum T3 levels change so much more quickly than serum T4 levels. There is also a metabolic block in very sick patients shifting 5′-deiodination to the production of inactive reverse T3 (Fig. 3). Hence, a fall in T3 is the dramatic expression of a metabolic problem, exacerbated by an increased distribution space between sick cells, and a fall in effective TSH levels and/or changes in TSH glycosylation, which also reduces its bioactivity. In practice, immunoassayable TSH levels can be quite variable and often marginally increased. Later, particularly as the serum protein levels fall because of inadequate hepatic production, there follows a marked fall in serum T4 levels, which often predicts a poor outlook for the patient (Fig. 7). During these swings in total T3 and T4 levels, the concentration of free hormone levels may remain normal. However, all results may be found depending on the speed of the metabolic changes with which the free hormone levels have to equilibrate. The presence of true thyroid disease during this phenomenon requires considerable expertise to assess.

11 URGENT SURGICAL ASSESSMENT OF THYROID FUNCTION

Most medical centers can now provide rapid thyroid function test results within a matter of hours. TSH, FT4, and T3 levels can all be obtained by automatic analyzers, allowing an early assessment of thyroid function in any situation. Only rarely is thyroid dysfunction sufficient to delay urgent surgery, but elective procedures should await the return to euthyroidism. The physician and the anesthesiologist will work with the surgical team to achieve this aim. The dangers of surgery in an uncontrolled hyperthyroid patient include

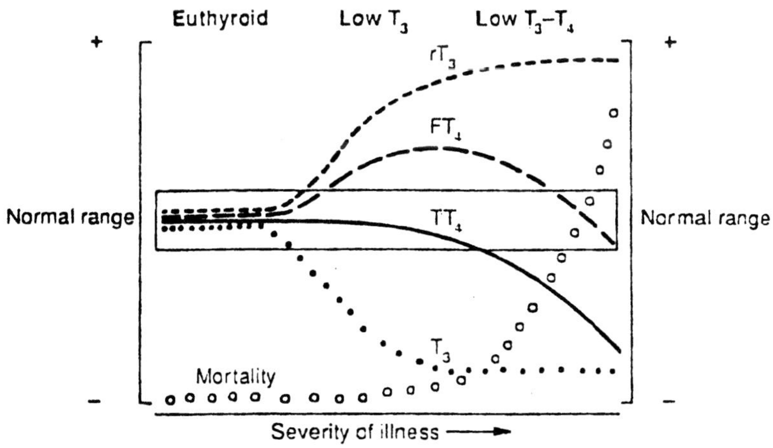

Figure 7 The sick euthyroid syndrome. A schematic representation of the changes in serum thyroid hormone values with increasing severity of nonthyroidal illness. A rapidly rising mortality rate accompanies the fall in serum TT4 and FT3 values. (From Ref. 31.)

increased cardiac risk, particularly in an elderly patient, and the occurrence of severely exacerbated hyperthyroidism after surgery ("thyroid storm").

REFERENCES

1. Larsen PR. Update on the human iodothyronine selenodeiodinases, the enzymes regulating the activation and inactivation of thyroid hormone. Biochem Soc Trans 1997; 25:588–592.
2. Riedel C, Dohan O, De I, V, Ginter CS, Carrasco N. Journey of the iodide transporter NIS: from its molecular identification to its clinical role in cancer. Trends Biochem Sci 2001; 26(8):490–496.
3. Dunn JT. What's happening to our iodine? J Clin Endocrinol Metab 1998; 83(10):3398–3400.
4. Delange F, de Benoist B, Pretell E, Dunn JT. Iodine deficiency in the world: where do we stand at the turn of the century? Thyroid 2001; 11(5):437–447.
5. Glinoer D. Pregnancy and iodine. Thyroid 2001; 11(5): 471–481.
6. Glinoer D. Potential consequences of maternal hypothyroidism on the offspring: evidence and implications. Horm Res 2001; 55(3):109–114.
7. Kraiem Z. Thoughts on the role of iodine in the emergence of modern humans. Thyroid 2001; 11(8): 807–808.
8. Moya CM, Mendive FM, Rivolta CM, Vassart G, Targovnik HM. Genomic organization of the 5′ region of the human thyroglobulin gene. Eur J Endocrinol 2000; 143(6):789–798.
9. Venkatesh SG, Deshpande V. A comparative review of the structure and biosynthesis of thyroglobulin. Comp Biochem Physiol C Pharmacol Toxicol Endocrinol 1999; 122(1):13–20.
10. Lamas L, Anderson PC, Fox JW, Dunn JT. Concensus sequences for early iodination and hormonogenesis in human thyroglobulin. J Biol Chem 1989; 264:13541–13545.
11. Dunn JT, Dunn AD. Update on intrathyroidal iodine metabolism. Thyroid 2001; 11(5):407–414.
12. Yen PM. Physiological and molecular basis of thyroid hormone action. Physiol Rev 2001; 81(3):1097–1142.
13. Forrest D, Vennstrom B. Functions of thyroid hormone receptors in mice. Thyroid 2000; 10(1):41–52.
14. Wikstrom L, Johansson C, Salto C, et al. Abnormal heart rate and body temperature in mice lacking thyroid hormone receptor alpha 1. EMBO J 1998; 17(2):455–461.
15. Weiss RE, Refetoff S. Resistance to thyroid hormone. Rev Endocr Metab Disord 2000; 1(1–2):97–108.
16. Arafah BM. Increased need for thyroxine in women with hypothyroidism during estrogen therapy. N Engl J Med 2001; 344(23):1743–1749.
17. Midgley JE. Direct and indirect free thyroxine assay methods: theory and practice. Clin Chem 2001; 47(8): 1353–1363.
18. Spencer CA, Takeuchi M, Kazarosyan M. Current status and performance goals for serum thyroglobulin assays. Clin Chem 1996; 42(1):164–173.
19. Stockigt JR. Free thyroid hormone measurement. A critical appraisal. Endocrinol Metab Clin North Am 2001; 30(2):265–289.
20. McGregor AM, Petersen MM, McLachlan SM, Rooke P, Smith BR, Hall R. Carbimazole and the autoimmune response in Graves' disease. N Engl J Med 1980; 303: 302–304.
21. Spencer CA, LoPresti JS, Fatemi S, Nicoloff JT. Detection of residual and recurrent differentiated thyroid carcinoma by serum thyroglobulin measurement. Thyroid 1999; 9(5):435–441.
22. Haugen BR, Pacini F, Reiners C, et al. A comparison of recombinant human thyrotropin and thyroid hormone withdrawal for the detection of thyroid remnant or cancer. J Clin Endocrinol Metab 1999; 84(11):3877–3885.
23. Vanderpump MPJ, Tunbridge WMG, French JM, et al. The incidence of thyroid disorders in the community: a twenty-year follow-up of the Whickham survey. Clin Endocrinol (Oxf) 1995; 43:55–68.
24. Davies TF. The pathogenesis of Graves' disease. In: Braverman LE, Utiger RD, eds. The Thyroid: A Fundamental Text. 8th ed. Philadelphia: Lippincott, 2000:525–536.
25. Davies TF. Thyroid-stimulating antibodies predict hyperthyroidism. J Clin Endocrinol Metab 1998; 83: 3777–3781.
26. Ludgate M, Perret J, Parmentier M, et al. Use of recombinant human thyrotropin receptor (TSH-R) expressed in mamalian cell lines to assay TSH-R autoantibodies. Mol Cell Endocrinol 1990; 73:R13–R18.
27. Camacho PM, Dwarkanathan AA. Sick euthyroid syndrome. What to do when thyroid function tests are abnormal in critically ill patients. Postgrad Med 1999; 105(4):215–219.
28. Griffin JE. The thyroid. In: Griffin JE, Ojeda SR, eds. Textbook of Endocrine Physiology. New York: Oxford, 1992:224–246.
29. Falk SA. Surgical treatment of hyperthyroidism. In: Falk SA, ed. Thyroid Disease. Philadelphia: Lippincott, 1997:319–340.
30. Refetoff S. In: De Groot LJ, ed. Endocrinology. Thyroid Hormone Transport. Grune & Stratton, 1979: 347–358.
31. Nicoloff JT. Abnormal measurements in nonendocrine illness. In: Hurst JW, ed. Medicine for the Practicing Physician. Butterworth-Heineman, 1991.

8

Thyroid Pathology

Margaret Brandwein-Gensler, Arthur E. Schwartz, and Pamela Unger

Mount Sinai School of Medicine, New York University, New York, New York, U.S.A.

1 BENIGN LESIONS

1.1 Goiter

Goiter (from the Latin *guttur*, or throat) is a clinical term used to describe any thyroid enlargement. The term generally refers to enlargement resulting from a variety of benign conditions: physiological (puberty, pregnancy), metabolic (dietary iodine deficiency, i.e., endemic goiter), abnormal iodine metabolism, or inflammatory/autoimmune diseases (Hashimoto's disease, Graves' disease). Since this term lacks specificity, thyroid malignancies also appear as a thyroid enlargement or mass. Early goiters may present as simple, smooth, or mildly enlarged palpable glands. Prolonged thyroid enlargement results in the formation of multiple adenomatous nodules, which may undergo hemorrhage and fibrosis, leading to a multinodular (adenomatous) goiter. Although adenomatous goiters are usually benign, they can cause serious clinical problems. The gland can be grossly disfiguring, encroach upon the trachea, or produce respiratory obstruction or hoarseness from recurrent laryngeal nerve paresis. Intrathoracic goiters can obstruct venous return (superior vena cava syndrome) as well as cause severe respiratory difficulties. As goiters increase in size, they can impinge upon and distort the trachea or esophagus, resulting in dyspnea and dysphagia.

On gross examination, a multinodular goiter may present as small nodules distributed diffusely or asymmetrically throughout the gland. Cut sections reveal multiple nodules, their glassy, pink/mahogany surface reflecting colloid storage. Histologically, one sees multiple follicles with flattened thyrocytes and colloid accumulation, with fibrosis, hemorrhage, calcification, and even ossification.

1.2 Adenomas

1.2.1 Follicular Adenoma

The most common solitary thyroid mass is an adenoma. These are encapsulated, benign, expansions of thyroid follicles, compressing adjacent thyroid parenchyma. On gross inspection, the capsule is usually thin and flimsy; a thickened capsule can raise the diagnostic possibility of a "minimally invasive follicular carcinoma" (this term is defined below) (1). Thyroid follicles can be large and distended by colloid or smaller with variable colloid content. Evidence of hyperactivity can be seen. If an adenoma is significantly hyperfunctional (e.g., toxic adenoma), then the histological distinction between it and an encapsulated papillary thyroid carcinoma can be difficult. This is because stimulated, hyperfunctioning thyroid will form hyperplastic pseudopapillae (see below). Adenomas may have a varied follicular architecture, which is of no prognostic significance. However, some variants of follicular adenomas require special mention.

1.2.2 Hürthle Cell Adenoma

Hürthle cells are thyrocytes that have undergone oncocytic metaplasia, a process of unknown significance that can occur in many endocrine and nonendocrine organs; it occurs in various processes: inflammatory (Hashimoto's thyroiditis), benign (Hürthle cell adenoma), or malignant (Hürthle cell carcinoma). Macroscopically, a Hürthle cell adenoma is an encapsulated mass with a deep mahogany hue. This color can be seen in any histologically oncocytic neoplasm (e.g., renal cell oncocytoma, parotid oncocytoma). Microscopically, the term oncocyte refers to cells with abundant, bright pink, granular cytoplasm due to increased mitochondria. Hürthle cells are large thyrocytes that have undergone oncocytic change. The cells can also be pleomorphic (i.e., atypical) and therefore worrisome. However, the criteria for malignancy remains the same for all follicular neoplasia: in the absence of capsular invasion or subcapsular vascular invasion, all follicular lesions, including all Hürthle cell adenomas, regardless of pleomorphism, are still benign adenomas. The distinction between Hürthle cell adenomas and carcinomas (as well as follicular adenomas and minimally invasive follicular carcinomas) relies on architecture (capsular or vascular invasion), not cytological features, such as cellular pleomorphism or mitoses. Neither fine needle aspiration nor frozen section examination can address this distinction. Fine needle aspiration permits only cytological evaluation. Frozen section examination allows only limited tissue sampling as compared to permanent section evaluation; focal diagnostic findings of invasion may not be observed. The size of Hürthle cell tumors may be helpful since it correlates strongly ($p < 0.005$) with the likelihood of malignancy. Large tumors (> 4 cm) are more likely to be malignant than small tumors (< 2 cm) (2,3).

1.2.3 Atypical Adenoma?

Historically, this term was applied to follicular adenomas (especially Hürthle cell adenomas) that possessed atypical features (nuclear atypia, necrosis) but fell short of the criteria required for malignancy (capsular invasion or subcapsular vascular invasion). They were often reported as "indeterminate" or "possibly malignant." Importantly, follow-up studies have shown that tumors classified as indeterminate behave in a clinically benign fashion, removing the need for this term (4).

1.2.4 Hyalinizing Trabecular Tumor

This uncommon subtype (also referred to as benign hyalinizing trabecular adenoma or malignant hyalinizing trabecular carcinoma) may be confused with thyroid malignancies; its own oncological potential has also been questioned. It appears as an encapsulated tan mass, microscopically composed of polygonal, oval, and elongated tumor cells arranged in cords (trabeculae) or clusters (Zellballen) with minimal follicle formation. The cellular cytoplasm is finely granular, oncocytic, or optically clear. Similar to papillary thyroid carcinoma, its nuclei are oval, elongated, with inclusions and grooves. Rare psammoma bodies can also be seen. The differential diagnosis includes medullary carcinoma and papillary thyroid carcinoma. Immunohistochemistry of hyalinizing trabecular adenoma confirms expression of thyroglobulin, but not calcitonin, distinguishing it from medullary carcinoma. The distinction between hyalinizing trabecular adenoma and papillary thyroid carcinoma can be difficult, and in fact bono fide papillary thyroid carcinoma can develop within hyalinizing trabecular adenoma, raising suspicions that hyalinizing trabecular adenoma may be a precursor of papillary thyroid carcinoma. To wit, RET/PTC gene rearrangements are common to papillary thyroid carcinoma and have also been detected in hyalinizing trabecular adenoma. To date, tumors reported as typical hyalinizing trabecular adenoma have followed benign courses (5–7).

1.3 Black Thyroid

Black thyroid is a curious incidental finding caused by injection of minocycline, a tetracycline derivative administered in the treatment of acne. Patients on long-term, high-dose minocycline therapy may develop pigment deposition in numerous organ systems, including the thyroid. This is thought to result from an oxidative interaction between minocycline and thyroid peroxidase; it may remain even after cessation of the drug. Grossly, the thyroid gland is black, and microscopically, the thyrocytes and colloid are pigmented. The pigmentation itself has no adverse affect on the thyroid gland. The incidental finding of thyroid pigmentation is usually limited to the surrounding gland and spares the adenoma or carcinoma that prompted surgery (8,9).

2 THYROIDITIS

2.1 Hashimoto's Thyroiditis

2.1.1 Diagnosis and Pathobiology

Hashimoto's thyroiditis is an autoimmune thyroiditis characterized by lymphocytic infiltration and destruction of thyroid with eventual loss of function. There is a marked female predominance; it is usually diagnosed during or after the fourth decade of life. Patients are usually euthyroid but may also present with hypothyroidism or hyperthyroidism (Hashitoxicosis). The usual presentation is that of a painless, firm thyroid mass. The gland may be asymmetrically enlarged, clinically simulating malignancy. Surgeons considering the diagnosis of Hashimoto's thyroiditis in these circumstances may avoid unnecessary thyroidectomies. The inflammation and fibrosis that often accompany Hashimoto's thyroiditis make surgical dissection especially difficult, with increased risk of damage to the recurrent laryngeal nerves and parathyroid glands. Fine needle aspiration and serological studies (see below) can lead to the diagnosis preoperatively. Serologically, patients with Hashimoto's thyroiditis have elevated antithyroid antibodies, mainly antithyroperoxidase, antithyroglobulin, and antimicrosomal antibodies. Antimicrosomal antibodies are specific but not sensitive in establishing the diagnosis (10). Cytological examination reveals abundant lymphocytes and Hürthle cells; fine needle aspiration may have good sensitivity to detect a diffuse process like Hashimoto's thyroiditis, but sampling limitations may fail to detect concomitant malignancy.

Hashimoto's thyroiditis is caused by abnormal activation of helper T lymphocytes within the thyroid. This may occur after viral infection or as a result of aberrant thyrocyte expression of major histocompatibility (MHC) class II proteins; these are the membrane glycoproteins responsible for immune distinction between "self" and "nonself". The activated T cells then recruit B lymphocytes, which produce a variety of antithyroid antibodies, and cytotoxic T cells that destroy thyrocytes. Thyroids affected by Hashimoto's thyroiditis are usually tan in color, reflecting the lymphocytic infiltrate. Microscopically, lymphocytes are seen infiltrating the thyroid and forming germinal centers. The thyrocytes may undergo oncocytic metaplasia (Hürthle cell change).

Eventually patients with Hashimoto's thyroiditis have depleted thyroid function, but they may remain euthyroid or develop episodic, fluctuating thyroid dysfunction. Less common complications include episodic hyperthyroidism or Hashimoto's encephalopathy. These patients are at risk for developing other autoimmune conditions, as well as thyroid malignancies (see below). Hashimoto's thyroiditis is managed by monitoring thyroid function and providing synthroid replacement for hypothyroidism (11).

2.1.2 Incidence of Neoplasia in Hashimoto's Thyroiditis

Lymphoma. There is a clear association between Hashimoto's thyroiditis and increased risk of thyroid lymphoma (12,13). The vast majority of thyroid lymphomas are encountered in patients with Hashimoto's thyroiditis. The usual presentation is that of a dramatically enlarging thyroid mass in an older woman, mimicking anaplastic carcinoma. The diagnosis may be established by fine-needle aspiration or core needle biopsy, avoiding unnecessary thyroidectomy in these cases. Histologically, most of these lymphomas are of B-cell origin, usually diffuse large B-cell lymphoma. Immunohistochemistry is routinely performed on such cases to make the distinction between lymphoma and other malignancies, (e.g., anaplastic carcinoma, undifferentiated squamous cell carcinoma) and then to further type the lymphoma. Many older literature reports of survivors of anaplastic thyroid carcinoma erroneously contained patients with large-cell malignant lymphoma, falsely improving the survival statistics.

Fine needle aspiration has the potential to establish the diagnosis preoperatively. The next diagnostic option includes core needle or open biopsy with frozen section analysis. This allows for fresh tissue to be saved for lymphoma markers. Only general lymphocyte, B-cell, and T-cell, markers can be immunohistochemically studied using formalin-fixed paraffin embedded tissue. The diagnostic sensitivity and specificity of fresh tissue studies is much greater: a vast array of lymphocyte markers can be detected, and B-cell clonality can be confirmed. Once a diagnosis of thyroid lymphoma is established, surgery is not a therapeutic option. Appropriate therapy is determined by clinical staging. The majority of cases present as either stage IE (confined to thyroid) or IIE disease (positive cervical and/or mediastinum lymph nodes). Radiotherapy is indicated for Stage IE disease, whereas adjuvant chemotherapy is preferred for patients with Stage II, III, and IV disease. Overall, thyroid lymphomas have a favorable outcome, but prognosis depends on clinical stage and histology: high-grade lymphomas or stage greater than IE have the greatest potential for a poor outcome. The overall relapse-free survival at 5 years is 72%, and the overall survival at 5 years is 88% (14–17).

Papillary Thyroid Carcinoma. The incidence of papillary thyroid carcinoma for patients with Hashimoto's thyroiditis is greater than expected, which initially suggested a causal relationship (18,19). But the burden of proving causality is a difficult task since both entities are relatively common, and their association may be considered merely coincidental. Lymphocytic infiltrate is common adjacent to papillary thyroid carcinoma and cannot be taken as evidence of Hashimoto's' thyroiditis. In addition, cytological atypia is common in Hashimoto's thyroiditis and may lead to the overdiagnosis of papillary thyroid carcinoma. Be that as it may, the RET/PTC1 and RET/PTC3 oncogenes, highly specific for thyroid malignancy, have been found in 95% of the Hashimoto's patients studied, without papillary thyroid carcinoma, suggesting a preneoplastic condition (20).

2.2 Graves' Disease

2.2.1 Diagnosis and Pathobiology

Graves' disease is an autoimmune thyroiditis resulting in hyperthyroidism. There is a female predominance of 6–10:1. Patients typically present with a goiter and hyperthyroidism. Radioactive iodine uptake is usually diffusely increased but may be localized to a dominant nodule ("toxic adenoma"). Opthalmopathy (exopthalmos, impaired ocular motility, diplopia) is frequently present and can alert the clinician to consider the diagnosis of Graves' disease. It is the most frequent cause of unilateral exopthalmos. In contrast to Hashimoto's thyroiditis, in which the thyroid parenchyma constitutes the actual lymphocytic battleground, Graves' disease can be considered as an "assault from afar." Host lymphocytes produce an array of antibodies that stimulate the TSH (thyroid-stimulating hormone) receptor, resulting in hyperthyroidism. However, the lymphocytic infiltration and mediated thyrocyte destruction present in Hashimoto's thyroiditis are not seen in Graves' disease. As in Hashimoto's thyroiditis, thyrocytes of Graves' disease also aberrantly express MHC antigens, thus stimulating immune reaction.

Graves' disease may be further complicated by pretibial myxedema, a nonpitting edema of the lower legs that invariably follows the hyperthyroidism and opthalmopathy and is probably a result of antithyroid antibodies cross-reacting and stimulating fibroblast receptors, resulting in glycosoaminoglycan overproduction. Graves' opthalmopathy is due to swelling of the extraocular muscles and retrobulbar fat. Similar to pretibial edema, it is due to excessive production of glycosoaminoglycans by orbital fibroblasts. The opthalmopathy is the result of a direct autoimmune targeting of orbital fibroblasts, probably through TSH receptor antibodies (21–23). After thyroid suppression or radioactive ablation, a Hashimoto's-like lymphocytic infiltrate remains; the aftermath of this battle is hypothyroidism, which will require synthroid replacement. The severe complications of Graves' opthalmopathy (corneal abrasion, impending blindness) require orbital decompression.

2.2.2 Diagnostic Differentiation from Papillary Thyroid Carcinoma

A thyroid gland affected by Graves' disease is enlarged, reddened, and "meaty," histologically manifesting colloid depletion and follicular hyperplasia. If colloid is present it is watery (nondense) or scalloped. The thyrocytes are tall and form pseudopapillae. A hyperfunctioning adenoma is an encapsulated lesion with the identical hyperplastic papillary histological findings. The distinction between the follicular hyperplasia of Graves' disease and papillary thyroid carcinoma may at times be difficult, especially during frozen section. The nuclear morphology, which aids in the recognition of papillary thyroid carcinoma (optically cleared nuclei, nuclear holes, nuclear grooves), is more reliably observed in the routine formalin-fixed "permanent sections" than in the nonfixed frozen section slides. In papillary thyroid carcinoma, the tumor nuclei are enlarged, oval, and overlapping, whereas the nuclei of hyperplastic thyrocytes remain smaller and rounded.

2.3 Subacute Thyroiditis—de Quervain's (Giant Cell) Thyroiditis

De Quervain's thyroiditis (giant cell, or granulomatous, or subacute granulomatous thyroiditis) is a transient thyroiditis. It is important to recognize this clinical entity, which is usually self-limiting, in order to avoid unnecessary surgery. Patients present with thyroid tenderness, referred ear pain, goiter, elevated serum T3, T4, and elevated erythrocyte sedimentation rate. The thyroid is diffusely enlarged and firm. There is a history of antecedent upper respiratory infection, but patients may also present with an acute, febrile illness with weakness and malaise. De Quervain's thyroiditis is considered a non-autoimmune, postviral thyroiditis.

The diagnosis can be established by clinical history, physical examination, and fine needle aspiration, which reveals plump transformed thyrocytes, epithelioid granulomas, multinucleated giant cells, and an acute and chronic inflammatory background, (24). Thyroid scintigraphy frequently reveals uniform decreased uptake, but at times the decreased uptake can be localized to one lobe or to a "cold spot." Thyroid ultrasound will demonstrate a diffusely enlarged, hypoechogenic gland, and this modality can be utilized to monitor patient course (25). Surgery is contraindicated. The goal of therapy is symptomatic relief; salicylates and nonsteroidal anti-inflammatory drugs are effective, but corticosteroids may be necessary for more severe forms (24,26).

2.4 Riedel's Thyroiditis

Riedel's thyroiditis (Riedel's struma) (invasive fibrous thyroiditis) is an extremely rare condition characterized by "invasive" fibrosis of the thyroid and a systemic inflammatory fibrosclerosing process. The usual presentation is that of a stony hard thyroid mass suggestive of malignancy. Patients may be dysphagic, dyspneic, hypothyroid, and even have vocal cord paralysis. Further systemic fibrosis may manifest as retroperitoneal fibrosis, sclerosing cholangitis, aortic sclerosis, renal cortical fibrosis, occlusive phlebitis, and lipidic endarteritis. The etiology is probably autoimmune. Riedel's thyroiditis is frequently associated with elevated antithyroid antibody titers and can be associated with concomitant Hashimoto's or Graves' disease. The mechanism of fibroblastic proliferation may relate to fibroblastic stimulation by anti-TSH receptor antibodies, as is seen with Graves' pretibial edema and opthalmopathy.

The clinical presentation can be indistinguishable from malignancy. Radiographic imaging (MRI or CT) will reveal a thyroid mass with obliterated fat planes. Fine needle aspiration is not likely to be diagnostic, since the fibroblastic proliferation makes aspiration difficult. Core or open biopsies should establish the correct diagnosis. Histologically, a dense fibrosclerotic process and extensive chronic inflammation is seen. Fibroinflammatory vascular changes may also be seen.

Riedel's thyroiditis is usually a self-limiting condition. High-dose prednisone can produce dramatic improvement, and continued glucocorticoid administration is recommended to prevent progressive multifocal fibrosclerosis (27–29).

3 ECTOPIC THYROID

3.1 Cervical Lymph Node Inclusions Versus Metastatic Disease

The issue of thyroid inclusions within cervical lymph node is controversial. Many pathologists consider the presence of any thyroid follicles in a lymph node to be evidence of metastasis, even in the absence of an established thyroid primary, since it is well known that papillary thyroid carcinoma is frequently announced by cervical metastasis. On the other hand, documented, benign, thyroid inclusions can, and do, occur within jugular lymph nodes (30–32). They represent entrapped remnants of thyroid tissue that have migrated during development. This gave rise to the term "lateral aberrant thyroid." Benign inclusions are extremely rare. Thyroid tissue within cervical lymph nodes is almost always more likely to be due to metastatic disease rather than developmental inclusion.

The diagnosis of benign inclusions requires defined, strict criteria:

1. Follicles should be located in only the lymph node capsule or subcapsular tissue.
2. There should be only a few follicles.
3. Cytologically, they should be identical to normal thyrocytes, lacking the nuclear features of papillary thyroid carcinoma.
4. The involved nodes should be from the jugular nodes, not paratracheal or supraclavicular.

If more than one third of the lymph node is replaced by thyroid tissue, if any psammoma bodies, papillary structures, or nuclear features of papillary thyroid carcinoma are seen, metastatic papillary thyroid carcinoma is likely. Of course, any incidental findings of thyroid follicles within cervical lymph nodes must be investigated further. Thyroid ultrasound with aspiration cytology or biopsy is an invaluable tool. If a thyroid nodule is found, lobectomy is required. If the work-up is negative and the above histological criteria for benignity are met, no further surgery may be needed, although this is a rare situation (33,34). If the thyroid inclusions meet the criteria for malignancy, ipsilateral thyroid lobectomy is mandatory whether or not a thyroid nodule is found. These cases almost always reveal occult microscopic papillary carcinomas (31,35). For this reason the term "lateral aberrant thyroid" should be avoided in the context of neoplasia because it does not remove the need to rule out primary carcinoma from the ipsilateral thyroid lobe (36,37). In rare instances the primary site may be in the opposite lobe.

3.2 Lingual Thyroid

Embryologically, the thyroid anlage originates from the foramen cecum, at the base of the tongue. This tissue descends as the thyroglossal duct, in the midline of the neck, reaching its normal position anterior to the trachea and larynx. Abnormalities in descent can occur anywhere along this route, and maldescent may also occur into the mediastinum. Lingual thyroid occurs when there is no, or only partial, descent of the thyroid from the foramen cecum. It is a rare clinical problem, but reported incidence varies from 1:10 to 1:100,000. Most cases occur in young women. Patients can present with dysphagia, dyspnea, and a hemorrhagic mass. Symptoms may increase with hormonal fluctuations (e.g., menstrual cycle) or may worsen with pregnancy. Patients are also frequently hypothyroid.

Grossly, the tissue has a spongy red appearance, and histologically, the follicles are similar to eutropic thyroid tissue but may be in a microfollicular arrangement. The follicles may appear to infiltrate into surrounding skeletal muscle but can be distinguished from follicular variant of papillary thyroid carcinoma by the lack of diagnostic nuclear findings (see below).

Lingual thyroid may be diagnosed by biopsy and further confirmed by thyroid scan. If the diagnosis is established clinically, no surgery may be required; this may be the only thyroid tissue present in the patient, and the incidence of malignancy within lingual thyroid is extremely low. Symptomatic lingual thyroid may be managed by thyroid suppression, which will decrease the size of the lingual mass, and also supplants endogenous thyroid function (38,39).

3.3 Thyroglossal Duct Cyst

Thyroglossal duct cysts are dilated remnants of the path of thyroid's descent. It is the most common cause of a midline mass of the upper neck. These cysts usually come to clinical attention in children or young adults, but they may also suddenly appear in older patients. Patients present with a soft cystic midline mass that moves with swallowing or thrusting the tongue forward. Sometimes, pressure upon the mass can result in discharge through communication with the foramen cecum, and patients will notice a bitter taste (dysgeusia) in their mouths. The cysts are almost always adherent to the hyoid bone, frequently penetrating it centrally and continuing upward to its lingual origins at the tongue base. They can also be present off the midline if the distal cystic portion is displaced laterally. The Sistrunk procedure, which includes resection of the central portion of the hyoid bone, is now standard practice and has virtually eliminated recurrences. Grossly, these cysts can average from 1 to 3 cm in diameter. The lining may have a shaggy appearance from repeated infections. Histologically, the cyst is epithelial lined with thyroid follicles in the cyst wall. Lymphoid infiltrate or fibrosis may obliterate the residual thyroid tissue. Approximately 1% of cases will contain a malignancy, usually papillary thyroid carcinoma (40–42).

3.4 Intratracheal Thyroid

Intratracheal thyroid rests represents the rarest form of thyroid ectopia. A 2% incidence of incidental, subglottic, submucosal thyroid tissue has been observed in 250 laryngectomy specimens, with a 4:1 preponderance for left-sided trachea. These subglottic rests can cause dyspnea or may be incidental findings in the setting of thyroid carcinoma. The latter situation can lead to some confusion regarding tumor staging; a neoplasm may be erroneously upstaged if incidental intratracheal rests are interpreted as tumor extension. Since the trachea is posterior to the path of the descending thyroid, the mechanism of intratracheal ectopia is not immediately obvious. There are two prevailing, nonexclusive theories. The malformation theory states that thyroidal descent and formation is completed prior to tracheal cartilage formation, allowing for thyroid tissue to become entrapped and displaced by developing trachea. The purported left-sided propensity of intratracheal thyroid has been thought to relate to migratory differences between the left and right lateral ultimobranchial contribution to the thyroid anlage. The invasion theory states that thyroid tissue continues to migrate, albeit along an aberrant pathway, and becomes situated in the trachea as a result of direct, yet oncologically benign invasion, as is seen quite frequently with mediastinal thyroid tissue (43–45).

3.5 Mediastinal Thyroid

Most cases of mediastinal (substernal) thyroid are inferior extensions of multinodular goiters and can be removed through the neck because their vascularization is derived cervically from the inferior thyroid artery. Truly aberrant mediastinal thyroid, which may be contained within the thymus or mediastinum, is rare, but these often have a separate vascularization from mediastinal vessels or branches of the internal mammary artery and therefore cannot be resected via cervical approach. Mediastinal goiter can compress the trachea or great vessels, causing respiratory failure or superior vena cava syndrome. Most patients are euthyroid but, uncommonly, can be hyperthyroid. The thyroid is usually markedly enlarged, multinodular, and histologically identical to typical multinodular goiters. In a small percentage of cases, a papillary carcinoma is present (46).

4 MALIGNANT THYROID NEOPLASIA

4.1 Papillary Carcinoma—Diagnosis, Pathobiology, and Variants

Papillary thyroid carcinoma is the most common form of thyroid malignancy, constituting 80% of all thyroid carcinomas. It occurs over a wide age range (5–95 years, median 39) with a female-to-male ratio of 3:1 (47). There are some genetic associations for papillary thyroid carcinoma; it may be associated with familial adenomatous polyposis (Gardner's syndrome) and also Cowden's syndrome (48–50). Ionizing radiation, particularly during childhood for benign conditions such as thymic "enlargement," eustachian tube obstruction, tinea capitus, etc., is a predisposing factor. This can occur with accumulation of lower sublethal energy doses, e.g., 0.2–40 rads (51). In vitro cell line studies have demonstrated that high doses (10, 50, and 100 Gy) of x-rays produce preferential activation of the RET/PTC1 oncogene (as compared with RET/PTC2, RET/PTC3 induction) in a dose-dependent manner, confirming the initiating potential of ionizing radiation as well as the significance of RET/PTC1 rearrangement in the early steps of thyroid carcinogenesis (52). Although low doses of beam therapy in children and adolescents incite future thyroid cancer, which usually develops one to two decades later, high-dose beam therapy to the neck or chest, such as that for Hodgkin's disease, does not do so. There have been no reports of an increased incidence of thyroid cancer after high-dose beam therapy, although an increased risk of lung, salivary, breast cancers, as well as sarcomas and other malignancies has been noted (53).

An increased risk for subsequent benign as well as malignant thyroid lesions is also seen after exposure to increased levels of radioactive I^{131} fallout. This has been observed in survivors of Hiroshima and Nagasaki, Marshall Islanders exposed to the Bikini atoll atomic bomb trail, and more recently survivors of Chernobyl (54,55). On the other hand, therapeutic doses of radioactive I^{131} has an ablative affect on the thyroid and is not associated with increased risk of subsequent thyroid malignancy (56).

Patients with papillary thyroid carcinoma may present with discrete thyroid masses, with or without adenopathy, or enlarged lymph nodes but no apparent thyroid mass. A frequent presentation in younger (5–19 years, mean 16 years) individuals is that of an unexplained enlarged jugular lymph node without an obvious site of primary disease (57). These pathological nodes characteristically represent metastasis from an occult, ipsilateral, localized sclerotic papillary thyroid carcinoma. Papillary carcinoma can have diverse appearances upon sectioning the gland: localized sclerotic nodules, diffusely sclerotic, infiltrative tumors, or encapsulated tumors mimicking follicular adenomata. Their interior can have a "furry," dull appearance, sometimes with yellow flecks, reflecting the relative lack of colloid and the presence of papillary projections (Fig. 1). The localized sclerotic form can be quite small (<1 cm), and nonpalpable ("occult"), coming to clinical attention because of the appearance of cervical metastases.

Papillary thyroid carcinoma has characteristic microscopic nuclear features. The nuclei are large and ovoid, as compared to normal thyrocytes, with a crowded overlapping appearance. Nuclear holes, grooves, and cleared nuclei are characteristic, but not specific or reliable, for the diagnosis. These findings are difficult to demonstrate at frozen section. The pathologist can rely only on the tumor architecture to make the diagnosis at that time (Fig. 2). Papillary thyroid carcinoma forms papillary structures, with fibrovascular cores, psammoma bodies, as well as follicular structures. If these follicular structures predominate histologically, the tumor is referred to as follicular variant of papillary thyroid carcinoma. While true tumor papillae can be discerned on frozen section analysis, the follicular variant of papillary carcinoma may be impossible to diagnose on frozen section, for not only are the diagnostic nuclear features lacking, the characteristic papillary architecture is now also lacking (Fig. 3). A previous aspiration cytology can be helpful if papillary thyroid carcinoma had been definitely diagnosed. Thus, most false-negative frozen section diagnoses for papillary thyroid carcinoma are, in fact, follicular variants of papillary thyroid carcinoma. Prior to the recognition of the follicular variant of papillary thyroid carcinoma, many of these tumors were misdiagnosed as follicular carcinomas.

Certain variants of papillary thyroid carcinoma deserve mention because they are associated with a poorer prognosis. A carcinoma that presents as a diffusely sclerotic tumor will invariably present at a higher stage (T3 or T4) and is more aggressive. The tall cell variant of papillary thyroid carcinoma represents approximately 10% of papillary carcinomas; it is defined as a tumor in which more than 30% of the cells are twice as tall as they are wide. It is frequently associated with high-grade features such as tumor necrosis, vascular invasion, solid areas, and increased mitotic figures. Several investigators found the tall cell variant to have a more aggressive behavior than ordinary well-differentiated papillary carcinoma (58,59). Columnar cell carcinoma is a rare variant, defined by tall tumor cells with stratified nuclei and subnuclear vacuoles, and is also associated with more aggressive behavior (60,61). Papillary thyroid carcinoma may also be an incidental synchronous finding of lobectomy performed for another nodule, such as an adenoma. These incidental occult tumors are usually small (< 1 cm). If confined to the thyroid parenchyma, lobectomy is curative and completion thyroidectomy is not necessary.

The overall survival statistics for patients with papillary thyroid carcinoma are excellent; the Surveillance, Epidemiology and End Results program (SEER) data reveal that overall 10-year survival is 98% (47). This deceptively rosy survival rate reflects a preponderance of "typical" papillary thyroid carcinomas, which are classified as "low-risk" cases. Low-risk patients are young (< 45 years), with small tumors (< 4 cm in diameter), and no distant metastasis. These tumors also lack high-grade histological features (diffuse sclerotic variant, tall cell variant) and do not extend into peri-thyroid soft tissue. The acronym AGES refers to variables impacting on prognosis (age > 45, male gender or tumor grade, extrathyroid extension, and patient stage). Histological features that define high grade for papillary thyroid carcinoma include extrathyroid extension, diffuse sclerotic type, tall cell variant, and columnar cell variant. A more in-depth discussion regarding treatment options with respect to risk category is presented in Chapter xx.

Twenty-year survival for intermediate-risk groups is 83% and for high-risk groups 43%. Distant metastases (such as lung) are associated with poor prognosis (62,63). The issue of regional, cervical metastases of papillary carcinoma is intriguing. Microscopic metastatic papillary carcinoma is common within cervical lymph nodes of patients with papillary carcinoma and has been documented in up to 80% of dissections, (64). Unlike other malignancies, in which survival dramatically drops by 50% with the presence of metastatic lymph nodes, positive nodal disease conveys no survival impact for patients with papillary thyroid carcinoma. This unique quirk of papillary carcinoma was confirmed in a report on approximately 12,000 National Cancer Institute study patients, which demonstrated that cervical lymph node metastasis was not an independent prognosticator and did not affect overall survival for patients with well-differentiated carcinoma (47). Performing jugular and central compartment lymph node dissection in the absence of clinical adenopathy has not been demonstrated to improve patient survival. The concept of "stagnant metastatic deposits" has been proposed, because in most patients papillary thyroid carcinoma almost never leaves the region of the neck (47,61,62,65–68). When papillary thyroid carcinoma does metastasize to distant sites, it usually involves the lungs or brain (62,69).

4.2 Follicular Carcinoma

Follicular carcinomas represents 17% of thyroid malignancies (47). There is a wide age range (8–98 years), but the mean patient age at diagnosis (48 years) is a decade older than that for papillary thyroid carcinoma (39 years). A female predominance (73%) is present. These carcinomas can be subdivided into two subgroups: minimally invasive well-differentiated encapsulated follicular carcinoma and invasive well to moderately differentiated follicular carcinoma. The presentation of a minimally invasive follicular carcinoma is identical to that of a follicular adenoma: patients present with a dominant nodule that is "cold" on radio-iodine scan. Fine needle aspiration is of no help in distinguishing between these two entities; the diagnosis must be made on architectural, not cytology features.

Patients with invasive follicular carcinoma can present with an irregular, firm, thyroid mass that may be fixed to the surrounding tissues. Occasionally, metastases may be the initial presentation, especially bony metastases. Here, preoperative cytology in the clinical setting of an obvious clinical malignancy can be helpful in distinguishing follicular carcinoma from papillary and anaplastic carcinomas.

4.2.1 Minimally Invasive Encapsulated Follicular Carcinoma

This is an encapsulated tumor, but the capsule is usually thicker than that of a routine adenoma. The interior of the tumor is usually mahogany colored, but glistening, not "furry" as in papillary carcinoma. Histologically, the thyroid follicles are usually small, but bland and indistinguishable from benign follicular adenomas. The diagnosis is established on permanent section by finding either complete penetration of the neoplasm through the capsule and/or subcapsular vascular/lymphatic

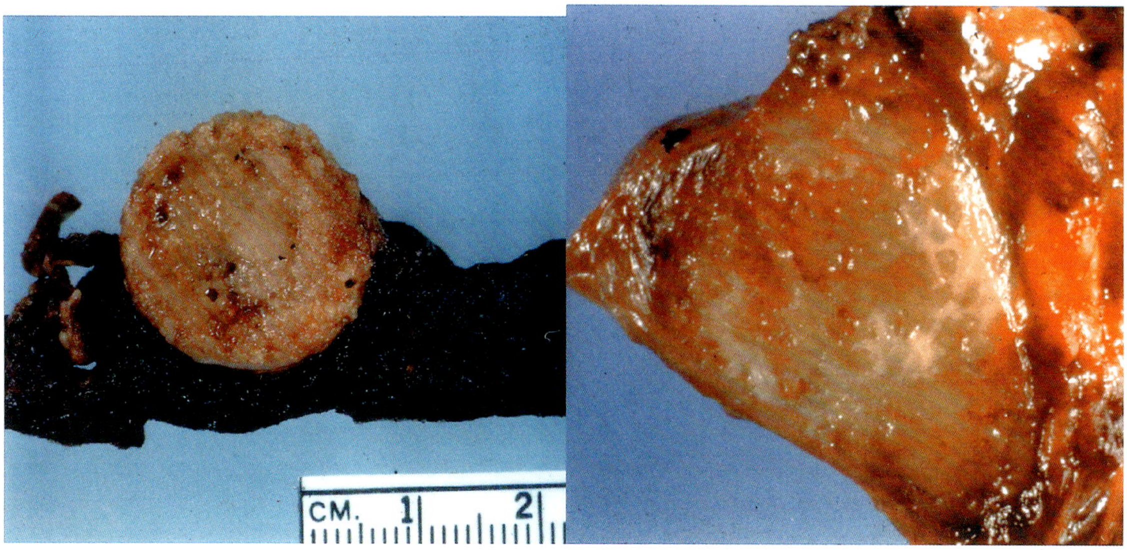

Figure 1 Papillary thyroid carcinoma. (Left) This circumscribed tumor has a characteristic "furry" cut surface, indicating papillae formation. (Right) This carcinoma has grown with an infiltrating scar-like appearance, indicative of sclerosis.

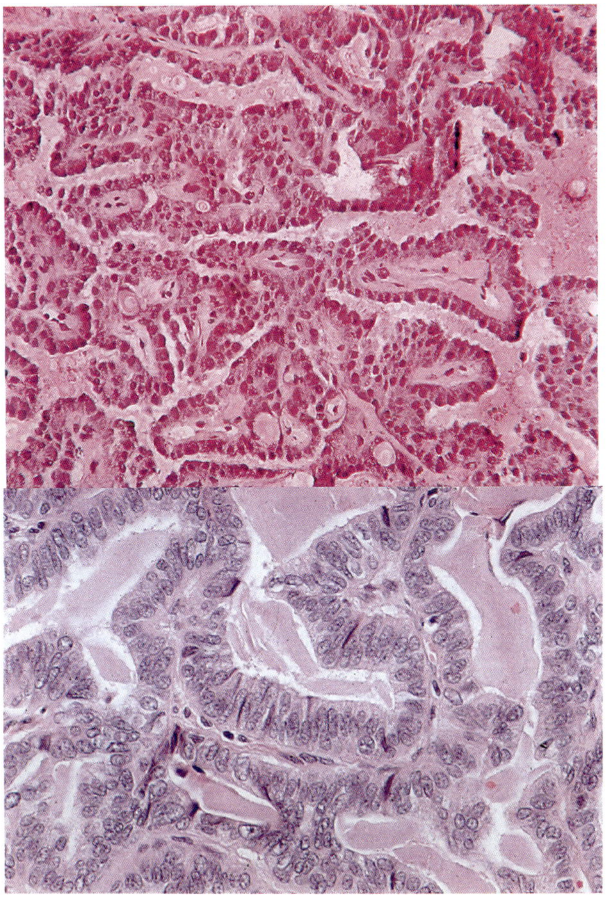

Figure 2 Papillary thyroid carcinoma. (Top) This frozen section is diagnostic for papillary thyroid carcinoma, as abundant "true" papillae are formed with fibrovascular cores. Note, however, that the tumor nuclei are condensed; no "Orphan Annie eye" cleared nuclei are seen. (Bottom) Formalin-fixed, paraffin-embedded ("permanent") sections from the same tumor specimen reveal characteristic oval overlapped nuclei with prominent grooves and optically cleared nuclei. (Hematoxylin and eosin)

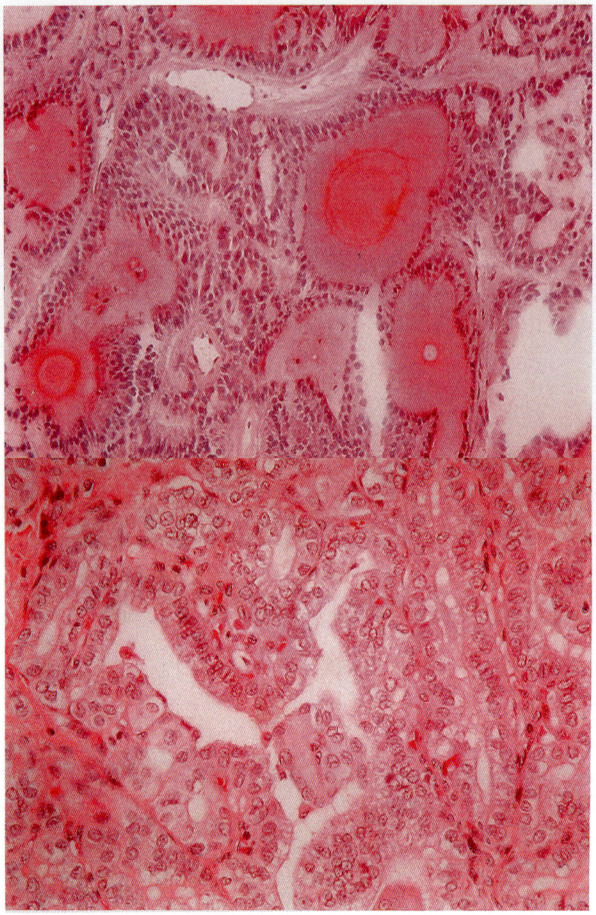

Figure 3 Papillary thyroid carcinoma, follicular variant. (Top) This frozen section reveals a neoplasm forming follicular structures. The absence of papillary structures and diagnostic nuclear features, render this image indistinguishable from a follicular adenoma. (Bottom) Permanent sections from this same neoplasm reveal follicular structures, but with nuclear features diagnostic for follicular variant papillary thyroid carcinoma.

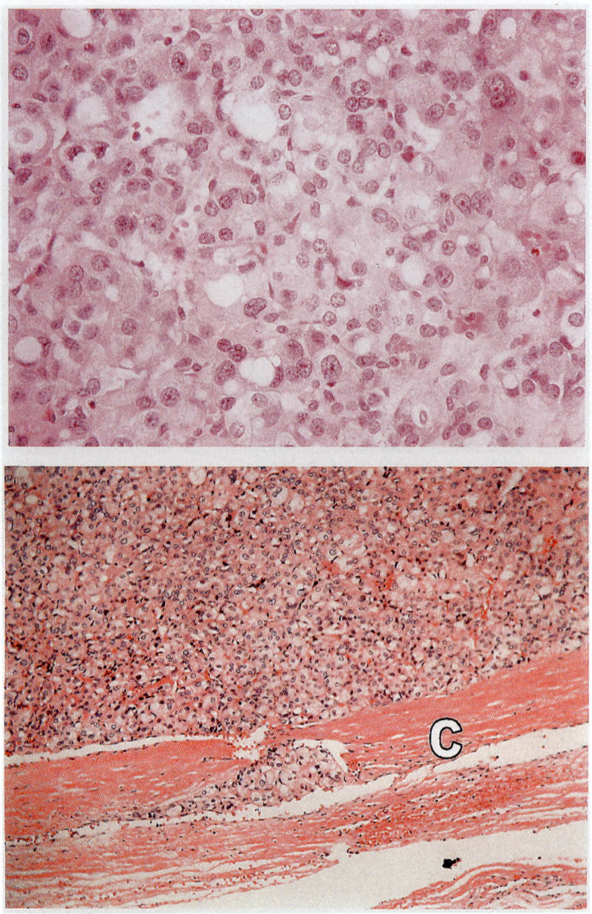

Figure 4 Hürthle cell carcinoma. (Top) Hürthle cells are characterized by abundant, granular eosinophilic cytoplasm and round nuclei with stippled chromatic and prominent nucleoli. The nuclear pleomorphism, that is, the degree of variation in shape and size among tumor nuclei, does not predict malignant potential. (Bottom) Tumor emboli can be seen within capsular (C) vascular spaces, a diagnostic feature of Hürthle cell carcinomas, and thyroid follicular carcinomas in general. (Hematoxylin and eosin)

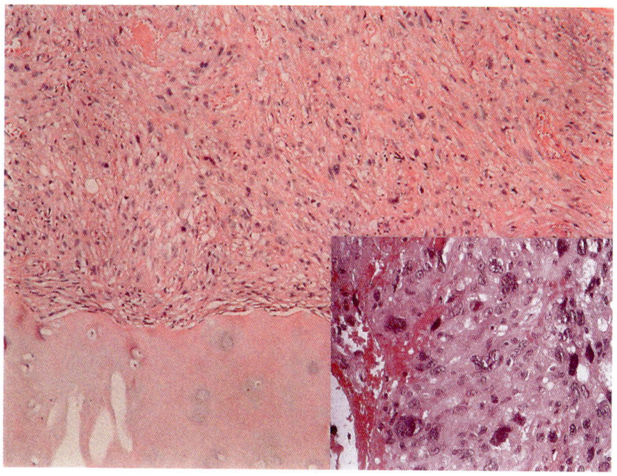

Figure 5 Anaplastic carcinoma. This highly malignant neoplasm can be seen invading laryngeal cricoid cartilage. (Inset) Anaplastic carcinoma is characterized by extreme nuclear pleomorphism, spindled and multinucleated tumor giant cells. (Hematoxylin and eosin)

invasion. If tumor extends into the thyroid parenchyma or necrosis is seen, then the tumor may be beyond "minimally invasive" and classified as invasive. Additional deeper sections from the paraffin block may be required for the diagnosis; the malignant thyrocytes may appear identical to benign thyrocytes and the pathologist cannot rely on the usual cytological indicators of malignancy.

In a large (n = 95) series of minimally invasive encapsulated follicular carcinomas reported from the Armed Forces Institute of Pathology, the female-to-male ratio was 2.4 : 1, and patient ages ranged from 20 to 95 years (average 42.0 years). The mean mass diameter was 2.8 cm. All of these patients were treated by surgical excision, and adjuvant radioactive iodine therapy was administered to 24 patients. The prognosis for minimally invasive encapsulated follicular carcinoma is excellent. The recurrence rate was 5% (mean 18.1 years), with no disease-related mortality. The remaining patients were disease-free after a significant follow-up period (mean 16.5 years) (70), which is significantly better than is seen for invasive follicular carcinoma (see below).

4.2.2 Invasive Follicular Carcinoma

Thyroid follicular carcinoma is the second most common thyroid malignancy after papillary carcinoma. Hürthle cell carcinoma, insular carcinoma, and trabecular-insular carcinoma are histological variants of invasive thyroid follicular carcinoma; all of these carcinomas have the same biological potential stage for stage. The true incidence of follicular carcinoma is difficult to determine from the older literature, because many cases of follicular variant papillary thyroid carcinoma (see above) had been previously classified as follicular carcinomas. One retrospective study documented that the ratio of papillary to follicular carcinomas diagnosed varied from 0.60 in 1974–76 to 6.88 in 1992–94 (71). This casts doubt on the survival statistics of follicular carcinoma in the older literature because the prognosis of follicular variant of papillary carcinoma is identical to that of papillary thyroid carcinoma, which is usually better than that of invasive follicular carcinoma. Marked geographical variations in the relative ratios between follicular and papillary thyroid carcinoma have been observed, probably relating to dietary iodine deficiencies (72–74).

On clinical examination, invasive follicular carcinoma presents as a firm thyroid mass. Fixation of the surrounding soft tissues raises the clinical suspicion of malignancy. A small percentage of patients (up to 11%) may present with metastatic disease (usually within bone, lungs, and soft tissues) (75). Histologically, this form of follicular carcinoma can be either well or moderately differentiated but invariably demonstrates frank invasion into the thyroid parenchyma, as well as vascular invasion. Invasion of extrathyroid soft tissue may also be seen and is a poor prognostic feature. The tumor cells of well-differentiated follicular carcinoma appear similar to normal thyrocytes, but they may be larger, with greater atypia. They can be distinguished from papillary thyroid carcinoma tumor cells since their nuclei are round and nonoverlapping. The tendency towards vascular invasion also suggests the diagnosis of follicular carcinoma. Histological variants of follicular carcinoma include trabecular-insular, Hürthle cell, clear cell, and mixed medullary-follicular carcinoma. These variants can be more solid and are moderately to poorly differentiated.

The issue of Hürthle cell carcinomas has historically been shrouded in some mystery due to some early publications by surgeons treating "Hurthle cell adenomas" that metastasized. Subsequent pathological studies have confirmed that the diagnostic criteria necessary to distinguish Hürthle cell adenoma from carcinoma are the same as in other follicular tumors: namely, capsular invasion and/or subcapsular vascular invasion (76) (Fig. 4). As mentioned, large Hürthle cell tumors (>4 cm) are more likely to be malignant than small tumors (<2 cm) (2,3).

Hürthle cell carcinomas do appear inherently different in some ways from follicular cancers; they rarely take up radioactive iodine but do make thyroglobulin, and they more commonly spread to lymph nodes (77). A review from Memorial Sloan-Kettering Cancer Center of over 1000 thyroid malignancies demonstrated that tumors diagnosed as Hürthle cell carcinoma have a greater likelihood of developing distant metastases than follicular carcinomas (78). However, regression analysis stratifying for tumor stage was lacking in this article, so further clinicopathological study is necessary before this issue can be confirmed. The data published from the SEER Program 1973–1991 do not address this issue (47). However, National Cancer Institute data actually stratify follicular thyroid carcinoma and Hürthle cell carcinoma by AJCC stage (79). This report finds that while Hürthle cell carcinomas are less likely to be encountered as Stage I malignancies, stage for stage patient survival appears similar for follicular carcinoma and Hürthle cell carcinoma.

Immunohistochemistry may be helpful in distinguishing some solid follicular carcinoma variants, such as trabecular-insular variant, which invariably express thyroglobulin, from medullary carcinoma, which will express calcitonin and possibly other neuroendocrine markers, but not thyroglobulin.

The prognosis of invasive follicular carcinoma is much poorer than that of minimally invasive follicular carcinoma or papillary thyroid carcinoma. The reported mortality rates vary from 16 to 60%. A number of studies have identified poor prognosticators. Older patients (>45 years), presence of distant metastases, thyroid capsular invasion, or tumor size greater than 2 cm are features invariably associated with a poorer prognosis (79,80).

4.3 Medullary Carcinoma

Medullary thyroid carcinoma represents approximately 3% of all thyroid malignancies (47). Most cases (80%) occur sporadically, whereas 20% of these tumors are familial, and may be associated with other endocrine pathologies such as pheochromocytoma and hyperparathyroidism (MEN 2A, MEN 2B, and isolated familial medullary thyroid carcinoma). The average age of presentation for sporadic tumors is 52.3 years, whereas the average age for index patients with hereditary tumors is 29 years, and for all screened patients is 23 years. Within this last group, the median age of diagnosis for hereditary tumors varies: 36 years for hereditary medullary carcinoma, 27.4 years for MEN IIa, and 17.2 years for MEN IIb (81). Patients with sporadic disease usually present with palpable thyroid masses. The index patient with familial disease (the first individual in a cohort to be identified) can also present with a thyroid mass but may also be hypertensive secondary to pheochromocytoma or hypercalcemic (with its attendant symptoms) due to hyperparathyroidism. Ultrasound and fine needle aspiration should then be performed for possible preoperative diagnosis of medullary carcinoma. Any suspicion of the diagnosis of medullary thyroid carcinoma should be relayed to the cytologist, so that provision can be made to perform immunohistochemistry for calcitonin. While immunohistochemistry can be performed retrospectively from the formalin-fixed paraffin embedded tissue blocks, cytology specimens require advance preparation of either additional unstained slides or a "spun-down" cytology block for immunohistochemistry.

The pentagastrin stimulation test can then confirm elevated calcitonin and hence the diagnosis. The provocative pentagastrin stimulation test is useful in distinguishing medullary carcinoma from false-positive, mild elevations in serum calcitonin (82). The preoperative diagnosis of medullary carcinoma should initiate investigations to distinguish sporadic tumors from index familial cases. The latter patients then require screening for other potential endocrine tumors as well as intensive familial screening. The identification of germline mutations in the proto-oncogene RET identifies these familial cases; this blood testing is especially important for all patients younger than 45 years. Within identified families, asymptomatic members can be screened and identified by elevated serum calcitonin. Medullary carcinoma is associated with an overall mild female predominance, which is more pronounced in sporadic cases (F:M = 1.84:1) than in hereditary cases (F:M = 1.18:1) (81).

Medullary carcinomas arise from the neuroendocrine parafollicular C cells (calcitonin-secreting C cells). These neural crest–derived cells are more concentrated within the lateral and superior aspects of the thyroid lobes. Not surprisingly, these tumors, especially the familial ones, have a predilection for the superior lateral thyroid lobes. Grossly, they are usually circumscribed, with a smooth cut surface, tan-white in color. Familial tumors may be smaller and multiple as compared to sporadic tumors, with adjacent C-cell hyperplasia (see below). Histologically, medullary carcinoma is composed of epithelioid or spindled neuroendocrine cells. Their nuclei have the fine, stippled chromatin characteristic of neuroendocrine tumors. Calcitonin deposition can be seen by light microscopy as amyloid and confirmed by immunohistochemistry. However, some medullary carcinomas can mimic oat cell (small cell) carcinomas, in that they appear as amyloid-poor, malignant, small, blue round cells. The diagnostic immunohistochemical profile for medullary carcinoma is expression of calcitonin and carcinoembryonic antigen, but no thyroglobin expression. C-cell hyperplasia represents a histologically benign proliferation of C cells and is the earliest thyroid manifestation of this endocrinopathy. It appears as nests of calcitonin-positive epithelial cells adjacent to follicles, the size and number of which are increased as compared to normal controls.

Total thyroidectomy and central neck dissection is the minimum therapy for patients with medullary carcinoma. In over 90% of cases, the disease is multicentric, and in contrast to well-differentiated thyroid cancer, positive nodes do have an adverse effect on survival. Prophylactic total thyroidectomy is recommended for all probands within identified families; it should be performed as soon as possible. Surgery is warranted as early as 6 years of age, and these thyroids usually reveal only C-cell hyperplasia. The prognosis of medullary thyroid carcinoma correlates with stage at presentation. Tumors detected by screening are identified at an earlier stage and are cured by total thyroidectomy and paratracheal lymph node dissection.

Conversely, the initial presence of systemic symptoms (diarrhea, bone pain, or flushing) is usually associated with widely metastatic, sporadic disease, and a significant (33.3%) 5-year mortality rate (83,84). Disease-free survival at 10 years is around 50% for sporadic medullary thyroid carcinoma.

4.4 Anaplastic Carcinoma

Anaplastic thyroid carcinoma comprises 5–15% of primary thyroid malignancies. It represents one of the most aggressive solid tumors in humans, usually presenting in the sixth and seventh decades of life, with a small female preponderance (84,85). The classic presentation is that of a rapidly growing neck mass causing hoarseness and airway obstruction. The acute symptoms frequently appear a short time before patients seek attention. More than half of patients will have a history of long-standing goiter. Leukocytosis and fever commonly accompany presentation. Distant metastases, usually to the lung, are common at presentation. Ultrasound and fine-needle aspiration cytology can usually establish the diagnosis preoperatively. If the aspiration is inconclusive, an open biopsy is required. Histologically, anaplastic thyroid carcinoma is composed of huge, bizarre, anaplastic, spindled cells and multinucleated tumor giant cells. The tumor cells are the most pleomorphic of any head and neck malignancies. The spindled cells resemble sarcoma (Fig. 5). Epithelioid tumor cells with squamous metaplasia can be present, which may be significant if a clinical differential diagnosis involves upper aerodigestive tract carcinomas. The majority of anaplastic thyroid carcinomas are found to contain foci of well-differentiated thyroid carcinoma, when adequately sectioned (86). Immunohistochemistry for thyroglobulin is usually negative in anaplastic carcinomas; thyroid transcription factor (TTF) is also usually negative or may be focally positive (87). If the anaplastic carcinoma is amenable to surgery, then it should be resected. Aggressive multimodality treatment radiation and chemotherapy should be offered in any case, but survival rates remain low and the median survival for most series is under 6 months.

5

5.1 Squamous Carcinoma—Primary Versus Secondary

Primary thyroid squamous carcinoma is rare, accounting for 0.7–3.4% of all thyroid malignancies. Approximately 130 cases have been reported in the English literature. It arises in either of two settings: either as a primary tumor or as a component of anaplastic or tall cell papillary thyroid carcinoma. There is a female predisposition with a female-to-male ratio of approximately 2 : 1. Most patients are in the fifth to sixth decades of life, similar to that of anaplastic thyroid carcinomas. Presentation is dramatic; patients have rapidly enlarging neck swelling, shortness of breath, and hoarseness. The tumors have been described as firm, necrotic, and extensively infiltrating the thyroid and peri-thyroidal soft tissue; they may extend to the larynx, trachea, and mediastinum. Positive cervical lymph nodes are common at presentation, and some patients may also have pulmonary metastases upon presentation (88,89).

Histologically, primary thyroid squamous carcinoma is composed of islands of malignant squamous cells with varying degrees of differentiation. Areas of well-differentiated or tall cell papillary carcinoma may be present, but not as the dominant histological component; it should comprise less than 30% of the carcinoma. A spindle cell component can also be present. The main differential diagnosis includes direct extension of a carcinoma from the larynx or esophagus or direct extension from a metastatic cervical lymph node from an upper aerodigestive tract primary. Clinical correlation, as well as finding papillary thyroid differentiation or immunohistochemical expression of thyroid transcription factor or thyroglobulin, can establish a carcinoma as being of thyroid origin.

Squamous cell carcinoma of the thyroid gland is a highly lethal tumor. Most patients die within a year despite combination therapy including surgery, radiation, and chemotherapy. The cause of death is often related to local recurrence or distant metastases (lungs, liver, heart, kidneys). The prognosis is similar to or even worse than anaplastic thyroid carcinoma.

One variant of thyroid squamous carcinoma that requires mention is CASTLE (carcinoma showing thymus-like differentiation). CASTLE tumors of the thyroid are rare and indolent with a favorable prognosis. Histologically, they are lobulated and expansive, with fibrous septa, indistinct cellular borders and possibly having foci of squamous differentiation.

5.2 Metastatic Disease to the Thyroid

Metastatic malignancies to the thyroid are relatively rare. In many cases the metastasis may be the initial manifestation of disease. The most common sources of primary disease are lung, gastrointestinal tract, and melanoma. Carcinomas from prostate, larynx, kidney and breast may also metastasize to the thyroid (91,92).

6 FROZEN SECTION ANALYSIS: STRENGTHS AND LIMITATIONS

Intraoperative tissue analysis involves sampling and rapidly freezing tissue that can be cryostat sectioned. The tissue sections are immediately stained and examined microscopically. The tissue-fixation step, which preserves morphology, is not technically feasible during frozen section.

Thus, the biggest limitation of frozen section analysis is suboptimal tissue morphology. Frozen section analysis will allow for the diagnosis of papillary thyroid carcinoma with typical papillary architecture, invasive follicular carcinoma, Hashimoto's thyroiditis, anaplastic carcinoma, and multinodular goiter. There are three common areas where frozen section analysis meets its limitations: (1) distinguishing follicular variant of papillary thyroid carcinoma from a follicular adenoma, (2) definitively identifying minimally invasive follicular carcinoma, and (3) distinguishing the papillary hyperplasia of Graves' disease from papillary carcinoma. As these first two issues are generally encountered while examining follicular adenomas, one can imagine just how often this differential diagnosis does arise.

When one reexamines false-positive or false-negative frozen section diagnoses regarding papillary thyroid carcinoma, these errors usually involve misdiagnosing follicular variant of papillary thyroid carcinoma (93, 94). As mentioned above, when papillary architecture is lacking, one can only base the diagnosis of follicular variant papillary thyroid carcinoma on nuclear morphology, which is compromised at frozen section analysis. The lack of formalin fixation obscures the nuclear holes, grooves, and cleared nuclei characteristic for the diagnosis. Hence, a surgeon wishing to perform a total thyroidectomy after a definitive diagnosis of papillary thyroid carcinoma must be patient and await the permanent section diagnosis 48 hours later.

Minimally invasive follicular carcinoma, as mentioned above, is an uncommon, low-grade malignancy. The diagnosis is based on observing either capsular invasion or subcapsular vascular invasion in a solitary follicular nodule. Grossly, these lesions resemble follicular adenomas. However, it has been noted that the fibrous capsules of these tumors can be thicker than those of conventional adenomas. Many histological samples may be necessary before a diagnosis of minimally invasive follicular carcinoma is made. However, sampling limitations at the time of frozen section usually preclude this diagnosis. Importantly, these minimally invasive follicular carcinomas are cytologically identical to follicular adenomas. Theoretically, any apparent follicular adenoma might yield diagnostic evidence of invasion after adequate sampling. For this reason, most pathologists will not definitely diagnose a benign follicular adenoma on frozen section. The diagnosis of "histologically benign follicular neoplasm" is used to imply a that the lesion is consistent with follicular adenoma, but that definitive diagnosis awaits the permanent sections.

Finally, Graves' disease is usually treated with thyroid suppression. Surgery may become necessary in the course of this illness if a thyroid nodule develops. Alternatively, a follicular adenoma may be hyperfunctioning (e.g., "hot"). The appearance of a hyperfunctioning adenoma is identical to Graves' disease with papillary hyperplasia. Under these conditions, the pathologist may histologically encounter the papillary hyperplasia of Graves' disease and need to distinguish it from papillary carcinoma. Again, the lack of nuclear details inherent to frozen section can lead the pathologist to defer definitive diagnosis until permanent section.

REFERENCES

1. Evans HL. Follicular neoplasms of the thyroid. A study of 44 cases followed for a minimum of 10 years, with emphasis on differential diagnosis. Cancer 1984; 54:535–540.
2. Chen H, Nicol TL, Zeiger MA, et al. Hürthle cell neoplasms of the thyroid: are there factors predictive of malignancy? Ann Surg 1998; 227:542–546.
3. Tallini G, Carcangiu ML, Rosai J. Oncocytic neoplasms of the thyroid gland. Acta Pathol Jpn 1992; 42:305–315.
4. Carcangiu ML, Bianchi S, Savino D, et al. Follicular Hürthle cell tumors of the thyroid gland. Cancer 1991; 68:1944–1953.
5. LiVolsi VA. Hyalinizing trabecular tumor of the thyroid: adenoma, carcinoma, or neoplasm of uncertain malignant potential? Am J Surg Pathol 2000; 24:1683–1684.
6. Cheung CC, Boerner SL, MacMillan CM, et al. Hyalinizing trabecular tumor of the thyroid: a variant of papillary carcinoma proved by molecular genetics. Am J Surg Pathol 2000; 24:1622–1666.
7. Carney JA, Ryan J, Goellner JR. Hyalinizing trabecular adenoma of the thyroid gland. Am J Surg Pathol 1987; 11:583–591.
8. Alexander CB, Herrera GA, Jaffe K, Yu H. Black thyroid. Clinical manifestations, ultrastructural findings and possible mechanisms. Hum Pathol 16: 1985: 72–78.
9. Pastolero GC, Asa SL. Drug related pigmentation of the thyroid associated with papillary carcinoma. Arch Pathol Lab Med 1994; 118:79–83.
10. Zophel K, Gruning T, Wunderlich G, Franke WG. Clinical value of a bispecific antibody binding to thyro-

globulin and thyroperoxidase (TGPO-aAb) in various thyroid diseases. Autoimmunity 1999; 29:257–262.
11. Jaruratanasirikul S, Leethanaporn K, Khuntigij P, Sriplung H. The clinical course of Hashimoto's thyroiditis in children and adolescents: 6 years longitudinal follow-up. J Pediatr Endocrinol Metab 2001; 14:177–184.
12. Pedersen RK, Pedersen NT. Primary non-Hodgkin's lymphoma of the thyroid gland: a population based study. Histopathology 1996; 28:25–32.
13. Kato I, Tajima K, Suchi T, et al. Chronic thyroiditis as a risk factor of B cell lymphoma in the thyroid gland. Jpn J Cancer Res 1985; 76:1085–1090.
14. Derringer GA, Thompson LD, Frommelt RA, et al. Malignant lymphoma of the thyroid gland: a clinicopathologic study of 108 cases. Am J Surg Pathol 2000; 24:623–639.
15. Belal AA, Allam A, Kandil A, et al. Primary thyroid lymphoma: a retrospective analysis of prognostic factors and treatment outcome for localized intermediate and high grade lymphoma. Am J Clin Oncol 2001; 24:299–305.
16. Scholefield JH, Quayle AR, Harris SC, Talbot CH. Primary lymphoma of the thyroid, the association with Hashimoto's thyroiditis. Eur J Surg Oncol 1992; 18:89–92.
17. Lam KY, Lo CY, Kwong DL, et al. Clinical aspects of primary thyroid lymphoma: diagnosis and treatment based on our experience of 119 cases. Thyroid 1993; 3:93–99.
18. Ott RA, McCall AR, McHenry C, et al. The incidence of thyroid carcinoma in Hashimoto's thyroiditis. Am Surg 1987; 53:442–445.
19. McLeod MK, East ME, Burney RE, et al. Hashimoto's thyroiditis revisited: the association with thyroid cancer remains obscure. World J Surg 1988; 12:509–516.
20. Wirtschafter A, Schmidt R, Rosen D, et al. Expression of the RET/PTC fusion gene as a marker for papillary carcinoma in Hashimoto's thyroiditis. Laryngoscope 1999; 109:1011–1015.
21. Koh LD, Napolitano G, Singer DS, et al. Graves' disease: a host defense mechanism gone awry. Int Rev Immunol 2000; 19:633–664.
22. Kriss JP. Pathogenesis and treatment of pretibial myxedema. Endocrinol Metab Clin North Am 1987; 16:409–415.
23. Wiersinga WM, Prummel MF. Pathogenesis of Graves' ophthalmopathy—current understanding. J Clin Endocrin Metabol 2001; 86:501–503.
24. Garcia Solano J, Gimenez Bascunana A, Sola Perez J, et al. Fine-needle aspiration of subacute granulomatous thyroiditis (De Quervain's thyroiditis): a clinico-cytologic review of 36 cases. Diagn Cytopathol 1997; 16: 214–220.
25. Bennedbaek FN, Hegedus L. The value of ultrasonography in the diagnosis and follow-up of subacute thyroiditis. Thyroid 1997; 7:45–50.
26. Volpe R. The management of subacute (DeQuervain's) thyroiditis. Thyroid 1993; 3:253–255.
27. Tutuncu NB, Erbas T, Bayraktar M, Gedik O. Multifocal idiopathic fibrosclerosis manifesting with Riedel's thyroiditis. Endocr Pract 2000; 6:447–449.
28. Julie C, Vieillefond A, Desligneres S, et al. Hashimoto's thyroiditis associated with Riedel's thyroiditis and retroperitoneal fibrosis. Pathol Res Pract 1997; 193: 573–577.
29. Heufelder AE, Hay ID. Evidence for autoimmune mechanisms in the evolution of invasive fibrous thyroiditis (Riedel's struma). Clin Investig 1994; 72:788–793.
30. Nicastri AD, Foote FW Jr, Frazell EL. Benign thyroid inclusions in cervical lymph nodes. JAMA 1965; 194: 1–4.
31. Meyer JS, Steinberg LS. Microscopically benign thyroid follicles in cervical lymph nodes. Serial section study of lymph node inclusions and entire thyroid gland in 5 cases. Cancer 1969; 24:302–311.
32. Fliegelman LJ, Genden EM, Brandwein M, et al. Significance and management of thyroid lesions in lymph nodes as an incidental finding during neck dissection. Head Neck 2001; 23:885–893.
33. Block MA, Wylie JH, Patton RB, Miller JM. Does benign thyroid tissue occur in the lateral part of the neck? Am J Surg 1966; 112:476–481.
34. Ward R. Relation of tumors of lateral aberrant thyroid tissue to malignant disease of the thyroid gland. Arch Surg 1940; 40:606–615.
35. Maceri DR, Babyak J. Lateral neck mass. Sole presenting sign of metastatic thyroid cancer. Arch Otolaryngol Head Neck Surg 1986; 112:47–49.
36. Rabinov CR, Ward PH, Pusheck T. Evolution and evaluation of lateral cystic neck masses containing thyroid tissue: "lateral aberrant thyroid" revisited. Am J Otolaryngol 1996; 17:12–15.
37. Paliaga A, Bianchelli G, Balercia G, et al. Contribution of the lateral anlage to the embryogenesis of the thyroid gland: evidence of a persisting thyrocarotid duct. Eur J Surg 1997; 163:795–797.
38. Baughman RA. Lingual thyroid and lingual thyroglossal tract remants. A clinical and histopthological study with a review of the literature. Oral Surg 1972; 34:781–799.
39. Casella A, Pisano R, Navarro Cuellar C, et al. Papillary carcinoma of the base of the tongue. Case Clin Minerva Stomatol 1999; 48:535–538.
40. Guimares SB, Uceda JE, Lynn HB. Thyroglossal duct remnants in infants and children. Mayo Clin Proc 1972; 47:117–120.
41. LiVolsi VA, Perzin KH, Savetsky L. Carcinoma arising in median ectopic thyroid (including thyroglossal duct tissue). Cancer 1974; 34:1303–1315.
42. O'Connell M, Grixti M, Harmer C. Thyroglossal duct carcinoma: presentation and management, including eight cases reports. Clin Oncol (R Coll Radiol) 1998; 10:186–190.

43. Donegan JO, Wood MD. Intratracheal thyroid—Familial occurrence. Laryngoscope 1985; 95:6–8.
44. Bone R, Biller HF, Irwin TM. Intralaryngotracheal thyroid. Ann Otol Rhinol Laryngol 1972; 81:424–428.
45. Brandwein M, Som PM, Urken M. Benign intratracheal thyroid: a possible cause for preoperative overstaging. Arch Otolaryngol Head Neck Surg 1998; 124:1266–1269.
46. Houck WV, Kaplan AJ, Reed CE, Cole DJ. Intrathoracic aberrant thyroid identification critical for appropriate operative approach. Ann Surg 1998; 64: 360–362.
47. Gilliland FD, Hunt WC, Morris DM, Key CR. Prognostic factors for thyroid carcinoma. A population-based study of 15,698 cases from the Surveillance, Epidemiology and End Results (SEER) program 1973–1991. Cancer 1997; 79:564–573.
48. Fenton PA, Clarke SE, Owen W, et al. Cribriform variant papillary thyroid cancer: characteristic of familial adenomatous polyposis. Thyroid 2001; 11:193–197.
49. Dahia PL, Marsh DJ, Zheng Z, et al. Somatic deletions and mutations in the Cowden disease gene, PTEN, in sporadic thyroid tumors. Cancer Res 1997; 57:4710–4713.
50. Loh KC. Familial nonmedullary thyroid carcinoma: a meta-review of case series. Thyroid 1997; 7:107–113.
51. Yoshida A, Noguchi S, Fukuda K, Hirohata T. Low-dose irradiation to head, neck, or chest during infancy as a possible cause of thyroid carcinoma in teen-agers: a matched case-control study. Jpn J Cancer Res 1987; 78:991–994.
52. Mizuno T, Iwamoto KS, Kyoizumi S, et al. Preferential induction of RET/PTC1 rearrangement by x-ray irradiation. Oncogene 2000; 19:438–4349.
53. Devita V, Hellman S, Rosenberg S. Cancer Principles and Practice of Oncology. 6th ed. Philadelphia: Lippincott, Williams and Wilkins, 2001:2378.
54. Takahashi T, Simon SL, Trott KR, et al. A progress report of the Marshall Islands nationwide thyroid study: an international cooperative scientific study. Tohoku J Exp Med 1999; 187:363–375.
55. Farahati J, Demidchik EP, Biko J, Reiners C. Inverse association between age at the time of radiation exposure and extent of disease in cases of radiation-induced childhood thyroid carcinoma in Belarus. Cancer 2000; 88:1470–1476.
56. Franklyn JA, Maisonneuve P, Sheppard M, et al. Cancer incidence and mortality after radioiodine treatment for hyperthyroidism: a population-based cohort study. Lancet 1999; 353:2111–2115.
57. Frankenthaler RA, Sellin RV, Cangir A, Goepfert H. Lymph node metastasis from papillary-follicular thyroid carcinoma in young patients. Am J Surg 1990; 160: 341–343.
58. Johnson T, Lloyd RV, Thompson NW, et al. Prognostic implications of the tall cell variant of papillary thyroid carcinoma. Am J Surg Pathol 1988; 12:22–27.
59. Ostrowski ML, Merino MJ. Tall cell variant of papillary thyroid carcinoma: a reassessment and immunohistochemical study with comparison to the usual type of papillary carcinoma of the thyroid. Am J Surg Pathol 1996; 20:964–974.
60. Wenig BM, Thompson LD, Adair CF, et al. Thyroid papillary carcinoma of columnar cell type: a clinicopathologic study of 16 cases. Cancer 1998; 82:740–753.
61. Ferreiro JA, Hay ID, Lloyd RV. Columnar cell carcinoma of the thyroid: report of three additional cases. Hum Pathol 1996; 27:1156–1160.
62. Shaha AR, Shah JP, Loree TR. Risk group stratification and prognostic factors in papillary carcinoma of thyroid. Ann Surg Oncol 1996; 3:534–538.
63. Shaha AR, Loree TR, Shah JP. Intermediate-risk group for differentiated carcinoma of thyroid. Surgery 1994; 116:1036–1040.
64. Clark OH. Predictors of thyroid tumor aggressiveness. West J Med 1996; 165:131–138.
65. Akslen LA, LiVolsi VA. Prognostic significance of histologic grading compared with subclassification of papillary thyroid carcinoma. Cancer 2000; 88:1902–1908.
66. Rüter A, Nishiyama R, Lennquist S. Tall-cell variant of papillary thyroid cancer: disregarded entity? World J. Surg 1997; 21:15–20.
67. Sebastian SO, Gonzalez JM, Paricio PP, et al. Papillary thyroid carcinoma: prognostic index for survival including the histological variety. Arch Surg 2000; 135: 272–277.
68. Shirahige Y, Ito M, Ashizawa K, Motomura T, et al. Childhood thyroid cancer: comparison of Japan and Belarus. Endocr J 1998; 45:203–209.
69. Ikekubo K, Hino M, Ito H, et al. Seven cases of brain metastasis from papillary thyroid carcinoma. Kaku Igaku 2000; 37:349–357.
70. Thompson LD, Wieneke JA, Paal E, et al. A clinicopathologic study of minimally invasive follicular carcinoma of the thyroid gland with a review of the English literature. Cancer 2001; 91:505–524.
71. Deandrea M, Gallone G, Veglio M, et al. Thyroid cancer histotype changes as observed in a major general hospital in a 21-year period. J Endocrinol Invest 1997; 20:52–58.
72. Fukunaga FH, Yatani R. Geographic pathology of occult thyroid carcinomas. Cancer 1975; 36:1095–1099.
73. Hedinger C. Geographic pathology of thyroid diseases. Pathol Res Pract 1981; 171:285–292.
74. Burgess JR, Dwyer T, McArdle K. The changing incidence and spectrum of thyroid carcinoma in Tasmania (1978–1998) during a transition from iodine sufficiency to iodine deficiency. J Clin Endocrinol Metab 2000; 85:1513–1517.
75. Shaha AR, Shah JP, Loree TR. Differentiated thyroid cancer presenting initially with distant metastasis. Am J Surg 1997; 174:474–476.

76. Stojadinovic A, Ghossein RA, Hoos A, et al. Hürthle cell carcinoma: a critical histopathologic appraisal. J Clin Oncol 2001; 19:2616–2625.
77. Schwartz MR. Pathology of the thyroid and parathyroid glands. Otolaryngol Clin North Am 1990; 23:175–215.
78. Shaha AR, Shah JP, Loree TR. Patterns of nodal and distant metastasis based on histologic varieties of differentiated carcinoma of the thyroid. Am J Surg 1996; 172:692–694.
79. Hundahl SA, Fleming ID, Fremgen AM, Menck HR. A National Cancer Data Base report on 53,856 cases of thyroid carcinoma treated in the U.S., 1985–1995. Cancer 1998; 83:2638–2648.
80. Zidan J, Kassem S, Kuten A. Follicular carcinoma of the thyroid gland: prognostic factors, treatment, and survival. Am J Clin Oncol 2000; 23:1–5.
81. Modigliani E, Cohen R, Campos JM, et al. Prognostic factors for survival and for biochemical cure in medullary thyroid carcinoma: results in 899 patients. The GETC Study Group. Groupe d'etude des tumeurs a calcitonine. Clin Endocrinol (Oxf) 1998; 48:265–273.
82. Hahm JR, Lee MS, Min YK, et al. Routine measurement of serum calcitonin is useful for early detection of medullary thyroid carcinoma in patients with nodular thyroid diseases. Thyroid 2001; 11:73–80.
83. Voutilainen PE, Multanen M, Haapiainen RK, et al. Long term prognosis of medullary thyroid carcinoma in 39 patients. Ann Chir Gynaecol 2000; 89:292–297.
84. Kebebew E, Ituarte PH, Siperstein AE, et al. Medullary thyroid carcinoma: clinical characteristics, treatment, prognostic factors, and a comparison of staging systems. Cancer 2000; 88:1139–1148.
84. Giuffrida D, Gharib H. Anaplastic thyroid carcinoma: current diagnosis and treatment. Ann Oncol 2000; 11:1083–1089.
85. Chang TC, Liaw KY, Kuo SH, et al. Anaplastic thyroid carcinoma: review of 24 cases, with emphasis on cytodiagnosis and leukocytosis. Taiwan Yi Xue Hui Za Zhi 1989; 88:551–556.
86. Nishiyama RH, Dunn EL, Thompson NW. Anaplastic spindle-cell and giant-cell tumors of the thyroid gland. Cancer 1972; 30:113–127.
87. Bejarano PA, Nikiforov YE, Swenson ES, Biddinger PW. Thyroid transcription factor-1, thyroglobulin, cytokeratin 7, and cytokeratin 20 in thyroid neoplasms. Appl Immunohistochem Molecul Morphol 2000; 8:189–194.
88. Kleer CG, Giordano TJ, Merino MJ. Squamous cell carcinoma of the thyroid: an aggressive tumor associated with tall cell variant of papillary thyroid carcinoma. Mod Pathol 2000; 13:742–746.
89. Lam KY, Lo CY, Liu MC. Primary squamous cell carcinoma of the thyroid gland: an entity with aggressive clinical behaviour and distinctive cytokeratin expression profiles. Histopathology 2001; 39:279–286.
90. Ng WK, Collins RJ, Shek WH, Ng IO. Cytologic diagnosis of "CASTLE" of thyroid gland: report of a case with histologic correlation. Diagn Cytopathol 1996; 15:224–227.
91. Michelow PM, Leiman G. Metastases to the thyroid gland: diagnosis by aspiration cytology. Diagn Cytopathol 1997; 16:94–95.
92. Ivy HK. Cancer metastatic to the thyroid: a diagnostic problem. Mayo Clin Proc 1984; 59:856–859.
93. Leteurtre E, Leroy X, Pattou F, et al. Why do frozen sections have limited value in encapsulated or minimally invasive follicular carcinoma of the thyroid? Am J Clin Pathol 2001; 115:370–374.
94. Lin HS, Komisar A, Opher E, Blaugrund SM. Follicular variant of papillary carcinoma: the diagnostic limitations of preoperative fine-needle aspiration and intraoperative frozen section evaluation. Laryngoscope 2000; 110:1431–1436.

9

Hyperthyroidism

Terry F. Davies and Arthur E. Schwartz

Mount Sinai School of Medicine, New York University, New York, New York, U.S.A.

1 INTRODUCTION

The clinical presentation of an overactive thyroid depends on the severity of the causative disease and the age of the patient. In younger patients thyroid overactivity may announce itself rapidly, with severe symptoms. In the elderly it usually progresses insidiously, perhaps with the development of unexplained cardiac arrhythmias. The frequency and intensity of the effects on many tissues may be influenced by the nature of the underlying disorder. The major causes of an overactive thyroid gland are summarized in Table 1. The vast majority of such patients, however, suffer from either hyperthyroid Graves' disease or a toxic multinodular goiter.

2 GRAVES' DISEASE

2.1 Presentation

Graves' disease is an autoimmune condition and one of the most common causes of an overactive thyroid gland. It is characterized by a diffuse goiter and hyperthyroidism, which is sometimes accompanied by a unique ophthalmopathy (Fig. 1), and a rare dermopathy, designated pretibial myxedema (1,2). The major signs and symptoms of hyperthyroidism are listed in Table 2. The hyperthyroidism may occur with or without Graves' eye disease. Less frequently the eye disease may present without thyroid involvement (euthyroid ophthalmopathy).

Graves' disease is most common in the third and fourth decades of life, is rare before the age of 10 years, and may occur in the elderly in an "apathetic" form without the typical signs and symptoms of hyperthyroidism. Like other thyroid disease, it is more common in women, with an overall prevalence of 2.7%, and a female:male ratio of approximately 7–10:1 The incidence in women has been estimated to be 1 case per 1000 per year over a 20-year follow-up (3).

The histology of Graves' disease is distinguished by the presence of a heterogeneous thyroiditis and evidence of hyperactive thyroid cells resulting in scalloping of the follicular lining. As a result of the infiltration, the disease may eventually change to thyroid failure because of the development of clinical autoimmune (Hashimoto's) thyroiditis. Furthermore, both these diseases may occur within the same family, indicating their close relationship.

2.2 Evidence for an Autoimmune Etiology

Most patients with Graves' disease display serum autoantibodies against thyroid peroxidase (TPO) (the "microsomal" antigen), thyroglobulin (Tg), and the TSH receptor (TSHR). T-cell–mediated autoimmunity can also be demonstrated against these three thyroid antigens. In addition, patients and their relatives may

Table 1 Causes of Hyperthyroidism

1. Graves' Disease
2. Nodular goiter (uninodular or multinodular)
3. Excess thyroid-stimulating hormone
Pituitary tumor
Trophoblastic tumor
Embryonal testicular carcinoma
Other malignant tumors
4. Ectopic thyroid-producing tissue
Metastatic thyroid carcinoma
Struma ovarii
5. Factitous hyperthyroidism
Excess thyroid hormone ingestion
6. Transient hyperthyroidism
Subacute (de Quervain's) thyroiditis
Autoimmune thyroiditis (postpartum thyroiditis)
Irradiation treatment

Table 2 Major Signs of Hyperthyroidism

Specific for Graves' disease
Eyes—proptosis, periorbital edema, muscle dysfunction
Diffuse, vascular goiter
Localized pretibial myxedma
Acropatchy
Splenomegaly and lymphadenopathy
Nonspecific
Eyes—stare, lid lag, tearing
Tachycardia and atrial fibrillation
Systolic hypertension
Apical systolic flow murmur
Weight loss
Proximal muscle weakness
Moist skin
Tremor
Brisk tendon reflexes
Hair loss

show an increased frequency of other autoimmune disorders, e.g., insulin-dependent diabetes (IDDM), myasthenia gravis, or rheumatoid arthritis. The autoantibodies specific to hyperthyroid Graves' disease are those directed against the TSH receptor (TSHRAb), which behave as TSH agonists and are referred to as thyroid-stimulating antibodies. These antibodies compete for the binding of TSH to the TSH receptor on the surface of the thyroid epithelial cells. Their direct stimulation of the gland removes the thyroid from pituitary TSH control (Fig. 2). Evidence suggests that the thyroid gland is itself the major site of thyroid

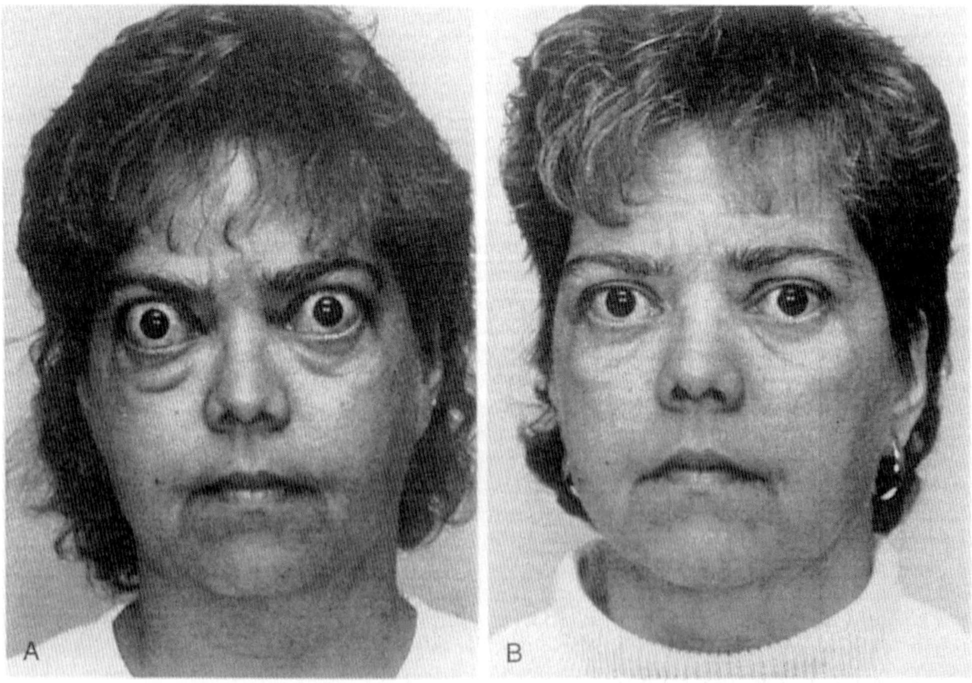

Figure 1 A Graves' patient with ophthalmopathy. (A) Note the proptosis and stare. (B) Following surgical orbital decompression. (From Ref. 1.)

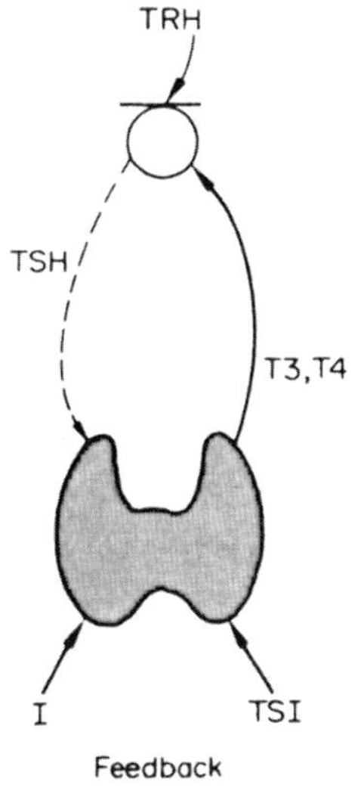

Figure 2 The loss of pituitary control of TSH function in Graves' disease. TSHR-Antibodies (thyroid-stimulating immunoglobulins, TSI) increase thyroid hormone synthesis and release which suppress the action of endogenous TRH on TSH and suppress TSH directly. Hence TSH levels are low but radioiodine uptake is high because it is under the control of TSI rather than TSH. (From Ref. 43.)

autoantibody secretion in Graves' disease, and the responsible B cells can be found among the intrathyroidal lymphocytic infiltrate.

2.3 Pathology

The thyroid in Graves' disease is typically a nonhomogeneous lymphocytic infiltration by T cells and B cells with an absence of follicular destruction (Fig. 3). Presurgical antithyroid drug treatment may reduce the relative degree of infiltration resulting in many pathological reports of sparse or absent infiltrate (4). Follicular epithelial cell size has been found to correlate with the intensity of the local infiltrate, and this could be explained by local production of thyroid-stimulating antibodies.

2.4 Pathogenesis of Graves' Ophthalmopathy and Dermopathy

The pathogenesis of the ophthalmopathy and dermopathy of Graves' disease is now better understood (5,6). Extraocular muscles and adipose tissue are swollen by the accumulation in the extracellular matrix of glycosaminoglycans. These are elaborated by fibroblasts under the influence of cytokines secreted by lymphocytes as part of the associated lymphocytic infiltration. This accumulation causes osmotic changes; the resulting swelling disrupts and impairs the function of the extraocular muscles, which eventually become fibrosed. A similar phenomenon has been proposed to explain pretibial myxedema. The antigen to which the infiltrating T cells react may be the TSH receptor itself. Evidence in support of this hypothesis includes the observation that TSHR mRNA and protein have been shown to be overexpressed in retroorbital fibroblasts and adipocytes when compared to many other sites and different cells where it is found.

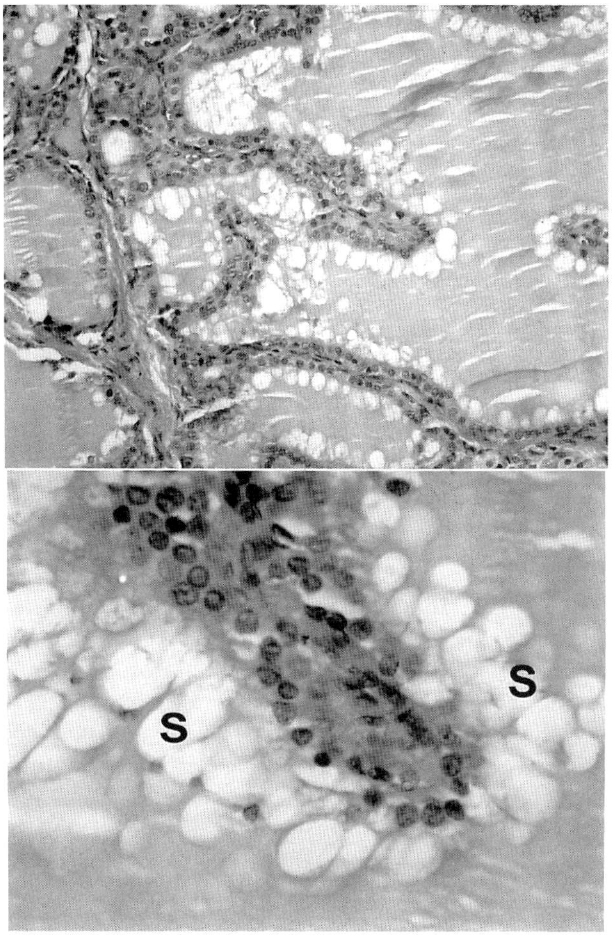

Figure 3 Histology of Graves' disease. (Top) Graves' hyperthyroidism is characterized by thyrocytic hyperplasia forming pseudopapillae that can mimic papillary thyroid carcinoma. (Bottom) The scalloped colloid (S) and thyrocyte nuclear morphology (small, round, nonoverlapped nuclei) distinguish Graves' disease from papillary thyroid carcinoma. (Hematoxylin and eosin)

3 TREATMENT OF GRAVES' HYPERTHYROIDISM

It is not yet possible to treat the basic immunopathogenic factors in Graves' disease. Existing therapies for the thyrotoxic and the ophthalmic manifestations are palliative in that they may relieve but do not cure the disorder. Furthermore, the lack of general agreement as to which therapy is best is evidence for the fact that none is ideal, as reflected in the treatment guidelines of the American Thyroid Association (7).

3.1 Antithyroid Drugs

The major agents for treating thyrotoxicosis are drugs of the thionamide class, most commonly propylthiouracil (PTU) and methimazole (Tapazole). These agents inhibit the oxidation and organic binding of thyroid iodide. In addition, large doses of PTU may impair the conversion of T_4 to T_3 by deiodinase type 1 in the peripheral tissues. The half-life of methimazole is about 6 hours, whereas that of propylthiouracil is about $1\frac{1}{2}$ hours. Hence, a single daily dose of methimazole may be sufficient. As mentioned earlier, thionamide drugs may also directly influence the immune response within the thyroid gland of patients with Graves' disease where the drugs are concentrated (8). The clinical importance of this immunosuppression and coincidental induction of apoptosis is unclear.

3.2 Use of Thionamides

The initial dose of propylthiouracil most commonly employed is 200 mg given orally every 8 hours. An equivalent dose of methimazole is 10–20 mg every 12 hours. Higher doses may be required in patients with severe thyrotoxicosis and large thyroid glands. The therapeutic response appears after a latent period because the agents inhibit the synthesis but not the release of preformed thyroid hormone. There appears to be little difference in the duration of the latent period when either of these agents is employed alone in the usual dosage. In a thyroid gland rich in iodine, as when the patient has received medications containing iodine, the clinical response to antithyroid agents may be delayed for months. Under normal circumstances, a return to euthyroidism is obtained within about 6 weeks. During antithyroid drug treatment the size of the thyroid decreases in many patients; a failure for this to be achieved may signal an intensification and prolongation of the disease process. Since the serum TSH concentration may remain subnormal for many months, presumably secondary to accelerated conversion of T4 to T3 within the pituitary gland, it is best to monitor the response to drug treatment using free T4 and T3 levels. It should also be noted that an enlarging thyroid gland in a treated patient with Graves' disease may signal the onset of tumor growth, requiring prompt sonographic investigation.

3.3 Adverse Reactions

Serious adverse reactions develop in only a small number of patients taking thionamide drugs. Agranulocytosis, occurring in less than 1% of the patients, is of most concern. Because of the frequency of lymphopenia in hyperthyroidism, a complete blood count and differential is recommended before starting antithyroid drug therapy. Serial leukocyte counts are prudent; if they display a downward trend the antithyroid drugs should be discontinued. Agranulocytosis, however, can appear suddenly without a gradual decline in the leukocyte count. The patient must be made alert to the appearance of a sore throat and fever, which can herald the condition, and immediately seek medical advice. A thionamide rash that can take many forms, including hives, occurs in less than 10% of patients. Less frequent reactions include arthralgia, myalgia, neuritis, hepatitis (with PTU), or cholestasis (with methimazole) and rare liver necrosis.

3.4 Predicting the Response to Drug Withdrawal

The persistence of high levels of circulating TSHR-Ab during treatment of Graves' disease portends a recurrence after withdrawal of antithyroid drugs (Table 3) (9). Factors preventing a recurrence include a change from TSHR stimulating antibody to blocking antibody (a rare occurrence), or the progression of concomitant thyroiditis and the onset of thyroid failure.

Table 3 Factors Predicting Recurrence of Graves' Disease

High titer of TSHR antibody
Continuing suppressed TSH levels
Failure to suppress radioiodine uptake or serum Tg on T3 (indirect measure of TSHR-Ab)
High T3 levels at diagnosis
Large thyroid size
Male sex
The postpartum period
Previous recurrence
Large iodine load
Major trauma—physical or mental

Furthermore, iodine deficiency itself may prevent the hyperthyroidism that is a consequence of recurrence of Graves' disease. Additional features associated with the likelihood of long-term remission after withdrawal of therapy include the initial presence of T3 toxicosis, a small thyroid or a decrease in size of the gland, and, in particular, return of the TSH concentration to normal during treatment. In practice, treatment should generally be continued for about 6–12 months and then withdrawn if the serum is TSHR-Ab negative. About three quarters of relapses occur in the first 6 months after withdrawal of therapy, and most of the remainder occur during the subsequent year. The frequency of long-term remission, after withdrawal of antithyroid therapy, has decreased over the past 30 years, perhaps because of the increase in dietary iodine intake. At present only about one third of patients experience a lasting remission. If antithyroid drugs fail, or adverse reactions ensue, radioactive iodine can be administered within a week or less following their discontinuation.

3.5 Iodine

Iodine is now rarely used as sole antithyroid therapy. Large doses of iodine inhibits hormone release rather than formation. Hence, the beneficial effect of iodine is evident more quickly than the effects of even large doses of agents that inhibit hormone synthesis. However, the addition to glandular organic iodine stores may retard the clinical response to subsequently administered thionamide drugs.

The decrease in radioiodine uptake produced by iodine prevents the use of radioiodine as treatment for many weeks. Therefore, aside from its use in preparation for subtotal thyroidectomy (see below), iodine is useful mainly in patients with accelerated thyrotoxicosis or severe thyrocardiac disease. Six mg of iodine daily is sufficient to control thyrotoxicosisis. This is the amount present in one eighth of a drop of saturated solution of potassium iodide (SSKI) or eight tenths of a drop of Lugol's solution. Large doses are more likely to produce adverse reactions. Three drops of SSKI three times daily is recommended. It should be administered with doses of a thionamide drug. Adverse reactions to iodine are unusual and are generally not serious. They include a rash that may be acneiform, drug fever, sialadenitis, conjunctivitis, and rhinitis.

3.6 Radioiodine

The advantage of radioiodine treatment is that it produces thyroid ablation without the potential complications of surgery. Attempts have been made to standardize the radiation delivered to the thyroid gland by varying the dose of radioiodine according to the size of the gland, the uptake of ^{131}I and its subsequent rate of release (a technique called dosimetry) (10). However, such calculations have not provided uniform results, probably because of variations in individual sensitivity secondary to the influence of TSHR-Ab. Hence, many physicians have settled on an arbitrary dose calculated to result in the delivery of 5–7 mCi of ^{131}I to the thyroid gland 24 hours after administration (or 5,000–10,000 rad/g). However, it remains impossible to predict the exact dose of radioactive iodine needed to effect euythyroidism in each specific patient, and repeat treatments may be required unless ablation is aimed for initially.

3.7 Complications of Radioiodine

In theory, radioiodine may affect extrathyroidal tissues that concentrate iodide, e.g., the salivary and gastric glands and the breasts. A radiation thyroiditis itself may lead to an exacerbation of thyrotoxicosis 10–14 days after the radioiodine is administered and has occasionally had serious consequences, including the precipitation of arrythmias or a thyrotoxic crisis. Radioiodine may also worsen Graves' ophthalmopathy, if only transiently (11). This treatment is also accompanied by a high frequency of late hypothyroidism. Many reports have documented that the incidence of hypothyroidism is significant during the first year or two after radioiodine treatment and continues to increase at a rate of approximately 5% per year thereafter. The incidence of postradioiodine hypothyroidism at 5 years has been reported up to 70% (1). For this reason, some physicians advocate an ablative approach to treatment. There is no evidence of a major increase in thyroid carcinoma, leukemia, or an increase of mutation rates, in patients followed many years after treatment (12). The conventional dose of radioiodine employed in the treatment of thyrotoxicosis delivers a radiation dose to the gonads that is roughly equivalent to that delivered by a barium enema examination or intravenous urogram. However, experience from the Chernobyl nuclear accident, which caused a large increase in the number of childhood thyroid cancers (13,14), has caused many physicians to think that the use of any radioactivity in children should be avoided despite some studies that have shown no higher incidence of thyroid carcinoma in adolescents and children treated with radioactive iodine (15). The available evidence supports the concept that, in children, low doses of radiation and fallout (6.5–1500 cGY) stimulate the development of thyroid nodules and cancer, while high doses (10,000 cGY), as in radioiodine therapy, which ablate thyroid tissue, are not associated with an increase in thyroid neoplasia.

3.8 Ophthalmopathy and Radioiodine

As discussed earlier, Graves' ophthalmopathy is most likely the result of crossover specificity between retro-orbital and thyroid antigens, perhaps to the TSH receptor itself. Following radioiodine therapy, the levels of circulating TSHR-Ab increase secondary to impairment of immune restraint caused by the intrathyroidal irradiation because regulatory T cells are especially sensitive to irradiation. Carefully conducted studies indicate that eye disease worsens in patients with Graves' ophthalmopathy who are treated with radioiodine, and some physicians advocate the use of glucocorticoids at the time of radiodine treatment to prevent such effects (16,17). As discussed later, some authors prefer surgical thyroidectomy for the management of Graves' disease with opthalmopathy, although no careful studies have proven this approach to be superior.

4 SURGERY FOR GRAVES' DISEASE

Subtotal thyroidectomy, for the appropriate patient with Graves' disease, offers swift and certain treatment, with a high degree of safety. It is an overnight procedure in most cases. In skilled hands the recurrence rate is 5% or less, the risk of recurrent nerve injury less than 1%, and the incidence of permanent hypocalcemia less than 1–1.5%.

4.1 History

Theodor Kocher, who in 1909 was awarded the Nobel Prize for Medicine or Physiology for his work on the thyroid gland, pioneered the development of thyroidectomy. The disastrous results of myxedema and tetany following total thyroid resection moved him to condemn the procedure. He noted, however, that patients fared better if only one lobe was removed or if the posterior capsule with a portion of the parenchyma of the thyroid lobe was left in place. The reasons were not understood at the time. He had performed 5000 thyroid resections by 1912, reducing the mortality of the operation from 18 to 0.5%.

Plummer's observation in 1923 that iodine blocked the release of thyroid hormone was a watershed event. The use of Lugol's solution for the preparation of hyperthyroid patients before surgery introduced a new era of reduced mortality and postoperative complications. It became the treatment of choice. Subtotal thyroidectomy was transformed from a hazardous endeavor to a safe and reliable procedure. In 1943 the advent of antithyroid drugs such as propylthiouracil and methimazole made it possible to render patients euthyroid before surgery. This was supplemented by iodine for 2–3 weeks before surgery because of its antithyroid activity and its additional value in decreasing the vascularity of the gland. The preparation of the patient in this fashion, as well as refinements in surgical technique, ushered in a new epoch of consistency and reliability in the treatment of hyperthyroidism. The use of adrenergic blocking agents such as propanolol and atenolol added to the safety of the operation. With modern preoperative preparation, the patient arrives in the operating room in a euthyroid state, and thyroid "storm" after surgery is almost never seen.

4.2 Indications for Surgery

Surgery is not a common choice of treatment for Graves' disease in the United States today. Sixty-nine percent of respondents to the American Thyroid Association preferred radioactive iodine ablation, whereas only 22% of European, 22% of Chinese, and 11% of Japanese and Korean physicians selected this method (18,19). Nevertheless, surgery retains a place in the therapeutic options for treatment of the condition. The indications are not precise, rigid, or absolute. Various approaches to treatment of hyperthyroidism have already been discussed, and each offers advantages and disadvantages. In some situations there is no evidence-based proof of superiority. Local custom, patient preference, and availability of medical or surgical expertise are important factors in making a choice. However, surgery achieves euthyroidism more rapidly than radioiodine, which requires 6 weeks or more to reach this status. In a situation when antithyroid drugs do not control hyperthyroidism or the patient becomes allergic to them, surgery can render the patient euthyroid in 10 days.

Currently, surgery is recommended for:

1. Patients with markedly enlarged glands that may encroach on the upper airway and digestive tract. In this situation there is often an accompanying cosmetic deformity that is simultaneously corrected.
2. Patients with accompanying thyroid nodules not designated benign on biopsy. Up to 20% of

nodules in patients with Grave's disease may be malignant.

3. Patients who wish to become pregnant within a year of treatment may be treated surgically to avoid any concern about the effect of radioiodine on the ovaries.
4. Already pregnant patients who cannot be adequately controlled by antithyroid drugs or who develop drug reactions may be considered for surgery. The optimum time is the second trimester.
5. Patients who are noncompliant in the use of antithyroid drugs and refuse radioactive iodine ablation.
6. Patients, especially children, who have a fear of radioactivity—although there is no definitive evidence to support an adverse effect.

Note: In recurrent or persistent hyperthyroidism radioactive iodine is the universal choice because of the vulnerability of the parathyroid glands and recurrent nerves in reoperation.

4.3 Surgery in Special Situations

4.3.1 Childhood

Many authors advise surgery for Grave's disease in children. Antithyroid drugs have a failure rate of 60% or higher and must be continued for a long period. There may be problems with side effects, allergies, and compliance (20). In many centers, however, radioactive iodine is the treatment of choice. If antithyroid drugs cannot be continued or radioactive iodine is declined, subtotal thyroidectomy offers effective and rapid management with few complications. In a series of 82 patients with a median age of 14 years treated by surgery and with a median follow-up of 8.3 years, there was a 6.1% incidence of recurrence, and no cases of permanent hypocalcemia or nerve palsy (21).

4.3.2 Ophthalmopathy

Although the issue is not settled, some authors believe that surgical thyroidectomy, rather than radioactive iodine and high-dose steroids, is the preferred management of hyperthyroid Grave's disease in the presence of ophthalmopathy (22,23). In a prospective randomized trial of total versus subtotal thyroidectomy on 150 patients for the control of Grave's orbitopathy, 70–74% improved after a period of 6–36 months regardless of whether total or subtotal thyroidectomy was performed (24).

4.4 Preparation for Surgery

The usual preparation of hyperthyroid patients for surgery can bring about a euthyroid state within 2–3 weeks. Propylthiouracil 100–200 mg three times a day or methimazole (which has a longer duration of effect) 10–40 mg per day is instituted to block iodination. Propranolol 10–20 mg up to four times a day can rapidly control overt thyrotoxic symptoms by blocking the catecholamine response in hyperthyroidism. Lugol's solution, 3 drops three times a day (disguised in tomato, apple, or orange juice), for 10 days before surgery blocks the release of thyroid hormone and has the additional advantage of decreasing the vascularity of the gland (25). In patients who cannot be given thionamides, iodine and blockers alone can be used for rapid preoperative preparation, with the caution that providing iodine in the absence of antithyroid drugs may worsen the hyperthyroidism in the longer term, since thyroid hormone synthesis has not been blocked. This regimen is not as reliable as the use of all three drugs but is usually effective in bringing thyroid function to normal within 10 days. No date for surgery should be set until a normal metabolic state has been restored. Much too often the operation is planned well in advance, and the patient is given a standardized regimen independent of the clinical progress. In addition, iodine should not be relied on to complete an as yet incomplete response to antithyroid therapy because iodine will enrich glandular hormone stores if the antithyroid drug is not entirely effective.

4.5 Choice of Operative Procedure in Graves' Disease

Surgery provides the best opportunity to leave the patient euthyroid; the figure of 70–80% is most often cited, but is highly dependent upon surgical skill. The most important factor determining postoperative thyroid function is the size of the remnant (26). The goal in surgical management is the removal of sufficient thyroid tissue to insure against recurrence, but that leaves the patient euthyroid. This cannot be consistently achieved because it is not possible to determine the exact amount of tissue that should remain. The figure of a 4–6 g total remnant of thyroid tissue is often given, but in fact is unreliable, because the functional activity is not necessarily related to the size of the remnant. The remnant is still the target of stimulation by TSHR-Abs that produce the disease, and it may hypertrophy under TSHR-Ab stimulation or lose function because of concomitant thyroiditis in an unpredictable way. In addition, the estimates of remnant weight at surgery are largely inaccurate, varying at least 30% above or below the actual weight (27). The objectives of removing sufficient tissue to cure the hyperthyroidism but not so much that the patient will become hypothyroid, compete with each other. Subtotal thyroidectomy is, therefore, a compromise between the risk of recurrent hyperthyroidism and hypothyroidism. Given this choice, recurrent hyperthyroidism is clearly the condition that is more undesirable. However, the remnant size cannot be relied upon to render the patient euthyroid in a predictable way. For this reason there are surgeons who recommend total thyroidectomy, claiming that the operation is equal in safety to subtotal thyroidectomy and can be completely relied upon to control hyperthyroidism (28).

If recurrence of Graves' disease develops, surgery cannot be safely repeated because of the scarring and distortion in the positions of the parathyroid glands and recurrent nerve, which make reoperation hazardous. The patient would be left with the choice of radioiodine, which may have been declined in the first place, or the use of antithyroid drugs. Since the first priority is control of disease, it is far more reasonable to err on the side of removing more, rather than less tissue. Hypothyroidism can be completely controlled and is easily managed by oral administration of thyroxine, which replaces all thyroid functions and is readily monitored by thyroid function studies.

4.6 Technique of Bilateral Subtotal Thyroidectomy

The traditional operation for Graves' disease is bilateral subtotal thyroidectomy. As in all procedures for hyperthyroidism, the main concern is permanent hypocalcemia because of devascularization or damage to the parathyroid glands and injury to the recurrent laryngeal nerve. After exposure of the thyroid lobe in the usual fashion, the middle thyroid vein and superior pole vessels are divided and ligated. The thyroid lobe is rotated medially; the lower parathyroid is identified and, if located towards the posterior aspect of the thyroid lobe, left in place. The upper parathyroid is almost always located posteriorly and also left in place. The recurrent nerve can most easily be identified at the level of the lower or midportion of the thyroid lobe. On the right side the course is more oblique because it comes in from a lateral position after recurring around the subclavian artery and may even be nonrecurrent, branching directly from the vagus at the level of the cricoid. The left nerve travels directly upward and is almost always recurrent. The lower portion is the easiest part of the nerve to identify. As the nerve courses upward it is usually anterior to the upper parathyroid; both may be enveloped by the fascia that anchors the upper thyroid pole to the upper two or three tracheal rings, cricoid cartilage, and pharynx (Berry's ligament). This fibrous sheet must then be dissected from the nerve as it courses superiorly to the point where it enters the larynx just below the cricothyroid muscle (Fig. 4). The superior parathyroid may be covered by this fibrous sheath, enveloped by it, or lie anteriorly. It usually drops posterior to the nerve as it is dissected from adjacent tissue. This is the most difficult part of the nerve dissection and where the superior parathyroid is most likely to be devascularized. The inferior parathyroid can usually be easily dissected from the thyroid and moved posteriorly. However, there are instances when it cannot be dissected free easily or it becomes devascularized during the surgery. To insure viability, such a gland should be removed, minced into 2 mm segments, and transplanted.

Subtotal thyroidectomy leaves the posterior capsule in place, eliminating the need to divide the branches of the inferior thyroid artery that provides the blood supply to the upper as well as the lower parathyroids (Fig. 4). In addition, if only the lower portion of the recurrent nerve is visualized in subtotal thyroidectomy (as is the preference of the authors), the dissection of the most vulnerable part of the nerve as it courses upward and under the cricothyoid muscle is avoided, as is the risk of devascularizing the superior parathyroid gland. In order to expose the upper portion of the nerve, the superior parathyroid frequently has to be dissected, with the attendant risk of damage to its blood supply. This hazard is also removed by leaving the posterior capsule of the thyroid undisturbed.

After the parathyroids and the recurrent nerve are protected, either by preserving the posterior capsule or by visualization and dissection, the ventral 80–90% of the thyroid parenchyma is removed by transecting anterior to the level of the parathyroids to preserve their blood supply. The thyroid capsule is finally sutured to the tracheal fascia creating a tamponade that controls any remaining bleeding (Fig. 5). The authors prefer to remove additional thyroid tissue from within the thyroid capsule after the gland has been transected, by the use of a cautery loop. This has the advantage of removing parenchymal tissue and does not endanger the nerve or the parathyroid gland (Figs. 5, 6). It also makes it easier to control the size of the remnant to be left in place.

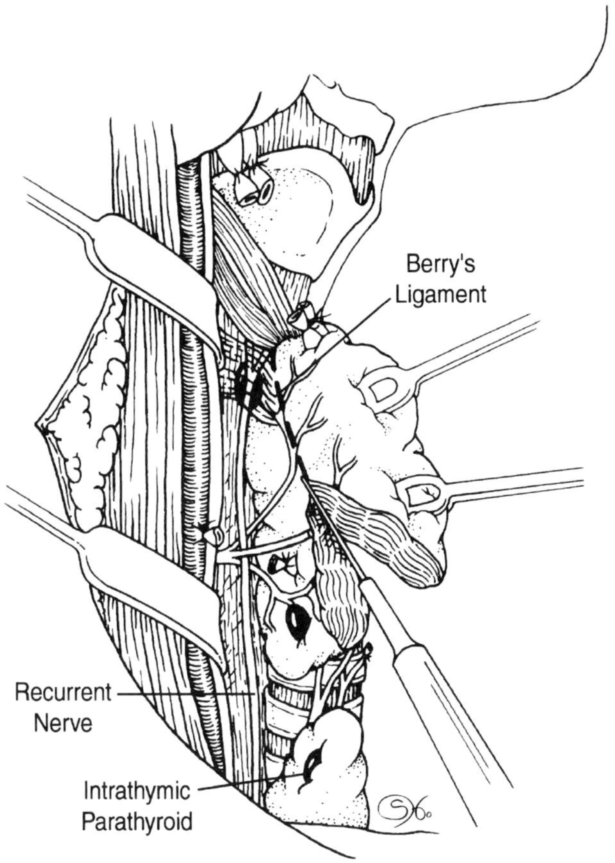

Figure 4 The superior pole vessels have been divided and ligated. The thyroid lobe is rotated medially and the lower portion of the recurrent nerve is identified. The inferior parathyroid gland can be seen in this patient; it is left in place. Berry's fascia is left intact. The recurrent nerve may or may not be visualized at its upper aspect; the upper parathyroid gland, similarly, need not be exposed. These structures are shielded by preserving a posterior rim of thyroid tissue as the thyroid lobe is transected from its lateral to medial side in an oblique direction toward the trachea. If the surgeon wishes to remove additional thyroid tissue, the gland can be transected at a deeper level, or additional parenchyma can be removed from within the capsule by a cautery loop. This facilitates inversion of the capsule of the thyroid into the tracheal fascia.

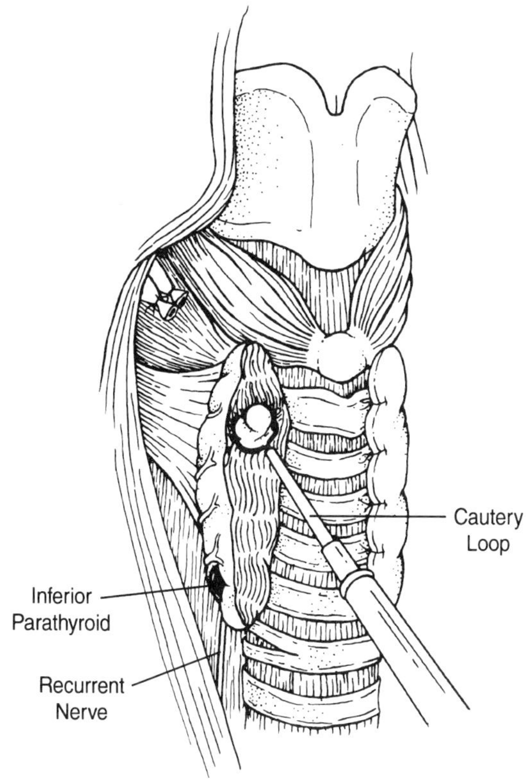

Figure 5 Eighty-five to 90% of the left thyroid lobe has been resected. The thyroid capsule has been sutured to the tracheal fascia, imbricating the remaining portion of the thyroid lobe. This also controls hemostasis by tamponading the residual thyroid tissue. The right thyroid lobe has been transected. Additional thyroid tissue will be removed from within the capsule by a cautery loop. This makes it possible to resect additional parenchymal tissue from within the thyroid capsule, avoiding the parathyroids and the recurrent nerve. It also facilitates more accurate measurement of the amount of tissue to be left in situ.

4.7 Near-Total Thyroidectomy

The technique of total thyroid lobectomy and contralateral near-total thyroidectomy for the opposite side (Hartley-Dunhill operation) is being used more frequently; it has valid reason to be considered. Lobectomy is undertaken on the side that is problematic, i.e., the one containing nodules or the one that is larger. The entire course of the recurrent nerve and superior parathyroid gland on the side of lobectomy are carefully dissected and preserved, but on the opposite side the upper portion of the nerve and the upper parathyroid are left in place, undisturbed, protected by the posterior capsule, and with less exposure to injury. The size of the remnant remaining on the near-total side can be more accurately controlled; approximately 4–5 g are recommended. Most studies show no higher rate of nerve injury or hypocalcemia than subtotal resection. This method is preferred by the authors.

4.8 Results of Surgery for Graves' Disease

The rate of recurrent or persistent hyperthyroidism after subtotal thyroidectomy is approximately 3–6%, when

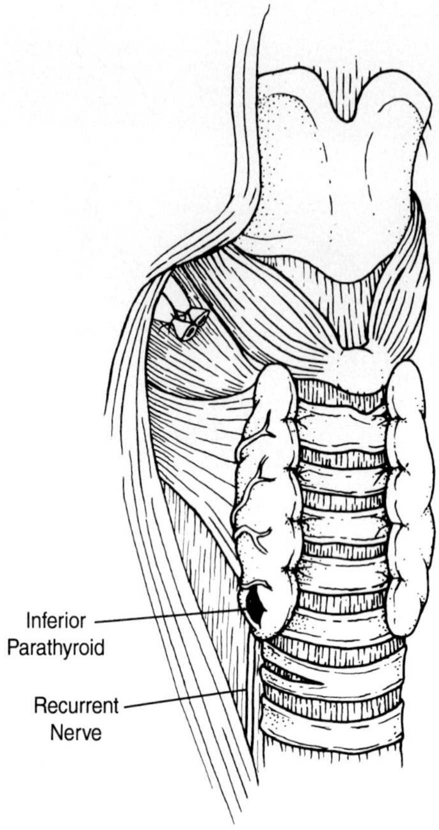

Figure 6 Classic subtotal thyroidectomy. Both thyroid lobes have been subtotally resected and their capsules sutured to the tracheal fascia. A total of 4–6 g of thyroid parenchyma is left in situ. A preserved inferior parathyroid is seen in the right lower pole.

the remnant size is 4–6 g. It is, of course not just a function of the amount of tissue left in place, because of the varying influence of TSH receptor antibodies and ongoing thyroiditis. The rate of hypothyroidism in subtotal thyroidectomy ranges around 30%, but again is a reflection of the remnant size and other variables. The incidence of hypothyroidism increases over the years since the remnant frequently becomes impaired by thyroiditis. There is 0% recurrence of hyperthyroidism for total thyroidectomy, but all patients become hypothyroid.

4.9 Complications of Surgery

The complications of surgery for hyperthyroidism are the same as for other thyroid surgery. Postoperative bleeding may require reopening the neck. The incidence is low, perhaps 1%, and usually easily controlled. Postoperatively bleeding into the neck creates pressure in a closed space that can threaten the airway and the life of the patient. In a hospital setting with close monitoring, experienced personnel can open the wound and preserve the airway. If bleeding occurs where trained help is not available, the result can be catastrophic. The authors believe that these patients should have overnight hospital surveillance (29). Recurrent nerve injury in thyroid surgery in experienced hands occurs in $<1\%$ of cases. The principle of exposure and dissection of the nerve has substantially reduced the incidence of palsy. Hypothyroidism cannot really be accepted as a complication of surgery because the object of the operation is to reduce thyroid parenchyma; the fine line between removing too much or too little is best resolved by taking a bit too much. Hypothyroidism is easily controlled, but recurrent or persistent hyperthyroidism is bad news.

4.10 Hypoparathyroidism

Although hypothyroidism can be readily controlled, permanent hypoparathyroidism is a more distressing problem. This condition produces serious metabolic problems that require lifelong surveillance. Despite treatment, cataracts occur in up to 70% of patients (30). Fatigue, paresthesias, and muscular irritability are continuing problems. Hypocalcemia is more frequent and severe after surgery for Graves' disease rather than other conditions. This is attributed to "hungry bones" as well as the effect of manipulation of the parathyroid glands and interference with their blood supply (31). This problem is usually transient, but there is a wide variation in the frequency of permanent hypoparathyroidism after thyroid surgery for Graves' disease. In experienced hands it is approximately 1–1.5% of patients, and there are some series reporting close to 0%. Temporary hypocalcemia is more common; it occurred in 14.6% of 150 Graves' patients managed by total, bilateral subtotal, or lobectomy with contralateral lobectomy (24).

5 TOXIC MULTINODULAR GOITER AND TOXIC SINGLE NODULES

Toxic multinodular goiter (TMG) is a disorder in which thyroid overactivity is secondary to thyroid nodules that secrete thyroid hormone autonomously, resulting in hyperthyroidism. On radiodine scanning these patients present as a mixture of "hot" and "cold" nodules. A single "hot" toxic adenoma (Plummer's disease) is a less common form of hyperthyroidism. It results from a single autonomous nodule of the thyroid gland, similar to the autonomous lesions seen in toxic multinodular goiter. The adenoma is usually palpable as a solitary mass, almost always over 2.5 cm in size, and can be confirmed by sonography.

5.1 Pathogenesis

Toxic multinodular goiter arises in patients with multinodular goiters of long duration. Thyroid hormone secretion is secondary to somatic mutations that result in constitutive activation of the TSH receptor or TSH receptor signal transduction pathways. The precise mutations in the TSH receptor itself may differ from nodule to nodule (32,33). A small number of autonomous adenomas have mutations in the G protein genes that lead to a similar state of constitutive activation (34). The constitutive activation of the TSHR results initially in functional autonomy of the nodules as shown by the lack of pituitary TSH control. Hyperthyroidism may develop quite suddenly after exposure to excess dietary iodine or iodine-containing contrast medium, which permits autonomous thyroid cells to increase hormone secretion to excessive levels. In addition, toxicity in patients with multinodular goiter may be the result of Graves' disease, which can develop within a multinodular gland or be the primary cause of the nodule formation (35). In the absence of Graves' disease, the remaining normal tissue between the nodules appears inactive as a result of the suppression of pituitary TSH by the excess thyroid hormones secreted by the active nodules. Hence, radioiodine scanning may distinguish between these conditions.

5.2 Clinical Presentation

Toxic multinodular goiter usually occurs after the age of 50 in patients who have had nontoxic multinodular goiter for many years; it is more frequent in women than in men. However, thyroid hormone excess in patients with multinodular goiters is usually less than that seen in Graves' disease. Since the hyperthyroidism is due to autonomously functioning adenomas rather than autoimmune disease, there are no spontaneous remissions; a continued growth of the adenomas and a progression of hyperthyroidism ensues. Eye and skin disease, a reflection of the autoimmune process seen in Graves' disease, are absent (Table 2). Serum T_4 and T_3 concentrations may be only slightly above normal, and a suppressed TSH may be the only finding. Cardiovascular manifestations, including tachycardia and atrial fibrillation, are more common than seen in Graves' disease because of the age of the patients with MNG. Furthermore, obstructive symptoms are not unusual in MNG because the enlarged thyroid gland may be retrosternal. On palpation the goiter is identical to a nontoxic multinodular goiter.

Single toxic adenomas occur in a younger age group than toxic multinodular goiter, frequently in patients in their third or fourth decade. Often there is a history of a longstanding, slowly growing lump in the anterior neck. It is unusual for adenomas to produce thyrotoxicosis until they have achieved a diameter of 2.5–3 cm. There may be progressive growth and increasing function over many years. At first the adenoma may present as a small nodule or may be nonpalpable, but it can be detected by sonography or radioidine scanning as a localized area of increased isotope accumulation. Ultimately the normal thyroid tissue is completely suppressed and atrophic, with a radioiodine scan revealing function limited to the adenoma ("hot nodule"). The mass is usually smooth, well defined, round or ovoid. It is firm and moves with swallowing. Often the remainder of the gland is not palpable. In contrast to Graves' disease, a bruit is never present.

5.3 Investigation

Serum thyroid function testing reveals a suppressed TSH and often an increased FT4 and FT3. However, a suppressed TSH may be the only abnormality, or it may be accompanied by an increased FT3 but a normal FT4. Other reasons for treatment may also be present, e.g., an accelerating loss of bone density or cardiac arrythmias. Ultrasonography offers accurate sizing of the major nodules present; radiodiodine scanning will reveal which of the nodules are toxic. A rapidly enlarging nodule may suggest the need for an aspiration biopsy, but cytology of active nodules can be difficult to interpret because they may simulate papillary carcinoma (36). An MRI or CT scan may be required to assess retrosternal extension and tracheal compression. Pulmonary flow studies can indicate the severity of tracheal obstruction.

6 TREATMENT OF TOXIC NODULES

Treatment of asymptomatic patients with functional nodules is best decided on an individual basis. Rather than thyroid hormone measurements, the degree of TSH suppression is an index of the progression of thyroid hormone production by the autonomous cells. Suppresion of TSH below the lower limits of normal indicates that hyperthyroidism is present and that therapy should be considered except in unusual situations.

Two therapies are most appropriate: radioiodine and surgery although in the very eldelry, antithyroid drugs may also be employed. Large nodules with concomitant physical symptoms are most readily treated with surgical excision. Surgical excision is also employed in patients younger than age 20, in whom radiation from ^{131}I to the perinodular normal thyroid tissue could theoretically predispose to the development of radiation related thyroid neoplasia, although there is no direct evidence for this caution. In addition, determining the dosage of radioactive iodine may be difficult, sometimes requiring repeat treatments.

6.1 Radioiodine

In terms of the specificity of treatment, multiple functioning thyroid nodules are ideal candidates for radioiodine therapy (37). The radiation is directed almost exclusively to the diseased tissue. Since TSH is suppressed, the normal thyroid tissue surrounding the nodule should not take up radioiodine, although in practice many patients develop thyroid failure. For the patient older than age 20 with a single autonomous nodule 3 cm in diameter or smaller, ^{131}I is an appropriate treatment if the risk of eventual hypothyroidism is acceptable. In general, higher doses of radioiodine are required than in Graves' disease, namely ~10 mCi deposited at 24 hours (38). Because of the potential for hypothyroidism with higher ^{131}I doses, prolonged follow-up is mandatory.

6.2 Surgery

When a toxic nodular goiter is sizable and enlarging, surgery can rapidly return the patient to a euthyroid state and simultaneously remove any suspicious "cold" nodules. In such patients a bilateral subtotal thyroidectomy ("near-total thyroidectomy") may be preferred. Surgery for a single autonomous adenoma has the advantage of avoiding the problem of hypothyroidism that may occur after radioiodine ablation. In this situation, a hemithyroidectomy is curative.

7 THYROTOXICOSIS IN SPECIAL CIRCUMSTANCES

7.1 Accelerated Thyrotoxicosis

Thyroid "storm," a severe and accelerated form of thyrotoxicosis, may be seen in postoperative thyrotoxic patients who were not adequately prepared for surgery (39). This condition has become a rarity because virtually every patient now arrives at the operating table in either a euthyroid state or with only mild persisting hyperthyroidism. Storm is usually abrupt in onset and characterized by symptoms of severe thyrotoxicosis and a change in mental status. Extreme hypermetabolism with body temperatures rising to 40°C or more are a distinguishing feature of the condition, which is most commonly precipitated by a medical complication such as infection rather than surgery. If not treated, the outcome can be lethal within 24–48 hours. Management is directed to stopping the synthesis and secretion of thyroid hormone and beta blocking their effects on peripheral tissues by inhibiting peripheral deiodination and adrenergic overactivity. Corticosteroids (dexamethasone 1–2 mg bid), blocking agents, thionamides, and Lugol's solution are used. A controlled cooling blanket is valuable in the attempt to decrease body temperature.

7.2 Amiodarone-Induced Thyrotoxicosis

This antiarrthymic drug has complex effects on the thyroid although the majority (~80%) of patients remain euthyroid (40). The drug resembles T4 and contains 37% iodine and has a half-life of 50–60 days and, therefore, remains available for a long period even after drug withdrawal. Amiodarone has a direct cytotoxic effect on thyroid cells, which may cause thyroid failure. However, the iodine load and/or the cell damage may also precipitate Graves' disease in susceptible individuals, particularly in areas of iodine deficiency. Amiodarone-induced hyperthyroidism may either develop rapidly in a patient or even after a few years of treatment. Antithyroid drugs and radioiodine may be ineffective because of the large intrathyroidal iodine load. Thyroidectomy is, therefore, the treatment of choice and allows the continuation of the drug (41,42).

REFERENCES

1. Davies TF, Larsen PR. Thyrotoxicosis. In: Wilson GM, Foster D, Kronenberg M, Larsen PR, eds. Williams Textbook of Endocrinology. Philadelphia: Saunders, 2002:374–442.
2. Davies TF. The pathogenesis of Graves' disease. In: Braverman LE, Utiger RD, eds. The Thyroid: A Fundamental Text. Philadelphia: Lipincott, 1996:525–536.
3. Vanderpump MPJ, Tunbridge WMG, French JM, Appleton D, Bates D, Clark F, Grimley Evans J, Hasan DM, Rodgers H, Tunbridge F, Young ET. The

incidence of thyroid disorders in the community: a twenty-year follow-up of the Whickham survey. Clin Endocrinol 1995; 43:55–68.
4. McGregor AM, Petersen MM, McLachlan SM, Rooke P, Smith BR, Hall R. Carbimazole and the autoimmune response in Graves' disease. N Engl J Med 1980; 303:302–304.
5. Bahn RS. Understanding the immunology of Graves' ophthalmopathy. Is it an autoimmune disease? Endocrinol Metab Clin North Am 2000; 29:287–296, vi.
6. Davies TF. Trauma and pressure explain the clinical presentation of the Graves' disease triad. Thyroid 2000; 10:629–630.
7. Singer PA, Cooper DS, Levy E, Ladenson PW, Braverman LE, Daniels G, Greenspan FS, McDougall R, Nikolai TF. Treatment guidelines for patients with hyperthyroidism and hypothyroidism. JAMA 1995; 273: 808–812.
8. Davies TF. A new role for methimazole in autoimmune thyroid disease: inducing T cell apoptosis. Thyroid 2000; 10:525–526.
9. Davies TF. Thyroid-stimulating antibodies predict hyperthyroidism. J Clin Endocrinol Metab 1998; 83: 3777–3781.
10. Wellman HN, Anger RT Jr. Radioiodine dosimetry and the use of radioiodines other than ^{131}I in thyroid diagnosis. Semin Nucl Med 1:1971; 356–378.
11. Bartalena L, Marcocci C, Bogazzi F, Manetti L, Tanda ML, Dell'Unto E, Bruno-Bossio G, Nardi M, Bartolomei MP, Lepri A, Rossi G, Martino E, Pinchera A. Relation between therapy for hyperthyroidism and the course of Graves' ophthalmopathy [see comments]. N Engl J Med 1998; 338:73–78.
12. Franklyn JA, Maisonneuve P, Sheppard M, Betteridge J, Boyle P. Cancer incidence and mortality after radioiodine treatment for hyperthyroidism: a population-based cohort study. Lancet 1999; 353:2111–2115.
13. Nikiforov Y, Gnepp DR. Pediatric thyroid cancer after the Chernobyl disaster. Pathomorphologic study of 84 cases (1991–1992) from the Republic of Belarus. Cancer 1994; 74:748–766.
14. Pacini F, Vorontsova T, Molinaro E, Shavrova E, Agate L, Kuchinskaya E, Elisei R, Demidchik EP, Pinchera A. Thyroid consequences of the Chernobyl nuclear accident. Acta Paediatr Suppl 1999; 88:23–27.
15. Hamburger JI. Management of hyperthyroidism in children and adolescents. J Clin Endocrinol Metab 1985; 60:1019–1024.
16. Bartalena L, Marcocci C, Bogazzi F, Panicucci M, Lepri A, Pinchera A. Use of corticosteroids to prevent progression of Graves' ophthalmopathy after radioiodine therapy for hyperthyroidism. N Engl J Med 1989; 321:1349–1352.
17. Bartalena L, Pinchera A, Marcocci C. Management of Graves' ophthalmopathy: reality and perspectives. Endocrinol Rev 2000; 21:168–199.
18. Alsanea O, Clark OH. Treatment of Graves' disease: the advantages of surgery. Endocrinol Metab Clin North Am 2000; 29:321–337.
19. Singer PA, Cooper DS, Levy E, Ladenson PW, Braverman LE, Daniels G, Greenspan FS, McDougall R, Nikolai TF. Treatment guidelines for patients with hyperthyroidism and hypothyroidism. JAMA 1995; 273:808–812.
20. Witte J, Goretzki PE, Roher HD. Surgery for Graves disease in childhood and adolescence. Exp Clin Endocrinol Diabetes 1997; 105(suppl 4):58–60.
21. Soreide JA, van Heerden JA, Lo CY, Grant CS, Zimmerman D, Ilstrup DM. Surgical treatment of Graves' disease in patients younger than 18 years. World J Surg 1996; 20:794–799.
22. Sridama V, DeGroot LJ. Treatment of Graves' disease and the course of ophthalmopathy. Am J Med 1989; 87:70–73.
23. Torring O, Tallstedt L, Wallin G, Lundell G, Ljunggren JG, Taube A, Saaf M, Hamberger B. Graves' hyperthyroidism: treatment with antithyroid drugs, surgery, or radioiodine—a prospective, randomized study. J Clin Endocrinol Metab 1996; 81:2986–2993.
24. Witte J, Goretzki PE, Dotzenrath C, Simon D, Felis P, Neubauer M, Roher HD. Surgery for Graves' disease: total versus subtotal thyroidectomy—results of a prospective randomized trial. World J Surg 2000; 24:1303–1311.
25. Chang DC, Wheeler MH, Woodcock JP, Curley I, Lazarus JR, Fung H, John R, Hall R, McGregor AM. The effect of preoperative Lugol's iodine on thyroid blood flow in patients with Graves' hyperthyroidism. Surgery 1987; 102:1055–1061.
26. Ozaki O, Ito K, Mimura T, Sugino K, Ito K. Factors affecting thyroid function after subtotal thyroidectomy for Graves' disease: case control study by remnant-weight matched-pair analysis. Thyroid 1997; 7: 555–559.
27. Falk SA. Surgical treatment of hyperthyroidism. In: Falk SA, ed. Thyroid Disease. Philadelphia: Lippincott, 1997:319–340.
28. Perzik S. The place of total thyroidectomy in the management of 909 patients with thyroid disease. Am J Surg 1976; 132:480–483.
29. Schwartz AE, Clark OH, Ituarte P, Lo GP. Therapeutic controversy: thyroid surgery—the choice. J Clin Endocrinol Metab 1998; 83:1097–1105.
30. Ireland AW, Hornbrook JW, Neale FC, Posen S. The crystalline lens in chronic surgical hypoparathyroidism. Arch Intern Med 1968; 122:408–411.
31. Yamashita H, Noguchi S, Tahara K, Watanabe S, Uchino S, Kawamoto H, Toda M, Murakami N. Postoperative tetany in patients with Graves' disease: a risk factor analysis. Clin Endocrinol (Oxf) 1997; 47:71–77.
32. Van Sande J, Parma J, Tonacchera M, Swillens S, Dumont J, Vassart G. Somatic and germline mutations

of the TSH receptor gene in thyroid diseases. J Clin Endocrinol Metab 1995; 80:2577–2585.
33. Tonacchera M, Chiovato L, Pinchera A, Agretti P, Fiore E, Cetani F, Rocchi R, Viacava P, Miccoli P, Vitti P. Hyperfunctioning thyroid nodules in toxic multinodular goiter share activating thyrotropin receptor mutations with solitary toxic adenoma. J Clin Endocrinol Metab 1998; 83:492–498.
34. Trulzsch B, Krohn K, Wonerow P, Chey S, Holzapfel HP, Ackermann F, Fuhrer D, Paschke R. Detection of thyroid-stimulating hormone receptor and Gsalpha mutations: in 75 toxic thyroid nodules by denaturing gradient gel electrophoresis. J Mol Med 2001; 78:684–691.
35. Kraiem Z, Glaser B, Yigla M, Pauker J, Sadeh O, Sheinfeld M. Toxic multinodular goiter: a variant of autoimmune hyperthyroidism. J Clin Endocrinol Metab 1987; 65:659–664.
36. Livolsi VA. Surgical Pathology of the Thyroid. Philadelphia: Saunders, 1990.
37. Nygaard B, Hegedus L, Gervil M, Hjalgrim H, Soe-Jensen P, Hansen JM. Radioiodine treatment of multinodular non-toxic goitre. Br Med J 1993; 307:828–832.
38. Bonnema SJ, Bennedbaek FN, Wiersinga WM, Hegedus L. Management of the nontoxic multinodular goitre: a European questionnaire study. Clin Endocrinol (Oxf) 2000; 53:5–12.
39. Ringel MD. Management of hypothyroidism and hyperthyroidism in the intensive care unit. Crit Care Clin 2001; 17:59–74.
40. Martino E, Bartalena L, Bogazzi F, Braverman LE. The effects of amiodarone on the thyroid. Endocr Rev 2001; 22:240–254.
41. Newman CM, Price A, Davies DW, Gray TA, Weetman AP. Amiodarone and the thyroid: a practical guide to the management of thyroid dysfunction induced by amiodarone therapy. Heart 1998; 79:121–127.
42. Eaton SE, Euinton HA, Newman CM, Weetman AP, Bennet WM. Clinical experience of amiodarone-induced thyrotoxicosis over a 3-year period: role of colour-flow Doppler sonography. Clin Endocrinol (Oxf) 2002; 56:33–38.
43. Hall R, Rees Smith B, Mukhtar E-D. Thyroid stimulators in health and disease. Clin Endocrinol 1975; 4:213–230.

10

Diagnosis and Management of Thyroid Nodules

Jeffrey I. Mechanick

Mount Sinai School of Medicine, New York University, New York, New York, U.S.A.

1 INTRODUCTION

Nodular thyroid disease refers to the presence of a solitary solid nodule, a multinodular gland, or one or more cystic lesions. The evolution of new concepts and technological advancements has had considerable impact on the management of nodular thyroid disease over the past decade. These include:

- Recognition of an increased prevalence of nodular thyroid disease and an increased potential for thyroid carcinoma in nodules traditionally thought to be at low risk (multinodular goiter, cystic, chronic, and those nodules associated with hyperthyroidism)
- Low lethality of papillary thyroid cancer, the most common type of thyroid cancer, based on long-term clinical data
- Popularization of office-based ultrasonography (US) and ultrasound-guided fine needle aspiration biopsy (UG-FNA)
- Development of highly sensitive thyroid-stimulating hormone (TSH) assays
- Demonstration of low sensitivity and specificity of L-thyroxine suppression therapy to differentiate benign from malignant nodules
- Use of minimally invasive thyroid surgical techniques

New thyroid nodules appear at an annual rate of 0.08% (1). There is a 5–10% lifetime risk for palpable nodular thyroid disease, which is increased in iodine deficient areas and decreased in iodine-sufficient areas (2). Also, 20–40% of patients with normal thyroid glands on palpation will have clinically significant ultrasound-demonstrable thyroid nodules (3,4) or additional nonpalpable nodules in a patient with a single palpable nodule (5). Furthermore, 50% of patients with thyroid glands that are normal by palpation will have small, subcentimetric nodules (6).

In contrast, thyroid cancer is relatively rare, affecting only 0.004% of Americans, with 12,000 new cases diagnosed each year, accounting for 1% of all malignancies and 0.5% of cancer mortality (7). Mortality from thyroid cancer is rare among patients with stage I disease, but increases with more extensive disease on presentation, hence providing the impetus for early detection of this potentially "curable" disease.

Solitary nodules or multinodular glands can harbor autonomously functioning tissue capable of producing a thyrotoxic state and a suppressed TSH level. Krohn and Paschke (8) hypothesized the following etiological sequence for the development of autonomous nodules: (1) diffuse thyroid hyperplasia in children in response to iodine deficiency, (2) increased risk of mutagenesis, (3) constitutive activation of the cAMP cascade via mutations in the TSH receptor and/or $G_s\alpha$ protein, and (4) selective growth of a mutant cell line which is independent of TSH stimulation. Nonfunctional (cold) nodules might be formed by a mutation in a gene favoring dedifferentiation, such as *ras* oncogene. Moreover, factors other than TSH, which crosstalk with TSH-dependent signaling pathways, have been implicated in thyroid cell growth and nodule formation. These include insulin, insulin-like growth factor 1, epidermal growth factor, basic fibroblast growth factor, and transforming growth factor-β.

Approximately 90–95% of solitary thyroid nodules are associated with normal TSH levels (9). Belfiore et al. (10) evaluated 5637 patients with nonfunctioning thyroid nodules from 1980 to 1990 and found an overall thyroid cancer frequency of 4.6% (5.3% in iodine-sufficient areas and 2.7% in iodine-deficient areas). Kuma et al. (1) found that most thyroid nodules decrease in size during a period of observation, with 38% actually disappearing and 13% enlarging. With subsequent evaluation, thyroid cancer was found by FNA in 26.3% of enlarging thyroid nodules, contrasted with only 6.4% of stable thyroid nodules. In a later study involving US and UG-FNA follow-up of 134 patients over a 9- to 11- year period, 92% of thyroid nodules remained benign, with 42–79% decreasing in size or disappearing altogether (12). However, 21–23% became larger, were referred to surgery, and found to harbor a malignancy in 4.5% of cases (12). The authors conclude that FNA-proven benign thyroid nodules remain benign over many years and do not require medical or surgical intervention unless there is growth.

Frequently, a palpable nodule represents a dominant nodule in a multinodular gland. These dominant nodules have an overall likelihood of malignancy comparable to truly solitary, solid nodules but less than simple cysts (10,13). Complex cysts, demonstrating both solid and cystic structures by ultrasound, and large (>3 cm) simple cysts that recur after aspiration have a similar risk of malignancy as purely solid nodules, since they may represent cystic degeneration of these solid lesions (14).

2 INITIAL EVALUATION

Patients with nodular thyroid disease are evaluated by a TSH level, neck US, and UG-FNA. This approach avoids unnecessary radiation exposure associated with scintigraphy and has also been associated with improved quality-adjusted life expectancy and cost-effectiveness when compared with an approach that would perform scintigraphy and/or immediate surgery on all thyroid nodules (15). An approach centered on the primacy of FNA increases the cancer yield 15–30% among solitary thyroid nodules while reducing unnecessary surgical procedures and decreasing the cost of care by 25% (16).

Historical features frequently guide the physician to the appropriate diagnostic algorithm. Certain clinical features are so significant with respect to risk that regardless of the FNA results, surgery should be seriously considered. These features include childhood and adolescence, age over 60 years, symptoms of tissue invasion in the neck resulting from the mechanical effects of tumor pressure or infiltration, history of radiation exposure to the head or neck, and family history of thyroid cancer. Thyroid nodules are more common in women. However, men and women have equal rates of thyroid cancer. Therefore, a thyroid nodule in a man is more likely to represent a malignancy. In fact, Belfiore et al (10) found that male patients over 70 years of age who had a nonfunctioning thyroid nodule had a 50% risk of thyroid cancer. Papillary thyroid cancer is more likely in iodine-sufficient regions (17), while follicular thyroid cancer is more likely in iodine-deficient regions (18).

In children with nodular thyroid disease and a history of radiation exposure to the head and neck, the incidence of thyroid cancer is 14–61% (19–21). These relatively high rates are principally due to the effects of radiation exposure on tumorigenesis in children. Therefore, patients should be questioned regarding possible radiation exposure for childhood conditions such as acne, thymic or tonsillar enlargement, tuberculous lymphadenopathy, and skin or scalp lesions. A patient who may have been exposed to Chernobyl radiation leakage as a child in Belarus or Ukraine is also at higher risk for thyroid cancer. Overall, the presence of a thyroid nodule and a history of radiation exposure is an indication for surgery.

With pregnancy, the thyroid gland enlarges physiologically and pre-existing nonpalpable thyroid nodules may become palpable. The evaluation of thyroid nodules in pregnancy is the same as in nonpregnant women with the exception that radioiodine studies are avoided. If a malignancy is discovered, surgery may be performed safely during the second trimester or deferred until after delivery.

Pain is generally not a feature of thyroid nodules, and when it does occur it is typically acute in onset, representing hemorrhage into a benign colloid nodule. In the elderly, a new or rapidly growing thyroid nodule could represent a malignancy, particularly an anaplastic lesion, and surgery should be considered promptly. Family history of thyroid cancer can suggest medullary thyroid cancer as part of the multiple endocrine neoplasia (MEN) syndromes (type 2a or 2b), non-MEN familial syndromes, familial papillary thyroid cancer that can also be associated with familial adenosis polyposis (Gardner's syndrome), and ataxia telangiectasia, or familial follicular carcinoma.

Physical examination of the thyroid gland should be performed with the patient seated upright, anteriorly and posteriorly (Fig. 1), as well as with the patient in the supine position with the neck fully extended. Since the thyroid gland is enveloped by the deep cervical fascia, which encompasses the thyroid cartilage and trachea, the gland will move with swallowing. This observation allows differentiation between a mass arising in the thyroid from lymph nodes and most other neck structures. One exception is a thyroglossal duct cyst, which will also move with swallowing because of its attachment to the hyoid bone. Whereas thyroid gland palpation is only possible through two layers of overlying strap muscles as well as the cervical fascia, the examination is relatively insensitive compared to office-based ultrasonography.

Generally, thyroid nodules greater than 1 cm in diameter are palpable unless they are situated deep in the neck. Though irregular and firm nodules are suspicious for cancer, papillary and follicular cancers can be soft; benign calcifications as well as thyroid cysts (if under tension) can be firm. Fixation of the nodule to underlying soft tissue is a sign of malignancy. Careful attention should be directed to the presence of lymphadenopathy, tracheal deviation, and clinical signs of hypo- or hyperthyroidism. Lateral thyroid nodules move with swallowing, whereas lymph nodes do not. Indirect laryngoscopy should be performed on all patients, especially those with large or symptomatic thyroid nodules, to assess vocal cord function. Recurrent nerve palsy is highly suspicious for malignancy

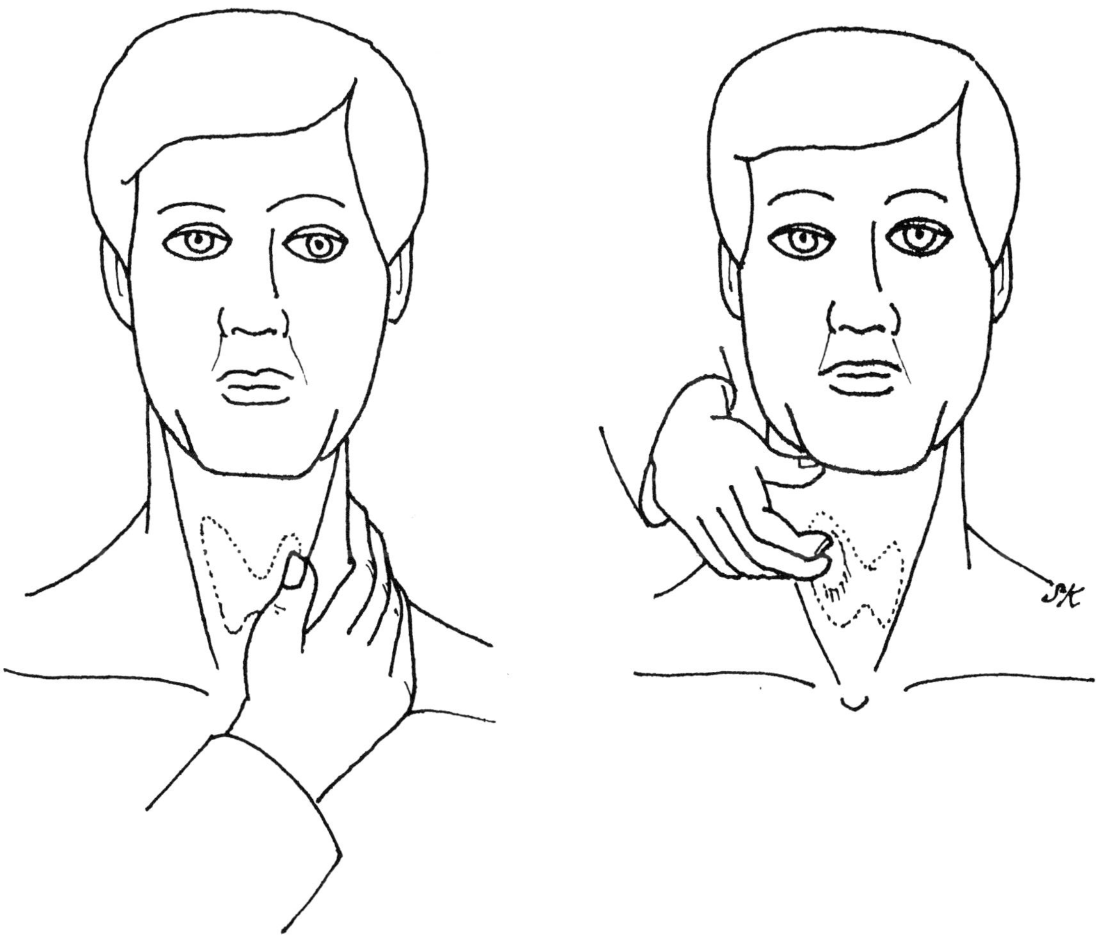

Figure 1 Physical examination of the thyroid gland: (left) anterior palpation using thumb; (right) posterior palpation using fingertips.

related to nerve invasion, though enlarging benign colloid nodules or even left atrial dilatation can elicit similar signs due to a direct pressure effect. Hamming et al. (22) studied 169 patients with nodular thyroid disease and found benign disease in 17% of patients with vocal cord paralysis, 29% with cervical lymphadenopathy, 29% with fixed nodules, and 50% with hard nodules. A summary of important history and physical findings in the evaluation of a patient with a thyroid nodule is given in Table 1.

If the TSH level is suppressed in a patient with nodular thyroid disease, hyperthyroidism is present and may be due to an autonomously functioning thyroid nodule (AFTN) or a nonfunctioning nodule in the setting of autoimmune or viral thyroiditis. Radioiodine scintigraphy can evaluate iodine transport and organification and is preferred over technetium scintigraphy, which can only evaluate iodine transport. Autonomously functioning thyroid nodules are seldom toxic when smaller than 2.5–3.5 cm. In general, AFTN are considered to be benign, though several studies have described significant malignancy rates when thyroidectomy is performed. Thyroid cancer is found in up to 6% of AFTN in adults and up to 11% of AFTN in children (23,24). Overall, Wong et al. (25) remark that 10% of warm nodules are malignant and 5% of hot nodules are malignant. These figures need to be confirmed in larger studies, but are comparable to the 4.6% overall incidence of carcinoma in nonfunctioning solitary thyroid nodules found by Belfiore et al. (10). These data support the use of UG-FNA, concomitant with drawing a TSH level, in all thyroid nodules at presentation. This is in considerable contrast to the previously held view that thyroid cancer is so rare in AFTN that UG-FNA is not necessary.

The presence of antithyroid antibodies can also support a diagnosis of Hashimoto's thyroiditis, which is frequently associated with benign nodularity due to lymphocytic infiltration. Nevertheless, an association between papillary thyroid cancer and Hashimoto's thyroiditis is well recognized in the literature (26). In a series of 136 patients with papillary thyroid cancer, 30% had chronic lymphocytic thyroiditis, 65% of whom had antithyroglobulin antibodies (27). Patients with both conditions were younger, female, and more likely to have multicentric tumors (27). Tumor-infiltrating lymphocytes were far more likely with papillary thyroid cancer when chronic lymphocytic thyroiditis existed (82.5% vs. 5%) (27). There is an improved prognosis in patients with papillary thyroid cancer when it is associated with Hashimoto's thyroiditis (27). Thyroid cancer may also be more frequent (28) and more aggressive (29) when associated with Graves' disease. However, recent studies argue against the association of thyroid cancer and Graves' disease (30,31).

A baseline serum thyroglobulin is of little help in the evaluation of nodular thyroid disease since it may be elevated in benign as well as malignant conditions. On the other hand, a baseline serum calcitonin level should be drawn as part of the routine screening in patients with a family history of medullary thyroid carcinoma (MTC) or multiple endocrine neoplasia type-2 (MEN-2). A diagnosis of MTC can be confirmed with pentagastrin-stimulated calcitonin levels and a diagnosis of MEN-2 with DNA analysis for *ret* mutations (32). In patients without a history of familial MTC or MEN-2, routine serum calcitonin screening for sporadic MTC in nodular thyroid disease has been controversial, though a recent study of 1448 patients by Hahm et al. (33) advocated this procedure. Proponents of routine screening simply argue that this rare tumor may be diagnosed preoperatively and therefore a more appropriate surgical procedure and lymph node dissection can be planned. Opponents argue that this screening test is

Table 1 History and Physical Findings in the Evaluation of Patients with Nodular Thyroid Disease

Favor benign disease	Favor malignant disease
Family history of autoimmune thyroid disease or benign nodular goiter	Previous or family history of thyroid cancer
Multinodular goiter without a dominant nodule	Age < 20 years or > 60 years
Symptoms of hypo- or hyperthyroidism	Male
Pain or tenderness associated with the nodule	Presence of dysphagia and hoarseness
The nodule is soft, smooth, and/or mobile	The nodule is firm, hard, and/or fixed
	Presence of cervical lymphadenopathy
	Childhood/adolescent radiation exposure to head/neck

not cost-effective and false elevations of calcitonin can occur with (1) single-site radioimmunoassays, (2) C-cell hyperplasia adjacent to a differentiated papillary or follicular carcinoma, (3) concurrent MTC and papillary carcinoma, (4) concurrent thyroiditis and C-cell hyperplasia, and (5) extrathyroidal calcitonin production in pulmonary Kulchitsky cells, pituitary gland, thymus, and cancers of lung, breast, liver, pancreas, and of neuroendocrine derivation.

3 RADIONUCLIDE SCANNING

Three commonly available radioisotopes are used for thyroid scintigraphy. ^{131}I is the most effective for whole body imaging for thyroid cancer follow-up, but the high energy of gamma emissions compromises the image resolution and the long half-life (8 days) increases radiation exposure. ^{123}I is used for routine evaluation of thyroid nodules because of the high ratio of detectable photons to radiation. It also has less overall thyroidal radiation exposure due to the absence of beta emissions and a short half-life (13 hr). ^{99m}Tc is trapped by thyroid tissue due to its similar charge and size as iodide, but it is not organified and therefore results that are not consistent with radioiodine images may occur. Technetium is frequently used because of its wide availability in nuclear medicine facilities, its low radiation exposure due to a very short half-life (6 hr), and ideal gamma energy with absence of beta emissions. Intense ^{99m}Tc-methoxyisobutylisonitrile (MIBI) uptake has also been associated with an increased likelihood of malignancy (34). In addition to the above, preliminary results with dual-phase ^{201}thallium imaging show promise as a potential discriminator between benign and malignant nodules, especially when FNA results prove to be equivocal (35).

Toxic autonomous nodules greater than 2.5 cm are usually associated with thyrotoxicosis, placing the patient at risk for osteoporosis, arrhythmia, and a variety of constitutional symptoms. These lesions should generally be treated with radioiodine, but surgery is appropriate for younger patients, those with larger, more symptomatic nodules or nodules with significant hemorrhage or cystic degeneration, or in those who simply prefer surgery after a thorough discussion with the physician. Percutaneous alcohol injection can also be considered as a safe alternative treatment. In elderly patients with subclinical hyperthyroidism due to an autonomously functioning nodule, there is an increased risk of atrial fibrillation, so radioiodine ablation should be considered (36). Scintigraphy may also be used as a complementary study to evaluate asymmetry, which may represent hemiagenesis, a hypertrophied lobe masquerading as a sonographically demonstrated nodule, substernal masses, and ectopic (usually lingual) or pedunculated thyroid tissue.

4 THYROID ULTRASONOGRAPHY

Ultrasonography is performed at baseline to (1) determine whether a palpable thyroid mass actually represents a discrete nodule, (2) assess malignant potential of the nodule (37), (3) determine whether additional, nonpalpable nodules are present, which may modify the risk of malignancy and guide the extent of surgery, (4) define the anatomy of the neck, especially vascular structures, when surgery seems likely, and (5) enable accurate cellular sampling with FNA. Nevertheless, US cannot diagnose a thyroid malignancy.

Sonographic features of benign nodules include normal or hyperechoic signal consistent with colloid, a "halo" sign (Fig. 2), or well-delineated margin, a thin-walled cyst, eggshell or amorphous calcifications, shadowing, decreasing size over time, lower intranodular blood flow using Doppler studies, and absence of lymphadenopathy. Alternatively, malignant nodules are generally hypoechoic, owing to increased cellularity, with an irregular border. Other features suggestive of malignant lesions are invasion of muscle or surrounding tissue, punctate microcalcifications, no shadowing, and higher intranodular blood flow. Metastatic lymph nodes are typically greater than 1 cm, rounded with an anterior-posterior/transverse ratio greater than 0.7, and without an echogenic hilar line.

The sensitivity of ultrasound is approximately 3 mm, well below the limits of palpation. Most of the sonographic features use to discriminate between benign and malignant lesions can be nonspecific or insensitive. For instance, Propper et al. (38) found the "halo" sign to be nonspecific and Takashima et al. (39) found that microcalcifications, which typically represent psammoma bodies in papillary thyroid carcinoma, had a 93% specificity, 70% positive predictive value, but a sensitivity of only 36%. Moreover, microcalcifications had the highest accuracy (76%) of any single sonographic sign (39). Roughly 15–25% of thyroid nodules are cystic, comprising simple cysts, hemorrhagic colloid nodules, and parathyroid cysts. However, papillary thyroid cancer with necrosis and hemorrhagic adenomas can also be cystic (40).

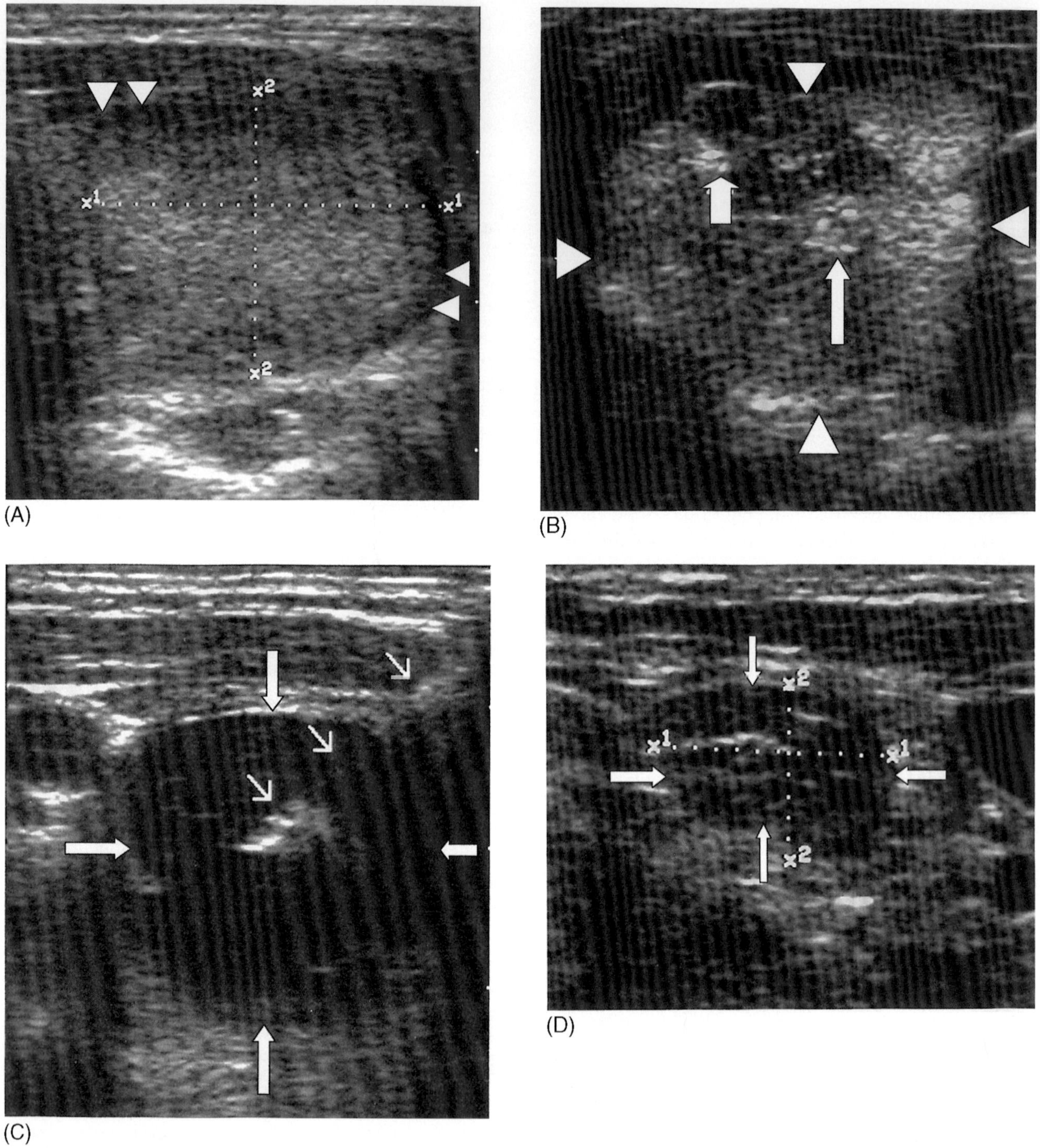

Figure 2 Thyroid ultrasonography. (A) Benign thyroid nodule representating a follicular adenoma which is isoechoic and solid, with a thin, regular halo (arrows), and measuring 2.5 cm × 1.9 cm. Halo sign is the presence of decreased echo signal along the periphery of the lesion corresponding to a capsule. (B) Papillary thyroid cancer with hypoechoic areas, an irregular border (arrowheads), and fine calcifications (long thin arrow). UG-FNA needle tip is indicated by the short wide arrow. (C) Thyroid cyst (large arrows) with UG-FNA needle (small arrows) inserted just prior to aspiration of fluid. Needle tip is more echogenic due to bevel. (Courtesy of Dr. Elise Brett, Mount Sinai School of Medicine.) (D) Pathological lymph node (arrows) in a patient with papillary thyroid cancer. Note that the ratio of anterior-posterior to transverse dimensions is 1.1 cm/1.4 cm = 0.8 (normal < 0.7), the node is hypoechoic, and there is no echogenic hilar line. (Courtesy of Dr. Elise Brett, Mount Sinai School of Medicine, New York, NY.)

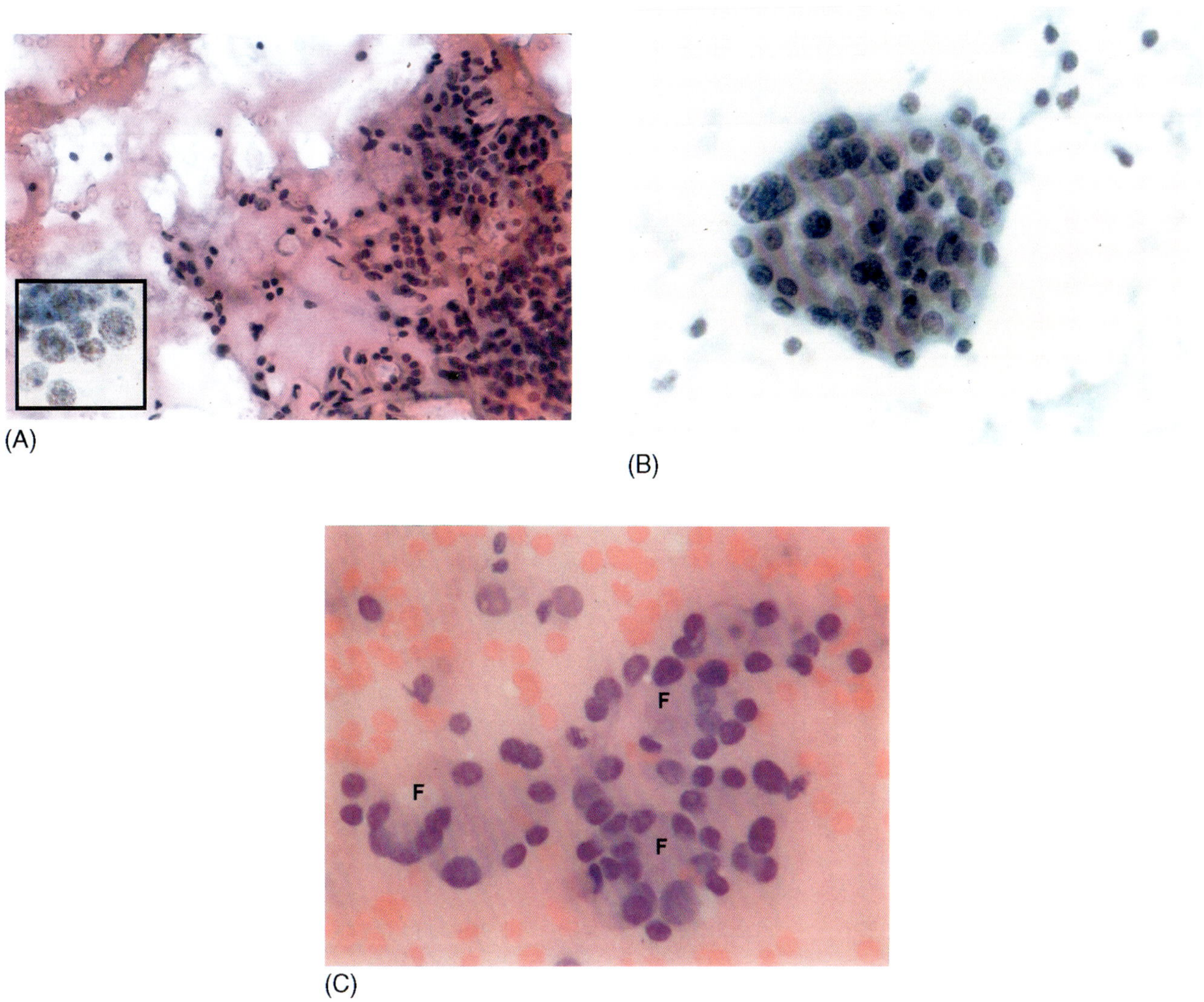

Figure 3 Cytologic features of benign and malignant thyroid fine needle aspirates. (A) nodular goiter—aspirates from colloid goiter showing clusters of follicular cells with uniform nuclei. There is abundant watery colloid in the background. Foamy macrophages (inset) indicating cystic degeneration (Papanicolaou stain). (B) Hashimoto's thyroiditis—an island of follicular epithelium, some of which are oncocytic (Hürthle cells, Ashkenazi cells). The nuclei of follicular cells can show anisonucleosis and pleomorphism, particularly in severe cases. Lymphoid cells are scattered in the background. Oncocytic changes are not specific to Hashimoto's thyroiditis, and can also be seen in goiter, follicular adenomas, Hürthle cell neoplasms, and even in oncocytic papillary thyroid carcinoma (Papanicolaou stain). (C) Follicular adenoma—follicular cells often arranged in thin layered flat sheets or clusters, with microfollicles (F). Follicular cells show uniform nuclei with fine chromatin and barely visible nucleoli. Colloid component can be present, though sometimes scantier than goiter (Diff-Quick Stain). (D) Papillary thyroid carcinoma—aspirates are usually cellular with papillary configuration. Follicular cells can have nuclear grooves (coffee bean shaped), intranuclear holes (insert), or occasionally intranuclear cytoplasmic vacuolation ("Orphan Annie eyes"). Colloid may be present. Multinucleated giant cells may be associated with epithelial clusters (Papanicolaou stain). (E) Anaplastic carcinoma—a highly pleomorphic tumor with markedly cytological atypia. Anisonucleosis is often accompanied by prominent nucleoli and mitotic figures. The background can be dirty due to tumor necrosis. Tumor cells can be spindly or squamoid. Clinically, metastatic lesions should be excluded before a diagnosis of anaplastic thyroid carcinoma can be made. (Papanicolaou stain). (Parts A–E courtesy of Dr. Beverly Wang, Mount Sinai School of Medicine, New York, NY.)

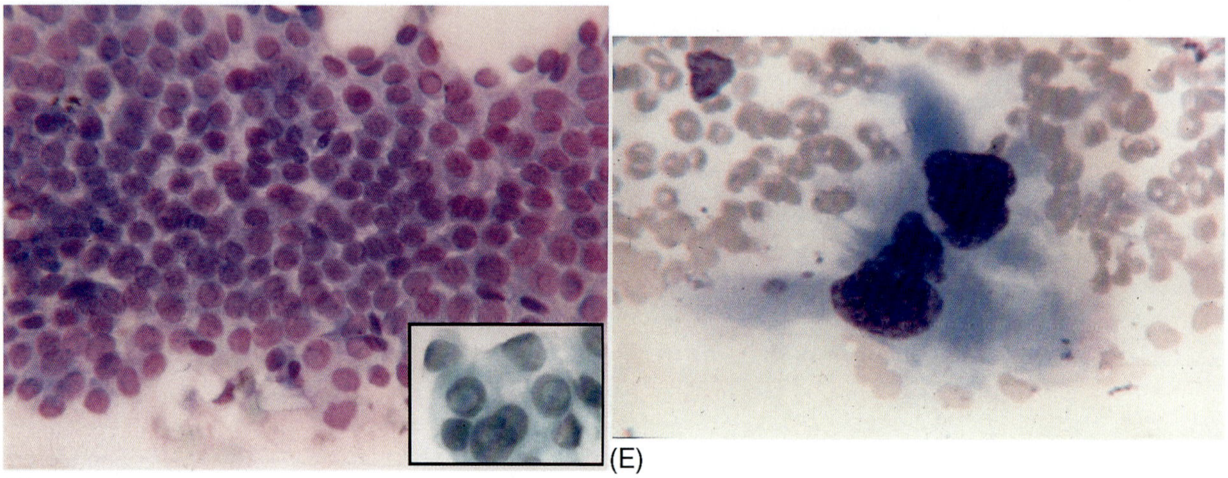

(D) (E)

Figure 3 Continued.

Additional reasons to perform a thyroid ultrasound include follow-up of thyroid nodular size, evaluation for thyroid cancer recurrence after hemithyroidectomy or total thyroidectomy, evaluation of potential pathogenic cervical lymph nodes, and confirmation of the presence of a thyroglossal duct cyst or other rare malformations mimicking thyroid pathology. Limitations of thyroid sonography are observer dependency and the inability to identify retrotracheal, retroclavicular, or substernal extensions of the thyroid due to acoustic shadowing from overlying air or bone (41).

Logistically, the patient is in the supine position with the neck extended. Transducing gel is applied to a high-frequency rectilinear transducer (typically 5–10 MHz) and the examiner proceeds to identify the right and left thyroid lobes, the isthmus, and adjacent structures, in the transverse and then longitudinal views (Fig. 2). Thyroidal volume for each lobe can be estimated by multiplying the length $\times$ width $\times$ thickness $\times$ $\pi/6$, based on a model of a rotation ellipsoid, and has an accuracy of 15–20%, with normal being 5–30 mL (37). Some ultrasound machines have the capability of color flow Doppler readings. This can identify vascular structures that might be mistaken for small nodules, as well as identify the high intrathyroidal blood flow seen with Graves' disease or low intrathyroidal blood flow seen with Hashimoto's thyroiditis.

Incidental thyroid nodules may be detected during routine US for parathyroid localization or during the evaluation of a dominant thyroid nodule. If there are sonographic features of malignancy as outlined above, or if an incidental nodule is larger than 1–1.5 cm in size, or if the patient has significant risk factors for thyroid cancer, UG-FNA of the incidental nodule is indicated. Otherwise, an appropriate follow-up ultrasound should be scheduled in 3–12 months depending on clinical features.

Thyroid US is also valuable for follow-up of patients with thyroid cancer. Patients with recurrent papillary thyroid cancer may have cervical lymphadenopathy, subcutaneous deposits of metastatic tissue, and/or growth of residual tumor in the thyroid bed after the primary surgical resection. These recurrent foci can be missed with physical examination, CT, MR imaging, or scintigraphy, but detected and biopsied with US. Ultrasound is particularly useful in cases of thyroglobulin-positive, radioiodine scan–negative patients. Sixteen of 63 such patients had sonographically demonstrable images suspicious for pathologic lymph nodes or local recurrences in a study by Antonelli et al. (41). Ultrasound-guided FNA was diagnostic in 49 of 52 (94%), postoperative thyroid cancer patients (42).

5 OTHER IMAGING TECHNIQUES

Even though CT or MR imaging for other problems may reveal thyroid nodules, these studies are rarely helpful in routine evaluation. This is because of the superior resolution afforded by neck ultrasound. However, CT and/or MR may prove useful in the evaluation of (1) substernal/mediastinal goiters, (2) thyroid cancer, (3) equivocal lesions by ultrasonography, (4) cervical, mediastinal, and retropharyngeal lymphadenopathy, and (5) tumors greater than 3 cm. In patients with thyroid cancer, CT and/or MR may also assist in the pre-operative evaluation of anatomy, definition of relationships with adjacent structures, and specific demonstration of the degree of invasion of the aerodigestive tract (43). Benign thyroid adenomas generally have a low signal intensity with T_1-weighted images on MR and enhance postgadolinium (43). Using two-dimensional proton MR spectroscopy, follicular adenomas may be differentiated from carcinomas (44).

6 FINE NEEDLE ASPIRATION

At present, fine needle biopsy, developed and popularized in Sweden, is the most effective procedure to discriminate between benign and malignant lesions in the thyroid gland. The accuracy of this method, however, is highly dependent on the expertise of the cytologist. It is recommended as part of the initial evaluation of all thyroid nodules in order to obtain a cytological diagnosis and level of clinical suspicion for malignancy (Fig. 3). Other uses of FNA include (1) establishing a cytological diagnosis when a previous FNA was nondiagnostic or inadequate, (2) establishing a cytological diagnosis in a patient already scheduled for surgery, based on the presence of clinical risk factors, to assist in planning the operative procedure, (3) to aspirate, or reaspirate, fluid from a symptomatic cyst, (4) to differentiate thyroid from nonthyroid (parathyroid or lymph node) nodules, (5) to obtain culturable material from a pyogenic cyst, and (6) to establish whether a new extrathyroidal mass in a thyroid cancer patient represents a pathological lymph node or subcutaneous metastatic deposit.

On occasion, rare tumors of the thyroid are discovered, such as lymphoma. Ancillary techniques have enabled more accurate diagnosis of thyroid lymphoma in the setting of a thyroid nodule in a patient with Hashimoto's thyroiditis. These methods include light chain restriction, flow cytometry, gene rearrangement, and immunohistochemical staining. In a series of 119 patients with primary thyroid lymphoma, in which all were associated with Hashimoto's thyroiditis, ultrasound demonstrated a characteristic asymmetric pseudocystic pattern in 43/46 (93%), and the FNA diagnosis was correct in 65/83 (78%), showing abundant monomorphic infiltration of lymphoid cells (45).

FNA has evolved considerably over the past 10 years. Freehand aspirations were adequate for larger, palpable, and completely solid nodules, but nonpalpable lesions were poorly sampled. Larger-bore needle aspirations (16–20 gauge) have the advantage of more cellular samples in solid nodules, without any increased diagnostic accuracy (46), and more effective draining of cystic fluid from symptomatic lesions. In a study by Carpi et al. (47) of microfollicular nodules that were nondiagnostic or suspicious for cancer by FNA, larger-needle aspiration biopsies found that the prevalence for cancer was 22% (14/63) among microfollicular and 4% (2/51) among combined microfollicular-macrofollicular nodules. Smaller bore needles (21–27 gauge), which are typically used for FNA, have the advantage of being associated with less pain and bleeding. Twenty-three to twenty-five gauge, 1 ½ inch needles furnish excellent results for most nodules. Hard or fibrotic nodules may require a larger needle.

Typically, the nodule is fixed by the fingers of the nonaspirating hand, and the needle, attached to a syringe (3–10 cc), is inserted perpendicularly to the anterior surface of the neck. Once the nodule is penetrated, a deliberate, vertical motion of the needle, back and forth over 1–2 mm, and then one or two 360 degree rotations, will jar loose cellular material. This material is then aspirated by applying negative pressure with the syringe. Great care must be taken to release the pressure once fluid, which is usually bloody, appears in the hub, so the cellular specimen is not overdiluted. If no fluid appears, the vertical and rotational motions can be repeated, and then suction reapplied. Occasionally suction is not needed since cells may flow into the needle by capillary action. After withdrawing the needle, the needle is detached and then reattached with air in the syringe. Air is then expelled, forcing the cellular contents within the needle onto a slide, which is then immediately smeared and fixed. The patient may apply pressure to gauze over the puncture site while the slides are being prepared. Additional aspirations are generally advised, especially without US guidance, to ensure cellular adequacy. The puncture site is dressed with an adhesive bandage after the slides are prepared. The patient should be observed for a few minutes to make sure there is no swelling, bleeding, or significant discomfort.

With the prevalence of FNA, and its incorporation into the initial evaluation of all thyroid nodules, several enhancements have appeared. First, performing FNA with US guidance increases the cellularity of the sampling and therefore the sensitivity and specificity of the procedure (Fig. 4). This is because the needle can be positioned at the solid periphery of complex cysts, or within a projection of solid tissue, where dividing cells reside, and away from fibrotic or calcified areas. Also, by directly visualizing the needle tip, the clinician can avoid traversing the nodule and sampling posterior extranodular tissue. Ultrasound guidance can also help avoid associated morbidity by steering the needle away from vascular structures or the trachea. Also, cystic structures can be drained and solid components sampled in less time, thus reducing discomfort to the patient.

In a study of 48 patients with nonpalpable thyroid nodules, there was a 100% accuracy for the diagnosis of occult papillary thyroid cancer by UG-FNA (48). Solymosi et al. (49) found that the implementation of US guidance, compared with nonguided FNA, improved the sensitivity (92% vs. 76%), specificity (87% vs. 65%), and diagnostic accuracy (87% vs. 66%) in 3446 vs. 1448 aspirates. In addition, UG-FNA reduced the rate of inadequate sampling from 16% to 7%. In a study by Yokozawa et al. (50) of 678 patients found to have benign nodules by standard FNA methods, 571 (84.2%) were confirmed to have benign cytology by UG-FNA, but 107 (15.8%) were found to have malignant cytology by UG-FNA. Of these 107 patients, surgery confirmed the presence of papillary thyroid cancer in 93, follicular carcinoma in 4, and medullary and anaplastic carcinoma in 1 each (50). Ultrasound-guided FNA has the potential disadvantage of greater cost, though this can be outweighed by the avoidance of repeated aspirations due to inadequate samples.

In addition, utilizing aspirator devices that allow one-handed insertion of the needle, aspiration of contents, and then purging the syringe enables more accurate placement of the needle and use of the nonaspirating hand to operate the US transducer. A foot-pedal to freeze images can also be incorporated. This allows single-person performance of the entire UG-FNA procedure, hence avoiding the need for an assistant. When draining larger cysts, a 20 cc syringe is attached to a special pistol grip (Cameco pistol) in order to create adequate suction.

Typically, the patient is first advised of the risks and benefits of the procedure. Specifically, the patient must be informed that the procedure is not 100% accurate

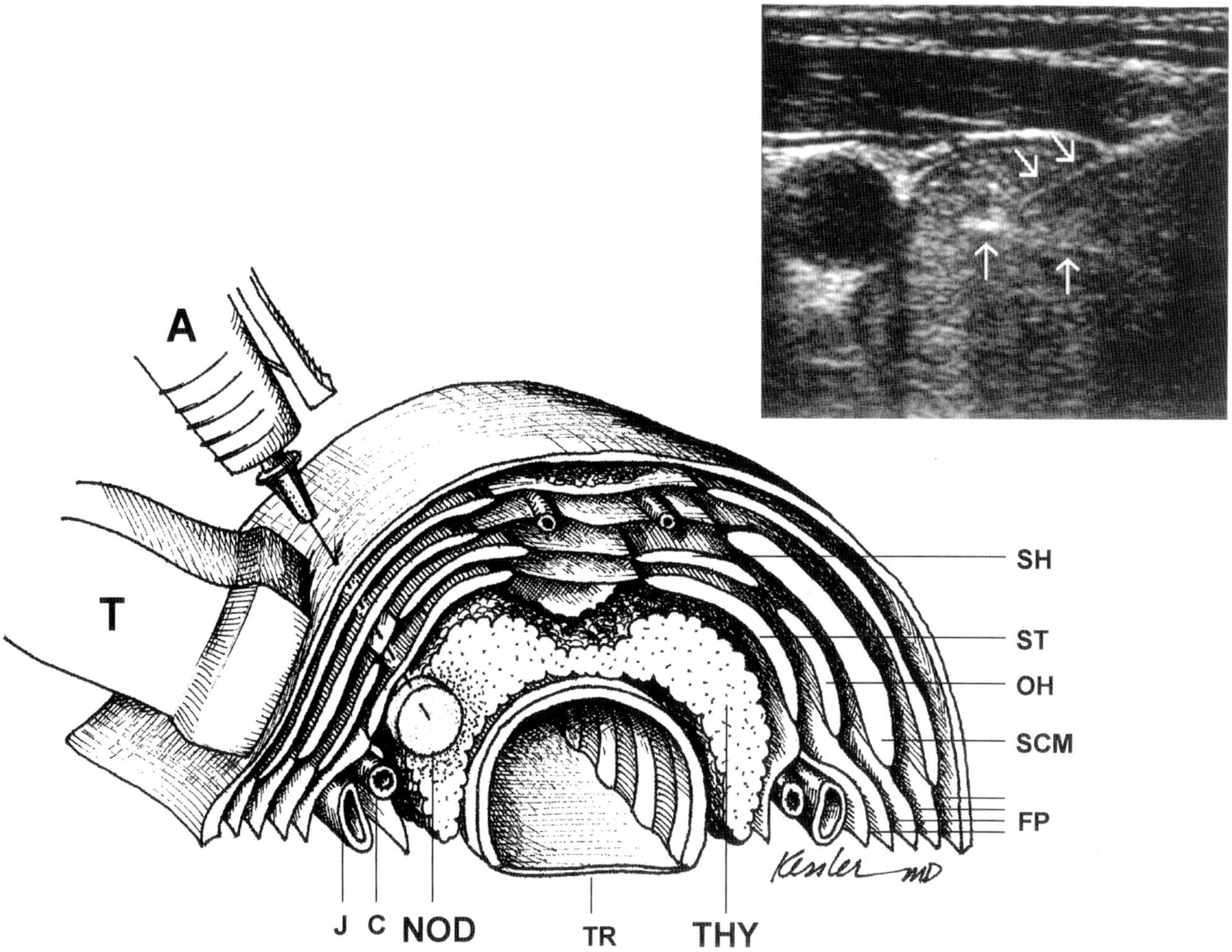

Figure 4 Single-person technique for ultrasound-guided fine needle aspiration of a thyroid nodule. The needle is inserted medial to the transducer and advanced within the plane of sound waves. (Insert) Sonogram of needle within a solid nodule (top arrows); the needle bevel is brighter than the needle shaft and casts a linear shadow angled away from the bevel (bottom arrows). The carotid artery (anechoic circular structure) is located to the left of the nodule in sonogram. Abbreviations: A, aspirator device (dominant hand); T, ultrasound transducer (nondominant hand); J, jugular vein; C, carotid artery; NOD, thyroid nodule; TR, trachea; THY, thyroid gland; FP, 4 fascial planes; SCM, sternocleidomastoid muscle; OH, omohyoid muscle; ST, sternothyroid muscle; SH, sternohyoid muscle.

for diagnosis of the thyroid nodule. Written consent is based on the discretion of the physician. No major complications have been associated with FNA, and risks generally consist of mild pain and bleeding. Persistence of either is very unusual and reassurance is frequently sufficient. Compression of the site if there is bleeding, even if a vascular structure is punctured or the patient is anticoagulated, is almost always adequate. However, whenever possible, anticoagulation should be held, and coagulapathies reversed, prior to the procedure. If the patient is too agitated, cannot be positioned properly with adequate neck extension, cannot remain still or refrain from speaking, coughing or swallowing, or if the anatomy is not clearly imaged due to ultrasound limitations, adiposity, overlying bony structures or shadows, tracheostomy, or a hyperdynamic vascular structure, then the procedure should be deferred and surgery considered.

Additional precautions include preparing the overlying skin with alcohol, or an equivalent antibacterial, using a topical anesthetic such as ethyl chloride, using proper gloves that can maintain adequate tactile sensation, and using a sterile conducting gel for the ultrasound tranducer. Some practitioners utilize skin-marking techniques to facilitate UG-FNA (51). Aspirated material should be expelled onto slides, smeared, and then, within a couple of seconds, sprayed with preservative. If immunostaining is desired, the smears are fixed with 95% ethanol or air-dried and then fixed with acetone. Alternatively, the sample may be expelled into a cytospin cell preparation in which erythrocytes are lysed and ThinPrep processing used. This latter method has the advantage of minimizing drying or crush artifact, providing more cellular slides for the cytologist, and improving nuclear and cytoplasmic staining with less background (52). Bidirectional feedback between the person performing the UG-FNA and the cytopathologist must occur in the interpretation of all samples. For example, some cytologists require 5–10 groups of 10–15 well-preserved cells/group for a smear to be considered adequate, whereas others require less rigorous criteria.

In a review by Gharib and Goellner (16), cytological results were diagnostic for benign (69%) or malignant disease (4%), indeterminate or suspicious for malignant disease (10%), or nondiagnostic due to inadequate cellularity (17%). In other studies, nondiagnostic aspirates occur in 7–25% of cases (53,54) (less than 8% with highly skilled clinicians) and are not included in determinations of specificity, sensitivity, or accuracy of the procedure. Inadequacy rates are also lower in nodules >2 cm (3%) compared with nodules <1 cm (13%), even with UG-FNA (55). Patients with inadequate aspirates of cystic fluid generally do not need to be reaspirated. When a solid nodule that has degenerated is aspirated in the center, inadequate cellularity is found in 16% (56). This rate decreases to 5.3, 4, and 2.6% with aspiration of two, three, or four areas distinct from the nodule center, respectively (56). Reaspiration of previously inadequate samples from solid nodules or complex cysts proves successful in 50% of patients (57,58) and can reduce the rate of false-negatives from 5.2% to <1.3% (59) but was found to be of limited utility in other studies (60,61). Alternatively, the clinician may examine the smears microscopically (using DiffQuick staining) at the time of the procedure for adequacy and repeat the procedure immediately if inadequate. Using this procedure with UG-FNA, the nondiagnostic rate can be reduced to only 2% (62), and when large needle aspirates are used with US and UG-FNA, the nondiagnostic rate becomes 0% (63). Since 9% of patients with persistently inadequate cytology specimens contain a malignancy, such patients with high-risk clinical and sonographic features should be referred to surgery (64).

Indeterminate findings account for 6–30% of nodules (53,54) and generally apply to follicular neoplasms, suggested by a microfollicular arrangement and scanty or absent colloid. This group is rather heterogeneous, consisting of true and false positives, with a cancer risk ranging from 10 to 80% (53). A recent study by Raber et al. (65) revealed an 18% malignancy rate among patients with indeterminate findings. Poller et al. (66) found that referring patients with indeterminate findings to surgery reduced false-negative FNA results thereby improving diagnostic efficacy. In a study of 368 patients by Kelman et al. (67) from Mount Sinai Hospital, there was a 31% overall malignancy rate. Lower malignancy rates occurred in nodules with frankly benign FNA (6.1% false-negatives) or indeterminate FNA without atypia (6.5%) (67). Indeterminate aspirates with atypia, with or without microfollicular cytology, had a malignancy rate of 60% (67). Similarly, Barbaro et al. (68) found that the presence of anisokaryosis, nuclear overlapping, and scant or absent colloid identified patients with microfollicular findings on cytology at higher risk for malignancy. Additionally, clinical features such as male gender, patients older than 40–50 years, or a nodule >3–4 cm identify patients with indeterminate findings at higher risk for malignancy and therefore warranting surgical management (10,69–73). When indeterminate findings are excluded from studies, accuracy rates are more relevant but only reflect 65% of nodules aspirated (53). Causes for false-positives are Hashimoto's thyroiditis, benign hot nodules, and Graves' disease.

Papillary carcinoma is diagnosed with much greater accuracy than follicular carcinoma owing to more specific cytological findings. When certain cytological features are present on ThinPrep preparations (intranuclear inclusions, papillary and/or sheet arrangements, nuclear grooves, powdery chromatin, nuclear molding, high cellularity, and small nucleoli), papillary thyroid cancer is diagnosed by FNA with 100% specificity and 70% sensitivity (74). However, the interpretation of nuclear grooves must be made cautiously. Even though 100% of papillary carcinomas studied had nuclear grooves, they were also seen in 70% of nonpapillary neoplasms and in 56% of nonneoplastic thyroid conditions (75). On the other hand, in the follicular variant of papillary thyroid cancer, malignant cells are found less often with FNA compared with papillary thyroid cancer (6.8% vs. 67.5%) and most FNA specimens are interpreted as "suspicious" or as a follicular neoplasm (76).

Sensitivity of FNA ranges from 65 to 98%, specificity from 52 to 100%, positive predictive value from 46 to 100% and negative predictive value from 83 to 99.5%. Overall accuracy ranges from 69 to 100%, with recent studies demonstrating a dramatic improvement in accuracy with UG-FNA compared to standard FNA using manual palpation.

An alternative to FNA and larger-bore aspirates is the core-needle or large-needle cutting biopsy that produces a sample to be evaluated by conventional histology. This offers the opportunity to study tissue architecture as well as cellular structure. The method employs a 14 gauge 2 3/8 inch or 3 1/8 inch Silverman needle or a 14 gauge 3 inch Tru-Cut disposable needle. Hematomas, tracheal puncture, and injury to the recurrent laryngeal nerve are potential hazards of the procedure but are quite rare if performed properly. Tumor seeding along the needle tract was not found in over 3000 biopsies by Miller (77). Sensitivity (84–96%), specificity (80–95%), and accuracy (90–91%) rates with an US-guided automated core biopsy procedure are comparable with rates associated with FNA (78,79). Core biopsies, especially when used in conjunction with FNA, are espoused by Quinn et al. (80), but the consensus opinion, based on clinical safety and performance, does not support their routine use (78,79,81,82).

Lastly, several molecular markers of malignancy used in cytological aspirates have been evaluated. Some are promising, such as galactin-3 (85), CD44v6 (85), thyroid peroxidase (TPO) (83), and human telomerase reverse transcriptase (hTERT) (84), though they have not yet been incorporated into the standard of care. In a prospective study by Bartolazzi et al. (85), coexpression of galactin-3 and CD44v6 among 1009 thyroid lesions by histology and 236 cytological samples yielded 98% specificity, 88% sensitivity, and 97% diagnostic accuracy for malignancy; the specificity and sensitivity of galactin-3 alone was 98% and 99%, respectively. In addition, galactin-3 immunostaining was significantly higher in Hürthle cell carcinomas (59%) compared with Hürthle cell adenomas (7.1%; $p < 0.05$) (86). When anti-TPO immunostaining is employed with FNA, the sensitivity, specificity, and accuracy for differentiating benign from malignant lesions is 100, 87, and 89%, respectively (87). The insular variant of follicular carcinoma demonstrates increased immunostaining with the neuroendocrine markers neuron-specific enolase and synaptophysin, despite the absence of endocrine granules histologically (88). Of note, chromogranin A immunostaining was not identified in nonmedullary thyroid tumors in this series (88). Elevated concentrations of immunoreactive thyroglobulin in nonthyroidal neck aspirates, such as suspicious lymph nodes, strongly suggest the presence of metastatic differentiated thyroid cancer (89).

7 LEVOTHYROXINE SUPPRESSION THERAPY

Many patients undergoing an evaluation for thyroid nodules have a nonmalignant FNA result or do not otherwise require surgical intervention. These patients need follow-up surveillance, and many physicians consider the use of suppressive therapy with levothyroxine. Successful suppression is defined as reduction in nodular size or volume by 50%, generally determined by ultrasonograpy. The rationale is predicated upon TSH serving as a growth stimulator of thyroid tissue. Poorly controlled studies have described reductions in thyroidal size from 0 to 68%, but recent controlled data have found no significant effect (90,91). In fact, spontaneous reductions in thyroid nodular size in placebo groups may be due to repeated diagnostic aspirations (92) and/or nodular degeneration, and only 10–20% of nodules in the treatment group respond (91). Conflicting reports demonstrate a beneficial effect of levothyroxine suppression therapy on the appearance of new nodules (93,94). However, in a patient exposed to head and neck irradiation, levothyroxine therapy may be indicated following partial thyroidectomy (91). The potential adverse effects of levothyroxine therapy are heart disease (95) and osteoporosis (96). Overall, levothyroxine suppression therapy should not be recommended as a routine measure to differentiate between benign and malignant thyroid nodules. It may be reserved for a small subset of patients with thyroid nodules who refuse surgery, have benign cytology, and complain of mild pressure symptoms. In these cases, the benefit may be related to perinodular, rather than nodular, shrinkage of tissue (97). The minimal dose of levothyroxine capable of suppressing TSH to the low-normal to frankly low range, while producing clinical benefit, should be used.

8 INTRAOPERATIVE PATHOLOGICAL METHODS TO EVALUATE THYROID NODULES

Some authors advocate lobectomy or total thyroidectomy in patients, based on FNA cytology results, without obtaining intraoperative frozen sections. Others disagree.

Although frozen sections are valuable in the diagnosis of frank thyroid malignancy, they are unlikely to detect capsular or vascular invasion in follicular carcinoma and are said to offer little advantage to a diagnostic aspirate in papillary carcinoma. In 1993, McHenry et al. (98) determined that frozen sections were unnecessary when a preoperative FNA was diagnostic for benign or malignant disease. In 1996, McHenry et al. (99) found the sensitivity, specificity, and accuracy of frozen sections to be 93, 100, and 97%, respectively, which was comparable to that of FNA. They further determined that the routine use of frozen sections was not cost-effective and should only be performed when FNA results are repeatedly nondiagnostic, to confirm the presence of lymph node involvement, or to evaluate thyroid nodules discovered incidentally at the time of surgery. Additional studies by Chang et al. (100), Hamming et al. (101), Lin et al. (102), Brooks et al. (103), and Mandell et al. (104) found that frozen section information affects the surgical procedure in less than 5% of cases and is generally unnecessary. Frozen sections, like FNA, are particularly insensitive for the diagnosis of the follicular variant of papillary carcinoma (105).

Although some authors depend entirely on FNA to determine surgical procedures, most institutions continue to rely on frozen sections. Additionally, frozen section can indicate the extent of tissue infiltration, which may influence the choice of surgical procedure. These methods often complement each other, though both fall short in distinguishing follicular adenoma from carcinoma. This differentiation must frequently await permanent sections.

Touch preparations represent a rapid, cost-effective alternative or complement to intraoperative frozen sections. They can recognize the follicular component of a papillary carcinoma but cannot differentiate a follicular adenoma from a follicular carcinoma. Alternatively, in two series of patients with thyroid nodules, chiefly composed of papillary thyroid carcinoma, Ultrafast Papanicolaou–stained scrape preparations (UFP) agreed with the final diagnosis in 89–98% of cases (106,107). This was compared with a 71% agreement between frozen sections and the final diagnosis (106). One explanation is that UFP are able to detect Orphan Annie–eyed clear nuclei, a more specific feature of papillary thyroid cancer than nuclear grooves or intranuclear cytoplasmic inclusions, better than conventionally processed touch preps or frozen sections (108).

9 CONCLUSIONS

The evaluation of thyroid nodules has been controversial, but with the accrual of clinical data and the popularization of UG-FNA, the following clinical algorithm emerges:

Once a thyroid nodule is detected by physical examination, or incidentally by an imaging technique, a TSH level is obtained and UG-FNA performed.

If the TSH is depressed, radioiodine scanning and uptake is undertaken to determine whether there are one or more nodules with autonomous function or one or more nonfunctioning nodules with internodular thyroiditis, such as Graves' disease (increased uptake) or Hashimoto's thyroiditis or viral thyroiditis (decreased uptake). Since recent data question the validity that AFTN are far less likely to be malignant compared with nonfunctioning nodules, UG-FNA may be considered in patients presenting with a thyroid nodule and a depressed TSH level, especially if other risk factors for malignancy are present.

If the TSH is normal or elevated, radioiodine scanning is not necessary. Thyroid hormone replacement therapy is started if the patient is hypothyroid.

Observation is indicated for asymptomatic, nonfunctioning thyroid nodules with benign cytology or if the cytology is indeterminate/nondiagnostic and the patient is at low risk for thyroid cancer. Repeat UG-FNA may be performed 3 months following initial evaluation, and then at regular intervals thereafter, to monitor for nodular growth and/or cytological changes.

Radioiodine therapy is reserved for AFTNs in adults who have benign cytology or a low risk for thyroid cancer. Children with AFTNs, and adults with AFTNs and suspicious cytology, should have surgery.

Surgery is also appropriate for patients when the thyroid nodule is: (1) symptomatic (dyspnea, dysphagia, or venous compression), enlarging, or at risk of becoming symptomatic, (2) autonomous, and radioactive iodine therapy is refused, (3) cosmetically a problem, (4) suspicious or diagnostic for a malignancy, or (5) none or the above, but the patient cannot tolerate the uncertainty of whether the nodule could represent a malignancy, despite extensive discussions with the physician. In this situation, offering a minimally invasive hemithyroidectomy/isthmusectomy un-

52. Weidman J, Chaubal A, Bibbo M. Cellular fixation. A study of CytoRich Red and cytospin collection fluid. Acta Cytol 1997; 41:182–187.
53. Belfiore A, La Rosa GL. Fine-needle aspiration biopsy of the thyroid. Endocr Metab Clin North Am 2001; 30:361–400.
54. Bakhos R, Selvaggi SM, DeJong S, Gordon DL, Pitale SU, Herrmann M, Wojcik EM. Fine-needle aspiration of the thyroid: rate and causes of cytohistopathologic discordance. Diagn Cytopathol 2000; 23:233–237.
55. Sabel MS, Haque D, Velasco JM, Staren ED. Use of ultrasound-guided fine needle aspiration biopsy in the management of thyroid disease [with discussion]. Am Surg 1998; 64:738–742.
56. Musgrave YM, Davey DD, Weeks JA. Assessment of fine-needle aspiration sampling technique in thyroid nodules. Diagn Cytopathol 1998; 18:76–80.
57. Gharib H, Goellner JR, Johnson DA. Fine-needle aspiration cytology of the thyroid: a 12 year experience with 11,000 biopsies. Clin Lab Med 1993; 13:699–709.
58. Goellner JR, Gharib H, Grant CS, Johnson DA. Fine needle aspiration cytology of the thyroid. 1980–1986. Acta Cytol 1987; 31:587–590.
59. Chehade JM, Silverberg AB, Kim J, Case C, Mooradian AD. Role of repeated fine-needle aspiration of thyroid nodules with benign cytologic features. Endocr Pract 2001; 7:237–243.
60. Merchant SH, Izquierdo R, Khurana KK. Is repeated fine-needle aspiration cytology useful in the management of patients with benign nodular thyroid disease? Thyroid 2000; 10:489–492.
61. Lucas A, Llatjos M, Salinas I, Reverter J, Pizarro E, Sanmarti A. Fine-needle aspiration cytology of benign nodular thyroid disease. Value of re-aspiration. Eur J Endocrinol 1995; 132:677–680.
62. Baloch ZW, Tam D, Langer J, Mandel S, LiVolsi VA, Gupta PK. Ultrasound-guided fine-needle aspiration biopsy of the thyroid: role of on-site assessment and multiple cytologic preparations. Diagn Cytopathol 2000; 23:425–429.
63. Karstrup S, Balslev E, Juul N, Eskildsen PC, Baumbach L. US-guided fine needle aspiration versus coarse needle biopsy of thyroid nodules. Eur J Ultrasound 2001; 13:1–5.
64. McHenry CR, Walfish PG, Rosen IB. Non-diagnostic fine needle aspiration biopsy: a dilemma in mangement of nodular thyroid disease. Am Surg 1993; 59: 415–419.
65. Raber W, Kaserer K, Niederle B, Vierhapper H. Risk factors for malignancy of thyroid nodules initially identified as follicular neoplasia by fine-needle aspiration: results of a prospective study of one hundred twenty patients. Thyroid 2000; 10:709–712.
66. Poller DN, Ibrahim AK, Cummings MH, Mikel JJ, Boote D, Perry M. Fine-needle aspiration of the thyroid. Cancer 2000; 90:239–244.
67. Kelman AS, Rathan A, Leibowitz J, Burstein DE, Haber RS. Thyroid cytology and the risk of malignancy in thyroid nodules: importance of nuclear atypia in indeterminate specimens. Thyroid 2001; 11:271–277.
68. Barbaro D, Simi U, Lopane P, Pallini S, Orsini P, Piazza F, Pasquini C, Soriani G. Thyroid nodules with microfollicular findings reported on fine-needle aspiration: invariably surgical treatment? Endocr Pract 2001; 7:352–357.
69. Baloch ZW, Fleisher S, LiVolsi VA, Gupta PK. Diagnosis of "follicular neoplasm": a gray zone in thyroid fine-needle aspiration cytology. Diagn Cytopathol 2002; 26:41–44.
70. Tuttle RM, Lemar H, Burch HB. Clinical features associated with an increased risk of thyroid malignancy in patients with follicular neoplasia by fine-needle aspiration. Thyroid 1998; 8:377–383.
71. Schlinkert RT, van Heerden JA, Goellner JR, Gharib H, Smith SL, Rosales RF, Weaver AL. Factors that predict malignant thyroid lesions when fine-needle aspiration is suspicious for follicular neoplasm. Mayo Clin Proc 1997; 72:913–916.
72. Tyler DS, Winchester DJ, Caraway NP, Hickey RC, Evans DB. Indeterminate fine-needle aspiration biopsy of the thyroid: identification of subgroups at high risk for invasive carcinoma. Surgery 1994; 116:1054–1060.
73. Davis NL, Gordon M, Germann E, Robins RE, McGregor GI. Clinical parameters predictive of malignancy of thyroid follicular neoplasms. Am J Surg 1991; 161:567–569.
74. Zhang Y, Fraser JL, Wang HH. Morphologic predictors of papillary carcinoma on fine-needle aspiration of thyroid with ThinPrep preparations. Diagn Cytopathol 2001; 24:378–383.
75. Gould E, Watzak L, Chamizo W, Albores-Saavedra J. Nuclear grooves in cytologic preparations. A study of the utility of this feature in the diagnosis of papillary carcinoma. Acta Cytol 1989; 3316–20.
76. Jain M, Khan A, Patwardhan N, Reale F, Safran M. Follicular variant of papillary thyroid carcinoma: a comparative study of histopathologic features and cytology results in 141 patients. Endocr Pract 2001; 7:79–84.
77. Miller JH. Needle biopsy of the thyroid: methods and recommendations. Thyroid Today 1982; 5:1–5.
78. Taki S, Kakuda K, Kakuma K, Annen Y, Katada S, Yamashita R, Kosugi M, Michigishi T, Tonami N. Thyroid nodules: evaluation with US-guided core biopsy with an automated biopsy gun. Radiology 1997; 202:874–877.
79. Liu Q, Castelli M, Gattuso P, Prinz RA. Simultaneous fine-needle aspiration and core-needle biopsy of thyroid nodules. Am Surg 1995; 61:628–632.

80. Quinn SF, Nelson HA, Demlow TA. Thyroid biopsies: fine-needle aspiration biopsy versus spring-activated core biopsy needle in 102 patients. J Vasc Interv Radiol 1994; 5:619–623.
81. Pisani T, Bononi M, Nagar C, Angelini M, Bezzi M, Vecchione A. Fine needle aspiration and core needle biopsy techniques in the diagnosis of nodular thyroid pathologies. Anticancer Res 2000; 20:3843–3847.
82. Silverman JF, West RL, Finley JL, Iarkin EW, Park HK, Swanson MS, Fore WW. Fine-needle aspiration versus large-needle biopsy or cutting biopsy in evaluation of thyroid nodules. Diagn Cytopathol 1986; 2:25–30.
83. De Micco C, Vassko V, Henry JF. The value of thyroid peroxidase immunohistochemistry for preoperative fine-needle aspiration diagnosis of the follicular variant of papillary thyroid cancer. Surgery 1999; 126: 1200–1204.
84. Siddiqui MT, Greene KL, Clark DP, Xydas S, Udelsman R, Smallridge RC, Ziegler MA, Saji M. Human telomerase reverse transcriptase expression in Diff-Quik-stained FNA samples from thyroid nodules. Diagn Mol Pathol 2001; 10:123–129.
85. Bartolazzi A, Gasbarri A, Papotti M, Bussolati G, Lucante T, Khan A, Inohara H, Marandino F, Orlandi F, Nardi F, Vecchione A, Tecce R, Larsson O, and the Thyroid Cancer Study Group. Application of an immunodiagnostic method for improving preoperative diagnosis of nodular thyroid lesions. Lancet 2001; 357:1644–1650.
86. Nascimento MCPA, Bisi H, Alves VAF, Longatto-Filho A, Kanamura CT, Medeiros-Neto G. Differential reactivity for galactin-3 in Hürthle cell adenomas and carcinomas. Endocr Pathol 2001; 12:275–279.
87. Henry JF, Denizot A, Porcelli A, Villafane M, Zoro P, Garcia S, De Micco C. Thyroperoxidase immunodetection for the diagnosis of malignancy on fine-needle aspiration of thyroid nodules. World J Surg 1994; 18:529–534.
88. Satoh F, Umemura S, Yasuda M, Osamura RY. Neuroendocrine marker expression in thyroid epithelial tumors. Endocr Pathol 2001; 12:291–299.
89. Pacini F, Fugazzola L, Lippi F, Ceccarelli C, Centoni R, Miccoli P, Elisei R, Pinchera A. Detection of thyroglobulin in fine-needle aspirates of nonthyroidal neck masses: a clue to the diagnosis of metastatic differentiated thyroid cancer. J Clin Endocrinol Metab 1992; 74:1401–1404.
90. Larijani B, Pajouhi M, Bastanhagh MH, Sadjadi A, Sedighi N, Eshraghian MR. Evaluation of suppressive therapy for cold thyroid nodules with levothyroxine: double-blind placebo-controlled clinical trial. Endocr Pract 1999; 5:251–256.
91. Gharib H, Mazzaferri EL. Thyroxine suppressive therapy in patients with nodular thyroid disease. Ann Intern Med 1998; 128:386–394.
92. Gordon DL, Flisak M, Fisher SG. Changes in thyroid nodule volume caused by fine-needle aspiration: a factor complicating the interpretation of the effect of thyrotropin suppression on nodule size. J Clin Endocrinol Metab 1999; 84:4566–4569.
93. Krouse RS, McCarty T, Weiss LM, Wagman LD. Postoperative suppressive therapy for thyroid adenomas. Am J Surg 2000; 66:751–755.
94. Papini E, Petrucci L, Guglielmi R, Panunzi C, Rinaldi R, Bacci V, Crescenzi A, Nardi F, Fabbrini R, Pacella CM. Long-term changes in nodular goiter: a 5-year prospective randomized trial of levothyroxine suppressive therapy for benign cold thyroid nodules. J Clin Endocrinol Metab 1998; 83:780–783.
95. Biondi B, Fazio S, Cuocolo A, Sabatini D, Nicolai E, Lombardi G, Salvatore M, Sacca L. Impaired cardiac reserve and exercise capacity in patients receiving long-term thyrotropin suppressive therapy with levothyroxine. J Clin Endocrinol Metab 1996; 81: 4224–4228.
96. Faber J, Galloe AM. Changes in bone mass during prolonged subclinical hyperthyroidism due to L-thyroxine treatment: a meta-analysis. Eur J Endocrinol 1994; 130:350–356.
97. Csako G, Byrd D, Wesley RA, Sarlis NJ, Skarulis MC, Nieman LK, Pucino F. Assessing the effects of thyroid suppression on benign solitary thyroid nodules. A model for using quantitative research synthesis. Medicine 2000; 79:9–26.
98. McHenry CR, Rosen IB, Walfish PG, Bedard Y. Influence of fine-needle aspiration biopsy and frozen section examination on the management of thyroid cancer. Am J Surg 1993; 166:353–356.
99. McHenry CR, Raeburn C, Strickland T, Marty JJ. The utility of routine frozen section examination for intraoperative diagnosis of thyroid cancer. Am J Surg 1996; 172:658–661.
100. Chang HY, Lin JD, Chen JF, Huang BY, Hseuh C, Jeng LB, Tsai JS. Correlation of fine needle aspiration cytology and frozen section biopsies in the diagnosis of thyroid nodules. J Clin Pathol 1997; 50:1005–1009.
101. Hamming JF, Vriens MR, Goslings BM, Songun I, Fleuren GJ, van de Velde CJ. Role of fine-needle aspiration biopsy and frozen section examination in determining the extent of thyroidectomy. World J Surg 1998; 22:575–579.
102. Lin HS, Komisar A, Opher E, Blaugrund SM. Surgical management of thyroid masses: assessing the need for frozen section evaluation. Laryngoscope 1999; 109:868–873.
103. Brooks AD, Shaha AR, DuMornay W, Huvos AG, Zakowski M, Brennan MF, Shah J. Role of fine-needle aspiration biopsy and frozen section analysis in the surgical management of thyroid tumors. Ann Surg Oncol 2001; 8:92–100.
104. Mandell DL, Genden EM, Mechanick JI, Bergman

DA, Biller HF, Urken ML. Diagnostic accuracy of fine-needle aspiration and frozen section in nodular thyroid disease. Otolaryngol Head Neck Surg 2001; 124:531–536.

105. Lin HS, Komisar A, Opher E, Blaugrund SM. Follicular variant of papillary carcinoma: the diagnostic limitations of preoperative fine-needle aspiration and intraoperative frozen section evaluation. Laryngoscope 2000; 110:1431–1436.

106. Basolo F, Baloch ZW, Baldanzi A, Miccoli P, LiVolsi VA. Usefulness of Ultrafast Papanicalaou-stained scrape preparations in intraoperative management of thyroid lesions. Mod Pathol 1999; 12:653–657.

107. Paessler M, LiVolsi VA, Baloch ZW. Role of Ultrafast Papanicolaou-stained scrape preparations as an adjunct to frozen sections in the surgical management of thyroid lesions. Endocr Pract 2001; 7:89–94.

108. Yang GC, Greenebaum E. Clear nuclei of papillary thyroid carcinoma conspicuous in fine-needle aspiration and intraoperative smears processed by Ultrafast Papanicolaou stain. Mod Pathol 1997; 10:552–555.

11

Mediastinal Goiter

Ashok Shaha

Memorial Sloan–Kettering Cancer Institute and Cornell Medical School, New York, New York, U.S.A.

1 INTRODUCTION

The management of mediastinal goiters is engrossing because of the complexity of surgical procedures and associated risks. Most frequently, surgery is advised to avoid problems related to airway, venous obstruction, and to rule out malignancy (1–7).

The etiology of thyroid adenomas remains unclear. In normal glands some areas of the follicles are more active than others in concentrating iodine and, presumably, in secreting thyroid hormones. This may be secondary to differences in cell response to thyroid-stimulating hormone (TSH). Variations occur in the frequency of mitoses within the same follicle. This follicular heterogeneity implies that clones of cells may divide at a higher rate than the remaining follicular cells and may give rise to adenomatous areas of growth (8).

The most common cause of goiter is iodine deficiency, usually seen in third world countries; it is one of the most common problems in mountainous regions such as the Alps and the Himalayas (8,9). Iodine deficiency, resulting in increased TSH output in an attempt to maintain the euthyroid state, is often associated with large multinodular goiters rather than a homogeneous expansion of all thyroid follicular cells. The incidence of goiter (colloid or endemic) is rare in the United States because of the compulsory use of iodized salt.

Thyroid tumors, of course, develop in the neck but can extend downward into the mediastinal region as they grow. Most enlarge over a long period of time and some occasionally remain asymptomatic. When symptoms are present, the most common are difficulty in breathing and an accompanying neck mass. The tumor may be almost entirely substernal at times, with no significant mass appearing in the neck. As a result of the bony confines of the thoracic inlet, mediastinal goiters lead to compression symptoms—mainly related to the trachea and esophagus but also at times producing venous obstruction (10,11).

Klein, a German surgeon, first reported in 1820 removal of a substernal goiter. The mortality from thyroid surgery before the Kocher era was almost 40%. Credit goes to Kocher, Halsted, and Lahey for perfecting the technique of thyroid surgery. As late as 1866, Samuel Gross from the University of Pennsylvania remarked that thyroid surgery was "butchery" and that "no honest and sensible surgeon would ever engage in thyroid surgery." Clearly, this was an era before antisepsis, hemostats, and the use of iodine to control hyperthyroidism! Kocher, with his vast experience in thyroid surgery, studied the physiology, improved the techniques of thyroid surgery, and was the first surgeon to receive the Nobel Prize for his contributions in thyroid diseases (12).

2 DEFINITION

There are several theories regarding substernal goiter, but the most popular is that the goiter represents an inferior growth from the cervical thyroid gland that is supplied by the vessels in the neck. The upright posture of human beings combined with normal swallowing and breathing mechanisms induce negative intrathoracic pressure. The weight of the enlarging mass allows the gland to grow and descend through the thoracic inlet into the substernal position. Inferiorly there is no anatomical structure that can restrict the growth of the thyroid gland. This leads to the path of least resistance—towards the thoracic inlet.

3 CLINICAL PRESENTATION AND SYMPTOMS

3.1 Respiratory

Most intrathoracic goiters present in the elderly and appear frequently in the sixth decade. Thirty to forty percent are asymptomatic, and in about 20% of patients there is no palpable neck mass. The diagnosis is sometimes made by a routine chest x-ray disclosing a mediastinal mass. Reeve et al. (13) reviewed 967,759 screening radiographs in Sydney, Australia, and reported the incidence of substernal goiter to be 1 in 5040. Seventy to eighty percent of all patients, however, can be demonstrated to be symptomatic at the time of initial evaluation, most usually due to displacement and narrowing of the trachea (Fig. 1).

Even though they may not be aware of a problem, dyspnea can often be provoked in approximately 85% of cases by raising both arms above the shoulders (Pemberton's sign). Hoarseness is a rare symptom. The recurrent nerve may be paralyzed due to the longstanding compression or stretching of a benign goiter, but the presence of hoarseness and a paretic recurrent nerve raises a suspicion of thyroid malignancy. Patients may be totally asymptomatic, but because of the bony confines of the thoracic inlet, the thyroid can act like an expanding mass within a rigid cage, leading to compression of vital structures. The most common symptom is related to compression of the upper airway. Ninety percent of symptomatic patients have mainly respiratory symptoms, including cough, hoarseness of voice, and shortness of breath. Symptoms range from mild to life threatening. Occasional dyspnea, cough, cyanosis, choking accompanied by suffocation, and respiratory collapse requiring emergency treatment may be seen. Shaha et al. (30) reported 24 patients with life-threatening respiratory symptoms, 9 of whom required intubation. Patients with acute airway obstruction require intervention on an urgent basis and should remain on a ventilator until surgery because acute asphyxia may result if it is discontinued (14–16).

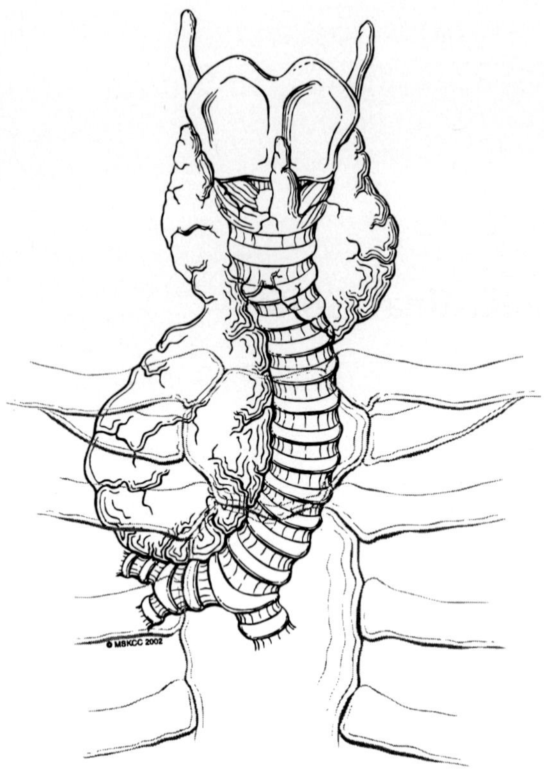

Figure 1 Schematic picture of mediastinal goiter with tracheal deviation. The bony confines of the thoracic inlet cause compression.

3.2 Esophageal

Approximately one third of patients will experience difficulty in swallowing as a result of pressure on the esophagus as it is displaced posteriorly and laterally by the goiter. This can be confirmed by esophagram. It is not usually a major problem.

3.3 Vascular Obstruction

Obstruction of venous return occurs in less 10% of cases. It may be minimal but can be demonstrated by elevating the patient's arms (Pemberton's sign) and observing the distention of neck veins. The symptoms and signs may become more severe as the intrathoracic mass becomes larger, progressing to a full-blown superior vena cava syndrome with dilatation of the veins of the neck, face, and descending collateral venous circulation, as well as cyanosis. The appearance of symptoms of venous obstruction is an urgent indication for surgery. The obstruction may be due to the encroaching bulk of a benign nodular goiter or the result of malignant infiltration.

Compression of the mediastinal great vessels can produce obstructive symptoms. Other rare symptoms may be related to superior vena cava syndrome, downward esophageal varices, Horner's syndrome, pleural effusion, and transient ischemic attacks secondary to the goiter stealing the blood from cerebral circulation (17–23).

3.4 Hyperthyroidism

Multinodular goiters, whether they are in the neck or in the mediastinum, can develop autonomous hyperfunctioning nodules, particularly if the goiter is long standing. Hyperthyroidism, as well as the presence of mediastinal goiter, is more common in elderly patients. Cougard reported an incidence of hyperthyroidism in 35% of 218 intrathoracic goiters in patients over 70 years if age. The cardiac effects of hyperthyroidism can be serious and often appear insidiously; arrhythmias, congestive failure, and ischemic heart disease carry a more serious implication in the elderly and may be life threatening.

Radioactive iodine (RAI) has been used to control the hyperthyroidism of large multinodular goiters, but it often requires repeated doses and a long time period to be effective. Radiation thyroiditis following RAI is also a risk in patients with compromised airway and may precipitate acute airway obstruction.

3.5 Malignancy

The incidence of overt cancer as well as incidental papillary carcinoma in mediastinal goiters ranges from 3 to 15% (14,15). If there is invasion of adjacent structures, a formidable surgical problem may result should laryngeal nerves or great vessels be involved. Lymphomas and thymomas are the most common malignant tumors following intrinsic thyroid carcinoma.

4 DIAGNOSTIC PROCEDURES

Many unsuspected intrathoracic goiters are revealed by routine AP and lateral chest x-rays. This can indicate the extent of substernal mass and its location in the mediastinum. It may also disclose tracheal displacement and or compression, calcifications, soft tissue masses, or displacement of the pleural reflection.

As noted previously, there may be no thyroid enlargement in the neck. But if a thyroid mass is present and the inferior margin cannot be defined, substernal extension is likely. Direct or fiberoptic laryngoscopy should be performed and may define laryngeal compression, distortion, or vocal cord paresis. However, airway compromise may be located well below the level of the larynx, requiring evaluation by imaging procedures.

Computerized tomography offers additional important information that is of great value in the management of the substernal goiter (24,25). It outlines the continuity of the intrathoracic mass with the cervical thyroid. The addition of contrast material increases its value. The extent, location, and borders of the intrathoracic goiter can be precisely defined. The integrity of the airway, as well as the presence and sites of distortion or compression, can be accurately evaluated. Calcifications and the homogeneity of the tumor can be easily assessed. By establishing the relationship of the goiter to the airway, esophagus, and great vessels, important information becomes available to the surgeon in determining the operative approach.

Magnetic resonance offers high-resolution imaging without the need for contrast agents. It offers a choice of tomographic cuts, and because of its greater accuracy in delineating soft tissue, it may more accurately delineate the goiter and adjacent structures such as trachea and vascular involvement.

Ultrasound, although of great help in the evaluation of cervical goiters, is not useful in substernal goiters because the bony thorax limits visibility. Barium swallow may evaluate and locate the position of the esophagus and determine if there is any major compression. Thyroid scanning is rarely helpful and may often be misleading due to the nonfunctional portion of the substernal goiter. Thyroid function tests are generally within normal limits, although hyperthyroidism may accompany toxic nodules.

Since most of the patients with substernal goiter are elderly, it is important not to assume that dyspnea is due solely to the goiter. Cardiac or pulmonary disease may account for part or even all of the symptoms. Pulmonary flow-loop studies can document the extent of pulmonary and extrapulmonary components of the dyspnea.

5 PATHOLOGY

The majority of substernal goiters are benign multinodular goiters or follicular adenomas. Perhaps 10–15% are malignant; papillary or follicular cancers and lymphomas predominate. Incidental papillary carcinomas are not unusual. Hyperplastic toxic nodules, lymphomas, and thyroiditis are also well recognized. Fifty percent of Hodgkin's and 20% of non-Hodgkin's lymphoma present as mediastinal masses. Due to the right-sided predominance of paratracheal nodes, superior vena cava (SVC) syndrome is present in 20% of patients, particularly in those with non-Hodgkin's lymphoma. Occasionally, anaplastic thyroid cancer may present as a substernal goiter; this condition produces rapid progression of disease and severe symptoms.

6 SURGICAL APPROACH

Most patients are symptomatic; the growth of the tumor is unpredictable. There is no satisfactory medical treatment for mediastinal goiter. The minimal regression seen with thyroid suppression offers no significant benefit, particularly if the mass is large. The majority of patients with substernal goiters should be considered for surgical intervention.

The overwhelming number of substernal goiters, even though may extend deep into the thorax, can be removed through a neck incision because of their cervical blood supply. Only 1–3% require exploration through the chest wall. Most substernal goiters are localized to the right or left lobes; only 7–10% are found to be bilaterally. The majority of intrathoracic goiters are in the anterior mediastinum. Perhaps 6–10% are found in the posterior mediastinum. A common location of goiters in the right mediastinum is between the superior vena cava and the vertebral bodies. Those on the left are more frequently anteriorly in the mediastinum, since the aorta acts as a posterior barrier.

Kocher was the first surgeon to develop a technique of surgery for substernal goiter and invented tools to facilitate its removal. He also described the technique of morcellation (piecemeal removal of the substernal goiter) in difficult cases. Lahey reported that nearly all the cases of substernal goiters could be easily removed through the neck (26–29). He stated: "It is a surprising fact that if the dissection is gentle and within the line of clearage, enormous masses may be removed into the neck with virtually no bleeding." Lahey also popularized the technique of morcellation for removal of large substernal goiters, as well as the use of modified sternal splitting or widening using wedges in difficult cases. Although there is still some debate regarding partial or complete sternal split, a lateral thoracotomy may occasionally be necessary. There is a high likelihood of patients developing acute airway distress and compromise, and as patients get older the surgery may be more difficult. Shaha et al. (30) reported a 22% incidence of acute airway symptoms, with 8% of the patients requiring emergent intubation.

7 SURGICAL TECHNIQUE

There are four main issues in the surgery for substernal goiter.

1. Retrieving the substernal portion of the thyroid in the neck
2. Avoiding major bleeding from inferior thyroid veins
3. Preserving the parathyroid glands
4. Careful identification and preservation of the recurrent laryngeal nerve

A variety of methods and technical details are described in the literature (31–33). The standard technique is as follows: a generous skin incision should be used. This is carried through the platysma and flaps are raised in the plane beneath this muscle. The dissection is continued in the midline. Generally the strap muscles are divided. At the minimum, the strap muscles should be transected on the side of a large substernal goiter. The middle thyroid vein is divided, ligated, and the superior thyroid vessels are divided and ligated close to the thyroid parenchyma. The identification of the recurrent laryngeal nerve may be quite difficult due to the large size of the substernal goiter and the displacement of the nerve. As the strap muscles are divided, they should be retracted away from the thyroid. A careful attempt is made to stay on the thyroid capsule and to be aware of the possibility that the recurrent nerve may be stretched over the thyroid mass in an unusual manner. Multiple inferior thyroid veins should be clamped and ligated carefully. Hemoclips may be helpful in this region. Special attention should be given to the identification and preservation of the superior parathyroid glands since the lower glands are more vulnerable to injury or devascularization as the goiter is delivered and removed from its substernal location. Gentle blunt dissection is helpful in the substernal area under the strap muscles; it is best approached starting laterally from the under aspect of the sternomastoid muscle and extending medially (Fig. 2). Occasionally the medial head of the sternomastoid may require transection for better exposure. Injury to the inferior thyroid veins can produce serious bleeding; retraction of these veins into the mediastinum or the tearing of veins

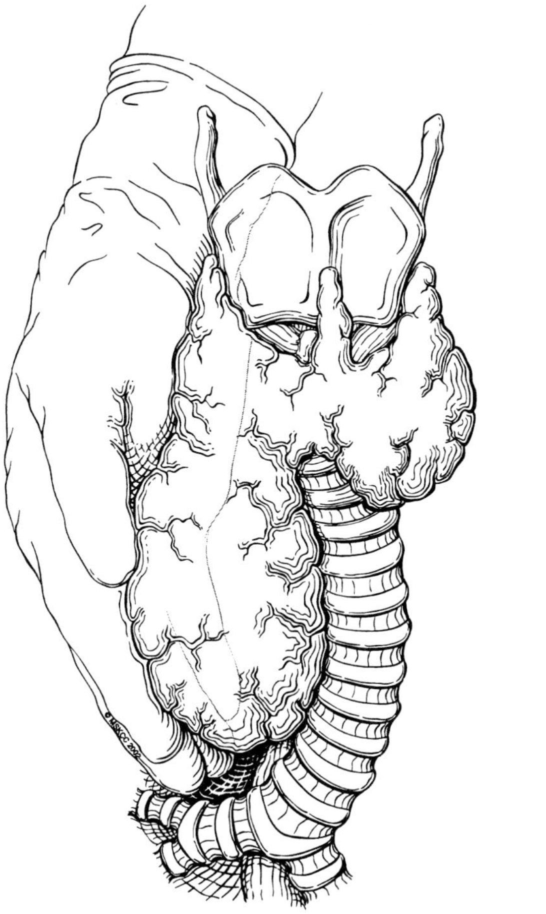

Figure 2 The technique of surgery for mediastinal goiter. Careful ligation of the inferior thyroid veins is necessary to avoid unexpected bleeding. Injury to the recurrent laryngeal nerve may be avoided by being aware of its location. The substernal goiter is retrieved by finger dissection.

below the level of the sternum can become a critical problem, sometimes requiring a sternotomy for control of the bleeding.

As the finger dissection is continued from the lateral surface and after ligation of multiple small inferior veins, the thyroid is generally delivered into the neck. At the beginning of the operation it is important to determine whether the goiter is in the posterior mediastinum with displacement and stretching of the recurrent laryngeal nerve anteriorly over the mass. If the thyroid mass is shelled out in this situation, the risk is that the overlying nerve will be avulsed with the specimen. It is advisable, whether the goiter is in the anterior or posterior mediastinum, to trace the course of the nerve, if possible, before removal of the substernal mass, protecting it from injury. If there is difficulty in finding the recurrent nerve inferiorly, a good alternative is to identify the nerve as it enters the trachea under the cricothyroid muscle at the junction of its middle and anterior third and then follow it downward. At times, however, identification and tracing of the recurrent laryngeal nerve may be difficult or impossible without delivering the substernal thyroid mass from the mediastinum and then dissecting laterally to find the nerve and the parathyroids. The dissecting hand is turned so that the palmar surface faces the sternum and blunt dissection is used to gently deliver the thyroid mass.

A variety of techniques have been described to find the recurrent laryngeal nerve and to carefully preserve it. The nerve may be considerably displaced in substernal goiter. It may be intimately adherent to the posterior capsule of the thyroid, displaced medially (along with displacement of the trachea and esophagus), or in very rare instances it may be displaced anteriorly—especially if the substernal goiter or a portion of it originates and extends into the posterior mediastinum. After taking down the superior thyroid pole and middle thyroid vein, the dissection proceeds on the posterior-medial surface of the goiter with careful identification of the inferior thyroid artery and recurrent laryngeal nerve. Sometimes, because of the large size of the thyroid, this may be impossible. Under these circumstances, it is more appropriate and easier to retrieve the thyroid from the substernal area and look for the recurrent laryngeal nerve in the tracheo-esophageal groove. It is extremely important to remain as close to the thyroid capsule as possible to avoid injury to the nerve, which may be intimately adherent to the posterior capsule of the thyroid. Once the thyroid is retrieved from the substernal portion, the recurrent laryngeal nerve can be easily identified majority of the time in the tracheo-esophageal groove, anterior to the inferior thyroid artery.

The nerve may be located behind the inferior thyroid artery. Charles Proye from Lille, France, has described a "toboggan technique," which is essentially finding the recurrent laryngeal nerve at the cricothyroid area and resecting on its surface, pushing the thyroid anteriorly. Once the nerve is found in the cricothyroid area, the remaining surgery becomes quite simple. The dissection is performed on the surface of the nerve, pushing the thyroid anteriorly and medially. In the author's judgment, this technique may be difficult, especially if there is a bulky thyroid substance in the cricothyroid area. However, one may sometimes use this technique profitably even when the goiter is quite large. After taking down the superior thyroid pole, the cricothyroid area can be easily exposed, leading to identification of the recurrent laryngeal nerve. On occasion, a small process of the thyroid substance (the tuberculum Zuckerkandl) is noted in the middle portion of the thyroid lobe, which is an out-pouching of the thyroid substance near the posterio-lateral area of the thyroid gland. This is seen in approximately 50–60% of the patients, and in our opinion careful dissection around the tuberculum Zuckerkandl will help identify the recurrent laryngeal nerve. One must keep in mind that occasionally the nerve may be anterior to the tuberculum Zuckerkandl and every attempt must be made to identify the nerve and preserve it carefully. At the upper pole the nerve makes an entry into the cricothyroid area just below the cricothyroideus. Berry's ligament, a thickening of the pretracheal fascia, frequently has to be dissected away from the nerve, but there may be small veins and arteries entering or adjacent to the ligament. Special care is needed in this region to avoid bleeding, which may be difficult to control, and occasionally leads to recurrent laryngeal nerve injury in an effort to control hemorrhage.

A subcapsular dissection may be done. The surgical procedure is usually a total thyroid lobectomy with excision of the substernal goiter. As previously noted, this is possible since most intrathoracic goiters originate from one thyroid lobe or the other, although at times a total thyroidectomy may be required if there is significant enlargement of the opposite lobe. In this circumstance, a near-total thyroidectomy on the lesser side may occasionally be advisable to avoid injury to the parathyroid glands if there is doubt about their integrity on the primary side. If a parathyroid gland is injured, it should be transplanted into the sternomastoid muscle. Although there is controversy about the use of drains in a routine thyroidectomy, the author prefers to use a suction drain such as a Hemovac or a Jackson-Pratt because of the extensive dead space following substernal thyroid surgery (3).

8 THORACIC APPROACH

Most substernal goiters can be easily retrieved using the above technique. However, a sternal split may sometimes be necessary, as well as other techniques such as the Drawer maneuver, where the substernal thyroid is held by two hands from the neck and pulled like a drawer. At times the mediastinal goiter is so large that it cannot be delivered through a cervical incision. Lahey popularized the morcellation and fragmentation of the mass as well as suctioning colloid from within the mass to facilitate its removal through the neck. Many authors advise against this method because of the risk of serious bleeding and the possibility of spilling and disseminating malignant disease. Nevertheless, it is still occasionally used with success.

9 STERNOTOMY

A sternal split is necessary in less than 2–8% of the patients. A partial or total sternal split may be considered. Sternotomy enlarges the thoracic inlet and provides access to the great vessels, offering a much safer dissection, and eases removal of the goiter. It may help in identifying the recurrent nerve. The vessels to the thyroid are divided and ligated prior to the sternal incision to reduce its blood supply, facilitating removal of the substernal mass. This is usually done prior to the sternal split. In the case of venous obstruction, however, the sternotomy is best performed initially to decompress the distended veins and make the dissection easier and safer.

Surgeons have drawn away from the thoracic approach in recent years. The anterior sternal-splitting incision has become the preferred choice because of the advantages it offers: it is easily combined with a neck incision and does not require re-positioning of the patient; In patients with an aberrant mediastinal thyroid, which is separate form the thyroid and derives its blood supply from intrathoracic mediastinal vessels, the sternal approach makes it possible to avoid avulsion of thoracic vessels and the severe hemorrhage that would result; there is excellent access to the large vessels of the chest, and it is usually possible to dissect the goiter free from its attachments under direct vision. Lateral thoracotomy incisions are reported to have a higher incidence of recurrent nerve injuries because of the difficulty in visualizing them through this approach.

10 ANESTHESIA

Preoperative evaluation of the laryngeo-tracheal tree will help locate the position and opening of the laryngeal aditus (2). Even though there may be considerable deviation of the trachea, the larynx will generally be in a normal position. Intubating these patients is usually not a difficult problem. Although there appears to be considerable enthusiasm for intubating these patients while awake, it may be more dangerous. Most of the time the airway is quite open and intubation with a small endotracheal tube is not difficult. Some anesthesiologists consider fiberoptic intubation, sometimes over a flexible bronchoscope, but any intubation in substernal goiter must be totally nontraumatic. The surgeon cannot undo the trauma caused by endotracheal injury. The internal trauma should be minimized in patients with substernal goiter. The cuff of the endotracheal tube should also be well below the vocal cords and the patient extubated smoothly to avoid any intrathoracic rise of pressure, causing postoperative bleeding.

11 COMPLICATIONS

The main complications are related to recurrent laryngeal nerve injury, generally occurring in less than 2 to 3% of cases. Important consideration should be given intraoperatively to localization of the parathyroid glands and careful preservation. As mentioned above, parathyroid autotransplantation may be necessary if the parathyroids are rendered avascular. Postoperative hematoma is a well-known complication and occurs in approximately 3% of the patients. Other complications such as pneumothorax and pneumonia are quite rare. Tracheomalacia may be the result of longstanding tracheal compression by the goiter; however, it appears to be an overstated condition. True tracheomalacia with disintegration of the tracheal rings is quite rare (34,35). A majority of the time, even with considerable deviation and compression of the trachea, the cartilage and rings of the trachea generally are intact, and in most cases the trachea returns to an almost normal position within 24–48 hours of surgery. If the trachea appears to be weak, a trachelopexy may occasionally be performed by suturing the tracheal wall to the surrounding musculature or sternal periosteum. Techniques such as support with silastic rings or a Gortex graft are well described in the literature. However, the clinical experience is limited to only a few patients. Most of the time the patients may be left intubated for 24–48 hours and extubated under close observation without any major problems related to tracheomalacia. Cattel and Hare (35) noted that compression of tracheal rings was rapidly reversed after removal of substernal goiters, but deviation of the trachea took months to return. Airway obstruction is more likely from kinking of an elongated trachea or injury on intubation. In rare instances a patient may require temporary tracheostomy.

The results of the surgery for substernal goiters are excellent, with a rare operative mortality. However, the risks to the recurrent laryngeal nerve and permanent hypoparathyroidism are slightly higher than in routine thyroidectomy. The extent of thyroidectomy is generally dictated by the size of the thyroid gland and the histopathology. Total thyroidectomy may be required because of the multiglandular nature of the disease and the absence of essentially normal thyroid tissue. A contralateral subtotal thyroidectomy may be considered to avoid injury to the parathyroids or recurrent laryngeal nerve. The sternoclavicular disarticulation, though described in the literature, is technically quite a difficult procedure and is not generally helpful in surgery for substernal goiter. A median sternotomy is preferred.

12 SUMMARY

Even though thyroid disease is very common, the incidence of substernal goiter is not high in the United States. However, it is a frequent condition noted in areas of endemic goiter. The main indication for surgery is tracheoesophageal compression and fear of malignancy. The preoperative work-up includes careful laryngoscopic evaluation, chest x-ray, and a computed tomography scan. The latter will give a better definition of the extent of the substernal goiter along with the location of the trachea. Substernal goiter is defined as the thyroid gland being more than 50% in the mediastinal location. The most common presenting and compelling symptom for treatment is airway compression. Since there is no effective medical treatment, surgical intervention is commonly indicated, with a majority of substernal goiters retrieved through the neck. In less than 1% of the patients, surgical intervention may include sternal split. The operative mortality is negligible and the incidence of life-threatening complications is very rare. The risk of injury to the recurrent laryngeal nerve or permanent hypoparathyroidism needs to be kept in mind and appropriate techniques used to minimize these distressing complications. Overall, surgery should be undertaken with a diagnosis of substernal goiter to avoid future problems related to the airway.

REFERENCES

1. Shaha AR, Alfonso AE, Jaffe BM. Operative treatment of substernal goiter. Head Neck 1988; 11:325–330.
2. Shaha AR. Surgery for benign thyroid disease causing tracheoesophageal compression. Otolaryngol Clin North Am 1990; 23:391–401.
3. Blum M, Biller B, Bergman DA. The thyroid cork: obstruction of the thoracic inlet due to retroclavicular goiter. JAMA 1974; 227:189–191.

4. Kelley TS, Mayors DJ, Boutsicaris PS. "Downhill" varices: a cause of upper gastrointestinal hemorrhage. Am Surg 1982; 48:35–38.
5. Parker DR, el-Shaboury AH. Fatal hematemesis due to benign retrosternal goiter. Postgrad Med J 1992; 68:756–757.
6. Cohen P, Bhat K, Song J, et al. Superior vena cava syndrome and right pleural effusion due to giant goiter. NY State J Med 1990; 90:467–468.
7. Cengiz K, Aykin A, Demirci A, Diren B. Intrathoracic goiter with hyperthyroidism, tracheal compression, superior vena cava syndrome and Horner's syndrome. Chest 1990; 97:1005–1006.
8. Gaitan E, Nelson NC, Poole GV. Endemic goiter and endemic thyroid disorders. World J Surg 1991; 15:205–215.
9. Kelly FC, Sneeden WW. Prevalence and geographical distribution of endemic goiter. In: World Health Organization. Endemic Goiter. Monograph Series 44 Geneva, 1960:9–25.
10. Shaha AR, Burnett C, Alfonso AE, Jaffe BM. Goiters and airway problems. Am J Surg 1989; 158:378–380.
11. Alfonso A, Christoudias G, Amaruddin Q, et al. Tracheal or esophageal compression due to benign thyroid disease. Am J Surg 1981; 142:350–353.
12. Becker WF. Pioneers in thyroid surgery. Ann Surg 1977; 185:493–504.
13. Reeve TS, Rubenstein C, Rundle FF. Intrathoracic goiter: its prevalence in Sydney metropolitan mass X-ray surveys. Med J Aust 1957; 2:149–152.
14. Newman E, Shaha AR. Substernal goiter. J Surg Oncol 1995; 60:207–212.
15. Singh B, Lucente FE, Shaha AR. Substernal goiter—a clinical review. Am J Otolaryngol 1994; 15:409–416.
16. Cougard P, Matet P, Goudet P, et al. Substernal goiters: 218 operated cases. Ann Endocrinol (Paris) 1992; 53:230.
17. Katlic MR, Wang C, Grillo HC. Substernal goiter. Ann Thor Surg 1985; 39:391–399.
18. Michel LA, Bradpiece HA. Surgical management of substernal goiter. Br J Surg 1988; 75:565–569.
19. Milliere D, Saada F, Etienne G, et al. Goiter with severe respiratory compromise: evaluation and treatment. Surgery 1988; 103:367–373.
20. Sanders LE, Rossi RL, Shahian DM, Williamson WA. Mediastinal goiter: the need for an aggressive approach. Arch Surg 1992; 127:609–613.
21. Cho HT, Cohen JP, Som ML. Management of substernal and intrathoracic goiters. Otolaryngol Head Neck Surg 1986; 94:282–287.
22. Wax MK, Briant DR. Management of substernal goiter. J Otolaryngol 1992; 21:165–170.
23. Manning PB, Thompson NW. Bilateral phrenic nerve palsy associated with benign thyroid goiter. Acta Chir Scand 1989; 155:429–431.
24. Bashist B, Ellis K, Gold RP. Computerized tomography of intrathoracic goiters. Am J Radiol 1983; 140:455–460.
25. Miller RD, Hyatt RE. Obstructive lesions of the larynx and trachea: clinical and physiologic characteristics. Mayo Clin Proc 1969; 44:145–161.
26. Lahey FH, Swinton NW. Intrathoracic goiter. Surg Gynecol Obstet 1934; 59:627–637.
27. Crile G. Intrathoracic goiter. Cleve Clin Quart 1939; 6: 313–322.
28. Lahey FH. Diagnosis and management of intrathoracic goiter. JAMA 1920; 75:163–166.
29. Lahey FH. Intrathoracic goiters. Surg Clin North Am 1945; 25:609–618.
30. Shaha AR, Alfonso AE, Jaffe BM. Acute airway distress due to thyroid pathology. Surgery 1987; 102:1068–1074.
31. Allo MD, Thompson NW. Rationale for the operative management of substernal goiter. Surgery 1983; 94:969–977.
32. Sand ME, Laws HL, McElevin RB. Substernal and intrathoracic goiter. Reconsideration of surgical approach. Am Surg 1983; 49:196–202.
33. DeSouza FM, Smith PE. Retrosternal goiter. J Otolaryngol 1983; 12:393–396.
34. Geelhoed GW. Tracheomalacia from compressing goiter: management after thyroidectomy. Surgery 1988; 104:1100–1108.
35. Cattel RB, Hare HF. The position of the trachea before and after removal of substernal goiter. Surg Clin North Am 1948; 28:781–792.

12

Medullary Thyroid Carcinoma

Lars-Erik Tisell and Håkan Ahlman
Sahlgrenska University Hospital, Göteborg, Sweden

1 BACKGROUND

In 1959 Hazard and colleagues defined medullary thyroid carcinoma (MTC) as a separate disease with specific clinical and pathological features. They found that the tumor was characterized by solid nonfollicular growth pattern, presence of amyloid in the stroma, and high incidence of lymph node metastases [1]. Within the next 10 years MTC was recognized to originate from the parafollicular C cells, secrete calcitonin, and occur in both sporadic and hereditary forms (2–6).The disease has a wide clinical spectrum ranging from aggressive tumors to rather indolent disease. In contrast to other thyroid diseases, MTC occurs almost equally in both sexes (7). In a study from the National Cancer Registry in Sweden, the age-standardized annual incidence of all MTC, sporadic and hereditary, was 2.1 per million inhabitants during 1970–1980. During this period MTC constituted 5.2% of all reported thyroid carcinomas in Sweden. Sporadic MTC was rather evenly distributed in the country, which speaks against environmental factors as causative agents. Hereditary MTC was more confined to certain regions, reflecting the location of identified families and differences in screening activity. Population-based surveys in the United States and Canada showed that MTC constituted 4–10% of the thyroid carcinomas. Data from the Thyroid Cancer Registry in Japan showed 1.55% of MTC among the patients with thyroid malignancies registered from 1977 to 1980. MTC can occur in four different settings: (1) in sporadic form, (2) as the single component in a hereditary disease, familial MTC (FMTC), (3) in the hereditary syndrome multiple endocrine neoplasia syndrome type 2A (MEN-2A), associated with parathyroid disease and pheochromocytoma, and (4) in the hereditary syndrome MEN-2B associated with pheochromocytoma and a specific phenotype characterized by marfanoid habitus, mucosal ganglioneuromas, and intestinal ganglioneuromatosis. Seventy-five percent of the patients with MTC have sporadic disease and 25% hereditary disease.

2 GENETICS

2.1 Hereditary MTC Syndromes

MEN-2 is an autosomal dominant genetic disorder, which can be clinically manifested as the MEN-2A syndrome (MTC 100%, pheochromocytoma 50%, and parathyroid neoplasia 10–20%). In 1961 Sipple (2) described six patients with both thyroid carcinoma and pheochromocytoma. Williams et al. (3) recognized that such thyroid tumors were of medullary type. In 1965 Schimke and Hartmann (4) suggested a single gene inheritance of MTC and pheochromocytoma, and 3 years later Steiner et al. (6) proposed that familial occurrence of MTC, pheochromocytoma, and parathyroid tumors should be designated MEN-2. Among the hereditary types of disease, MEN-2A is the most frequent syndrome (68%), followed by the MTC-only syndrome (FMTC) (21%) (8). A minority of patients suffer from the MEN-2B syndrome (11%). Later, variants of the MEN-2A syndrome were recognized, i.e., MEN-2A associated with cutaneous lichen amyloidosis or with Hirschsprung's disease (9–11). In 1966 Williams and Pollock (12) described the MEN-2B syndrome (MTC 100%, marfanoid habitus and intestinal ganglioneuromatosis/mucosal neuromas nearly 100%, and pheochromocytoma 50%) (Fig. 1). These patients have no parathyroid disease. All these syndromes are caused by germline mutations of the *RET* proto-oncogene, and affected individuals will develop multifocal bilateral MTC with almost complete penetrance usually at a young age. The other syndrome features have incomplete penetrance.

2.2 Genetic Background

In 1987 the causative *RET* proto-oncogene was mapped to chromosome 10 (13,14), and several *RET* mutations were thereafter described in kindreds with MEN-2 syndromes and FMTC (15–20). The large *RET* proto-oncogene comprises 21 exons and codes for a tyrosine kinase receptor with a cadherin-like extracellular region, which is cysteine-rich close to the cell membrane, and an intracellular tyrosine kinase domain (21). Hereditary MTC is mainly caused by mutations in the cysteine-rich extracellular region or in the intracellular kinase domain and involves 6 exons (Fig. 2). The classic MEN-2A syndrome is usually associated with mutations in the extracellular region of *RET*, i.e., codon 634 (75–85%) and codons 609, 611, 618, and 620 (altogether 10–15%). On the other hand, the MEN-2B syndrome is associated with mutations in the intracellular kinase domain, i.e., codon 918 (95%) and rarely codon 883 (Fig. 2) (22).

Somatic point mutations of *RET* are rather unusual in sporadic MTC (25–30%) (23). Codon 918 is most commonly affected. Patients with this mutation have aggressive tumors and short survival in analogy with its germline counterpart, which causes the MEN-2B syndrome (24). The codon 918 mutation may be of importance for tumor progression, frequently combined with a codon 836 polymorphism (25). Somatic point mutations have also been reported for exons 10, 11, 13, 14, and 15 at low frequency (23). Furthermore, base pair deletions of exon 11 seem to be common in sporadic MTC, which may lead to impaired *RET* function (26,27). If mutation analysis was regularly performed in cases with apparently sporadic MTC, hereditary disease may be revealed in 6–8% (28). The molecular basis for development of sporadic MTC is still largely unknown. The diverging clinical courses seen in spo-

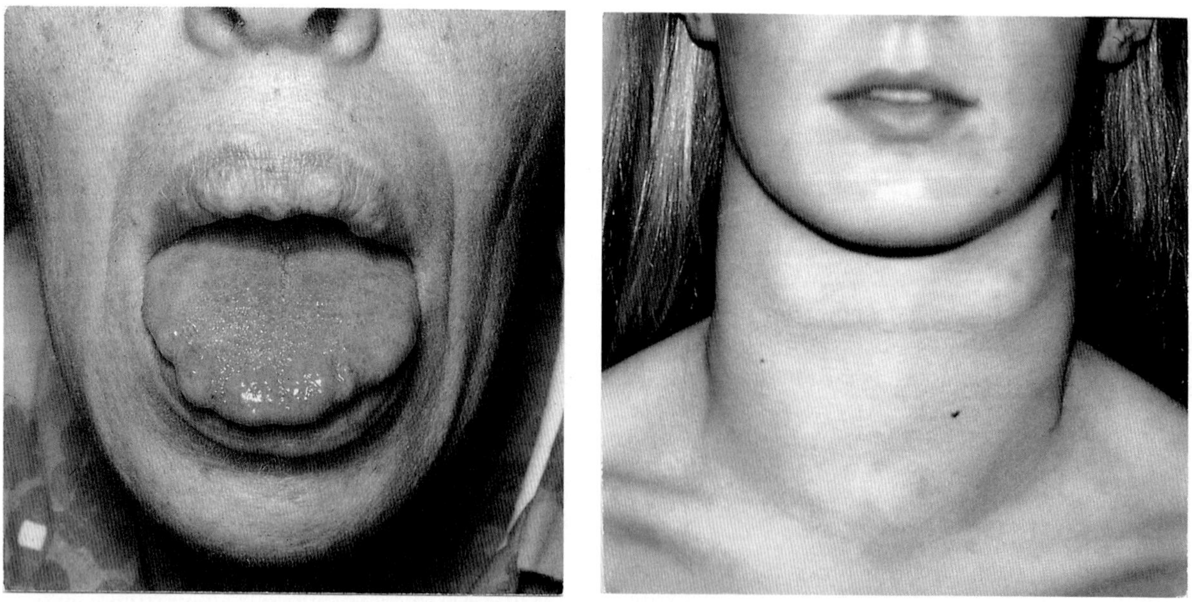

Figure 1 Two patients with the MEN-2B syndrome (codon 918 mutation) with (left) or without (right) phenotypic features. The left panel shows characteristic mucosal ganglioneuromas of the lips and tongue. The right panel shows a massive MTC at clinical presentation in a young patient.

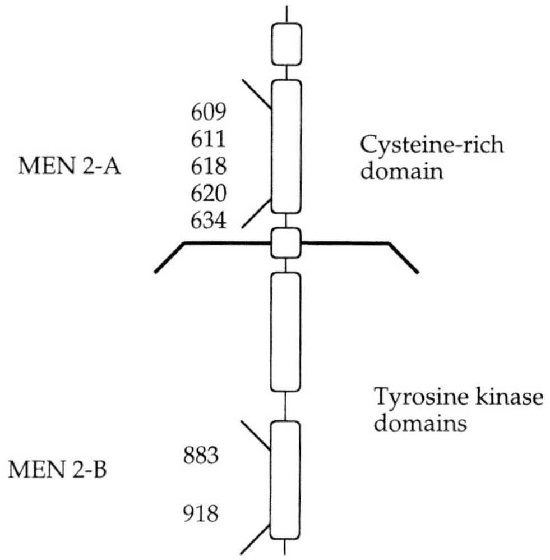

Figure 2 Schematic illustration of *RET* with mutations associated with MEN-2A and -2B indicated. FMTC and MEN-2A are mainly associated with the same mutations in the cysteine-rich domain. FMTC can also be associated with mutations in codons 768, 791, and 891 in the tyrosine kinase domains (not shown).

radic MTC patients may indicate a complex multifactorial pathogenesis.

2.3 RET/GFR α Receptor

Under physiological circumstances the ligand glial cell derived neurotrophic factor (GDNF) binds to a receptor system, consisting of the GDNF receptor (= GFR α-1) and the extracellular domain of *RET*, which in turn triggers dimerization of the receptor, autophosphorylation of *RET*, and activation of two intracellular kinase signaling pathways (22). Mutations of *RET* can cause tumor transformation via at least two mechanisms: (1) gain of function, e.g., the most common extracellular mutation at codon 634 causes dimerization of the *RET*/GFR α-1 receptor in the absence of ligand leading to continuous intracellular signaling; (2) altered substrate recognition, e.g., the most common intracellular mutation at codon 918 causes activation of the intracellular signaling pathways in the absence of receptor dimerization.

To date, three additional GFR-like receptors and three additional ligands (neurturin, perseptin, and artemin) have been identified as important for nerve growth and maturation (29). Like GDNF, they bind to *RET* in complex with the membrane-bound components GFRα-2 to -4. Mutations of GDNF homologues and their receptors do not seem to be involved in MEN-2A (30), but occur frequently in both sporadic and familial Hirschsprung's disease (31).

2.4 Consequences of Genetic Testing

With the rapid progress of our knowledge about *RET* mutations and hereditary MTC, the concept of prophylactic total thyroidectomy in individuals at risk has developed. The timing of this surgical procedure has been much discussed and also relates to more aggressive clinical phenotypes seen with certain genotypes. It must be emphasized that the clinical experience with some of these rare mutations is still limited and guidelines for treatment are only tentative at this stage. An attempt to stratify the risks in variants of hereditary MTC according to the experience of M.D. Anderson Cancer Center is presented in Table 1 together with treatment recommendations discussed at the international MEN workshops (32). The ideal age for intervention has not been settled unequivocally, but in general most experts want to intervene arround the age of 5 years in patients with MEN-2A or FMTC, but in infancy in MEN-2B patients

Table 1

Risk score	Clinical manifestation/RET mutation	Recommended treatment
High	MEN-2B[a]/codon 883, 918 or 922	Total thyroidectomy + central node dissection mandatory within the first year of life
Intermediate	Codon 611, 618, 620, or 634	Total thyroidectomy + central node dissection recommended within the first 5 years of life
Low	Codon 609, 768, 790[b], 791[b], 804 or 891	No consensus: Total thyroidectomy can be performed within the first 5 years of life, or at later age, or at the first abnormalities at continued provocation tests

[a]Germline transmission through several generations is less common, but testing recommended on all children at risk irrespective of presence of the MEN-2B phenotype, or not. Since individuals with de novo mutations have no family history of MEN-2B, testing is recommended on all subjects with phenotypic features.

[b]No deaths from MTC have been observed in patients with these mutations.

(33,34). In patients with MEN-2A, the clinical course of MTC is quite variable and resembles sporadic MTC, e.g., patients with metastases can have stable disease while others rather rapidly develop skeletal metastases and hormonally induced diarrhea and die of metastatic growth in the central neck and airways. On the other hand, the onset of MTC in MEN-2B is very early, and young patients may present with a cervical mass and incurable metastatic disease. Patients with FMTC have more indolent tumor disease and may live well even with elevated calcitonin levels. Many are cured by thyroidectomy alone.

In several series on preventive thyroidectomy it was shown that *RET* mutation carriers had foci of MTC despite normal calcitonin levels, i.e., provocation tests underestimated the histopathological findings. Some of the surgical procedures should therefore be considered therapeutic rather than preventive. Furthermore, children with abnormal provocation tests frequently had microscopic MTC at surgery, a tumor entity with metastatic potential. Accordingly, 15–20% recurrent disease may appear after long-term follow-up in children subject to thyroidectomy due to early diagnosed MTC by biochemical standards (35–37). In one series from the Netherlands gene-carrying children (5–18 years old) from MEN-2A kindreds with normal calcitonin testing all had foci of MTC in their surgical specimens (38). In a large MEN-2A screening study from 7 kindreds, the gene carriers were offered total thyroidectomy. Among the operated patients, all with elevated calcitonin levels had macro/microscopic MTC and all with normal calcitonin had macro/microscopic MTC or C-cell hyperplasia. No metastases were identified in any of the central lymph nodes dissected in the entire patient material, and the stimulated calcitonin levels were normal after surgery (39). In early series on prophylactic thyroidectomy in children with verified *RET* mutations, no signs of recurrent disease have been noted with an observation up to 3 years (34).

There is now consensus that children at risk should undergo genetic testing at an early age. The testing should rely on two peripheral blood samples, drawn and analyzed on separate occasions to avoid testing errors and sample mix-up. After extraction of DNA from lymphocytes, *RET* regions are amplified by PCR and mutations detected by direct sequencing, analyses of restriction sites, and gel shifts. The future follow-up will be focused on recurrence rates after prophylactic thyroidectomy, i.e., stimulated calcitonin levels at regular intervals should be performed combined with screening for pheochromocytoma and hyperparathyroidism. We still recommend that FMTC patients be medically managed like MEN-2A patients with attention to development of pheochromocytoma and parathyroid disease, since FMTC may potentially represent one end of the MEN-2A spectrum with low penetrance of the disease mutation (40).

3 PATHOLOGY

The typical tumor presents as a firm, gray-white mass, usually well demarcated and sometimes encapsulated. The cell of origin for MTC is the C cell which, can be identified by immunohistochemical staining for calcitonin. C cells comprise about 0.1% of the thyroid epithelial cells (41). The C cells are located within individual follicles, being sandwiched between the basement membrane and the follicular epithelium either as single cells or in small groups (41,42). The tumor may grow in trabecular sheets or in insular nests, separated by fibrous tissue. Most of the normal C cells are located deep within the lateral thyroid lobes along the upper two thirds of their central axis. The C-cell hyperplasia includes focal, diffuse, and nodular hyperplasia. Nod-

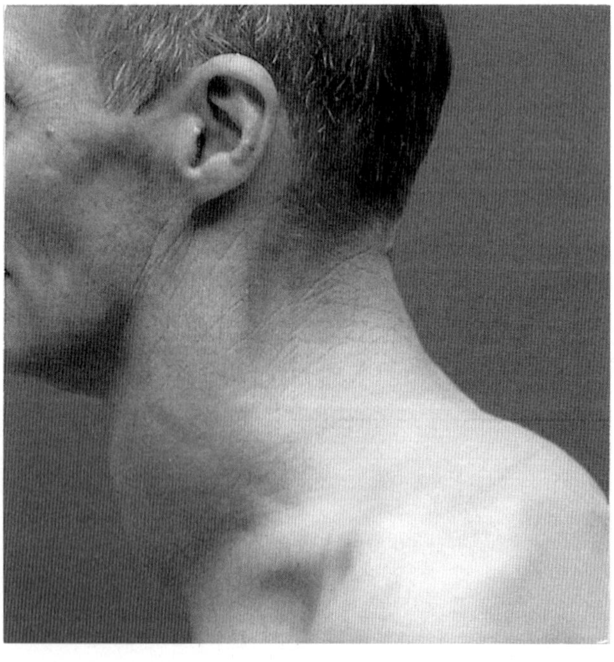

Figure 3 The proband of a family with the MEN-2A syndrome (codon 618 mutation) at clinical presentation with an advanced MTC, lymph node metastases, and infiltrating growth in structures of the neck and mediastinum.

ular hyperplasia is present when the lumen of the follicle is obliterated by proliferating C cells. Early MTC represents the stage when C cells break through the basement membrane and invade the interstitium (41,42). The size of a MTC at clinical presentation can vary from a few mm to large tumors that extend from the mandible down into mediastinum (Fig. 3). In most cases MTC is initially located within the regions of highest C-cell concentration. In familial MTC the tumors are often bilateral and multicentric and associated with bilateral C-cell hyperplasia. Microscopically, MTC is composed of polygonal, or spindle-shaped, cells with granular eosinophilic cytoplasm. Amyloid (a calcitonin gene product) may occur in the stroma but is no prerequisite for the diagnosis. The method to establish the diagnosis is immunocytochemical staining for calcitonin, but the tumor also stains for the carcinoembryonic antigen CEA and chromogranin A and several other substances, e.g., histaminase, serotonin, adrenocorticotropic hormone (ACTH), calcitonin gene-related peptide (CGRP), corticotropin-releasing factor (CRF), and vasoactive intestinal peptide (VIP). Deposits of calcium in the stroma can occur in the thyroid tumor, and in exceptional cases calcified hepatic metastases can be revealed on plain abdominal films (Fig. 4). Calcified tumor masses are usually associated with advanced disease, but even with this sign long survival may occur. Mixed tumor variants (MTC–follicular thyroid carcinoma and MTC–papillary thyroid carcinoma) are rare. The diagnosis can be made when two independent tumors are ruled out. The clonal properties of the two components differ, and some tumors can be regarded as MTC with surrounding thyroid hyperplasia (43). Except for bilaterality and multicentricity, there are no histological or histochemical differences between hereditary and sporadic MTC.

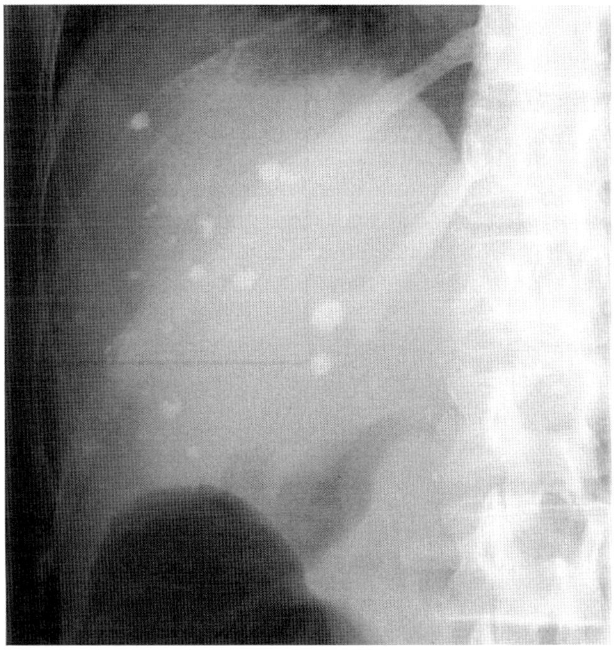

Figure 4 Plain abdominal films of a MEN-2B patient with calcified MTC metastases in the liver.

4 CALCITONIN AND CEA, PHYSIOLOGY, AND TUMOR MARKERS

The existence of a calcium-lowering factor was first postulated by Coop and colleagues (44). Experimentally they perfused the regional neck vessels, supplying the parathyroids and thyroids, with blood of varying calcium concentrations and found that hypercalcemic perfusion suppressed the systemic calcium levels. First they believed that the parathyroids produced this new factor. Further studies showed that the hypocalcemic factor, now termed calcitonin, was a thyroid hormone originating from the parafollicular C cells. There is a close correlation between the number of C cells and the tissue content of calcitonin. Acute elevations of the serum calcium concentration stimulate the release of stored calcitonin. Calcitonin is a 32-amino-acid peptide hormone, which suppresses the serum calcium concentration, presumably through its action on osteoclast activity. Hypercalcemia increases the circulating levels of gastrin, which also elicits release of calcitonin in order to maintain normocalcemia. Pentagastrin is a synthetic peptide, sharing the active carboxy-terminal tetrapeptide of gastrin, which is used for pharmacological release of calcitonin (45). MTC cells express gastrin (CCK-B) receptors, which is a prerequisite for both the physiological and the pharmacological stimulation of the calcitonin release (46). Determination of serum concentrations of calcitonin is used as a diagnostic test for MTC. To increase the sensitivity of this test, the calcitonin concentrations are determined both before and after i.v. infusion of calcium (2 mg/kg/min) followed by a bolus dose of pentagastrin (0.6 μg/kg). After introduction of the more reliable immunoradiometric assays (with a detection limit of 2–4 ng/L and an upper normal reference limit of 20 ng/L), we routinely use the pentagastrin test, but still use the combined stimulation test in cases with borderline elevations of calcitonin concentrations after stimulation with pentagastrin alone.

4.1 False-Negative Calcitonin Tests

In patients with residual MTC after earlier operations, 63% had undetectable basal serum calcitonin concentrations, although their stimulated calcitonin values were elevated (47). Therefore, when serum calcitonin concentrations are tested, the stimulation test should be used to avoid false-negative tests. False-negative calcitonin tests can also occur in patients with less differentiated MTC. The calcitonin values of such a patient are given in Table 2. He presented with a large sporadic MTC that was visualized by somatostatin receptor scintigraphy. In our experience, patients with positive somatostatin receptor scintigraphies have aggressive tumors and poor prognosis (48). The preoperative test showed a high basal serum calcitonin concentration, which was increased by only 12% after injection of calcium and pentagastrin. The CEA levels were raised to 6 μg/L. At operation a large tumor (75 g) was found that infiltrated structures in the neck and upper mediastinum, including one inferior laryngeal nerve, the esophagus, and the cervical and brachial nerve plexa. A total thyroidectomy was done with an extensive microdissection of the neck and upper mediastinum (see below). Forty-six out of 82 lymph nodes contained tumor with perinodal growth. Tumor tissue remained after the operation. Microscopic examination revealed the typical features of a less differentiated MTC, i.e., cellular and nuclear polymorphism, frequent mitoses, areas with necrosis, no amyloid, and a heterogeneous distribution of calcitonin-poor C cells. To our surprise, the postoperative calcitonin test was normal and at later check-ups the CEA value was normalized. CEA has a long half-life; it takes at least 2 months after a tumor reduction before CEA is normal. During the following 4 years the calcitonin values increased very little. No stimulation of serum calcitonin concentrations was noted by combined i.v. injections of calcium and pentagastrin. In 1991 a small increase in the stimulated serum calcitonin concentration occurred. The following year the patient developed distant metastases in the lungs and liver, and he died shortly thereafter. In this patient the severity of disease was better reflected by the CEA values than by the calcitonin concentrations. It must be noted that CEA is not MTC-specific; normal and hyperplastic C cells do not contain CEA, and not all MTC cells stain for CEA. In patients with aggressive MTC, an increase in serum concentrations of CEA can occur despite stable serum calcitonin concentrations; an increase in CEA can even be associated with decreased calcitonin levels. The calcitonin tests are usually the most efficient for the diagnosis and follow-up of patients with MTC, but CEA may be useful to identify a subset of patients with poor prognosis.

Table 2 False-Negative Calcitonin Stimulation Test in a Patient with Less Differentiated MTC and Residual Disease After Surgery

	Serum calcitonin (ng/L)		
Month/year	Basal	Peak	CEA (μg/L)[c]
2/86	17,000[a]	19,000[a]	6
2/86	300[a]	290[a]	-
10/86	440[a]	420[a]	5
5/87	470[a]	400[a]	5.3
4/88	840[a]	800[a]	5.5
5/89	860[a]	880[a]	12
9/90	31[b]	52[b]	25
11/91	64[b]	146[b]	85
3/92	356[b]	732[b]	240

[a] Values determined by a radioimmunoassay, upper normal limit 300 ng/L.
[b] Values determined by an immunoradiometric assay, upper normal limit 20 ng/L.
[c] CEA determined with an immunofluorometric assay, upper normal limit 5 μg/L.

4.2 False-Positive Calcitonin Tests

C-cell hyperplasia not related to MEN-2 occurs in 5–10% of the normal population and is especially common in children younger than 6 years and in individuals older than 50 years. Such individuals can have borderline increased calcitonin levels that cannot be distinguished from the neoplastic state that precedes MTC (49). After the introduction of genetic testing, it was revealed that a few MEN-2A family members with C-cell hyperplasia had undergone thyroidectomy due to false-positive stimulated calcitonin tests. The genetic analysis proved that they were not gene carriers (50). Patient serum may contain anti-IgG antibodies (heterophilic antibodies), which are capable of reacting with antibodies used in the assay. This may cause spuriously elevated calcitonin values in an immunoradiometric assay. The interference can be eliminated by addition of nonimmune mouse or bovine serum. Therefore, when a patient presents with unexpectedly high serum calcitonin concentrations, the laboratory should be consulted (51).

4.3 Other Pitfalls

Hypercalcitoninemia can occur in patients with neuroendocrine tumors other than MTC, e.g., gastroenteropancreatic endocrine tumors, pheochromocytomas, and paragangliomas. Contrary to previous opinion, it has been found that the calcitonin release from these tumors can be enhanced by i.v. injections of pentagastrin to a similar degree as seen in MTC. These tumors were indicated as the source of calcitonin by immunocytochemical studies and by normalization of the serum calcitonin concentration after tumor excision (52,53). It is thus important to know that pentagastrin-stimulated calcitonin release does not always indicate the presence of MTC. Nowadays the screening programs for early detection of MTC in members of families with hereditary disease are based on genetic testing (34,39). However, the stimulated calcitonin tests still have an important role in the diagnosis of sporadic MTC (75% of all cases) and in the follow-up after surgery in all MTC patients.

5 PROGNOSIS AND RISK FACTORS

In one series with 116 MEN-2A patients, 36 family members had been diagnosed before the screening era; 29 of these patients died of pheochromocytoma and the other 7 died of MTC. Out of 80 patients who had been diagnosed by screening, 2 died of pheochromocytoma and 7 of MTC (38). This shows that the proportion of deaths by pheochromocytoma was substantially reduced by the screening programs. Nowadays, very few patients with hereditary disease die of pheochromocytoma, and most of the disease-specific mortality in MEN-2A and MEN-2B is due to MTC.

5.1 Patient-Related Prognostic Factors

According to the study by Saad et al. (7), the most important factors that influence the prognosis are the type and stage of MTC. MEN-2A patients had a better survival rate than those with sporadic disease (Table 3). MEN-2B is known to be the most aggressive form of MTC, while FMTC has the most favorable prognosis of all types of MTC (8). In a large study including 741 patients from the German MTC Register (54), the 5- and 10-year adjusted survival rates for all stages of MTC were 81% and 64%, respectively (Table 4); similar figures have been reported by other investigators. In a univariate analysis the stage of disease at diagnosis, type of disease (sporadic or familial), age at diagnosis, and gender were relevant prognostic factors to identify groups with high or low risk, respectively, e.g., young female patients with familial disease diagnosed at early stage had the best prognosis. The most essential factor that influenced survival was the stage of disease at the time of diagnosis. In a multivariate analysis adjusted for tumor stage, the significant difference in relative hazard between patients with sporadic and those with familial disease disappeared. From these findings it was suggested that once a MTC has become clinically manifest, its course may not differ biologically between sporadic and familial cases. The generally better prognosis seen in MEN-2A patients than in sporadic cases may be related to the stage at which the disease was detected rather than to inherent differences in biological behavior of the tumor. The mean age at diagnosis for the sporadic cases was 50 years, with the highest incidence in the fifth decade and the mean age for the familial cases was 33 years, with the highest incidence in the fourth decade (54). The MEN-2B patients may thus have the most malignant MTC tumors partly as a result of the early onset of disease. Screening of MEN-2B families has led to earlier MTC operations; consequently, in recent MEN-2B series the MTC appeared to be less aggressive than predicted from earlier experience (55,56).

5.2 Morphological Prognostic Factors

In a study of 241 patients the histopathological characteristics and nuclear DNA content of MTC tumors were evaluated as prognostic factors (57). The following tumor characteristics indicate good prognosis: high frequency (> 50%) of calcitonin-immunoreactive cells,

Table 3 Importance of MTC Type to Postoperative Survival

Authors (Ref.)	Treatment period	Type of MTC	No. of patients	Age (yr) at presentation	5- and 10-year survival (%)
Saad et al. (7)	1944–83	Sporadic	125 (81%)	46	74 and 55
		Familial	30 (19%)[a]	32	100 and 94
		Sporadic	559 (75%)	50	79 and 62
Raue et al. (54)	1967–91	Familial	182 (25%)	33	88 and 72

[a] Five patients with MEN-2B syndromes excluded.

Table 4 Importance of MTC Stage to Postoperative Survival

Authors (Ref)	No. of patients	Treatment period	Survival rates (%) I	II	III	IV	All
Saad et al. (7)[a]	161	1944–83					
Survival after 5 years			92	89	58	40	78
Survival after 10 years			82	80	23	25	61
Raue et al. (54)[b]	741	1967–91					
Survival after 5 years			100	81	75	50	81
Survival after 10 years			74	77	60	37	64

[a] Mean age at diagnosis = 44 years.
[b] Mean age at diagnosis = 46 years.

presence of amyloid in the tumor, and intact tumor capsule. There were two- or threefold differences in hazard rate between patients with, or without, these tumor characteristics. Also the nuclear DNA content is a strong predictor of the outcome in MTC. The importance of calcitonin immunoreactivity and the amyloid content was tested in multivariate analyses adjusted for the mentioned prognostic factors and also for stage of the disease, heredity, age, sex, tumor size, and treatment. According to these analyses, the relative hazard for calcitonin immunoreactivity and amyloid content changed only marginally, which indicates that these parameters are independent prognostic factors. Now that gene carriers of the MEN-2A and FMTC syndromes can be identified in childhood and even in infancy by genetic testing, thyroidectomy can be done before MTC has developed and the prognosis for these cases of familial MTC will be excellent (34). About half of the MEN-2B gene carriers who have inherited the mutation will benefit from the early genetic testing. The diagnosis of the sporadic cases and the MEN-2B cases with de novo mutations will be discussed in Sec. 7.

6 ECTOPIC CUSHING'S SYNDROME

An ectopic Cushing's syndrome occurs in about 4% of patients with MTC (58). In two thirds of these patients the diagnosis of MTC precedes with several years the discovery of the Cushing's syndrome. In the other patients the two diseases are detected simultaneously. At presentation they have the signs and symptoms usually seen with the nonectopic Cushing's syndrome; in addition, about a third of the cases have watery diarrhea, often with 10–15 stools a day. Such diarrhea can also occur in other MTC patients with large tumor burden. The exact cause of the diarrhea is not known, but calcitonin, prostaglandins, serotonin, and VIP have been suggested as etiological substances. In some cases the diarrhea can be abolished, or palliated, by tumor reduction (59). Also, medication with the somatostatin analogue octreotide can palliate the diarrhea (60–62). Patients with the ectopic Cushing's syndrome are characterized by rapid onset of symptoms, progressive clinical course, and often radiographically evident tumors. They usually have hypokalemic alkalosis and severe muscle wasting and weakness. The diagnosis is established by very high levels of serum and urinary cortisol and no suppression of ACTH secretion by the high dose (8 mg) of dexamethasone. In preparation for surgery the hypokalemic alkalosis should be corrected. In patients with hypercortisolism the risk for thromboembolic complications is high and prophylactic measures should be taken. Radical extirpation of the MTC with metastases would be the optimal solution, but this can be done only in exceptional cases. Ectopic Cushing is in the great majority of cases a late symptom associated with advanced dissemination of the tumor. Therefore, in most patients the treatment of choice is laparoscopic bilateral adrenalectomy. Most patients have been exposed to high levels of corticosteroids. Therefore, they need high-dose glucocorticoid coverage during surgery and postoperatively. The corticosteroid dose should be tapered over several weeks. After the patients have recovered from adrenalectomy, cytoreductive surgery can be considered. In individual cases we have seen survival exceeding 5 years after liver resection, but on the whole the prognosis is dismal. The long duration of hypercortisolism before diagnosis of a Cushing's syndrome would be shortened and the prognosis improved if all MTC patients with persistent disease after surgery were not only regularly checked for the serum concentrations of calcitonin and CEA, but also for serum potassium and urinary levels of steroids. Ectopic Cushing can occur in both sporadic and hereditary MTC; one of our patients had a cysteine-to-glycine mutation at codon 634 of the *RET* protooncogene. She was 31 years old when diagnosed with ectopic Cushing.

7 PREOPERATIVE DIAGNOSIS

7.1 Fine Needle Aspiration Biopsy

With routine stains most MTC cells are polygonal, or spindle-shaped, often with eccentric nuclei, and appear larger than normal follicular cells. With May-Grünwald–Giemsa staining, characteristic red granulation of the cytoplasm can be found in a minority of the cells. Amyloid can be seen both intra- and extracellularly, staining bluish-grey or violet (63). To establish the MTC diagnosis, immunocytochemical staining for calcitonin should be done. No examination of a thyroid nodule is complete without fine needle aspiration biopsy (FNAB). This examination is especially important in the diagnostic work-up of sporadic MTC. With correct diagnosis, an appropriate thyroid operation can be planned. In patients with recurrent MTC, FNAB can verify the nature of lesions that have been detected by other means. In case of nonpalpable metastases, the biopsies can be guided by ultrasonography or by CT. A cytological diagnosis of MTC necessitates calcitonin and calcium studies as well as biochemical testing to rule out pheochromocytoma and hyperparathyroidism.

7.2 Sporadic MTC

The diagnosis of sporadic MTC must continue to rely on clinical observations and the awareness of the physician. Up to 90% of the patients with palpable MTC have lymph node metastases (64). Therefore MTC should be suspected in patients with palpable thyroid tumors and lymph node metastases. A few patients with sporadic MTC are incidentally diagnosed at surgery for colloid goiter or hyperparathyroidism. Such tumors are usually small (<1 cm). More than 95% of sporadic MTC are palpable, and they can be diagnosed by FNAB, complemented with basal and pentagastrin-stimulated calcitonin tests. Forty percent of MEN-2A gene carriers will not have presented with symptoms before the age of 70 (65). Therefore, the family history is not always reliable. This is one reason why genetic tests should also be recommended to patients with apparently sporadic MTC. Some MEN-2A patients have de novo mutations; such patients will also benefit from a policy with genetic testing for all patients with apparently sporadic MTC (28).

7.3 MTC as Part of MEN-2B Syndrome

The MEN-2B syndrome is a rare condition (11% of familial MTC). About half of the patients with MEN-2B syndromes have hereditary disease and can be diagnosed by genetic screening of affected kindreds. Half of the MEN-2B patients have de novo mutations (66), and many of them will be diagnosed first when they have got symptoms of MTC or pheochromocytoma. Others will be diagnosed due to the characteristic phenotype or due to other symptoms that may occur in the MEN-2B syndrome, e.g, intestinal problems. These symptoms can start during infancy first as constipation, later as constipation, diarrhea, and megacolon. They can also present with symptoms of skeletal abnormalities, e.g., scoliosis, or with problems from oral and ocular ganglioneuromas. Delayed puberty is another symptom of MEN-2B. The physician who attends patients with these symptoms should be aware of the MEN-2B syndrome so that these patients can be be diagnosed earlier by genetic testing and be offered a thyroidectomy leading to less morbidity and longer survival. The sooner MEN-2B patients are diagnosed, the better the outcome; the optimum time for surgery is during infancy. However, that early it is difficult to clinically diagnose a patient with de novo mutations, since the typical phenotype is not yet so apparent. Figure 1 shows the typical sign of thick bumpy lips due to mucosal ganglioneuromas in an adult patient; these signs were still absent in the teenage patient. Samaan et al. (67) reported an infant case who had thyroid surgery at the age of 3 months; in this case the suspicion of a MEN-2B syndrome came up because of failure to thrive, possible intestinal obstruction, and a rectal biopsy showing ganglioneuromas. The diagnosis was further strengthened when thickening of the corneal nerves was detected. This is a typical sign of MEN-2B that usually does not appear before 2 years of age. On suspicion of MEN-2B syndrome, the diagnosis can today be done directly by genetic testing.

8 PREOPERATIVE WORK-UP

8.1 Work-Up Before a Primary Operation

The routine work-up before surgery for patients with MTC includes genetic testing to identify patients with hereditary disease. Calcitonin tests are done to roughly estimate the amount of tumor tissue and to establish the diagnosis in sporadic cases. Serum concentrations of CEA are determined to alert the physician if the disease takes a more aggressive turn. Cytological verification of the tumor type is done in all sporadic cases. Since a vocal cord paralysis can occur preoperatively as a result of aggressive tumor growth, a laryngoscopy with examination of the vocal cord movements should be performed. Our ambition is to do neck operations even in patients with distant metastases in order to avoid, or delay, tumor infiltration into vital structures. In patients with advanced primary tumors, preoperative tracheoscopies and esophagoscopies are done with possibility for biopsies. In advanced primary cases, many of the studies discussed in the next section will be used.

8.2 Work-Up Before a Repeat Operation

Before a repeat operation an investigation of the vocal cord movements is mandatory, because the finding of a palsy of an inferior laryngeal nerve will influence the design of the operation towards a less radical operation on the nonaffected side. Before surgery for persistent or recurrent MTC, we try to localize the tumors and diagnose possible distant metastases. The first localizing procedure is a careful palpation of the neck and FNAB of all suspect lesions. Ultrasonography can be used preoperatively and intraoperatively in the neck to localize hypoechoic metastases down to a size of 5 mm. For preoperative morphological verification, FNAB should be performed on suspect lesions. These investigations are complemented by contrast-enhanced CT and/or MRI, especially when searching for liver, lung, and skeletal metastases. High sensitivity has been reported for selective venous catheterization with blood samplings for determination of serum calcitonin concentrations. However, this procedure can localize a tumor to a region, but not to a distinct site. MTC may have high expression of somatostatin receptors and can therefore be visualized by octreotide scintigraphy. In one study, 22 MTC patients who had persistently increased serum calcitonin concentrations after previous surgery were investigated by octreotide scintigraphy. Fifteen tumor sites were localized by octreotide scintigraphy in 11 of the patients. The smallest tumor that was visualized by the scintigraphy had a volume of 0.5 cm^3. Nine other tumor sites were found by other means. Half of the known lymph node metastases in the neck and upper mediastinum and 6 of 7 distant metastases were visualized by scintigraphy. Because of its capacity to detect distant metastases, we recommend octreotide scintigraphy before repeat operations. The growth rate of MTC can be monitored by measuring the increase in serum calcitonin concentrations over time. The patients with positive scintigraphies had a higher annual increase in

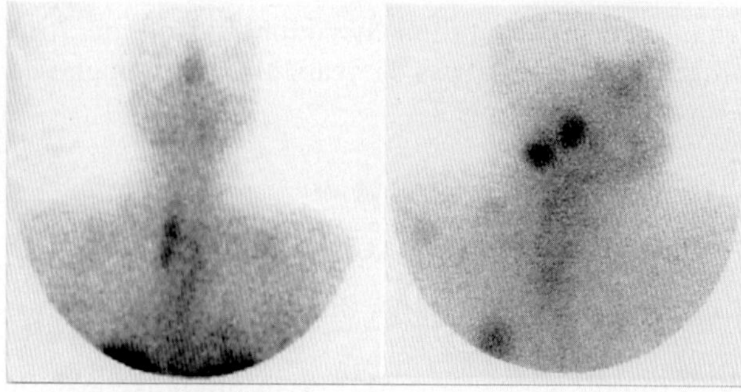

Figure 5 Octreotide scintigraphy in two patients with aggressive MTC. Left panel shows unilateral uptake of the radionuclide after primary surgery and several reoperations. After scintigraphy the surgical exploration was limited to the right side. Right panel shows multifocal uptakes in the right upper neck, mediastinum, and along the right clavicle.

calcitonin than the other patients. This shows that a high density of somatostatin receptors is compatible with a high tumor growth rate. Tumor-associated symptoms and death of MTC occurred only in patients with scintigraphically visualized tumors. This means that a positive octreotide scintigraphy is a bad prognostic factor (48) (Fig. 5).

In an interesting study, Tung et al. (68) found by laparoscopy small (<5 mm) liver metastases in 7 of 36 examined patients who had persistent high calcitonin values after previous MTC operations. These metastases had not been revealed by CT and MRI scans. In a patient with such small metastases, we should not hesitate to do a neck operation if there were macroscopic tumors in the neck. We should further evaluate the liver lesions with the intention to perform cytoreduction if possible.

9 SURGICAL TREATMENT

9.1 Primary Operations

As prophylaxis against thrombosis, all patients have s.c. injections with low molecular weight heparin. For surgery the patient is placed in the supine position with a large piece of foam padding placed under the shoulders and upper chest to avoid pressure sores. For optimal access during the operation, the head and neck are bent moderately backwards and placed on a vacuum pillow with adjustable pressure. The arms are positioned along the body and the anesthesiologist stationed at the foot of the operation table. These arrangements make it possible for the surgeon to shift position from the head of the patient or to the right or left side when needed in order to get optimal access to the operation field. To facilitate the dissection, magnifying glasses can be used.

The operation is started with a transverse incision about 4–5 cm above the jugulum. The superior and inferior flaps are created. The superior flap is freed up to the hyoid bone and the inferior down to the sternum. The flaps are freed laterally on both sides. We almost never use longitudinal incisions, since they are associated with a worse cosmetic result. Both recurrent nerves should be dissected free to their entrance into the larynx and the lymph nodes close to the nerves are excised. The whole thyroid with the pyramidal lobe and adjacent lymph nodes down to the innominate vein should be removed en bloc. After this has been done, the operation field is thoroughly searched for remaining lymph nodes; it is checked that no thyroid tissue or lymph nodes remain on the trachea. We also clean the anterior surface of the carotid artery and jugular vein from lymph nodes and soft tissue. Lateral neck dissections are done in case of palpable primary tumors or palpable lymph node metastases. Then the fascia over the carotid artery and the anterior jugular vein is opened, the vagus exposed, and the lymph nodes along the two vessels extirpated. This dissection continues up to the level where the accessory nerve passes over the internal jugular vein beneath the posterior belly of the digastric muscle. The lower limit for this dissection are the subclavian vessels. Sometimes it is possible to extirpate lymph node metastases located in the mediastinum below the right subclavian artery from the cervical incision. In these cases we continue the mediastinal clearance after a sternal split has been done. After the jugular vein and carotid artery have been cleaned, we dissect laterally from the jugular vein under the sternocleidomastoid muscle and over the cervical plexus down to the supraclavicular fossa. We also follow the accessory nerve to clean the posterior triangle. All tissue specimens are sent for histopathological examination with information about the exact site of each specimen. If a reoperation becomes necessary, the pathology report is a valuable tool for the planning of a new operation. Four parathyroids are identified, if possible, and they are usually autotransplanted into muscle tissue.

9.2 Reoperations

Few patients with lymph node metastases have their calcitonin values normalized by a lymph node dissection (33). Many patients with residual MTC do well for many years. However, MTC is generally a progressive disease, as shown by a mean annual increase in calcitonin concentrations of about 100% in 36 of 40 patients with residual MTC followed over 6 years (47). It is not unusual that patients with residual MTC survive for more than 20 years but still ultimately die of MTC. It has been shown that patients with residual MTC can have their increased serum calcitonin conentrations normalized by a repeat operation in about 30% of cases (59,64,69–71). In a study by Moley et al. (59) reoperation resulted in normalization of the plasma calcitonin concentrations in 28% of the patients and in a decrease of calcitonin by 40% or more in another 42%.

The design of the repeat operation depends on the information from the localization studies, from the operative notes, and from the pathology report of the previous operation. If the previous operation was done by a nonspecialized surgeon, we usually do a systematic reoperation on both sides of the neck; in other cases the operation can be done more selectively. A repeat operation for MTC is much more demanding than a primary operation mainly due to scar tissue. The operation starts with a laborious dissection to restore the anatomy. To be successful the surgeon must have an anatomical knowledge out of the ordinary. The best chance to cure the patient is at the first operation. Therefore, this operation should be done by a surgeon with experience of thyroidectomy and extensive lymph node dissections.

The young girl with a hereditary MEN-2B syndrome shown in Figure 1 had primary surgery for MTC 15 years ago. She had bilateral thyroid tumors, and a total thyroidectomy was done with central and lateral lymph node clearance on both sides of the neck; 129 lymph nodes were excised, including 8 metastases with perinodal growth. Two parathyroids were identified and transplanted into muscle tissue. Her serum calcitonin concentrations dropped from about 110,000 to 230 ng/L (upper normal limit < 300 ng/L). Eight years ago she was diagnosed with bilateral pheochromocytomas; she had bilateral resections of the tumors leaving in situ the normal parts of the adrenals. Today, 15 years after the thyroid operation, she still has normal stimulated serum calcitonin concentrations, normal adrenocortical function, and no signs of recurrent pheochromocytoma. She also has a normal serum concentration of parathyroid hormone but regularly takes some extra calcium.

10 NONSURGICAL TREATMENT

Surgical treatment is always the primary choice. In cases with local recurrence reoperation is recommended. MTC is not responsive to radioiodine, since the tumor cells are not derived from the thyroid follicle and lack the iodine pump. MTC is not very sensitive to external irradiation; prospective studies are lacking. In one large retrospective series, patients with this type of treatment actually had worse outcome (72). External irradiation is frequently associated with long-term side effects, e.g., dryness of airway and oral mucosa. Futhermore, surgical treatment after external irradiation can be very difficult to perform. On the other hand, external irradiation can be valuable in the treatment of skeletal metastases (73). Chemotherapy with single agents has no proven effect in patients with advanced disease. Combinations of cytotoxic agents used for other types of neuroendocrine tumors also had limited success (74,75). The best partial response rate (15%) was seen for 5-FU and streptozotocin alternating with dacarbazine (76).

Since MTC can be visualized scintigraphically by anti-CEA antibodies labeled with radionuclide, radioimmunotherapy with ^{131}I antibodies has been attempted. Antiproliferative effects were seen in half of the patients with acceptable side effects from the bone marrow (77). In our own diagnostic studies of thyroid neoplasias, we used ^{111}In-labeled octreotide with preferential binding to somatostatin receptors of subtypes 2 and 5. The MTC tumors with the worst prognosis were the ones that were visualized scintigraphically (48). The tumor-to-blood activity concentration ratios were favourable for radiotherapy as well as for lymph node metastases studied after dissection into tumor-free or tumor-bearing parts (78). Octreotide can also be used to alleviate hormonal symptoms in advanced disease, but tachyphylaxis may develop rather rapidly (62). Addition of interferon α-2b can potentiate the therapeutic effects at the cost of drug-related toxicity (79). Novel medical or radiopharmaceutical treatment strategies are clearly required.

11 FINAL COMMENTS

Pentagastrin tests will identify children with hereditary MTC at an average age of 15 years (38). In the two series discussed (Table 3) the mean age at diagnosis was 33 years. One reason for this late diagnosis is probably the fact that the series included patients diagnosed either before or after the introduction of screening programs; i.e., the survival data will underestimate the potential survival advantage in a series with biochemically screened patients. The introduction of genetic testing as screening will further improve the prognosis for the familial cases. To improve the prognosis for sporadic MTC, these patients should be referred for primary surgery to centers with expertise in the disease.

ACKNOWLEDGMENT

This work was supported by grants from the Swedish MRC (5220).

REFERENCES

1. Hazard JB, Hawk WA, Crile G. Medullary (solid) carcinoma of the thyroid: a clinicopathologic entity. J Clin Endocrinol Metab 1959; 19:152–161.
2. Sipple JH. The association of pheochromocytoma with carcinoma of the thyroid gland. Am J Med 1961; 163–166.
3. Williams ED, Brown CL, Doniach I. Pathological and clinical findings in a series of 67 cases of medullary carcinoma of the thyroid. J Clin Pathol 1966; 19:103–113.
4. Schimke RN, Hartmann WH. Familial amyloid-producing medullary thyroid carcinoma and pheochromocytoma. A distinct genetic entity. Ann Intern Med 1965; 63:1027–1039.
5. Schimke RN, Hartmann WH, Prout TE, Rimoin DL. Syndrome of bilateral pheochromocytoma, medullary thyroid carcinoma and multiple neuromas. N Engl J Med 1968; 279:1–7.
6. Steiner AL, Goodman AD, Powers SR. Study of a kindred with pheochromocytoma, medullary thyroid carcinoma, hyperparathyroidism and Cushing's disease; multiple endocrine neoplasia type 2. Medicine 1968; 47:371–409.
7. Saad MF, Ordonez NG, Rashid RK, Guido JJ, Hill CS, Hicky RC, Samaan NA. Medullary carcinoma of the thyroid. A study of the clinical features and prognostic factors in 161 patients. Medicine 1984; 63:319–342.
8. Farndon JR, Leight GS, Dilley WG, Baylin SB, Smallridge RC, Harrison TS, Wells SA Jr. Familial medullary thyroid carcinoma without associated endocrinopathies: a distinct clinical entity. Br J Surg 1986; 73:278–281.
9. Gagel RF, Levy ML, Donovan DT, Alford BR, Wheeler T, Tschen JA. Multiple endocrine neoplasia type 2a associated with cutaneous lichen amyloidosis. Ann Intern Med 1989; 111:802–806.
10. Verdy M, Weber AM, Roy CC, Morin CL, Cadotte M, Brochu P. Hirschsprung's disease in a family with multiple endocrine neoplasia type 2. J Pediatr Gastroenterol Nutr 1982; 1:603–607.
11. Decker RA, Peacock ML, Watson P. Hirschsprung's disease in MEN-2A: increased spectrum of RET exon 10 genotypes and strong genotype-phenotype correlation. Hum Mol Genet 1998; 7:129–134.

12. Williams ED, Pollock DJ. Multiple mucosal neuromata with endocrine tumors: a syndrome allied to Von Recklinghausen's disease. J Pathol Bacteriol 1966; 91:71–80.
13. Simpson NE, Kidd KK, Goodfellow PJ, McDermid H, Myers S, Kidd JR, Jackson CE, Duncan AM, Farrer LA, Brasch, et al. Assignment of multiple endocrine neoplasia type 2 A on chromosome 10 by linkage. Nature 1987; 328:528–530.
14. Mathew CG, Chin KS, Easton DF, Thorpe K, Carter C, Liou GI, Fong SL, Bridges CD, Haak H, Kruseman AC, et al. A linked genetic marker for multiple endocrine neoplasia type 2 A on chromosome 10. Nature 1987; 328:527–528.
15. Mulligan LM, Kwok JB, Healy CS, Elsdon MJ, Eng C, Gardner E, Love DR, Mote SE, Moore JK, Papi L, et al. Germ-line mutations of the RET proto-oncogene in multiple endocrine neoplasia type 2 A. Nature 1993; 6428:458–460.
16. Donis-Keller H, Dou S, Chi D, Carlson KM, Toshima K, Lairmore TC, Howe JR, Moley JF, Goodfellow P, Wells SA Jr. Mutations in the RET proto-oncogene are associated with MEN-2A and FMTC. Hum Mol Genet 1993; 7:851–856.
17. Mulligan LM, Eng C, Attie T, Lyonnet S, Marsh DJ, Hyland VJ, Robinson BG, Frilling A, Verellen-Dumoulin C, Safar A, et al. Diverse phenotypes associated with exon 10 mutations of the RET proto-oncogene. Hum Mol Genet 1994; 12:2163–2167.
18. Carlson KM, Dou S, Chi D, Scavarda N, Toshima K, Jackson CE, Wells SA Jr, Goodfellow P, Donis-Keller H. Single missense mutation in the tyrosine kinase catalytic domain of the RET protooncogene is associated with multiple endocrine neoplasia type 2B. Proc Natl Acad Sci USA 1994; 4:1579–1583.
19. Hofstra RM, Landvater RM, Ceccherini I, Stulp RP, Stelwagen T, Luo Y, Pasini B, Hoppener JW, van Amstel HK, Romeo G. A mutation in the RET proto-oncogene associated with multiple endocrine neoplasia type 2 B and sporadic medullary thyroid carcinoma (see comments). Nature 1994; 6461:375–376.
20. Eng C, Clayton D, Schuffenecker I, Lenoir G, Cote G, Gagel RF, van Amstel HK, Lips CJ, Nishisho I, Takai SI, Marsh DJ, et al. The relationship between specific RET proto-oncogene mutations and disease phenotype in multiple endocrine neoplasia type 2. International RET Mutation Consortium analysis. JAMA 1996; 276:1575–1579.
21. Takahashi M. Structure and expression of the ret transforming gene. IARC Sci Publ 1988; 92:189–197.
22. Hansford JR, Mulligan LM. Multiple endocrine neoplasia type 2 and RET: from neoplasia to neurogenesis. J Med Genet 2000; 37:817–827.
23. Dralle H, Gimm O, Machens A. Sporadic medullary thyroid carcinoma. In: Doherty GM, Skogseid B, eds. Surgical Endocrinology. Philadelphia: Lippincott Williams & Wilkins, 2001:109–126.
24. Zedenius J, Larsson C, Bergholm U, Bovee J, Svensson A, Hallengren B, Grimelius L, Bäckdahl M, Weber G, Wallin G. Mutations of codon 918 in the RET proto-oncogene correlate to poor prognosis in sporadic medullary thyroid carcinomas. J Clin Endocrinol Metab 1995; 80:3088–3090.
25. Gimm O, Neuberg DS, March DJ, Dahia PL, Hoang-Vu C, Raue F, Hinze R, Dralle H, Eng C. Over-representation of a germline RET sequence variant in patients with sporadic medullary thyroid carcinoma and somatic RET codon 918 mutation. Oncogene 1999; 18:1369–1373.
26. Alemi M, Lucas SD, Sällström JF, Bergholm U, Åkerström G, Wilander E. A complex nine base pair deletion in RET exon 11 common in sporadic medullary thyroid carcinoma. Oncogene 1997; 14:2041–2045.
27. Kalinin V, Frilling A. 27-Bp deletion in the ret proto-oncogene as a somatic mutation associated with medullary thyroid carcinoma. J Mol Med 1998; 76:365–367.
28. Wohllk N, Cote GJ, Bugalho MM, Ordonez N, Evans DB, Doepfert H, Khorana S, Schultz P, Richards CS, Gagel RF. Relevance of RET proto-oncogene mutations in sporadic medullary thyroid carcinoma. J Clin Endocrinol Metab 1996; 81:3740–3745.
29. Baloh RH, Enomoto H, Johnson EM Jr, Milbrandt J. The GDNF family ligands and receptors—implications for neural development. Curr Opinion Neurobiol 2000; 10:103–110.
30. Marsh DJ, Zheng Z, Arnold A, Andrew SD, Learoyd D, Frilling A, Komminoth P, Neumann HP, Ponder BA, Rollins BJ, et al. Mutation analysis of glial cell line-derived neurotrophic factor, a ligand for an RET/co-receptor complex, in multiple endocrine neoplasia type 2 and sporadic neuroendocrine tumors. J Clin Endocrinol Metab 1997; 82:3025–3028.
31. Eng C, Mulligan LM. Mutations of the RET proto-oncogene in the multiple endocrine neoplasia type 2 syndromes, related sporadic tumors, and Hirschsprung disease. Hum Mutat 1997; 9:97–109.
32. Kikumori T, Evans D, Lee JE, Cote GJ, Gagel RF. Genetic abnormalities in MEN-2. In: Doherty GM, Skogseid B, eds. Surgical Endocrinology. Philadelphia: Lippincott Williams & Wilkins, 2001:531–540.
33. O'Riordain DS, O'Brien T, Weaver AL, Gharib H, Hay ID, Grant CS, van Heerden JA. Medullary thyroid carcinoma in multiple endocrine neoplasia types 2A and 2B. Surgery 1994; 116:1017–1023.
34. Wells SA Jr, Skinner MA. Prophylactic thyroidectomy, based on direct genetic testing, in patients at risk for the MEN-2 syndromes. Exp Clin Endocrinol Diabetes 1998; 106:29–34.
35. Graham SM, Genel M, Touloukian RJ, Barwick KW, Gertner JM, Torony C. Provocative testing for occult medullary carcinoma of the thyroid; findings in seven children with multiple endocrine neoplasia type IIa. J Pediatr Surg 1987; 22:501–503.

36. Skinner MA, DeBenedetti MK, Moley JF, Norton JA, Wells SA Jr. Medullary thyroid carcinoma in children with multiple endocrine neoplasia types 2A and 2B. J Pediatr Surg 1996; 31:177–181.
37. Gagel RF, Cote GJ, Martins, Bugalho MJ, Boyd AE III, Cummings T, Goepfert H, Evans DB, Cangir A, Khorana S, Schultz PN. Clinical use of molecular information in the management of multiple endocrine neoplasia type 2A. J Intern Med 1995; 238:333–341.
38. Lips CJ, Landsvater RM, Hoppener JW, Geerdink RA, Blijham G, van Veen JM, van Gils AP, de Wit MJ, Zewald RA, Berends MJ, et al. Clinical screening as compared with DNA analysis in families with multiple endocrine neoplasia type 2 A. N Engl J Med 1994; 331: 828–835.
39. Wells SA Jr, Chi DD, Toshima K, Dehner LP, Coffin CM, Dowton SB, Ivanovich JL, DeBenedetti MK, Dilley WG, Moley JF, et al. Predictive DNA testing and prophylactic thyroidectomy in patients at risk for multiple endocrine neoplasia type 2A. Ann Surg 1994; 220:237–250.
40. Nilsson O, Tisell LE, Jansson S, Ahlman H, Gimm O, Eng C. Adrenal and extraadrenal pheochromocytomas in a family with germline RET V804 mutation. JAMA 1999; 281:1587–1588.
41. Wolfe HJ, DeLellis RA. Familial medullary thyroid carcinoma and C-cell hyperplasia. Clin Endocrinol Metab 1981; 10:351–365.
42. DeLellis RA, Nunnemacher G, Wolfe HJ. C-cell hyperplasia an ultrastructural analysis. Lab Invest 1977; 36:237–248.
43. Volante M, Papotti M, Roth J, Saremaslani P, Speel EJ, Lloyd RV, Carney JA, Heitz PU, Bussolati G, Komminoth P. Mixed medullary-follicular thyroid carcinoma. Molecular evidence for a dual origin of tumor components. Am J Pathol 1999; 155:1449–1509.
44. Coop DH, Cameron EC, Cheney BA, Davidson AGF, Henze KG. Evidence for calcitonin—a new hormone from the parathyroid that lowers blood calcium. Endocrinology 1962; 70:638–649.
45. Cooper CW, Schwesinger WH, Mahgoub AM, Ontjes DA. Thyrocalcitonin: stimulation of secretion by pentagastrin. Science 1971; 172:1238–1240.
46. Amiri-Mosavi A, Ahlman H, Tisell LE, Wängberg B, Kölby L, Forsell-Aronsson E, Lundberg PA, Lindstedt G, Nilsson O. Expression of cholecystokinin-B/gastrin receptors in medullary thyroid cancer. Eur J Surg 1999; 165:628–631.
47. Tisell LE, Dilley WG, Wells SA Jr. Progression of postoperative residual medullary thyroid carcinoma as monitored by plasma calcitonin levels. Surgery 1996; 119:34–39.
48. Tisell LE, Ahlman H, Wängberg B, Hansson G, Mölne J, Nilsson O, Lindstedt G, Fjälling M, Forssell-Aronsson E. Somatostatin receptor scintigraphy in medullary thyroid carcinoma. Br J Surg 1997; 84:543–547.
49. Lips CJM, Leo JR, Berends MJH, Minder WH, Blok APR, Geerdink RA, Hackeng WHL, Roelofs JMM, Vasen HFA, Vette JK. Thyroid C-cell hyperplasia and micronodules in close relatives of MEN-2A patients: Pitfalls in early diagnosis and reevaluation of criteria for surgery. Henry Ford Hosp J Med 1987; 35:133–138.
50. Landsvater RM, Rombouts AGM, Meerman GJ, Schillhorn-van Veen JMJ, Berends MJH, Geerdink RA, Struyvenberg A, Buys C, Lips CJM. The clinical implication of a positive calcitonin test for C-cell hyperplasia in genetically unaffected members of an MEN 2A kindred. Am J Hum Genet 1993; 52:335–342.
51. Weber TH, Käpyaho KI, Tanner P. Endogenous interference in immunoassays in clinical chemistry. A review. Scand J Clin Lab Invest 1990; 50:77–82.
52. Hein MD, Monchik JM, Jackson IMD. Pentagastrin stimulation of calcitonin in pheochromocytoma does not always indicate multiple endocrine neoplasia type II. J Endocrinol Invest 1989; 12:265–267.
53. McLeod MK, Vinik AI. Calcitonin immunoreactivity and hypercalcitoninemia in two patients with sporadic, nonfamilial, gastroenteropancreatic neuroendocrine tumors. Surgery 1992; 111:484–488.
54. Raue F, Kotzerke J, Reinwein D, Schröder S, Röher HD, Deckart H, Höfer R, Ritter M, Seif F, Buhr H, et al. Prognostic factors in medullary thyroid carcinoma: evaluation of 741 patients from the German Medullary Thyroid Carcinoma Register. Clin Invest 1993; 71:7–12.
55. Vasen HFA, van der Feltz M, Raue F, Kruseman AN, Koppeschaar HPF, Pieters G, Seif FJ, Blum WF, Lips CJM. The natural course of multiple endocrine neoplasia type IIb. A study of 18 cases. Arch Intern Med 1992; 152:1250–1252.
56. Sizemore GW, Carney JA, Gharib H, Capen CC. Multiple endocrine neoplasia Type 2B: Eighteen-year follow-up of a four-generation family. Henry Ford Hosp Med J 1992; 40:236–244.
57. Bergholm U, Adami HO, Auer G, Bergström R, Bäckdal M, Grimelius L, Hansson G, Ljungberg O, Wilander E. Histopathologic characteristics and nuclear DNA content as prognostic factors in medullary thyroid carcinoma. Cancer 1989; 64:135–142.
58. Keusch G, Binswanger U, Dambacher MA, Fischer JA. Ectopic ACTH syndrome and medullary thyroid carcinoma. Acta Endocrinol (Copenh) 1977; 86:306–316.
59. Moley JF, Wells SA, Dilley WG, Tisell LE. Reoperation for recurrent or persistent medullary thyroid cancer. Surgery 1993; 114:1090–1096.
60. Ahlman H, Tisell L-E. The use of a long-acting somatostatin analogue in the treatment of advanced endocrine malignancies with gastrointestinal symptoms. Scand J Gastroenterol 1987; 22:938–942.
61. Smid WM, Dullaart RPF. Octreotide for medullary thyroid carcinoma associated diarrhoea. Neth J Med 1992; 40:240–243.

62. Mahler C, Verhelst J, de Longueville M, Harris A. Long-term treatment of metastatic medullary thyroid carcinoma with the somatostatin analogue octreotide. Clin Endocrinol 1990; 33:261–269.
63. Söderström N, Telenius-Berg M, Åkerman M. Diagnosis of medullary carcinoma of the thyroid by fine needle aspiration biopsy. Acta Med Scand 1975; 197: 71–76.
64. Tisell LE, Hansson G, Jansson S. Surgical treatment of medullary carcinoma of the thyroid. Horm Metab Res Suppl 1989; 21:29–31.
65. Ponder BAJ, Finer N, Coffey R, Harmer CL, Maisey M, Ormerod MG, Pembrey ME, Ponder MA, Rosswick P, Chalet S. Family screening in medullary thyroid carcinoma presenting without a family history. Q J Med 1988; 252:299–308.
66. Carlson KM, Bracamontes J, Jackson CE, Clark R, Lacroix A, Wells SA Jr, Goodfellow PJ. Parent-of-origin effects in multiple endocrine neoplasia type 2 B. Am J Hum Genet 1994; 55:1076–1082.
67. Samaan NA, Draznin MB, Halpin RE, Bloss RS, Hawkins E, Lewis RA. Multiple endocrine syndrome type IIb in early childhood. Cancer 1991; 68:1832–1834.
68. Tung WS, Vesely TM, Moley JF. Laparoscopic detection of hepatic metastases in patients with residual and recurrent medullary thyroid cancer. Surgery 1995; 118:1024–1029.
69. Tisell LE, Hansson G, Jansson S, Salander H. Reoperation in the treatment of asymptomatic metastasizing medullary thyroid carcinoma. Surgery 1986; 99:60–66.
70. Gimm O, Ukkat J, Dralle H. Determinative factors of biochemical cure after primary and reoperative surgery for sporadic medullary thyroid carcinoma. World J Surg 1998; 22:562–568.
71. Moley JF, Debenedetti MK, Dilley WG, Tisell LE, Wells SA. Surgical management of patients with persistent or recurrent medullary thyroid cancer. J Intern Med 1998; 243:521–526.
72. Samaan NA, Schultz PN, Hickey RC. Medullary thyroid carcinoma: prognosis of familial vs. nonfamilial disease and the role of radiotherapy. Horm Metab Res Suppl 1989; 21:21–25.
73. Simpson WJ. Radioiodine and radiotherapy in the management of thyroid cancers. Otolaryngol Clin North Am 1990; 23:509–521.
74. Scherubl H, Raue F, Ziegler R. Combination chemotherapy of advanced medullary and differentiated thyroid cancer. Phase II study. J Cancer Res Clin Oncol 1990; 116:21–23.
75. Wu LT, Averbuch SD, Ball DW, de Bustros A, Baylin SB, McGuire WP III. Treatment of advanced medullary thyroid carcinoma with a combination of cyclophosphamide, vincristin, and dacarbazine. Cancer 1994; 73:432–436.
76. Schlumberger M, Abdelmoumene N, Delisle MJ, Coucette JE. Treatment of advanced medullary thyroid cancer with an alternating combination of 5-FU-streptozotocin and U-darcarbazine. Br J Cancer 1995; 71:363–365.
77. Juweid M, Sharkey RM, Behr T, Swayne LC, Herskovic T, Pereira M, Rubin AD, Hanley D, Dunn R. Radioimmunotherapy of medullary thyroid cancer with ^{131}I-labelled anti-CEA antibodies. J Nucl Med 1996; 37:905–911.
78. Forssell-Aronsson EB, Nilsson O, Benjegård SA, Kölby L, Bernhardt P, Mölne J, Hashemi SH, Wängberg B, Tisell LE, Ahlman H. 111-In-DTPA-D-Phe1-octreotide binding and somatostatin receptor subtypes in thyroid tumors. J Nucl Med 2000; 41:636–642.
79. Lupoli G, Cascome E, Arlotta F, Vitale G, Celentano L, Salvatore M, Lombardi G. Treatment of advanced medullary thyroid carcinoma with a combination of recombinant interferon α-2B and octreotide. Cancer 2000; 78:1114–1118.

13

Management of Papillary and Follicular Thyroid Cancer

Ernest L. Mazzaferri

The Ohio State University, Columbus, Ohio, and University of Florida, Gainesville, Florida, U.S.A.

1 INTRODUCTION

Papillary and follicular thyroid cancer, together termed differentiated thyroid cancer (DTC), is usually curable when it is discovered at an early stage and is treated appropriately. Derived from follicular epithelial cells that normally trap iodine and secrete thyroid hormone, these tumors usually have receptors for and grow in response to thyrotropin (TSH). They are the only malignant tumors that respond to a combination of thyroid surgery, radioiodine (^{131}I), and thyroxine (T4) suppression of TSH and that synthesize and secrete thyroglobulin (Tg), a senistive marker that is elevated by small amounts of tumor. Indeed, in the absence of normal thyroid tissue, early detection of persistent tumor is made possible by an elevation of the serum Tg level. Papillary cancer comprises the majority of thyroid malignancies (90%) and has the best 10-year relative survival rate (93%), responding better to treatment than other thyroid tumors. Nonetheless, it accounts for over half the deaths from thyroid cancer (Table 1) (1), killing more patients than all other forms of thyroid cancer.

Multiple factors affect the long-term prognosis of DTC (2), but it is mainly determined by interactions between the patient and the tumor—intrinsic constants in the prognostic equation that cannot be modified—and by therapy and follow-up paradigms, which in the final analysis stand as the only modifiable variables that have an impact upon outcome. Appropriate treatment applied early can completely eradicate the tumor in most cases. This is the main goal of therapy.

Management of DTC poses some problems because there have been no prospective randomized trials of therapy and none are likely to be done, given its typically prolonged course and relative infrequency. Instead, clinicians rely on large patient cohort studies in which therapy has not been randomized, resulting in some debate about management. Nonetheless, mortality rates of thyroid cancer fell significantly in the United States between 1973 and 1996 (20%; $p < 0.05$) (3), almost certainly as a result of early diagnosis and effective treatment of DTC. This decline in mortality, however, occurred only in women (3), perhaps because they seek medical attention earlier than men, whose tumors are typically discovered about three decades later in life than they are in women, when tumors are at a more advanced stage (3).

Much of the following discussion refers to treatment of DTC because the management of papillary and follicular thyroid cancer is similar (2). Two general approaches to management of DTC have been promoted. Although both use surgery and T4 suppression of TSH, they are otherwise quite different. One simply relies upon resection of the primary tumor by hemithyroidectomy, with no use of sensitive postoperative testing because the tumor is considered so indolent as to pose no threat to survival. The other and more common approach, used for tumors larger than 1 cm, employs

Table 1 Incidence and 10-Year Relative Survival of 53,856 Patients with Thyroid Cancer

Type of thyroid cancer (N)	Number	Incidence (%)	10-year relative survival (%)	Proportion of all cancer deaths (%)
Papillary	42,686	80	93	53
Follicular	6,764	11	85	16
Hürthle	1,585	3	76	7
Medullary	1,928	4	75	10
Anaplastic	893	2	14	14

Source: Ref. 1.

total thyroidectomy and ^{131}I ablation and sensitive follow-up tests to identify persistent tumor.

2 MEASURING OUTCOME

Analyzing outcome only in terms of cancer death gives an incomplete picture because fatality rates from DTC are low (Table 1) while recurrence rates are high, often resulting in persistent disease that cannot be eradicated. At 45-year follow-up, the cancer death rate in our patients was only about 8%, whereas the recurrence rate was 47% (Fig. 1) (2). Most of the adverse outcomes, nearly 68% of the deaths, and 78% of the recurrences happened within the first decade after initial therapy; however, cancer deaths occurred as late as 35 years and recurrences as late as 45 years after therapy (Fig. 2A) (2). Recurrence is more common under age 20 and over age 60* (Fig. 2B) (2). Local tumor comprised 68% of the recurrences in our study (2). The other 32% were mostly in lung, which over 40 years caused half the patients with them to die (2). The 30-year cancer mortality rate was almost twice as high with recurrence in soft tissues of the neck (30%) compared with cervical lymph nodes or the contralateral thyroid (16%; $p < 0.05$).

2.1 Long-Term Impact of Tumor Recurrence

Recurrence of thyroid cancer is often regarded as a trivial event, yet it is commonly the harbinger of a bad outcome. In the latest analysis (2) of our group with DTC, most (69%) of the cancer deaths occurred among a subgroup of 359 patients with recurrent tumor, while the remaining deaths occurred among the 2% with known persistent disease after surgery. About 15% of patients with recurrent cancer died of disease. However, serum Tg measurements were not available during the early years of this study, and many patients thought to have a recurrence undoubtedly had unrecognized persistent tumor after surgery that would now be promptly recognized with TSH-stimulated serum Tg measurements. Regional lymph node recurrence alone was found in 130 (8.5%) of our patients, and among this group 18 patients (14%) eventually died of cancer. This presentation represented 36% of the recurrences (2) and 23% of the cancer deaths. The median age of those who died was 49.5 years (range 16–75 yr); 11% (2/18) were under age 30 years, and 89% (16/18) were over 30 years. Another study (4) of 58 patients with lymph node recurrence found that the 10-year relative survival was almost 99% for patients under age 45 years but only 43% for older patients ($p = 0.0014$); multivariate analysis showed that lymph node recurrence had an independent and highly significant negative effect on survival ($p < 0.001$) in patients over age 45 years. Three (5.5%) of 55 patients in our study (2) with recurrence in the contralateral thyroid lobe, with or without regional lymph node metastases, died of cancer. Their median age was 42 years (range 39–58 yr). Seven of 13 patients (54%) in our study with muscle or aerodigestive recurrences died of thyroid cancer; their

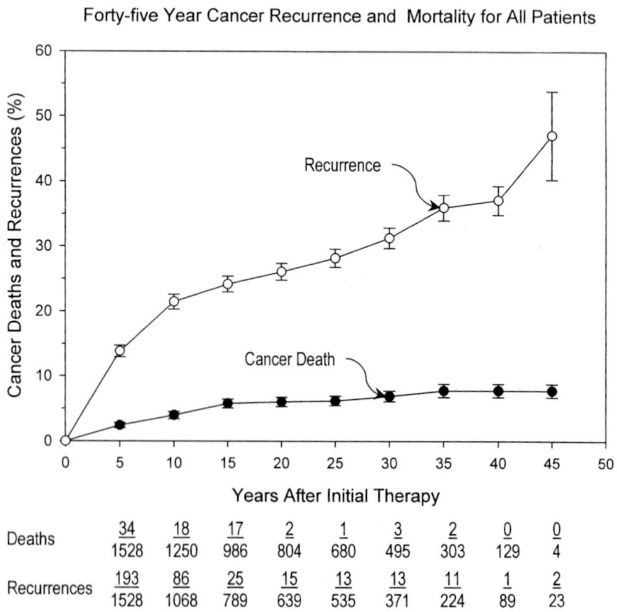

Figure 1 Forty-five year tumor recurrence and mortality rates in a cohort of 1528 patients after a median follow-up of 16.6 years. Here and elsewhere the data are from a cohort of patients published in 1994 (6) and updated in 2001 (2).

*Here and elsewhere, age refers to patient age at the time of initial therapy.

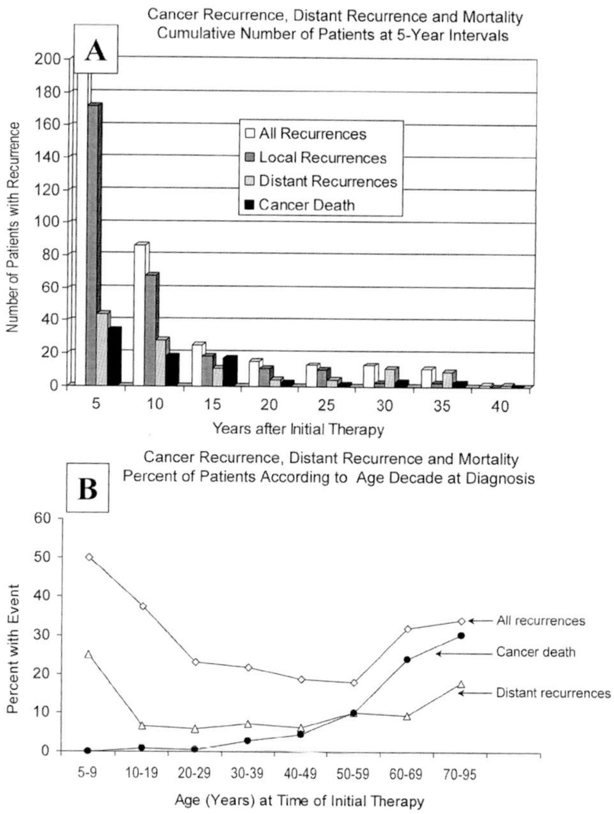

Figure 2 Tumor recurrence rates in 1,528 patients after a median of 16.6 years of follow-up. There were 359 recurrences (23.5% of patients). Local recurrence ($n = 272$, 17.8%) is cervical or mediastinal; distant recurrence ($n = 114$, 7.5%) is sites outside the neck. (A) Number of patients with recurrences at 5-year intervals. (B) 40-year recurrence, distant recurrence, and cancer death rates stratified by age at the time of initial therapy. Patients ($n = 27$) with both local and distant recurrences are shown as distant recurrence. (Modified from Ref. 2.)

median age was 55 years (range 39–72 yr). Among our 114 patients with recurrences in the lung or other distant sites, 34 (30%) have died of cancer and others are likely to do so in the future. The median age of those with distant metastases who died of cancer was 53.5 years (range 21–75 yr) compared with a median age of 35 years (range 7–91 yr; $p = 0.0001$) for patients with distant metastases who did not die of thyroid cancer.

3 FACTORS INFLUENCING CHOICE OF THERAPY

It is important to understand how risk factors affect outcome because it is here that most clinicians disagree, recommending therapy and follow-up according to their view of risk. Some prognostic features indicate how aggressively DTC might grow or respond to treatment, setting the stage for long-term prognosis (Table 2) (5). The first group comprises patient characteristics—mainly age, gender, and genetic features (6). The second group of variables comprises gross and histological features of the tumor (Table 2) (5,7). The third set of independent prognostic variables relates to treatment (Table 3).

3.1 Patient Variables

3.1.1 Age

Age over 40 years is a powerful independent prognosticator of death from thyroid cancer, with fatality rates rising increasingly thereafter (Fig. 2B) (6,8). The lowest morality rates are in children and young adults, except under the age of 10 years, when they are higher (9–11). Paradoxically, children have tumors of more advanced stage at the time of diagnosis, with more local and distant metastases and higher recurrence rates (40%) than those in middle-aged adults (20%) (Fig. 2B) (9,11–13). Over 20% of children develop pulmonary metastases during the course of their disease (6,8,12).

3.1.2 Gender

The incidence of DTC in men is about half that in women, but their cancer death rates are twice those of women (Table 2) (3,6). At the time of diagnosis, men are about three decades older than women and have twice the frequency of distant metastases and about 30% more local metastases than do women (3).

3.1.3 Family History of Papillary Thyroid Cancer

About 5% of papillary cancers are inherited as an autosomal dominant trait, although the responsible gene(s) has not been identified. They are more aggressive cancers with a less favorable prognosis than sporadic papillary cancer (14,15) unless they occur with certain heritable syndromes such as familial adenomatous polyposis (Gardner's syndrome) (16), Cowden disease (17, 18), or Carney complex (19). Papillary cancer in these syndromes occurs at a young age, is bilateral and multicentric, and has an excellent prognosis (20). Early diagnosis of thyroid cancer is possible in affected kindred members.

3.2 Tumor Variables

Certain tumor and histological features have an important bearing on prognosis, particularly tumor size,

Table 2 Risk Stratification of Variables Influencing Cancer Recurrence and Cancer Death

Factors predictive of high risk	Factors predictive of moderate-to-low risk
Patient variables	
Age < 15 years or > 45 years	Age 15–45 years
Male sex	Female sex
Family history of thyroid cancer	No family history of thyroid cancer
Tumor variables	
Tumor > 4 cm in diameter	Tumor < 4 cm in diameter
Bilateral disease	Unilateral disease
Extrathyroidal extension	No extrathyroidal extension
Vascular invasion (papillary and follicular cancer)	Absence of vascular invasion
Cervical or mediastinal lymph node metastases	No lymph node metastases
Certain tumor subtypes: Hürthle cell, tall cell, columnar cell, diffuse sclerosis, insular variants	Encapsulated papillary thyroid cancer, papillary microcancer
High histological grade: marked nuclear atypia, tumor necrosis, and vascular invasion	Low histological grade: absence of nuclear atypia, tumor necrosis, and vascular invasion
Tumors or metastases that concentrate radioiodine poorly or not at all	Tumors or metastases that concentrate radioiodine well
Distant metastases	No distant metastases

Source: Modified from the National Comprehensive Cancer Network Guidelines for the diagnosis and treatment of thyroid cancer (5,6).

invasion of the thyroid capsule, vascular invasion, and histology.

3.2.1 Genetic Aspects of the Tumor

Several oncogenes are found in DTC, but the most frequent are a group of somatic rearrangements of the RET proto-oncogene (21,22). Found in 40–60% of cases, these oncogenes are primary causal events in the development of both naturally occurring and radiation-induced papillary cancer (23–26) and are found in many of the tumors from the children of Chernobyl (27), especially RET/PTC3. A comprehensive study (23), however, found that RET rearrangements were not restricted to malignant or radiation-induced tumors. Earlier studies had suggested that RET/PTC rearrangements might predict prognosis, but no significant correlation was found in this study between RET/PTC and clinical features or stage of the tumor (23). Others (28) also have found RET/PTC in benign Hürthle cell tumors. Nonetheless, its presence in microscopic papillary tumors in humans (29) and laboratory animals (23) supports an early role for RET/PTC in papillary carcinogenesis without a tight link to disease progression. Because RET expression is not strictly limited to papillary cancer and has no clear effect on outcome, it has little use as a diagnostic or prognostic marker (30).

3.2.2 Tumor Size

An isolated primary tumor smaller than about 1.0 cm in diameter, a microcarcinoma, rarely recurs or causes death (8). Such tumors often have a stellate appearance, and when found by serendipity pose no risk; however, multiple, invasive, and metastatic microscopic tumors have a less favorable outcome (31). There is a direct relationship between tumor size and outcome that independently predicts the risk of recurrence (Fig. 3A), distant metastases, and death (Fig. 3B) from papillary and follicular cancer (Table 3) (2,6). Tumor stratified as 1.5 cm, 1.5–4.4 cm, and $\geq$4.5 cm caused distant metastases, respectively, in 4, 10, and 17% of our patients and 30-year cancer-specific mortality rates, respectively, of 0.5, 8, and 22% (6). A tumor larger than 4.0 cm portens a particularly poor outcome, whether it is of papillary (6,8), follicular (32,33), or Hürthle cell histology (34,35), and a tumor larger than 5.0 cm is highly likely to produce distant metastases (6). However, the size of a follicular or Hürthle cell tumor cannot be used to predict its benign or malignant nature and is of no value in making intraoperative decisions about the extent of thyroid resection. For example, a case-control study (36) found no significant difference in tumor size between follicular cancers (31.5 $\pm$ 1.7 mm) and adenomas (30.8 $\pm$ 1.5 mm). It is not uncommon for small follicular cancers to produce distant metastases.

Table 3 Cox Regression Model on Cancer Recurrence, Distant Metastasis Recurrence, and Death Due to Thyroid Cancer in 1501 Patients Without Distant Metastases at the Time of Initial Therapy

Variable	Hazard ratio	p-Value	95% Confidence interval
All cancer recurrence (N = 1501)			
Age[a]	1.0	0.2	0.9–1.3
Local tumor invasion	1.4	0.01	1.1–2.2
Lymph node metastases[b]	1.3	0.01	1.1–1.6
Follicular histology	0.8	0.012	0.7–0.96
Tumor size[c]	1.2	0.0001	1.1–1.3
Thyroid remnant ^{131}I ablation[d]	0.8	0.016	0.7–0.97
Therapy with ^{131}I[d]	0.5	0.0001	0.4–0.6
Surgery more than lobectomy[e]	0.7	0.0001	0.6–0.9
Distant metastasis recurrence (N = 1501)			
Age[a]	1.3	0.0001	1.2–1.5
Follicular histology	1.0	0.864	.8–1.2
Lymph node metastases[b]	1.6	0.002	1.2–2.2
Local tumor invasion	1.6	0.927	0.9–2.7
Tumor size[c]	1.2	0.001	1.1–1.3
Thyroid remnant ^{131}I ablation[d]	0.6	0.002	0.5–0.8
Therapy with ^{131}I[d]	0.4	0.0001	0.2–0.6
Surgery more than lobectomy[e]	0.8	0.379	0.6–1.2
Cancer mortality (N = 1501)			
Age[a]	9.5	0.0001	5.3–17.1
Time to treatment[f]	2.4	0.0001	1.5–4.0
Follicular histology	1.4	0.003	1.1–1.8
Lymph node metastases[b]	2.0	0.006	1.2–3.4
Tumor size[c]	1.2	0.025	1.02–1.3
Local tumor invasion	1.1	0.002	1.0–1.2
Female (vs. male)	0.6	0.046	0.4–0.99
Thyroid remnant ^{131}I ablation[d]	0.5	0.0001	0.4–0.7
Surgery more than lobectomy[e]	0.5	0.0001	0.4–0.7
Therapy with ^{131}I[d]	0.4	0.010	0.2–0.8

[a] Age stratified as 40 years vs. ≥40 for cancer mortality, and by decade for recurrences and distant recurrences.
[b] Lymph node metastases present vs. absent.
[c] Tumor diameter stratified into 1 cm increments from tumors of size 1 cm to >5 cm.
[d] Remnant ablation is the use of ^{131}I in patients with uptake only in the thyroid bed and no evidence of residual tumor; therapy with ^{131}I is postoperative treatment of patients with known residual disease.
[e] Bilateral thyroid surgery vs. lobectomy with or without isthmusectomy.
[f] Time to treatment ≤12 months vs. >12 months.
Source: Ref. 2.

3.2.3 Papillary Microcarcinoma

Histologically malignant, solitary microscopic papillary cancers are clinically benign when they are found by serendipity in specimens obtained during surgery for benign thyroid disease (37,38) and require no further therapy. The recurrence and mortality rates of such papillary microcancers are near zero (31,39). However, this tumor must be distinguished from the 20% that are microscopic multifocal tumors that metastasize to cervical lymph nodes in as many as 60% of the cases (31,40,41). This is a distinctly different entity than tumor discovered by serendipity. Extracapsular lymph node invasion, which is particularly poor prognostic sign, may occur in patients with thyroid microcarcinoma, which may lead to distant metastases and death, even without undifferentiation of the tumor (31,42). Aggressive microcarcinomas that occur in a familial setting (14) are multifocal bilateral tumors with vascular invasion, capable of causing

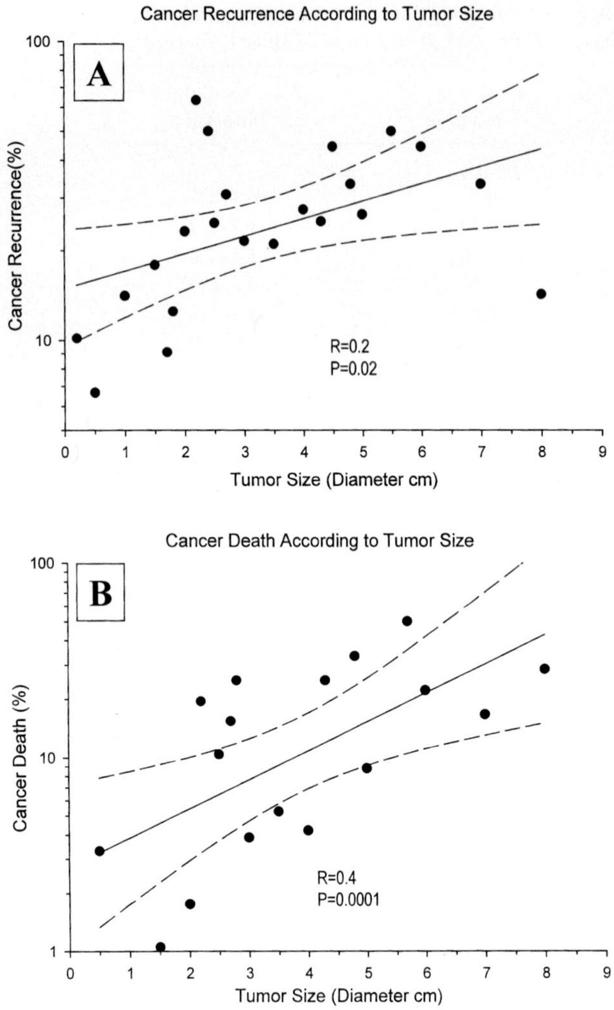

Figure 3 Tumor size correlates with (A) cancer recurrence and (B) cancer-specific mortality. (Updated from Ref. 6.)

recurrence, pulmonary metastases, and death. More aggressive treatment and careful follow-up are required in such cases.

3.2.4 Tumor Invasion of the Thyroid Capsule or Tumor Capsule

Tumor invading the neck is the second most common cause of death from DTC, the first being lung metastases. Eight percent of papillary and 12% of follicular cancers breached the thyroid capsule in our patients (6), which was an independent predictor of recurrence and mortality (Table 3) (2). Up to one third of papillary cancers microscopically penetrate the thyroid capsule (6,43). Gross invasion typically causes death within a few years of its discovery. It commonly involves neck muscles and vessels, recurrent laryngeal nerves, larynx, pharynx, and esophagus, and may extend into the spinal cord and brachial plexus. Invasive tumors have recurrence rates that are twice as high and mortality rates that are nearly 10-fold higher during the first 10 years than those among patients without this feature (Fig. 4) (6,8,44,45).

3.2.5 Tumor Multicentricity

Multiple microscopic intraglandular tumors occur in about 20% of patients with papillary thyroid cancer when the thyroid is examined routinely and in up to 80% if it is examined with great care (46). Long held to be intrathyroidal metastases, evidence now shows that they arise independently in a background of tissue that is environmentally or genetically susceptible, producing tumors with different RET/PTC arrangements in the same gland (29). The implication is that residual thyroid tissue remaining after initial therapy is highly susceptible to developing new tumor.

Although its prognostic importance is debated, microscopic tumor multicentricity—a finding that is not apparent until the final histological sections have been studied—has a bearing upon prognosis and the decision to forgo contralateral thyroid lobe resection and remnant ablation (31). It is impossible to predict the presence of bilateral tumor preoperatively because its rate

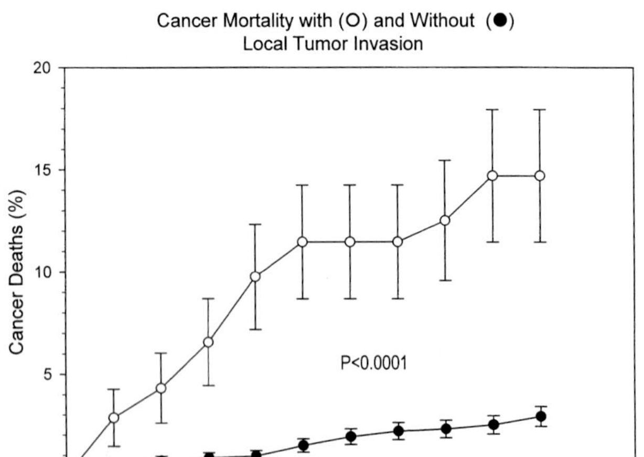

Figure 4 Cancer deaths according to the presence or absence of local tumor invasion. There are 77 cancer-specific deaths in this analysis. (Updated from Ref. 6.)

is the same with low- and high-risk tumors* (47,48). Multifocal disease in one thyroid lobe is almost always associated with contralateral tumor (43,47,49–57) and has rates of nodal and distant metastases and a likelihood of developing persistent disease that are two to three times higher than with single tumors (6,57,58). These data provide strong evidence that multiple intrathyroidal tumors are common with both papillary and follicular thyroid cancer and that their presence is unpredictable and prognostically unfavorable, leading to higher rates of tumor persistence and cancer mortality.

3.2.6 Papillary Histology

This is typically an unencapsulated, invasive tumor with ill-defined margins (8), but about 10% are fully encapsulated and associated with an especially good prognosis (59). The tumor may develop hemorrhagic necrosis, making it soft to palpation and yielding a thick brownish fluid on fine needle aspiration (FNA) that may be mistaken for a benign cyst (60). Most have a typical architectural appearance with complex branching papillae and a fibrovascular core covered by a single layer of tumor cells intermingled with follicular structures, although some have a pure follicular or trabecular appearance (61). The term "mixed papillary-follicular cancer" has no clinical value because the follicular component does not alter ^{131}I uptake or prognosis (62). Nuclear features are more important than the architectural appearance in establishing a diagnosis of papillary cancer. Tumors with a pure follicular pattern but typical cellular features of papillary cancer are termed follicular variant papillary cancer, which some pathologists argue comprise most of the cancers diagnosed as follicular cancer (63). The distinctive cellular features of papillary cancer permit its diagnosis by FNA histology (64). Intrathyroidal vascular invasion, which has long been recognized as an important feature predicting poor survival with follicular and Hürthle cell cancer, is also prognostically important in papillary cancer (7). One study (65) found that it was more likely to be associated with distant metastasis at the time of diagnosis (26.1% vs. 2.2%; $p = 0.001$) and to cause distant recurrence (20% vs. 3%; $p = 0.002$) than tumors without vascular invasion and that extrathyroidal vascular invasion was associated with an even higher incidence of distant metastases at the time of diagnosis (40%).

Subclassification of Papillary Histology. Histological subclassifications have a bearing upon prognosis (Table 2). One study found that 55% of the cases of DTC were of the usual type, whereas 27% showed complex histological features with different histological components and 18% were diagnosed as specific subtypes (7). Tall cell cancers often show tumor necrosis and vascular invasion. Tumors with solid areas also have an increased incidence of mitotic figures and vascular invasion (7). Patients with tall cell or columnar cell tumors usually have reduced survival. One multivariate analysis showed, however, that tumor size and histological grade (marked nuc- lear atypia, tumor necrosis, and vascular invasion) were prognostically more important than tumor subtype (7).

Follicular Variant Papillary Thyroid Cancer. About 10% of papillary cancers have microfollicular pattern indistinguishable from follicular cancer with nuclear features of papillary cancer on FNA cytology and histological sections (46,64). Its prognosis is reported by some to be similar to that of typical papillary cancer by others to be more unfavorable with more metastases (64,66,67).

Diffuse Follicular Variant Papillary Thyroid Cancer. This uncommon tumor may be confused with multinodular goiter or macrofollicular adenoma on frozen section (67). It occurs in women with goiter, often with hyperthyroidism. Most have distant metastases with very high mortality rates (67).

Tall Cell Variant. About 10% of papillary cancers have papillae with cells that are twice as tall as they are wide and that comprise 30% or more of the tumor (67). Compared with typical papillary cancer, this tumor appears about two decades later (mid-50s), is larger and more often associated with local invasion and distant metastases that lack ^{131}I uptake, and has mortality rates up to threefold higher (17,64,67). It can be identified by FNA cytology and often expresses the p53 oncogene (17).

Columnar Cell Variant. Found mainly in men, this rare tumor is composed of rectangular cells with clear cytoplasm (67). Over 90% have metastases that are unresponsive to ^{131}I, resulting in death in most patients (64,67). Encapsulated tumors have a better prognosis (59).

*In this study (47) low risk was defined as tumor confined to the thyroid gland, age less than 45 years, tumor smaller than 2 cm, and no lymph nodes, and high risk as age over 45 years, tumor 2 cm or larger, or positive lymph nodes.

Diffuse Sclerosing Variant. About 5% of spontaneously occurring papillary cancers and about 10% of tumors among the children of Chernobyl are of this type (64,67,68). It usually presents as a goiter with extensive squamous metaplasia, sclerosis, psammoma bodies, and abundant lymphatic invasion involving the entire thyroid. Metastases to cervical nodes occur in almost all patients and to lung in about 25% of patients (64,67). FNA cytology shows squamous metaplasia, inflammatory cells, and psammoma bodies, but may be mistaken for thyroiditis. Although local and pulmonary metastases are more frequent than usual, there is some disagreement about whether its long-term prognosis is worse than that of typical papillary thyroid cancer (64,67).

Solid or Trabecular Variant. This tumor has a predominantly (>75%) solid architectural pattern but maintains the typical nuclear features of papillary thyroid cancer. It has a tendency for extrathyroidal spread and lung metastases that impart a poor prognosis (64,67), but some find it more common in children in whom its prognosis is the same as that of typical papillary thyroid cancer (69).

Oxyphilic (Hürthle Cell) Papillary Variant. About 2% of papillary thyroid cancers have Hürthle cell (oxyphilic) features (70). Some have a familial occurrence and are multicentric (71). It cannot be identified as papillary cancer by FNA but is recognize by its papillary architecture on the histological sections. Compared with typical papillary cancer, it has higher recurrence and mortality rates (64,70).

3.2.7 Follicular Histology

Usually a solitary encapsulated tumor with a microfollicular histological pattern, its malignant nature is identified by capsular and vascular invasion by tumor, but this applies only to vessels in or beyond the tumor capsule, since tumor in capillaries within the tumor has no diagnostic or prognostic importance (72). Highly invasive tumors extend into surrounding tissues, causing metastases in 80% of patients and producing high mortality rates (73). Most, however, are encapsulated, minimally invasive cancers that closely resemble follicular adenomas. FNA is often not diagnostic, showing normal or atypical follicular cells with little or no colloid that is reported as indeterminate or as a follicular neoplasm, requiring surgery to establish the diagnosis (5). The distinction between follicular adenoma and cancer usually is made only on the permanent histological sections of 10 or more samples of the tumor periphery and not by frozen section study (72).

Vascular invasion has a worse prognosis than capsular invasion alone (74), and minimally invasive tumors almost neer metastasize or cause death (33,43,73), although there is disagreement about the diagnostic criteria for this tumor. LiVolsi (72) indicates that for this diagnosis the minimum criteria are invasion of the capsule, invasion through the capsule, and invasion into veins in or beyond the capsule. Others (75) base the diagnosis on small-to-medium vessel invasion or capsular invasion up to full thickness, without parenchymal tumor extension or necrosis; however, patients meeting these criteria developed recurrent disease, and one died with disease. Thus, diagnostic uncertainty often exists that may require multiple opinions to resolve, which poses a serious management predicament at the time of initial surgery (76,77).

3.2.8 Hürthle Cell Histology

Although often considered variants of follicular cancer (78,79), a malignant tumor consisting mainly (75% or more) of Hürthle (oncocytic) cells is usually classified as Hürthle cell cancer (80), the diagnostic criteria for which are identical to those of follicular cancer except for its cellular features (72). A subset exhibits RET/PTC rearrangements, supporting classification of Hürthle cell tumors into three groups: Hürthle adenomas, Hürthle cancers, and Hürthle cell papillary thyroid cancers (28). Because Hürthle cell cancers comprise only about 3% of thyroid cancers (Table 1), relatively few large series have been reported to provide guidance about therapy (70,79,81–89). Some consider them to be aggressive and unpredictable tumors with mortality rates as high as 25% (90), whereas others find them no more aggressive than similarly staged follicular cancers (79,89). However, most data support the latter view. Large series report pulmonary metastases in 25–35% of Hürthle cell cancers, about twice the rate of follicular cancer (91,92). Ten-year relative survival was 76% for 1585 patients with Hürthle cell cancer compared with 85% for 6764 patients with follicular cancer (Table 1) (1). Hürthle cell papillary cancer, which is uncommon, has higher than usual recurrence and mortality rates (70).

Management difficulties are highlighted by reports of recurrent Hürthle cancer from tumors first classified as adenomas (83). Cytology specimens typically show clusters of Hürthle cells with no colloid and are reported as indeterminate or suspicious, which also can be seen in Hashimoto's thyroiditis. Many are minimally invasive encapsulated Hürthle cell cancers that closely resemble Hürthle cell adenomas (76). One large study (82) categorized Hürthle cell tumors into three groups: tumors of uncertain malignant or benign status with partial tumor capsular invasion but no vascular invasion, minimally invasive cancers with a single focus of complete capsular invasion or vascular invasion or both, and widely invasive cancers with more than one focus of complete capsular or vascular invasion or both. After a median follow-up of 8 years only those with widely invasive cancers had local recurrences (73%), metastases (64%), or died of cancer (54%). The median size of invasive tumors was 4.5 cm, compared with 3.0 cm in the others. Factors associated with a poor survival were extrathyroidal extension of the tumor and lymph node metastases (82).

3.2.9 Insular Thyroid Cancer

About 5% of thyroid cancers have solid clusters of cells with small follicles that resemble pancreatic islet cells but contain Tg. This should be considered as a separate follicular epithelial tumor rather than a variant of papillary or follicular cancer (72). It is unusually large and invasive, and compared with papillary cancer it occurs at an older age with fewer neck metastases but more distant metastases and has about a threefold higher mortality rate (17). It displays aggressive behavior in children but in young patients is usually is responsive to thyroidectomy and ^{131}I therapy (93).

3.2.10 Thyroglossal Duct Tumors

Tyroglossal duct cysts are common in children but also are estimated to occur in about 7% of adults (94). Found anywhere from the base of the tongue to the manubrium, they are usually in the midline superior to the thyroid or less frequently in the lateral anterior neck (95) or rarely within the thyroid gland itself (96,97). About 1% are complicated by malignancy (98), usually in adults (99). Only about 150 cases have been reported (100), but 90% are papillary cancers and the rest are Hürthle cell, squamous, follicular, insular, epidermoid, or anaplastic thyroid cancers (98,101). When the thyroid gland is also resected, about 10% contain malignant foci, indicating that some thyroglossal tumors are metastases from the thyroid (98). Malignant tumors are almost always small and confined to the thyroglossal cyst, with clinical characteristic of a small incidental microcarcinoma. Nonetheless, a few are large and invasive (102,103) or metastatic to regional lymph nodes (101,104,105), and at least one has been reported in a 44-year old woman with a thyroglossal papillary thyroid cancer who developed metastases and died of disease despite having undergone a Sistrunk operation, local excision of a recurrence, and thyroidectomy, although her thyroid showed no histological foci of cancer (106).

Malignancy should be suspected when the thyroglossal cyst is hard, fixed, or associated with cervical lymph node enlargement. Neck CT, MRI, or ultrasonography may show a small mass within the wall of a cyst, a solid mass in the course of a thyroglossal duct, or a complex invasive midline neck mass, or calcification in a thyroglossal papillary thyroid cancer or metastatic node (102). The diagnosis can be made with FNA; however, diagnostic difficulties are common despite the well defined criteria for identifying papillary cancer within a thyroglossal cyst (94). In one review (94) of 17 cases of in which an FNA diagnosis of thyroglossal cyst papillary cancer had been made, the true-positive rate was 53% and the false-negative rate was 47%. In many false-negative cases fluid was simply aspirated without further study.

3.2.11 Regional Metastases

In one review (8) lymph node metastases were reported in 36% of 8029 adults with papillary cancer and in 17% of 1540 patients with follicular cancer, although some were likely follicular variant papillary cancers. Nodal metastases occur in up to 80% of children with papillary cancer (9,13,107). A palpable cervical lymph node, often the first sign of malignancy, is usually associated with multiple nodal metastases at surgery (108).

The prognostic importance of regional lymph node metastases is debated. Some find they have no impact on recurrence or survival (32,109–112), whereas many others find nodal metastases are a risk for tumor recurrence and cancer-specific mortality and that they correlate well distant metastases, especially if they are bilateral cervical or metastases or if tumor invades the lymph node capsule (6,41,113–119). One study found that 15% of patients with and none without cervical node metastases died of disease (120). Another study of patients with distant metastases from papillary cancer found that 80% had mediastinal node metastases when cancer was first diagnosed (121). Patients with DTC in our study who had cervical or mediastinal lymph node metastases had higher 30-year cancer mortality rates than those without them (10% vs. 6%; $p < 0.01$) (6). Nodal metastases were an independent and significant variable predicting tumor recurrence, distant recurrence, and cancer-specific mortality (Table 3) (6).

3.2.12 Distant Metastases

Distant metastases are the main cause of death from DTC. Almost 10% of papillary cancers and 25% of follicular cancers cause distant metastases, half of which are present when the cancer is diagnosed (8). They occur most often with Hürthle cell cancer (35%) and after age 40 (92,122). Among 1231 patients in 13 studies, the metastatic sites were lung (49%), bone (25%), or both (15%), and central nervous system or other soft tissues (10%) (8). Bone metastases are more common after age 45 and are usually multicentric (123). The causes of cancer death in one study (124) were respiratory insufficiency from lung metastasis (43%), massive hemorrhage (15%), airway obstruction (13%) by tumor, and circulatory failure (15%) and from compression of the vena cava by mediastinal or sternal metastases. In our study, 27% of the distant metastases were found at the time of initial diagnosis of cancer, and 73% were detected 1 to 48 years later (6).

Although some patients with distant metastases survive for decades, especially younger patients, about half die within 5 years regardless of tumor histology (8). A patient's age, metastatic sites, and whether the tumor concentrates ^{131}I influence outcome (92,122,125–127). In one study (128) survival rates with distant metastases were 53% at 5 years, 38% at 10 years, and 30% at 15 years but were longest in young patients with lung metastases (128). In another study (129) half the patients were alive at 10 years when distant metastases were confined to the lung. Finding lung metastases at an early stage is associated with an even longer survival (130). Tumor bulk is second only to patient age as a predictor of death (131). Large tumors tend not to concentrate ^{131}I. For example, one study (131) found that tumor concentrated ^{131}I in 95% of patients with lung metastases associated with a normal chest x-ray, in 88% of patients with micronodular disease seen on x-ray, and in 37% with macronodular disease (131). Survival is best when diffuse lung metastases are seen only on a post–^{131}I imaging, especially if seen only on a post-^{131}I treatment whole-body scan (RxWBS) (125,126,128,132). Survival with small (< 1 cm) lung metastases is intermediate when they are seen chest x-ray and concentrate ^{131}I and is worst when they are larger and do not concentrate ^{131}I (92,122,125). One study (131) found that complete responses to treatment occurred in 82% of patients with pulmonary or bone metastases with a normal radiograph compared with only 15% with an abnormal radiograph. Together these observations provide a strong argument for early detection and treatment of metastases.

4 CURRENT TRENDS AND OTHER IMPORTANT FACTORS RELATED TO SELECTION AND TIMING OF THERAPY

4.1 Delay in Therapy

There is wide agreement that FNA should be the first test to do in a euthyroid patient with a thyroid nodule (5); however, it was not done in about 40% of 5584 thyroid cancer cases undergoing surgery in the United States (133) during 1996 and was obtained in only 27.4% of 2537 patients treated in Germany (134). Surveys of North American endocrinologists, however, show that they regularly perform FNA early and rely heavily on its results to make a decision (135), but they choose surgery when there is a strong clinical suspicion of thyroid cancer even if the FNA is negative. However, patients managed by primary care physicians and surgeons may undergo a delay in diagnosis, which in one study (136) was 12 months or longer in almost 30% of the cases, which has the potential to increase mortality rates in those with malignant thyroid nodules.

A strong correlation exists between delay in diagnosis and cancer mortality rates (Fig. 5). Median time from the first clinical manifestation of a malignant nodule to initial therapy in our study (6) was 4 months among those who survived and 18 months in patients who died of cancer ($p < 0.001$); when therapy was delayed longer

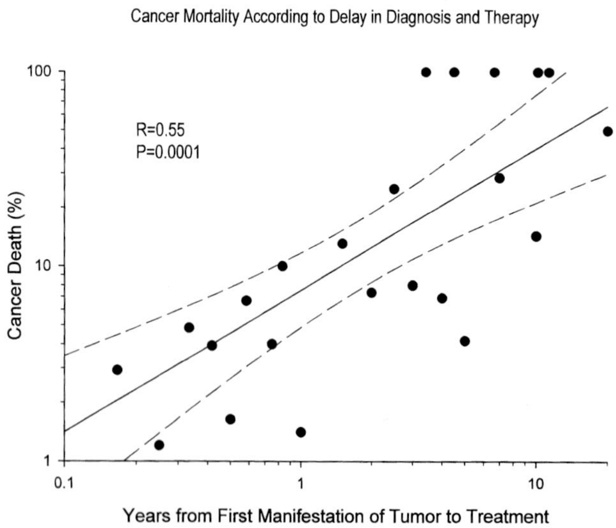

Figure 5 Cancer deaths according to time elapsed from first clinical manifestation of the tumor to initial therapy. There are 77 cancer-specific deaths in this analysis, and each data point represents 1 or more patients. (Updated from Ref. 6.)

than a year, 30-year cancer mortality rates more than doubled compared with the rates in patients without a delay in therapy (13% vs. 6%; $p < 0.001$), tumor stage was more advanced, and the incidence of distant metastases found at the time of diagnosis more than doubled. A delay longer than 12 months was an independent risk factor related to tumor recurrence, distant metastases, and survival (6). In another study (54), when completion thyroidectomy was delayed for more than 6 months, mortality rates were significantly higher than when it was done within 6 months of initial surgery.

4.2 Tumor Staging and Clinical Staging Systems

Clinical staging systems designed to assess risk of thyroid cancer mortality—mainly derived from multivariate analyses of tumor stage and age—accurately predict risk of cancer death in some patients (111,137–143). Important examples* are the EORTC (European Organization for Research on Treatment of Cancer) scheme (144), the American Joint Committee on Cancer/International Union Against Cancer (AJCC/UICC TNM) (Table 4) system, the AMES (Age-Metastasis-Extent-Size) system (145) the AGES (Age-Grade-Extent-Size) system (142), and MACIS systems (Metastasis-Age-Completeness of resection, Invasion-Size) (111). When applied to papillary cancer data, four of the schemes that use age (EORTC, TNM, AMES, AGES) clearly separated 20-year cancer mortality rates among low-risk patients (1%) and high-risk patients (30–40%) (142), reflecting low cancer mortality rates under age 40 years (Fig. 2B) (139,146). A study that classified 269 patients with papillary cancer according to five prognostic scoring schemes found that some patients in the lowest risk group for each scheme died of cancer (139). Another study (124) found that over 10% of the patients dying of DTC had a TNM classification of 1 or 2 according to the AJCC/UICC staging system (137). This is an especially serious problem when risk is simply dichotomously categorized as low or high (137). When mortality risk in 1528 of our patients (median age 34 yr) was assessed according to the AMES criteria, 45-year mortality rates of low-risk and high-risk patients were 4.8% and 33.1%, respectively ($p <$ 0.0001) (Fig. 6A). As noted by the authors (145) of this prognostic scoring system, almost all patients are low risk by AMES criteria (Fig. 6B) and the actuarial death rates are low, but as seen in our analysis the numbers of deaths in the low-risk ($n = 37$) and high-risk groups ($n = 40$) are nearly identical (Fig. 6B, lower panel).

EORTC: Age in years +12 if male, +10 if medullary, +10 if poorly differentiated follicular, +45 if anaplastic, +10 if extending beyond thyroid, +15 if one distant metastasis, +30 if multiple distant metastases. *TNM*: see Table 4. *AMES*: High risk is female > 50 years, male > 40 years, tumor > 5 cm (if older age), distant metastases, substantial extension beyond tumor capsule (follicular) or gland capsule (papillary). *AGES* is calculated from 0.5 × age in years (if >40), +1 (if grade 2), +3 (if grade 3 or 4), +1 (if extrathyroidal), +3 (if distant spread), +0.2 × maximum tumor diameter. *MACIS* is equal to 3.1 if aged ≤39 years or 0.08 x age if aged ≥40 years, +0.3 × tumor size in centimeters, +1 if incompletely resected, +1 (if locally invasive), +3 (if distant metastases present).

Table 4 AJCC/UICC TNM Staging System

Stage	Papillary or follicular < 45 years	Papillary or follicular ≥45 years	Medullary
I	M_0	T_1	T_1
II	M_1	$T_{2\text{–}3}$	$T_{2\text{–}4}$
III		T_4 or N_1	N_1
IV		M_1	M_1

T, primary tumor, T_1, < 1 cm; T_2, ≥1–4 cm; T_3, > 4 cm; T_4, extention beyond thyroid capsule; N, regional lymph nodes; N_1, regional lymph node metastases (cervical and upper mediastinal nodes); M, distant metastases; M_0, no distant metastases; M_1, distant metastases present.
Source: Ref. 137.

A second serious problem using age to assess risk is that cancer-free survival cannot be accurately predicted because young patients have high rates of cancer recurrence, often in the lung (Fig. 2B). Using AMES staging criteria, 35-year cancer recurrence rates were higher among our patients at low risk than those at high risk (56.8% vs. 35.2%; $p < 0.001$) (Fig. 6A, lower panel). There were 302 recurrences in low-risk patients and only 57 among high-risk patients (Fig. 6B, upper panel), of which 89 and 25 were distant metastases in the two groups, respectively (Fig. 6C). The AJCC/UICC staging system yields similar results for cancer deaths and recurrences; distant metastases after initial therapy, for example, occurred in 53, 29, and 21 patients stratified, respectively, as stage 1, 2, or 3 according to this classification (Fig. 6C).

Almost none of the multivariate analyses used to construct the various clinical staging systems take into account the effects of therapy, tacitly assuming that treatment does not alter outcome. This shortcoming was recognized by the authors of the original EORTC staging system for thyroid cancer (141), who stated: "Since we have ignored therapy in these analyses, we

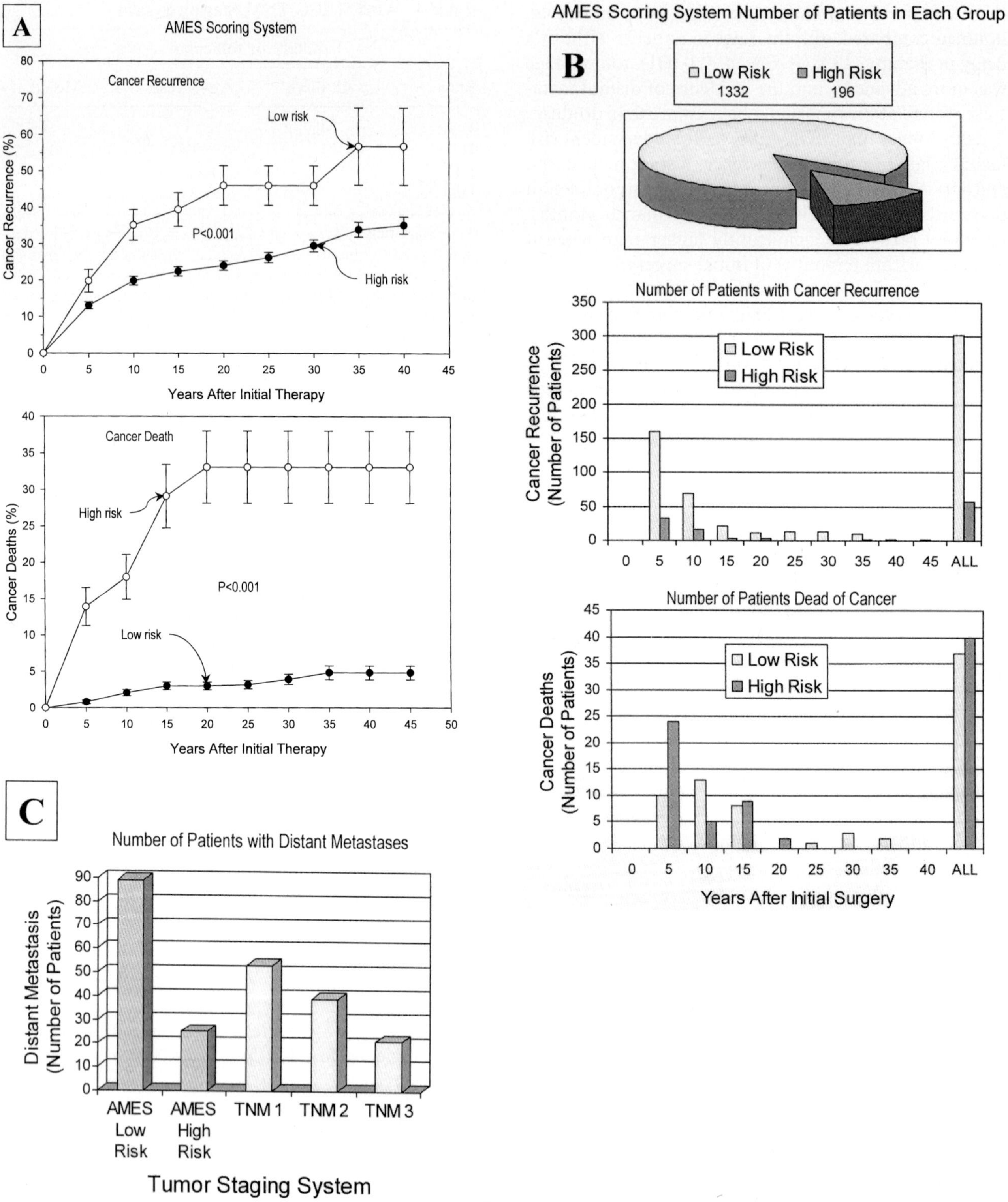

Figure 6 Outcome according to AMES Scoring System (see text) in 1528 patients reported in Ref. 6. (A) Cumulative cancer recurrence rates (upper) and cancer-specific mortality (lower). (B) Proportion of patients categorized as low risk and high risk by AMES criteria (upper panel); number of patients experiencing cancer recurrence (middle panel) and cancer death (lower panel). (C) Number of patients developing distant metastases according to AMES or AJCC/UICC (TNM) clinical staging systems.

must admit the possibility that the effects of therapy, if taken into account, might alter the importance of some prognostic factors. Technically, one is entitled to ignore therapy in studying prognostic factors only if it is known that therapy has no effect on the natural history of the disease. This is probably not the case in thyroid cancer." Subsequent authors have largely ignored this (32,111,142,143). Thus, prognostic staging schemes do not permit the surgeon to make meaningful decisions for individual patients at the time of surgery based on risk group.

4.3 Current Practice in the United States and Europe

Six studies shed light upon current practice in the United States and Europe. At an international symposium held in 1987 in The Netherlands, 160 surgeons, endocrinologists, pathologists, and nuclear medicine specialists recommended total thyroidectomy followed by postoperative ^{131}I thyroid remnant ablation for most patients with DTC, regardless of their age (147). Hemithyroidectomy alone was considered sufficient therapy only for tumors confined to one lobe if they were papillary cancers with or without ipsilateral nodal metastases or follicular cancers with minimal capsular invasion.

The second study was based upon the responses of 157 thyroid experts from around the world to a questionnaire concerning management of a patient with a solitary thyroid nodule (148). Total or near-total thyroidectomy was recommended for papillary cancer by 60% and for follicular cancer by 74% of the respondents. Most did not alter the extent of surgery according to the histological type of the tumor. Thyroid remnant ablation with ^{131}I was advised for papillary cancer by 81% and for follicular thyroid cancer by 97% of the respondents. Almost all recommended postoperative suppression of TSH with T4 and serum Tg determinations during follow-up.

The third study was based upon the responses of the clinical members of the American Thyroid Association to a questionnaire about their long-term management of a patient with papillary thyroid cancer (149). Most recommended near-total thyroidectomy and ^{131}I ablation, and almost everyone preferred long-term T4 therapy in doses sufficient to lower the TSH levels from 0.01 to 0.5 μU/mL. The majority did not alter treatment for any of the following: a history of radiation, extremes of age, nodule smaller than 1 cm, multiple tumor foci in the contralateral lobe, or nodule capsular invasion.

The fourth study reviewed 5584 cases of thyroid cancer treated in the United States during 1996 (133). The vast majority of patients presented with AJCC/UICC stage 1 or 2 tumors (72% of papillary and 70.7% of follicular cancers). Near-total or total thyroidectomy without lymph node dissection (LND) was performed in 77.4% of papillary, 68.2% of follicular, and 75% of Hürthle cell cancers. The frequency of T4 suppression of TSH and radioiodine therapy was uncertain because outpatient follow-up was incomplete. Surgeons in the United States thus choose total or near-total thyroidectomy for most patients with DTC, regardless of tumor stage.

The sixth study (134) analyzed patterns of care for 2537 patients with DTC treated in Germany during 1996. Patients were staged according to the AJCC/UICC clinical staging system. More than 50% of the patients with papillary cancer were at stage 1, and 37–39% of the follicular cancer patients were, respectively, at stages 1 and 2. The single most common procedure was near-total thyroidectomy without LND. Total or near-total thyroidectomy, with or without LND, was done for 90% of papillary and 89% of follicular cancers. Paradoxically, 2% of patients at stage 1 were treated with a lobectomy, but 23% underwent a radica neck dissection, whereas 33% at stage 4 underwent a total thyroidectomy without LND. After surgery ^{131}I was used in 80% of patients with stage 1, almost 90% with stages 2–4 papillary thyroid cancer, and in over 90% with follicular cancer, regardless of stage. External beam radiation was added to the treatment regimen for many patients diagnosed as having stage 3 or 4 (30% with papillary cancer and 33% with follicular cancer).

4.4 National Comprehensive Cancer Network Guidelines

A panel of experts from 17 National Comprehensive Cancer Network (NCCN) institutions, who first convened in 1998–1999 to discuss the diagnosis and treatment of thyroid cancer, wrote the most explicit clinical guidelines for the management this disease (5). Offered in lieu of prospective randomized trials, the guidelines reflect some disagreement about the initial management of T2N0 papillary cancers (single primary tumor 1–4 cm without regional lymph node metastases), mainly because several members (32) are strong proponents of lobectomy without ^{131}I therapy for such patients, a position held by the minority of the panelists. Nonetheless, this review must be considered when addressing a choice of surgical and medical therapy.

5 INITIAL SURGERY

Debate continues to center on the extent of thyroidectomy that is optimal, particularly for patient for patients with single primary tumors between 1 and 3 cm confined to the thyroid gland and without histological characteristics threatening a poor prognosis (113). In most cases this decision must be made preoperatively, which leaves the surgeon vulnerable to performing surgery on the basis of incomplete information about the histological characteristics of the tumor, particularly if FNA has not been performed.

5.1 Frozen Section Studies at Surgery

FNA has a high sensitivity and specificity for the diagnosis of papillary (150) but not for follicular cancer (85). Thus, total thyroidectomy can be done without frozen section (FS) when the FNA is positive for cancer (151,152). One study (152) of 240 patients who underwent surgery for nodular thyroid disease found that the test characteristics of FNA and FS were equally accurate for identifying thyroid cancer: the sensitivity of FNAB and FS was 67%, the specificity 99%, and the accuracy 89%; the positive predictive value was 96% for FNAB and 98% for FS; the negative predictive values were 88% and 87%, respectively. FNA cytology, designated as a "follicular neoplasm," is rarely resolved by FS study (153). A prospective randomized study (154) in which FS was or was not performed found that for vast majority of patients (96.4%) with follicular neoplasms, FS was neither informative nor cost-effective, nor were there significant differences in surgical times or total hospital charges; however, the cost attributable to each diagnosis FS was about $12,470. These analyses show that FS is not necessary when FNA cytology is malignant, and when the result is uncertain, routine FS should be omitted and patients should undergo completion thyroidectomy based on the final histology (152,155,156).

5.2 Subtotal Lobectomy

Resection of less than a thyroid lobe, sometimes done as a nodulectomy, is inadequate therapy for a thyroid nodule and is not the current standard of practice (64,157). Even microscopic thyroid cancer requires more surgery than subtotal lobectomy (31,37,39).

5.3 Ipsilateral Lobectomy and Isthmusectomy Versus Total

Although many surgeons perform a procedure called near-total thyroidectomy, its definition is open-ended, leaving much doubt as to the actual extent of surgery and the amount of thyroid tissue left behind. This is why the NCCN guidelines avoid this term (5). As a practical matter, a small amount of thyroid tissue almost always remains in the thyroid bed after total thyroidectomy, most commonly on the contralateral side in the tracheoesophageal grove. A thyroid remnant of 1 or 2 cm^2 (1–2 g) does not interfere with thyroid ^{131}I ablation, but larger amounts are more difficult to ablate with ^{131}I.

The debate concerning the extent of surgery centers on the importance assigned to patient age in prognosis scoring systems (see tumor staging above) (158). For example, Hay et al. (159) reported in 1987 that survival was not demonstrably improved when patients underwent more than ipsilateral lobectomy at the Mayo Clinic for low-risk papillary cancers (MACIS score $<$ 3.99) and concluded that such extensive surgery was indicated only for those with higher MACIS scores. In 1998, however, Hay et al. (160) changed this recommendation after comparing outcome with unilateral or bilateral lobectomy for low-risk papillary cancer according to the AMES criteria. Although there were no significant differences in cancer mortality or distant metastasis rates between the two surgical groups, 20-year rates for local recurrence and nodal metastasis after unilateral lobectomy were high—respectively, 14% and 19%—significantly more ($p = 0.0001$) than the 2% and 6% rates seen after bilateral thyroid lobe resection. On the basis of this study, Hay et al. concluded that bilateral thyroid resection is the preferable initial surgical approach to patients with low-risk papillary cancer. Some do not concur with this view, justifying unilateral lobectomy for nearly all patients with papillary and follicular thyroid cancer simply on the basis of the low mortality rates in patients categorized as low risk by the AMES, TNM, or other classification schemes (which is the majority of patients) and the high complication rates with more extensive thyroidectomy (32,145).

It is a bit more difficult to demonstrate that the extent of surgery influences survival with DTC, although there is considerable proof that it influences disease-free survival (139,160). Patients with primary tumors larger than 1.5 cm in our study who underwent total or near-total thyroidectomy or less surgery, respectively, had 30-year recurrence rates of 28.3.1% and 43.7%, (p = 0.003) (Fig. 7A) and 30-year cancer-specific mortality rates, respectively, of 6.6% and 13.5% ($p = 0.03$) (Fig. 7B). Multivariate analysis disclosed that the extent of surgery was an independent variable that significantly influenced tumor recurrence and cancer-specific mortality rates (Table 3) (2,6). Many others also report the rate of tumor recurrence or locally persistent disease is higher following surgery involving less than near-total thyroidectomy (161).

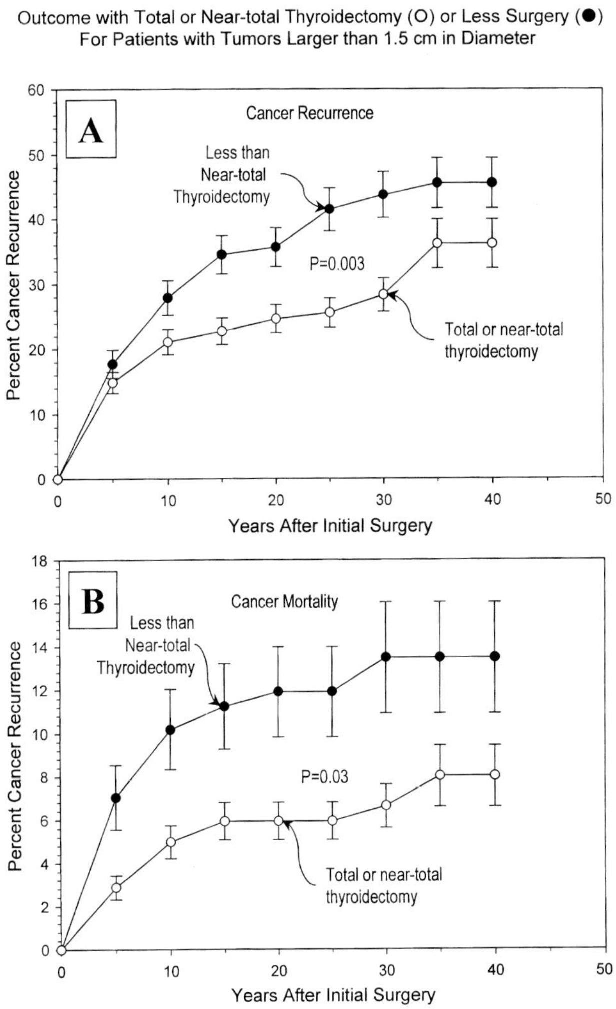

Figure 7 (A) Cancer recurrence and (B) cancer-specific mortality in 939 patients undergoing total or near-total thyroidectomy compared with patients undergoing less surgery. p-Values are from log rank analysis of life table data. (Updated from Ref. 6.)

Most physicians and surgeons believe that the primary treatment of DTC is total or near-total thyroidectomy followed by ^{131}I ablation of uptake in the thyroid bed for any patient in whom papillary, follicular, or Hürthle cell cancer is diagnosed preoperatively or at surgery (see contemporary views above) (2,162–164), even in children and young adults with low-risk tumors (160,165–167). Exceptions are isolated papillary thyroid cancers confined to the thyroid that are smaller than about 1 cm and minimally invasive follicular or Hürthle cell cancers smaller than about 4 cm. Lobectomy is adequate surgery when a papillary microcarcinoma is discovered serendipitously on thefinal pathology studies of surgery done for benign disease, providing the patient has not been exposed to radiation and has no other risk factors and has a truly low-risk cancer, i.e., a tumor smaller than 1 cm that is unifocal and confined to the thyroid without vascular invasion (6,31,37). Complications with lobectomyare few, and survival in this latter group is virtually assured (6,31,37,39).

Postoperative treatment with ^{131}I obscures the therapeutic influence of surgery (139); however, when the extent of thyroidectomy with and without the use of ^{131}I ablation was analyzed in our patients, treatment with total thyroidectomy with ^{131}I therapy was associated with the lowest recurrence rates (Fig. 8).

5.4 Surgery for Follicular and Hürthle Cell Neoplasms

Although some find frozen section study at the time of surgery helpful in the diagnosis follicular or Hürthle cell cancer (168), it has not proved useful in the hands of most pathologists, mainly because it is specific but not sensitive in diagnosing follicular or Hürthle cell cancer (72,169–171). Because the distinction between follicular or Hürthle cell adenomas and cancers can be made only by review of the permanent histological sections, most guidelines call for lobectomy with the caveat that com-

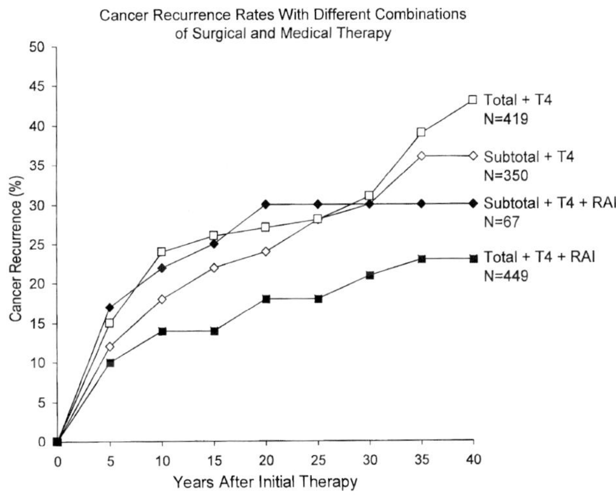

Figure 8 Tumor recurrence after thyroid surgery and thyroid hormone therapy with and without ^{131}I therapy. Total thyroidectomy includes subtotal thyroidectomy (ipsilateral lobectomy, isthmusectomy, and near-total contralateral lobectomy); subtotal thyroidectomy is lobectomy within or without isthmusectomy. Patients undergoing total thyroidectomy had more advanced tumor stage than those undergoing subtotal thyroidectomy (ANOVA $p < 0.001$). (Modified from Ref. 2.)

pletion thyroidectomy may be necessary for some minimally invasive follicular and Hürthle cell cancers (5).

To help solve the problem of clinical management of minimally invasive follicular and Hürthle cancers, attempts have been made to predict malignancy based upon the clinical and pathological feature of a tumor. Although some believe that patient age and tumor size are not different enough in minimally invasive cancers and adenomas to reliably select patients for more extensive thyroidectomy on this basis (83,84), others suggest that tumor size is especially important in making intraoperative decisions. In one study, however, patients with Hürthle cell adenomas and cancers did not differ with respect to the patient's age, sex, or history of head and neck irradiation, though patients with cancer had significantly larger tumors (4.0 ± 0.4 vs. 2.4 ± 0.2 cm; $p < 0.005$) (85). Although the incidence of malignancy in this study was 65% among tumors 4 cm or larger, it was 17% for tumors 1 cm or smaller and 23% for tumors 1–4 cm, emphasizing that small tumor size does not exclude cancer, but suggesting that resection of both thyroid lobes during the initial surgery should be considered for tumors with indeterminate cytology that are larger than 4 cm because they are so likely to be malignant (85).

5.5 Surgery for Thyroglossal Duct Neoplasms

There is some controversy concerning the optimal treatment of papillary cancer within a thyroglossal duct. Because the cancer is almost always small and usually has a benign course (172), many suggest that if the thyroid is normal and there are no other risk factors for recurrence, then the thyroglossal duct remnant should be removed by local excision using a Sistrunk procedure (100,173,174). Others argue for a more aggressive approach with total thyroidectomy and Sistrunk procedure because nodal metastases, local invasion, and microscopic intrathyroidal tumor aae not infrequently present (101,175). Microcancers require only local excision; however, thyroidectomy should be considered for tumors larger than 1 cm or if the histology is other than papillary thyroid cancer and if it is invasive or metastatic.

5.6 Completion Thyroidectomy

A large thyroid remnant hampers long-term follow-up with serum Tg determinations and whole-body ^{131}I scans, and the decision to forgo completion thyroidectomy must be discussed with the patient in this light. In practice, many patients have substantial thyroid remnants when evaluated by DxWBS (176) and Tg measurements, even after reportedly undergoing total or near-total thyroidectomy. Thyroid ultrasound is particularly useful when the extent of surgery is uncertain, since leaving a thyroid remnant smaller than 2 g (2 cm^2) facilitates postoperative ^{131}I ablation (177).

Residual tumor in the contralateral lobe cannot be predicted on the basis of a patient's clinical stage, and its prompt resection with completion of the thyroidectomy plays an important role in outcome. Contralateral papillary cancer is found frequently at completion thyroidectomy regardless of whether the patient appears to be at low or high risk of a poor outcome. A study (47) of 182 patients with papillary cancer undergoing completion thyroidectomy found that 44% had one or more tumor foci in the contralateral resected lobe, which was associated with ipsilateral lymph node metastases in 22 cases; however, 10 others had contralateral lymph node metastases without tumor foci in the contralateral lobe. The presence of lymph node metastases in the first surgical specimen and the time interval between the first surgery and completion thyroidectomy (6 months) in this study correlated with a higher frequency of bilaterality ($p = 0.033$ and $p = 0.044$, respectively). Postsurgical ^{131}I WBSs in this study (47) revealed persistent lymph node metastases in 7 patients and diffuse micronodular lung metastases in 6 that were inapparent before the patients underwent completion thyroidectomy. Another study (54) showed that patients who underwent completion thyroidectomy within 6 months of their primary operation developed significantly fewer lymph node metastases and hematogenous recurrences and survived significantly longer than those in whom the second operation was delayed for longer than 6 months. Accordingly, tumor in the contralateral lobe cannot be regarded as a clinically benign finding akin to microscopic papillary cancer found by serendipity during thyroidectomy for benign disease. When completion thyroidectomy is performed for any primary tumor larger than 1 cm, residual cancer is found in the contralateral lobe in over half the papillary cancers and almost 40% of follicular cancers, whether or not the ipsilateral lobe tumor appeared multicentric (Table 5) (178). Although some find few recurrences in the contralateral lobe and argue that multiple microscopic tumors are inconsequencial (32,179), others report recurrence rates of 5–20% in the contralateral lobe and a higher incidence of pulmonary metastases after hemithyroidectomy than after total thyroidectomy (113). In our study (2) almost 4% (55 patients) had recurrence in the contralateral thyroid lobe, with or without regional lymph node metastases, and 5% (3 patients) of this group died of cancer.

Table 5 Results of Completion Thyroidectomy in Patients with Differentiated Thyroid Cancer

Authors (ref.)	Papillary (*N*)	Papillary cancer in contralateral (*N*)	Follicular (*N*)	Follicular cancer in contralateral lobe (*N*)	Hürthle (*N*)	Hürthle cell cancer in contralateral lobe (*N*)	All patients (*N*)	All patients cancer in contralateral lobe (*N*)
Auguste and Attie (178)	58	ND[a]	17	ND	5	ND	80	38% (30)[a]
Calabro et al. (49)	51	ND	12	ND	3	ND	66	44% (28)[a]
DeGroot and Kaplan (50)	18	33% (6)	8	25% (2)	0	0	26	31% (8)
Krausz et al. (51)	70	47% (33)	30	33% (10)	0	0	100	43% (43)
Emerick et al. (43)	0	0	19	11% (2)	0	0	19	11% (2)
Kawaura et al. (48)	165	56% (93)	0	0	0	0	165	56% (93)
Pacini et al. (47)	182	44% (80)	0	0	0	0	182	44% (80)
Pasieka et al. (52)	41	68% (28)	12	42% (5)	7	57% (4)	60	62% (37)
Rao et al. (53)	75	61% (46)	54	52% (28)	0	0	129	57% (74)
Scheumann et al. (54)	65	ND	66	ND	ND	0	131	77% (101)[a]
Total	725	52%[b] (286/551)	218	38%[b] (47/123)	15	57%[b] (4/7)	958	52% (496)

[a] Data not broken down according to papillary, follicular, or Hürthle cell cancer.
[b] Weighted average.

Thus, when subtotal thyroidectomy has been performed, it is best to consider completion thyroidectomy for lesions that are anticipated to have any potential for recurrence. Treatment with ^{131}I is a poor substitute for surgery on the contralateral lobe because large thyroid remnants are difficult to ablate with ^{131}I (177). Completion thyroidectomy has a low complication rate and is thus appropriate to perform routinely for aggressive thyroid cancer variants, for patients with metastatic disease, or with papillary cancers larger than 1 cm, or minimally invasive follicular or Hürthle tumors larger than 4.0 cm and for those with follicular tumors with more than minimal capsular invasion, or multifocal cancers of any size because so many patients have residual cancer in the contralateral thyroid lobe (43,50, 54,178,180–183). When there has been a local or distant tumor recurrence following subtotal thyroidectomy, cancer is found in over 60% of the excised contralateral lobes (183). A study of children from Chernobyl found that completion thyroidectomy permitted the diagnosis and treatment of recurrent cancer and lung or lymph node metastases in 61% of patients in whom residual cancer was not recognized preoperatively (167).

5.7 Lymph Node Surgery

Although lymph node recurrence occurs in 10–14% of patients, some do not regard it with concern, especially when it occurs in young patients. However, this is not true (see regional metastases above). We found that lymph node metastases, especially bilateral cervical and mediastinal, were an independent variable that affected recurrence and survival even in younger patients (Table 3). Others report that systematic compartment-oriented dissection of lymph node metastases significantly improves recurrence ($p < 0.0001$) and survival ($p < 0.005$) rates in patients with T1–T3 tumors (184).

The NCCN guidelines recommend bilateral central compartment dissection or lateral modified radical neck dissection if lymph nodes are involved (Table 2) (5). A study (185) of 199 patients with papillary cancer who had undergone total thyroidectomy and bilateral cervical lymph node dissection found that although 21% had clinically apparent nodal involvement prior to surgery, 61% had cervical lymph node metastases at surgery, which were bilateral in 24% (40% of the patients with positive cervical nodes). The main ipsilateral sites of involvement were paratracheal (50%), midjugular (37%), and supraclavicular (22%); the main contralateral sites were paratracheal (21%) and midjugular (10%) (185).

A sentinel lymph node was found in 91% (20 of 22 patients) with nodal metastases in one study that used isosulfan blue dye (186). A sentinel node tumor was identified in 60% by hematoxylin-eosin and in 100% by immunohistochemical staining (186). Eleven patients

(55%) with a positive sentinel node had other nodal metastases—9 in the central compartment, 1 in the jugular compartment and 1 in both areas; the 2 patients with negative sentinel nodes had lymph node metastases elsewhere (186). In another study, giving 100 mCi ^{131}I and locating functioning lymph node metastases with the aid of an intraoperative probe improved the completeness of surgical excision of persistent thyroid cancer (187). Suspected and unsuspected metastases were detected in 56% of the patients in one study, but another 25% had nodal metastases that were undetected by this and other techniques (187).

5.8 Surgery for Invasive Tumor

DTC infrequently invades the upper aerodigestive tract, but when it does it often has undifferentiated areas and causes significant morbidity. Computed tomographic, ultrasonography, and endoscopic examinations are useful in providing accurate assessment of the extent of tumor invasion. In a study (188) of 262 patients with invasive papillary cancer in which complete tumor removal was achieved in 56%, the sites of invasion were muscle 53%, trachea 37%, laryngeal nerve 47%, esophagus 21%, larynx 12%, and other sites 30%. The overall survival rate, which was 79% at 5 years, 63% at 10 years, and 54% at 15 years, was significantly influenced by invasion of the trachea and esophagus, and to a lesser extent by completeness of resection, but not by invasion of muscle, larynx, and recurrent laryngeal nerves (188).

Although survival may be improved by complete surgical excision of the tumor, the extent of surgery that is required to do this requires prudent clinical judgment and a fully informed patient. In one study (189) only 46 of 1098 patients with thyroid cancer required resection of some portion of the upper aerodigestive tract, including 35 who had a history of prior surgical treatment with or without radiation or ^{131}I therapy. Treatment included total (n = 27) or partial (n = 5) laryngectomies, circumferential or partial tracheal resections, and circumferential or partial esophagectomies, or some combinations of these procedures and postoperative external beam radiation or ^{131}I in some cases. Five-year survival rate for all patients exceeded 50%; more than 70% with papillary and follicular cancers survived for 5 years, and a few lived for 30 years (189).

Aggressive resection appears to be justified in some patients for control of locally advanced DTC and seems to be of greatest benefit to those over about 45 years. In one study (90) of 40 patients with locally invasive papillary cancer in which 19 underwent complete resection and 21 did not, 15-year survival rates were 100% after complete and 74.2% with incomplete resection, but were 100% among patients younger than 45 years even after incomplete resection. Another study (191) reported the results of radical surgery in 18 elderly patients with locally invasive papillary cancer. One was a patient whose larynx and a portion of the trachea and esophagus were resected and reconstructed using a forearm free flap for the digestive tract. Nine others had a sleeve or a window resection of the trachea with immediate end-to-end anastomosis in all but one, two underwent partial esophagectomy, and six had a resection of the outer layer of the trachea or esophagus. One patient died of rupture of the carotid artery and one died of cancer in 4 years and another died of an unrelated disease; the other 15 patients were living and well 1–5 years postoperatively.

Tracheostomy should be considered in patients with tumor that is locally invasive. One study (192) of 515 patients with thyroid cancer found that 33% (170 patients) had local infiltration of tumor, about 40% of which (69 patients) required tracheostomy, 55% for laryngeal nerve invasion or intratracheal bleeding and 45% as a prophylactic intraoperative procedure to avoid later death from asphyxiation. However, tracheostomy did not influence the outcome of patients with DTC, and in some cases its complications delayed or prohibited postoperative external radiotherapy. Nonetheless, tracheostomy must be carefully considered in patients with invasive tumor that is threatening the airway.

5.9 Surgical Complications

The main complications of thyroidectomy, which are most common after total thyroidectomy, are hypoparathyroidism and recurrent laryngeal nerve damage. The rates of hypoparathyroidism immediately after surgery are as high as 5% in adults (193) and are even higher in children (67,194) undergoing total thyroidectomy. However, the rates of persistent hypocalcemia are much lower. Among seven surgical series, the average rates of permanent recurrent laryngeal nerve injury and hypoparathyroidism, respectively, were 3% and 2.6% after total thyroidectomy and 1.9% and 0.2% after subtotal thyroidectomy (195). The rates of persistent hoarseness and hypoparathyroidism are even lower. A study (196) reported a 0.5% one-year rate of persistent hypocalcemia after total thyroidectomy compared with a rate of 5.4% immediately after total thyroidectomy. When experienced surgeons perform the surgery and the posterior thyroid capsule is left intact on the contralateral side, hypoparathyroidism occurs at a low rate. A study of 5860 patients treated in Maryland found that surgeons who performed more than 100 thyroidectomies a year had the lowest overall complication rates (4.3%), which were fourfold lower than those of surgeons who performed fewer than 10 cases annually (197).

5.10 Thyroidectomy During Pregnancy

Thyroid cancer may occasionally progress rapidly during pregnancy, perhaps due to high maternal β-hCG, which has a TSH-like effect (198). Most DTCs nonetheless grow slowly and have an excellent prognosis during pregnancy, and surgery usually can be delayed until after delivery (199) or may be done safely during the second trimester (199,200).

6 RADIOIODINE ABLATION OF RESIDUAL NORMAL THYROID TISSUE

Remnant ablation refers to the ^{131}I destruction of residual macroscopically normal thyroid tissue that remains after removal of all normal and malignant thyroid tissue. Although total or near-total thyroidectomy is performed in an attempt to remove all or nearly all thyroid tissue, some ^{131}I uptake usually remains in the thyroid bed (176), which must be ablated before residual tumor can be optimally identified and ^{131}I will fully concentrate in metastases (167). The standard preparation is to render the patient hypothyroid in order to stimulate endogenous TSH secretion and sodium iodide symporter (NIS) activity. An alternative approac is to prescribe T4 after thyroidectomy and to stimulate NIS with exogenous rhTSH, which was done in one study (201) of 10 patients, resulting in complete resolution of all visible ^{131}I thyroid bed uptake on follow-up 5–13 months later. This approach has the potential to successfully ablate thyroid remnants without the need to induce hypothyroidism, but the FDA has not yet approved this specific use of the drug.

6.1 Rationale for Thyroid Remnant Ablation

Although there is some debate about ^{131}I remnant ablation after near-total thyroidectomy (56,142), there are at least five compelling reasons to consider doing it (2). First, a large remnant can obscure ^{131}I uptake in cervical or lung metastases (132,167). Second, high TSH levels necessary to enhance tumor ^{131}I uptake for diagnosis, and treatment cannot be achieved when a large thyroid remnant is present (202); in fact, large remnants should be surgically removed. Third, Tg measurement made under TSH stimulation is the most sensitive test for cancer only when there is no normal thyroid tissue present, which usually requires ablation of thyroid bed uptake (203). Fourth, remnant ablation may destroy residual normal follicular cells destined to become malignant (29) and occult cancer that might recur years later (Fig. 9). Lastly, and perhaps the most compelling reason, lung metastases may be seen only on the DxWBS or RxWBS after remnant ablation (204,205).

6.2 Indications for Thyroid ^{131}I Remnant Ablation

This decision is tightly linked to that for performing total or near-total thyroidectomy. Remnant ablation

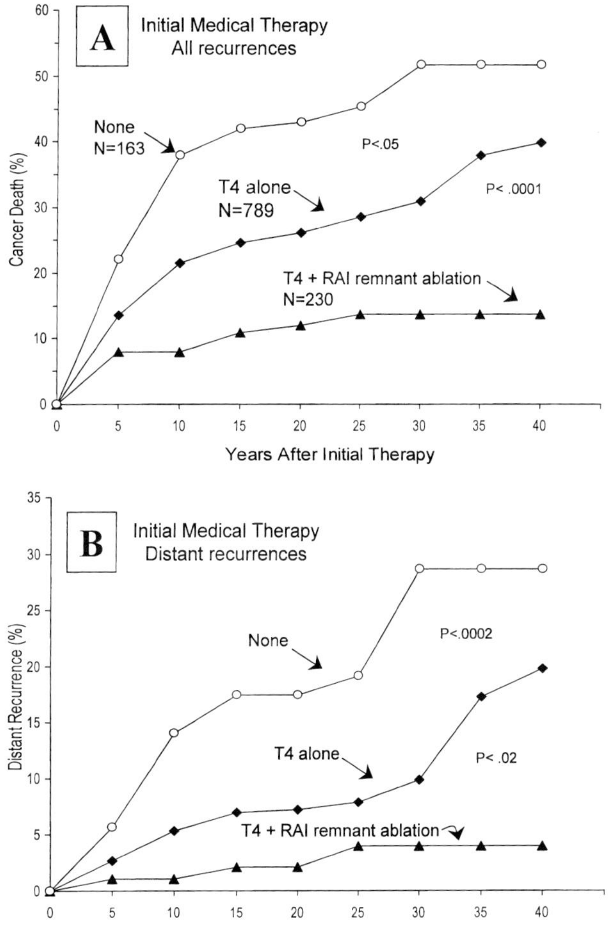

Figure 9 Tumor recurrence 16.7 years (median) after thyroid surgery and ^{131}I ablation of uptake in the thyroid bed compared to those treated with thyroid hormone alone: (A) all recurrences; (B) distant metastases recurrences. *p*-Values are log rank statistical analysis of 40-years life-table data. (Modified from Ref. 2.)

should be done when the patient has ^{131}I uptake in the thyroid bed and no known foci of cancer after resection of a tumor that has the potential for recurrence (56). If 6–12 months after ^{131}I ablation thyroid bed uptake is less than 0.5% at 48 hours, a second ablation is unlikely to be of further benefit since such a small amount of uptake is unlikely to represent residual cancer if the Tg is low and is unlikely to be the sole source of a high serum Tg level [>2 ng/mL after recombinant human thyrotropin (rhTSH) (2) or > 10 after T4 withdrawal (2,206)]. As a practical matter most patients who have undergone total or near-total thyroidectomy have thyroid bed ^{131}I uptake that requires ablation. Although some advise a more selective approach for ^{131}I ablation based on tumor stage (207), the same authors report that 38% of the patients undergoing ablation in their clinic have low-risk tumors (T1 or T2 and N0) (208). Once T4 has been withdrawn and the patient has followed a low iodine diet for imaging, remnant ablation can be done as a outpatient on the same day that DxWBS is performed (6,55,114,139).

6.3 Therapeutic Impact of ^{131}I Remnant Ablation

Recurrence rates are lower after ^{131}I ablation (56), sometimes with reduced cancer mortality rates (2), but not all find this, perhaps because more extensive thyroidectomy had been done (142). One study (113) found that remnant ablation decreased recurrence rates of tumors larger than 1 cm, including those localized to the thyroid gland or metastatic to regional lymph nodes predicted to have a good prognosis; however, it reduced the risk of death only in those with more advanced disease. In another study, the rates of pulmonary metastases among 58 patients with DTC were 11% after partial thyroidectomy, 5% after subtotal thyroidectomy and ^{131}I, 3% after total thyroidectomy, and only 1.3% after total thyroidectomy and ^{131}I (57). In a study (209) of 321 patients treated in 13 Canadian hospitals with ^{131}I, mainly to ablate residual normal and microscopic tumor tissue in those with microscopic residual papillary or follicular cancer, local disease was controlled more often with either postoperative external radiotherapy or ^{131}I therapy, or both, than with T4 alone ($p < 0.001$) (209). The 20-year survival with microscopic residual disease treated by surgery alone was less favorable (about 40%) than after treatment with either ^{131}I or external radiation (about 90%; $p < 0.01$), whereas ^{131}I treatment without obvious residual disease did not increase survival (209). In a later and somewhat contradictory study from Canada of 382 patients with DTC, total thyroidectomy and ^{131}I ablation was associated with a significantly lower rate of local relapse regardless of tumor stage (114).

We previously reported that among 1004 patients, tumor recurrence, distant metastases, and cancer deaths were significantly lower following remnant ^{131}I ablation and T4 treatment compared with T4 treatment alone or no postoperative therapy (56). In the latest analysis of this cohort (2), 1182 patients with DTC had undergone thyroid remnant ^{131}I ablation (230 patients) or were either treated with T4 alone (789 patients) or no postoperative medical therapy (163 patients). After a median follow-up time of 20.8 years for patients treated with T4 alone and 14.7 years for those undergoing thyroid remnant ablation, outcomes were as follows: after treatment with T4 alone, the tumor recurrence rate was about fourfold ($p < 0.0001$) (Fig. 9A) and the distant metastasis rate was about fivefold ($p < 0.02$) (Fig. 9B) that of thyroid ^{131}I ablation. When ^{131}I ablation doses were stratified into two groups: 29–50 mCi (42.7 ± 1.2 SE) in 62 (46%) patients and 51–200 mCi (114.6 ± 4.0) in 72 (54%) patients, both groups experienced similar 30-year recurrence rates (4% and 6%, respectively; $p = 0.1$). Among patients over age 40 years at the time of diagnosis with tumors 1 cm or larger, there were fewer cancer deaths 40 years after thyroid remnant ablation than after the other treatment strategies (20% vs. 2%; $p < 0.001$).

In the past, many used 30 mCi ^{131}I to ablate a thyroid remnant if only a small amount of thyroid tissue remained after surgery, mainly to avoid hospitalization; however, hospitalization for the use of larger doses is no longer necessary in most states (210). Radiation exposures to household members of patients given more than 30 mCi are well below the limit (5.0 mSv) mandated by NRC regulations (211). Small ^{131}I doses still have some appeal because of the lower cost and the lower whole-body radiation dose, which has been estimated to be 6.1 rem for 30 mCi, 8.5 rem for a 50 mCi, and 12.2 rem for a 60 mCi (212). Moreover, 100 mCi of ^{131}I may cause salivary injury and transient testicular damage. However, some prefer larger ^{131}I doses to ablate thyroid tissue and to treat residual microscopic cancer (213). A meta-analysis found that a single administration of about 30 ^{131}I failed to fully ablate the remnant (46%) more often than did 77–100 mCi (27%; $p < 0.001$) (214). However, a wide range of failure occurred among the low-dose cases, mainly from variation in the extent of surgery. After near-total thyroidectomy, both high and low ^{131}I activities were most likely to completely ablate the remnant (214).

7 POSTTREATMENT FOLLOW-UP VIEWED FROM THE PERSPECTIVE OF CHOICE OF THERAPY

Performing a DxWBS and measuring serum Tg is the standard of care in the initial phases of follow-up of patients with DTC (2,215), but it cannot be done adequately in the face of large amounts of residual thyroid tissue. Whether it is best to perform a DxWBS before ^{131}I therapy is uncertain. The experts that formulated the NCCN thyroid cancer guidelines could not reach a consensus on recommending a DxWBS in leu of RxWBS in postsurgical evaluations (5). During follow-up after ^{131}I ablation, a DxWBS is usually unnecessary, although one retrospective study (216) of 76 patients undergoing follow-up after initial thyroid ablation suggested that two consecutive negative ^{131}I DxWBSs had a greater likelihood of predicting relapse-free survival than did one such study; however, serum Tg levels were not measured under TSH stimulation, which is a considerably more sensitive test than DxWBS (217,218). Another study (208) of 256 patients found that a 2–5 mCi ^{131}I DxWBS performed 6 months to 1 year after thyroid ablation did not correlate with the serum Tg but only confirmed the completeness of thyroid ablation; patients with a Tg level exceeding 10 ng/mL after T4 withdrawal were selected for RxWBS after 100 mCi of ^{131}I. Furthermore, tumor amenable to early therapy may be found when recombinant human TSH (rhTSH)-stimulated serum Tg rises above 2 ng/mL without performing a DxWBS, which merely provides data concerning the completeness of thyroid ablation but not persistent tumor (217). Thus, rhTSH-stimulated Tg > 2 ng/mL warrants further diagnostic study.

7.1 Recombinant Human TSH

Periodic elevation of serum TSH levels must be done to stimulate Tg release and ^{131}I uptake because this is the optimal way to detect persistent cancer during follow-up. T4 may be withdrawn, which causes symptomatic hypothyroidism, or rhTSH may be given intramuscularly, which stimulates thyroidal ^{131}I uptake and Tg release while the patient continues taking T4, thus avoiding clinically symptomatic hypothyroidism (219). A large international multicenter study proved that rhTSH stimulates ^{131}I uptake for DxWBS and that the combination of WBS and Tg measurements could detect 100% of the patients with metastatic DTC (217). The recommended dose of rhTSH, 0.9 mg, is given intramuscularly on 2 consecutive days followed by at least 4 mCi of ^{131}I on the third day and a DxWBS and Tg measurement on the fifth day. Whole-body images are acquired after 30 minutes of scanning or after 40,000 counts, whichever occurs first. This is necessary because 4 mCi of ^{131}I after rhTSH has about the same effect as 2 mCi given during hypothyroidism, which reduces renal clearance and raises body ^{131}I retention (220). After thyroid ablation a serum Tg of 2.0 ng/mL or higher 72 hours after the last rhTSH injection usually indicates that persistent tumor is present. Although tumor may be identified on the rhTSH-stimulated DxWBS providing the recommended scanning procedure is followed (217), more often the DxWBS is negative after remnant ablation both during T4 withdrawal (208) and after rhTSH (221), even in patients with residual cancer. The drug is well tolerated. Transient headache (7.3%) and nausea (10.5%) are its main adverse effects (217), with almost no other symptoms and no dysphoric mood states as occur with hypothyroidism (219).

7.2 Diagnostic ^{131}I Whole-Body Scans

DxWBS is done to detect areas of uptake following diagnostic or therapeutic amounts of ^{131}I; however, scanning is not very useful when there are large amounts of normal thyroid tissue remaining after surgery that prevent the TSH from rising above 30 μU/mL. High ^{131}I uptake in a remnant may produce a starburst effect that makes visualizing tumor impossible.

7.2.1 Thyroid Stunning

Administering more than 2 mCi of ^{131}I for DxWBS may have a sufficiently harmful effect upon the tissue in which it concentrates to interfere with subsequent uptake of ^{131}I for several weeks (222–224), which may be avoided by using 2 or 3 mCi of ^{131}I or 500 μCi of ^{123}I, but this is less sensitive than using larger ^{131}I or ^{123}I doses in identifying remnants or metastases (223,225). Using higher doses of ^{123}I may improve DxWBS images, but the cost is great. Delaying ^{131}I therapy for some time after the DxWBS may be responsible for the stunning effect (223,224), which did not occur in 172 patients treated with ^{131}I within 72 hours of having received 5 mCi for a diagnostic scan (176). Of greater importance to the debate, recent studies (226,227) show that the therapeutic effect of ^{131}I ablation is unimpaired after DxWBS thyroid stunning.

7.2.2 Posttreatment Whole Body Scans

Although a DxWBS is usually done postoperatively to help determine the optimal ^{131}I dose to ablate residual thyroid tissue or cancer, another approach is to perform an RxWBS after administering ^{131}I given on the basis of a high postoperative serum Tg level. This often yields critical information when the serum Tg level is high and tumor cannot be found on examination or by DxWBS, neck ultrasonography, CT, or MRI. About 4–7 days after ^{131}I therapy is given, an RxWBS may show ^{131}I uptake by lesions not detected on the DxWBS (204,208).

7.2.3 Serum Thyroglobulin Measurements

Measuring the serum Tg concentration is the best way to detect normal and malignant thyroid tissue because there are no other sources to falsely elevate it. Patients who are free of disease have undetectable serum Tg levels during T4 therapy and with TSH stimulation (208,228). Antithyroglobulin antibodies (TgAb), which are found in up to 25% of patients with DTC compared with about 10% of the general population, must be measured in the same serum sample in which Tg is determined because the presence of TgAb usually invalidates the Tg result (203). Immunometric assay (IMA) methods are prone to underestimating the serum Tg level when TgAb is detectable, increasing the risk of a false-negative test (203). Conversely, when Tg remains high when measured by IMA in the presence of TgAb, residual cancer may be present (203).

Postablation serum TgAb levels correlate directly with the presence or absence of disease (203). The first serum Tg after surgery is a good prognosticator of long-term outcome. One study (229) found that an initial Tg value higher than 70 ng/mL had a 90% positive predictive value for metastases; however, the Tg may remain detectable for up to a year after initial treatment before becoming undetectable (208). Thereafter, Tg should be measured when TSH has been stimulated by T4 withdrawal or rhTSH stimulation, which lowers the false-negative rate well below that of DxWBS (208,217, 230). A Tg mRNA method is more sensitive than the IMA method, particularly during T4 treatment or when TgAb are present, but the test is not yet widely available and there is a problem with mRNA degradation in improperly handled blood samples (231).

Tg and WBS are usually considered complementary (232). However, persistent DTC is rarely present when serum Tg values are less than 2 ng/mL during rhTSH stimulation (217) or less than 5 ng/mL after T4 withdrawal (228); however, results of Tg assays vary in different laboratories, even if an international standard (CRM 457) is used (233). Nevertheless, cancer is rarely found with low or undetectable TSH-stimulated Tg levels (208) unless tumor is undifferentiated. In lieu of performing a DxWBS 6 months to 1 year after thyroid ablation, measuring a serum TSH-stimulated Tg after T4 withdrawal or rhTSH injection serves as a better guide for the selection of patients who might have persistent disease (208). A DxWBS done with 2–5 mCi after T4 withdrawal is relatively useless compared with administering 100 mCi or more and performing an RxWBS when the Tg rises above some arbitrary limit that suggests the presence of metastases—usually around 10 ng/mL after T4 withdrawal or 2 ng/mL after rhTSH stimulation (204,208).

Ten percent of 107 patients who were clinically free of disease and who mostly (95%) had undetectable serum Tg levels during T4 therapy had persistent tumor in lung (4 patients), and lymph nodes (5 patients; 3 with central compartment, 1 bilateral cervical, and 1 mediastinal nodes) identified by an rhTSH-stimulated Tg above 2 ng/mL (221). Similar to T4 withdrawal (208), rhTSH-stimulated DxWBS failed to reveal the site of metastases in every case (221). Thus, tumor amenable to early therapy may be found when rhTSH-stimulated serum Tg rises above 2 ng/mL, long before the DxWBS is abnormal. The sensitivity of rhTSH-stimulated Tg for detecting residual cancer in this study (221) was 100%, while the false-negative rates were 64% for Tg > 0.5 ng/mL on T4 therapy, 73% for rhTSH-stimulated DxWBS, and zero for an rhTSH-stimulated Tg > 2 ng/mL. An elevated rhTSH-stimulated Tg > 2 ng/mL warrants further study with other imaging modalities.

7.3 Thyroglobulin-Positive, Diagnostic WBS-Negative Patients

Lung metastases sometimes are found only on RxWBS after administrating large doses of ^{131}I. (204) One study of 283 patients found that 6% of those with high serum Tg levels treated with 100 mCi of ^{131}I had distant metastases detected on RxWBS that were not detected on a 2 mCi DxWBS. (128) Another study (234) found that all but one of 17 patients with elevated serum Tg levels and a negative 5 mCi DxWBS had ^{131}I uptake after 75 to 140 mCi of ^{131}I; more than half had lung metastases. Among 89 consecutive pairs of ^{131}I DxWBS and RxWBS studies done on 79 patients in patients with negative 4 to 5 mCi ^{131}I DxWBS studies had an RxWBS study revealing distant metastases; all had a serum Tg level above 15 ng/mL when the T4 withdrawal TSH was > 30 μU/mL (2). This can only be done when compete thyroid ablation has been done.

7.3.1 Whole-Body Positron Emission Tomography Scanning with F-18-Fluorodeoxyglucose

FDG-PET scanning should be considered when tumor is suspected on the basis of high serum Tg levels but RxWBS and neck ultrasonography are negative. Poorly differentiated thyroid cancer often loses the ability to concentrate ^{131}I and exhibits increased metabolic activity, as evidenced by enhanced glucose uptake. FDG-PET scanning thus may identify DTC metastasis that cannot be identified by ^{131}I or ^{99m}Tc scintigraphy, because FDG uptake is an indicator of poor functional differentiation and of more aggressive tumor growth (235). Patients who are at risk of dying of cancer can thus be identified by FDG-PET scanning. For instance, one study (236) showed that the strongest predictor of survival was the volume of FDG-avid disease; only 1 death (of leukemia) occurred in PET-negative patients (n = 66), whereas patients over 45 years with distant metastases that concentrated FDG were at the highest risk and those with FDG volume greater than 125 had the worst short-term survival (236). High-dose ^{131}I therapy has little or no effect on the viability of metastatic disease that avidly concentrations FDG.

Although PET has better sensitivity, resolution imaging, and spatial localization, these features must be balance against its higher cost compared with thallium scintigraphy (237). False-positive F-18-FDG uptake may occur with benign lung disease and artifactually (238) PET scanning is of most value in patients with high serum Tg levels and negative imaging studies, including ^{131}I RxWBS, because it gives information about prognosis.

7.3.2 Treatment of Patients with Tg-Positive, DxWBS-Negative Studies

The exact Tg level that is used for recommending treatment of patients with negative DxWBS studies and a high Tg has been coming down; it was about 30 or 40 ng/mL about a decade ago but now is about 10 ng/mL after thyroid hormone withdrawal (5,204, 239), but this remains an arbitrary cut-off. Although some skepticism has been voiced about this therapeutic maneuver, it is beneficial. The prognostic importance of finding lung metastasis at an early stage was shown by Schlumberger (240), who reported 100% 10-year survival with lung metastases detected only by elevated Tg levels and confirmed by RxWBS; however, survival fell to 91% when chest x-rays were normal but DxWBS was positive, falling to 63% when the chest x-ray showed lung micronodules and 11% when it showed macronodules. Multivariate analysis has shown the independent prognostic significance of the size of pulmonary metastases at the time of therapy (131). Another multivariate analysis in 134 patients with pulmonary metastases showed that an early diagnosis (a normal chest x-ray with pulmonary metastases found only on ^{131}I scintigraphy) and treatment of the metastases with ^{131}I were the most important elements giving rise to a significant improvement in survival rate and a prolonged disease-free survival (130). Treatment of pulmonary metastases found only on RxWBS usually reduces the tumor burden, but complete eradication of metastases may be difficult to achieve (241). Two to 4 years after receiving a total of 350–700 mCi of ^{131}I, 3 of 10 patients treated in our clinic had no ^{131}I uptake on the RxWBS scan and serum Tg levels less than 5 ng/mL while off T4. Two other studies (241,242) found clearly beneficial effects of ^{131}I therapy for such patients: 80% achieved a negative whole-body ^{131}I posttherapy scan, 60% had a serum Tg less than 5 ng/mL off thyroid hormone, and 6 of 8 patients had normalization of the CT scan, and 2 had negative lung biopsies. Improvement sometimes occurs with one or two ^{131}I treatment (12), but when a partial reduction of metastatic disease is achieved, patients usually have a good quality of life with little disease progression and a low mortality rate (12).

8 THYROID HORMONE SUPPRESSION OF THYROTROPIN

Recurrence rates, including those of distant metastases, are significantly reduced with T4 therapy (6,56), but the optimal TSH level required to achieve this is uncertain. A retrospective study (243) found that relapse-free survival was significantly better with a consistently suppressed TSH ($\leq$0.05 μU/mL) than when serum TSH levels were always 1 μU/mL or higher. In this study, the level of TSH suppression was an independent predictor of recurrence (243). However, a prospective study of 617 patients in the National Thyroid Cancer Treatment Cooperative Study (244) found that disease stage, patient age, and ^{131}I therapy independently predicted disease progression, but that the degree of TSH suppression did not. When the TSH is suppressed to about 0.1 μU/mL, suppressing it into thyrotoxic ranges usually does not further lower the Tg level (245). Thus, suppressing TSH to an undetectable (e.g., $<$ 0.1 μU/mL) thyrotoxic range in patients who have no evidence of disease is likely not to confer greater therapeutic benefit.

As a practical matter, the most appropriate T4 dose usually is that which reduces the serum TSH to just below the lower limit of the normal range for the assay being used, unless there is persistent disease when TSH levels of about 0.1 μU/mL may be necessary (162).

9 EXTERNAL RADIATION THERAPY

Disease-free survival may be improved by external beam radiation therapy administered to patients over age 40 with invasive papillary cancer (T4 tumor) (114,246). Patients with residual microscopic papillary cancer are more commonly rendered disease-free by external radiotherapy (90%) than without it (26%) (209). Patients with microscopically invasive follicular cancer also are more likely to be rendered disease-free when postoperative external radiation is given (53%) than when it is not (38%) (209). Radiotherapy is also useful in the treatment of isolated bone metastases (131).

10 CHOICE OF THERAPY FOR RECURRENT DISEASE

The first choice of therapy for recurrent disease is surgery if the tumor can be localized and is resectable. For locoregional recurrences that are not amenable to surgery ^{131}I therapy is recommended for those that concentrate it and external beam radiotherapy for those that do not, or both may be used. Up to 75% of DTCs and their metastases and about one third of Hürthle cel l cancers concentrate ^{131}I (209). For disseminated tumor, ^{131}I dosimetry should be considered if the tumor concentrates ^{131}I; however, the larger the tumor mass is, the less likely that ^{131}I therapy will ablate it, but depends upon the site and number of tumor foci (5). Surgery should be considered for symptomatic bone metastases or those in weight-bearing extremities or vertebral tumors impinging upon the spinal cord. The most common sites of bone metastases in one large study were vertebrae (29%), pelvis (22%), ribs (17%), and femur (11%), 53% of which were multiple tumors (247). The 10-year survival rate from the time of diagnosis of bone metastasis was 13%, which by multivariate analysis was favorably influenced by their uptake of ^{131}I and the absence of nonosseous metastases (247). Patients with bone metastases experience serious morbidity: during the course of the disease a pathological fracture occurred in 27% and cord compression from vertebral metastases occurred in 14% (247). Another study (127) of 109 patients with bone metastases reported survival rates at 5 and 10 years of 41% and 15%, respectively. Features associated with an improved survival were bone metastases as the presenting symptom of thyroid cancer ($p < 0.0005$), the absence of metastasis in other organs ($p < 0.03$), the cumulative dose of ^{131}I ($p < 0.0001$), and complete surgical removal of bone metastases surgery in young patients ($p < 0.04$).

Surgical resection should be considered for CNS metastases, which pose a special problem because ^{131}I therapy may induce cerebral edema. In a study (247) of 47 cases of brain metastases, they were a primary clinical feature at initial presentation in 15% of the cases, were identified during the subsequent course of the disease in 68%, and were only discovered at autopsy in 23%. Once brain metastases are diagnosed, disease-specific mortality is very high—78% with a median survival of 12.4 months in one retrospective study (247)—but this was significantly improved by surgical resection of one or more tumor foci. The median disease-specific survival from diagnosis of brain metastases was 16.7 months for patients who underwent local excision of one or more brain metastases, compared with 3.4 months for those who did not ($p < 0.05$). Brain metastases from thyroid cancer are an extremely poor prognostic sign. Inoperable brain metastases should be treated with gamma knife rather than external radiation if possible (247).

10.1 Adjuvant Chemotherapy

Life-threatening tumor refractory to all other forms of therapy may be palliatively treated with doxorubicin (Adriamycin), although the response rate is poor (8). Chemotherapy is used for tumors that are not amenable to surgery or external beam radiotherapy and are unresponsive to ^{131}I. Among 49 patients with metastatic DTC treated with five chemotherapy protocols, only two (3%) patients had objective responses (248). A review of published series found that 38% of patients had a response to doxorubicin defined as a reduction in tumor mass (249). Combination chemotherapy is not clearly superior to doxorubicin therapy alone (8).

11 TREATMENT OF CHILDREN

Children with DTC can be divided into two groups: prepubertal children under about age 10–12 years whose tumors seem to have a somewhat different biological behavior than those in adults, and adolescents between about 13 and 18 years of age whose tumors are similar to those in young adults and for whom treatment is generally regarded to be similar to that in young adults. There is some disagreement about the appropriate treatment of prepubertal children, with some disputing the use of total thyroidectomy and questioning the routine application of ^{131}I thyroid ablation, mainly because of higher complication rates of aggressive therapy in children and the lack of prospective studies. Compared with adults, thyroid cancer in children is more advanced at diagnosis, but paradoxically has a better prognosis (Fig. 2B). Their tumors are mainly papillary cancers but a few are follicular cancers (250). Compared with adults, more children have lymph node metastases (60–90%) and distant metastases (10–20%), about half of which are present at the time of diagnosis (8,66,250–252). Extrathyroidal tumor extension occurs in up to half of children (8,251), causing as many as 25% to have microscopic or gross residual disease after surgery, and resulting in disease-free survival rates as low as 76% at 5 years and 66% at 10 years (251). Recurrence is often found years after the initial therapy. For example, in a study (251) of 30 children under age 16, who mostly (66%) underwent total thyroidectomy and ^{131}I ablation, the median time to recurrence was 7 years but adverse events occurred a late as 44 years after surgery. Recurrence rates are higher in children under age 10 years, particularly with multifocal or metastatic tumors at the time of diagnosis (252), which have the poorest survival rates (251).

Nonetheless, studies show that children and adolescents with DTC live for many years, regardless of tumor stage at the time of diagnosis or the development of recurrence, which has led many to regard DTC in children as a relatively indolent disease that rarely causes death. This is not entirely correct. Long-term follow-up is necessary to know the eventual outcome of children with metastases. For example, a study (253) of 14 children with papillary cancer metastatic to lung who were followed for an average of 19.3 years (1–45 yr) found that none had died of metastatic disease, but half continued to have manifestations of residual cancer. In a longer-term study (254) overall survival was 100% at 10 years even in children with distant metastases; however, one fourth developed recurrent disease and six died of thyroid cancer at age 40 ± 2.1 years, 26 ± 3.1 years after the initial diagnosis. Among these cases, one patient had invasive disease and lung metastases at diagnosis and died of progressive lung metastases after 36 years. The other five children initially had local/regional disease but developed lung and skeletal metastases after a 2- to 20-year disease-free interval (254). In three cases, the cause of death was related to initial radiotherapy: one developed tracheal necrosis 26 years after diagnosis and died of upper airway complications, whereas two others developed sarcomas of the cervical region 22 and 29 years after the diagnosis of thyroid cancer (254). Another study from France (255) of 72 children with DTC followed a median of 13 years after having undergone treatment at age 16 years or younger for DTC, which had metastasized to lung in 18% and to lymph nodes in 90% and that had invaded the thyroid capsule in 67%, found that only 60% had a complete remission after initial treatment. Children without distant metastases for whom surgery was macroscopically incomplete had a relapse rate five times that in patients whose surgery was complete. Six patients died from thyroid cancer at ages ranging from 19 to 44 years 12–33 years after initial treatment (255). Despite a favorable long-term survival rate (90.3% at 20 yr), the standardized mortality ratio was equal to 8.1 (255), underscoring the need for complete surgical treatment and fastidious long-term follow-up.

Treatment of children with DTC is controversial because few large series have been reported. Many recommend total or near-total thyroidectomy and ^{131}I ablation, especially for tumors that are large, multiple, or metastatic (256–258), or for familial papillary cancer (259). Although some withhold ^{131}I ablation for children over age 10 year with low tumor stage and node-negative disease (251), modified neck dissection is generally recommended for children with clinically positive neck lymph nodes (250). Data provide support for total thyroidectomy and ^{131}I therapy in children with DTC. A study (260) of 109 children with DTC (aged 6–17 yr), in which the primary treatment comprised total thyroidectomy in 82% and ^{131}I ablation in 78% with T4 suppression of TSH in all patients, found that the survival rate was 100% but that the 5- 10-year disease-free survival rates were only 80% and 61%, respectively. Multivariate analysis showed that total thyroidectomy was the most significant factor ($p = 0.007$) for disease-free survival, while less than total thyroidectomy increased the relative risk of relapse by a factor of 10 and that ^{131}I treatment decreased the relative risk of relapse by a factor of 5 (260). However, the rate of permanent postoperative complications was relatively high, including laryngeal nerve palsy (9%) and hypoparathyroidism (5.5%) and both (1%). The authors (260) nonetheless concluded that this treatment should be routinely applied even in younger children. Another study (261) of 37 patients with papillary cancer confined to the thyroid found that patients treated with lobectomy with or without isthmusectomy were more likely to have recurrence than those treated with subtotal or total thyroidectomy (odds ratio 8.7; 95% CI 1.4–54). Although the incidence of complications was statistically similar among the several surgical groups, 3 patients treated with more extensive surgery had permanent hypoparathyroidism. A comprehensive review (262) of the literature of the current treatment strategies for pediatric patients with non-medullary DTC concluded that, for the majority of children, total or near-total thyroidectomy is the standard initial therapy for DTC, that this is commonly followed by the administration of ^{131}I postoperatively to ablate the thyroid remnant, and that the duration of follow-up is life-long, even if the patient appears to be clinically free of disease.

Completion thyroidectomy may be necessary in children. Almost half of 47 children from Chernobyl with thyroid cancer who had undergone lobectomy were subject to completion thyroidectomy after undergoing neck ultrasonography and FNA to identify thyroid nodules in the contralateral lobe and suspicious lymph nodes (167). Papillary cancer was found in nearly 29% of the surgical specimens: half in the remaining thyroid lobe and half in metastatic lymph nodes. Moreover, posttherapy whole-body scans demonstrated lung metastases in 28% and lymph node metastases in 33% of the children. However, 21% developed hypoparathyroidism and 5.2% unilateral laryngeal nerve palsy. Thus, completion thyroidectomy allowed for the diagnosis and treatment of persistent thyroid cancer and lung or lymph node metastases in 61% of the patients in whom residual disease was not previously recognized, but the high complication rate of surgery underscores that highly trained and experience surgeons must perform thyroidectomy in children.

REFERENCES

1. Hundahl SA, Fleming ID, Fremgen AM, Menck HR. Two hundred eighty-six cases of parathyroid carcinoma treated in the US between 1985–1995—A National Cancer Date Base report. Cancer 1999; 86:538–544.
2. Mazzaferri EL, Kloos RT. Current approaches to primary therapy for papillary and follicular thyroid cancer. J Clin Endocrinol Metab 2001; 86(4):1447–1463.
3. Ries LAG, Eisner MP, Kosary CL, Hankey BF, Miller AB, Cleeg L, et al. SEER Cancer Statistics Review, 1973–1997. Bethesda, MD: National Cancer Institute, 2000.
4. Voutilainen PE, Multanen MM, Leppaniemi AK, Haglund CH, Haapiainen RK, Franssila KO. Prognosis after lymph node recurrence in papillary thyroid carcinoma depends on age. Thyroid 2001; 11(10):953–957.
5. Mazzaferri EL. NCCN thyroid carcinoma practice guidelines. Oncology 1999; 13 (suppl 11A):391–442.
6. Mazzaferri EL, Jhiang SM. Long-term impact of initial surgical and medical therapy on papillary and follicular thyroid cancer. Am J Med 1994; 97:418–428.
7. Akslen LA, LiVolsi VA. Prognostic significance of histologic grading compared with subclassification of papillary thyroid carcinoma. Cancer 2000; 88(8):1902–1908.
8. Mazzaferri EL. Thyroid carcinoma: papillary and follicular. In: Mazzaferri EL, Samaan N, editors. Endocrine Tumors. Cambridge: Blackwell Scientific Publications Inc., 1993: 278–333.
9. Dottorini ME, Vignati A, Mazzucchelli L, Lomuscio G, Colombo L. Differentiated thyroid carcinoma in children and adolescents: a 37-year experience in 85 patients. J Nucl Med 1997; 38:669–675.
10. Harach HR, Williams ED. Childhood thyroid cancer in England and Wales. Br J Cancer 1995; 72:777–783.
11. Hung W. Well-differentiated thyroid carcinomas in children and adolescents: a review. Endocrinologist 1994; 4:117–126.
12. Samuel AM, Rajashekharrao B, Shah DH. Pulmonary metastases in children and adolescents with well-differentiated thyroid cancer. J Nucl Med 1998; 39:1531–1536.
13. Zimmerman D, Hay ID, Gough IR, Goellner JR, Ryan JJ, Grant CS, McConahey WM. Papillary thyroid carcinoma in children and adults: long-term follow-up of 1039 patients conservatively treated at one institution during three decades. Surgery 1988; 104:1157–1166.
14. Lupoli G, Vitale G, Caraglia M, Fittipaldi MR, Abbruzzese A, Tagliaferri P, Bianco AR. Familial papillary thyroid microcarcinoma: a new clinical entity. Lancet 1999; 353:637–639.
15. Rios A, Rodriguez JM, Illana J, Torregrosa NM, Parrilla P. Familial papillary carcinoma of the thyroid: report of three families. Eur J Surg 2001; 167(5):339–343.
16. Bell B, Mazzaferri EL. Familial adenomatous polyposis (Gardner's syndrome) and thyroid carcinoma: a case report and review of the literature. Dig Dis Sci 1993; 38:185–190.
17. Burman KD, Ringel MD, Wartofsky L. Unusual types of thyroid neoplasms. Endocrinol Metabol Clin North Am 1996; 25:49–68.
18. Dahia PLM, Marsh DJ, Zheng ZM, Zedenius J, Komminoth P, Frisk T, Wallin G, Parsons R, Longy M, Larsson C, Eng C. Somatic deletions and mutations in the Cowden disease gene, *PTEN*, in sporadic thyroid tumors. Cancer Res 1997; 57:4710–4713.
19. Stratakis CA, Courcoutsakis NA, Abati A, Filie A, Doppman JL, Carney JA, Shawker T. Thyroid gland abnormalities in patients with the syndrome of spotty skin pigmentation, myxomas, endocrine overactivity, and schwannomas (Carney complex). J Clin Endocrinol Metab 1997; 82:2037–2043.
20. Cetta F, Olschwang S, Petracci M, Montalto G, Baldi

C, Zuckermann M, Costantini RM, Fusco A. Genetic alterations in thyroid carcinoma associated with familial adenomatous polyposis: clinical implications and suggestions for early detection. World J Surg 1998; 22:1231–1236.
21. Donghi R, Sozzi G, Pierotti MA, Biunno I, Miozzo M, Fusco A, Grieco M, Santoro M, Vecchio G, Spurr NK, et al. The oncogene associated with human papillary thyroid carcinoma (PTC) is assigned to chromosome 10 q11–q12 in the same region as multiple endocrine neoplasia type 2A (MEN2A). Oncogene 1989; 4:521–523.
22. Smanik PA, Furminger TL, Mazzaferri EL, Jhiang SM. Breakpoint characterization of the ret/PTC oncogene in human papillary thyroid carcinoma. Hum Mol Genet 1995; 4:2313–2318.
23. Elisei R, Romei C, Vorontsova T, Cosci B, Veremeychik V, Kuchinskaya E, Basolo F, Demidchik EP, Miccoli P, Pinchera A, Pacini F. Ret/ptc rearrangements in thyroid nodules: studies in irradiated and not irradiated, malignant and benign thyroid lesions in children and adults. J Clin Endocrinol Metab 2001; 86(7):3211–3216.
24. Jhiang SM, Mazzaferri EL. The ret/PTC oncogene in papillary thyroid carcinoma. J Lab Clin Med 1994; 123:331–337.
25. Jhiang SM, Cho JY, Furminger TL, Sagartz J, Tong Q, Capen CC, Mazzaferri EL. Thyroid carcinomas in RET/PTC transgenic mice. Recent Results Cancer Res 1999; 154:265–270.
26. Santoro M, Chiappetta G, Cerrato A, Salvatore D, Zhang L, Manzo G, Picone A, Portella G, Santelli G, Vecchio G, Fusco A. Development of thyroid papillary carcinomas secondary to tissue-specific expression of the RET/PTC1 oncogene in transgenic mice. Oncogene 1996; 12:1821–1826.
27. Nikiforov YE, Nikiforova M, Fagin JA. Radiation-induced post-Chernobyl pediatric thyroid carcinomas. Oncogene 1998; 17:1983–1988.
28. Cheung CC, Ezzat S, Ramyar L, Freeman JL, Asa SL. Molecular basis of Hürthle cell papillary thyroid carcinoma. J Clin Endocrinol Metab 2000; 85(2):878–882.
29. Sugg SL, Ezzat S, Rosen IB, Freeman JL, Asa SL. Distinct multiple *RET*/PTC gene rearrangements in multifocal papillary thyroid neoplasia. J Clin Endocrinol Metab 1998; 83:4116–4122.
30. Basolo F, Molinaro E, Agate L, Pinchera A, Pollina L, Chiappetta G, Monaco C, Santoro M, Fusco A, Miccoli P, Elisei R, Capezzone M, Pacini F. RET protein expression has no prognostic impact on the long-term outcome of papillary thyroid carcinoma. Eur J Endocrinol 2001; 145(5):599–604.
31. Baudin E, Travagli JP, Ropers J, Mancusi F, Bruno-Bossio G, Caillou B, Cailleux AF, Lumbroso JD, Parmentier C, Schlumberger M. Microcarcinoma of the thyroid gland—the Gustave-Roussy Institute experience. Cancer 1998; 83:553–559.
32. Shaha AR, Loree TR, Shah JP. Prognostic factors and risk group analysis in follicular carcinoma of the thyroid. Surgery 1995; 118:1131–1138.
33. Brennan MD, Bergstralh EJ, van Heerden JA, McConahey WM. Follicular thyroid cancer treated at the Mayo Clinic, 1946 through 1970: initial manifestations, pathologic findings, therapy, and outcome. Mayo Clin Proc 1991; 66:11–22.
34. Sanders LE, Silverman M. Follicular and Hürthle cell carcinoma: predicting outcome and directing therapy. Surgery 1998; 124:967–974.
35. Khafif A, Khafif RA, attie JN. Hürthle cell carcinoma: a malignancy of low-grade potential Head Neck 1999; 21:506–511.
36. Gauger PG, Reeve TS, Delbridge LW. Intraoperative decision making in follicular lesions of the thyroid: Is tumor size important? J Am Coll Surgeons 1999; 189:253–258.
37. Tourniaire J, Bernard MH, Bizollon-Roblin MH, Bertholon-Gregoire M, Berger-Dutrieux N. Thyroid papillary microcarcinoma: 179 cases since 1973. Presse Med 1998; 27:1467–1469.
38. Rodriguez JM, Moreno A, Parrilla P, Sola J, Soria T, Tebar FJ, Aranda F. Papillary thyroid microcarcinoma: clinical study and prognosis. Eur J Surg 1997; 163:255–259.
39. Moosa M, Mazzaferri EL. Occult thyroid carcinoma. Cancer J 1997; 10:180–188.
40. Sugino K, Ito K Jr, Ozaki O, Mimura T, Iwasaki H, Ito K. Papillary microcarcinoma of the thyroid. J Endocrinol Invest 1998; 21:445–448.
41. Sugitani I, Yanagisawa A, Shimizu A, Kato M, Fujimoto Y. Clinicopathologic and immunohistochemical studies of papillary thyroid microcarcinoma presenting with cervical lymphadenopathy. World J Surg 1998; 22:731–737.
42. Yamashita H, Noguchi S, Murakami N, Toda M, Uchino S, Watanabe S, Kawamoto H. Extracapsular invasion of lymph node metastasis—a good indicator of disease recurrence and poor prognosis in patients with thyroid microcarcinoma. Cancer 1999; 86:842–849.
43. Emerick GT, Duh Q-Y, Siperstein AE, Burrow GN, Clark OH. Diagnosis, treatment, and outcome of follicular thyroid carcinoma. Cancer 1993; 72:3287–3295.
44. Carcangiu ML, Zampi G, Pupi A, Castagnoli A, Rosai J. Papillary carcinoma of the thyroid. A clinicopathologic study of 241 cases treated at the University of Florence, Italy. Cancer 1985; 55:805–828.
45. Salvesen H, Njolstad PR, Akslen LA, Albrektsen G, Soreide O, Varhaug JE. Papillary thyroid carcinoma: a multivariate analysis of prognostic factors including an evaluation of the p-TNM staging system. Eur J Surg 1992; 158:583—589.
46. LiVolsi VA. Papillary lesions of the thyroid. In: LiVolsi VA, ed. Surgical Pathology of the Thyroid. Philadelphia: W.B. Saunders Company, 1990: 136—172.
47. Pacini F, Elisei R, Capezzone M, Miccoli P, Molinaro

E, Basolo F, Agate L, Bottici V, Raffaelli M, Pinchera A. Contralateral papillary thyroid cancer is frequent at completion thyroidectomy with no difference in low- and high-risk patients. Thyroid 2001; 11(9):877–881.
48. Kawaura M, Pathak I, Gullane PJ, Mancer K, Irish J, Brown D, Rotstein L. Multicentricity in papillary thyroid carcinoma: analysis of predictive factors. J Otolaryngol 2001; 30(2):102–105.
49. Calabro S, Auguste L, Attie JN. Morbidity of completion thyroidectomy for initially misdiagnosed thyroid carcinoma. Head Neck Surg 1988; 10.
50. DeGroot LJ, Kaplan EL. Second operations for "completion" of thyroidectomy in treatment of differentiated thyroid cancer. Surgery 1991; 110:936–940.
51. Krausz Y, Ish-Shalom S, Dejong RBJ, Shibley N, Lapidot M, Maaravi Y, Glaser B. Somatostatin-receptor imaging of medullary thyroid carcinoma. Clin Nucl Med 1994; 19:416–421.
52. Pasieka JL, Zedenius J, Auer G, Grimelius L, Höög A, Lundell G, Wallin G, Bäckdahl M. Addition of nuclear DNA content to the AMES risk-group classification for papillary thyroid cancer. Surgery 1992; 112:1154–1160.
53. Rao RS, Fakih AR, Mehta AR, Agarwal R, Raghavan A, Shrikhande SS. Completion thyroidectomy for thyroid carcinoma. Head Neck Surg 1987; 9:284–286.
54. Scheumann GFW, Seeliger H, Musholt TJ, Gimm O, Wegener G, Dralle H, Hundeshagen H, Pichlmayr R. Completion thyroidectomy in 131 patients with differentiated thyroid carcinoma. Eur J Surg 1996; 162:677–684.
55. Taylor T, Specker B, Robbins J, Sperling M, Ho M, Ain K, Bigos ST, Brierley J, Cooper D, Haugen B, Hay I, Hertzberg V, Klein I, Klein H, Ladenson P, Nishiyama R, Ross D, Sherman S, Maxon HR. Outcome after treatment of high-risk papillary and non-Hürthle-cell follicular thyroid carcinoma. Ann Intern Med 1998; 129:622–627.
56. Mazzaferri EL. Thyroid remnant ^{131}I ablation for papillary and follicular thyroid carcinoma. Thyroid 1997; 7:265–271.
57. Massin JP, Savoie JC, Garnier H, Guiraudon G, Leger FA, Bacourt F. Pulmonary metastases in differentiated thyroid carcinoma. Study of 58 cases with implications for the primary tumor treatment. Cancer 1984; 53: 982–992.
58. Loh KC, Greenspan FS, Gee L, Miller TR, Yeo PPB. Pathological tumor-node-metastasis (pTNM) staging for papillary and follicular thyroid carcinomas: a retrospective analysis of 700 patients. J Clin Endocrinol Metab 1997; 82:3553–3562.
59. Evans HL. Encapsulated columnar-cell neoplasms of the thyroid—a report of four cases suggesting a favorable prognosis. Am J Surg Pathol 1996; 20:1205–1211.
60. de los Santos ET, Keyhani-Rofagha S, Cunningham JJ, Mazzaferri EL. Cystic thyroid nodules: the dilemma of malignant lesions. Arch Intern Med 1990; 150:1422–1427.
61. Hedinger C, Williams ED, Sobin LH. The WHO histological classification of thyroid tumors: a commentary on the second edition. Cancer 1989; 63:908–911.
62. Mazzaferri EL, Young RL, Oertel JE, Kemmerer WT, Page CP. Papillary thyroid carcinoma: the impact of therapy in 576 patients. Medicine (Baltimore) 1977; 56:171–196.
63. LiVolsi V, Asa SL. The demise of follicular carcinoma of the thyroid gland. Thyroid 1994; 4:233–236.
64. Ain KB. Papillary thyroid carcinoma etiology, assessment, and therapy. Endocrinol Metabol Clin North Am 1995; 24:711–760.
65. Gardner RE, Tuttle RM, Burman KD, Haddady S, Truman C, Sparling YH, Wartofsky L, Sessions RB, Ringel MD. Prognostic importance of vascular invasion in papillary thyroid carcinoma. Arch Otolaryngol Head Neck Surg 2000; 126(3):309–312.
66. Sobrinho-Simoes M, Soares J, Carneiro F. Diffuse follicular variant of papillary carcinoma of the thyroid: report of eight cases of a distinct aggressive type of tumor. Surg Path 1990; 3:189–203.
67. LiVolsi VA. Unusual variants of papillary thyroid carcinoma. In: Mazzaferri EL, Kreisberg RA, Bar RS, eds. Advances in Endocrinology and Metabolism. St. Louis: Mosby-Year Book, Inc., 1995: 39–54.
68. Nikiforov Y, Gnepp DR. Pediatric thyroid cancer after the Chernobyl disaster: pathomorphologic study of 84 cases (1991–1992) from the Republic of Belarus. Cancer 1994; 74:748–766.
69. Rosai J. Papillary carcinoma. Monogr Pathol 1993; 138–165.
70. Herrera MF, Hay ID, Wu PS, Goellner JR, Ryan JJ, Ebersold JR, Bergstralh EJ, Grant CS. Hürthle cell (oxyphyilic) papillary thyroid carcinoma: a variant with more aggresive biologic behavior. World J Surg 1994; 16:669–674.
71. Katoh R, Harach HR, Williams ED. Solitary, multiple, and familial oxyphil tumours of the thyroid gland. J Pathol 1998; 186:292–299.
72. LiVolsi VA. Follicular lesions of the thyroid. In: LiVolsi VA, ed. Surgical Pathology of the Thyroid. Philadelphia: W.B. Saunders Company, 1990: 173–212.
73. Lang W, Choritz H, Hundeshagen H. Risk factors in follicular thyroid carcinomas: a retrospective follow-up study covering a 14-year period with emphasis on morphologic findings. Am J Surg Pathol 1986; 10:246–255.
74. van Heerden JA, Hay ID, Goellner JR, Salomao D, Ebersold JR, Bergstralh EJ, Grant CS. Follicular thyroid carcinoma with capsular invasion alone: a nonthreatening malignancy. Surgery 1992; 112:1130–1138.

75. Thompson LD, Wieneke JA, Paal E, Frommelt RA, Adair CF, Heffess CS. A clinicopathologic study of minimally invasive follicular carcinoma of the thyroid gland with a review of the English literature 2. Cancer 2001; 91(3)505–524.
76. Mazzaferri EL. Management of a solitary thyroid nodule. N Engl J Med 1993; 328:553–559.
77. Tielens ET, Sherman SI, Hruban RH, Ladenson PW. Follicular variant of papillary thyroid carcinoma: a clinicopathologic study. Cancer 1994; 73:424–431.
78. Hedinger CE. Problems of classification of thyroid tumors and their bearing on prognosis and therapy. Schweiz Med Wochenschr 1993; 123:1673–1681.
79. Watson RG, Brennan MD, van Heerden JA, McConahey WM, Taylor WF. Invasive Hürthle cell carcinoma of the thyroid: natural history and management. Mayo Clin Proc 1984; 59:851–855.
80. LiVolsi VA. Hürthle Cell Lesions. Surgical Pathology of the Thyroid. Philadelphia: W.B.Saunders Co., 1990: 275–288.
81. Rosen IB, Luk S, Katz I. Hürthle cell tumor behavior: dilemma and resolution. Surgery 1985; 98: 777–783.
82. Stojadinovic A, Ghossein RA, Hoos A, Urist MJ, Spiro RH, Shah JP, Brennan MF, Shaha AR, Singh B. Hürthle cell carcinoma: a critical histopathologic appraisal. J Clin Oncol 2001; 19(10):2616–2625.
83. Sugino K, Ito K, Mimura T, Kameyama K, Iwasaki H, Ito K. Hürthle cell tumor of the thyroid: analysis of 188 cases. World J Surg 2001; 25(9):1160–1163.
84. McHenry CR, Thomas SR, Slusarczyk SJ, Khiyami A. Follicular or Hürthle cell neoplasm of the thyroid: Can clinical factors be used to predict carcinoma and determine extent of thyroidectomy? Surgery 1999; 126: 798–802.
85. Chen H, Nicol TL, Zeiger MA, Dooley WC, Ladenson PW, Cooper DS, Ringel M, Parkerson S, Allo M, Udelsman R. Hürthle cell neoplasms of the thyroid—Are there factors predictive of malignancy? Ann Surg 1998; 227:542–546.
86. Evans HL, Vassilopoulou-Sellin R. Follicular and Hürthle cell carcinomas of the thyroid—a comparative study. Am J Surg Pathol 1998; 22:1512–1520.
87. McDonald MP, Sanders LE, Silverman ML, Chan HS, Buyske J. Hürthle cell carcinoma of the thyroid gland: prognostic factors and results of surgical treatment. Surgery 1996; 120:1000–1004.
88. Papotti M, Torchio B, Grassi L, Favero A, Bussolati G. Poorly differentiated oxyphilic (Hürthle cell) carcinomas of the thyroid. Am J Surg Pathol 1996; 20:686–694.
89. Arganini M, Behar R, Wu TC, Straus F2d, McCormick M, DeGroot LJ, Kaplan EL. Hürthle cell tumors: a twenty-five-year experience. Surgery 1986; 100:1108–1115.
90. Thompson NW, Dunn EL, Batsakis JG, Nishiyama RH. Hürthle cell lesions of the thyroid gland. Surg Gynecol Obstet 1973; 139:555–560.
91. Samaan NA, Schultz PN, Hickey RC, Haynie TP, Johnston DA, Ordonez NG. Well-differentiated thyroid carcinoma and the results of various modalities of treatment. A retrospective review of 1599 patients. J Clin Endocrinol Metab 1992; 75:714–720.
92. Ruegemer JJ, Hay ID, Bergstralh EJ, Ryan JJ, Offord KP, Gorman CA. Distant metastases in differentiated thyroid carcinoma: a multivariate analysis of prognostic variables. J Clin Endocrinol Metab 1988; 67:501–558.
93. Hassoun AAK, Hay ID, Goellner JR, Zimmerman D. Insular thyroid carcinoma in adolescents—a potentially lethal endocrine malignancy. Cancer 1997; 79:1044–1048.
94. Yang YJ, Haghir S, Wanamaker JR, Powers CN. Diagnosis of papillary carcinoma in a thyroglossal duct cyst by fine-needle aspiration biopsy. Arch Pathol Lab Med 2000; 124(1):139–142.
95. McHenry CR, Danish R, Murphy T, Marty JJ. Atypical thyroglossal duct cyst: a rare cause for a solitary cold thyroid nodule in childhood. Am Surg 1993; 59(4):223–228.
96. Hatada T, Ichii S, Sagayama K, Ishii H, Sugihara A, Terada N, Yamamura T. Intrathyroid thyroglossal duct cyst simulating a thyroid nodule. Tumori 2000; 86(3):250–252.
97. North JH Jr, Foley AM, Hamill RL. Intrathyroid cysts of thyroglossal duct origin. Am Surg 1998; 64(9):886–888.
98. Weiss SD, Orlich CC. Primary papillary carcinoma of a thyroglossal duct cyst: report of a case and literature review. Br J Surg 1991; 78:87–89.
99. Ewing CA, Kornblut A, Greeley C, Manz H. Presentations of thyroglossal duct cysts in adults. Eur Arch Otorhinolaryngol 1999; 256 (3):136–138.
100. Montero GC, Keituqwa YT, Alvarez DJ, Marques RL, Blasco HA. [Papillary carcinoma on thyroglossal duct cyst]. Acta Otorrinolaringol Esp 2001; 52(1):75–78.
101. Miccoli P, Pacini F, Basolo S, Iacconi P, Puccini M, Pinchera A. [Thyroid carcinoma in a thyroglossal duct cyst: tumor resection alone or a total thyroidectomy?]. Ann Chir 1998; 52(5):452–454.
102. Glastonbury CM, Davidson HC, Haller JR, Harnsberger HR. The CT and MR imaging features of carcinoma arising in thyroglossal duct remnants. Am J Neuroradiol 2000; 21(4):770–774.
103. Kaplan HJ, Tamkin JA. Invasive thyroglossal duct carcinoma in childhood. Ear Nose Throat J 1989; 68(6):460–462, 464.
104. Kurzen F, Flugel W, Brauer CF, Schneider W, Adler D. [Papillary carcinoma of the thyroid in a thyroglossal duct cyst with metastasis to an ipsilateral cervical lymph node]. HNO 1999; 47(8):741–744.

105. Page CP, Kemmerer WT, Haff RC, Mazzaferri EL. Thyroid carcinomas arising in thyroglossal ducts. Ann Surg 1974; 180:799–803.
106. Cervera-Paz FJ, Roquette GJ, Bartual PJ. [Ectopic primitive thyroid papillary carcinoma: report of a fatal case and review of literature]. Acta Otorrinolaringol Esp 1994; 45(2):124–127.
107. Danese D, Gardini A, Farsetti A, Sciacchitano S, Andreoli M, Pontecorvi A. Thyroid carcinoma in children and adolescents. Eur J Pediatr 1997; 156:190–194.
108. Attie JN, Setzin M, Klein I. Thyroid carcinoma presenting as an enlarged cervical lymph node. Am J Surg 1993; 166:428–430.
109. Shah JP, Loree TR, Dharker D, Strong EW, Begg C, Vlamis V. Prognostic factors in differentiated carcinoma of the thyroid gland. Am J Surg 1992; 164:658–661.
110. Frankenthaler RA, Sellin RV, Cangir A, Goepfert H. Lymph node metastasis from papillary-follicular thyroid carcinoma in youngpatients. Am J Surg 1990; 160:341–343.
111. Hay ID, Bergstralh EJ, Goellner JR, Ebersold JR, Grant CS. Predicting outcome in papillary thyroid carcinoma: development of a reliable prognostic scoring system in a cohort of 1779 patients surgically treated at one institution during 1940 through 1989. Surgery 1993; 114:1050–1058.
112. Cady B. Staging in thyroid carcinoma. Cancer 1998; 83:844–847.
113. DeGroot LJ, Kaplan EL, McCormick M, Straus FH. Natural history, treatment, and course of papillary thyroid carcinoma. J Clin Endocrinol Metab 1990; 71:414–424.
114. Tsang TW, Brierley JD, Simpson WJ, Panzarella T, Gospodarowicz MK, Sutcliffe SB. The effects of surgery, radioiodine, and external radiation therapy on the clinical outcome of patients with differentiated thyroid carcinoma. Cancer 1998; 82:375–388.
115. Simpson WJ, McKinney SE, Carruthers JS, Gospodarowicz MK, Sutcliffe SB, Panzarella T. Papillary and follicular thyroid cancer. Prognostic factors in 1,578 patients. Am J Med 1987; 83:479–488.
116. Herrera MF, López-Graniel CM, Saldaña J, Gamboa-Dominguez A, Richaud-Patín Y, Vargas-Vorackova F, Angeles-Angeles A, Llorente L, Castillo C, Pérez B, Rivera R, González O, Rull J. Papillary thyroid carcinoma in Mexican patients: clinical aspects and prognostic factors. World J Surg 1996; 20:94–100.
117. Yamashita H, Noguchi S, Murakami N, Kawamoto H, Watanabe S. Extracapsular invasion of lymph node metastasis is an indicator of distant metastasis and poor prognosis in patients with thyroid papillary carcinoma. Cancer 1997; 80:2268–2272.
118. Kurozumi K, Nakao I, Nishida T, Nakahara M, Ogino N, Tsujimoto M. Significance of biologic aggressiveness and proliferating activityin papillary thyroid carcinoma. World J Surg 1998; 22:1237–1242.
119. Akslen LA, Varhaug JE. Oncoproteins and tumor progression in papillary thyroid carcinoma—presence of epidermal growth factor receptor, c-erbB-2 protein, estrogen receptor related protein, p21-ras protein, and proliferation indicators in relation to tumor recurrences and patient survival. Cancer 1995; 76:1643–1654.
120. Sellers M, Beenken S, Blankenship A, Soong S, Turbat-Herrera E, Urist M, Maddox W. Prognostic significance of cervical lymph node metastases in differentiated thyroid cancer. Am J Surg 1992; 164: 578–581.
121. Lindegaard MW, Paus E, Hie J, Kullman G, Stenwig AE. Thyroglobulin radioimmunoassay and 131I scintiraphy in patients with differentiated thyroid carcinoma. Acta Chir Scand 1988; 154:141–215.
122. Samaan NA, Schultz PN, Haynie TP, Ordonez NG. Pulmonary metastasis of differentiated thyroid carcinoma: treatment results in 101 patients. J Clin Endocrinol Metab 1985; 60:376–380.
123. Pittas AG, Adler M, Fazzari M, Tickoo S, Rosai J, Larson SM, Robbins RJ. Bone metastases from thyroid carcinoma: clinical characteristics and prognostic variables in one hundred forty-six patients. Thyroid 2000; 10(3):261–268.
124. Kitamura Y, Shimizu K, Nagahama M, Sugino K, Ozaki O, Mimura T, Ito K, Tanaka S. Immediate causes of death in thyroid carcinoma: clinicopathological analysis of 161 fatal cases. J Clin Endocrinol Metab 1999; 84:4043–4049.
125. Schlumberger M, Challeton C, De Vathaire F, Parmentier C. Treatment of distant metastases of differentiated thyroid carcinoma. J Endocrinol Invest 1995; 18:170–172
126. Sisson JC, Giordano TJ, Jamadar DA, Kazerooni EA, Shapiro B, Gross MD, Zempel SA, Spaulding SA. 131-I treatment of micronodular pulmonary metastases from papillary thyroid carcinoma. Cancer 1996; 78:2184–2192.
127. Bernier MO, Leenhardt L, Hoang C, Aurengo A, Mary JY, Menegaux F, Enkaoua E, Turpin G, Chiras J, Saillant G, Hejblum G. Survival and therapeutic modalities in patients with bone metastases of differentiated thyroid carcinomas. J Clin Endocrinol Metab 2001; 86(4):1568–1573.
128. Schlumberger M, Tubiana M, De Vathaire F, Hill C, Gardet P, Travagli JP, Fragu P, Lumbroso J, Caillou B, Parmentier C. Long-term results of treatment of 283 patients with lung and bone metastases from differentiated thyroid carcinoma. J Clin Endocrinol Metab 1986; 63:960–967.
129. Brown AP, Greening WP, McCready VR, Shaw HJ, Harmer CL. Radioiodine treatment of metastatic thyroid carcinoma: the Royal Marsden Hospital experience. Br J Radiol 1984; 57:323–327.

130. Casara D, Rubello D, Saladini G, Masarotto G, Favero A, Girelli ME, Busnardo B. Different features of pulmonary metastases in differentiated thyroid cancer: natural history and multivariate statistical analysis of prognostic variables. J Nucl Med 1993; 34:1626–1631.
131. Schlumberger M, Challeton C, De Vathaire F, Travagli JP, Gardet P, Lumbroso JD, Francese C, Fontaine F, Ricard M, Parmentier C. Radioactive iodine treatment and external radiotherapy for lung and bone metastases from thyroid carcinoma. J Nucl Med 1996; 37:598–605.
132. Vassilopoulou-Sellin R, Klein MJ, Smith TH, Samaan NA, Frankenthaler RA, Goepfert H, Cangir A, Haynie TP. Pulmonary metastases in children and young adults with differentiated thyroid cancer. Cancer 1993; 71:1348–1352.
133. Hundahl SA, Cady B, Cunningham MP, Mazzaferri E, McKee RF, Rosai J, Shah JP, Fremgen AM, Stewart AK, Holzer S. Initial results from a prospective cohort study of 5583 cases of thyroid carcinoma treated in the united states during 1996. U.S. and German Thyroid Cancer Study Group. An American College of Surgeons Commission on Cancer Patient Care Evaluation study. Cancer 2000; 89(1):202–217.
134. Holzer S, Reiners C, Mann K, Bamberg M, Rothmund M, Dudeck J, Stewart AK, Hundahl SA. Patterns of care for patients with primary differentiated carcinoma of the thyroid gland treated in Germany during 1996. U.S. and German Thyroid Cancer Group. Cancer 2000; 89(1):192–201.
135. Bennedbaek FN, Hegedus L. Management of the solitary thyroid nodule: results of a North American survey. J Clin Endocrinol Metab 2000; 85(7):2493–2498.
136. Ortiz R, Hupart KH, DeFesi CR, Surks MI. Effect of early referral to an endocrinologist on efficiency and cost of evaluation and development of treatment plan in patients with thyroid nodules. J Clin Endocrinol Metab 1998; 83(11):3803–3807.
137. American Joint Committee on Cancer. Head and neck tumors. Thyroid gland. In: Beahrs OH, Henson DE, Hutter RVP, Myers MH, ed. Manual for Staging of Cancer. Philadelphia: J.B. Lippincott, 1992: 53–54.
138. Cady B, Sedgwick CE, Meissner WA, Wool MS, Salzman FA, Werber J. Risk factor analysis in differentiated thyroid cancer. Cancer 1979; 43:810–820.
139. DeGroot LJ, Kaplan EL, Straus FH, Shukla MS. Does the method of management of papillary thyroid carcinoma make a difference in outcome? World J Surg 1994; 18:123–130.
140. Sherman SI, Brierley JD, Sperling M, Ain KB, Bigos ST, Cooper DS, Haugen BR, Ho MN, Klein I, Ladenson PW, Robbins J, Ross DS, Specker B, Taylor T, Maxon HR III, National Thyroid Cancer Treatment Cooperative Study Registry Group. Prospective multicenter study of thyroid carcinoma treatment–initial analysis of staging and outcome. Cancer 1998; 83:1012–1021.
141. Byar DP, Green SB, Dor P, Williams D, Colon J, van Gilse.H.A., Mayer M, Sylvester RF, Van Glabbede M. A prognostic index for thyroid carcinoma. A study of the E.O.R.T.C. Thyroid Cancer Cooperative Group. Eur J Cancer 1979; 15:1033–1041.
142. Hay ID. Papillary thyroid carcinoma. Endocrinol Metabol Clin North Am 1990; 19:545–576.
143. Cady B, Rossi R. An expanded view of risk-group definition in differentiated thyroid carcinoma. Surgery 1988; 104:947–953.
144. Tennvall J, Biorklund A, Moller T, Ranstam J, Akerman M. Is the EORTC prognostic index of thyroid cancer valid in differentiated thyroid carcinoma? Retrospective multivariate analysis of differentiated thyroid carcinoma with long follow-up. Cancer 1986; 57:1405–1414.
145. Cady B. Our AMES is true: how an old concept still hits the mark: or, risk group assignment points the arrow to rational therapy selection in differentiated thyroid cancer. Am J Surg 1997; 174:462–468.
146. Hundahl SA, Fleming ID, Fremgen AM, Menck HR. A National Cancer Data Base report on 53,856 cases of thyroid carcinoma treated in the US, 1985–1995. Cancer 1998; 83:2638–2648.
147. Van De Velde CJH, Hamming JF, Goslings BM, Schelfhout LJDM, Clark OH, Smeds S, Bruining HA, Krenning EP, Cady B. Report of the consensus development conference on the management of differntiated thyroid cancer in the Netherlands. Eur J CancerClin Oncol 1988; 24:287–292.
148. Baldet L, Manderscheid JC, Glinoer D, Jaffiol C, Coste Seignovert B, Percheron C. The management of differentiated thyroid cancer in Europe in 1988. Results of an international survey. Acta Endocrinol (Copenh) 1989; 120:547–558.
149. Solomon BL, Wartofsky L, Burman KD. Current trends in the management of well differentiated papillary thyroid carcinoma. J Clin Endocrinol Metab 1996; 81:333–339.
150. Yang GC, Liebeskind D, Messina AV. Ultrasound-guided fine-needle aspiration of the thyroid assessed by Ultrafast Papanicolaou stain: data from 1135 biopsies with a two- to six-year follow-up. Thyroid 2001; 11(6):581–589.
151. Boyd LA, Earnhardt RC, Dunn JT, Frierson HF, Hanks JB. Preoperative evaluation and predictive value of fine-needle aspiration and frozen section of thyroid nodules. J Am Coll Surgeons 1998; 187:494–502.
152. Hamming JF, Vriens MR, Goslings BM, Songun I, Fleuren GJ, Van De Velde CJH. Role of fine-needle aspiration biopsy and frozen section examination in determining the extent of thyroidectomy. World J Surg 1998; 22:575–580.

153. Mulcahy MM, Cohen JI, Anderson PE, Ditamasso J, Schmidt W. Relative accuracy of fine-needle aspiration and frozen section in the diagnosis of well-differentiated thyroid cancer. Laryngoscope 1998; 108:494–496.
154. Udelsman R, Westra WH, Donovan PI, Sohn TA, Cameron JL. Randomized prospective evaluation of frozen-section analysis for follicular neoplasms of the thyroid. Ann Surg 2001; 233(5):716–722.
155. McHenry CR, Raeburn C, Strickland T, Marty JJ. The utility of routine frozen section examination for intraoperative diagnosis of thyroid cancer. Am J Surg 1996; 172:658–661.
156. Lin HS, Komisar A, Opher E, Blaugrund SM. Surgical management of thyroid masses: assessing the need for frozen section evaluation. Laryngoscope 1999; 109(6):868–873.
157. Pasieka JL, Rotstein LE. Consensus conference on well-differentiated thyroid cancer: a summary. Can J Surg 1999; 36:298–301.
158. Cady B, Hay ID, Shaha AR, Clark OH, Rossi R, Dudley N. Unilateral total lobectomy: Is it sufficient surgical treatment for patients with AMES low-risk papillary thyroid carcinoma? Discussion. Surgery 1998; 124:964–966.
159. Hay ID, Grant CS, Taylor WF, McConahey WM. Ipsilateral lobectomy versus bilateral lobar resection in papillary thyroid carcinoma: a retrospective analysis of surgical outcome using a novel prognostic scoring system. Surgery 1987; 102:1088–1095.
160. Hay ID, Grant CS, Bergstralh EJ, Thompson GB, van Heerden JA. Unilateral total lobectomy: Is it sufficient surgical treatment for patients with AMES low-risk papillary thyroid carcinoma? Surgery 1998; 124:958–966.
161. Sarda AK, Bal S, Kapur MM. Near-total thyroidectomy for carcinoma of the thyroid. Br J Surg 1989; 76:90–92.
162. Mazzaferri EL. Carcinoma of follicular epithelium: radioiodine and other treatment outcomes. In: Braverman LE, Utiger RD, eds. The Thyroid: A Fundamental and Clinical Text. Philadelphia: Lippincott Williams & Wilkins., 2000: 904–929.
163. Mazzaferri EL. An overview of the management of papillar and follicular thyroid carcinoma. Thyroid 1999; 9:421–427.
164. Schlumberger MJ. Medical progress—papillary and follicular thyroid carcinoma. N Engl J Med 1998; 338:297–306.
165. Mazzaferri EL. Treating differentiated thyroid carcinoma: Where do we draw the line? Mayo Clin Proc 1991; 66:105–111.
166. Newman KD, Black T, Heller G, Azizkhan RG, Holcomb GW III, Sklar C, Vlamis V, Haase GM, La Quaglia MP. Differentiated thyroid cancer: determinants of disease progression in patients <21 years of age at diagnosis—a report from the Surgical Discipline Committee of the Children's Cancer Group. Ann Surg 1998; 227:533–541.
167. Miccoli P, Antonelli A, Spinelli C, Ferdeghini M, Fallahi P, Baschieri L. Completion total thyroidectomy in children with thyroid cancer secondary to the Chernobyl accident. Arch Surg 1998; 133:89–93.
168. Paphavasit A, Thompson GB, Hay ID, Grant CS, van Heerden JA, Ilstrup DM, Schleck C, Goellner JR. Follicular and Hürthle cell thyroid neoplasms—Is frozen-section evaluation worthwhile? Arch Surg 1997; 132:674–679.
169. Hamburger JI, Hamburger SW. Declining role of frozen section in surgical planning for thyroid nodules. Surgery 1985; 98:307–312.
170. Keller MP, Grabbe MM, Norwood SH. Accuracy and significance of fine-needle aspiration and frozen section in determining the extent of thyroid resection. Surgery 1987; 101:632–635.
171. Bugis SP, Young JE, Archibald SD, Chen VS. Diagnostic accuracy of fine-needle aspiration biopsy versus frozen section in solitary thyroid nodules. Am J Surg 1986; 152(4):411–416.
172. Yoo KS, Chengazi VU, O'Mara RE. Thyroglossal duct cyst with papillary carcinoma in an 11-year-old girl. J Pediatr Surg 1998; 33:745–746.
173. Tradati N, DePaoli F, Benazzo M, Andrle J, Calabrese L, Giugliano G, Gibelli B, Zurrida S, Chiesa F. Papillary carcinoma in thyroglossal duct remnants: presentation ofour cases and decision procedure for prophylactic thyroid gland dissection. Oncol Rep 2000; 7(6):1349–1353.
174. Falconieri G, Della LD, Zanella M. Papillar thyroid carcinoma of the thyroglossal duct cyst: comparative cytohistologic and immunochemical study of 2 new cases and review of the literature. Int J Surg Pathol 2001; 9(1):65–71.
175. Sisson GA, Feldman DE. The management of thyroid carcinoma metastatic to theneck and mediastinum. Otolaryngol Clin North Am 1980; 13:119–126.
176. Cholewinski SP, Yoo KS, Klieger PS, O'Mara RE. Absence of thyroid stunning after diagnostic whole-body scanning with 185 MBq 131I. J Nucl Med 2000; 41(7):1198–1202.
177. Maxon HR, Englaro EE, Thomas SR, Hertzberg VS, Hinnefeld JD, Chen LS, Smith H, Cummings D, Aden MD. Radioiodine-131 therapy for well-differentiated thyroid cancer—a quantitative radiation dosimetric approach: outcome and validation in 85 patients. J Nucl Med 1992; 33:1132–1136.
178. Auguste LJ, Attie JN. Completion thyroidectomy for initially misdiagnosed thyroid cancer. Otolaryngol Clin North Am 1990; 23:429–439.
179. Sanders LE, Cady B. Differentiated thyroid cancer—reexamination of risk groups and outcome of treatment. Arch Surg 1998; 133:419–424.

180. Chao TC, Jeng LB, Lin JD, Chen MF. Completion thyroidectomy for differentiated thyroid carcinoma. Otolaryngol Head Neck Surg 1998; 118:896–899.
181. Mettlin C, Lee F, Drago J, Murphy GP. The American Cancer Society National Prostate Cancer Detection Project. Cancer 1991; 67(12):2929–2958.
182. De Jong SA, Demeter JG, Lawrence AM, Paloyan E. Necessity and safety of completion thyroidectomy for differentiated thyroid carcinoma. Surgery 1992; 112:734–737.
183. Pasieka JL, Thompson NW, McLeod MK, Burney RE, Macha M. The incidence of bilateral well-differentiated thyroid cancer found at completion thyroidectomy. World J Surg 1992; 16:711–716.
184. Scheumann GFW, Gimm O, Wegener G, Hundeshagen H, Dralle H. Prognostic significance and surgical management of locoregional lymph node metastases in papillar thyroid cancer. World J Surg 1994; 18:559–568.
185. Mirallie E, Visset J, Sagan C, Hamy A, Le Bodic MF, Paineau J. Localization of cervical node metastasis of papillary thyroid carcinoma. World J Surg 1999; 23 (9):970–973.
186. Arch-Ferrer J, Velazquez D, Fajardo R, Gamboa-Dominguez A, Herrera MF. Accuracy of sentinel lymph node in papillar thyroid carcinoma. Surgery 2001; 130(6):907–913.
187. Travagli JP, Cailleux AF, Ricard M, Baudin E, Caillou B, Parmentier C, Schlumberger M. Combination of radioiodine (131I) and probe-guided surgery for persistent or recurrent thyroid carcinoma. J Clin Endocrinol Metab 1998; 83(8):2675–2680.
188. McCaffrey TV, Bergstralh EJ, Hay ID. Locally invasive papillary thyroid carcinoma: 1940–1990. Head Neck 1994; 16(2):165–172.
189. Ballantyne AJ. Resections of the upper aerodigestive tract for locally invasive thyroid cancer. Am J Surg 1994; 168:636–639.
190. Tanaka K, Sonoo H, Yamamoto Y, Udagawa K, Arime I, Kunisue H, Yamamoto S, Kurebayashi J, Shimozuma K. Analyses of the outcome of locally invasive papillary thyroid carcinomas. Thyroid 1999; 9(10):1017–1022.
191. Fujimoto Y, Obara T, Ito Y, Kodama T, Yashiro T, Yamashita T, Nozaki M, Suzuki K. Aggressive surgical approach for locally invasive papillary carcinoma of the thyroid in patients over forty-five years of age. Surgery 1986; 100:1098–1106.
192. Holting T, Meybier H, Buhr H. [Problems of tracheotomy in locally invasive anaplastic thyroid cancer]. Langenbecks Arch Chir 1989; 374:72–76.
193. Burge MR, Zeise TM, Johnsen MW, Conway MJ, Qualls CR. Risks of complication following thyroidectomy. J Gen Intern Med 1998; 13:24–31.
194. Dralle H, Gimm O, Simon D, Frank-Raue K, Görtz G, Niederle B, Wahl RA, Koch B, Walgenbach S, Hampel R, Ritter MM, Spelsberg F, Heiss A, Hinze R, Höppner W. Prophylactic thyroidectomy in 75 children and adolescents with hereditary medullary thyroid carcinoma: German and Austrian experience. World J Surg 1998; 22:744–751.
195. Udelsman R, Lakatos E, Ladenson P. Optimal surgery for papillary thyroid carcinoma. World J Surg 1996; 20:88–93.
196. Pattou F, Combemale F, Fabre S, Carnaille B, Decoulx M, Wemeau JL, Racadot A, Proye C. Hypocalcemia following thyroid surgery: Incidence and prediction of outcome. World J Surg 1998; 22:718–724.
197. Sosa JA, Bowman HM, Tielsch JM, Powe NR, Gordon TA, Udelsman R. The importance of surgeon experience for clinical and economic outcomes from thyroidectomy. Ann Surg 1998; 228:320–328.
198. Driggers RW, Kopelman JN, Satin AJ. Delaying surgery for thyroid cancer in pregnancy—a case report. J Reprod Med 1998; 43:909–912.
199. Moosa M, Mazzaferri EL. Outcome of differentiated thyroid cancer diagnosed in pregnant women. J Clin Endocrinol Metab 1997; 82:2862–2866.
200. Vini L, Hyer S, Pratt B, Harmer C. Management of differentiated thyroid cancer diagnosed during pregnancy. Eur J Endocrinol 1999; 140:404–406.
201. Robbins RJ, Tuttle RM, Sonenberg M, Shaha A, Sharaf R, Robbins H, Fleisher M, Larson SM. Radioiodine ablation of thyroid remnants after preparation with recombinant human thyrotropin. Thyroid 2001; 11(9):865–869.
202. Goldman JM, Line BR, Aamodt RL, Robbins J. Influence of triiodothyronine withdrawal time on 131-I uptake postthyroidectomy for thyroid cancer. J Clin Endocrinol Metab 1980; 50:734–739.
203. Spencer CA, Takeuchi M, Kazarosyan M, Wang CC, Guttler RB, Singer PA, Fatemi S, LoPresti JS, Nicoloff JT. Serum thyroglobulin autoantibodies: prevalence, influence on serum thyroglobulin measurement, and prognostic significance in patients with differentiated thyroid carcinoma. J Clin Endocrinol Metab 1998; 83:1121–1127.
204. Schlumberger M, Mancusi F, Baudin E, Pacini F. 131–I therapy for elevated thyroglobulin levels. Thyroid 1997; 7:273–276.
205. Wartofsky L, Sherman SI, Gopal J, Schlumberger M, Hay ID. The use of radioactive iodine in patients with papillary and follicular thyroid cancer. J Clin Endocrinol Metab 1998; 83:4195–4199.
206. Grünwald F, Menzel C, Fimmers R, Zamora PO, Biersack HJ. Prognostic value of thyroglobulin after thyroidectomy before ablative radioiodine therapy in thyroid cancer. J Nucl Med 1996; 37:1962–1964.
207. Schlumberger M. Use of radioactive iodine in patients with papillary and follicular thyroid cancer: towards a selective approach. J Clin Endocrinol Metab 1998; 83:4201–4203.

HP. Thyroid carcinoma in childhood: management and follow up of 11 cases. Eur J Pediatr 1994; 153:17–22.

258. Samuel AM, Sharma SM. Differentiated thyroid carcinomas in children and adolescents. Cancer 1991; 67:2186–2190.
259. Musholt TJ, Musholt PB, Petrich T, Oetting G, Knapp WH, Klempnauer J. Familial papillary thyroid carcinoma: genetics, criteria for diagnosis, clinical features, and surgical treatment. World J Surg 2000; 24(11):1409–1417.
260. Jarzab B, Handkiewicz JD, Wloch J, Kalemba B, Roskosz J, Kukulska A, Puch Z. Multivariate analysis of prognostic factors for differentiated thyroid carcinoma in children. Eur J Nucl Med 2000; 27(7):833–841.
261. Welch Dinauer DA, Tuttle RM, Robie DK, McClellan DR, Francis GL. Extensive surgery improves recurrence-free survival for children and young patients with class I papillary thyroid carcinoma. J Pediatr Surg 1999; 34(12):1799–1804.
262. Hung W, Sarlis NJ. Current controversies in the management of pediatric patients with well-differentiated non-medullary thyroid cancer: a review. Thyroid 2002; 12:1490–1498.

14

Anaplastic Thyroid Carcinoma

Arthur E. Schwartz and Margaret Brandwein-Gensler

Mount Sinai School of Medicine, New York University, New York, New York, U.S.A.

Anaplastic thyroid carcinoma (ATC) is the dark side of thyroid malignancy. One can only wonder why the thyrocyte, the progenitor of the usually easily controlled well-differentiated thyroid cancers, also gives rise to virulent, relentless, and almost universally lethal anaplastic thyroid cancer (Fig. 1). Although only 2–5% of thyroid carcinomas are anaplastic, they account for approximately 50% of the 1200 annual deaths in the United States from thyroid malignancy (1). In the United States from 1973 to 1991, ATC constituted 1.4% of thyroid cancer with an estimated yearly incidence of 1.6%. This represents an annual incidence of 300 cases (2).

The outlook for survival is poor. In most series life expectancy is measured in months from the time of diagnosis. The overall average is 3–6 months, but some patients survive 2 or more years (Fig. 2). Despite aggressive treatment, the cause of death is frequently the inability to control local neck disease.

1 DEMOGRAPHICS

As in most thyroid conditions, benign and malignant, the incidence of ATC is more prevalent in women than men. Some series report a ratio of 3 or 2 to 1, as in most other thyroid disease, while others find anaplastic carcinoma to have less of a predilection for women, citing a ratio of 1.5 female to 1 male (1,3). Anaplastic thyroid cancer is usually an affliction of the elderly, from the seventh to ninth decades of life; it is rarely diagnosed in individuals younger than 50 years of age (Fig. 3). In contrast to differentiated thyroid cancer, the prognosis is not closely related to the age of onset, although younger patient are said by some to survive somewhat longer than those of advanced age. Despite the aging of the general population as a result of increased life expectancy, the incidence of ATC appears to be decreasing. Although some of the observed decline may be the result of more stringent histological requirements, the trend appears real. The proportion of ATC in Bombay decreased from 7.7 to 4.2% from the period of 1969–73 to 1989–93, although the number of thyroid cancers more than tripled during this period (4). A similar decrease in the proportion of anaplastic thyroid carcinoma to well-differentiated thyroid cancer has been reported from Italy (5).

2 CLINICAL PRESENTATION

A rapidly expanding neck mass, often painful, heralds the disease in almost all patients. In most cases the tumor is already substantial in size (5–6 cm) at the time of presentation. The most common symptoms are directly due to the expansion and infiltration of the tumor in the neck. Difficulties in swallowing, speaking, and breathing appear in over 30% of patients. Hoarseness, which may be a reflection of recurrent nerve involvement, is present in a similar proportion. Neck pain, weight loss, and cough are common companions to these symptoms. These findings are rare in patients

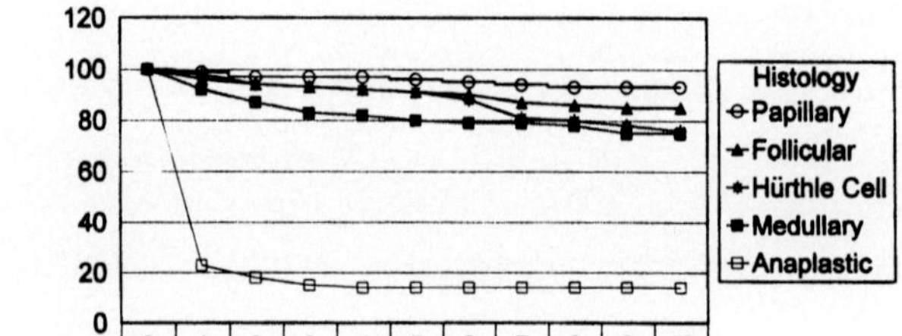

	0	1	2	3	4	5	6	7	8	9	10
Papillary	100	99	97	97	97	96	95	94	93	93	93
Follicular	100	96	94	93	92	91	90	87	86	85	85
Hürthle Cell	100	98	94	93	92	91	88	81	80	78	76
Medullary	100	92	87	83	82	80	79	79	78	75	75
Anaplastic	100	23	18	15	14	14	14	14	14	14	14

Years after Diagnosis

Figure 1 Relative survival by histology of thyroid carcinomas diagnosed between 1985–1990. (From Ref. 36.)

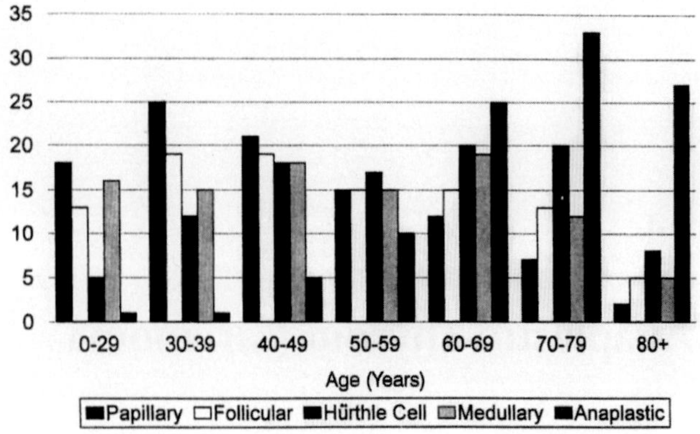

Figure 3 Age distribution (in percent) of thyroid carcinoma by histology. (From Ref. 36.)

with well-differentiated thyroid cancer and are therefore ominous signs when they present in an older patient.

Half of the patients have disseminated metastases at presentation: 90% in lungs, 15% in bone, and 15% in brain (6). Neck nodes are usually involved, but this may not be clinically apparent because fascial planes do not restrain the primary tumor. It may impossible to identify the lymph nodes in the overall mass (Fig. 4). Tumor quickly invades the thyroid capsule and adjacent structures. Soft tissues of the neck, cervical musculature, as well as trachea and esophagus are penetrated by direct extension; the initial finding is often a large inclusive irregular mass. Direct tracheal invasion is not unusual (Fig. 5) (see also Chapter 8). Tracheostomy is often required for survival; it was performed in 42 of 82 cases, as reported by Nel et al., sometimes as a prelude to radiotherapy (7). Pulmonary metastases were found in 87% of fatal cases reported by Silverberg et al. (8). Although metasases appear most frequently in the lungs and bones, pleura, liver, adrenal, pancreas, and other distant sites may also be involved (9). In an autopsy study of 15 patients who died from ATC, all had pulmonary metastases, 80% had metastases in bone, 60% in soft tissues of the neck, 27% in the trachea, and more than half to other soft tissues of the body (10). The

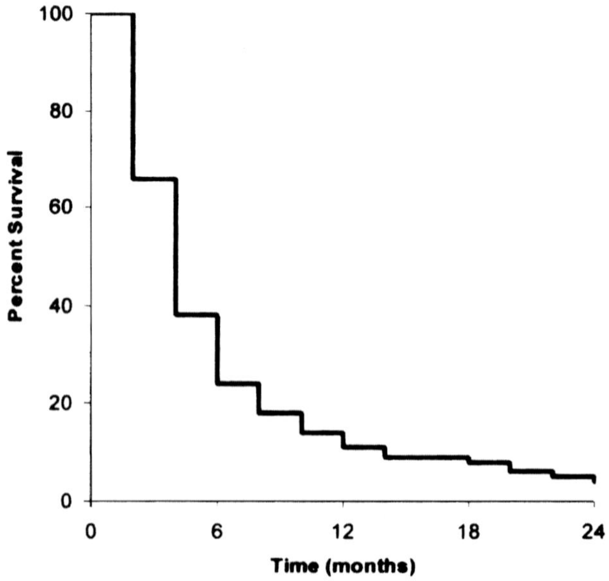

Figure 2 Overall survival after a diagnosis of anaplastic thyroid carcinoma. (From Ref. 1.)

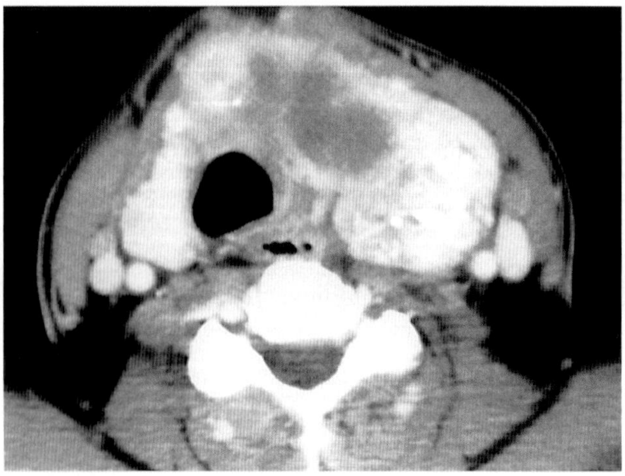

Figure 4 CT scan showing a large invasive anaplastic thyroid carcinoma extending into adjacent tissues and displacing the trachea. (Courtesy of Dr. Peter Sam.)

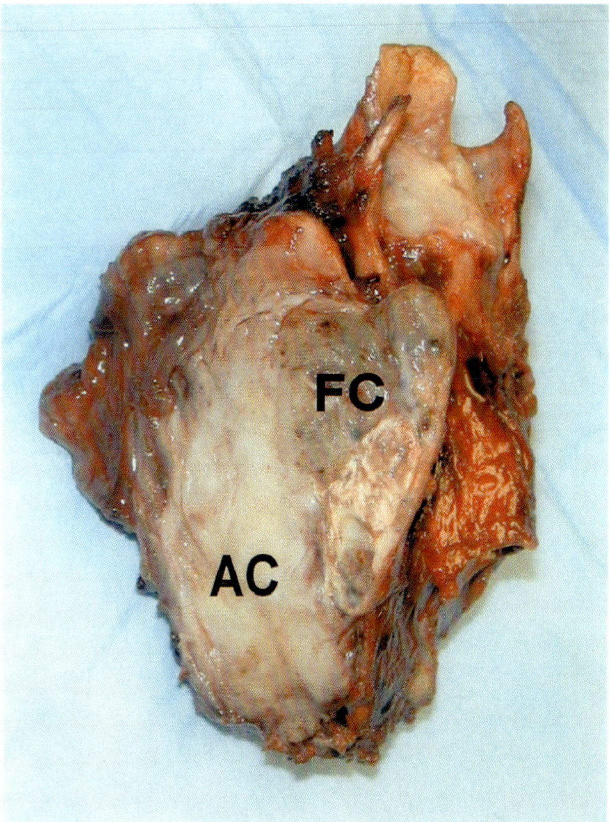

Figure 5 Total laryngectomy with anaplastic thyroid carcinoma (AC), transformation from follicular carcinoma (FC). Distinct differences can be appreciated on gross examination between these two malignant components.

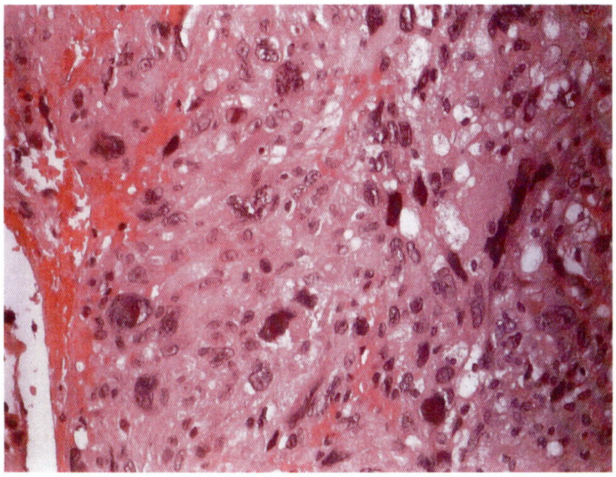

Figure 7 Anaplastic thyroid carcinoma composed of highly pleomorphic tumor cells.

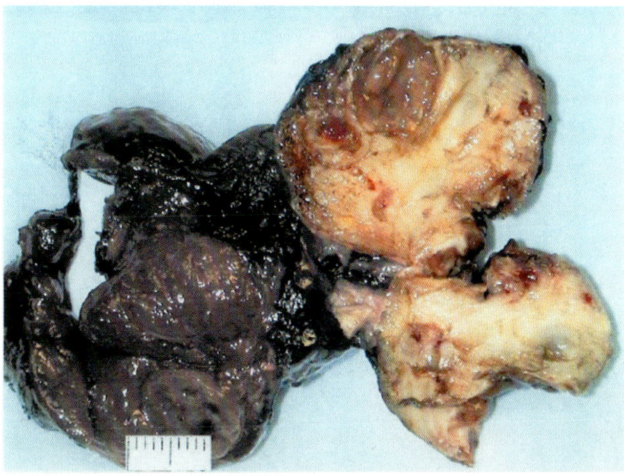

Figure 6 Thyroidectomy resection specimen showing a localized, scar-like example of anaplastic thyroid carcinoma.

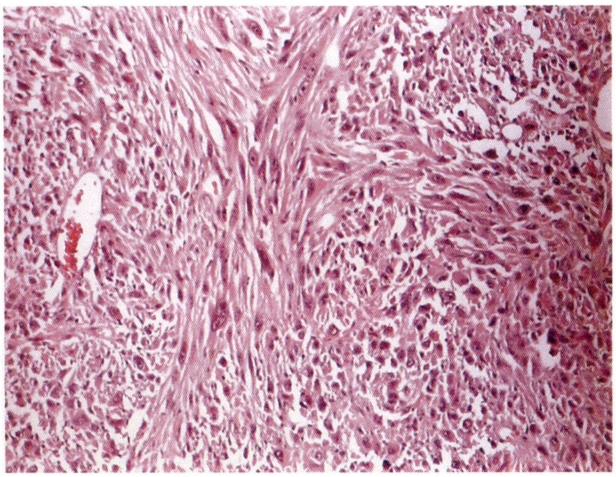

Figure 8 Anaplastic thyroid carcinoma with sarcomatoid spindle cells.

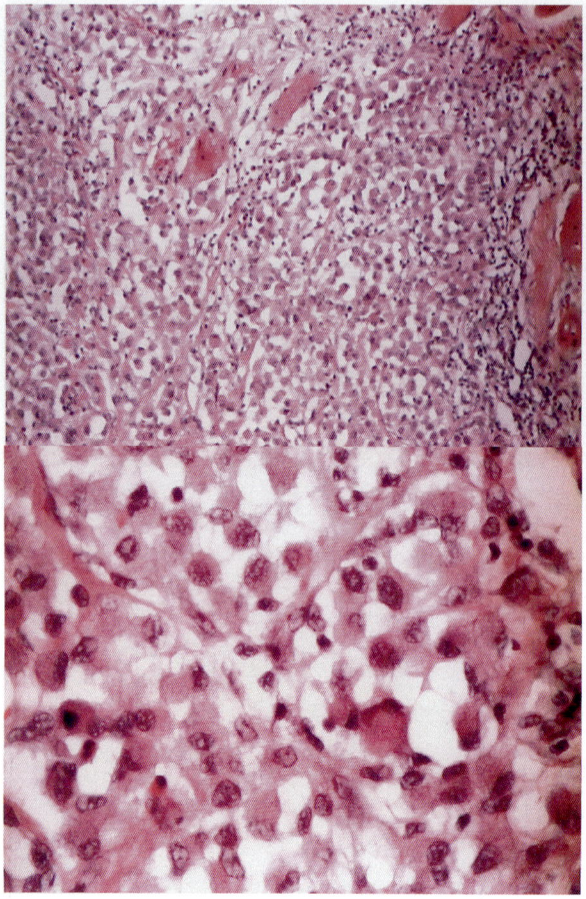

Figure 9 Anaplastic thyroid carcinoma composed of discohesive malignant round cells. This appearance may lead to the misdiagnosis of malignant lymphoma. Conversely some large or small cell lymphomas can be misdiagnosed as anaplastic thyroid cancer: (top) low power; (bottom) high power.

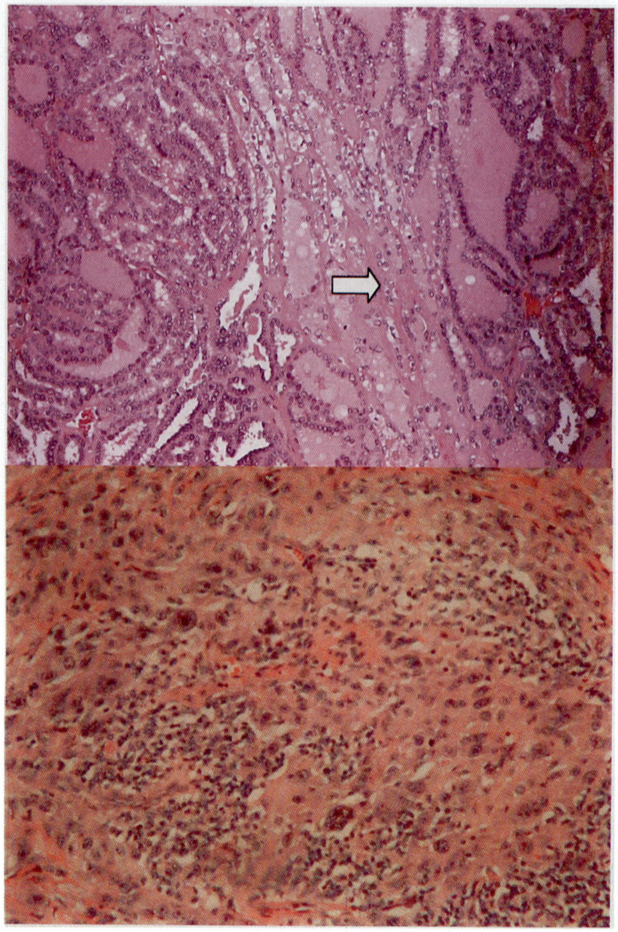

Figure 10 Papillary thyroid carcinoma with progression to anaplastic thyroid carcinoma: (top) Papillary thyroid carcinoma with necrosis (arrow), an unusually finding for papillary carcinoma; (bottom) pleomorphic tumor cells indicating progression to anaplastic thyroid carcinoma, taken from the same specimen.

disease is almost always widely disseminated at the time it presents, and the lethal outcome already determined. It is not surprising that anaplastic thyroid carcinoma is classified Stage IV, regardless of tumor size, nodes, or metastases (11).

3 DIAGNOSIS

3.1 Clinical

A thyroid tumor in an older patient that is painful, growing rapidly, and presents an indurated irregular mass fixed to the adjacent tissues is suspicious for ATC. Cervical nodes are frequently involved and hoarseness may be present.

Evaluation of the extent of the tumor and particularly the invasion of muscles and trachea is critical in considering therapeutic decision choices. Magnetic resonance imaging (MRI) is the most useful diagnostic technique because it evaluates soft tissues accurately and can offer the surgeon information about the possible resection of the tumor and the extent of surgery that would be required.

3.2 Pathology

On gross examination, anaplastic thyroid carcinoma give rise to large, obviously invasive tumors that may contain necrotic and hemorrhagic foci (Fig. 6). Vascular invasion is a common finding, as is necrosis. The tumor is composed of malignant spindle cells, multinucleated tumor giant cells, and polygonal squamoid cells in varying proportions (Fig. 7). Spindle cell predominant ATC can therefore resemble sarcoma, or vice versa (Fig. 8). The multinucleated tumor giant cells can be accompanied by osteoclast-like cells and in this way simulate metastatic breast carcinoma. In addition, ATC with a prominent squamoid component can mimic aggressive upper aerodigestive squamous carcinomas that have metastasized to the cervical soft tissues.

Foci of well-differentiated thyroid carcinoma (papillary or follicular) are commonly found within anaplastic cancer; this transformation supports the diagnosis of anaplastic thyroid carcinoma. It speaks for "dedifferentiation" of well-differentiated thyroid cancer into anaplastic cancer (12–14).

3.3 Fine Needle Biopsy

As in most thyroid tumors, fine needle aspiration biopsy is the diagnostic option of first choice and has the highest yield. Since the tumor is most frequently disseminated widely throughout the gland rather than constituting a local focus, needle biopsy is usually an effective method to make the diagnosis (see Chapter 10). A core or open biopsy may be required to rule out other tumors such as lymphomas, undifferentiated medullary carcinoma, or poorly differentiated insular cancers that can mimic anaplastic cancer histologically.

The classic case of ATC, usually strongly suspected from the physical findings, is easily confirmed in most instances by cytology from a fine needle biopsy. The procedure can be performed readily at the initial examination of the patient, as an office or bedside procedure. The finding of bizarre spindle cells, multinucleated giant cells, and irregular pleomorphic cells validates the diagnosis. If the tumor appears unresectable, the patient may be spared an unnecessary and futile operation.

Fine needle aspiration biopsy allows for greater cell sampling and is less invasive than open or core biopsy. It is a cytological technique, however, allowing only the aspiration and examination of thyroid cells; it does not afford the opportunity to study the architecture of the lesion. If a "cell block" is generated from a cytology specimen it can be paraffin embedded and is available for immunological study. Should the mass be the result of a paucicellular or fibrotic process such as Riedel's struma, the aspiration may yield little material, constituting a "dry tap." In this situation, a true-cut needle biopsy or open biopsy is the logical next step.

There are limitations, nevertheless, to the fine needle diagnosis of ATC. If necrosis and inflammation predominate, the findings may mimic acute thyroiditis. Rarely, a soft tissue sarcoma may metastasize to the thyroid or a rare primary thyroid sarcoma may arise. Fine needle biopsy in this situation may also yield bizarre malignant spindle cells, leading to the erroneous diagnosis of ATC (15). The possibility of a sampling error must also be considered. It is not unusual for ATC to be mixed with elements of papillary or follicular carcinoma. The cytological diagnosis of papillary or follicular thyroid carcinoma in a clinical setting that is suspicious for anaplastic thyroid cancer does not exclude the possibility that that these conditions may be accompanied by anaplastic carcinoma.

3.4 Immunochemistry

The differential diagnosis of ATC importantly includes lymphoma as well as rare primary and metastatic carcinomas, sqamous carcinoma, melanoma, and sarcomas. Historically small and large cell lymphomas were frequently misdiagnosed as ATC, producing a falsely optimistic survival rate for ATC (Fig. 9). It is probable that 20–25% of previously diagnosed anaplastic thyroid cancers actually represent other entities such as lymphoma, medullary and insular carcinoma, as well as other malignancies (16). Today, with immunochemical markers for T cells and B cells widely available, the distinction between lymphoma and ATC is relatively straightforward.

Immunohistochemical studies developed and employed over the last 2 decades are routinely performed in the evaluation of poorly differentiated thyroid cancers. These have removed lymphomas and other malignancies from ATC survival statistics, resulting in a more realistic understanding of the prognosis. These immunochemical techniques can be performed retrospectively on formalin-fixed, paraffin-embedded tissue sections of previously diagnosed cases, enabling researchers to reevaluate the outlook for ATC.

Thyroglobulin protein is rarely expressed for ATC. Thyroid transcription factor-1 (TTF-1), a member of the NKx2 family of transcription factors, is a mediator of thyroid-specific transcription of the thyroglobulin (TG) gene. It is a more sensitive marker of thyroid differentiation, but its expression in ATC as detected by immunohistochemistry is still relatively rare. ATC also expresses vimentin, S-100, and cytokeratins (17–19).

This profile is not specific and does not allow for the exclusion of other diagnoses such as metastatic squamous carcinoma. In situ hybridization for thyroglobulin mRNA is a more sensitive means of confirming ATC as being of thyroid origin, though it is not as routinely available as an ancillary diagnostic test (20).

Although thyroglobulin and TTF-1 expression can be negative in ATC as well as lymphoma, lymphoma expresses lymphocyte markers and seldom expresses keratins.

In a study of 30 tumors from M.D. Anderson Hospital, Venkatesh and colleagues (9) found the expression of keratin to be the single most useful epithelial marker in confirming the diagnosis of anaplastic thyroid cancer, differentiating it from other tumors including sarcomas, melanomas, and lymphomas. Keratin was present in 24 of 30 tumors studied (80%). In 9 of these cases, staining occurring in over 50% of the cells. In addition, 10 tumors (33%) stained for epithelial membrane antigen (EMA); all of these also reacted for keratin. The expression of keratin is valuable in distinguishing ATC from malignancies of nonthyroid origin such as lymphomas, sarcoma, and melanoma. Epithelial membrane antigen (present in 33% of ATC, as noted) can also assist in the differential diagnosis.

Although 28 tumors in this study stained for vimentin (93.3%), with a pattern similar to that of keratin, vimentin is present in so many diverse tumors, e.g., lung, ovary, endometrium, and aerodigestive tract, as well as in normal endometrium, that it is not useful in the diagnosis of ATC (9).

When long-term survivors of ATC are evaluated and the pathology is reviewed, it is often found that some of these patiens actually had lymphomas that responded to radiotherapy or chemotherapy, or medullary carcinomas that classically have a slow progression. Indeed, in "ATC" patients who survive more than 2 years, careful histological and immunological review is required. When cases of lymphoma are excluded, survival is far less.

The differential diagnosis of ATC also includes squamous carcinoma, small-cell variant of medullary carcinoma, and insular-type follicular carcinoma. As previously noted, immunohistochemistry may not be able to distinguish ATC from primary or secondary squamous carcinoma. Medullary carcinoma can be distinguished from ATC by the expression of calcitonin and carcinoembryonic antigen (CEA). Insular-type follicular carcinoma (poorly differentiated carcinoma) can be distinguished by its diffuse and abundant thyroglobulin and TTF expression, as well as careful histological study.

3.5 Anaplastic Carcinoma Arising Within Well-Differentiated Thyroid Cancer

The presence of well-differentiated thyroid carcinoma in association with ATC can be helpful in confirming the diagnosis of ATC and also supports the hypothesis that the disease may arise as a terminal dedifferentiation of well-differentiated thyroid cancer, (Fig. 10). In the report from M.D. Anderson Hospital, 89% of the 74 cases of ATC with sufficient tissue for histological examination demonstrated areas of transformation of differentiated carcinoma to ATC (3). The frequent presence of foci of well-differentiated thyroid carcinoma within ATC may be considered evidence of transformation, suggesting "dedifferentiation" of well- differentiated thyroid carcinoma into ATC (14,21,22).

Current models of thyroid carcinogenesis demonstrate a stepwise process of progressive loss of tumor suppressor genes. Transgenic mice with the ret/PTC1 rearrangement all developed thyroid carcinomas. Crossbreeding with p53 knockout mice resulted in some offspring with ret/PTC1 p53-negative homozyous genotypes. Those mice with homozygous p53 deletions

The use of doxorubicin as a radiosensitizer accompanied by hyperfractional radiotherapy, introduced by Kim and Leeper from Memorial Hospital, was said to offer an improvement in control of local disease. They reported achieving local control in 68% of 19 patients (32). The biological advantage of dose fractionation is that it affects rapidly growing tumors producing an early response and spares slowly responding normal tissues, thereby offering a therapeutic gain (33). The use of chemotherapeutic agents such as doxorubicin and cisplatin is unfortunately accompanied by severe tracheitis, pharyngitis and esophagitis, especially since they are usually combined with radiotherapy. The addition of chemotherapy and radiotherapy certainly reduces the patient's remaining quality of life.

In a recent report, Tennvall et al. (34) from the Lund University Hospital in Sweden reported on evolving protocols (three were described) of hyperfractionated radiotherapy in combination with doxorubicin and surgery when feasible. Chemotherapy consisted entirely of preoperative doxorubicin (they identify it as the most effective drug) and fractionated radiotherapy. In two protocols radiation was given pre- and postoperatively, and in the third it was given entirely preoperatively at an accelerated rate of 1.6 Gy twice daily. In this group a total dose of 46 Gy was administered in 2 weeks followed by surgery 2 weeks later. None of the 17 patients in this group died of local recurrence in the neck, although additional surgery was sometimes required. The authors attributed this to the accelerated radiotherapy. Of a total of 55 patients in the three groups, 40% developed local recurrence, although death was attributed to local failure "in only 24% of patients." Nine percent survived more than 2 years. Overall median survival was in the area of 3 months (34).

5 SURVIVAL

No standard protocol of surgery, radiotherapy, or chemotherapy has been proved to increase survival. The median life expectancy from the time of diagnosis is approximately 3–4 months. Indeed a long survival brings the original diagnosis under suspicion and mandates a review of the slides.

Perhaps 10 percent of patients survive more than a year with some patients living 2 or more years (Fig. 2). There are rare long-term survivors. Two-year survivals range from almost none (35) to 14% (9). In a report of 82 patients, Nel and colleagues found that 8 were alive at 2 years, but at 3 years only 3 had survived (7).

In trying to define favorable factors, dividing patients into short-term and long-term (over 2 years) survivors, Venkatesh and colleagues found that long-term survivors (54.1 ± 13.7 years) were significantly younger at diagnosis than short-term survivors (63.9 ± 10.5 years), but this did not reach statistical significance. As noted ealier, complete tumor resection also improved the outlook in this report, but again was not statistically significant (9).

It is thought that favorable factors are minimal lesions that are completely resected, the addition of radiotherapy and chemotherapy, and an onset below 45 years of age.

6 CONCLUSION

Our inability to influence the course of ATC is humbling. It reminds us that as much as we have learned, there is more that we do not know. This merciless condition will require an understanding of disease processes that are as yet unknown and will yield to therapy we have yet to discover.

REFERENCES

1. McIver B, Hay ID, Giuffrida DF, et al. Anaplastic thyroid carcinoma: a 50-year experience at a single institution. Surgery 2001; 130:1028–1034.
2. Gilliland FD, Hunt WC, Morris DM, et al. Prognostic factors for thyroid carcinoma. A population-based study of 15,698 cases from the Surveillance, Epidemiology and End Results (SEER) program 1973-1991. Cancer 1997; 79:564–573.
3. Aldinger KA, Samaan NA, Ibinez M, et al. ATC of the thyroid: a review of 84 cases of spindle and giant cell carcinoma of the thyroid. Cancer 1978; 41:2267–2275.
4. Agrawal S, Rao RS, Parikh DM, et al. Histologic trends in thyroid cancer 1969–1993: a clinico-pathologic analysis of the relative proportion of ATC of the thyroid. J Surg Oncol 1996; 63:251–255.
5. Lampertico P. Anaplastic (sarcomatoid) carcinoma of the thyroid gland. Semin Diagn Pathol 1993; 10:159–168.
6. Ain KB. Anaplastic thyroid carcinoma: a therapeutic challenge. Semin Sur Oncol 1999; 16:64–69.
7. Nel CJ, van Heerdon JA, Goelinger JR, et al. ATC of the thyroid: a clinico-pathologic study of 82 cases. Mayo Clin Proc 1985; 60:51–58.
8. Silverberg SG, Hutter RV, Foote FW. Fatal carcinoma of the thyroid: histology, metastases, and causes of death. Cancer 1970; 25:792–802.
9. Venkatesh YS, Ordonez NG, Schultz PN, et al. ATC of

the thyroid. A clinicopathologic study of 121 cases. Cancer 1990; 66:321–330.

10. Thomas CG Jr, Buckwalter JA. Poorly differentiated neoplasms of the thyroid gland. Ann Surg 1973; 177: 632–642.
11. Fleming D, et al. eds. American Joint Committee on Cancer Manual for Staging of Cancer. 5th ed. Philadelphia: Lippincott-Raven, 1997.
12. Carcangiu ML, Steeper T, Zampi G, et al. Anaplastic thyroid carcinoma. A study of 70 cases. Am J Clin Pathol 1985; 83:135–158.
13. Spires JR, Schwartz MR, Miller RH. Anaplastic thyroid carcinoma. Association with differentiated thyroid cancer. Arch Otolaryngol Head Neck Surg 1991; 1988 114: 40–44.
14. Ordonez NG, El-Naggar AK, Hickey RC, et al. Anaplastic thyroid carcinoma. Immunocytochemical study of 32 cases. Am J Clin Pathol 1991; 96:15–24.
15. Andrion A, Gaglio A, Dogliani N, et al. Liposarcoma of the thyroid gland. Fine-needle aspiration cytology, immunohistology, and ultrastructure. Am J Clin Pathol 1991; 95:675–679.
16. Holting T, Moller P, Tschahargane C, et al. Immunohistochemical reclassification of anaplastic carcinoma reveals small and giant cell lymphoma. World J Surg 1990; 14:291–295.
17. Bejarano PA, Nikiforov YE, Swenson ES, et al. Thyroid transcription factor-1, thyroglobulin, cytokeratin 7, and cytokeratin 20 in thyroid neoplasms. Appl Immunohistochem Mol Morphol 2000; 8:189–194.
18. Miettinen M, Franssila KO. Variable expression of keratins and nearly uniform lack of thyroid transcription factor 1 in thyroid anaplastic carcinoma. Hum Pathol 2000; 31:1139–1145.
19. Sierra M, Gamboa-Dominguez A, Herrera MF, et al. Anaplastic carcinoma of the thyroid at the Instituto Nacional de la Nutricion Salvador Zubiran. Rev Invest Clin 1997; 49:97–103.
20. Papotti M, Volante M, Negro F, et al. Thyroglobulin mRNA expression helps to distinguish anaplastic carcinoma from angiosarcoma of the thyroid. Virchows Arch 2000; 437:635–642.
21. Carcangiu ML, Steeper T, Zampi G, et al. J. Anaplastic thyroid carcinoma. A study of 70 cases. Am J Clin Pathol 1985; 83:135–158.
22. Spires JR, Schwartz MR, Miller RH. Anaplastic thyroid carcinoma. Association with differentiated thyroid cancer. Arch Otolaryngol Head Neck Surg Jan 1988; 114:40–44.
23. La Perle KM, Jhiang SM, Capen CC. Loss of p53 promotes anaplasia and local invasion in ret/PTC1-induced thyroid carcinomas. Am J Pathol 2000; 157: 671–677.
24. Wierzchowski W, Szybinski P, Nowak W, et al. Poorly differentiated carcinoma of the thyroid—immunohistochemical evaluation of p53 and p27 protein expression. Wiad Lek 2001; 54(suppl)1:79–87.
25. Lam KY, Lo CY, Chan KW, et al. Insular and anaplastic carcinoma of the thyroid: a 45-year comparative study at a single institution and a review of the significance of p53 and p21. Ann Surg 2000; 231:329–338.
26. Holting T, Meybier H, Buhr H. Status of trachoestomy in treatment of respiratory emergency in anaplastic thyroid cancer. Wien Klin Wochenschr 1990; 102:264–266.
27. Tan RK, Finley RK, Driscoll D, et al. Anaplastic carcinoma of the thyroid: a 24-year experience. Head Neck 1995; 17:41–48.
28. Haigh PI, Ituarte PH, Wu HS, et al. Completely resected (ATC) combined with adjuvant chemotherapy is associated with prolonged survival. Cancer 2001; 91:2335–2342.
29. Junor EJ, Paul J, Reed NS. Anaplastic thyroid carcinoma: 91 patients treated by surgery and radiotherapy. Eur J Sur Oncol 1992; 18:83–88.
30. Tollefsen RH, De Cosse JJ, Hutter VP. Papillary carcinoma of the thyroid: a clinical and pathological study of 70 fatal cases. Cancer 1964; 17:1035–1044.
31. Sugino K, Koichi I, Mimura T, et al. The importance of operations in the management of anaplastic thyroid carcinoma. Surgery 2002; 131:245–248.
32. Kim J, Leeper R. Treatment of locally advanced thyroid carcinoma with combination doxorubicin and radiation therapy. Cancer 1987; 60:2372–2375.
33. Withers HR. Biologic basis for altered fractionation schemes. Cancer 1985; 55:2086–2095.
34. Tennvall J, Lundell G, Wahlberg P, et al. Anaplatic thyroid carcinoma: three protocols combining doxorubicin, hyperfractionated radiotherapy and surgery. Br.J Cancer 2002; 86:1848–1853.
35. Norton J, Doppman J, Jensen R. Cancer of the endocrine system. In: DeVita A, Hellmann S, Rosenberg S, eds. Cancer, 4th edition. Philadelphia: JB Lippincott, 1989:1337.
36. Hundahl SA, Fleming ID, Fremgen AM. A national cancer data base report on 58,856 cases of thyroid carcinoma treated in the U.S., 1985-1995. Cancer 1998; 83:2638–2649.

15

Endoscopic Thyroid Surgery

Laurent Biertho

Les Cliniques Saint Joseph, Liege, Belgium

Michel Gagner

Mount Sinai School of Medicine, New York University, New York, New York, U.S.A.

1 INTRODUCTION

Thyroid resection is one of the most common operations performed throughout the world. This procedure is classically realized through a transverse cervical incision and is associated with a very low morbidity and mortality rate. However, the visible scar on the anterior surface of the neck is disliked by many patients, especially by young women in which this operation is commonly performed.

With the general tendency to perform a less invasive surgery, an endoscopic approach has been applied to neck surgery. The first endoscopic neck exploration was performed in 1995 for parathyroidectomy (1). Since then, endoscopic parathyroid resections have been performed worldwide, and large series have been reported (2,3).

After experimentation on animal models (4) showing the feasibility of the technique, Hüscher performed the first endoscopic thyroid resection in 1997 (5). Nonetheless, endoscopic thyroid surgery is more technically challenging, compared to parathyroidectomy, due to the size of the thyroid gland, the extent of the dissection required, and the higher rate of malignancy.

The current indications, techniques, and results of endoscopic thyroid surgery are described in this chapter.

2 PREOPERATIVE WORKUP

In addition to a detailed history, physical examination, and thyroid function tests, the following exams are usually realized.

Ultrasonography is performed to define the dimension, nature and localization of the thyroid pathology and to evaluate the contralateral lobe. A Doppler study is also used to assess the vascularization of the gland in case of thyroiditis.

Fine needle aspiration is used to define the histology of "cold" nodules and, before endoscopic thyroid surgery, to rule out a carcinoma. Atypical or suspicious cytology are currently considered as a contraindication for an endoscopic resection. One concern about fine needle aspiration is that subclinical hemorrhage can create substantial adhesions, making endoscopic dissection difficult (6).

Other preoperative imaging studies (scintigraphy, computed tomography (CT) scanner, magnetic resonance) are performed according to the suspected lesion and are similar to the classical workup used for thyroid pathologies.

3 INDICATIONS

The ideal indication for endoscopic thyroid surgery is a solitary, nonfunctioning thyroid nodule of less than 30 mm in diameter. Other current indications include solitary toxic nodule, recurrent thyroid cyst, and small multinodular goiters. Moreover, a thin patient, with a long narrow neck is more suited for an endoscopic approach.

4 CONTRAINDICATIONS

Contraindications to an endoscopic approach include nodules larger than 3 cm in diameter, a large multinodular goiter, history of prior neck surgery, thyroiditis, and patients with recent infection, inflammation, irradiation, or burn to the neck (6,7). Graves' disease, with enlarged and highly vascular thyroid gland, is also considered a contraindication by most surgeons, due to the higher risk of bleeding. Obesity associated with a short, wide neck is also a relative contraindication, as space and exposure can be reduced. Patients with atypical, highly suspicious, or malignant cytology should be excluded, as endoscopic surgery may not allow a correct grading of the tumor. Finally, elderly patients or those with severe associated pathologies may not tolerate CO2 insufflation and should be excluded.

5 PROCEDURE

After induction of a general anesthesia, the patient is positioned with the neck slightly extended, or even slightly folded (8), with the table in a reversed Trendelenburg position (Fig. 1). The sternal notch, anterior border of the sternocleidomastoid muscle (SCM), and external jugular veins are marked with a pen. The procedure requires a 5 mm endoscope, instruments, and trocars (Karl Storz Endoscopy, Tuttlingen, Germany) (Figs. 2, 3). Three main endoscopic approaches have been described: the cervical, the axillary, and the breast approach.

5.1 Cervical Approach

5.1.1 Incision and Creation of the Working Space

A 10-mm incision is made at the sternal notch or just above it, and the cervical fascia is opened. A subplatysmal space is created by blunt dissection and introduction of a swab in the opening. A 5 mm trocar is inserted and secured in place with a Prolene purse string suture. CO_2 insufflation is started to a pressure of 8–12 mmHg. Initial dissection is made with the tip of a 0°, 5 mm endoscope (Karl Storz Endoscopy, Tuttlingen, Germany), along the anterior border of the SCM. Once a sufficient space is obtained, three additional trocars are inserted under visual control, and a 30° or occasionally 45° endoscope is used to perform the rest of the procedure (Fig. 4).

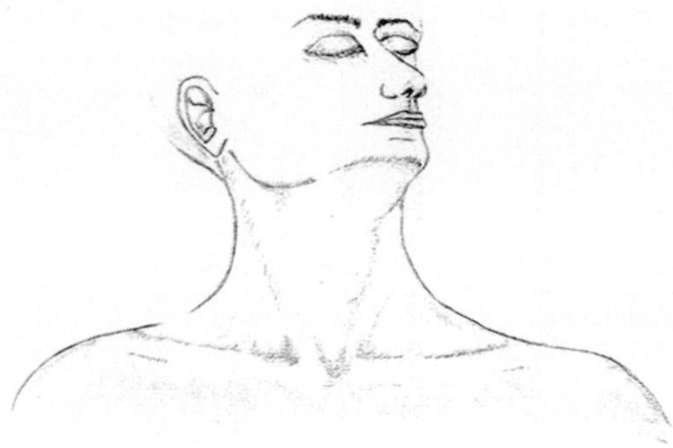

Figure 1 Position of the patient for a right thyroidectomy.

5.1.2 Dissection of the Thyroid Lobe

The strap muscles are mobilized from the anterior surface of the thyroid gland. The use of electrocautery is usually avoided when laryngeal nerve is not yet exposed. Vascular clips, 5 mm (US Surgical, Norwalk, CT), or 5-mm ultrasonic scalpel (US Surgical, Norwalk, CT) are used for hemostasis. The middle thyroid vein is first dissected and divided between clips or with ultrasonic shear.

5.1.3 Dissection of the Recurrent Laryngeal Nerve and Parathyroid Gland

The inferior thyroid artery, inferior parathyroid, and recurrent laryngeal nerve (RLN) are identified (Figs. 5, 6). With the nerve under visual control, the inferior thyroid artery is divided between clips. If the laryngeal nerve cannot be localized, the procedure should be converted to a classical, open approach. The laryngeal nerve is then separated from the posterior aspect of the thyroid gland using blunt dissection. The inferior and superior parathyroids glands are also mobilized and preserved. The superior thyroid vessels are dissected and transected between clips after identification of the superior laryngeal nerve (Fig. 7). The thyroid gland is retracted in the anteromedial direction, and the ligament of Berry and isthmus are divided using ultrasonic

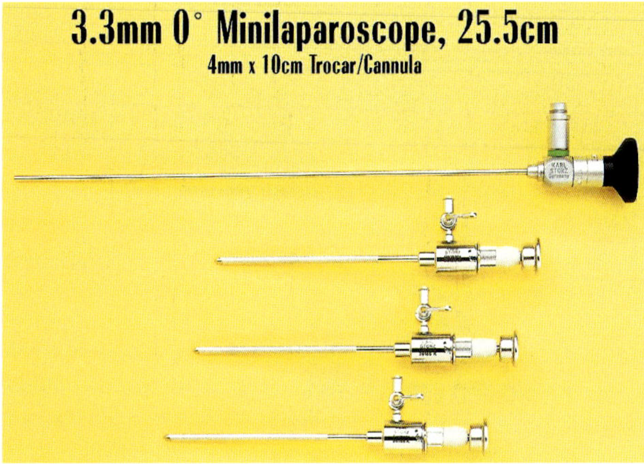

Figure 2 5-mm endoscope and trocars.

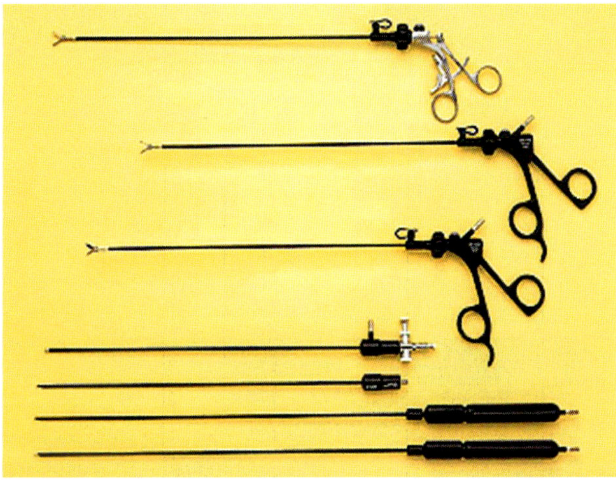

Figure 3 5-mm endoscopic instruments.

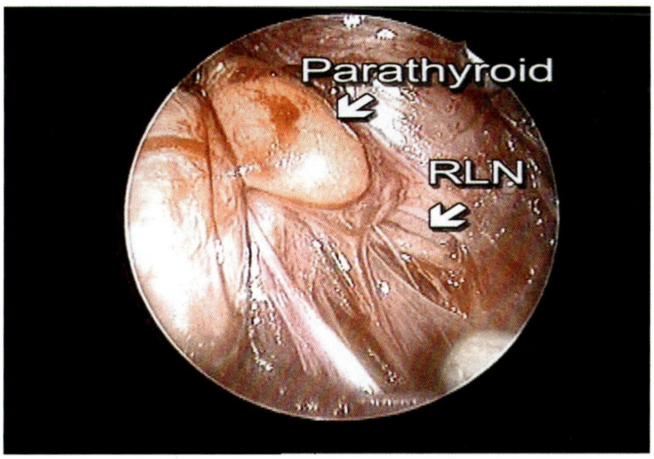

Figure 5 Endoscopic aspect of the recurrent laryngeal nerve and inferior parathyroid gland.

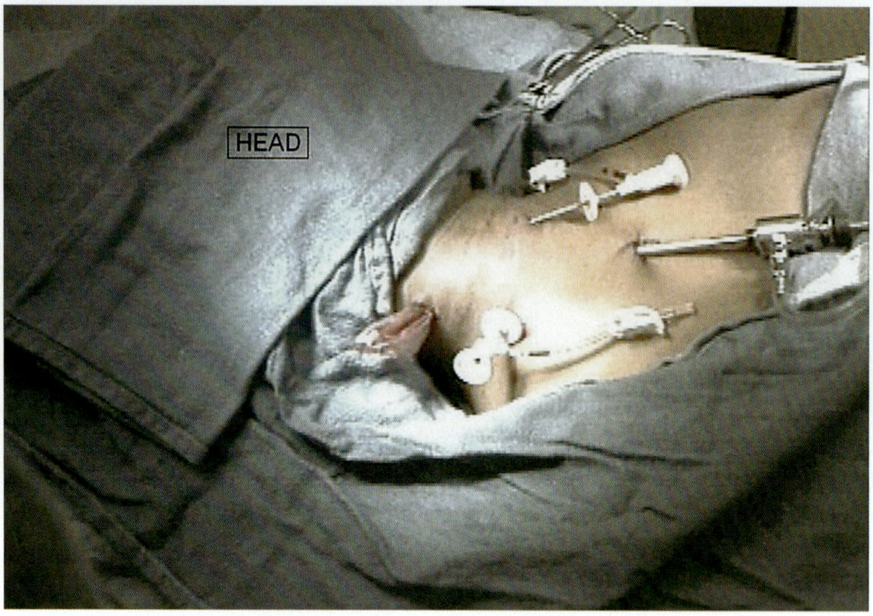

Figure 8 Extraction of the specimen.

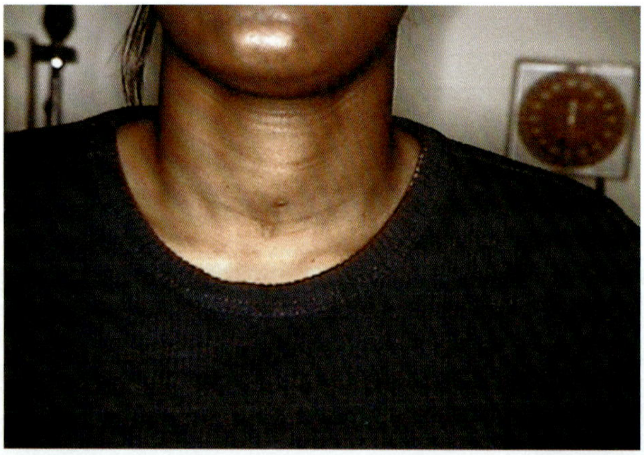

Figure 9 Cosmetic results after endoscopic thyroidectomy using a cervical approach.

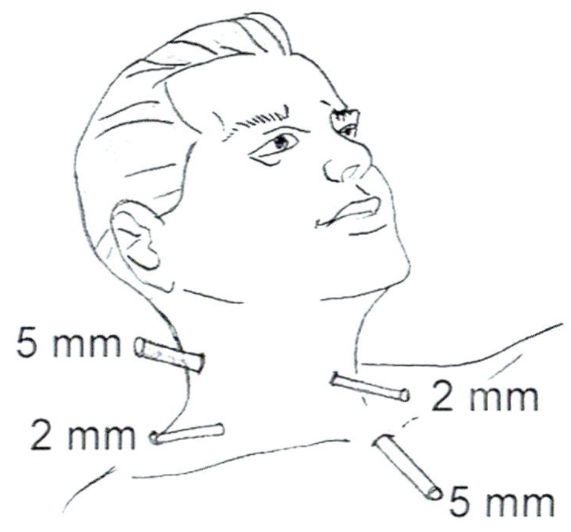

Figure 4 Trocars position for a right thyroidectomy using a cervical approach.

scalpel. The specimen is then placed in a retrieval bag and extracted through the supero-lateral trocar site (Fig. 8).

5.2 Transaxillary Approach

In order to avoid any visible scars in the neck, Ikeda et al. (9,10) performed endoscopic thyroid resections using an axillary approach. A 30 mm incision is made in the axillar, and the lower layer of the platysma muscle is dissected through the upper layer of the pectoralis major. A 12 mm trocar is inserted, and CO_2 is insufflated with a pressure of 4 mmHg. Two other trocars are then inserted below the first one. Access to the thyroid is then gained through the subplatysmal space. The thyroid gland is exposed by dividing the sternothyroid muscle. The recurrent laryngeal nerve is then identified, as are the parathyroid glands. The inferior and superior pedicles are then controlled as described above. A closed suction drain is usually left in place at the end of the procedure. The advantages of this technique include

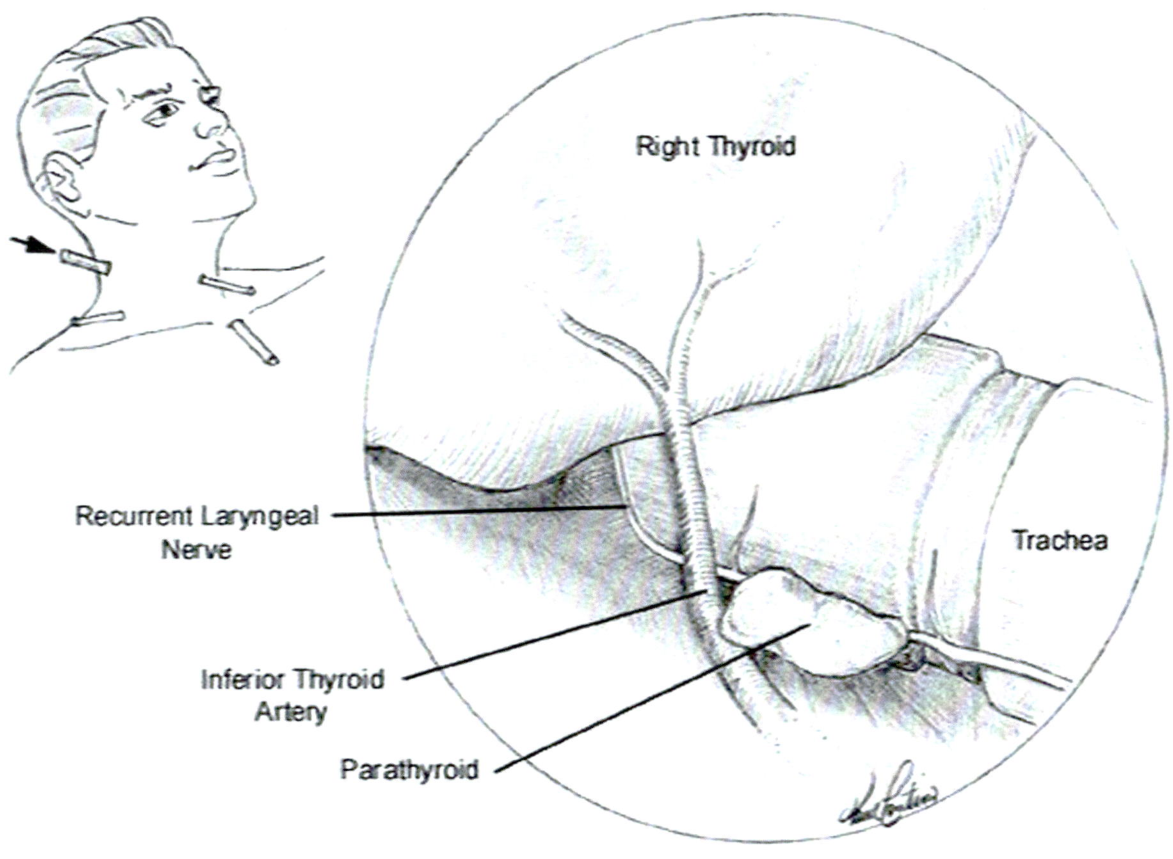

Figure 6 Inferior thyroid artery, inferior parathyroid gland, and recurrent laryngeal nerve.

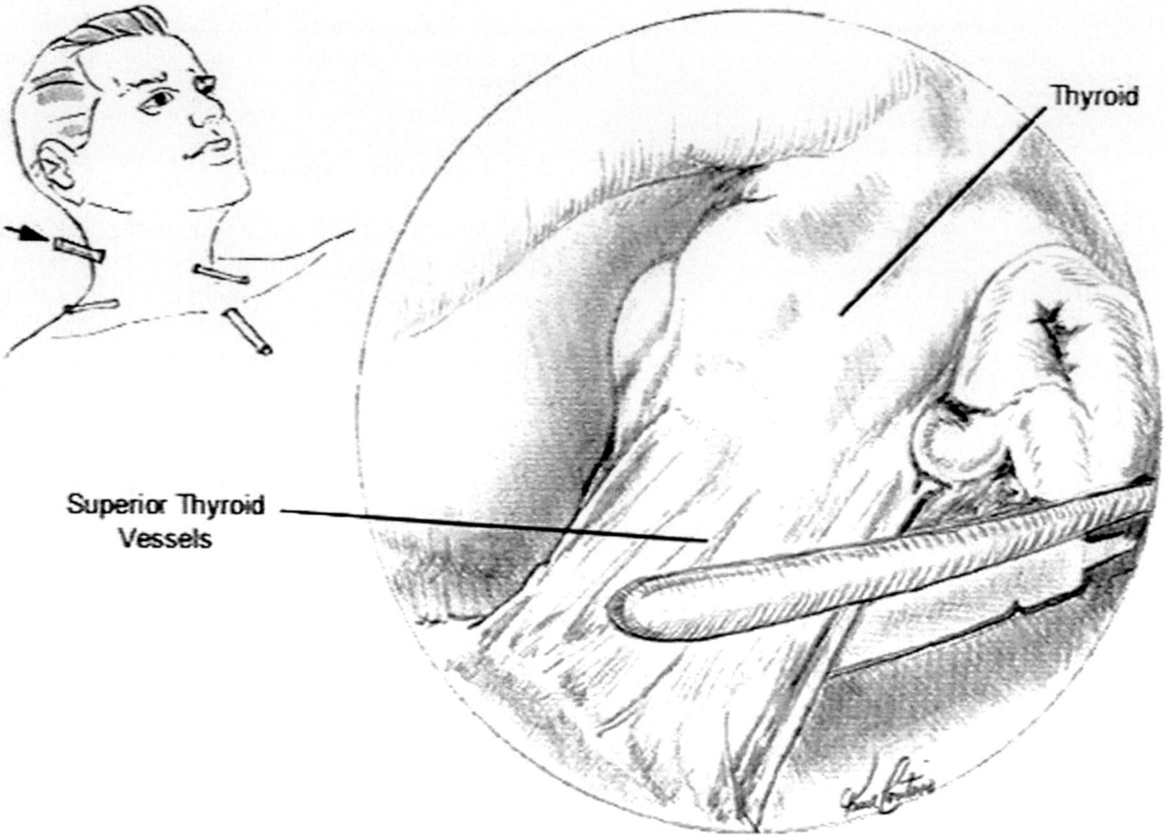

Figure 7 Control of the superior thyroid pedicle.

avoidance of any scars in the neck, the lateral approach to the thyroidal bed (similar to a classical approach), an easier dissection of the superior and inferior poles, and an easier access to the perithyroid fascia, which can be opened without injury to the glands or to the recurrent laryngeal nerve. The main disadvantages of this technique are probably the technical difficulties, the extent of the dissection, and the duration of the procedure (about 3 hr).

5.3 Breast Approach

In 1998, Ishii et al. (11) described a technique of thyroid resection using a breast approach. The aim of this technique is also to avoid the presence of any scars in the neck. A 15 mm incision is made in the right or left parasternal border at the level of the nipples. A subcutaneous tunnel is created using blunt dissection, and a subplatysmal space is created. A 12 mm trocar is first inserted, and CO_2 insufflation is started, with a pressure of 5 mmHg. A subplatysmal space is developed from the superior margin of the thyroid cartilage to the lateral borders of the SCM. Two additional 5 mm trocars are then inserted at the upper margin of both mammary areolas. Dissection is started at the lower pole and proceeds to the posterior and lateral aspects of the gland. The recurrent laryngeal nerve and parathyroid glands are usually identified. Main disadvantages of this technique are the risk of keloid scars associated with incision in the chest, the technical difficulty of the procedure, the risk of hematoma due to the extent of the dissection, and the impossibility to use any of the incisions if a conversion is required.

5.4 Gasless Endoscopy

Intracranial pressure is increased when CO_2 insufflation of 15 mmHg is used to perform neck surgery in animal models (12). On the opposite, pressures of 10 mmHg do not seem to increase the intracranial pressure. However, other complications due to CO_2 insufflation in the neck can occur (e.g, hypercapnia, respiratory acidosis, or subcutaneous emphysema). In order to reduce those complications, Hüscher et al. (5) described the use of a lifting device to perform an endoscopic thyroid surgery, with reduced CO_2 pressure (6 mmHg). Shimizu et al.

(13,14) have also performed totally gasless endoscopic thyroid resections using Kirschner wires inserted horizontally in the subcutaneous layer of the anterior part of the neck. Those wires are lifted up and fixed to a L-shaped pole to create a tent-like working space. They have performed more than 40 cases using this technique and conclude that this procedure is safe and can be used in selected cases.

Miccoli et al. (15,16) have also described a video-assisted thyroidectomy (VAT). Dissection of the thyroid lobe is performed through a 15 mm medial incision using a 5 mm 30° endoscope with classical instruments. Working space is maintained using an external retractor.

6 RESULTS

The current reports of endoscopic thyroid resections involve mainly small series of cases. There was only one prospective randomized trial (16), and the largest series included 67 patients (15). The results, conversion rate, and morbidity in these series of endoscopic thyroid resections have been reviewed (Tables 1 and 2).

More than 130 endoscopic thyroid resections have been reported. Among these, 31 were total or subtotal thyroidectomies, 87 lobectomies, and 13 partial lobectomies. Most of the operations were performed for benign tumors (86.3%), including 12 cases of Graves' diseases. Malignant tumors are considered, for most authors, a contraindication to an endoscopic resection. However, Miccoli et al. (15,16) consider small, low-risk (T1) papillary carcinomas an indication for a video-assisted resection.

Operative time was globally increased compared to an open procedure, with a mean 136.4 minutes. However, it should decrease as experience is gained.

The global conversion rate was 7.6% (10 cases). The causes of conversion were:

- Carcinoma diagnosed on the frozen section that required an open completion in three cases.
- Insufficient working space in three cases. The two causes of conversion in Gagner et al.'s study (7) were a 7 cm cyst and a 4 cm nodule, leading to the conclusion that endoscopic thyroid resections should not be attempted for tumors larger than 3 cm in diameter.
- Hemorrhage in two cases. Both conversions were due to bleeding from the superior pole, illustrating the difficulty in controlling bleeding in such a small working space, especially when the superior pedicle is involved.

Table 1 Endoscopic Thyroid Resections: Histological Results

Authors (Ref.)	*N*	Procedure	*N*	Histology	*N*	Mean size/mean weight
Yeung (6)	8	Lobectomies	8	Benign tumors	8	1.98 cm (0.4–3.8)
Gagner and Inabnet (7)	18	Lobectomies	10	Adenoma	13	2.7 cm (0.6–7)
		Subtotal thyroidectomy	4	Cyst	2	
		Isthmusectomy	4	Multinodular goiter	1	
				Papillary thyroid carcinoma	2	
Ishii et al. (11)	5	Lobectomies	4	Follicular adenoma	5	4 × 5 cm (3–7)
		Partial thyroidectomy	1			
Shimizu et al. (13)	5	Lobectomies	2	Follicular adenoma	4	3.2 cm (2–4.5)
		Extirpation	3	Follicular carcinoma	1	
Miccoli et al. (15)	67	Lobectomies	52	Follicular adenomas	43	2.1 cm (0.9–3)
		Total thyroidectomies	15	Toxic adenoma	6	
				Toxic multinodular goiter	3	
				Papillary carcinoma	15	
Yamamoto et al. (18)	12	Subtotal thyroidectomy	12	Graves' disease	12	44 g (18–92)
Yeh et al. (19)	16	Lobectomy	13	Nodular hyperplasia	8	5.8 cm (3.5–8.0)
		Tumorectomy	3	Follicular adenoma	6	
				Hurthle tumor	1	
				Cyst	1	
Total	131	Total or subtotal thyroidectomies	31	Benign tumors	113	
				Carcinoma	18	
		Lobectomies	87			
		Less than one lobe	13			

Table 2 Endoscopic Thyroid Resections: Operative Results

Authors (Ref.)	Operative time (min)	Conversion	Morbidity
Yeung et al. (6)	241 (180–330)	37.5% (1 failure to define anatomy, 1 adhesion, 1 insufficient space)	0
Gagner et al. (7)	220 (120–330)	11.1% (2 insufficient working space)	5.6% (1 incidental parathyroidectomy)
Ishii et al. (11)	226 (177–281)	0	0
Shimizu et al. (13)	126 (90–150)	0	0
Miccoli et al. (15)	Lobectomy: 73.6 Thyroidectomy: 110	3% (1 hemorrhage, 1 conversion for carcinoma)	4.48% (2 transient postop hypocalcemia, 1 transient RLN palsy)
Yamamoto et al. (18)	259.8 (175–420)	8.33% (1 bleeding from sup. pole)	8.33% (1 RLN palsy with hypoparathyoidism)
Yeh et al. (19)	102 (28–300)	11.1% (2 conversions for carcinoma)	0
Total	136.4 (28–420)	10 (7.6%)	5 (3.8%)

The two last conversions were due to (1) the difficulties in recognizing the normal anatomy, which is considerably different from the classical approach, and (2) adhesions.

There were no preoperative or postoperative deaths.

Global morbidity was 3.8% (5 cases). Four cases involved minor complications (two transient hypocalcemias, one transient RLN palsy, and one incidental parathyroidectomy). There was one case of RLN palsy with hypocalcemia after a subtotal thyroidectomy for Graves' disease. However, the technique used was to dissect the thyroid in contact with the thyroid capsule, without any attempt to localize the RLN or the parathyroid glands.

7 DISCUSSION

The results reported in Table 2 suggest that endoscopic thyroid surgery is feasible and safe. In a series of 6702 classical thyroidectomies, the overall complication rate was 3.8%, with an incidence of permanent laryngeal nerve palsy of 0.7% (17). These rates seem to be similar to those reported after endoscopic resections (a 3.8% morbidity rate with a 0.75% rate of laryngeal nerve palsy).

This approach could offer different potential advantages:

A better cosmetic result. Most people dislike having a scar on the anterior surface of the neck, especially as thyroid pathologies are frequently found in young women. The shorter skin incision and absence of musculo-cutaneous flap offer a better cosmetic result after endoscopic resection (Fig. 9). In a prospective randomized trial comparing a group of 25 patients undergoing a video-assisted thyroidectomy to another group of 24 patients undergoing a classical thyroidectomy, Miccoli et al. (16) found a better cosmetic result in the endoscopic group ($p < 0.01$). Gagner and Inabnet (7) found the same results in a study comparing endoscopic versus conventional thyroid resections ($p < 0.005$).

Reduction in postoperative pain. This point is difficult to assess due to the low analgesic requirement after both classical and endoscopic thyroid surgery. Post-operative convalescence could be reduced after an endoscopic thyroidectomy, as trauma to the tissues is decreased. However, the difference was not statistically significant in the study by Gagner and Inabnet (7).

Potential reduction of RLN or parathyroid glands lesions: The endoscopic magnification may enhance the identification and reduce the risk of lesion to the important neurovascular structures, laryngeal nerves, and parathyroid glands with their blood supply. However, this point has to be evaluated by large, prospective, randomized trials.

Concerns associated with endoscopic thyroidectomies have also been expressed:

These procedures are technically complex and associated with an increased operative time. However, operative time should decrease as experience is gained and with the development of new instruments and techniques. This approach also requires a very careful selection of patients in that the safety and feasibility of the operation is dependent on that selection.

An increasing number of classical thyroidectomies are performed under local or loco-regional anesthesia in an outpatient hospitalization. Endoscopic resections still require general anesthesia, which is not minimally invasive and usually requires an overnight stay. Even if video-assisted parathyroidectomies have been performed under local anesthesia (20), when CO_2 insufflation is used for endoscopic resection, general anesthesia is required. The length of hospital stay for endoscopic thyroid surgery ranges from 1 to 7 days and is usually increased compared to a classical approach.

A thyroid carcinoma cannot be totally ruled out by the preoperative work-up, and we still ignore the outcomes when resection is performed by endoscopy. Canalar carcinoma diagnosed on a frozen section should be converted to radicalize the thyroidectomy. For follicular carcinoma, a final histopathological exam should be required, and the patient should be reoperated using a classical approach if the diagnosis is confirmed. However, for some authors (15), a low-risk (T1) small papillary carcinoma can be resected by endoscopy, as lymphadenomectomy is not required and resection is judged adequate.

8 CONCLUSION

Endoscopic thyroid resections are feasible and safe given very careful selection of patients. Potential advantages include better cosmetic results and reduced postoperative pain and morbidity rate. It is, however, technically complex and requires increased operative time, a general anesthesia, and a longer hospital stay. Large prospective randomized studies are still needed to refine the indications for endoscopic thyroid surgery and to confirm its safety and efficacy.

REFERENCES

1. Gagner M. Endoscopic subtotal parathyroidectomy in patients with primary hyperparathyroidism. Br J Surg 1996; 83:875.
2. Miccoli P, Berti P, Conte M, Raffaelli M, Materazzi G. Minimally invasive videoassisted parathyroidectomy: lesson learned from 137 cases. J Am Coll Surg 2000; 191:613–618.
3. Howe JR. Minimally invasive surgery: minimally invasive parathyroid surgery. Surg Clin North Am 2000; 80:1346–1399.
4. Jones DB, Quasebarth MA, Brunt LM. Videoendoscopic thyroidectomy: experimental development of a new Technique. Surg Laparosc Endosc 1999; 9: 167.
5. Hüscher CSG, Chiodini S, Napolitano C, Rcher A. Endoscopic right thyroid lobectomy. Surg Endosc 1997; 11: 877.
6. Yeung GH. Endoscopic surgery of the neck: a new frontier. Surg Laparosc Endosc 1998; 8:227–232.
7. Gagner M, Inabnet WB III. Endoscopic thyroidectomy for solitary thyroid nodules. Thyroid 2001; 11:161–163.
8. Yeung HC, Ng WT, Kong CK. Endoscopic thyroid and parathyroid surgery. Surg Endosc 1997; 11: 1135.
9. Ikeda Y, Takami H, Sasaki Y, Kan S, Niimi M. Endoscopic resection of thyroid tumors by the axillary approach. J Cardiovasc Surg 2000; 41:791–792.
10. Ikeda Y, Takami H, Sasaki Y, Kan S, Niimi M. Endoscopic neck surgery by the axillary approach. J Am Coll Surg 2000; 191:336–340.
11. Ishii S, Oghami M, Arisawa Y, Ohmori T, Noga K, Kitajima M. Endoscopic thyroidectomy with anterior chest wall approach. Surg Endosc 1998; 12:611.
12. Rubino F, Pamoukian VN, Zhu JF, Deutsch H, Inabnet WB, Gagner M. Endoscopic endocrine neck surgery with carbon dioxide insufflation: the effect on intracranial pressure in a large animal model. Surgery 2000; 128:1035–1042.
13. Shimizu K, Akira S, Jasmi AY, Kitamura Y, Kitagawa W, Akasu H, Tanaka S. Videoassisted neck surgery: endoscopic resection of thyroid tumors with a very minimal neck wound. J Am Coll Surg 1999; 188:697–703.
14. Shimizu K, Kitagawa W, Akasu H, Tanaka S. Endoscopic hemithyroidectomy and prophylactic lymph node dissection for micropapillary carcinoma of the thyroid by using a totally gasless anterior neck skin lifting method. J Surg Oncol 2001; 77:217–220.
15. Miccoli P, Berti P, Raffaelli M, Conte M, Materazzi G, Galleri D. Minimally invasive video-assisted thyroidectomy. Am J Surg 2001; 181:567–570.
16. Miccoli P, Berti P, Raffaelli M, Materazzi G, Baldacci S, Rossi G. Comparison between minimally invasive video-assisted thyroidectomy and conventional thyroidectomy: a prospective randomized study. Surgery 2001; 130:1039–1043.
17. Bliss RD, Gauger P, Delbridge LW. Surgeon's approach to the thyroid gland: surgical anatomy and the

importance of technique. World J Surg 2000; 24:891–897.
18. Yamamoto M, Sasaki A, Asahi H, Shimada Y, Sato N, Nakajima J, Mashima R, Saito K. Endoscopic subtotal thyroidectomy for patients with Graves' disease. Surg Today 2001; 31:1–4.
19. Yeh TS, Jan YY, Hsu BRS, Chen KW, Chen MF. Video-assisted endoscopic thyroidectomy. Am J Surg 2000; 180:82–85.
20. Miccoli P, Bendinelli C, Berti P, Vignali E, Pinchera A, Marcocci C. Video-assisted versus conventional parathyroidectomy in primary hyperparathyroidism: a prospective randomized study. Surgery 1999; 126:1117–1121.

16

Video-Assisted Thyroid Surgery

Paolo Miccoli, Piero Berti, and Gabriele Materazzi

University of Pisa, Pisa, Italy

1 INTRODUCTION

The first minimally invasive procedure ever performed in the neck district was an endoscopic parathyroidectomy carried out by Gagner in 1995 (1). Parathyroid pathology seemed in fact very viable to be treated endoscopically: indeed parathyroid adenomas are almost always benign, their volume rarely exceeds 3 cm, and they do not present important vascular connections.

The success obtained with this and other similar procedures (2,3) convinced several surgeons to remove small thyroid nodules as well as parathyroid adenomas; in spite of the concern expressed by some endocrine surgeons, both endoscopic and video-assisted thyroidectomy soon became quite popular. This trend is expressed in the papers that appeared or are about to appear on surgical reviews (4–7).

2 MINIMALLY INVASIVE VIDEO-ASSISTED THYROIDECTOMY

This technique, in its present from, is characterized by the absence of any gas insufflation and by the external retraction. It was first described in 1999 (8), at which time a short insufflation was used to create the operative space. Later a blunt dissection proved to be sufficient to create a good space between the thyroid and the strap muscles so as to rely only on external retraction (4). Since that time more than 240 procedures have been performed by the authors and the operation has been adopted in several centers (9).

3 INDICATIONS

A careful selection of patients is of paramount importance to assure a good outcome for this operation: the greatest limit is represented by the volume of the nodule and even more of the gland to be operated on. The lobe in fact has to be removed without disrupting its capsule because of the necessity of an accurate histological evaluation in that these nodules are often suspect for carcinoma (either follicular or papillary). Other important limits are represented by the presence of adhesions that can make it difficult to recognize the most important structures, such as the recurrent nerve. Therefore, redo surgery is considered a contraindication for this procedure, but great caution should also be addressed to thyroiditis. For this reason an accurate evaluation of thyroid antibodies, characteristically increased in this disease, must be obtained before operating on these patients. Also, operative ultrasonographic study should be the most accurate because it is important to correctly evaluate thyroid and nodule volume and because it can help to recognize echographic aspects of thyroiditis.

General indications might be summarized as follows:

1. Thyroid nodules < 30 mm at largest diameter
2. Thyroid gland volume < 20 mL, as estimated by ultrasound

3. No history of thyroiditis
4. No previous neck surgery or irradiation
5. Presence of benign, follicular, or "low-risk" papillary carcinoma determined by cytological examination

4 TECHNIQUE

The procedure can be divided into four separate steps.

4.1 Preparation of the Operative Space

The patient, under general endotracheal anesthesia, is in supine position with the neck not extended: hyperextension must be avoided because it would reduce the operative space. The skin is protected by means of a sterile film (Tegaderm®). A 1.5 cm horizontal skin incision is performed 2 cm above the sternal notch in the central cervical area (Fig. 1). Subcutaneous fat and platysma are carefully dissected so as to avoid any minimum bleeding. Two small retractors (army-navy type) (Fig. 2) are used to expose the midline, which has to be incised for 2–3 cm on an absolutely bloodless plane.

The blunt dissection of the thyroid lobe from the strap muscles is completely carried out through the skin incision by gentle retraction and using tiny spatulas. The same small retractors maintain the operative space in which a 30° 5 or 7 mm endoscope is inserted through the skin incision: from this moment on the procedure is entirely endoscopic until the extraction of the affected lobe. Preparation of the thyro-tracheal groove is completed under endoscopic vision by using small (2 mm in diameter) instruments (Fig. 3).

4.2 Ligature of the Main Thyroid Vessels

Neither clips nor ligatures are currently used to achieve hemostasis. A Harmonic Scalpel device (Ultracision®) is utilized for all the vessels. The first one to be separated is the middle vein, if present, or the small veins between jugular vein and thyroid capsule. Their section allows a beter exposure of the thyroid space. The upper pedicle is then prepared by retracting the thyroid lobe downward and medially (Fig. 4). The spatula is used to retract the vessels laterally. This also allows the external branch of the superior laryngeal nerve (Fig. 5) to be easily identified during most procedures. Injury can be avoided by keeping the inactive blade of the Ultracision device in the posterior position so as to not transmit heat to this delicate structure.

4.3 Visualization and Dissection of the Recurrent Nerve and Parathyroid

When retracting medially and lifting up the thyroid lobe by means of retractors, the cervical fascia can be opened by gentle spatula retraction and the recurrent nerve appears in the groove between trachea and thyroid. A good anatomical landmark for its visualization is the Zuckerkandl lobe of the thyroid. Superior parathyroid gland can be easily visualized thanks to endoscopic magnification and dissected by Ultracision. Both of these structures must be carefully separated from the thyroid lobe before it is extracted (Fig. 6).

4.4 Extraction of the Lobe and Resection

At this point in time the lobe is completely freed. The endoscope and retractors can be removed and the upper portion of the gland rotated and pulled out using conventional forceps. Gentle traction over the upper pole allows the thyroid lobe to be completely extracted (Fig. 7). The operation is now conducted as in open surgery under direct vision. The lobe is freed from the trachea by dissecting Berry's ligament. It is very important to check the laryngeal nerve once again so as to avoid its injury before the final step. The isthmus is then dissected from the trachea and divided by means of Ultracision.

Drainage is not necessary. The midline is then approached by a single stitch; the platysma is closed by a subcuticular readsorbable suture, and a cyanoacrylate sealant is used for the skin (Fig. 8).

Surgical follow-up should include direct laryngoscopy to check vocal cord mobility and neck ultrasonography in all cases. Serum calcium measurement is obtained in those patients submitted to total thyroidectomy in order to evaluate their parathyroid function.

5 RESULTS

Our experience consists of 241 patients operated on since June 1998. Female-to-male ratio was 4:1. Lobectomy was carried out in 148 (61.4%) patients, total thyroidectomy in 93 (38.6%) patients. Mean operative time of lobectomy was 49.4 (range 20–120) minutes, while total thyroidectomy was accomplished in 61.8 (30–130) minutes. Preoperative diagnosis is shown in Table 1. Conversion to traditional cervicotomy was required in 4 cases (1,6%). Two cases occurred at the beginning of the experience. In the first one conversion was due to intraoperative bleeding from the upper vascular ped-

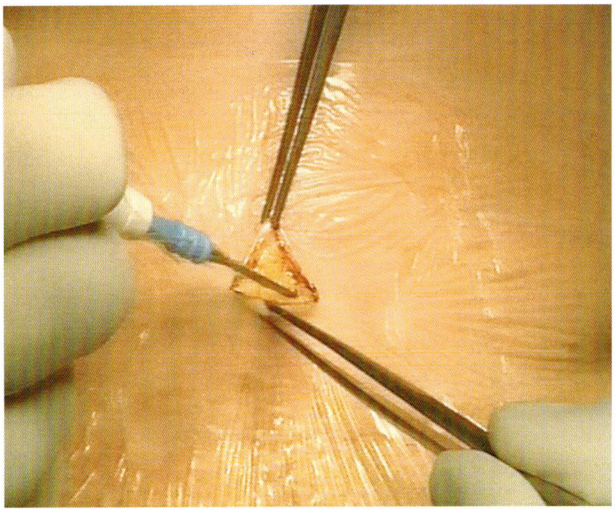

Figure 1 A 1.5 cm horizontal skin incision is performed 2 cm above the sternal notch.

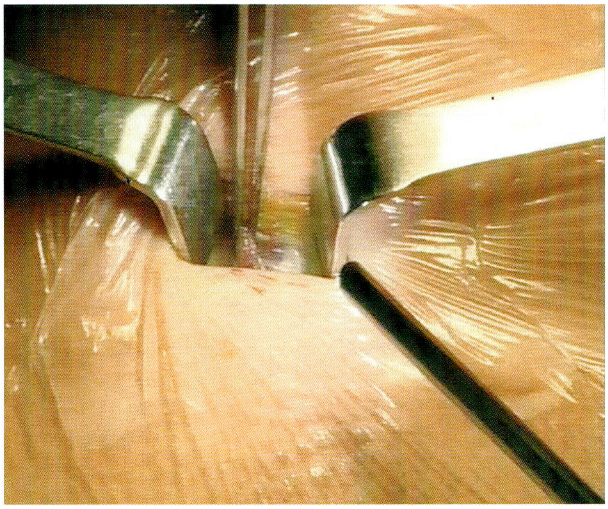

Figure 2 Two small retractors are used to expose the midline.

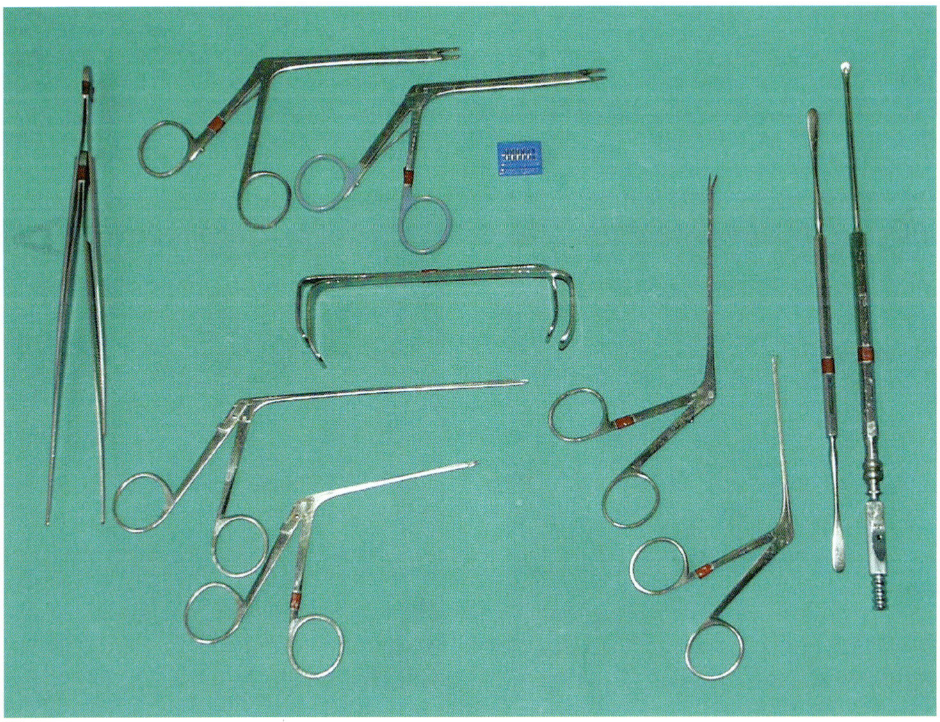

Figure 3 Instruments for MIVAT.

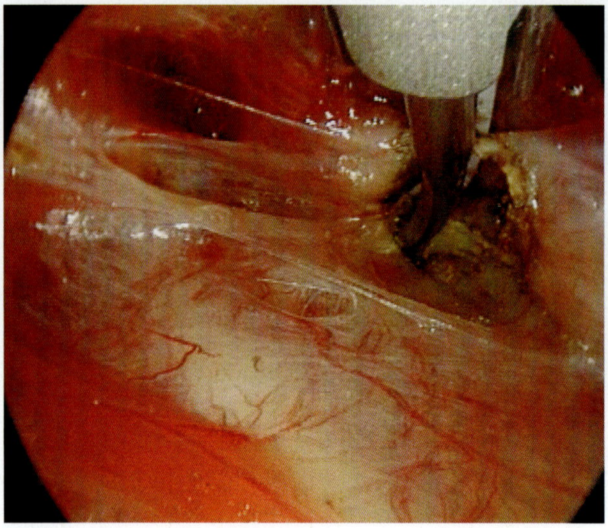

Figure 4 The upper pedicle is prepared and transected by ultracision.

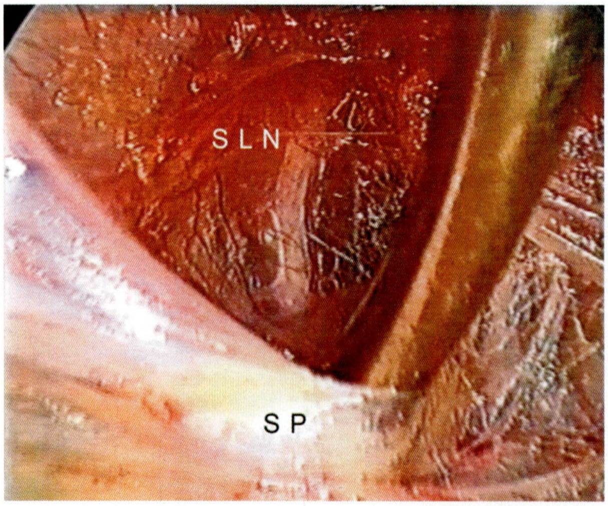

Figure 5 The external branch of the superior laryngeal nerve is easily visualized during section of the upper pedicle.

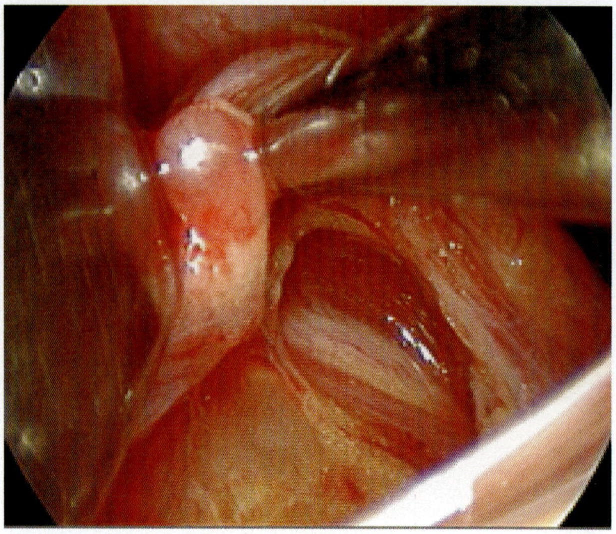

Figure 6 Endoscopic magnification allows good visualization of parathyroid glands and recurrent laryngeal nerve.

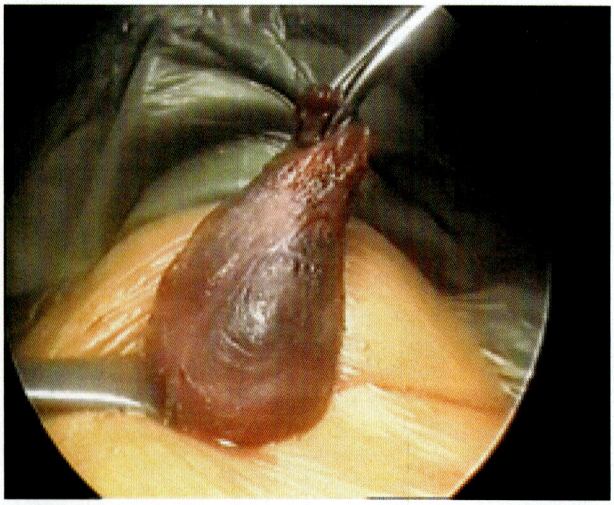

Figure 7 Gentle retraction over the upper pole allows the thyroid lobe to be completely extracted.

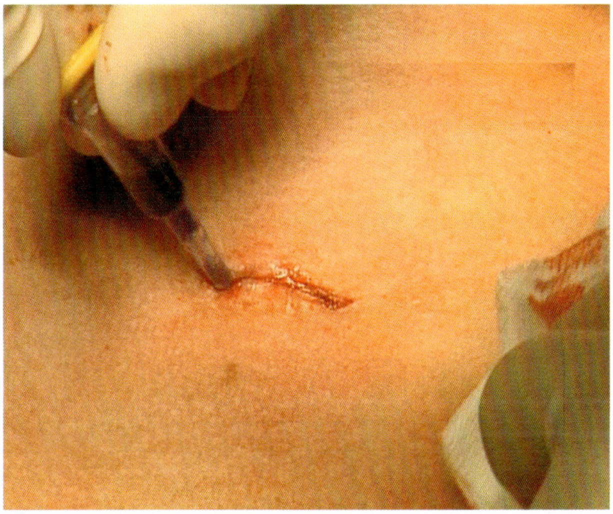

Figure 8 Sealant is used to close the skin.

Table 1 Preoperative Diagnosis

	N (%)
Follicular nodule	89 (36.9)
Papillary carcinoma	68 (28.3)
Multinodular goiter	44 (18.2)
Hürtle cell nodule	25 (10.3)
Toxic adenoma	11 (4.6)
Graves' disease	1 (0.4)
Toxic multinodular goiter	3 (1.2)
Total	241 (100%)

icle. In the second one we chose to perform completion thyroidectomy by an open approach in a patient with positive frozen section (papillary cancer) because we were concerned about the duration of the procedure by the video-assisted approach. Since then we have always performed a total video-assisted thyroidectomy in similar cases. In the third case conversion was due to unexpected esophageal infiltration by a small papillary carcinoma, and in the last case we converted because of difficult dissection caused by thyroiditis. In an even larger series of 336 cases operated on with this technique and described in a multicentric study (9), the first reason for conversion was in fact the difficulty of the lobe dissection because it rendered uncertain the identification of the most important structures such as the recurrent nerve.

Postoperative hospital stay was the same as in all other patients who underwent traditional surgery (overnight discharge). No postoperative bleeding was registered in our series. All patients were satisfied with the cosmetic results. In a recent prospective randomized study (10) on a limited series of patients comparing MIVAT to traditional thyroidectomy, we demonstrated that cosmetic results, evaluated by verbal response scale and numeric scale as well as postoperative distress, were significantly better in patients who underwent MIVAT; patients in the MIVAT group experienced significantly less pain than patients in the conventional thyroidectomy group at 6, 24, and 48 hours after operation as evaluated by visual analogue scale ($p = 0.003$). Similarly, patients in the MIVAT group were more satisfied with the cosmetic result as evaluated by a verbal response scale and a numerical scale ($p = 0.003$ and $p = 0.01$, respectively).

Complications experienced in the entire series of 241 patients consisted of one recurrent nerve palsy, 4 transient recurrent nerve injuries, 1 definitive hypoparathyroidism, and 2 transient hypocalcemias.

6 COMPLICATIONS

Potential complications of video-assisted thyroidectomy are roughly the same as in open surgery: nerve injuries, hemorrhage, and hypoparathyroidism are the most important. The magnification of the endoscope allows easy identification of both superior (external branch) and inferior laryngeal nerves and parathyroid glands. One could argue that preservation of these delicate structures should be adequately obtained during MIVAT.

In our series consisting of 241 patients operated on for benign and malignant disease we registered one definitive inferior laryngeal nerve palsy (0.4%) and four transient injuries (1.6%). The low percentage of laryngeal nerve injury is the best proof that MIVAT is as safe as standard thyroidectomy. Furthermore, the endoscope magnification gives a view of these structures which, particularly for the external branch of the superior laryngeal nerve, is far better than that obtained in the open operation.

The incidence of hypoparathyroidism was no greater in our series than in traditional surgery. We registered one case of definitive hypoparathyroidism (0.4%) and two cases of transient hypocalcemia (0.8%).

Only once did we experience bleeding that forced us to convert the procedure. It happened in the earlier period of our experience during the upper pedicle ligature where a clip was displaced from the artery and control of bleeding was difficult. In the last 150 cases we used the harmonic scalpel (Ultracision), which avoided the utilization of clips in most of cases. Since its introduction we have not experienced either postoperative or intraoperative bleedings requiring conversion. No patients have complained of complications at the cervical wound level: neither sepsis nor infiltration has occurred in the present series.

Even when performed in different surgical settings MIVAT proved to be a safe surgical procedure. In the previously mentioned multicentric study (336 cases) (9), the complication rate was comparable to if not lower than in conventional surgery: operative complications were represented by recurrent nerve palsy in 8 cases (2.1%): only one patient showed a permanent lesion (0.3%), while in 7 patients the lesion was transient and always lasted for less than 1 month. Eleven patients exhibited hypoparathyroidism, which corresponds to 9.8% of the 112 total thyroidectomies performed, but only two complained of a permanent hypocalcemia that necessitated a substitutive therapy, reducing the rate of permanent hypoparathyroidism to only 1.8%. Three patients experienced hemorrhage with conversion required in only one case (bleeding from the upper pedicle too hazardous to manage via endoscopic procedure). The hemorrhage resolved into a postoperative hematoma in two cases where only conservative therapy was necessary; a wound sepsis occurred in one case.

7 CONCLUSIONS

MIVAT has proven to be a safe procedure when performed in different surgical settings (9), and it is a valid therapeutic option as long as indications are strictly followed, because some advantages in terms of cosmetic result and postoperative pain can be demonstrated (10). Some concern exists about the radical nature of this minimally invasive procedure because "low risk" papillary carcinoma accounts for almost 20% of all cases. We evaluated whole body scans (WBS) and serum thyroglobulin (sTg) dosage in these patients in a previous series (11). The results were comparable to those of traditional surgery both in terms of I^{131} uptake and sTg levels, demonstrating that a satisfying outcome can be achieved in this kind of carcinoma occurring frequently in young females who are particularly concerned about the operation's cosmetic outcome.

REFERENCES

1. Gagner M. Endoscopic parathyroidectomy (lett). Br J Surg 1996; 83:875.
2. Henry JF, Defechereux T, Gramatica L, de Boissezon C. Minimally invasive videoscopic parathyroidectomy by lateral approach. Langenbecks Arch Surg 1999; 384: 298–301.
3. Miccoli P, Bendinelli C, Vignali E, Mazzeo S, Cecchini G, Pinchera A, Marcocci C. Endoscopic parathyroidectomy: report of an initial experience. Surgery 1998; 124: 1077–1080.
4. Miccoli P, Berti P, Raffaelli M, Conte M, Materazzi G, Galleri D. Minimally invasive video-assisted parathyroidectomy. Am J Surg 2001; 181(6):567–570.
5. Shimizu K, Akira S, Jasmi AY, et al. Video-assisted neck surgery: endoscopic resection of thyroid tumors with a very minimal neck wound. J Am Coll Surg 1999; 188:697–703.
6. Ohgami M, Ishii S, Ohmori T, Noga K, Furukawa T, Kitajima M. Scarless endoscopic thyroidectomy: breast approach better cosmesis. Surg Laparosc Endosc Percutan Tech 2000; 10:1–4.
7. Ikeda Y, Takami H, Sasaky Y, Kan S, Niimi M. Endoscopic neck surgery by the axillary approach. J Am Coll Surg 2000; 191:849–851.
8. Miccoli P, Berti P, Conte M, et al. Minimally invasive surgery for small thyroid nodules: preliminary report. J Endocrinol Invest 1999; 22:849–851.
9. Miccoli P, Bellantone R, Mourad M, Walz M, Raffaelli M, Berti P. Minimally invasive video-assisted thyroidectomy (MIVAT): a multi-institutional experience. World J Surg 2002; 26:972–975.
10. Miccoli P, Berti P, Raffaelli M, Materazzi G, Baldacci S, Rossi G. Comparison between minimally invasive video-assisted thyroidectomy and conventional thyroidectomy: a prospective randomized study. Surgery 2001; 130.
11. Miccoli P, Elisei R, Materazzi G, Capezzone M, Galleri D, Pacini F, Berti P, Pinchera A. Minimally invasive video-assisted thyroidectomy for papillary carcinoma: a prospective study of its completeness. Surgery 2002; 132:1070–1074.

17

Physiology of the Parathyroid Glands and Pathophysiology of Primary Hyperparathyroidism

John P. Bilezikian and Shonni J. Silverberg

Columbia University, New York, New York, U.S.A.

1 INTRODUCTION

The subject of this chapter is the parathyroid glands both with regard to their important role in governing calcium homeostasis and to abnormalities associated with syndromes of overproduction of parathyroid hormone, hyperparathyroidism. While the chapters that follow in this section deal with surgical considerations of this subject matter, the material in this chapter provides key background information for the parathyroid surgeon.

2 REGULATION OF CALCIUM HOMEOSTASIS BY THE PARATHYROID GLANDS

The parathyroid glands play a key role in maintaining normal extracellular calcium concentration by virtue of their capacity to register with exquisite sensitivity small changes in this divalent cation (1). Parathyroid hormone (PTH), the principal product of the parathyroid gland, acts on its two target organs, bone and kidney, to maintain normal extracellular calcium levels. A small reduction in the extracellular calcium concentration is associated with a virtually simultaneous increase in parathyroid hormone secretion. PTH mobilizes skeletal calcium. At the kidney, PTH conserves calcium at the distal tubule. It also stimulates the conversion of 25-hydroxyvitamin D to the active metabolite of vitamin D, 1,25-dihydroxyvitamin D. 1,25-Dihdroxyvitamin D, in turn, acts on the gastrointestinal tract to facilitate calcium absorption. The net effect of these physiological adjustments is a return of the reduced extracellular calcium concentration to normal. When the extracellular calcium concentration rises for any reason not related to an intrinsic abnormalitiy of the parathyroid glands, a reverse series of physiological events occurs. Secretion of PTH is immediately halted. A sharp decline in PTH concentration reduces skeletal calcium mobilization, facilitates urinary calcium excretion, and reduces the production of 1,25-dihydroxyvitamin D. The net effect of these physiological adjustments is a return of the elevated extracellular calcium concentration to normal.

When these physiological control mechanisms react to a pathophysiological stimulus, namely in renal insufficiency or in settings of hypercalcemia not related to a primary abnormality of the parathyroids, the glands still behave in the same manner, namely with an increase or a decrease in PTH, but often the glands cannot compensate adequately. In renal failure, therefore, the serum calcium will be low in association with a compensatory elevated PTH level. In non–parathyroid-dependent hypercalcemia, PTH will be suppressed but the serum calcium is still elevated. Understanding this pathophysiology helps in the differential diagnosis of states associated with hypercalcemia and hypocalcemia (see below).

The calcium-sensing receptor (CaR) is a key mediator of parathyroid responsiveness to changes in extracellular calcium. The CaR recognizes its cognate ligand, calcium ion, in the same manner that a hormone receptor recognizes its ligand. In fact, similar to a hormone receptor, the CaR is located in the outer plasma membrane of the parathyroid cell. It is also present on a variety of other cell types, such as the kidney (2,3). Like a hormone, therefore, calcium acts as a first messenger and stimulates the cell machinery to either increase or decrease transcription and ultimately secretion of PTH. In the disorder familial hypocalciuric hypercalcemia (FHH), also termed familial benign hypocalciuric hypercalcemia (FBHH), there is often a mutation in the CaR causing a reduction in the sensitivity of the parathyroid cell to extracellular calcium (4,5). It is important to distinguish this disorder (FHH/FBHH) from primary hyperparathyroidism because the management of these two disorders is quite different. The CaR receptor can also be the site of a mutation in which the receptor is activated (5). In this case sensitivity of the parathyroid cell to extracellular calcium is heightened. The patient has hypocalcemia but completely normal levels of PTH.

3 DIFFERENTIAL DIAGNOSIS OF HYPERCALCEMIA

The diagnosis of primary hyperparathyroidism is made with due consideration for the differential diagnosis of hypercalcemia. Primary hyperparathyroidism is one of the two most common causes of hypercalcemia. The other is malignancy. These two etiologies account for over 90% of all patients with hypercalcemia (6). A much longer, complete list of potential causes of hypercalcemia is considered after these two etiologies are ruled out or if there is reason to believe that a different cause is likely. The clinical presentation of hypercalcemia associated with primary hyperparathyroidism or malignancy gives a convenient clue as to which one is more likely. The modern presentation of primary hyperparathyroidism is essentially an asymptomatic disorder discovered most often in the course of routine biochemical testing (7). In contrast, hypercalcemia of malignancy occurs in the latter stages of advanced malignancy. Patients with hypercalcemia of malignancy are usually symptomatic both of the advanced malignancy and the hypercalcemia. The biochemical distinction between primary hyperparathyroidism and malignancy is firmly established by measuring the PTH level. With the two-site immunoradiometric or immunochemiluminometric assay for PTH, patients with primary hyperparathyroidism will have frank elevations 75–90% of the time. In the small percentage of patients whose parathyroid hormone level is normal, it tends to be in the upper range of normal and, thus, clearly "abnormal" when hypercalcemia is simultaneously present. Although the IRMA assay current in commercial use is called "intact," work by Broussard et al. demonstrated that a large non-(1–84)PTH fragment is detected by this assay (8). This large amino-terminal truncated fragment(s), missing the first 4–6 N-terminal amino acids, has 100% cross-reactivity with the commercially available "intact" assay for PTH. Recently, a newer IRMA assay for PTH has been developed in which the recognition sites on the PTH molecule are at 39–84 and 1–6, thus giving this assay a specificity for the full-length biologically active region of the molecule exclusively (9). Studies by Silverberg et al. (10) have applied this new assay to a group of subjects with surgically proven primary hyperparathyroidism. In comparison to the intact assay and the older radioimmunoassay for mid-molecule PTH, the newer assay performed better with respect to a higher percentage of patients with frankly elevated levels (96%) in comparison to the intact (73%) and mid-molecule (63%) assays. It remains to be seen whether this newer assay for the whole molecule will be more clinically useful than the one that is currently available.

As a rule, therefore, patients with hypercalcemia and elevated PTH levels have primary hyperparathyroidism. Exceptions to this rule are associated with two medications, lithium and thiazide diuretics, that can cause hypercalcemia. Actually, many of these patients do have primary hyperparathyroidism, but the only way to be sure is to withdraw the medication and to monitor the serum calcium and PTH after 3 months. In someone who is dependent upon lithium therapy for their mental well-being, withdrawal may be difficult or unwise. Another exception is tertiary hyperparathyroidism in which hypercalcemia and elevated parathyroid hormone can be seen together. Tertiary hyperparathyroidism is an end result of longstanding, poorly controlled renal insufficiency. This usually does not present a problem in differential diagnosis because the advanced renal failure is clearly evident. In these cases there is a change from mechanisms of parathyroid gland compensation (i.e., to normalize the tendency for hypocalcemia to develop; a secondary hyperparathyroidism—see discussion above) to mechanisms of parathyroid gland autonomy (i.e., a tertiary hyperparathyroidism) with attendant hypercalcemia (11,12). It is of interest that some of these patients are actually found, at surgery, to have primary hyperparathyroidism, that is, a single adenomatous gland superimposed upon a background of hyperplastic tissue (13). Patients who develop hypercalcemia after longstanding renal insufficiency may show evidence for monoclonality of individual, hyperactive parathyroid glands (14). A final exception to the rule that patients with elevated levels of calcium and PTH have primary hyperparathyroidism is FHH/FBHH (see discussion above).

In contrast to the hypercalcemia of primary hyperparathyroidism, the hypercalcemia of malignancy is invariably associated with suppressed levels of parathyroid hormone. This is even true in humoral hypercalcemia of malignancy in which the tumor (lung cancer, esophagus, cervix, vulva, head and neck, breast, renal, and HTLV-1 T-cell lymphoma) elaborates parathyroid hormone–related protein (PTHRP). PTHRP is the product of a gene that retains lingering similarity to the PTH gene. PTHRP shares with PTH only a limited region of primary sequence homology, the first 13–15 amino acids at the amino-terminal end of the molecule. This limited but important sequence homology, along with similarities in spatial configuration for sequences up to amino acids 30–34, probably explains why PTHRP shares with PTH some key biological properties such as the ability to resorb bone and to conserve renal calcium (15). Commercially available assays for PTH do not detect PTHRP in the circulation because the two require antigenic determinants for PTH are not shared by PTHRP. Thus, in the distinction between hypercalcemia of malignancy and hypercalcemia of primary hyperparathroidism, the PTH assay is a key biochemical point. It is elevated in primary hyperparathyroidism and suppressed in malignancy-associated hypercalcemia.

Table 1 Differential Diagnosis of Hypercalcemia

Primary hyperparathyroidism
Malignancy
Hyperthyroidism
Pheochromocytoma
VIPoma
Adrenal insufficiency
Lithium
Thiazide diuretics
Thyroid hormone
Vitamin A
Vitamin D
Tuberculosis
Sarcoidosis
Lymphoma
Familial hypocalciuric hypercalcemia
Immobilization
Acute or chronic renal disease

The remainder of the differential diagnosis of hypercalcemia is long but becomes important clinically when the two most common causes of hypercalcemia have been ruled out (Table 1). Of course, one would be more likely to think of hyperthyroidism, for example, in the hypercalcemic patient who is overtly thyrotoxic. Similarly, if a patient has known sarcoidosis or other granulomatous disorder, one should think more quickly about those potential etiologies even though they are unlikely from a statistical point of view.

4 EPIDEMIOLOGY OF PRIMARY HYPERPARATHYROIDISM

Primary hyperparathyroidism is a common endocrine disorder due in large part to the widespread use of the multichannel autoanalyzer, which was introduced in the early 1970s (16). Prior to that time, however, primary hyperparathyroidism was not a common endocrine disease (17). Despite its rarity, as described in older reports, the frequency with which it was diagnosed was, in large measure, a function of one's index of suspicion. For example, Raymond Keating, whose work at the Mayo Clinic helped to establish modern concepts of the disease, began to recognize primary hyperparathyroidism with regularity only after he was made more acute aware of it by Aub, Bauer, and Albright (18). This experience was the clue that primary hyperparathyroidism was much more prevalent in the population at large than its incidence would have suggested. With the advent of the autoanalyzer it was rather quickly apparent that there were many individuals with primary hyperparathyroidsm whose disease was not being recognized simply because calcium determinations were not being routinely obtained. Incidence figures rose dramatically when calcium determinations were obtained in the context of the multichannel biochemistry profile. Reporting its experience before and after the introduction of the autoanalyzer, the Mayo Clinic saw a four- to fivefold increase in the incidence of primary hyperparathyroidism to approximately 100,000 new cases per year or about 27.7 cases per 100,000 person-years (16,19). Apart from these reports, most other population-based studies on the prevalence of primary hyperparathyroidism are Scandinavian (20,21). Epidemiological uncertainties with the extensive Scandinavian databases include the fact that persistent hypercalcemia has been the primary identification marker without clear documentation of parathyroid disease by concomitant parathyroid hormone determinations (22,23). Postmortem examination of the parathyroid glands do not help to solidify the database because such studies are not accompanied by functional evidence for hyperparathyroidism during life (24). More recently, using serum parathyroid hormone values along with the serum calcium concentration, Lundgren et al. showed that 2.6% of the postmenopausal population in Sweden had primary hyperparathyroidism (25,26). On follow-up testing, however, only two thirds had confirmation of the diagnosis. These results, nevertheless, help to underscore the point that primary hyperparathyroidism is a common endocrine disorder. It increases with age and is much more common in women by a ratio of approximately 3:1 (16,22,23, 26–28).

Reports from the United States and Europe have suggested that the incidence of primary hyperparathyroidism may be declining (22,25,29). Such reports are surprising and have not been widely confirmed. In fact, the incidence of primary hyperparathyroidism would appear to be, in the experience of most endocrinologists, unchanged. If it is demonstrated that the incidence of primary hyperparathyroidism is declining, this could well be due to efforts on the part of health care insurers to control costs by restricting access to the multichannel screening test. In the sporadic form of primary hyperparathyroidism, by far the most common presentation seen, no clearly definable risk factors can be identified. A history of childhood irradiation to the face or neck is obtained in a small number of individuals (30,31).

5 MOLECULAR PATHOGENESIS OF PRIMARY HYPERPARATHYROIDISM

In primary hyperparathyroidism, clones of abnormal parathyroid cells emerge that dominate the homeostatic system such that the usual steep inverse relationship between PTH release and calcium ion is altered or shifted to the right. For a given extracellular calcium concentration, PTH is higher. Although in large measure the underlying defect is altered sensitivity of a clone of parathyroid cells to calcium, increases in the mass of abnormal parathyroid tissues also contribute to excessive secretion of PTH (32–34). No specific mutations of the CaR have been described in primary hyperparathyroidism.

The molecular pathogenetic abnormalities in primary hyperparathyroidism involve several candidate genes that have variably been implicated as causal in the disorder. Two genes have been established as etiologically important. The first gene to be associated with primary hyperparathyroidism is cyclin D1/PRAD 1 (or CCND1). This parathyroid oncogene on human chromosome 11q13 is activated by a tumor-specific DNA rearrangement with the PTH gene locus in some patients with primary hyperparathyroidism (35–38). The rearrangement leads to transcriptional activation and overexpression of structurally normal cyclin D1 by bringing this gene into proximity with regulatory regions of the PTH gene. Thus, when the PTH gene is active or activated, the cyclin D1 gene is also stimulated, leading to growth of the clone that harbors the genetic abnormality. According to Arnold, as many as 20–40% of parathyroid adenomas may overexpress cyclin D1, although the exact mechanisms for this overexpression is likely to vary greatly (39–42).

The second genetic abnormality that has been decribed as etiologically important in primary hyperparathyroidism is the gene associated with multiple endocrine neoplasia, type 1 (MEN1) (43,44). The MEN1 gene product is a tumor suppressor. In primary hyperparathyroidism, or in any mechanism of tumorogenesis due to a tumor suppressor gene, complete inactivation (biallelic dysfunction) is required. As many as 12–20% of patients with sporadic primary hyperparathyroidism, that is, those who do not have the multiple endocrine neoplasia syndrome, have been shown to harbor biallelic defects in the MEN1 gene (44–46).

Although clearly much more information is needed about the molecular pathogenesis of primary hyperparathyroidism, the implication of at least two genes so far suggests that perhaps most patients with this order will ultimately be shown to have some underlying molecular defect for the abnormal setpoint for calcium in this disorder. A number of other candidate gene defects have been described and are currently under investigation (47–49).

6 PATHOLOGY OF PRIMARY HYPERPARATHYROIDISM

By far the most common lesion found in patients with primary hyperparathyroidism is the solitary parathyroid adenoma, occurring in 80% of patients. While in most cases a single adenoma is found, multiple parathyroid adenomas have been reported in 2–4% of cases (50–52). These may be familial or sporadic. Parathyroid adenomas can be discovered in many unexpected anatomical locations. Embryonal migration patterns of parathyroid tissue account for a plethora of possible sites for ectopic parathyroid adenomas. The most common sites for ectopic adenomas are within the thyroid gland, the superior mediastinum, and the thymus. Occasionally, the adenoma may ultimately be identified in the retroesophageal space, the pharynx, the lateral neck, and even the alimentary submucosa of the esophagus.

In approximately 15% of patients with primary hyperparathyroidism, all four parathyroid glands are involved. There are no clinical features that differentiate single versus multiglandular disease. The etiology of four-gland parathyroid hyperplasia is multifactorial. It may be associated with a familial hereditary syndrome, such as multiple endocrine neoplasia, Types 1 and 2a. As in the case of parathyroid adenomas, underlying molecular mechanisms are heterogeneous.

7 BIOCHEMICAL FEATURES OF PRIMARY HYPERPARATHYROIDISM

Typical biochemical indices associated with primary hyperparathyroidism are shown in Table 2. The serum calcium determination is typically not greater than 1 mg/dL above the upper limits of normal. The serum phosphorus is in the lower range of normal, with only approximately 25% of patients showing phosphorus levels that are frankly low. Total alkaline phosphatase activity is in the high normal range, as is the case for more specific markers of bone turnover, bone-specific alkaline phosphatase activity, osteocalcin, or collagen breakdown products (*N*-telopeptide, deoxypyridinoline). The 25-hydroxyvitamin D level tends to be in the lower range of normal, while the 1,25-dihydroxyvitamin D level tends to be in the upper range of normal. Approximately 25% of patients with primary hyperparathyroidism will have levels of 1,25-dihydroxyvitamin D that are frankly elevated (53). The pattern of 25-hydroxyvitamin D and 1,25-dihydroxyvitamin D concentrations in primary hyperparathyroidism is due to the property of parathyroid hormone to facilitate the conversion of the monohydroxylated precursor to the dihydroxylated active vitamin D product. Urinary calcium excretion is typically in the upper range of normal, with as many as 40% of individuals showing frank hypercalciuria. Curiously, the presence of hypercalciuria in those without a history of kidney stones does not have predictive value for the development of nephrolithiasis (54).

Table 2 Biochemical Indices in Primary Hyperparathyroidism

	Patient values	Normal reference ranges
Calcium (mg/dL)	10.7 ± 0.1	8.4–10.2
Phosphorus (mg/dL)	2.9 ± 0.1	2.5–4.5
Alk Phos (IU/L)	114 ± 4	< 100
PTH (pg/mL)	121 ± 7	10–65
25-OH Vit D (ng/mL)	21 ± 1	9–52
1,25-OH_2 Vit D (ng/mL)	59 ± 2	15–60
Urinary calcium (mg)	248 ± 12	250–300
DPD (nmol/mmol Cr)	17 ± 6	4–21

The values for this table are obtained from the cohort of patients followed by Silverberg, Bilezikikian et al. over the past 15 years.

8 CLINICAL FEATURES OF PRIMARY HYPERPARATHYROIDISM

It is not surprising that with more widespread recognition of primary hyperparathyroidism, the classical signs and symptoms of the disease would change (55).

8.1 The Skeleton

The frequency of specific radiological manifestations of primary hyperparathyroidism has fallen from 23% in the Cope series (17) to less than 2% in the series of Silverberg et al. (56,57). In fact, overt skeletal disease in primary hyperparathyroidism is so infrequent that skeletal x-rays are rarely indicated. Although osteitis fibrosa cystica is distinctly unusual in patients who present with primary hyperparathyroidism in the United States, this does not imply that the skeleton is unaffected in those with asymptomatic disease. The availability of sensitive techniques to monitor the skeleton has given us an opportunity to address these issues in patients who have asymptomatic primary hyperparathyroidism.

8.2 Bone Densitometry

The advent of bone mineral densitometry as a major diagnostic tool for osteoporosis occurred at a time when the clinical profile of primary hyperparathyroidism was changing from a symptomatic to an asymptomatic disease. Questions about skeletal involvement in primary hyperparathyroidism could be addressed, therefore, despite the absence of overt radiological features of primary hyperparathyroidism. Bone mass measurement, now an integral element of the evaluation of all patients with primary hyperparathyroidism, typically shows evidence for skeletal involvement (56). Parathyroid hormone is known to be catabolic at sites of cortical bone. The distal 1/3 site of the radius provides a convenient cortical site for bone density evaluation in primary hyperparathyroidism to investigate the possibility that this site would be preferentially affected. Another physiological property of parathyroid hormone is an anabolic one, at cancellous sites, such as the lumbar spine. In primary hyperparathyroidism, as expected from physiological considerations, bone density at the distal radius (1/3 site) is diminished (55,56). Bone density at the lumbar spine is only minimally reduced, typically within 5% of age-matched mean values. The hip region, containing a relatively equal admixture of cortical and cancellous elements, shows bone density that is intermediate between the cortical and cancellous sites (Fig. 1). The results support not only the notion that parathyroid hormone is catabolic in cortical bone, but also the view that parathyroid hormone can be, under certain circumstances, anabolic for cancellous bone (58–60). In postmenopausal women, the same pattern was observed (56). Postmenopausal women with primary hyperparathyroidism, therefore, show a reversal of the pattern typically associated with postmenopausal estrogen deficiency, namely preferential loss of cancellous bone. These observations suggest that primary hyperparathyroidism may help to protect postmenopausal women from bone loss due to estrogen deficiency.

The bone density profile in which there is relative preservation of skeletal mass at the spine and diminution at the more cortical radial site is not always seen in primary hyperparathyroidsm. A small group of patients with primary hyperparathyroidism have evidence of vertebral osteopenia at the time of presentation. In our natural history study, approximately 15% of patients had a lumbar spine Z-score of ≤1.5 at the time of diagnosis (61).

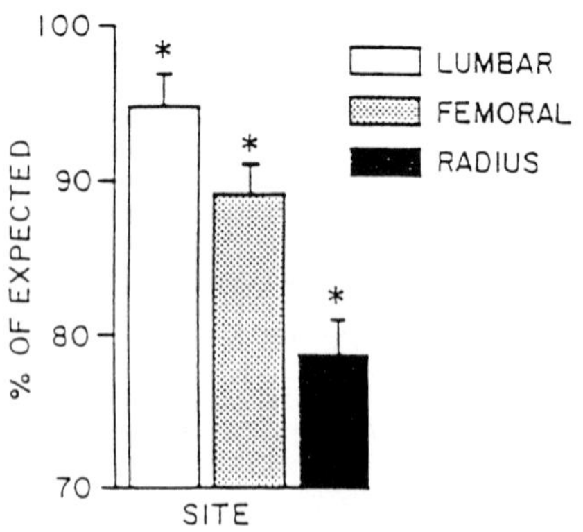

Figure 1 A typical pattern of bone loss is seen in asymptomatic patients with primary hyperparathyroidism. The lumbar spine is relatively well preserved, while the distal radius (1/3 site) is preferentially affected. (From Ref. 56.)

8.3 Histomorphometry of Bone

Analyses of percutaneous bone biopsies from patients with primary hyperparathyroidism demonstrate cortical thinning, maintenance of cancellous bone volume, and a very dynamic process associated with high turnover and accelerated bone remodeling. Confirming the results by bone densitometry, cancellous bone volume is clearly well preserved in primary hyperparathyroidism. This is seen in the group of all subjects we studied as well as among the subcohort of postmenopausal women with primary hyperparathyroidism. Several studies have shown that cancellous bone is actually increased in primary hyperparathyroidism as compared to normal subjects (62–64). Preservation of cancellous bone volume extends to comparisons with the expected losses associated with the effects of aging on cancellous bone physiology. In patients with primary hyperparathyroidism, there is no relationship between trabecular number or separation and age, suggesting that the actual plates and their connections are maintained over time more effectively than in normal aging individuals. Thus, primary hyperparathyroidism seems to retard the normal age-related processes associated with trabecular loss (65). One of the mechanisms by which cancellous bone is preserved in primary hyperparathyroidism is through the maintenance of interconnected trabecular plates (66).

8.4 Fracture Risk

Since bone mineral density is an important predictor of fracture risk, the densitometric data in primary hyperparathyroidism suggest certain expectations about fracture incidence. One would expect, for example, that fracture incidence would be increased in the forearm and reduced in the lumbar spine. However, the data are not conclusive; rather they are highly controversial. Dauphine et al. (67) and Khosla et al. (68) reported that vertebral fractures were increased, but other observations have failed to confirm these reports (69–72). When vertebral fracture is the starting point for case finding, primary hyperparathyroidism is rarely found, although measurement of the serum calcium is recommended by many as part of the evaluation of all newly diagnosed cases of osteoporosis. Expectations for increased fracture risk at cortical sites such as the forearm are also not supported by available data, although it would seem logical to anticipate more long bone fractures. But primary hyperparathyroidism is not a dominant feature in most series of hip fracture patients (72). Khosla et al. have analyzed retrospectively the incidence of fractures in primary hyperparathyroidism over a 28-year period (1965–1992). Fracture rate was reported to be increased among the 407 cases of primary hyperparathyroidism at the forearm (68).

Also noteworthy with regard to the changing clinical profile of the disease is the reduction in the incidence of kidney stone disease from approximately 60% in the preautoanalyzer era to current series in which the incidence is less than 20% (54,73). Still, renal stone disease is the most common overt complication of primary hyperparathyroidism.

Attempts to link carbohydrate intolerance and frank diabetes mellitus to primary hyperparathyroidism have been made (74–76), but the association is even more tenuous than other associations that have been alleged, such as hypertension (see below). Peptic ulcer disease and pancreatitis do not appear to be part of the syndrome of modern primary hyperparathyroidism (77–79).

Neuromuscular complications of classic primary hyperparathyroidism are not seen anymore. In a detailed neurological study of 42 patients with a mean serum calcium concentration of 11.1 ± 0.1 mg/dL, Turken et al. (80) found no consistent pattern of abnormalities either on physical examination or on electromyography. Joborn et al. (81) studied 18 randomly selected patients with primary hyperparathyroidism and concluded that, as a group, patients had slight, but significant impairment of muscle function, a finding that the authors speculated might be responsible for the "fatigue" of which some patients complain.

Quite apart from the potential for neuromuscular involvement in primary hyperparathyroidism, neuropsychiatric abnormalities have yet to be thoroughly characterized, although it remains an area of active interest (82–85). Many patients, families, and physicians note features of depression, cognitive difficulties, and anxiety in those with the disease. Although many of these complaints have been described as being reversible after parathyroidectomy, appropriately controlled studies are lacking.

In these and other potential complications of primary hyperparathyroidism, it has not been possible to ascertain with any degree of certainty that they are seen over and above what one would expect in the general population. A problem confounding epidemiological studies is that these associated disorders are also common in the population. Their linkage, therefore, could reflect no more than the likelihood that common disorders will be associated with a certain frequency by chance alone. Moreover, well-controlled prospective studies evaluating these potential complications of primary hyperparathyroidism are lacking (see below).

There are several reports of more cancers in patients with primary hyperparathyroidism (86,87). Many of these reports, however, are subject to selection bias. In patients with hypercalcemia detected unexpectedly on a biochemical profile, the most important cause to exclude is hypercalcemia associated with malignancy. Thus, the association between primary hyperparathyroidism and malignancy may be due simply to a more diligent search for cancer in patients with hypercalcemia. Another possible mechanism for a chance association between primary hyperparathyroidism and cancer results from the frequency with which clinically silent thyroid malignancies are found during neck exploration for parathyroid disease (88,89). Wermers et al. have reported, on the other hand, that following the diagnosis of primary hyperparathyroidism there was no increase in the incidence of malignancy (90).

In the United States, mortality does not seem to be increased in primary hyperparathyroidism, according to the epidemiology data of the Mayo Clinic experience (90). On the other hand, reports of increased mortality from the Scandinavian literature (91–98) and from Germany (99) are available. The reason for this difference may again be explained by the level of activity of the primary hyperparathyroidism, in that mortality in the Scandinavian experience did correlate with the extent of hypercalcemia and the weight of the parathyroid adenoma (21). Also consistent with this idea, in the Rochester, Minnesota experience, those whose serum calcium was in the highest quartile did have higher mortality in comparison to those in the lower three quartiles (90). On the whole, these observations suggest that mild, asymptomatic primary hyperparathyroidism is not associated with increased mortality rates. On the other hand, when the disease presents in more symptomatic forms, data from series in which mortality was increased in more symptomatic subjects become pertinent.

Most patients with primary hyperparathyroidism are asymptomatic. They have neither symptoms nor complications that are clearly and commonly associated with hypercalcemia or excessive parathyroid hormone. An exception to this statement is the experience in countries such as India, Brazil, and China, in which primary hyperparathyroidism still can present predominantly as a symptomatic disorder (100,101). To a certain extent these countries may not have as ready access to multichannel screening as western countries. The disease, therefore, could be discovered in a more advanced state. This does not account for the fact, however, that when patients with asymptomatic primary hyperparathyroidism are monitored conservatively, without surgical or medical intervention, they do not typically show progression to the more symptomatic form of the disease. Therefore, there are likely to be other explanations for why, in these countries, the disease still presents with such overt symptomatology. One possibility is that patients with symptomatic primary hyperparathyroidism are invariably vitamin D deficient. Based upon the actions of vitamin D to help control parathyroid function, its deficiency could fuel the parathyroid process to become even more active. Even in our experience, patients with mild hyperparathyroidism whose 25-hydroxyvitamin D levels are in the lowest tertile have evidence of more active disease (102).

9 INDICATIONS FOR SURGERY

Primary hyperparathyroidism is cured when the abnormal parathyroid tissue is removed. The decision to recommend surgery is tempered by the realization that the majority of patients with primary hyperparathyroidism are asymptomatic. Moreover, we lack predictive indices that indicate who among the asymptomatic are at risk for experiencing complications of this disease (84). The NIH Consensus Development Conference on the Management of Asymptomatic Primary Hyperparathyroidism issued guidelines for surgery to aid the clinician faced with the hyperparathyroid patient (79,103). At that time there was essentially no information in asymptomatic primary hyperparathyroidism as to who was at risk for the complications of this disease. After considering the information that was available, a set of guidelines was issued and has been used, with some modification over the past 12 years, by many endocrinologists (103). Certainly anyone with overt complications (radiological bone disease, kidney stones, classical neuromuscular symptoms) should have surgery. Among those with asymptomatic primary hyperparathyroidism, the following guidelines were recommended: (1) serum calcium concentration >1–1.6 mg/dL above the upper limit of normal; (2) marked hypercalciuria (>400 mg daily excretion); (3) bone density more than 2 standard deviations below age- and sex-matched control subjects (Z-score ≤ -2.0); (4) relatively young patients (<50 years old); (5) inability or unwillingness to be followed without surgery. Using these guidelines, approximately 60% of patients with primary hyperparathyroidism will meet at least one criterion and thereby become a candidate for surgery. Again, it should noted that only a small percentage of these patients are frankly symptomatic. The majority are asymptomatic but become surgical candidates by virtue of age, the serum or urinary calcium concentration, or because of reduced bone mass.

These guidelines for surgery, however, are subject to modification by the physician and the patient. Some physicians will recommend surgery for all patients with primary hyperparathyroidism; other physicians will not recommend surgery unless clear-cut complications of primary hyperparathyroidism are present. The patient enters into this therapeutic dialogue as well. Some patients cannot tolerate the idea of living with a curable disease and will seek surgery in the absence of any of the aforementioned criteria. Other patients with coexisting medical problems may not wish to face the risks of surgery even though surgical indications are present.

In April 2002, the National Institutes of Health (NIH) convened a Workshop on Asymptomatic Primary Hyperparathyroidism. During this 2-day conference, experts in virtually every aspect of the disease—medical and surgical—focused upon developments in the field since the 1990 Consensus Development Con-

Table 3 Comparison of New and Old Guidelines for Parathyroid Surgery[a] in Asymptomatic Primary Hyperparathyroidism

Measurement	Guidelines, 1990	Guidelines, 2002[b]
Serum calcium above upper limit of normal	1–1.6 mg/dL	1.0 mg/dL
24-hour urinary calcium	400 mg	Not recommended
Creatinine clearance	Reduced by 30%	Not recommended
Serum creatinine	Not recommended	If abnormal
Bone mineral density	Z-score ≤ -2.0 (forearm)	T-score ≤ -2.5 at any site
Age	<50	<50

[a] Surgery is also indicated in patients for whom medical surveillance is neither desired nor possible.
[b] *Source*: Ref. 104.

ference. The results of this workshop led to a new set of recommendations for management of patients with this disease (104) (Table 3). The newer recommendations set the upper limit of tolerance for serum calcium at 1 mg/dL above the upper limit of normal; serum creatinine has replaced the urinary calcium as an index; three-site bone densitometry is advocated with a lower limit set as a T-score (no longer Z-score) of ≤ -2.5 at any site. The recommendation for surgery in persons under 50 years was sustained in light of recent data of Silverberg et al. (105).

10 IMAGING OF ABNORMAL PARATHYROID GLANDS

Surgery in primary hyperparathyroidism is covered in subsequent chapters. Parathyroid surgery requires exceptional expertise and experience (106). The glands are notoriously variable in location, requiring knowledge by the surgeon of typical ectopic sites such as intrathyroidal, retroesophageal, the lateral neck, and the mediastinum. Because of potential difficulties in locating abnormal parathyroid tissue, preoperative approaches have been developed. Noninvasive imaging of the parathyroids include technetium-99m (Tc-99m) sestamibi with or without single photon emission computed tomography (SPECT), ultrasound (US), computed tomography (CT), and magnetic resonance imaging (MRI). Although each of these approaches has advantages and disadvantages, the Tc-99m sestamibi procedure appears at this time to enjoy the greatest popularity. Tc-99m sestamibi imaging can be conducted with another imaging agent, ^{123}Iodine, so that the thyroid gland image can be "subtracted" from the image obtained with Tc-99m sestamibi. Another approach is to use Tc-99m sestamibi only, taking advantage of the fact that the thyroid gland discharges the radionuclide more rapidly than the abnormal parathyroid gland. A delayed image, 2 hours after administration, compared with the initial image might therefore show selective retention in parathyroid tissue. Tc-99m sestamibi has another advantage in that the entire mediastinal and cervical regions can be visualized. The sensitivities for parathyroid localization using Tc-99m sestamibi techniques have been reported in many series (107,111). Overall, the success rate of Tc-99m sestamibi imaging is 60–70%. In patients who have not had previous parathyroid surgery, some centers report an even higher success rate.

Invasive localization tests with arteriography and selective venous sampling for parathyroid hormone in the draining thyroid veins are available when noninvasive studies have not been successful (112). When combined with arteriographic demonstration of the tumor, complete identification is established. Unfortunately, arteriography and selective venous catheterization are time-consuming, expensive, and difficult procedures. Their success is dependent upon the skill of the angiographer. When the need for these tests arises in a patient, referral is usually made to one of the few sites in the United States that do these studies on a regular basis.

The value of localization tests prior to parathyroid surgery is controversial. It has been claimed that localization of gland(s) leads to greater operative success and that operating time is diminished. In patients who have not had prior neck surgery, expert parathyroid surgeons claim that these tests do not prevent failed operations and do not shorten operating time (113). In the patient who has not had previous neck surgery, an experienced parathyroid surgeon will find the abnormal parathyroid gland(s) well over 90% of the time (114). Successful localization with any of these localization procedures is not better than 80%. Nevertheless, there is an understandable desire to have as much information regarding the location of the presumed parathyroid adenoma prior to surgery as possible. Thus, these localization tests are becoming more widely used. This is particularly true as surgical approaches, described in subsequent chapters, are beginning to rely on preoperative localization in order to minimize neck exposure. The minimally invasive parathyroidectomy (MIP), for example, requires successful preoperative localization (115).

In patients who have had prior neck surgery, preoperative localization tests become more compelling, even to the expert parathyroid surgeon. The general approach is to utilize noninvasive studies first. Tc-99m with SPECT imaging along with US are best for parathyroid tissue that is located in proximity to the thyroid, whereas CT and MRI testing are better for ectopically located parathyroid tissue. In view of the substantial incidence of false-positive studies with all the noninvasive localization procedures, confirmation with two approaches is useful in order to be confident of accurate localization.

11 CLINICAL COURSE OF PRIMARY HYPERPARATHYROIDISM

The change in clinical presentation of primary hyperparathyroidism from a symptomatic to an asymptomatic disease has required longitudinal studies to assess the extent to which any features progress or complications appear over time. Attempts to document the natural history of primary hyperparathyroidism extend back to an earlier generation through the work of Scholz and Purnell (116). Although this study had limitations, there did seem to be evidence from their series that primary hyperparathyroidism could be associated with lack of progression. The first truly long-term prospective study of the natural history of primary hyperparathyroidism with or without surgery has been provided by Silverberg and colleagues over a 10-year period of surveillance (117).

11.1 Natural History Without Surgery

Biochemical abnormalities associated with primary hyperparathyroidism are stable during long-term follow-up of mild, asymptomatic patients. The serum calcium, phosphorus, urinary calcium, and bone markers do not change over time. Similarly, parathyroid hormone levels are stable. There is no evidence that mild primary hyperparathyroidism is associated with progressive renal impairment, at least as measured by the serum creatinine, blood urea nitrogen, or creatinine clearance. Yearly bone mass measurements did not reveal that the group as a whole showed any declines at the lumbar spine, hip, or distal radius (Fig. 2). The relative stability of bone mineral density is supported by histomorphometric data from bone biopsies showing that age-related declines in indices of trabecular connectivity are not evident (118). Thus, despite advancing age, patients with primary hyperparathyroidism maintain their cancellous microarchitecture.

Although most patients with primary hyperparathyroidism exhibit remarkable stability, a small proportion of patients do have evidence of disease progression over time. Four percent of our patients developed substantial worsening of their hypercalcemia (serum calcium >12 mg/dL) and 15% developed marked hypercalciuria (urinary calcium excretion >400 mg/day). Approximately 12% of patients did demonstrate progressive declines in bone mineral density to the point where they met NIH guidelines for surgery (cortical Z-score ≤ 2.0). No clinical, biochemical, or densitometric predictors of disease progression could be identified, except for the observation that those patients who tended to show

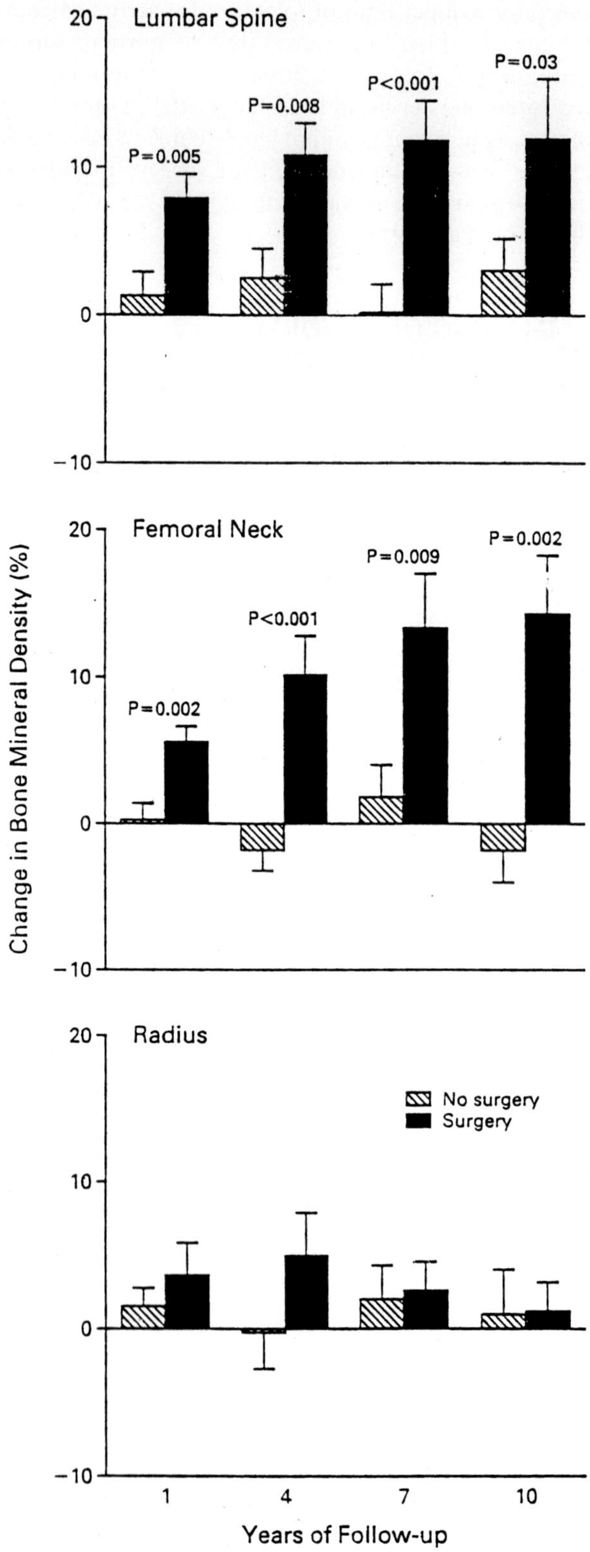

Figure 2 Conservative versus surgical management of primary hyperparathyroidism: changes in bone mineral density. Data shown are the cumulative percentage changes from baseline at each site after 1, 4, 7, and 10 years of follow-up in patients who did not undergo parathyroidectomy and in those who underwent parathyroidectomy. (From Ref. 117.)

evidence for progression were younger, on average, than those who did not progress over time (52 vs. 60 years old).

Although relative stability is the rule and progression is the exception, the fact that one quarter of subjects with asymptomatic primary hyperparathyroidism will show progression (25–27%) means that it is important to monitor patients who do not undergo parathyroid surgery. Serum calcium should be measured twice yearly; urinary calcium excretion yearly. Bone mineral density should also be monitored annually.

In all patients with symptomatic disease, such as nephrolithiasis, and chose not to undergo parathyroid surgery, the disease clearly continued to progress, as demonstrated by recurrent nephrolithiasis or other complications of primary hyperparathyroidism. Although we did not follow many patients in this category without surgery, the fact that all of them showed evidence of progression argues that such patients are best advised to undergo parathyroidectomy.

11.2 Natural History with Surgery

Most patients who met surgical guidelines underwent parathyroid surgery. After surgery they were monitored for 10 years. Following parathyroid surgery there is a prompt return to normal serum and urinary calcium levels along with the parathyroid hormone level per se. Studies of bone markers are limited but indicate a reduction in these markers of bone turnover following successful surgery. Although the choice of markers in individual studies varied, our group (119), Guo et al. (120), and Tanaka et al. (121) all reported declining levels of bone markers following surgery. Data are also available concerning the kinetics of change in bone resorption versus bone formation following parathyroidectomy. Markers of bone resorption decline rapidly following successful parathyroid surgery, but indices of bone formation decline more gradually (119). Urinary pyridinoline and deoxypyridinoline fell as early as 2 weeks post-operatively, preceding reductions in alkaline phosphatase. Similar data were reported by Tanaka et al. (121), who demonstrated a difference beween changes in osteocalcin and urinary N-telopeptide following parathyroid surgery; Minisola et al. reported a decrease in bone resorption markers without any significant change in alkaline phosphatase or osteocalcin (122). The persistence of elevated bone formation markers coupled with rapid declines in bone resorption markers indicates a shift in the coupling between bone formation and bone resorption toward an anabolic accrual of bone mineral after surgery.

In fact, bone density does increase following parathyroid surgery (117,123,124). Parathyroid surgery leads to a 10–12% increase in bone density at the lumbar spine and hip (Fig. 2). The increase at the lumbar spine and femoral neck is prompt, with the greatest increment in the first postoperative year. The trend towards a further increase after year 1 is significant only at the femoral neck. The increase at the lumbar spine and femoral neck sites, which contain a significant amount of cancellous bone, is sustained over a decade following surgery, despite the tendency of advancing age to be associated with a decline in bone mass over time. Lumbar spine and femoral neck bone density increased to the same extent in a subgroup of postmenopausal women with primary hyperparathyroidism who underwent parathyroid surgery. In the group as a whole, as well as in the cohort of postmenopausal women, there was no significant change at the site enriched in cortical bone, the distal radius. This is a curious observation in view of the fact that the lumbar spine, enriched in cancellous bone, appears to be relatively well protected by parathyroid hormone. The higher turnover rate of cancellous bone and the filling in, postoperatively, of the expanded remodeling space at this region could account, at least in part, for these observations (125). In patients who have vertebral osteopenia or frank osteoporosis (15% of the population of our hyperparathyroid subjects), the postoperative increase in bone density is even greater than the group as a whole, reaching an average of 20% higher after surgery (126). The marked improvement seen in patients with low vertebral bone density argues for surgery in those who present with cancellous as well as cortical bone loss.

In patients who underwent parathyroid surgery because of their renal stone disease, there were no recurrences of nephrolithiasis over a decade of observation. This is consistent with other published reports in which a reduction in stone incidence of 90% is typically seen after successful surgery. The 5–10% of patients who continue to form stones after parathyroidectomy may well have a nonparathyroid cause for their stone disease, which persists despite cure of their primary hyperparathyroidism (117,127,128). Alternatively, previous stone disease could have damaged the kidney such that the local environment continues to be hospitable for recurrent stones even after successful surgery.

The course of nontraditional manifestations of primary hyperparathyroidism is more difficult to document after successful parathyroid surgery. The neuropsychological manifestations of primary hyperparathyroidism have been the most difficult to follow because verifiable instruments in well-controlled prospective studies are still lacking. In 1987 Brown et al. reported on 34 patients who had a formal psychiatric and neuropsychological testing (129). Follow-up observations were obtained in 10 patients 6 months after successful parathyroidectomy and after 6 months of conservative follow-up without surgery. No postoperative improvement was observed. Similar observations were made by Cogan et al. (130). In contrast, Joborn et al. (131), using a self-rating scale, reported improvements following successful surgery. The study of Solomon et al. is perhaps the best attempt to date to document changes in neuropsychological functioning before and after parathyroid surgery (85). The author saw improvements in patients who underwent parathyroid surgery, but she also observed improvements in the control group of patients who underwent neck surgery for thyroid disease. It is evident that prospective, well-controlled studies with verifiable instruments will be needed not only to document whether or not neuropsychological functioning is impaired in primary hyperparathyroidism but also whether it is improved following successful surgery.

The cardiovascular system has also been a focus of attention before and after parathyroid surgery. When hypertension is associated with primary hyperparathyroidism, it does not seem to improve (132–135) despite a minority of reports to the contrary (136–138). Stefenelli et al. have considered possible adverse effects of primary hyperparathyroidism on valvular and myocardial calcification (139). They showed that myocardial and valvular calcifications were present in a greater number of patients with primary hyperparathyroidism than controls. They also showed that among those who were not hypertensive, left ventricular hypertrophy had a tendency to regress one year after successful surgery. These observations are of interest, but it is important to note that the patients studied by Stefenelli et al. had more advanced disease than is typically seen in many centers at this time. The more active nature of the primary hyperparathyroidism in the Stefenelli series may restrict the applicability of these observations to the more typical patients with asymptomatic disease.

11.3 NONSURGICAL APPROACHES TO PRIMARY HYPERPARATHYROIDISM

Patients with primary hyperparathyroidism should be encouraged to maintain a normal intake of calcium, despite the temptation to place constraints on dietary calcium. Calcium excretion is not different when individuals on high or low calcium intakes are compared (116). On the other hand, in those with elevated levels of 1,25-dihydroxyvitamin D_3, high-calcium diets were associated with worsening hypercalciuria. This observation suggests that dietary calcium intake in primary hyperparathyroid patients can be liberalized to 1000 mg/day if 1,25-dihydroxyvitamin D_3 levels are not increased, but should be more tightly controlled if 1,25-dihydroxyvitamin D levels are elevated. However, there is no evidence in individuals without a history of nephrolithiasis that they are more at risk for a kidney stone if hypercalciuria is present.

Oral phosphate can lower the serum calcium by up to 1 mg/dL (140,141). Problems with oral phosphate included limited gastrointestinal tolerance, possible further increase in parathyroid hormone levels, and the possibility of soft tissue calcifications after long-term use (141). This agent is no longer advisable as a chronic treatment for primary hyperparathyroidism.

Bisphosphonates are antiresorptive agents with an overall effect to reduce bone turnover. Although they do not affect parathyroid hormone secretion directly, bisphosphonates could reduce serum and urinary calcium levels. Early studies with the first-generation bisphosphonates (etidronate aand clodronate) were disappointing (142,143). The amino-substituted bisphosphonates, such as alendronate and risedronate, have been the subject of limited investigation so far. In a very short 7-day study of 19 patients with primary hyperparathyroidism, risedronate lowered the serum and urinary calcium as well as the hydroxyproline excretion significantly while the parathyroid hormone concentration rose (144). A randomized, controlled study of 26 patients with primary hyperparathyroidism (145) evaluated effects on bone mineral density after a 2-year study with 10 mg every other day (5 mg/d) of alendronate. Alendronate was associated with a reduction in bone turnover and an increase in bone mineral density over baseline by 8.6 ± 3.0%, in the hip by 4.8 ± 3.9%, and in the total body by 1.2 ± 1.4%. The control group that did not received alendronate lost about 1.5% bone mineral density (BMD) in the femoral neck. Hassani et al. (146) investigated 45 patients with asymptomatic primary hyperparathyroidism with alendronate, 10 mg daily, in a studied that was not randomized. Nevertheless, the results also showed that alendronate was associated with increases in bone mineral density of the lumbar spine and femoral neck (146). A similar positive response to alendronate has been observed by Kahn et al. (147), who are conducting an ongoing study on 44 patients with primary hyperparathyroidism. This is a randomized, placebo-controlled, double-blinded study. After one year of therapy, the alendronate treatment group is showing a significant 5.3% increase in lumbar spine and 3.7% increase in total hip bone mineral density. Bone resorption and bone formation markers decreased by 74% and 49%, respectively, in treated patients. There were no changes in ionized calcium, phosphorus, or PTH.

Estrogen use is associated with a 0.5–1.0 mg/dL reduction in total serum calcium levels in postmenopausal women with primary hyperparathyroidism who receive estrogen replacement therapy, although parathyroid hormone levels do not change (148–150). Bone mineral density in estrogen-treated patients with primary hyperparathyroidism have also documented a salutary effect of treatment on BMD at the femoral neck and lumbar spine (151). This makes estrogen replacement therapy an attractive approach in the postmenopausal woman with very mild primary hyperparathyroidism who does not have any contraindications to such therapy. The selective estrogen receptor modifier raloxifene has been studied by Rubin et al. (151a). In preliminary observations, raloxifene has been associated with modest reductions in serum calcium concentration.

Calcimimetics consist of a family of molecules that act on the parathyroid cell calcium-sensing receptor. By interacting at an allosteric site on the calcium receptor, these compounds mimic the effect of extracellular calcium and thereby act as agonists. Similar to calcium, therefore, these calcimimetics lead to an increase in intracellular calcium and inhibit inhibit parathyroid cell function. The phenylalkylamine (*R*)-*N*-(3-methoxy-α-phenylethyl)-3-(2-chlorophenyl)-1- propylamine (R-568) is one such calcimimetic compound, which is known to increase cytoplasmic calcium and reduce parathyroid hormone secretion in vitro (152). This calcimimetic inhibited parathyroid hormone secretion and serum calcium in a dose-related fashion among postmenopausal women with primary hyperparathyroidism (153). A more potent calcimimetic, AMG 073, has been the subject of additional studies and has shown further efficacy to reduce serum calcium and the PTH level in patients with primary hyperparathyroidism (154–156). If further studies confirm the potential utility of calcimimetics in primary hyperparathyroidism, it is possible that such an agent might be effective in inducing sustained reductions in parathyroid hormone and serum calcium without the need for parathyroidectomy.

REFERENCES

1. Brown EM. Extracellular Ca-sensing, regulation of parathyroid cell function, and role of calcium and other ions as extracellular (first) messengers. Physiol Rev 1991; 71:371–411.
2. Hebert SC, Brown EM, Harris HW. Role of the Ca-sensing receptor in divalent mineral ion homeostasis. J Exp Biol 1997; 200:295–302.
3. Quamme GA. Efect of hypercalcemia on renal tubular handling of calcium and magnesium. Can J Physiol Pharmacol 1982; 60:1275–1280.
4. Brown EM, Pollak M, Seidman CE, Seidman JG, Chou YH, Riccardi D, Hebert SC. Calcium-ion-sensing cell-surface receptors. N Engl J Med 1995; 333: 234–240.
5. Bai M, Quinn nS, Trivedi S, Kifor O, Pearce SH, Pollak M, Kvapcho K, Hebert SC, Brown EM. Expression and characterization of inactivating and activating mutations in the human Ca-sensing receptor. J Biol Chem 1996; 271:19537–19545.
6. Silverberg SJ, Fitzpatrick LA, Bilezikian JP. Hyperparathyroidism. In: Becker KL, ed. Principles and Practice of Endocrinology and Metabolism. 3rd ed. Philadelphia: JB Lippincott, Williams and Wilkins, 2001:548–556.
7. Bilezikian JP, Silverberg SJ, Gartenberg F, Kim TS, Jacobs TP, Siris ES, Shane E. Clinical presentation of primary hyperparathyroidism in the United Staates. In: Bilezikian JP, Marcus R, Levine MA, eds. The Parathyroids. 2nd ed. San Diego: Academic Press, 2001:349–360.
8. Broussard J, Lepage R, Cardinal H, Roy L, Rousseau L, Dorias C, d'Amour P. Influence of glomerular filtration rate on non-(1–84) parathyroid hormone (PTH) detected by intact PTH assays. Clin Chem 2000; 46: 697–703.
9. Gao P, Scheibel S, D'Amour P, John M, Rao S, Schmidt-Gayk H, Cantor T. Development of a novel immunoradiometric assay exclusively for biologically active whole parathyroid hormone 1–84: implications for improvement of accurate assessment of parathyroid function. J Bone Min Res 2001; 16:605–614.
10. Silverberg SJ, Brown IN, Bilezikian JP, Deftos LJ. A new highly sensitive assay for parathyroid hormone in primary hyperparathyroidism. J Bone Min Res 2000; 15(suppl I): S167.
11. Hruska KA, Teitelbaum SL. Renal osteodystrophy. N Engl J Med 1995; 333:166–174.
12. Martin KJ, Slatopolsky E. The parathyroids in renal disease: pathophysiology. In: Bilezikian JP, Marcus R, Levine MA, eds. The Parathyroids. 2nd ed. San Diego: Academic Press, 2001:625–634.
13. Falchetti A, Bale AE, Amorosi A, Bordi C, Cicchi P, Bandini S, Marx SJ, Brandi ML. Progression of uremic hyperparathyroidism involves allelic loss on chromosome 11. J Clin Endocrinol Metab 1993; 76:139–144.
14. Arnold A, Brown MF, Urena P, Randall RG, Sarfati E, Drueke TB. Monoclonality of parathyroid tumors in chronic renal failure and in primary parathyroid hyperplasia. J Clin Invest 1995; 95:2047–2053.
15. Goltzman D, Henderson JE. Expression of PTHrP in disease. In: Bilezikian JP, Raisz LR, Rodan GA, eds.

Principles of Bone Biology 2nd ed. San Diego: Academic Press, 2002:1079–1092.

16. Heath H III, Hodgson SF, Kennedy M. Primary hyperparathyroidism: incidence, morbidity and potential economic impact in a community. N Engl J Med 1980; 302:189–193.
17. Cope O. The story of hyperparathyroidism at the Massachusetts General Hospital. N Engl J Med 1966; 21(1):174–182.
18. Keating FR Jr, Cook EN. Recognition of primary hyperparathyroidism: analysis of 24 cases. J Am Med Assoc 1945; 129:994–1002.
19. Melton LJ III. Epidemiology of primary hyperparathyroidism. J Bone Mineral Res 1991; 6(suppl 2):S25–S30.
20. Stenstrom G, Heedman P. Clinical findings in patients with hypercalcemia: a final investigation based on biochemical screening. Acta Med Scand 1974; 195:473–477.
21. Rastad J, Lundgren E, Ljunghall S. Clinical presentation of primary hyperparathyroidism. In: Bilezikian JP, Marcus R, Levine MA, eds. The Parathyroids. 2n ed. San Diego, CA: Academic Press, 2001:361–374.
22. Palmer M, Jacobsson G, Akerstrom G, Ljunghall S. Prevalence of hypercalcemia in a health survey: a 14-year follow-up study of serum calcium values. Eur J Clin Invest 1988; 18:39–46.
23. Christensson T, Hellstrom K, Wengle B, Alveryd A, Wikland B. Prevalence of hypercalcemia in a health screening in Stockholm. Acta Med Scand 1976; 200: 131–137.
24. Akerstrom G, Rudberg C, Grimelius L, Bergstrom R, Johansson H, Ljunghall S, Rastad J. Histologic parathyroid abnormalities in an autopsy series. Hum Pathol 1986; 17:520–527.
25. Lundgren E, Rastad J, Thurfjell E, Akerstrom G, Ljunghall S. Population-based screening for primary hyperparathyroidism with serum calcium and parathyroid hormone values in menopausal women. Surgery 1997; 121:287–294.
26. Lundgren E. Primary hyperparathyroidism of postmenopausal females. Prospective case-control analysis on prevalence, clinical characteristics and treatment. Compr Sum Ups Fac Med 1999; 820:1–51.
27. Lindstedt G, Nystrom E, Lundberg P-A, Johansson E, Eggertsen R. Screening of an elderly population in primary care for primary hyperparathyroidism. Scand J Prim Health Care 1992; 10:192–197.
28. Sorva A, Valvanne J, Tilvis RS. Serum ionized calcium and the prevalence of primary hyperparathyroidism in age cohorts of 75, 80 and 85 years. J Intern Med 1992; 231:309–312.
29. Wermers RA, Khosla S, Atkinson EJ, Hodgson SF, O'Fallon WM, Melton LJ III. The rise and fall of primary hyperparathyroidism: a population-based study in Rochester, Minnesota, 1965–1992. Ann Intern Med 1997; 126:433–440.
30. Cohen J, Gierlowski TC, Schneider AB. A prospective study of hyperparathyroidism in individuals exposed to radiation in childhood. JAMA 1990; 264: 581–584.
31. Bondeson AG, Bondeson L, Thompson NW. Hyperparathyroidism after treatment with radioactive iodine: not only a coincidence? Surgery 1989; 106:1025–1027.
32. Brown EM. Four parameter model of the sigmoidal relationship between parathyroid hormone release and extracellular calcium concentration in normal and abnormal parathyroid tissue. J Clin Endocrinol Metab 1983; 56:572–581.
33. Gittes RF, Radde IC. Experimental model for hyperparathyroidism: effect of excessive numbers of transplanted isologous parathyroid glands. J Urol 1996; 95: 595–603.
34. Parfitt M. Parathyroid growth: normal and abnormal. In: Bilezikian JP, Marcus R, Levine MA, eds. The Parathyroids. 2nd ed. San Diego: Academic Press, 2001:293–330.
35. Arnold A. Molecular basis of primary hyperparathyroidism. In: Bilezikian JP, Marcus R, Levine MA, eds. The Parathyroids. 2nd ed. San Diego: Academic Press, 2001:331–347.
36. Arnold A, Kim HG, Gaz RD, et al. Molecular cloning and chromosomal mapping of DNA rearranged with the parathyroid hormone gene in a parathyroid adenoma. J Clin Invest 1989; 83:2034–2040.
37. Rosenberg CL, Kim HG, Shows TB, et al. Rearrangement and overexpression of D11S287E, a candidate oncogene on chromosome 11q13 in benign parathyroid tumors. Oncogene 1991; 6:449–453.
38. Motokura T, Bloom T, Kim HG, et al. A novel cyclin encoded by a bc11-linked candidate oncogene. Nature 1991; 350:512–515.
39. Hemmer S, Wasenius VM, Haglund C, et al. Deletion of 11q23 and cyclin D1 overexpression are frequent aberrations in parathyroid adenomas. Am J Path 2001; 158:1355–1362.
40. His ED, Zukerberg LR, Yang WI, et al. Cyclin D1/PRAD1 expression in parathyroid adenomas: an immunohistochemical study. J Clin Endocrinol Metab 1996; 81:1736–1739.
41. Tominaa Y, Tsuzuki T, Uchinda K, et al. Expression of PRAD1/cyclin D1, retinoblastoma gene products, and Ki67 in parathyroid hyperplasia caused by chronic renal failure versus primary adenoma. Kidney Int 1999; 55:1375–1383.
42. Vasef MA, Brynes RK, Sturm M, et al. Expression of cyclin D1 in parathyroid carcinomas, adenomas, and hyperplasias: a paraffin immunohistochemical study. Mod Pathol 1999; 12:412–416.
43. Chandrasekharappa SC, Guru SC, Manickam P, et al. Positional cloning of the gene for multiple endocrine neoplasia-type 1. Science 1997; 276:404–407.
44. European Consortium on MEN1. Identification of the multiple endocrine neoplasia type 1 (MEN1) gene. Hum Mol Genet 1997; 6:1177–1183.
45. Carling T, Correa P, Hessman O, et al. Parathyroid

MEN1 gene mutations in relation to clinical characteristics of nonfamilial primary hyperparathyroidism. J Clin Endocrinol Metab 1998; 83:2960–2963.
46. Farnebo F, The BT, Hytola S, et al. Alterations of the MEN1 gene in sporadic parathyroid tumors. J Clin Endocrinol Metab 1998; 83:2627–2630.
47. Tahara H, Smith AP, Gas RD, et al. Genomic localization of novel candidate tumor suppressor gene loci in human parathyroid adenomas. Cancer Res 1996; 56:599–605.
48. Palanisamy N, Imanishi Y, Rao PH, et al. Novel chromosomal abnormalities identified by comparative genomic hybridization in parathyroid adenomas. J Clin Endocrinol Metab 1998; 83:1766–1770.
49. Farnebo F, Kytola S, The BT, et al. Alternative genetic pathways in parathyroid tumorigenesis. J Clin Endocrinol Metab 1999; 84:3775–3780.
50. Verdonk CA, Edis AJ. Parathyroid "double adenomas": fact or fiction? Surgery 1981; 90:523–526.
51. Harness JK, Ramsburg Sr, Nishiyama RH, Thompson NW. Multiple adenomas of the parathyroids: do they exist? Arch Surg 1979; 114:468–474.
52. Attie JN, Bock G, Auguste L. Multiple parathyroid adenomas: report of thirty-three cases. Surgery 1990; 108:1014–1102.
53. Silverberg SJ, Bilezikian JP. Primary hyperparathyroidism. In: Becker KL, ed. Principles and Practice of Endocrinology and Metabolism. Philadelphia: Lippincott-Willliams & Wilkins, 2001:564–573.
54. Bilezikian JP. Nephrolithiasis in primary hyperparathyroidism. In: Coe FL, Favus MJ, Pak CYC, Parks JH, Preminger GM, eds. Kidney Stones: Medical and Surgical Treatment. Philadelphia: Lippincott-Raven, 1996:783–802.
55. Bilezikian JP, Silverberg SJ, Shane E, Parisien M, Dempster DW. Characterization and evaluation of asymptomatic primary hyperparathyroidism. J Bone Mineral Res 1991; 6(suppl I):585–589.
56. Silverberg SJ, Shane E, DeLaCruz L, et al. Skeletal disease in primary hyperparathyroidism. J Bone Mineral Res 1989; 4:283–291.
57. Bilezikian JP, Silverberg SJ. Clinical spectrum of primary hyperparathyroidism. Rev Endocr Metab Disord 2000; 1:237–245.
58. Dempster DW, Cosman F, Parisien M, Shen V, Lindsay R. Anabolic actions of parathyroid hormone on bone. Endocr Rev 1993; 14:690–709.
59. Canalis E, Hock JM, Raisz LG. Anabolic and catabolic effects of PTH on bone and interactions with growth factors. In: Bilezikian JP, ed. The Parathyroids: Basic and Clinical Concepts. San Diego: Academic Press, 2001:183–198.
60. Slovik DM, Rosenthal DI, Doppelt SH, Potts JT, Daly MA, Neer RM. Restoration of spinal bone in osteoporotic men by treatment with human PTH (1–34) and vitamin D. J Bone Mineral Res 1986; 1:377–381.
61. Silverberg SJ, Locker FG, Bilezikian JP. Vertebral osteopenia: a new indication for surgery in primary hyperparathyroidism. J Clin Endocrinol Metab 1996; 81:4007–4012.
62. Parisien M, Silverberg SJ, Shane E, et al. The histomorphometry of bone in primary hyperparathyroidism: preservation of cancellous bone structure. J Clin Endocrinol Metab 1990; 70:930–938.
63. Parisien M, Silverberg SJ, Shane E, de la Cruz L, Lindsay R, Bilezikian JP, Dempster DW. The histomorphometry of bone in primary hyperparathyroidism: preservation of cancellous bone. J Clin Endo-crinol Metab 1990; 70:930–938.
64. Dempster DW, Parisien M, Silverberg SJ, Liang X-G, Schnitzer M, Shen V, Shane E, Kimmel DB, Recker R, Lindsay R, Bilezikian JP. On the mechanism of cancellous bone preservation in postmenopausal women with mild primary hyperparathyroidism. J Clin Endocrinol Metab 1999; 84:1562–1566.
65. Parisien M, Cosman F, Mellish RWE, Schnitzer M, Nieves J, Silverberg SJ, Shane E, Kimmel K, Recker R, Bilezikian JP, Lindsay R, Dempster DW. Bone struc ture in postmenopausal hyperparathyroid, osteoporotic and normal women. J Bone Min Res 1995; 10:1393–1399.
66. Parisien M, Mellish RWE, Silverberg SJ, Shane E, Lindsay R, Bilezikian JP, Dempster DW. Maintenance of cancellous bone connectivity in primary hyperparathyroidism: trabecular and strut analysis. J Bone Min Res 1992; 7:913–920.
67. Dauphine RT, Riggs BL, Scholz DA. Back pain and vertebral crush fractures: an unrecognized mode of presentation for primary hyperparathyroidism. Ann Intern Med 1975; 83:365–367.
68. Khosla S, Melton LJ III, Wermers RA, Crowson CS, O'Fallon WM, Riggs BL. Primary hyperparathyroidism and the risk of fracture: a population based study. J Bone Min Res 1999; 14:1700–1707.
69. Rao DS, Ellis B, Kleerekoper M, Parfitt AM. Mild asymptomatic primary hyperparathyroidism is not a risk factor for vertebral fractures. Ann Intern Med 1988; 109:959–962.
70. Melton LJ III, Atkinson EJ, O'Fallon WM, Heath H III. Risk of age-related fractures in patients with primary hyperparathyroidism. Arch Intern Med 1992; 152:2269–2273.
71. Kleerekoper M, Peterson E, Nelson D, et al. Identification of women at risk for developing postmenopausal osteoporosis with vertebral compression fractures: role of history and single photon absorptiometry. Bone Mineral 1989; 7:171–186.
72. Johnson BE, Lucasey B, Robinson RG, Lukert BP. Contributing diagnoses in osteoporosis. Arch Intern Med 1989; 149:1069–1072.
73. Silverberg SJ, Bilezikian JP. Primary hyperparathyroidism. In: De Groot LJ, Jameson JL, eds. Endocrinology. 4th ed. Philadelphia: WB Saunders, 2001: 1075–1093.

74. Ljunghall S, Palmer M, Akerstrom G, Wide L. Diabetes mellitus, glucose tolerance and insulin response to glucose in patients with primary hyperparathyroidism before and after parathyroidectomy. Eur J Clin Invest 1983; 13:373–377.
75. Bannon MP, vanHeerden JA, Palumbo PJ, Ilstrup DM. The relationship between primary hyperparathyroidism and diabetes mellitus. Ann Surg 1988; 207:430–433.
76. Silverberg SJ, Bilezikian JP. Clinical course of primary hyperparathyroidism. In: Bilezikian JP, Marcus R, Levine MA, eds. The Parathyroids. 2nd ed. San Diego: Academic Press, 2001:387–398.
77. Sitges-Serra A, Alonso M, deLecea C, Gores PF, Sutherland DE. Pancreatitis and hyperparathyroidism. Br J Surg 1988; 75:158–160.
78. Prinz RA, Aranha GV. The association of primary hyperparathyroidism and pancreatitis. Am Surg 1985; 51:325–329.
79. Bess MA, Edis AJ, van Heerden JA. Hyperparathyroidism and pancreatitis. Chance or a causal association? JAMA 1980; 243:246–247.
80. Turken SA, Cafferty M, Silverberg SJ, et al. Neuromuscular involvement in mild, asymptomatic primary hyperparathyroidism. Am J Med 1989; 87:553–557.
81. Joborn C, Rastad J, Stalberg E, Akerstrom G, Ljunghall S. Muscle function in patients with primary hyperparathyroidism. Muscle Nerve 1989; 12:87–94.
82. Joborn C, Hetta J, Johansson H, et al. Psychiatric morbidity in primary hyperparathyroidism. World J Surg 1988; 12:476–481.
83. Ljunghall S, Jakobsson S, Joborn C, Palmer M, Rastad J, Akerstrom G. Longitudinal studies of mild primary hyperparathyroidism. J Bone Mineral Res 1991; 6(suppl 2):S111–S116.
84. Silverberg SJ, Bilezikian JP. Clinical course of primary hyperparthyroidism. In: Bilezikian JP, Marcus R, Levine MA, eds. The Parathyroids. 2nd ed. San Diego: Academic Press, 2001:387–398.
85. Solomon BL, Schaaf M, Smallridge RC. Psychologic symptoms before and after parathyroid surgery. Am J Med 1994; 96:101–106.
86. Wajngot A, Werner S, Granberg PO, Lindvall N. Occurrence of pituitary adenomas and other neoplastic diseases in primary hyperparathyroidism. Surg Gynecol Obstet 1980; 151:401–403.
87. Farr HW, Fahey TJ Jr, Nash AG, Farr CM. Primary hyperparathyroidism and cancer. Am J Surg 1973; 126: 539–543.
88. Attie JN, Vardhan R. Association of hyperparathyroidism with nonmedullary thyroid carcinoma: Review of 31 cases. Head Neck 1993; 15:20–23.
89. Kambouris AA, Ansari MR, Talpos GT. Primary hyperparathyroidism and associated neoplasms. Henry Ford Med J 1987; 35:207–210.
90. Wermers RA, Khosla S, Atkinson EJ, Grant CS, Hodgson SF, O'Fallon M, Melton LJ. Survival after the diagnosis of hyperparathyroidism. Am J Med 1998; 104:115–122.
91. Palmer M, Adami H-O, Bergstrom R, Akerstroom G, Ljunghall S. Mortality after surgery for primary hyperparathyroidism: a follow-up of 441 patients operated on from 1956 to 1979. Surgery 1987; 102:1–7.
92. Hedback G, Tisell L-E, Bengtsson B-A, Hedman I, Oden A. Premature death in patients operated on for primary hyperparathyroidism. World J Surg 1990; 14: 829–836.
93. Hedback G, Oden A. Increased risk of death from primary hyperparathyroidism—an update. Eur J Clin Invest 1998; 28:271–276.
94. Hedback G, Oden A. Death risk factor analysis in primary hyperparathyroidism. Eur J Clin Invest 1998; 28:1011–1018.
95. Ronni-Sivula H, Sivula A. Long-term effect of surgical treatment on the symptoms of primary hyperparathyroidism. Ann Clin Res 1985; 17:141–147.
96. Walgenbach S, Hommel G, Junginger T. Outcome after surgery for primary hyperparathyroidism: ten-year prospective follow-up study. World J Surg 2000; 24: 564–569.
97. Hedback G, Oden A. The influence of surgery on the risk of death in patients with primary hyperparathyroidism. World J Surg 1991; 15:399–407.
98. Hedback G, Oden A, Tisell L-E. Parathyroid adenoma weight and the risk of death after treatment for primary hyperparathyroidism. Surgery 1995; 117:134–139.
99. Hedback G, Oden A. Survival of patients operated on for primary hyperparathyroidism (lett). Surgery 1999; 125: 240–241.
100. Bilezikian JP, Meng X, Shi Y, Silverberg SJ. Primary hyperparathyroidism in women: New York and Beijing (a tale of two cities). Int J Fertil Women's Health 2000; 45:158–165.
101. Mithal A, Bandeira F, Meng X, Silverberg S, Shi Y, Mishra SK, Griz L, Macedo G, Celdas G, Bandeira C, Bilezikian JP, Rao DS. Primary hyperparathyroidism in India, Brazil and China. In: Bilezikian JP, Marcus R, Levine MA, eds. The Parathyroids. 2nd ed. San Diego: Academic Press, 2001:375–386.
102. Silverberg SJ, Shane E, Dempster DW, Bilezikian JP. Vitamin D insufficiency in primary hyperparathyroidism. Am J Med 1999; 107:561–567.
103. Consensus Development Conference Panel. Diagnosis and management of asymptomatic primary hyperparathyroidism: Consensus Development Conference Statement. Ann Intern Med 1991; 114:593–597.
104. Bilezikian JP, Potts JT Jr, El-Hajj Fuleihan G, Kleerekoper M, Neer R, Peacock M, Rastad J, Silverberg SJ, Udelsman R, Wells SA. Summary statement from a workshop on asymptomatic primary hyperparathyroidism: a perspective for the 21st century. J Bone Min Res 2002; 1752:N2–N11.

105. Silverberg SJ, Brown I, Bilezikian JP. Age as a criterion for surgery in primary hyperparathyroidism. Am J Med, 2002; 113:681–684.
106. Wells SA Jr, Doherty GM. The surgical management of hyperparathyroidism. In: Bilezikian JP, Marcus R, Levine MA, eds. The Parathyroids. 2d ed. San Diego: Academic Press, 2001:487–498.
107. Chen CC, Skarulis MC, Fraker DL, Alexander HR, Marx SJ, Spiegel AM. Technetium-99m-sestamibi imaging before reopration for primary hyperparathyroidism. J Nucl Med 1995; 36:2186–2191.
108. Wei JP, Burke GH, Mansberger AR Jr. Prospective evaluation of the efficacy of technetium 99m sestamibi and iodine 123 radionuclide imaging of abnormal parathyroid glands. Surgery 1992; 112:1111–1116.
109. Ishibashi M, Nishida H, Hiromatsu Y, Kojima K, Uchida M, Hayabuchi N. Localization of ectopic parathyroid glands using technetium-99m sestamibi imaging: comparison with magnetic resonance and computed tomographic imagine. Eur J Nucl Med 1997; 24:197–201.
110. MacFarlane MP, Fraker DL, Shawker TH, Norton JA, Doppman JL, Chang RA, Skarulis M, Marx SJ, Speigel AM, Alexander HR. Use of preoperative fine needle aspiration in patients undergoing reoperations for primary hyperparathyroidism. Surgery 1994; 116:959–965.
111. Neumann DR, Esselstyn CB, Macintyre WJ, Go RT, Obuchowski NA, Chen EQ, Licata AA. Comparison of FDG-PET and sestamibi-SPECT in primary hyperparathyroidism. J Nucl Med 1996; 37:1809–1815.
112. Doppman JL. Preoperative localization of parathyroid tissue in primary hyperparathyroidism. In: Bilezikian JP, Marcus R, Levine MA, eds. The Parathyroids. 2nd ed. San Diego: Academic Press, 2001: 475–486.
113. Roe SM, Burns RP, Graham LD, Brock WB, Russell WL. Cost-effectiveness of preoperative localization studies in primary hyperparathyroid disease. Ann Surg 1994; 219:582–586.
114. Kaplan EL, Yoshiro T, Salti G. Primary hyperparathyroidism in the 1990s. Ann Surg 1992; 215:300–317.
115. Udelsman R. Unilateral neck exploration under local or regional anesthesia. In: Gaganer M, Inaback WB III, eds. Minimally Invasive Endocrine Surgery. Philadelphia: Lippincott, Williams and Wilkins, 2002:94–101.
116. Scholz DA, Purnell DC. Asymptomatic primary hyperparathyroidism. Mayo Clin Proc 1981; 56:473–478.
117. Silverberg SJ, Shane E, Jacobs TP, Siris E, Bilezikian JP. The natural history of treated and untreated asymptomatic primary hyperparathyroidism: a ten year prospective study. N Engl J Med 1999; 341: 1249–1255.
118. Parisien M, Dempster DW, Shane E, Bilezikian JP. Histomorphometric analysis of bone in primary hyperparathyroidism. In: Bilezikian JP, Marcus R, Levine M, eds. The Parathyroids. 2nd ed. San Diego: Academic Press, 2001:423–436.
119. Seibel MJ, Gartenberg F, Silverberg SJ, et al. Urinary hydroxypyridinium crosslinks of collagen in primary hyperparathyroidism. J Clin Endocrinol Metab 1992; 74:481–486.
120. Guo CY, Thomas WER, Al-Dehaimi AW, Assiri AMA, Eastell R. Longitudinal changes in bone mineral density and bone turnover in women with primary hyperparathyroidism. J Clin Endocrinol Metab 1996; 81:3487–3491.
121. Tanaka Y, Funahashi H, Imai T, Tominga Y, Takagi H. Parathyroid function and bone metabolic markers in primary and secondary hyperparathyroidism. Semin Surg Oncol 1997; 13:125–133.
122. Minisola S, Romagnoli E, Scarnecchia L, et al. Serum CITP in patients with primary hyperparathyroidism: studies in basal conditions and after parathyroid surgery. Eur J Endocrinol 1994; 130:587–591.
123. Martin P, Bermann P, Sillet C. Partially reversible osteopenia after surgery for primary hyperparathyroidism. Arch Intern Med 1986; 146:689–691.
124. Fuleihan GEH, Moore F Jr, LeBoff MS, Hurwitz S, Gundberg CM, Angell J, Scott J. Longitudinal changes in bone density in hyperparathyroidism. J Clin Densitometry 1999; 2:153–162.
125. Silverberg SJ, Locker FG, Bilezikian JP. Vertebral osteopenia: a new indication for surgery in primary hyperparathyroidism. J Clin Endocrinol Metab 1996; 81:4007–4012.
126. Silverberg SJ, Locker FG, Bilezikian JP. Vertebral osteopenia: a new indication for surgery in primary hyperparathyroidism. J Clin Endocrinol Metab 1996; 81:4007–4012.
127. Deaconson TF, Wilson SD, Lemann J. The effect of parathyroidectomy on the recurrence of nephrolithiasis. Surgery 1987; 215:241–251.
128. Kaplan RA, Snyder WH, Stewart A, et al. Metabolic effects of parathyroidectomy in asymptomatic primary hyperparathyroidism. J Clin Endocrinol Metab 1976; 42:415–426.
129. Brown GG, Preisman RC, Kleerekoper MD. Neurobehavioral symptoms in mild primary hyperparathyroidism: related to hypercalcemia but not improved by parathyroidectomy. Henry Ford Med J 1987; 35:211–215.
130. Cogan MG, Covey CM, Arieff AI, Wisniewski A, Clark OH. Central nervous system manifestations of hyperparathyroidism. Am J Med 1978; 65:963–970.
131. Joborn C, Hetta J, Lind L, Rastad J, Akerstrom G, Ljunghall S. Self-rated psychiatric symptoms in patients operated on because of primary hyperparathyroidism and in patients with longstanding mild hypercalcemia. Surgery 1989; 105:72–78.
132. Jones DB, Jones JH, Lloyd HJ, Lucas PA, Wilkins WE, Walker DA. Changes in blood pressure and renal function after parathyroidectomy in primary hyperparathyroidism. Postgrad Med J 1983; 59:350–353.

133. Bradley EL III, Wells JO. Primary hyperparathyroidism and hypertension. Am Surg 1983; 49:569–570.
134. Rapado A. Arterial hypertension and primary hyperparathyroidism. Am J Nephrol 1986; 6(suppl I):49–50.
135. Dominiczak AF, Lyall F, Morton JJ, et al. Blood pressure, left ventricular mass and intracellular calcium in primary hyperparathyroidism. Clin Sci 1990; 78:127–132.
136. Diamond TW, Botha JR, Wing J, Meyers AM, Kalk WJ. Parathyroid hypertension. A reversible disorder. Arch Intern Med 1986; 146:1709–1712.
137. Broulik PD, Horky K, Pacovsky V. Blood pressure in patients with primary hyperparathyroidism before and after parathyroidectomy. Exp Clin Endocrinol 1985; 86:346–352.
138. Ringe JD. Reversible hypertension in primary hyperparathyroidism pre- and postoperative blood pressur in 75 cases. Klin Wochenschr 1984; 62:465–469.
139. Stefanelli T, Mayr H, Bergler-Klein J, Globits S, Woloszczuk W, Niederle B. Primary hyperparathyroidism: incidence of cardiac abnormalities and partial reversibility after successful parathyroidectomy. Am J Med 1993; 95:197–202.
140. Locker FG, Silverberg SJ, Bilezikian JP. Optimal dietary calcium intake in primary hyperparathyroidism. Am J Medicine 1997; 102:543–550.
141. Stock JL, Marcus R. Medical management of primary hyperparathyroidism. In: Bilezikian JP, Marcus R, Levine MA, eds. The Parathyroids. 2nd ed. San Diego: Academic Press, 2001:459–474.
142. Kaplan RA, Geho WB, Poindexter C, Haussler M, Dietz GW, Pak CYC. Metabolic effects of diphosphonate in primary hyperparathyroidism. J Clin Pharmacol 1977; 17:410–419.
143. Shane E, Baquiran DC, Bilezikian JP. Effects of dichloromethylene diphosphonate on serum and urinary calcium in primary hyperparathyroidism. Ann Int Med 1981; 95:23–27.
144. Reasner CA, Stone MD, Hosking DJ, Ballah A, Mundy GR. Acute changes in calcium homeostasis during treatment of primary hyperparathyroidism with risedronate. J Clin Endocrinol Metab 1993; 77: 1067–1071.
145. Adami S. Effects of oral alendronate in elderly patients with osteoporosis and mild primary hyperparathyroidism. 2001; 16:113–119.
146. Hassani S, Braunstein GD, Seibel MJ, Brickman AS, Geola F, Pekay AE, Hershman JM. Alendronate therapy of primary hyperparathyroidism. Endocrinologist 2001; 11:459–464.
147. Khan AA, Bilezikian JP, Kung AWC, Ahmed MM, Dubois SJ, Ho AYY, Motagally Z, Rubin M, Silverberg SJ, Standish TIM, Syed ZA. A double blind randomized placebo controlled trial of alendronate in primary hyperparathyroidism. J Bone Miner Res 2001; 16:S226.
148. Gallagher JC, Nordin BEC. Treatment with estrogens of primary hyperparathyroidism in post-menopausal women. The Lancet, 1972; 503–507.
149. Marcus R, Madvig P, Crim M, Pont A, Kosek J. Conjugated estrogens in the treatment of postmenopausal women with hyperparathyroidism. Ann Intern Med 1984; 100:633–640.
150. Selby PL, Peacock M. Ethinyl estradiol and norethindrone in the treatment of primary hyperparathyroidism in postmenopausal women. N Engl J Med 1986; 314: 1481–1485.
151. Grey AB, Stapleton JP, Evans MC, Tatnell MA, Reid IR. Effect of hormone replacement therapy on BMD in post-menopausal women with primary hyperparathyroidism. Ann Int Med 1996; 125:360–368.
151a. Rubia MR, Lee K, McMahon DJ, Silverberg SJ. Raloxifene lowers serum calcium and markers of bone turnover in primary hyperparathyroidism. J Clin Endocrinol Metab 2003; 83:1174–1178.
152. Steffey ME, Fox J, Van Wagenen BC, DelMar EG, Balandrin MF, Nemeth EF. Calcimimetics: structurally and mechanistically novel compounds that inhibit hormone secretion from parathyroid cells. J Bone Mineral Res 1993; 8:s17.
153. Silverberg SJ, Marriott TB, Bone HG III, Locker FG, Thys-Jacobs S, Dziem G, Sanguinetti ES, Bilezikian JP. Short term inhibition of parathyroid hormone secretion by a calcium receptor agonist in primary hyperparathyroidism. N Engl J Med 1997; 307:1506–1510.
154. Shoback DM, Bilezikian JP, Binder TA, Graves T, Turner SA, Peacock M. Calcimimetic AMG073 normalizes total serum calcium in patients with primary hyperparathyroidism. J Bone Min Res 2000; 15(suppl I):S210.
155. Shoback DM, Firek AF, Mims RB, Binder TA, Graves T, Turner SA, Peacock M. An evaluation of the calcimimetic AMG 073 in patients with hypercalcemia and primary hyperparathyroidism. J Bone Min Res 2001; 16(suppl I):S303.
156. Peacock M, Shoback DM, Greth WE, Binder TA, Graves T, Brenner RM, Turner SA, Marcus. The calcimimetic AMG 073 reduces serum calcium in patients with primary hyperparathyroidism. J Bone Min Res 2001; 16(suppl I):S163.

18

Sestamibi Scintigraphy and Ultrasonography in Primary Hyperparathyroidism

Chun Ki Kim and Richard S. Haber

Mount Sinai School of Medicine, New York University, New York, New York, U.S.A.

1 INTRODUCTION

Surgical removal of solitary parathyroid adenomas or hyperplastic parathyroid glands is the current accepted treatment for primary hyperparathyroidism (1). Approximately 95% of patients with primary hyperparathyroidism are cured in the course of initial bilateral neck exploration performed by an experienced surgeon (1,2). A recent meta-analysis showed that 87% of 6331 patients with primary hyperparathyroidism had a solitary adenoma (3). Because patients with a solitary lesion may be cured by less extensive surgery, numerous imaging techniques for a preoperative localization of the lesion were developed in the 1980s. However, the vast majority of these techniques did not have a sufficiently high accuracy, and in 1991 the National Institutes of Health (NIH) consensus panel stated that routine imaging of the parathyroid glands before an initial neck exploration was not necessary. Subsequently, during the 1990s sestamibi parathyroid scintigraphy, first introduced in 1989, as well as high-resolution ultrasonography gained popularity as a preoperative parathyroid localization tool for directing a unilateral neck exploration or even more targeted surgery.

This chapter discusses issues related to the two imaging modalities and the impact of the techniques on surgical approach/patient management. The utility of these techniques in patients with secondary or tertiary hyperparathyroidism will not be discussed.

2 SESTAMIBI SCINTIGRAPHY

2.1 Radiotracer and Imaging Technique

Technetium-99m (Tc-99m) sestamibi is a lipophilic cationic complex. The cellular uptake of this tracer is proportional to blood flow. Cellular retention of sestamibi is related to mitochondrial metabolism and transmembrane potential (4). Tc-99m sestamibi has been found to be a transport substrate for multidrug-resistant P-glycoprotein. The degree of P-glycoprotein expression in various tissues may affect the degree of sestamibi retention/washout (5).

2.1.1 Dual Isotope [Tc-99m sestamibi/iodine-123 (or Tc-99m pertechnetate)] Subtraction Protocol

Sestamibi, after intravenous injection, is taken up by both the enlarged parathyroid glands and the thyroid (6,7). Therefore, another radiopharmaceutical that is concentrated only by the thyroid [either iodine-123 (I-123) sodium iodide given orally, or Tc-99m-pertechnetate given intravenously] is administered. The I-123 (or Tc-99m pertechnetate) images are visually compared with and/or digitally subtracted from the sestamibi images.

I-123 thyroid imaging is typically performed before sestamibi is injected. Tc-99m pertechnetate imaging can be performed either before or after a sestamibi study, provided that the doses of pertechnetate and sestamibi are adjusted to not affect each other.

In many cases the outline of the thyroid may not be clearly visualized on the delayed sestamibi view because of rapid sestamibi washout from the thyroid. For this reason, the I-123 (or Tc-99m pertechnetate) image should be subtracted from the early sestamibi image rather than from the delayed image (Figs. 1, 2) (8). I-123 and Tc-99m sestamibi images may be acquired simultaneously using dual energy window (159 and 140 keV, respectively) setting. Some authors have found this protocol useful because errors due to patient's motion between two images (when obtained in sequence) can be eliminated (9,10).

2.1.2 Single Isotope [Tc-99m sestamibi] Double-Phase Protocol

Following the initial uptake phase, washout of sestamibi from abnormal parathyroid tissue is usually slower than from normal thyroid tissue. Based on this differential washout, a single isotope (Tc-99m sestamibi) double-phase protocol was introduced (12). Using this protocol, images are obtained at 10 minutes (early images) and at 1.5–2.5 hours (delayed images) after injection of sestamibi. On the early images, activity of the enlarged parathyroid gland may be more intense than (Fig. 1), as intense as (Fig. 2), or possibly less intense than (Fig. 3) the thyroid activity. Because washout of sestamibi from the enlarged parathyroid gland is usually slower than that from the thyroid, parathyroid-to-thyroid activity ratio on the delayed images is generally higher than that on the early images (Fig. 1), which is often used as indicative of a positive study. However, washout from the enlarged parathyroid gland compared with the thyroid may also vary. It may be similar to that from the thyroid (Fig. 2) or even faster (Fig. 3).

2.1.3 Additional Images

For both protocols it is important to obtain an image of the chest/mediastinum. If a parallel hole collimator is used for planar imaging or SPECT, the mediastinum is usually included within a field of view together with the neck. Therefore, no additional view will be necessary. However, if a pinhole collimator is used for neck imaging with a relatively small field of view, then a separate chest image should be obtained, either in all patients or only in those with a negative neck finding depending on the logistics of each laboratory. Mediastinal images can be particularly helpful before second operation in patients with persistent or recurrent disease because the likelihood of ectopic tissue in this group is higher.

SPECT images (Fig. 4) or anterior oblique views can be helpful for more precise localization of the lesions (3,8,11). We have found the SPECT technique very useful for identifying descended retroesophageal superior parathyroid adenoma, which mimicks an inferior lesion on the planar views (Fig. 5) (12). Our data suggest

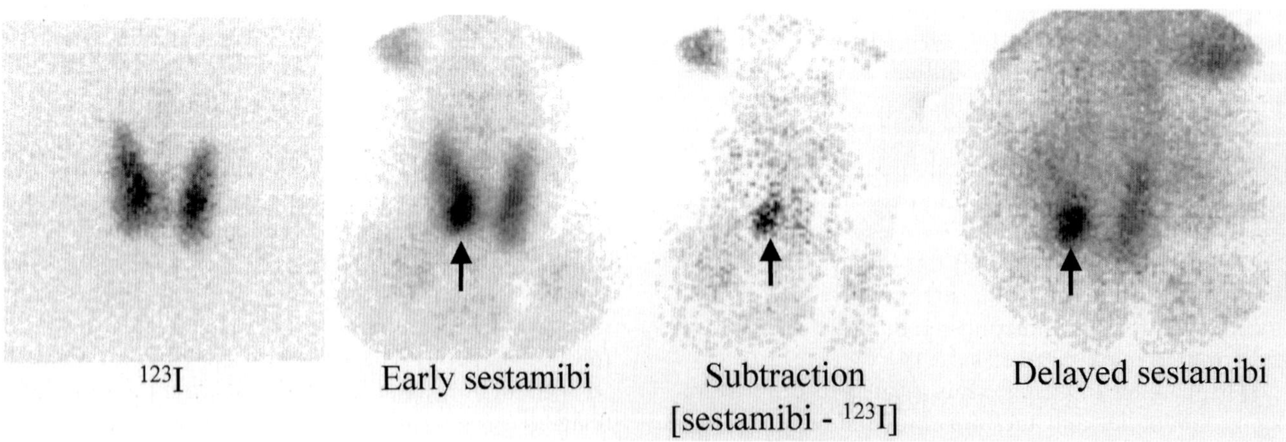

Figure 1 A typical example of a parathyroid adenoma. The I-123 scan shows a normal thyroid gland. The early sestamibi and subtraction images demonstrate a lesion (arrow) in the right lower pole of the thyroid. The delayed sestamibi image shows more delayed washout of radioactivity from the lesion than from the thyroid, resulting in increased contrast. A pinhole collimator was used.

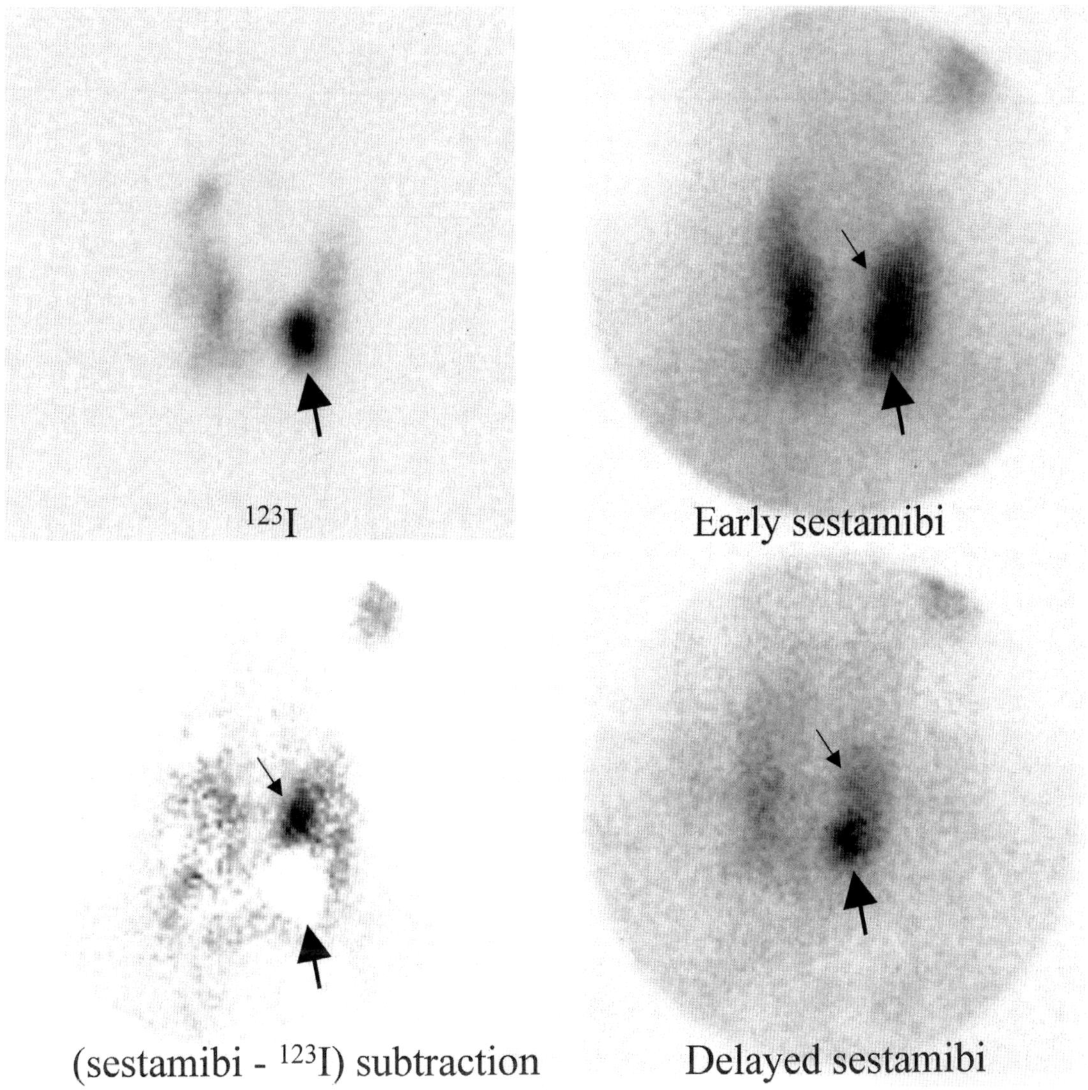

Figure 2 The I-123 image shows heterogeneous tracer uptake in the thyroid gland with a hot thyroid nodule in the left lower pole (thick arrow). The subtraction image reveals a focus of mismatched increased sestamibi activity on the medial side of the left upper pole (thin arrow). The delayed sestamibi image shows retention of activity in the hot thyroid nodule (thick arrow), but no significant retention in the left upper pole focus. A parathyroid adenoma in the left upper pole and multiple thyroid nodules (the hot nodule in the left lower pole noted on the scan being the largest one) were found at surgery. Based on the early and delayed sestamibi images alone without the I-123 image, the hot thyroid nodule in the left lower pole could have been interpreted as a parathyroid adenoma, and the actual parathyroid adenoma in the upper pole would have been missed.

that the more posteriorly located (at the lower thyroid pole level) on the SPECT images an abnormal focus is, the higher the probability of descended retroesophageal solitary parathyroid adenoma. This observation could have an impact on planning surgical route and potentially reduce the extent of exploratory dissection.

Readers interested in details of the imaging protocol, such as collimators, doses of each tracer, image acquisition parameters, etc., are referred to a publication by the Society of Nuclear Medicine (13).

2.1.4 Dual Isotope Subtraction Protocol Versus Single Isotope Double-Phase Protocol

There appears to be no consensus as yet regarding which protocol (sestamibi dual phase vs. dual isotope subtrac-

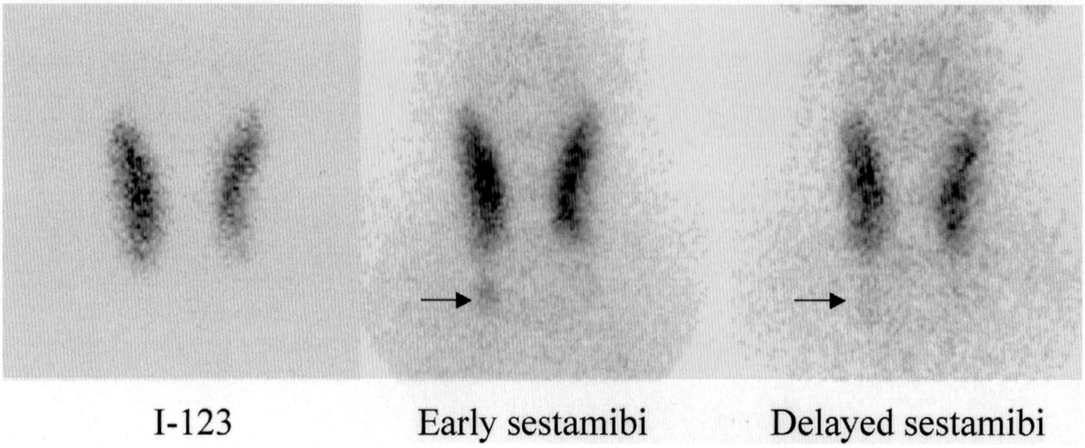

Figure 3 This patient had a 460 mg parathyroid adenoma in the right lower pole. The early sestamibi image demonstrate a lesion that is clearly outside the boundary of thyroid, and a subtraction image is not even necessary. However, the lesion shows even faster washout than the thyroid (arrows). If the lesion was immediately adjacent to the thyroid, it would not have been diagnosed correctly based on the double phase protocol alone.

tion) should be used. The combined sensitivity of dual isotope subtraction imaging and dual-phase sestamibi imaging protocols from pooled data from articles published in the early 1990s were 87% and 73%, respectively, for abnormal parathyroid glands (14). A few recent reports have directly compared the accuracy of the two imaging protocols in their own patient groups. The dual isotope subtraction technique indeed appears to have a higher sensitivity (8–10, 15) as well as a lower false-positive rate (9,10).

We have found the dual isotope subtraction technique to be slightly more accurate for localization. How-

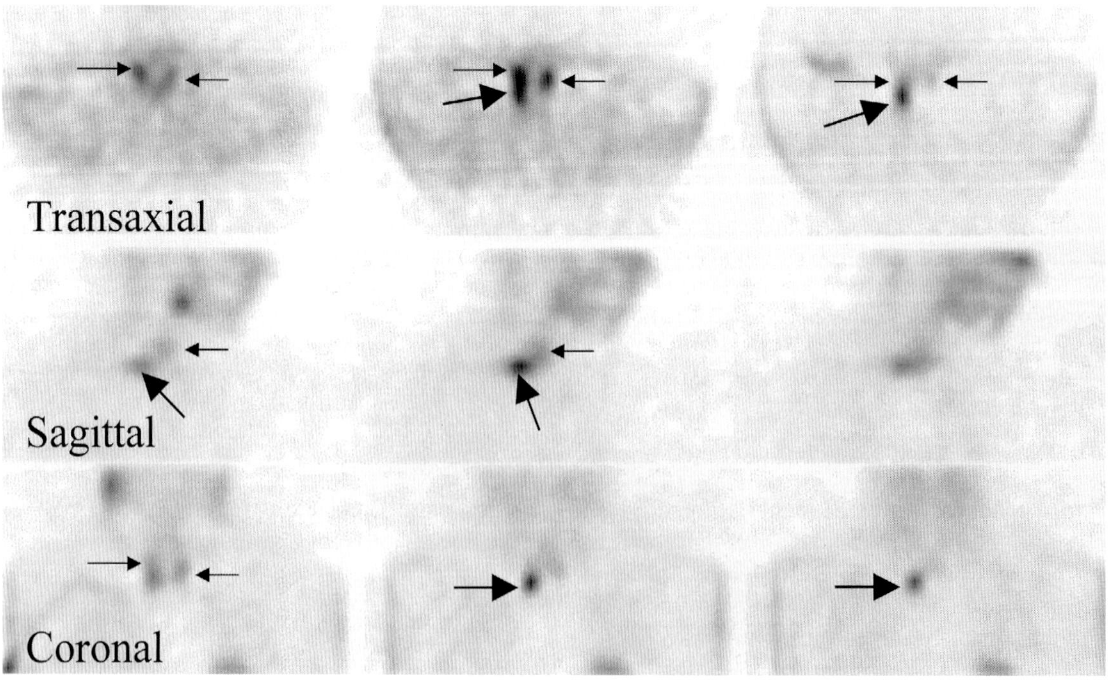

Figure 4 SPECT sestamibi images nicely demonstrate the depth of a parathyroid adenoma (large arrows) near the right lower pole. Small arrows indicate the thyroid.

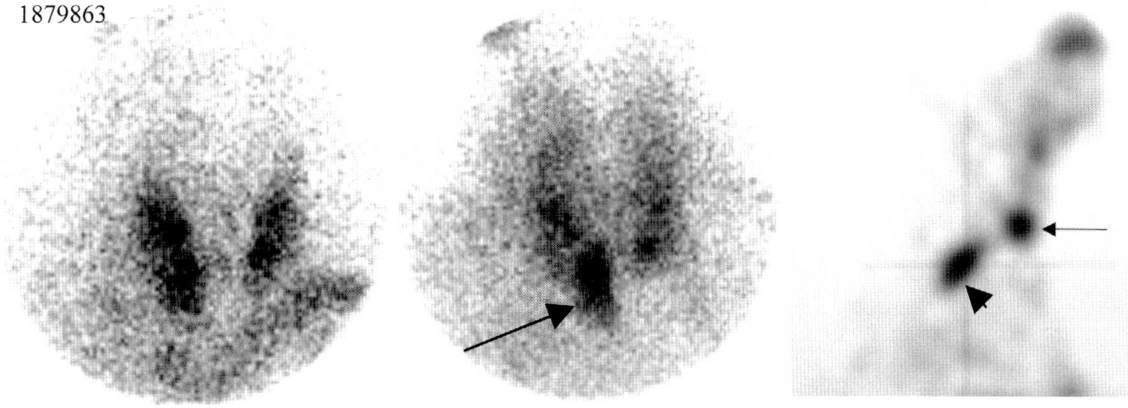

Figure 5 On the delayed sestamibi images, retention of activity is noted in a large focus (large arrow) just inferomedial to the lower pole of the right thyroid lobe, which would normally be interpreted as a inferior parathyroid adenoma. However, a selected sagittal SPECT image demonstrates that the location of the lesion (arrow head) is significantly more posterior than usual. The thin arrow indicated the lower pole of the right thyroid lobe. A descended retroesophageal superior parathyroid adenoma was found at surgery.

ever, the two protocols were essentially complementary (16), and both I-123/sestamibi subtraction and dual phase (early and delayed sestamibi) imaging are performed in our laboratory. Patients on thyroid hormone replacement therapy would be an exception to this. I-123 scan is not performed in these patients because the thyroid may not be visualized due to suppression. Instead, dual phase sestamibi imaging is performed first. If the result is unclear, then Tc-99m pertechnetate imaging may be performed since uptake of this tracer is usually affected to a lesser degree by suppression than is I-123.

2.2 Efficacy of Sestamibi Scintigraphy

The reported sensitivity and specificity ranges are approximately 50–100% and 75–100%, respectively. It has been suggested in a review article (3) that the average sensitivity and specificity from "qualified" reports, when an optimal technique is utilized, were 90.7% and 98.7%, respectively. However, it is not possible to get a really representative sensitivity and specificity because, in addition to the differences in the imaging protocol discussed above, several other variations exist. These include administered sestamibi dose (4–25 mCi), time of imaging after tracer administration (particularly delayed imaging), collimator (pinhole, converging and/or parallel hole) used, and image interpretation criteria for the positive sestamibi study. For example, patient 2 in Figure 3 has a parathyroid adenoma that is less intense than the thyroid on the early image even with faster washout. According to the criteria adopted by many authors, this would be a negative study.

Some authors reported the sensitivity and specificity on the basis of the number of the abnormal parathyroid glands, and others did on a patient basis. More importantly, if the sestamibi scan is used for directing a unilateral exploration or more targeted parathyroidectomy, a study showing no abnormal gland in the presence of multiglandular disease should be interpreted as true negative for a solitary adenoma rather than false negative for multigland disease. Likewise, a study showing two or more abnormal glands in a patient with multiglandular disease should be interpreted as true negative for a solitary adenoma rather than true positive for multigland disease. Based on these modified interpretation criteria, we have found that the positive-predictive value of sestamibi study demonstrating a single lesion for directing the surgical approach (not for detecting individual lesions) is greater than 95% (17). At any rate, all of the issues and variations discussed above need to be standardized to obtain a truly clinically relevant efficacy of sestamibi imaging.

2.3 False-Positive Studies

The most common cause of false-positive studies is benign thyroid nodules (Fig. 2). Thyroid carcinoma and thymoma may also cause false-positive studies. Reactive lymph nodes have also been reported to create false-positive studies, although some authors dispute this finding (3).

Kim et al. (18) reported that the right auricle is often seen as an isolated right paramediastinal focus (in the right parasternal region at the level of the top of the left ventricular myocardium on the anterior sestamibi image) and that, less frequently, the superoanterior right ventricular wall also appears as a focus in the inferior mediastinum. These findings should not be interpreted as an ectopic parathyroid lesion in the mediastinum.

2.4 Clinical Impact of Sestamibi Scintigraphy

The NIH Consensus Development Conference Panel concluded in 1991 that preoperative localization in patients without previous neck operation is rarely indicated and has not proved to be cost effective (1). One of the arguments used to support this conclusion was that no single pre-operative localization technique (or even in combination) used during the 1980s had a higher sensitivity than the 95% success rate of bilateral neck exploration by experienced surgeons.

2.4.1 Impact on Surgical Approach

Despite the fact that the average sensitivity of sestamibi imaging in recent literature still does not exceed 95%, this technique has gained popularity among surgeons in the 1990s. It is clearly because the information obtained from the scan is now used in a different way: whether the scan finding can guide surgeons for a targeted surgery is a clinically more relevant issue than its sensitivity in detecting all abnormal glands. It may also partly be due to improved imaging technique and improved interpretation with longer experience.

Controversy still persists. Some centers still seem to prefer bilateral exploration (19,20). Greene et al. (19) reported that sestamibi-guided parathyroidectomy may not offer any advantage over the standard bilateral exploration because a bilateral neck exploration can be performed on an outpatient basis and at low cost, with a high success rate and minimal morbidity. However, they did not compare the two techniques directly in their own patient group. Shen et al. (20) concluded that sestamibi imaging is inadequate for directing unilateral neck exploration for first-time parathyroidectomy because parathyroidectomy would have failed in 10% of their patients if unilateral neck explorations had been performed on the basis of sestamibi scan results. However, the prevalence of multiple abnormal parathyroid glands in their population was unusually high (30%) compared to others (10–20%). A high prevalence of multigland disease will naturally decrease the positive-predictive value of a study showing a single abnormal focus for a solitary adenoma. If only 15% of their patients had multiple abnormal glands, unilateral neck exploration would have failed in only 5% of patients.

The failure rate of surgery can be further reduced with an intraoperative PTH assay. The majority of recent investigations regarding this issue have found sestamibi imaging (alone or in combination with ultrasonography and/or intraoperative PTH assay) useful in directing unilateral exploration or more targeted minimally invasive (with or without radioguidance) surgery (21–25). We cetainly have found the positive-predictive value of sestamibi study demonstrating a single lesion for directing the surgical approach (not for detecting individual lesions) to be very high (17).

Norman et al. (24) emphasized the importance of radioguided parathyroidectomy. They studied 17 patients who were referred for persistent primary hyperparathyroidism after undergoing at least one neck exploration. All patients had a sestamibi scan prior to their initial operation that was interpreted as clearly positive and then, during or after an unsuccessful operation, deemed false-positive. The authors repeated sestamibi scintigraphy, which demonstrated the same single focus in all patients. During minimally invasive radioguided parathyroidectomy, an adenoma was successfully located and removed in all patients. This series indicates that radioguided surgery should increase the success rate of parathyroidectomy even more and that the false-positive rate of sestamibi imaging may be even lower than that reported in the literature. However, controversy exists, and some authors feel that radioguided parathyroidectomy does not add any significant advantage (26).

2.4.2 Other Impacts

Denham and Norman (3) reported that the average operative time for a standard bilateral exploration in 15 articles (753 patients) was 109.3 ± 29 minutes compared with 49 ± 5.0 minutes for a limited resection using sestamibi localization in 3 articles plus their unpublished data ($p < 0.0001$). A direct comparison between the two surgical approaches in a single series is also available. In the series by Norman et al. (23), surgery times for the two approached were 127 minutes and 90 minutes, respectively. Hindie et al. (9) also reported that average surgery time was reduced from 120 to 90 minutes with the guidance of sestamibi imaging. Gupta et al. reported the total operative time of 49 ± 21 minutes for unilatreal neck exploration guided by preoperative sestamibi imaging compared to 103 ± 45 minutes for bilateral neck exploration (27).

Other benefits associated with sestamibi guided parathyroidectomy include a decrease in the number of specimens submitted to pathology for frozen section analysis, local anesthesia instead of general anesthesia resulting in a shorter recovery room time and shorter hospital stay after surgery. All of these factors contribute to the cost saving even after adding the cost of sestamibi scintigraphy (3). However, adding the cost of preoperative ultrasonography and intraoperative PTH measurement, if also used, complicates the issue related to cost-effectiveness. The controversy certainly has not been resolved.

Aside from all these issues, sestamibi imaging in patients with persistent or recurrent hyperparathyroidism clearly appears to be useful in localizing previously unidentified parathyroid lesions in the neck or in ectopic locations before a second operation (28–31).

3 ULTRASONOGRAPHIC IMAGING OF ENLARGED PARATHYROID GLANDS

High-resolution ultrasonography is an excellent technique for the preoperative localization of enlarged parathyroid glands in primary hyperparathyroidism. Its advantages include simplicity and convenience, lack of radiation exposure, low cost, precise anatomical detail, and ability to detect coexisting nodular thyroid disease.

3.1 Technique of Parathyroid Ultrasonography

The superficial location of the parathyroid glands in the anterior neck facilitates their examination by high-resolution ultrasonography, since there is an inverse relationship between ultrasound frequency and depth of penetration. Most parathyroid adenomas lie at a depth of 1.0–1.5 cm beneath the skin, permitting clear imaging with high-frequency high-resolution ultrasound transducers. A variety of "small parts" ultrasound transducers may be used, including linear, convex, and sector-type phased-array probes with frequencies of 7.5–10 mHz. Such transducers yield two-dimensional views with a resolution as low as 1–2 mm.

Ultrasound examination of the anterior neck should be performed as a "real-time" examination analogous to a physical examination, rather than by reviewing static images obtained beforehand. The examination is performed with the patient in the supine position with the neck maximally extended to optimize visualization of the upper mediastinum. A pad under the shoulder blades may be used for this purpose. Ultrasound transmission gel is applied to the skin. Beginning with the thyroid region the examiner moves the probe over the central compartment of the neck on each side from the level of the submandibular glands to the clavicles. In the majority of patients with primary hyperparathyroidism, enlarged parathyroid glands are immediately apparent to experienced ultrasound operators. If an enlarged parathyroid gland is identified, the examiner notes the precise location with respect to surrounding structures such as the thyroid gland and great vessels, the depth from the skin, and the size in three dimensions.

3.2 Location and Ultrasonographic Appearance of Enlarged Parathyroid Glands

Enlarged parathyroid glands appear as hypoechoic structures, in sharp contrast to the hyperechoic thyroid tissue to which they are usually juxtaposed (Fig. 6). In

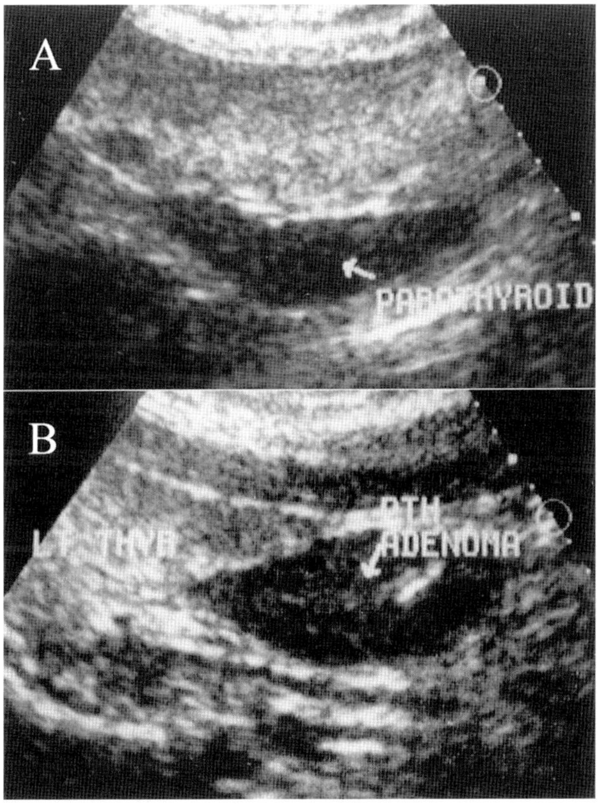

Figure 6 (A) Sagittal ultrasonographic view of enlarged upper parathyroid gland posterior to the mid-upper left lobe of the thyroid. The sharply demarcated hypoechoic adenoma (0.8 × 2 cm) lies posterior and adjacent to the more hyperechoic thyroid tissue. (B) Sagittal ultrasonographic view of a lower left parathyroid adenoma (1 × 2 cm). The hypoechoic adenoma lies immediately adjacent to the hyperechoic lower left pole of the thyroid, seen at the upper left.

most cases they are elongated in the sagittal dimension and oval in shape. Normal parathyroid glands are only occasionally detectable by ultrasonography due to their small size.

Enlarged superior parathyroid glands are usually found posterior and adjacent to the upper one third of a thyroid lobe (Fig. 6A). Enlarged superior parathyroid glands lying posterolateral to the trachea may be hidden by the acoustic shadow of the tracheal cartilage, but their detection may be facilitated by asking the patient to turn the head to the opposite side, causing protrusion of such deep parathyroid adenomas from the acoustic shadow. Enlarged inferior parathyroid glands are usually found immediately adjacent to the lower pole of a thyroid lobe (Fig. 6B). It is, however, common for enlarged inferior parathyroid glands to lie at a variable inferior distance from the lower pole of a thyroid lobe, often within the mediastinum. By orienting the ultrasound transducer inferiorly and posteriorly above the clavicles, the uppermost mediastinum down to the level of the innominate and subclavicular veins can be visualized in most patients, permitting localization of some ectopic mediastinal parathyroid adenomas. Although ectopic inferior parathyroid adenomas lying within 2–3 cm of a lower thyroid pole may be successfully imaged using this technique, many cannot be imaged by ultrasonography due to the acoustic shadows cast by the bony structures of the chest.

Either the superior or inferior parathyroid glands may occasionally be partly or entirely intrathyroidal. Intrathyroidal parathyroid adenomas are easily detected by ultrasonography, since their hypoechoic ultrasound image stands out against the surrounding hyperechoic normal thyroid tissue (Fig. 7). Although easily detected by ultrasonography, intrathyroidal parathyroid adenomas have an ultrasonographic appearance indistinguishable from that of thyroid nodules, which are commonly hypoechoic as well. The true nature of intrathyroidal parathyroid adenomas may be suspected when their location is immediately adjacent to the usual extrathyroidal parathyroid position, i.e., within the posterior aspect of an upper thyroid lobe or at the extreme lower pole of the thyroid. The diagnosis can be confirmed by ultrasound-guided fine needle aspiration of the suspected parathyroid adenoma, with subsequent demonstration of high levels of parathyroid hormone in the diluted aspirate by immunoassay (32). Because intrathyroidal parathyroid adenomas may lie entirely within the thyroid capsule and may not be evident during surgical exploration, their demonstration by ultrasonography can prevent unsuccessful operations for hyperparathyroidism.

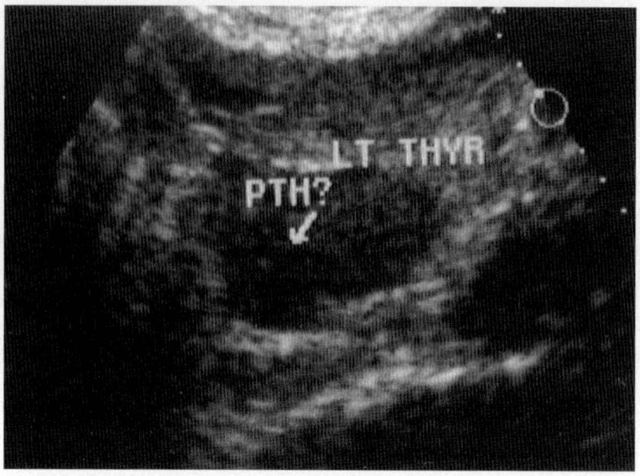

Figure 7 Transverse ultrasonographic view of a 1 cm intrathyroidal parathyroid adenoma lying within the upper left pole of the thyroid. The hypoechoic adenoma is entirely surrounded by hyperechoic thyroid tissue. Material obtained by ultrasound-guided fine needle aspiration yielded high levels of parathyroid hormone by immunoassay, distinguishing the mass from a thyroid nodule.

When only a single enlarged parathyroid gland is detected, a presumptive diagnosis of a solitary adenoma is made. The detection of more than one enlarged parathyroid gland suggests the presence of parathyroid hyperplasia or less commonly multiple adenomas.

3.3 Diagnostic Weaknesses of Ultrasonography

The major weakness of ultrasonography is the frequent failure to localize enlarged parathyroid glands in patients with primary hyperparathyroidism. Common causes of such false-negative examinations include ectopic parathyroid adenomas obscured by the acoustic shadows of the trachea or mediastinum and the presence of parathyroid hyperplasia (33,34), in which enlargement of individual glands may be minimal. In addition, the presence of multinodular thyroid enlargement decreases the sensitivity of ultrasonography for detecting enlarged parathyroid glands (35,36), probably because of diminished resolution of ultrasound imaging deep to large goiters.

Ultrasonography may also yield false-positive results. First, patients with apparently solitary parathyroid adenomas demonstrated by ultrasonography may in fact harbor multigland disease, and ultrasonography has poor sensitivity for diagnosing the presence of parathyroid hyperplasia (33,34). Second, nonparathyroid anatomical structures may be mistaken for parathyroid adenomas. The hypoechoic appearance and elongated shape of cervical lymph nodes is similar to that of parathyroid adenomas, although the presence of linear hilar echoes in lymph nodes is a distinguishing feature. Occasionally posterior or inferior thyroid nodules may be difficult to distinguish from extrathyroidal parathyroid adenomas, although this distinction is evident to experienced observers in most cases. In static ultrasonographic images the anechoic thyroid veins in cross section may mimic parathyroid adenomas, but vascular structures are easily recognized in a "real-time" examination with multiple viewing angles or by color-flow Doppler ultrasonography when this technology is available.

3.4 Diagnostic Accuracy of Parathyroid Ultrasonography

The reported ability of ultrasonography to correctly localize enlarged parathyroid glands in primary hyperparathyroidism ranges from 44 to 87% (33,35–43), with most recent series reporting sensitivities of 67–87% in patients without prior parathyroid surgery (33,35,37,38,43). However, the reliability of positive test results is high, with reported positive predictive values of 89–97% based on anatomical findings at surgery (33,35,38,42,43).

It is likely that the reported accuracy of ultrasonography for preoperative localization of enlarged parathyroid glands is highly dependent on the skill and experience of the examiner (43,44). Other factors that may explain the variable reported accuracy of ultrasonography in primary hyperparathyroidism include (1) the inclusion of patients with persistent or recurrent disease after prior surgery, since these patients are likely to have a high incidence of ectopic mediastinal parathyroid adenomas not detectable by ultrasonography (45), (2) the number of patients with parathyroid hyperplasia, and (3) the frequency of multinodular thyroid disease.

3.5 Coexisting Nodular Thyroid Disease

Since nodular thyroid disease is common in the general population (46), ultrasonography will detect thyroid nodules in many patients undergoing evaluation for primary hyperparathyroidism. The majority of such nodules are nonpalpable nodules measuring less than 1 cm (46), and most such small nodules are probably not clinically significant since they are so common. However larger thyroid nodules, often not palpable, are reported to be associated with hyperparathyroidism (47). Moreover, an association of hyperparathyroidism with thyroid cancer has been reported by several authors (reviewed in Ref. 47). In the present authors' experience, 3 of 86 patients undergoing preoperative ultrasonography for hyperparathyroidism were found to have thyroid cancer at surgery. In all three the thyroid cancer was nonpalpable and was detected by ultrasonography. Two of these patients underwent fine needle aspiration using ultrasound guidance, leading to a preoperative diagnosis of thyroid cancer.

3.6 Intraoperative Ultrasonography

Several studies have reported the use of intraoperative ultrasonography for the localization of parathyroid adenomas in reoperative cases after failed initial surgery for hyperparathyroidism. Either a dedicated sterile intraoperative transducer or one draped in a sterile sheath can be used. Norton et al. (48) reported a series of 25 consecutive patients undergoing reoperation and found that intraoperative ultrasonography was more likely to correctly localize abnormal parathyroid glands (correct in 76% of cases) than preoperative ultrasonography (correct in 36% of cases) and had a much lower false-positive rate. The intraoperative imaging was felt to limit the dissection and to shorten the length of the operation by 50%, but was not deemed essential for localizing abnormal glands. It was more likely to localize abnormal inferior and intrathyroidal glands than abnormal superior glands. A second report by this group confirmed these findings (49). Feingold et al. (50) reported the results of a series of 52 reoperations for primary hyperparathyroidism in which intraoperative ultrasonography was available and used at the discretion of the surgeon in 34 cases. In six of these cases intraoperative ultrasonography was deemed essential for localizing the parathyroid adenoma: in five cases because the adenoma was hidden in dense scar tissue despite successful preoperative imaging with sestamibi scintigraphy or ultrasonography, and in one case because it lay within a strap muscle.

4 SESTAMIBI SCINTIGRAPHY VERSUS ULTRASONOGRAPHY FOR PARATHYROID IMAGING

Among previous reports that have directly compared ultrasonography and sestamibi scintigraphy in patients undergoing initial parathyroid surgery, Mazzeo et al. (38) and De Feo et al. (43) reported that the two methods were similar in their ability to correctly predict the surgical findings, while Casas et al. (51) and Lumachi et al. (52) found that sestamibi imaging was superior. In a large series including ultrasonography in 447 patients and sestamibi scintigraphy in 70 of these patients, Chapuis et al. (37) found that ultrasonography provided better results. In the present authors' experience with parathyroid imaging using both methods in 74 patients undergoing initial surgery for primary hyperparathyroidism, the likelihood of a positive test, the likelihood of a correct positive test, and the positive predictive value were 80%, 74%, and 93%, respectively; for ultrasonography and 92%, 82%, and 90%, respectively, for sestamibi scintigraphy (53). These differences were not statistically significant except for the slightly higher likelihood of a positive test with sestamibi scintigraphy, which was attributable to much better sensitivity for detecting ectopic substernal parathyroid adenomas.

On the other hand, five series, which included patients with prior failed parathyroid surgery, showed superior imaging results with sestamibi imaging (36,41, 42,54,55), as well as a series that did not specify whether such patients were included (40). In one such study sestamibi imaging was correct in all six patients with prior unsuccessful parathyroid surgery, while ultrasonography provided correct imaging in only three of the six (42). Because patients with failed prior surgery are likely to have a high incidence of ectopic parathyroid adenomas in the upper mediastinum, which are relatively inaccessible to ultrasonography (52,56), sestamibi imaging would be expected to yield superior results in such patients. However, one recent study that focussed exclusively on such reoperative cases found that preoperative ultrasonography provided superior sensitivity to sestamibi scintigraphy (50).

The accuracy of ultrasonography may be more operator-dependent. In our recent series, accuracy of one sonographer specializing in thyroid and parathyroid ultrasonography was 80%, while combined accuracy of other general sonographers was 64% ($p = 0.04$) (57). There was no significant difference in accuracy of sestamibi scan reading among three readers.

5 SUMMARY

There are still some issues in parathyroid scintigraphy that have not been resolved completely, including which dual isotope (I-123/sestamibi vs. Tc-99m pertechnetate/sestamibi) and/or double-phase imaging methods or combined methods are most efficatious. We believe that the dual isotope subtraction technique and the sestamibi double-phase technique complement each other. There are different views on the image acquisition details and cost-effectiveness.

Sestamibi imaging and high-resolution ultrasonography have been shown to achieve high accuracy in localizing parathyroid adenomas. Numerous reports published during the past decade support the use of one or both of these techniques for directing a unilateral neck exploration or more targeted parathyroidectomy.

REFERENCES

1. Consensus Development Conference Panel. Diagnosis and management of asymptomatic primary hyperparathyroidism: consensus development conference statement. Ann Intern Med 1991; 114:593–597.
2. Wells SA Jr, Ashley SW. The parathyroid glands. In: Sabiston DC Jr, ed. Textbook of Surgery: The Biological Basis of Modern Surgical Practice. 14th ed. Philadelphia: WB Saunders Company, 1991:598–615.
3. Denham DW, Norman J. Cost-effectiveness of preoperative sestamibi scan for primary hyperparathyroidism is dependent solely upon the surgeon's choice of operative procedure. J Am Coll Surg 1998; 186:293–305.
4. Piwnica-Worms D, Kronauge JF, Chiu ML. Uptake and retention of hexakis (2-methoxyisobutyl isonitrile) technetium(I) in cultured chick myocardial cells. Mitochondrial and plasma membrane potential dependence. Circulation 1990; 82:1826–1838.
5. Piwnica-Worms D, Chiu ML, Budding M, Kronauge JF, Kramer RA, Croop JM. Functional imaging of multidrug-resistant P-glycoprotein with an organotechnetium Complex. Cancer Res 1993; 53:977–984.
6. Coakley AJ, Kettle AG, Wells CP, O'Doherty MJ, Collins RE. ^{99}Tcm sestamibi—a new agent for parathyroid imaging. Nucl Med Commun 1989; 10:791–794.
7. O'Doherty MJ, Kettle AG, Wells P, Collins RE, Coakley AJ. Parathyroid imaging with technetium-99m-sestamibi: preoperative localization and tissue uptake studies. J Nucl Med 1992; 33:313–318.
8. Chen CC, Skarulis MC, Fraker DL, Alexander R, Marx SJ, Spiegel AM. Technetium-99m-sestamibi imaging before reoperation for primary hyperparathyroidism. J Nucl Med 1995; 36:2186–2191.
9. Hindie E, Melliere D, Jeanguillaume C, Perlemuter L, Chehade F, Galle P. Parathyroid imaging using simultaneous double-window recording of technetium-99m-sestamibi and iodine-123. J Nucl Med 1998; 39:1100–1105.
10. Neumann DR, Esselstyn CB Jr, Go RT, Wong CO, Rice TW, Obuchowski NA. Comparison of double-phase 99mTc-sestamibi with 123I-99mTc-sestamibi subtraction SPECT in hyperparathyroidism. AJR 1997; 169: 1671–1674.

11. Taillefer R, Boucher Y, Potvin C, Lambert R. Detection and localization of parathyroid adenomas in patients with hyperparathyroidism using a single radionuclide imaging procedure with technetium-99m-sestamibi (double-phase study). J Nucl Med 1992; 33:1801–1807.
12. Kim CK, Kim S, Eskandar Y, Krynyckyi BR, Zhang Z, Knesaurek K, Inabnet WB, Machac J. Appearance of descended superior parathyroid adenoma on SPECT parathyroid imaging [abstr]. J Nucl Med 2002; 43:326.
13. Greenspan BS, Brown ML, Dillehay GL, et al. Procedure guideline for parathyroid scintigraphy. J Nucl Med 1998; 39:1111–1114.
14. McBiles M, Lambert AT, Cote MG, Kim SY. Sestamibi parathyroid imaging. Semin Nucl Med 1995; 25: 221–234.
15. Chen CC, Holder LE, Scovill WA, Tehan AM, Gann DS. Comparison of parathyroid imaging with technetium-99m-pertechnetate/sestamibi subtraction, double-phase technetium-99m-sestamibi and technetium-99m-sestamibi SPECT. J Nucl Med 1997; 38:834–849.
16. Kim CK, Lim J, Lorberboym M, Elgazzar A, Machac J. Parathyroid scintigraphy: dual (I-123 and Tc-99m MIBI) vs single (early and delayed MIBI) isotope imaging [abstr]. J Nucl Med 1996; 37:16.
17. Kim CK, Kim S, Krynyckyi BR, Machac J, Inabnet WB. Efficacy of sestamibi parathyroid scintigraphy for directing surgical approaches based on modified interpretation criteria. Clin Nucl Med 2002; 27:246–248.
18. Kim CK, Jung E, Yun M, Lorberboym M, Mechanick JI, Bergman D, Inabnet WB, Krynyckyi BR, Machac J. A normal variant on thallium/Tc-99m MIBI whole body imaging: the superior right atrial wall (auricle) and superoanterior right ventricular wall are often seen as mediastinal lesions. Clin Nucl Med 2001; 26:412–418.
19. Greene AK, Mowschenson P, Hodin RA. Is sestamibi-guided parathyroidectomy really cost-effective? Surgery 1999; 126:1036–1040.
20. Shen W, Sabancı U, Morita ET, Siperstein AE, Duh QY, Clark OH. Sestamibi scanning is inadequate for directing unilateral neck exploration for first-time parathyroidectomy. Arch Surg 1997; 132:969–974.
21. Pattou F, Torres G, Mondragon-Sanchez A, Huglo D, N'Guyen H, Carnaille B, Proye C. Correlation of parathyroid scanning and anatomy in 261 unselected patients with sporadic primary hyperparathyroidism. Surgery 1999; 126:1123–1131.
22. Purcell GP, Dirbas FM, Jeffrey RB, Lane MJ, Desser T, McDougall IR, Weigel RJ. Parathyroid localization with high-resolution ultrasound and technetium Tc 99m sestamibi. Arch Surg 1999; 134:824–828.
23. Norman J, Chheda H, Farrell C. Minimally invasive parathyroidectomy for primary hyperparathyroidism: decreasing operative time and potential complications while improving cosmetic results. Am Surg 1998; 64: 391–395.
24. Norman JG, Jaffray CE, Chheda H. The false-positive parathyroid sestamibi: a real or perceived problem and a case for radioguided parathyroidectomy. Ann Surg 2000; 231:31–37.
25. Bonjer HJ, Bruining HA, Pols HA, de Herder WW, van Eijck CH, Breeman WA, Krenning EP. Intraoperative nuclear guidance in benign hyperparathyroidism and parathyroid cancer. Eur J Nucl Med 1997; 24:246–251.
26. Inabnet WB III, Kim CK, Haber RS, Lopchinsky RA. Radioguidance is not necessary during parathyroidectomy. Arch Surg 2002; 137:967–970.
27. Gupta VK, Yeh KA, Burke GJ, Wei JP. 99m-Technetium sestamibi localized solitary parathyroid adenoma as an indication for limited unilateral surgical exploration. Am J Surg 1998; 176:409–412.
28. Ishibashi M, Nishida H, Hiromatsu Y, Kojima K, Uchida M, Hayabuchi N. Localization of ectopic parathyroid glands using technetium-99m sestamibi imaging: comparison with magnetic resonance and computed tomographic imaging. Eur J Nucl Med 1997; 24:197–201.
29. Cheung AH, Wheeler MS, Madanay LD, Hew E, Coel MN, Wong LM. Multi-center sestamibi parathyroid imaging study in Hawaii. Hawaii Med J 1997; 56:114–117.
30. Fayet P, Hoeffel C, Fulla Y, Legmann P, Hazebroucq V, Luton JP, Chapuis Y, Richard B, Bonnin A. Technetium-99m sestamibi scintigraphy, magnetic resonance imaging and venous blood sampling in persistent and recurrent hyperparathyroidism. Br J Radiol 1997; 70: 459–464.
31. Caixas A, Berna L, Hernandez A, Tebar FJ, Madariaga P, Vegazo O, Bittini AL, Moreno B, Faure E, Abos D, Piera J, Rodriguez JM, Farrerons J, Puig-Domingo M. Efficacy of preoperative diagnostic imaging localization of technetium 99m-sestamibi scintigraphy in hyperparathyroidism. Surgery 1997; 121:535–541.
32. Sacks BA, Pallotta JA, Cole A, Hurwitz J. Diagnosis of parathyroid adenomas: efficacy of measuring parathormone levels in needle aspirates of cervical masses. Am J Roentgenol 1994; 163:1223–1226.
33. Tziakouri C, Eracleous E, Skannavis S, Pierides A, Symeonides P, Gourtsoyiannis N. Value of ultrasonography, CT, and MR imaging in the diagnosis of primary hyperparathyroidism. Acta Radiol 1996; 37:720–726.
34. Doppman JL, Miller DL. Localization of parathyroid tumors in patients with asymptomatic hyperparathyroidism and no previous surgery. J Bone Mineral Res 1991; 6(suppl 2):S153.
35. Gofrit ON, Lebensart PD, Pikarsky A, Lackstein D, Gross DJ, Shiloni E. High-resolution ultrasonography: highly sensitive specific technique for preoperative localization of parathyroid adenoma in the absence of multinodular thyroid disease. World J Surg 1997; 21: 287–291.
36. Staudenherz A, Abela C, Niederle B, Steiner E, Helbich T, Puig S, Kaserer K, Becherer A, Leitha T, Kletter K. Comparison and histopathological correlation of three parathyroid imaging methods in a population with a

high prevalence of concomitant thyroid disease. Eur J Nucl Med 1997; 24:143–149.
37. Chapuis Y, Fulla Y, Bonnichon P, Tarla E, Abboud B, Pitre J, Richard B. Values of ultrasonography, sestamibi scintigraphy, and intraoperative measurement of 1-84 PTH for unilateral neck exploration of primary hyperparathyroidism. World J Surg 1996; 20:835–840.
38. Mazzeo S, Caramella D, Lencioni R, Molea N, De Liperi A, Marcocci C, Miccoli P, Iacconi P, Bossio GB, Viacava P, Lazzeri E, Bartolozzi C. Comparison among sonography, double-tracer subtraction scintigraphy, and double-phase scintigraphy in the detection of parathyroid lesions. Am J Roentgenol 1996; 166:1465–1470.
39. Kohri K, Tozawa K, Hayashi Y, Sasaki S, Ueda K, Sonoda T, Kurita K. Clinical features of primary hyperparathyroidism: preoperative localization and parathyroidectomy. Biomed Pharmacother 2000; 54(suppl 1):69–71.
40. Hindie E, Melliere D, Simon D, Perlemuter L, Galle P. Primary hyperparathyroidism: is technetium ^{99m}-sestamibi/iodine-123 subtraction scanning the best procedure to locate enlarged parathyroid glands before surgery? J Clin Endocrinol Metab 1995; 80:302–307.
41. Geatti O, Shapiro B, Orsolon PG, Proto G, Guerra UP, Antonucci F, Gasparini D. Localization of parathyroid enlargement: experience with technetium-99m methoxyisobutylisonitrile and thallium-201 scintigraphy, ultrasonography and computed tomography. Eur J Nucl Med 1994; 21:17–22.
42. Bonjer HJ, Bruining HA, Valkema R, Lameris JS, de Herder WW, van der Harst E, Pols HAP. Single radionuclide scintigraphy with ^{99m}technetium-sestamibi and ultrasonography in hyperparathyroidism. Eur J Surg 1997; 163:27–32.
43. De Feo ML, Colagrande S, Biagini C, Tonarelli A, Bisi G, Vaggelli L, Borrelli D, Cicchi P, Tonelli F, Amorosi A, Serio M, Brandi ML. Parathyroid glands: combination of (99m)Tc MIBI scintigraphy and US for demonstration of parathyroid glands and nodules. Radiology 2000; 214:393–402.
44. Lloyd MN, Lees WR, Milroy EJ. Preoperative localization in primary hyperparathyroidism. Clin Radiol 1990; 41:239–243.
45. Akerström G, Rudberg C, Grimelius L, Johansson H, Lundström B, Rastad J. Causes of failed primary exploration and technical aspects of re-operation in primary hyperparathyroidism. World J Surg 1992; 16:562–569.
46. Mazzaferri EL. Management of a solitary thyroid nodule. N Engl J Med 1993; 328:553–559.
47. Regal M, Paramo C, Luna Cano R, Perez Mendez LF, Sierra JM, Rodriguez I, Garcia-Mayor RV. Coexistence of primary hyperparathyroidism and thyroid disease. J Endocrinol Invest 1999; 22:191–197.
48. Norton JA, Shawker TH, Jones BL, Spiegel AM, Marx SJ, Fitzpatrick L, Aurbach GD, Doppman JL. Intraoperative ultrasound and reoperative parathyroid surgery: an initial evaluation. World J Surg 1986; 10:631–639.
49. Kern KA, Shawker TH, Doppman JL, Miller DL, Marx SJ, Spiegel AM, Aurbach GD, Norton JA. The use of high-resolution ultrasound to locate parathyroid tumors during reoperations for primary hyperparathyroidism. World J Surg 1987; 11:579–585.
50. Feingold DL, Alexander HR, Chen CC, Libutti SK, Shawker TH, Simonds WF, Marx SJ, Skarulis MC, Doppman JL, Schrump DS, Bartlett DL. Ultrasound and sestamibi scan as the only preoperative imaging tests in reoperation for parathyroid adenomas. Surgery 2000; 128:1103–1109.
51. Casas AT, Burke GJ, Sathyanarayana, Mansberger AR, Wei JP. Prospective comparison of technetium-99m-sestamibi/iodine-123 radionuclide scan versus high-resolution ultrasonography for the preoperative localization of abnormal parathyroid glands in patients with previously unoperated primary hyperparathyroidism. Am J Surg 1993; 166:369–373.
52. Lumachi F, Zucchetta P, Marzola MC, Boccagni P, Angelini F, Bui F DF, D'Amico F, Favia G. Advantages of combined technetium-99m-sestamibi scintigraphy and high-resolution ultrasonography in parathyroid localization: comparative study in 91 patients with primary hyperparathyroidism. Eur J Endocrinol 2000; 143:755–760.
53. Haber RS, Kim CK, Inabnet WB. Ultrasonography for pre-operative localization of enlarged parathyroid glands in primary hyperparathyroidism: comparison with technetium-99m sestamibi scintigraphy. Clin Endocrinol 2002; 57:241–249.
54. Light VL, McHenry CR, Jarjoura D, Sodee DB, Miron SD. Prospective comparison of dual-phase technetium-99m-sestamibi scintigraphy and high resolution ultrasonography in the evaluation of abnormal parathyroid glands. Am Surg 1996; 62:562–567.
55. Peeler BB, Martin WH, Sandler MP, Goldstein RE. Sestamibi parathyroid scanning and preoperative localization studies for patients with recurrent/persistent hyperparathyroidism or significant comorbid conditions: development of an optimal localization strategy. Am Surg 1997; 63:37–46.
56. Shawker TH, Avila NA, Premkumar A, Bradford MH, Doppman JL. Ultrasound evaluation of primary hyperparathyroidism. Ultrasound Q 2000; 16:73–87.
57. Kim CK, Kim S, Eskandar Y, Krynyckyi BR, Haber R, Machac J, Inabnet WB. Efficacy of parathyroid scintigraphy (PS) vs ultrasonography (U) for directing targeted surgery (DTS) [abstr]. J Nucl Med 2002; 43:330–331.

19

Surgical Management of Hyperparathyroidism

Arthur E. Schwartz

Mount Sinai School of Medicine, New York University, New York, New York, U.S.A.

1 INTRODUCTION

The presentation, diagnosis, and operative approach to hyperparathyroidism have undergone great changes since it was first recognized as a clinical entity in 1925. The classic case of Captain Charles Martell offers guidance that is still useful (1). This previously vigorous sea captain had decreased 7 inches in height, developed the multiple skeletal deformities of osteitis fibrosis cystica, and passed gravel at the end of urination. In the course of six operations for hyperparathyroidism at the Massachusetts General Hospital, at least two normal parathyroids were removed. At a seventh procedure an adenoma in the anterior mediastinum was discovered and removed through a sternal splitting incision. Postoperatively he became hypocalcemic. Six weeks thereafter he died of tetany and laryngospasm during an attempt to remove a kidney stone. The lessons from this case remain with us today—the limited ability to predict ectopic parathyroid adenomas that may be beyond the reach of a neck incision, and the realization that the removal of normal parathyroid glands can be devastating.

The classical syndrome of skeletal deformity with cysts and bone depletion no longer pertains. Nor are recurrent kidney stones and severe kidney damage needed to suspect the diagnosis. Hyperparathyroidism is now diagnosed with close to 100% accuracy; it is commonly identified in its silent stage when routine chemistries demonstrate hypercalemia. The discussion at present concerns the timing and the need for operative intervention in the management of asymptomatic disease, as well as the surgical approach.

The diagnosis of hyperparathyroidism has changed from that of requiring the physician to suspect the disease from a constellation of diverse symptoms. Routine blood tests now make the diagnosis. We know the structure of parathormone, understand its variations, and are able to identify its active component by immunochemistry.

The surgical approach to the disease is changing with the introduction of more accurate localizing techniques and the ability to monitor parathyroid hormone (PTH) levels during the operative procedure. This makes it possible to approach the operation in a more focused manner and with new techniques.

Neck exploration for hyperparathyroidism offers a 95% or better rate of success, a mortality rate that approaches zero, and a morbidity rate that is less than 1%. Few other procedures offer this ratio of benefit to risk.

2 EMBRYOLOGY

A valuable key to successful parathyroid surgery lies in understanding the embryology. The central portion of the thyroid arises from a diverticulum in the floor of the pharynx. The lateral portions of the thyroid as well as the superior parathyroids and parafollicular C cells (derived from the ultimobranchial body) originate in the 4th branchial pouch; they do not usually stray far from each other as they descend into the neck. It is intriguing that the superior parathyroid and parafollicular C cells, each intimately involved in the metabolism of calcium, share a common primordium (Fig. 1). The inferior parathyroid glands and the thymus have a common origin from the 3rd branchial pouch, but occasionally do not completely part company on their downward journey. They may be found accompanying each other in the low neck or superior mediastinum. It is not surprising therefore, that 85% of mediastinal parathyroid tumors are found within or close to the thymus. The inferior glands may be contained within the parenchyma of the thymus, adjacent to it, or be present in the nearby fatty and areolar tissue. They travel a longer distance than the superior glands and are more prone to anatomical ectopia. As the glands become larger and heavier because of adenomatous or hyperplastic change, they are more likely to become displaced downward in the tissue planes that offer least resistance. This migration may be increased by gravity, negative intrathoracic pressure, or swallowing. Enlarged superior glands tend to be displaced downward and posteriorly, along the tracheoesophageal groove and into the

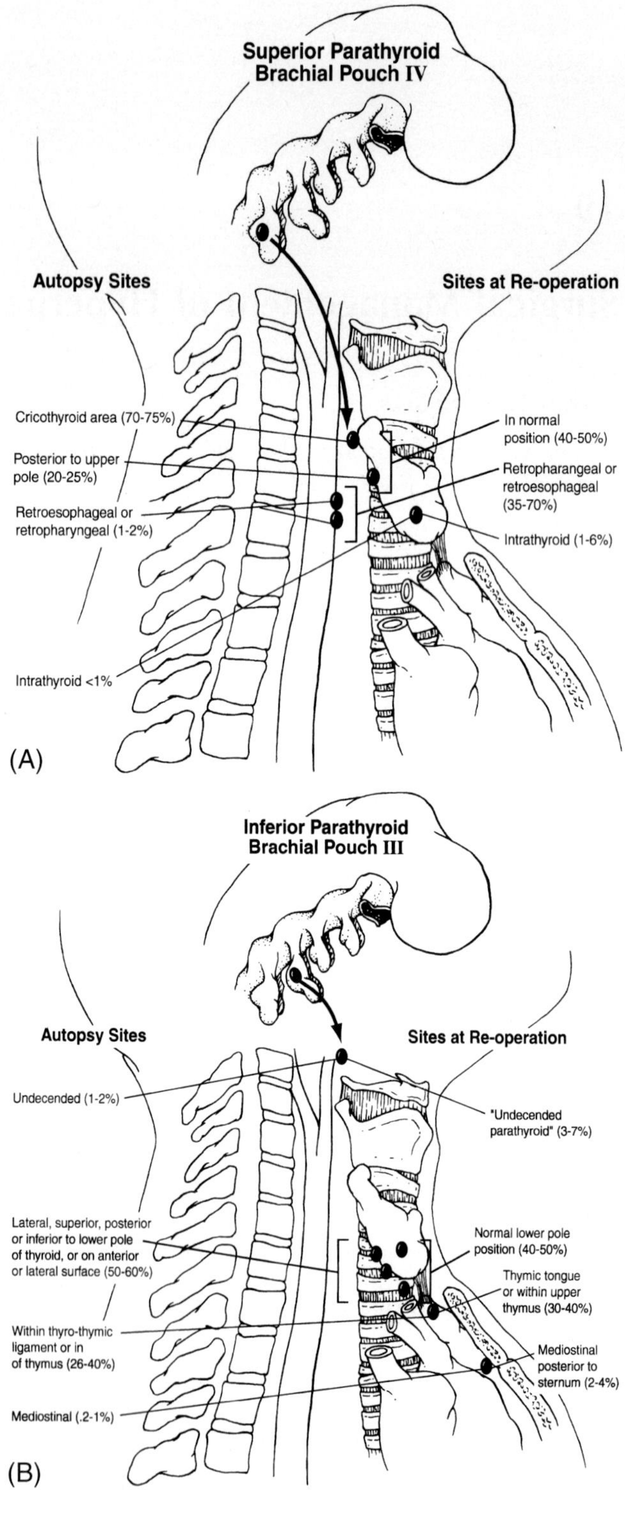

Figure 2 Position and percentage distribution of superior (A) and inferior (B) parathyroid gland: at autopsy, and on reexploration after initial failed surgery for hyperparathyroidism. Intrathyroid parathyroid glands are assumed to originate in the superior glands. Statistics are approximate. (Refs. 2, 3, 68, 69, 93.)

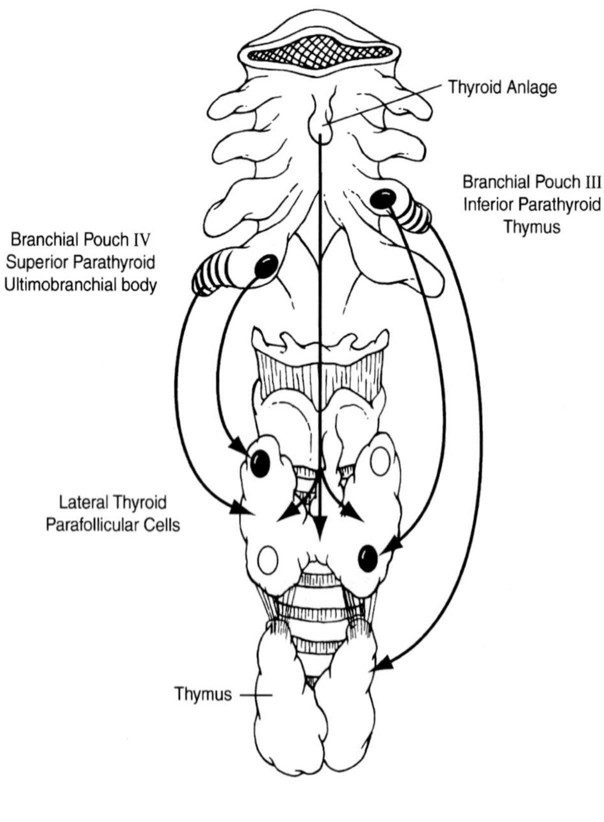

Figure 1 Embryological derivation, descent, and final location of thyroid and parathyroid glands.

posterior mediastinum (Fig. 2A). Displaced inferior glands are more likely to be found in the anterior mediastinum (Fig. 2B).

3 SURGICAL ANATOMY

In a dissection of 503 autopsy cases, Åkerström et al. found 84% to have four parathyroid glands. In 3% of the persons examined, only three glands could be identified. Supernumery glands were present in 13% of individuals, usually a fifth gland located in the thymus (2). This is in approximate agreement with other authors.

3.1 Superior Parathyroid Glands (Branchial Pouch IV)

The superior parathyroid glands are more constant in location, presumably because there is minimal migration in their embryological development. In a postmortem study by Wang (3), 77% of 312 superior parathyroid glands were found posteriorly at the cricoid junction. They were intimately associated with, and occasionally hidden by the recurrent laryngeal nerve and the adjacent vascular branches. Twenty-two percent of the 312 superior glands were located behind the upper pole of the thyroid. The superior parathyroids were almost always located beneath the capsule of the thyroid. One percent of glands were found behind the junction of the lower pharynx and upper esophagus.

These findings are in general conformity with the previously noted study of 503 autopsy cases reported by Åkerström and associates from the University of Uppsala, Sweden (2). They found that 80% of superior glands were located within a circumscribed area 2 cm in diameter, approximately 1 cm above the intersection of the recurrent laryngeal nerve and the inferior thy-

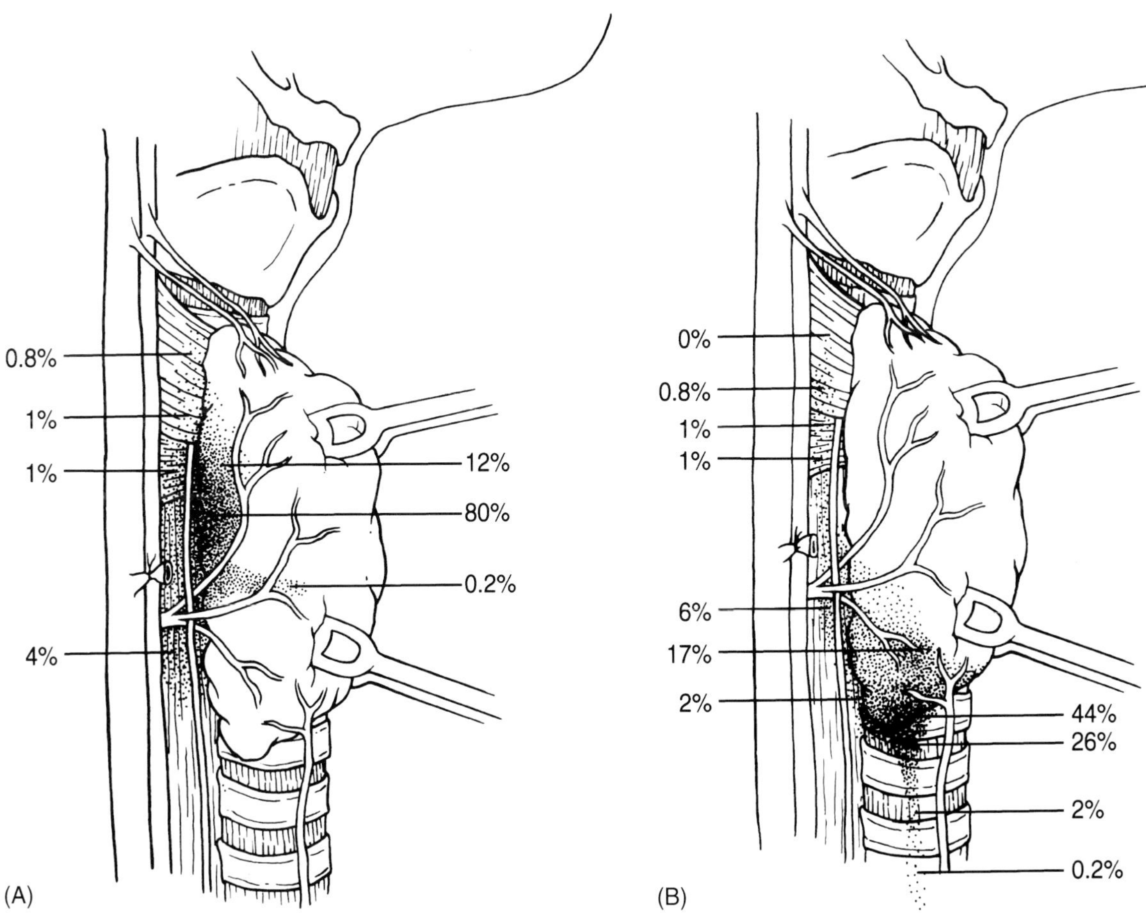

Figure 3 Location of superior (A) and inferior (B) parathyroid glands. The numbers represent the percentages of glands found at different locations in an autopsy study of 503 cases. More frequent locations are indicated by darker shading. (Adapted from Ref. 2.)

roid artery, lying posterior to the superior portion of the thyroid or applied to it (Fig. 3A).

The superior parathyroid glands are characteristically positioned behind the recurrent nerve but may be found within the fascia attaching the upper pole of the thyroid to the pharyngeal wall and trachea (Berry's ligament), or anterior to it. Care must be taken not to damage the gland when dissecting this fascia. As superior glands descend, they follow a posterior plane; the usual ectopic positions are along the tracheoesophageal groove or the posterior mediastinum (Fig. 2A).

3.2 Inferior Parathyroid Glands (Branchial Pouch III)

Inferior parathyroid glands are not distributed in as constant a position as the superior glands. They originate from the 3rd branchial pouch in association with the thymus and travel much further downward in their embryological development. Classically, they appear anterior to the recurrent nerve and applied to the thyroid gland. Their more widely dispersed distribution is likely an embryological consequence of their journey further downward than the superior glands and their common origin with the thymus (Fig. 1). This may be responsible for the approximately 30% of lower glands that are found in the tissue inferior to the thyroid, adjacent to, or within the thymus. When inferior glands descend or are in ectopic positions, they rest in an anterior plane and are frequently located in the thyrothymic ligaments, the thymus, or lower in the anterior mediastinum.

Wang (3), in a study of 160 cadavers, found inferior glands to be more widely dispersed than the upper glands, located somewhat evenly between the lower pole of the thyroid and the thymus. Forty-two percent were located on the anterior or posterior lateral surface of the lower pole of the thyroid, frequently hidden in thyroid creases. Thirty-nine percent were located in the lower neck within the thymic tongues. The mediastinum was the site of 2% of the inferior glands. Fifteen percent were situated at some distance lateral to the lower pole of the thyroid lobe; most were suspended by vascular pedicles. Of six glands that were ectopic, three were found high at the carotid bifurcation, and three in the mid-thyroid area close to, but outside the carotid sheath. Åkerström et al. observed that 61% of inferior parathyroid glands were found just below, posterior, or lateral to the lower pole of the thyroid. The next most common location (26%) was the region inferior to the thyroid lobes, in close association with the fibrous tissue connecting the lower thyroid pole and the thymus, or within the cervical portion of the thymus (Fig. 3B). If the third pharyngeal pouch fails to descend, the "inferior parathyroid" may remain trapped high in the neck, in the parapharyngeal area along the carotid artery as high as the base of the skull. A small amount of thymus is often attached to the gland, confirming the embryology, and explaining the use of the term: "undescended parathymus" (4) (Figs. 1, 2B).

Bilateral symmetry is common in the location of the parathyroid glands, extending a helping hand to the surgeon. It is present in 80% of the superior and 70% of the inferior glands, but less frequently in those glands found in aberrant locations. Relative symmetry in the position of all four glands is present in 60% of cases (2).

Since the parathyroids arise and travel downward separately from the thyroid, they typically have their own capsule. A normal or enlarged parathyroid gland can be suspected at surgery if a nodule on the surface of the thyroid moves separately when nudged by a "peanut" sponge placed on the end of a hemostat. This mobility is especially evident when the gland is enlarged by an adenoma; these will usually shell out easily from the surface of the thyroid, or from the location to which they have migrated.

4 SURGICAL PATHOLOGY

4.1 Features of Normal Parathyroid Glands

In 1800 Ivar Sanström, a Swedish medical student, first described the human parathyroid glands. It was not recognized until 1815, 15 years later, that excision of the parathyroid glands, rather than the removal of the thyroid, was the cause of tetany (5). In 1907 Halsted commented, "it seems hardly credible that the loss of bodies so tiny should be followed by a result so disastrous" (6).

A normal parathyroid gland measures approximately 5 × 4 × 2 mm, the size of a lentil. It is light tan in color, oval or bean shaped, concave on the side applied to the thyroid, convex on the exposed side, and is often embedded within or cradled by a small fat pad (Fig. 4). It is frequently shaped by the pressure of neighboring structures because of its soft consistency. In most cases it is bean-shaped, but occasionally it may be elongated, bilobed, or multilobate. When the parathyroid becomes adenomatous or hyperplasic, the flattened shape becomes globular. The color is a function of stromal fat content; it progresses from a yellowish-light brown or tan in a normal gland, to a reddish-brown as the fat content decreases in the abnormal gland. Adenomas and hyperplastic glands usually contain less stromal fat, a factor in their histological diagnosis.

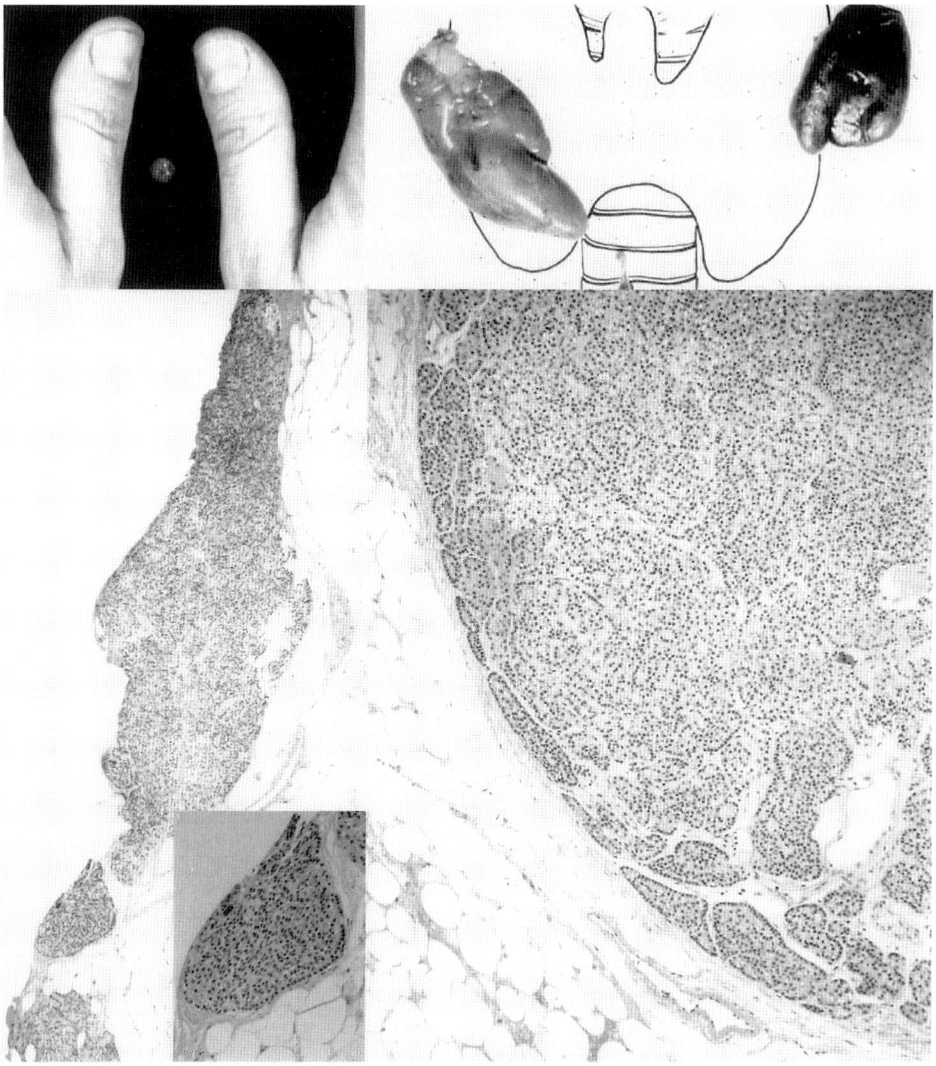

Figure 4 Parathyroid: normal and adenoma. (Top left) The normal parathyroid gland is roughly the shape and size of a lentil. It is shown between the thumbs of the pathologist. (Top right) Two enlarged inferior parathyroid glands, part of a four-gland water-clear hyperplasia. The size of the glands is in scale with the thyroid drawing. (Bottom left) Normal parathyroid gland consisting of a mixture of chief cells, clear cells and oncocytic cells, with a variable amount of adipose tissue. (Inset) All of these endocrine cells have characteristic round nuclei and prominent cell membranes. (Bottom right) Compare normal parathyroid histology with that of an enlarged parathyroid. While the cytological components remain the same, the cellular abundance is indicative of hyperplasia. Histologically, there are no features that can consistently distinguish an adenoma from glandular hyperplasia (hematoxylin and eosin). (Courtesy of Dr. Michael Klein, Mount Sinai School of Medicine.)

A single gland may weigh between 20 and 70 mg; the combined weight of all four glands is usually between 120 and 160 mg and should be less than 210 mg (7). Ghandur- Mnaymneh, in a study of 100 individuals who died from other causes, found that the high range of individual gland weight was 72.6 mg in whites and 91.6 mg in blacks, more than in previous reports (8). The weight of a gland is the most useful indication in determining whether it is abnormally enlarged. Parathormone secretion is a direct reflection of the mass of the gland. Therefore, gland weight is a crucial component of any surgical pathology report.

Approximately 80–100 mg of parathyroid tissue (two normal sized glands) is usually enough to maintain normal calcium levels, an important guide to the surgeon performing parathyroid or thyroid surgery.

4.2 Cellular Structure

The parathyroid gland is composed mainly of "chief cells," the most important functional component. Clear cells and oxyphil cells are functional modifications of the chief cells. Oxyphil cells are larger than chief cells, distinguished by their granular eosinophilic cytoplasm, the result of abundant mitochondria. Clear cells are the largest parathyroid cells, characterized by clear cytoplasm containing many small vacuoles.

4.3 Adenoma

Adenomas are almost always solitary and are more frequently found in the inferior glands. The cut surface ranges from a mahogany red-brown to a tan or light brown; cystic areas may be present. They are usually composed of chief cells but may also contain a variable mixture of oxyphilic or water-clear cells. Chief cells in adenomas are usually large and variable in size, hyperchromatic with nuclear pleomorphism, and may be multinucleated. As in many endocrine entities, nuclear pleomorphism should not be regarded as a sign of malignancy; it constitutes a second criterion used in discriminating adenomas from hyperplastic glands (9). Occasional mitotic figures can be seen but are usually fewer than 1 per 10 high power fields. More numerous mitotic figures should raise the suspicion of carcinoma. The size of the glands corresponds roughly to the degree of hypercalcemia (10). The remaining parathyroids are frequently suppressed, often containing increased intracellular and stromal fat, but this cannot be grossly distinguished at surgery. The other glands may also appear entirely normal. Studies have confirmed that adenomas are the result of clonal proliferation derived from a single mutated cell or as a result of a constitutive (somatic) mutation in chromosome 11, in the region of the MEN1 gene. Generally, chromosomal mutations can be present only in the diseased tissue (acquired) or within all the cells of an individual (germline). Mutations within chromosome 11 can be confined to the parathyroid cells (sporadic or nonfamilial hyperparathyroidism) or may be a constitutive, somatic mutation (e.g., familial, syndromic hyperparathyroidism) (11).

4.4 Hyperplasia

Typically all glands are enlarged, hypercellular, and contain decreased intracellular and stromal fat. Chief cells usually predominate. Parathyroid hyperplasia may be sporadic or a component of familial hyperplasia, MEN 1, 2a, or 2b, although hyperparathyroidism is rare in type 2b. Usually all four glands are enlarged and hyperplastic, but the hyperplasia may be asymmetrical, with one or two glands enlarged and the others apparently normal in size. There may be a uniform cellular hyperplasia, or a multinodular hyperplasia, with adjacent gland compression and admixed adipose tissue. This nodularity can easily mimic an adenoma. In fact, parathyroid hyperplasia and adenomas are not as distinct and mutually exclusive, as was once previously conceptualized. Adenomas can evolve within diffuse hyperplasia, giving rise to asymmetrical enlargement. Genetic studies of allelic loss within chromosome 11 further support this concept (12).

Histologically, parathyroid hyperplasia can be composed uniformly of chief cells or be of mixed cellularity. Water-clear hyperplasia is less common and sporadic; there is no genetic component.

4.5 Distinguishing Adenoma from Hyperplasia

When one gland is enlarged and the others are normal, it is obvious that the pathology is that of an adenoma. However when there are two or even three enlarged glands and the remaining gland(s) are normal in size, the surgeon confronts a dilemma: Is this a case of multiple adenomas or of hyperplasia? The decision can be difficult or even impossible at the operating table. The differentiation between adenoma and hyperplasia leads to a difference in management. Aggressive resection of additional glands if an adenoma is misdiagnosed as hyperplasia can result in postoperative hypocalcemia. When a single gland is enlarged, the diagnosis is almost certainly adenoma. If this finding were an early stage of hyperplasia, recurrence after excision would be expected. This is not the case. Recurrent hypercalcemia following removal of a single enlarged gland is approximately 1% (13).

None of the histological features said to distinguish hyperplasia from adenoma have survived after evaluation of large numbers of cases. Historically, the distinction was guided by the doctrine that an encapsulated mass compressing adjacent parathyroid tissue defined an adenoma. This has not proved reliable; some adenomas lack discernable capsules, and some hyperplasias have a nodular nature, compressing surrounding parathyroid tissue (14,15). Additionally, there may be considerable variation in the size of the glands in parathyroid hyperplasia. The dictum that adenomas can be distinguished from hyperplastic glands by the presence of a rim of normal tissue is no longer valid. The absence of specific histological features to differentiate adenomas from hyperplasia has led to the use of the more practical terms "single gland" or "multiple gland" disease (16).

Double adenomas, though unusual, are real entities, occurring in 2–8% of patients with primary hyperparathyroidism; they appear more often in patients over 60 years of age and are frequently missed by localizing procedures (17,18). Although the generally accepted incidence is approximately 2%, Moore et al. (89) found a frequency of 13% and Tezelman et al. (18) reported a 12% incidence. Overaggressive management, assuming that this represents an early stage of hyperplasia, can lead to hypocalcemia. Some authorities maintain that these are misinterpreted nodular hyperplasia (19). The surgeon at the operating table, rather than the pathologist at the microscope, is the best judge of the distinction between adenomas and hyperplasia. The size of the gland conforms roughly to the degree of hypercalcemia. From the clinical point of view, only one guide has withstood the test of time: removal of only the enlarged glands. This approach has produced a high rate of cure and a very low rate of postoperative hypoparathyroidism (20).

When a single enlarged gland is removed, the hypercalcemia will be corrected. If more than one gland is enlarged, removal of the enlarged ones and sparing those that are small and apparently normal may result in mild elevation of parathormone, but not clinical hypercalcemia. Whether this condition represents asymmetrical hyperplasia or multiple adenomas has not been determined. In contrast to primary hyperplasia, the parathyroid glands in renal failure are uniformly enlarged.

4.6 Role of Biopsies During Surgery

In spite of frozen section techniques to differentiate adenomas from hyperplasia based on the assessment of stromal fat, which is depleted in hyperplastic glands that may appear normal in size and appearance, this method has not proved to be of practical help to the surgeon in the operating room. Stromal fat can be unevenly distributed, varies with patient age, and may be distorted when frozen, producing specimens that appear falsely hyperplasic when biopsied. The irregular distribution of fat and parenchymal cells renders gland biopsies inadequate as an indicator of function (21). Although some authors feel that adenomas can be distinguished from hyperplasia by intraoperative parathyroid biopsy, using methods such as saline density or intracellular lipid stains similar to Sudan black and oil-red, no histological feature has been found reliable (22,23). The surgeon must decide whether a parathyroid gland is normal, relying on size, shape, color, and the appearance of the other glands. The pathologist can only reliably confirm that the specimen is or is not parathyroid tissue (24). The weight of the resected gland is the most reliable indication of abnormality.

At our institution the usual frozen section report on an enlarged gland removed in an exploration for hyperparathyroidism is "enlarged parathyroid gland." We do not biopsy grossly normal parathyroid glands.

4.7 Parathyroid Carcinoma

This condition is rare, occurring in approximately 2% of cases of hyperparathyroidism. The malignancy is also remarkable in that it is usually functional, producing large amounts of parathormone. Presenting serum cal-

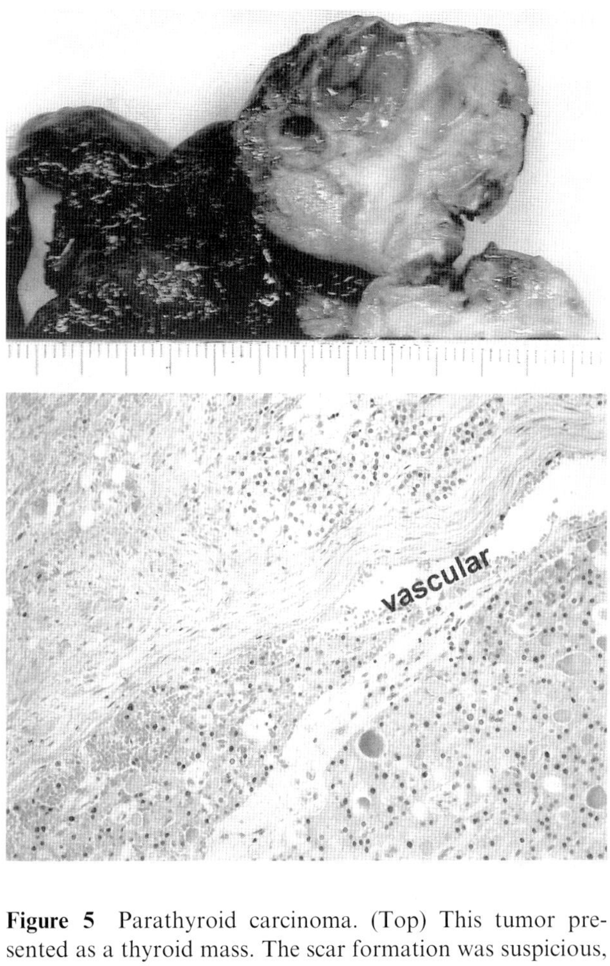

Figure 5 Parathyroid carcinoma. (Top) This tumor presented as a thyroid mass. The scar formation was suspicious, though not diagnostic for malignancy. (Bottom) Histologically, the carcinoma is seen invading vascular spaces. Immunohistochemistry for parathyroid hormone confirmed this tumor was of parathyroid origin (hematoxylin and eosin).

cium levels are often high (>12 mg%). The tumors are frequently large. The combination of a high PTH level and a palpable mass raises the suspicion of parathyroid carcinoma. The usual parathyroid adenoma is not palpable.

At surgery the tumor frequently presents a gray or whitish appearance, with obvious infiltration of adjacent tissue. The histological diagnosis cannot be made without evidence of invasion of adjoining tissue, blood vessel involvement, or metastases (Fig. 5). Although mitotic figures are usually present, they are not diagnostic; they may also, on occasion, be seen in adenomas. The disease progresses slowly; metastases appear late. Neck node metastases are rare. Widespread systemic involvement is unusual; the lungs, with a 25% incidence of involvement, are the most common sites of visceral involvement.

Although occasionally the carcinoma may be nonfunctioning, the patient usually suffers from the metabolic disturbances of increased parathyroid hormone: hypercalcemia, bone disease, and the other consequences of uncontrolled hypercalcemia. If the carcinoma cannot be controlled, complications of hypercalcemia are the usual cause of mortality.

5 INDICATION FOR SURGERY IN PRIMARY HYPERPARATHYROIDISM

The most common cause of elevated serum calcium is primary hyperparathyroidism due to an adenoma or four-gland hyperplasia. In 85–90% of patients the condition is due to a single adenoma. The condition is more common than previously realized, with an incidence of 1 in 500 women and 1 in 2000 men every year. In some patients hyperplasia is the result of genetic conditions such as familial hyperparathyroidism or multiple endocrine neoplasia (MEN I, MEN 2a, but rarely MEN 2b). In these situations all parathyroid glands are hyperplastic. Although there are diverse causes of hypercalcemia, hyperparathyroidism and malignancy account for 90% of cases. If PTH assays are within normal limits, other entities must be considered. Endocrine disorders such as thyrotoxicosis or acute adrenal insufficiency can result in hypercalcemia. Malignancy may elevate serum calcium as a result of bone metastases; metastatic breast cancer accounts for 80% of these cases. Cancers that involve bone marrow, e.g., myeloma, leukemia, lymphoma, may also produce elevation of serum calcium. Excess intake of calcium (e.g., milk products), vitamin A, or vitamin D can also be responsible for hypercalcemia. Granulomatous conditions such as sarcoidosis and tuberculosis must be excluded. Prolonged immobilization, Paget's disease, and intake of certain drugs such as thiazide diuretics or estrogens must be considered as well.

Some tumors (e.g. lung, renal cancer) secrete a PTH-like substance that induces hypercalcemia. The intact or two-site PTH assay is preferred for diagnosis because it does not crossreact with parathyroid hormone-related peptides secreted by nonparathyroid cancers (25). The majority of patients with hyperparathyroidism are now diagnosed by routine blood chemistries revealing increased serum calcium and are confirmed by PTH assays that are exquisitely accurate.

Familial hypocalciuric hypercalcemia, an autosomal dominant condition with high penetration, must be differentiated from primary hyperparathyroidism. Despite mean calcium levels of 12 mg/dL, these patients do not suffer from the clinical consequences of hyperparathyroidism and do not require surgery. Importantly, serum parathormone and urine calcium are normal. A family history of hypercalcemia suggests hypocalcalciuric hypercalcemia, familial hyperparathyroidism, or a multiple endocrine neoplasia syndrome; hence the hypercalcemia of familial hypocalciuric hypercalcemia must be distinguished from that of other hereditary conditions. Mean calcium excretion is in the area of 100 mg/day compared to elevations of 300 mg or more in hyperparathyroidism. Calcium to creatinine clearance ratio is less than 0.01 compared to hyperparathyroidism, where it is greater than 0.1 (26).

Patients with minimal elevations of serum calcium are now diagnosed at an early stage of primary hyperparathyroidism, leading to controversy concerning the indications for surgical management. A prescient study by Scholtz and Purnell (27) foretold that hyperparathyroidism, even when silent, is a condition with future serious consequences. In a prospective evaluation of 142 asymptomatic patients with mild elevations in serum calcium (10.2–11.0 mg/dL), 33 patients (23%) followed for 10 years required surgery for progressive disease. This rate increases to 36% if those who died of other causes, declined follow-up, or could not be traced are taken into account (27). It was not possible to predict which patients with asymptomatic hyperparathyroidism would ultimately require surgery. It is interesting to note that 12 patients who initially presented with mild hypercalcemia could not be demonstrated to have hypercalcemia 10 years later.

There is agreement by most authors that surgery is indicated for asymptomatic patients with serum calcium levels above 11.5–12 mg/dL. Still, a substantial number of patients with limited elevation of serum calcium and PTH are "asymptomatic" and are increasingly being considered for surgery. Vague protean symptoms such as fatigue, back pain, memory loss, depression, polyuria, and polydipsia now invite the diagnosis of hyperparathyroidism. Low levels of dopamine, serotoninin, and norepinephrine derivatives have been demonstrated in the cerebrospinal fluid of patients who have parathyroid disease accompanied by neuropsychiatric symptoms. These metabolites return to normal levels following successful parathyroidectomy. Similar depressed levels are present in patients with endogenous depression who do not have parathyroid disease (28). In a study of reoperation for persistent hyperparathyroidism, 37% of patients felt depressed before reoperation; 12% remained depressed after successful surgery (29).

Many observers believe that true asymptomatic hyperparathyroidism is rare and that on careful investigation less than 5% of patients are completely free of symptoms or related difficulties. After detailed questioning and investigation, most report some symptom or problem related to primary hyperparathyroidism, and in 80% of cases these conditions improve after successful parathyroidectomy (30–32). More information is being acquired. Recent studies demonstrate that correction of hyperparathyroidism markedly benefits cancellous bone density in the spine (33). Scandinavian population-based studies indicate that patients with untreated hyperparathyroidism have an increased risk of death, mainly from cardiovascular disease and malignancy, compared to a control group in the normal population; the higher the hypercalcemia, the higher the death rate (34). Another assessment showed that surgery decreases the risk of premature death (35).

Medical opinion is gradually shifting to the opinion that patients with proved hyperparathyroidism should be offered surgical treatment, even though they appear to be asymptomatic. The disease has an invisible morbidity and mortality.

6 PREOPERATIVE LOCALIZATION

Before localization techniques were available, the success rate for the qualified surgeon operating on a patient diagnosed with hyperparathyroidism was over 95%. It is still frequently maintained that the next step after diagnosis is to locate an experienced parathyroid surgeon. There are respected authors who advise against preoperative localization in initial explorations because of the significant numbers of false positives and negatives, stating that it is not cost effective (36–39). This view is shared by the 1991 NIH consensus statement (40) (Table 1).

Table 1 Cost of Diagnostic Procedures at Mt. Sinai Medical Center

Ultrasound	\$200
Sestamibi scan	\$1206
MRI (with gadolinium)	\$1700
CT (with gadolinium)	\$1075
Intraoperative parathormone assay	\$150 per sample[a]

[a] An uncomplicated operation at MSH requires four samples.

We prefer preoperative localization studies because they do no harm and often provide valuable information; they are essential in unilateral approaches. It is disheartening when, in order to cut costs, a failed initial procedure has been performed without testing, and later, an accessible parathyroid adenoma is identified by a localization procedure.

All non-invasive imaging procedures are sensitive to the size of the abnormal gland, offering help in a large adenoma but little assistance in multiglandular disease, where it is most needed. Since each noninvasive test is dependent upon a specific physical or metabolic characteristic of the abnormal parathyroid gland, results are different for each technique, but the methods may complement each other. Nevertheless, false positives are a significant problem and false negatives are not uncommon. No testing method can be relied upon for the diagnosis and localization of hyperplastic glands or multiple adenomas. Ultrasound is most useful for abnormal glands adjacent to or within the thyroid; it can reveal thyroid pathology that is non-palpable and unsuspected, enabling treatment at the same time as parathyroid exploration. Nuclear scanning is more effective for ectopic locations in the neck or mediastinum.

It is possible to combine the anatomical localization of CT and MRI with the functional identification of nuclear imaging. Although the use of a battery of tests is not cost-effective overall in primary explorations, it can offer a huge advantage to the patient who has a mediastinal or deep cervical gland.

6.1 Localization in Secondary Explorations

There is a great difference between the location of abnormal glands removed on initial exploration and those removed at reoperation for failed procedures.

Forty percent of abnormal parathyroid glands missed at initial explorations are found in their usual position in relationship to the thyroid at reoperation, casting a shadow on the experience of the surgeon and raising the question of whether localization procedures might have helped (68).

Mediastinal glands below the level of the thymus are normally present in from 0.2–2% of cases. (2,3). At reoperation Shen and associates found 28% missed glands to be located in this position (mediastinal but not in the thymus) (29).

Parathyroid glands are normally present in the retropharyngeal or retroesophageal space in only 1% of cases (2). However, Brennan et al., at reexploration for failed initial explorations, found 39% at this location (68). Carty and Norton found 72% of missing superior glands to be in this area on reexploration (69).

Since the majority of parathyroid glands in their classic locations adjacent to the thyroid are removed at the initial surgery, the incidence of abnormal parathyroid glands at ectopic sites is markedly increased at reoperation. Hence the increased importance of localizing those in uncommon positions, e.g., undescended inferior glands stranded high in the neck, those adjacent to or within the carotid sheath, adenomas located in the paratracheal and paraesophageal areas, intrathyroid glands, and those within or adjoining the thymus; this can be critical for the surgeon undertaking a second exploration. There is virtually universal agreement that localization procedures are required in patients undergoing reoperation.

6.2 Ultrasound

Ultrasound is cost-effective; it is most useful for locating adenomas in intrathyroidal or juxtathyroid positions, but less reliable in patients with concomitant thyroid disease. It can also reveal unsuspected thyroid pathology. There is a wide range in reported sensitivity. In large measure, accuracy is a reflection of the skill and experience of the operator. Efficacy is related to the location and size of the glands; inferior glands and those adjacent to, or within the thyroid, are more easily recognized than superior or deep glands (41). A negative study suggests the possibility of multiple gland disease, a tumor located posteriorly behind the trachea and esophagus, or retrosternal in the thymus and mediastinum; the latter are difficult to visualize because overlying bone or air create their own acoustic shadows. In this situation nuclear scanning is complementary. Ultrasound is simple and noninvasive, and the cost is miniscule in relation to the overall expense of parathyroid surgery. It is a good first choice (Table 1).

Intraoperative ultrasound as well as intraoperative nuclear scanning have been found helpful by some surgeons, but they are not in general use. In a recent report by Jaskowiak et al. (42), intraoperative gamma probe localization was reported to be particularly valuable in reoperative surgery for missed parathyroid adenomas, with dense scarring and obscured anatomy. However, there are limitations to this method since thyroid adenomas may also retain sestamibi and it is not useful for multiple gland disease. (see also Chapter 18).

6.3 Computerized Tomography and Magnetic Resonance

MRI is replacing CT as a diagnostic tool, particularly in recurrent cases; it is particularly valuable for ectopic glands because of its increased sensitivity (43). When employed with gadolinium, sensitivity is further improved (up to 87%) (44) (Fig. 6). MRI is especially useful in locating superior mediastinal and ectopic adenomas. The similarity of the signal to thyroid and fat can be overcome by various modifications of the signal that suppress the image produced by fat (45).

6.4 Nuclear Imaging

Technetium sestamibi scanning has displaced thallium-technetium subtraction techniques because of its improved resolution and sensitivity (46). The relative amount of oncocytic cells within an adenoma or hyperplasia correlates directly with sestamibi uptake (47). Poor uptake in hyperplasia and multiple adenomas are limitations. Sestamibi scanning has the ability to offer planar anterior and lateral views without the need for subtraction. Sestamibi-single photon emission computerized tomography (SEPT) offers three-dimensional images that can visualize the gland in the anterior/posterior plane and can locate adenomas deep in the neck and in the mediastinum.

Fine needle aspiration can confirm that lesions identified by imaging studies are indeed parathyroid in nature. It is documented by cytology, PTH assay, and immunohistochemical staining for PTH (48).

6.5 Angiography and Venous Sampling

Angiography and venous sampling are reserved for secondary procedures because of their invasive nature but can be of great value in this situation. They are capable of identifying an adenoma in approximately two thirds of cases, with less than 5% false-positives (49). Venous sampling offers similar results; for greater accuracy it is usually used in combination with arteriography. Angiography can also be helpful because it

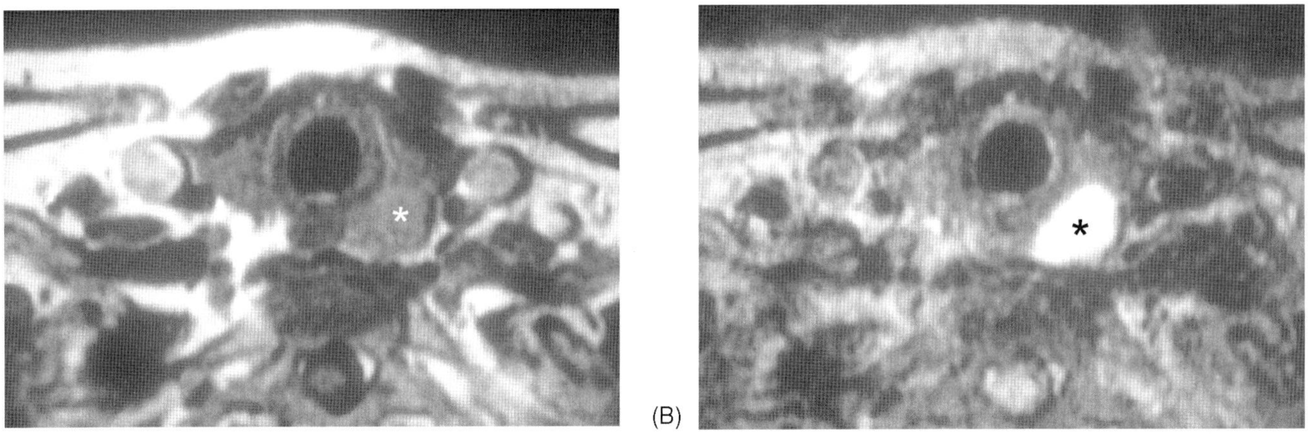

(A) (B)

Figure 6 Diagnosis of parathyroid adenoma: MRI with gadolinium. (A) Axial T_1-weighted MR image shows a low signal intensity, ovoid mass in the left tracheoesophageal groove. (B) Axial T_2-weighted MR image shows the mass to have homogeneous high signal intensity that enhances after gadolinium contrast administration, confirming that this is a parathyroid adenoma. (Courtesy of Dr. Peter Som, Mount Sinai School of Medicine.)

facilitates ablation techniques that can treat mediastinal adenomas without operative intervention (50). Since there is a risk of cerebrovascular complications, these methods are extremely dependent on user expertise and experience (51). In experienced hands they can be of great value.

7 SURGERY FOR PRIMARY HYPERPARATHYROIDISM

The usual goal in the surgery of hyperparathyroidism is the removal of a single enlarged gland and identification of the other normal glands to confirm the diagnosis of adenoma. This is the most common finding and the gold standard in treatment.

The recognition and treatment of parathyroid hyperplasia offers satisfactory results but is beset by a higher incidence of persistent and recurrent disease. The situation becomes difficult when more than one but fewer than four glands are enlarged. The dilemma of differentiating asymmetrical hyperplasia from multiple adenomas at surgery has not yet been solved.

Experienced surgeons achieve success in 95–97% of patients. Failure is usually due to inability to locate, identify, and excise an adenoma or to recognize and treat multiple gland disease. The main difficulty is the recognition of multiglandular disease. Removal of a single adenoma, when it is the etiology of hyperparathyroidism, is curative. Double adenomas, however, are clinical realities, although there is controversy differentiating this condition from hyperplasia (83).

8 RENAL FAILURE (SECONDARY HYPERPARATHYROIDISM)

Continuing renal failure stimulates hyperplasia of the parathyroid glands. With kidney failure, an insufficient amount of the active form of vitamin D (calcitriol) is produced by the kidneys; deceased absorption of calcium ensues. Hypocalcemia stimulates the parathyroids to increase the production of PTH, resulting in hyperplasia of all glands. The total weight and degree of enlargement is proportional to the duration and degree of functional renal impairment (52). Lower serum calcium and higher serum phosphate levels follow. This eventuates in "secondary" hyperparathyroidism with progressive bone disease that can be symptomatic and severe and is reflected in elevated alkaline phosphatase and serum PTH levels. A serum calcium-phosphate product of more than 70–75, despite limitation of phosphate intake, confirms the presence of serious disease. The hypercalcemia can usually be controlled by medical means, but when these measures fail, operative intervention is indicated for continuing vascular and extraskeletal calcifications, severe intractable pruritis, or progressive bone disease that does not respond to medical therapy or dialysis.

9 SURGERY FOR PARATHYROID HYPERPLASIA

Parathyroid hyperplasia constitutes a diverse group of conditions, which may be sporadic, familial, the result of MEN syndromes, or the consequence of renal failure. Fifteen to 20% of sporadic hyperparathyroidism and 80% of familial hyperparathyroidism is due to multiglandular hyperplasic disease; the hypercalcemia of multiple endocrine neoplasia is invariably due to hyperplastic disease. The goal in the surgical management of hyperplasia is more difficult than that of adenoma because all parathyroid glands must be identified and a sufficient amount of parathyroid tissue must be preserved to sustain normocalcemia. Renal failure stimulates all parathyroid tissue and is characterized by enlargement of all glands, whereas in sporadic or familial hyperplasia enlargement may be varied and uneven. A scrupulous search for all the parathyroid glands is the most important part of the operation. The most common cause of persistent or recurrent hyperparathyroidism after surgery for hyperplasia is an undiscovered gland in the neck or the anterior mediastinum (53). Since the presence of only three glands is rare, occurring in only 3% of patients, if four glands are not found in their usual positions, it is wise to assume that there is an ectopic fourth gland and to conduct a thorough search. The search includes exploration and resection of nodal and fatty tissue from the lower poles of the thyroid to the manubrium of the sternum, and if a fourth gland is not found, thymectomy through the cervical incision is indicated.

The majority of patients have four parathyroid glands but supernumary glands are present in about 13% of individuals (2). They are frequently located in the upper mediastinum in association with the thymus. Failure to find these glands frequently accounts for the persistence of hypercalcemia after surgery for hyperplasia.

Adenomas and hyperplasia are different conditions. Recurrence after removal of a single adenoma occurs in less than 5% of patients, but persistent or recurrent hyperparathyroidism occurs in 20–44% of patients with familial hyperparathyroidism (54,55). Differing approaches to the surgery of hyperplasia are in use, each with their proponents.

9.1 Subtotal Parathyroidectomy

Oliver Cope was the first to observe that that hyperparathyroidism could result from either single adenomas or multiglandular disease. He recommended the resection of adenomas and subtotal parathyroidectomy for multiple gland disease (1). This method consists of resection of 3½ parathyroid glands and preservation, in situ, of approximately 50 mg of the fourth, with its blood supply intact. The preserved remnant is marked with a vascular clip so that it can be identified if reexploration is required. It is essential that this remnant remain viable. A prudent approach is to divide the gland to be left in situ early in the procedure and observe it carefully. If it becomes devascularized during the course of the surgery, another parathyroid can still be used. This avoids the discouraging experience of completing the gland excisions and finding that the only remaining half gland is not viable. Thymectomy should be included with the procedure.

Parathyroid tissue should be cryopreserved for future use, if needed.

9.2 Total Parathyroidectomy and Autotransplantation

Since its introduction by Wells in 1973, total parathyroidectomy with autotransplantation of 50 mg of parathyroid tissue to the forearm has been the choice of many surgeons (56). The advantage is that the risk of devasculaization of the parathyroid remnant in subtotal resection is eliminated. Easy access to the forearm under local anesthesia is available should hypercalcemia persist or recur, rather than a more difficult reexploration of the neck.

The disadvantage of autotransplation is the possibility of the loss of all parathyroid function should the graft fail. It is critical, therefore, that the remaining parathyroid tissue at the time of excisional surgery be cryopreserved for future use in the event of graft failure. Reimplantantation of cryopreserved tissue is not as successful as immediate grafting of fresh tissue. As many as 92% of fresh autotransplanted grafts will function, whereas only two thirds of transplanted cryopreserved grafts succeed (57). Graft viability can be conveniently monitored by comparing PTH levels from the transplanted arm to that of the opposite side. Vascular ingrowth and function develops in 10–20 days (61). A PTH gradient of 1.5–2.0 or greater between the grafted and nongrafted forearm is evidence of graft function (57). Prolonged calcium and vitamin D supplementation (4–8 weeks or more) is required in patients who undergo total parathyroidectomy and autotransplantation.

Although hyperfunction of the graft may develop, producing nodularity or a palpable mass at the forearm transplant site, a partial reexcision can easily be performed under local anesthesia.

Others have not experienced equally beneficial results. Feldman et al. (58), in an NIH follow-up study of 46 autografts (20 immediate and 26 cryopreserved) with a mean follow-up of 35 months, found that 33% of grafts were fully functional (normocalcemic with no medication) and 20% were partially functional (normocalcemic on calcium alone). Forty percent of patients derived no benefit from the procedure. The authors cite other studies, including the original reports from the NIH, showing similar results. There was no difference between the use of fresh or cryopreserved tissue. In their opinion, these findings justify a 3 ½ gland resection rather than 4-gland parathyroidectomy and autotransplantation for parathyroid hyperplasia (58).

Authors who prefer total parathyroid resection and forearm autotransplant rather than subtotal 3 ½ gland resection refer to reports of high rates of persistent or recurrent hypercalcemia in patients with familial disease and the more difficult access to the gland remnant in the neck.

Controversy persists over the choice of total parathyroidectomy with forearm transplantation versus 3½ gland resection for parathyroid hyperplasia, with no clear conclusion. Advocates of subtotal parathyroidectomy point out that it eliminates the period of temporary hypocalcemia in the postoperative period and refer to a 5% risk of permanent hypocalcemia in total parathyroidectomy with auto transplantation (59). They note that preserved cryografts function in only 60% of patients (58,60). There is no clear evidence that one method is superior to the other. Statistics can support either approach. Respected authorities disagree: Wells et al. (61) prefer total parathyroidectomy and forearm transplant, whereas Kraimps and Barbier (62) endorses 3½ gland resection; both report good results. Either technique should include transcervical thymectomy and removal of nodal and fatty tissue in the central neck compartment above the sternum to insure the removal of ectopic or supernumery parathyroid glands. In addition, it is essential that parathyroid tissue be cryopreserved for future use in the event of postoperative hypoparathyroidism (63).

9.3 Technique of Autotransplantation

Grafting can be facilitated by cooling the gland in a bath of iced saline for 20–30 minutes until it becomes firm and easier to handle. Forty or 50 mg (the weight of a normal gland) is then minced into 1 × 2 mm segments and transplanting in groups of three to four segments each, into the brachioradialis muscle of the forearm. The muscle is carefully spread apart in the direction of its fibers by a curved clamp, and pockets are created to receive the fragments. Each packet of fragments is placed into a separate area of the muscle. Care is needed to avoid hemorrhage, since accumulation of blood would not permit the fragments to adhere to the adjacent muscle, preventing vascularization of the grafts. Three to five fragments are inserted into each of these pockets and the overlying fascia is approximated. Transplantation into the sternomastoid muscle is performed in a similar manner (Fig. 7).

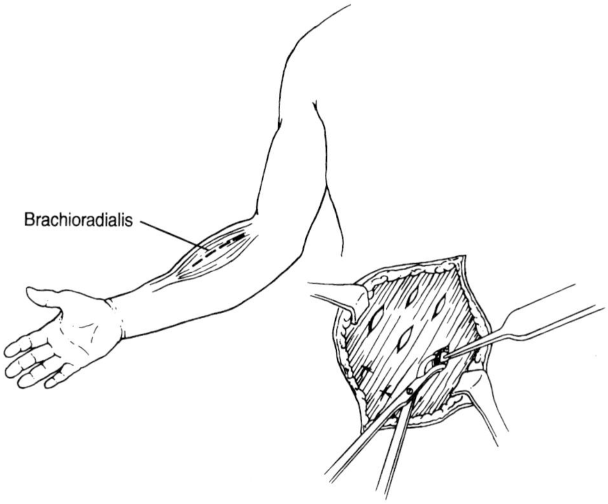

Figure 7 Forearm transplantation of the parathyroid gland.

10 CONSERVATIVE VERSUS AGGRESSIVE APPROACH TO MULTIPLE ENLARGED GLANDS

Hyperfunction of endocrine glands is almost always accompanied by hyperplasia, hypertrophy, and gland enlargement. Parathyroid hyperplasia is usually associated with the enlargement four glands. If two enlarged glands are present, the surgeon must decide whether this represents a double adenoma or an uneven early development of hyperplasia that requires more aggressive treatment. Biopsy is not helpful in this situation because there are no absolute criteria to differentiate adenomas from hyperplastic glands. Furthermore, the excessive use of biopsies may damage the parathyroids, resulting in postoperative hypocalcemia.

Frozen section can only confirm that a suspected nodule is parathyroid tissue rather than a lymph node, fat, or thymus. It is much less reliable than an experienced surgeon in differentiating adenoma from hyperplasia (64). The decision must be made on clinical grounds.

Our approach to parathyroid surgery is to remove only the enlarged glands and to avoid parathyroid biopsies. This practice has been demonstrated to be the most successful with the least risk. In a classic report, Edis et al. (65) reported a prospective study comparing the removal of only enlarged glands with that of a more "liberal" aggressive approach. In 50 patients the "liberal" approach included frequent removal of two glands, resection of 3 ½ glands when more than one gland was enlarged, and extensive use of biopsy identification. This resulted in symptomatic hypocalcemia in 24% of patients. In another group of 50 patients the "conservative" approach of removing only enlarged glands resulted in a 2% incidence of symptomatic hypercalcemia. The cure rate was identical. The value of a conservative approach was validated (65). Using the conservative approach for the management of adenomas, a success rate of over 95% can be expected. Recurrent or persistent hypercalcemia is usually the result of failure to locate an abnormal gland or to discern multiple gland disease. Wideranging dissection and the removal of more parathyroid tissue than required is frequently associated with postoperative hypocalcemia.

11 OPERATIVE TECHNIQUE

The careful surgeon will be more successful. Hemostasis must be scrupulous; blood will interfere with the visualization of normal or abnormal parathyroids and will prevent the surgeon from observing the nuances of color and texture that help differentiate fat, thyroid nodules, lymph nodes, and thymus from normal or abnormal parathyroid glands.

A transverse neck incision is made. Flaps are developed cephelad and caudad just beneath the platysma. The strap muscles are separated in the midline. If additional exposure is needed, the medial third of the sternohyoid muscles are divided transversely near their insertions and retracted laterally. After carefully elevating and separating the sternothyroid muscles from the thyroid gland, they can be completely or partially divided in a transverse manner (a cautery knife may be useful for this). This offers excellent access to the thyroid and parathyroid glands (see Chapter 6). The initial operative approach is similar to that for thyroid surgery.

Halsted and Evans, using vascular cast injections, demonstrated that the inferior thyroid arteries are the main blood supply of the inferior as well as the superior parathyroid glands, although the superior thyroid artery contributes in about 10% of cases. They also found that the glands were supplied by a single delicate end artery and that there were no capsular collaterals; they stressed that tetany was more likely from interference with circulation than excision of the parathyroid glands (66). It is critical, therefore, not to disturb normal glands. Tracking the branches of the inferior arteries may lead the surgeon to a gland in an abnormal location. Shen et al. (67) reported that 90% of parathyroid tumors found at reoperation were removed through the neck, even though 26% of these were located in the mediastinum. Cervical excision was feasible because the usual blood supply of inferior parathyroid glands, even those located in the mediastinum, is from the inferior thyroid arteries. When glands are located lower in the mediastinum and supplied by thymic branches of the internal mammary artery, a sternal splitting incision is usually required.

Though a normal parathyroid is difficult to feel, one that is enlarged, firm, or misshaped by tumor can sometimes be identified by palpation. Gentle exploration with a finger downward along the tracheoesophageal groove, the retrotracheal and retroesophageal areas, and the superior mediastinum can be rewarding (Fig. 2A). This is the location of 30–70 % of ectopic superior parathyroid glands that are missed at initial surgery and found on reoperation (68,69).

12 STEPS IN PARATHYROID EXPLORATION

The search for the parathyroids begins by seeking them in their normal position. A quick look for all four glands is more rewarding than an exhaustive search of each location before proceeding to the next.

Division of the middle thyroid vein is required to facilitate rotation of the thyroid lobe.

The thyroid lobe can be rotated medially to search for an enlarged inferior gland. It is often necessary to divide the superior thyroid vessels to adequately inspect the normal position of the superior parathyroid gland.

Locate all normal glands, and then begin the search for a missing gland. Symmetry of position is often helpful. If all four glands cannot be found, the next step is to repeat the search, carefully returning to the usual locations. The usual position of a missing gland is within 1 or 2 cm of its normal location. This is where 30–50% of missing glands are found on reexploration of failed initial procedures (68).

A quick inspection of the upper mediastinal area may uncover a missing lower gland adjacent to or within the thymus, frequently within the ligaments that descend from the lower poles of the thyroid lobes to the thymus at the thoracic inlet (thyrothymic ligaments). Twenty-six to 39% of normal lower parathyroid glands are found in this location (2,3).

If no obvious enlarged gland is discovered, the area inferior to the thyroid should be cleared, and the portion of the thymus accessible through the neck should be resected. Thymectomy is especially important in the management of hyperplasia; a 5th parathyroid occurs in approximately 13% of patients, usually in this location.

Look for a missing superior parathyroid inferior to the inferior glands. It may have descended downward into the posterior mediastinum and be discovered by exploring the parapharyngeal, paralaryngeal, and retrotracheal areas visually and by palpation. One percent of normal parathyroid glands are situated in the posterior superior mediastinum, but on reexploration after initial failure, 30–40% of missing glands are discovered in this location (67–69). Open the carotid sheath completely for evaluation. Explore up to and beyond the carotid bifurcation. Palpation alone will miss even enlarged glands within the sheath.

A missing inferior gland may be found superior to the superior glands. It may be located adjacent to the carotid vessels or in the parapharyngeal area, as high as the base of the skull. This would represent an "undescended parathyroid" (4) (Fig. 2B).

If the missing abnormal parathyroid gland cannot be found, a thyroid lobectomy on the side of the missing gland is undertaken. The gland may be located within the thyroid lobe or, more usually, folded into a recess that cannot be identified on gross examination. This accounts for perhaps 1–2% of abnormally situated parathyroid glands. When present it may represent a true intrathyroid superior gland that has been trapped between the median and lateral lobe of the thyroid, since the superior parathyroid and the lateral portion of the thyroid share a common origin from the fourth branchial pouch.

If an adenoma cannot be found, mediastinal exploration through a sternal split is not undertaken at the initial operation. A period of observation and further diagnostic tests are indicated. In addition, the neck exploration may have devascularized the adenoma.

Valuable guidance for parathyroid exploration is available in the literature. As is frequently the case, the most useful lessons are those learned from failure. Shen and colleagues (67), in a report on 102 reoperations for persistent or recurrent hyperparathyroidism, which roughly parallels the experience of others, found the most common reasons for failure at the original surgery were ectopic locations of tumors (53%), incomplete resection of multiple abnormal glands (37%), and adenomas missed in their normal locations (7%) (though most others report 40–50%). Of the ectopic glands, 28% were paraesophageal, 26% were in the mediastinum (but not in the thymus), 24% intrathymic, 11% intrathyroidal, 9% in the carotid sheath, and 2% undescended in the high neck. Eighty-three percent were accessible through a cervical incision.

13 COMPLICATIONS OF SURGERY

13.1 Hypocalcemia

Resection of a parathyroid adenoma or hyperplastic glands is followed by a decline in the serum calcium level, usually within 6 hours and progressing up to 48 hours or more after surgery. This does not require treatment unless symptoms develop. The most vulnerable patients are those with bone disease from longstanding calcium depletion. In the classic case of Captain Charles Martell, tetany resulted when normal parathyroid glands had been removed in six previous operations and a mediastinal adenoma—the patient's only source of parathormone—was discovered and resected (1). Muscle cramps, paresthesias, perioral numbness, tingling of the fingertips or hands, muscle spasms, and carpopedal spasm are characteristic symptoms of hypocalcemia that may occur postoperatively. Chvostek's sign (tapping the parotid area to demonstrate facial spasm as the result of seventh nerve hyperactivity) is a useful test for early hypocalcemia, but is positive in a small percentage of normal individuals. Trousseau's sign, or carpopedal spasm, which can be demonstrated when a blood pressure cuff is inflated between systolic and diastolic pressure, is evidence of severe hypocalcemic. Untreated hypocalcemia can result in tetany with lethal consequences as the result of convulsions, stridor, or respiratory arrest.

Although transient hypocalcemia is common after parathyroid surgery, it is rarely permanent. In 379 patients surgically treated at the Mayo Clinic for primary hyperparathyroidism, the incidence of permanent hypocalcemia was 0.3% (70).

The practice of routine preoperative prophylaxis with oral calcium and calcitriol has been advocated and is reported to markedly decrease the incidence of postoperative symptomatic hypocalcemia (71). Mild hypocalcemia that is asymptomatic or transient does not require treatment. Serum calcium should be checked every 8–12 hours until it is stable at 8 mg/dL or the patient is asymptomatic. Ionized calcium levels are a more accurate measure of the physiological calcium level, though more expensive. Serum calcium is lowered by 0.8 mg for each decrease of 1.0 g in serum albumen. Symptomatic hypocalcemia, depending on the severity, requires oral or intravenous calcium replacement. Calcitriol, the active fraction of vitamin D needed for the absorption and metabolism of calcium, should also be provided. Acute symptoms of hypocalcemia require intravenous calcium: 1–2 ampules of calcium gluconate in 10% solution can be administered as a drip in 250 mL of isotonic saline every 8 hours, as needed.

Oral maintainence of serum calcium can be provided with Os-Cal 500™: (500 mg elemental calcium as calcium carbonate), or Tums™, which offers the same amount of elemental calcium in the form of calcium carbonate at one-third the price. Two to 5 g of calcium per day can be given.

Vitamin D [1,25-$(OH)_2D_3$] is supplied as calcitriol (Rocaltrol™) 0.25–0.5 μg one to four times per day. This should be regulated to conform to serum calcium levels.

Hypomagnesemia may account for persistent hypocalcemia that is refractory to calcium and vitamin D. In this situation parenteral magnesium replacement will contribute to a normal serum calcium (72).

13.2 Recurrent Nerve Injury

In 379 patients surgically treated at the Mayo Clinic for primary hyperparathyroidism, the operative mortality was 0.3%, and the incidence of persistent vocal cord paralysis was 0.8% (70). Although some surgeons advise dissecting the recurrent nerve as a routine, many feel that it is not necessary for a primary uncomplicated exploration. If the search becomes difficult, however, it is good judgment to identify the nerve. Secondary operations require exposure of the nerve because of the increased risk of injury. Patow reported a 6.6% incidence of vocal cord paralysis in 163 patients undergoing parathyroid reoperation (73).

13.3 Postoperative Hemorrhage

Bleeding into the closed space of the neck is always serious because it may herald respiratory obstruction. Dressings should be minimal so that the wound can be observed. Any sign of increasing swelling in the neck requires immediate opening of the wound to relieve pressure.

14 MINIMALLY INVASIVE SURGERY

Although the traditional approach to parathyroid exploration by an experienced surgeon offers a 95% or greater prospect of success, the advent of new techniques has encouraged surgeons to perform more focused and less invasive operations, exploring the neck unilaterally through small incisions and using local anesthesia with intravenous sedation. Most notable has been the availability of quick intraoperative parathormone levels (QPTH) and sestamibi-SPECT (single proton emission computerized tomography) scanning, which offers three-dimensional reconstruction. In a study of 303 patients operated upon for hyperparathyroidism, a solitary tumor was identified in 105 cases by ultrasonography and confirmed to be at the same site by technetium 99m-sestamibi scanning; at surgery the tests proved accurate in 101 of 105 patients (96%) (83). At present, the combination of improved localization techniques and biochemical confirmation of success offers great promise for minimal access surgery.

The benchmark of parathyroid surgery has been the visualization of all parathyroid glands at surgery, using the criteria of appearance, size, color, and configuration to determine which to remove. This method has proven extremely effective and has yielded excellent results.

The availability of a rapid PTH assay, introduced in 1988 by Wang, has taken parathyroid surgery to a new level of quantifiable accuracy, making it possible to establish "biochemical proof of cure" while the patient is still on the operating table (74). Although this method is a valuable adjunct in standard parathyroidectomy, it constitutes the anchor for limited exploration (74,75). The half-life of intact PTH has been calculated to be 3.3 minutes for adenomas and 7.1 minutes after subtotal parathyroidectomy for multiglandular disease (76). The assay can be performed in 15–20 minutes. A drop by 50% in the venous PTH, 10 minutes after excision of an adenoma is considered the measure of success. In multiglandular disease, failure of the PTH assay to fall within 10 minutes is an indication that abnormal tissue remains; some authors advise that a drop of 70% in 10–20 minutes is a preferred benchmark. The assay is also an indicator of success in the treatment of multiglandular disease because if additional abnormal tissue remains, it will not fall within 10 minutes (89). Sensitivity is reported to be 94–97%, with specificity of 100% (77). Al-

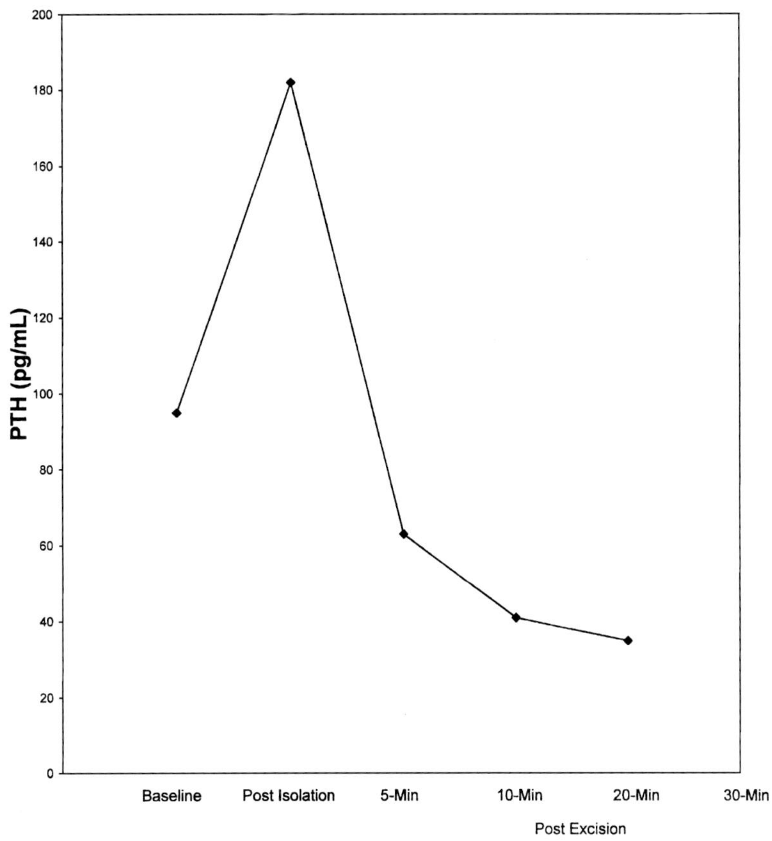

Figure 8 The essential measure of success is a decrease in PTH level by 50% within 10–20 minutes after resection, although some authors use different sampling times. Note that the level of hormone is highest just prior to excision, the result of a surge of hormone released during manipulation of the gland. Serum parathyroid hormone levels during resection of a parathyroid adenoma. (Courtesy of Dr. Edward Diamond, Mount Sinai School of Medicine.)

though some surgeons convert to a bilateral exploration if the PTH does not fall after the first sample, other authors wait for a repeat sample before undertaking this change in procedure (89). At our institution a base sample is taken, another after identification of the parathyroid and just prior to its excision (manipulation sample), followed by samples at 10 and 20 minutes postresection (Fig. 8).

The enduring benefit of this assay is not a smaller skin incision or the saving of operative time; it is the intraoperative confirmation that the hypercalcemia has been corrected. This assurance was not previously possible, even after exhaustive exploration.

The other pillar sustaining limited access surgery is the continuing improvement of localization techniques. Ultrasound, more useful in the neck, and sestamibi scanning, which can sometimes identify mediastinal glands or those in ectopic sites, have a mutual complementary benefit; each has an advantages where the other is weak. They constitute the most useful preoperative workup at this time.

15 BENEFITS OF UNILATERAL SURGERY

Decreased operating time is cited as a benefit of unilateral explorations. It resulted in a mean saving of 23 minutes in operating time as compared to bilateral exploration in a series of 371 patients undergoing surgery for sporadic hyperparathyroidism (69 unilateral, 92 bilateral) (78). Most authors report similar results or better.

These studies do not take into consideration the time spent when local anesthesia has to be converted to general anesthesia or time lost when unilateral procedures have to be converted to bilateral explorations. In this situation operating time is increased; there is a 30-minute wait to find out that the PTH level has not dropped, and then an additional loss of time when abnormal tissue is removed from the opposite side and a repeat assay is performed (89). The fact that unilateral explorations are performed on selected patients contributes substantially to the reduction in operative time.

Local or regional anesthesia in limited access parathyroid surgery is said to improve the postoperative course, reduce postoperative pain, and facilitate early hospital discharge. This is not easy to quantify. Local anesthesia is not new; it was employed by Dr. Felix Mandl in performing the first successful parathyroidectomy on the streetcar conductor Albert Ghane for severe bone disease in Vienna in 1925 (79). It can also be employed for bilateral neck exploration with or without sestamibi scanning; Lo Gerfo reported a series of 236 such patients who underwent bilateral neck explorations for hyperparathyroidism under local anesthesia; the cure rate was 98%, and the average operating time was 43 minutes for patients who had parathyroid procedures alone and 66 minutes in those who had thyroid procedures in addition. One recurrent nerve was excised because of concomitant thyroid cancer; no others were injured. Overall, 70% of patients were discharged within 6 hours (80).

Most unilateral explorations are scheduled as outpatient procedures, in contrast to bilateral exploration patients, who are usually observed overnight, thereby increasing cost. This is a discretionary decision; it is possible to perform many bilateral explorations as outpatient procedures or "23-hour admissions." Indeed, some institutions perform thyroidectomy on an outpatient basis, although the author does not recommend it (81).

Bilateral exploration can be performed through a 4–5 cm incision. Unilateral limited access surgery requires only half this length, although some may require enlargement. A more substantial benefit is that if contralateral reoperation is required later, it can be approached through an undisturbed clean field, removing the hazard of dissecting a recurrent nerve and parathyroid glands whose positions may be distorted by scarring.

Decreased morbidity is sometimes cited as a benefit of unilateral exploration. This is problematic. Persistent vocal cord paralysis occurred in 0.8% of 384 consecutive patients who had bilateral open exploration at the Mayo Clinic (82). Arici and associates report that in 2000 cases they have never observed a recurrent nerve injury in a patient having an initial open parathyroid operation without other procedures (83). Recurrent nerve injuries occur in minimal access explorations (84,85). There are reports of significant numbers of patients explored unilaterally without any incidence of nerve damage, but the fact that these are single side procedures in previously unexplored patients must be considered. It seems unreasonable that the risk for recurrent nerve injury would be less in unilateral limited access surgery than in bilateral open surgery, when the identical operation is performed through a smaller incision with less exposure.

Cost-effectiveness is difficult to evaluate. It depends on the use or omission of preoperative scanning, the use of intraoperative parathormone assays requiring a dedicated machine and technician in the operating room, whether frozen section examinations are employed, and if general or local anesthesia is employed. The greatest saving is from avoiding overnight admissions; this can be duplicated in the bilateral open approach.

16 SURGICAL TECHNIQUE

The surgical approach can be through the midline, retracting or transecting the strap muscles, dividing the middle thyroid vein, and rotating the thyroid medially to expose the parathyroid locations. This method is most suitable for inferior glands.

We prefer a lateral approach that is useful for inferior glands and especially so for superior glands; it is particularly valuable when there is midline scarring from previous neck procedures. The sternomastoid and strap

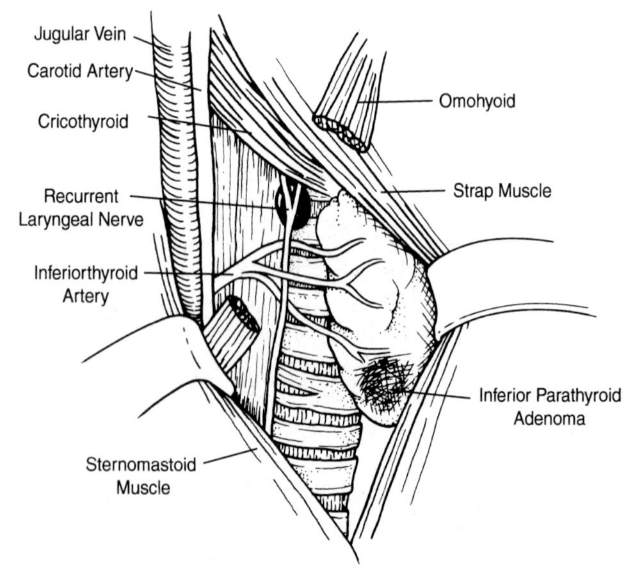

Figure 9 An enlarged inferior parathyroid gland and the presence of a normal superior gland suggest an inferior parathyroid adenoma. Lateral approach to the parathyroid glands.

muscles are retracted in opposite directions. Division of the strap muscles or the omohyoid may help to increase exposure, offering excellent access to the thyroid and the usual locations of the parathyroids (Fig. 9).

17 LIMITATIONS OF MINIMAL ACCESS SURGERY

Results of unilateral parathyroid exploration are restricted by the intrinsic rate of 15% or more of multiglandular disease as well as the limitations of preoperative localization methods. Proye et al., in a review of 918 bilateral neck explorations, reported a 19.7% incidence of multiglandular disease (86). The best noninvasive studies have sensitivities of only 80%, often missing multiglandular disease and ectopic glands (89). Although sestamibi scans can localize up to 90% of adenomas, they cannot be relied upon to identify multiple gland disease or hyperplasia (87). In an effort to extend the envelope of unilateral exploration when preoperative scanning and sonograms are negative, some authors advocate a bilateral jugular fine needle aspiration on the operating table to determine whether there is a step up in hormone level on either side (88). An 85% success rate can theoretically be achieved by unilateral exploration, but these problems make 70% a more reasonable expectation (89).

In 15–30% of cases, unilateral explorations have to be converted into traditional open bilateral explorations because of difficulty in locating adenomas or problems in managing hyperplasia (89). The surgeon who undertakes this approach must be prepared to handle this possibility.

Limited access surgery is an evolving concept. Future development of reliable methods of identifying abnormal parathyroid glands, particularly in multiple gland disease and those beyond the range of cervical incisions, will be the pathway to an expanding use of this method. The combination of ultrasound and 99m sestamibi scanning is the choice of most surgeons at this time.

At present the unilateral approach is most useful for selected cases: single gland disease accurately located preoperatively and conveniently available through a neck incision. When ultrasonography and SPECT-sestamibi scans identify the same solitary parathyroid tumor, the success rate is virtually the same as that of bilateral surgery, justifying a focused approach in such patients (83).

Patients whose localization studies are negative or who demonstrate more than one lesion on preoperative localizations studies, those with parathyroid hyperplasia that is sporadic or related to familial disease or renal failure, and individuals who have coexistent thyroid pathology that may require surgical intervention are best managed by bilateral exploration.

18 ENDOSCOPIC APPROACH

In 1994 Prinz et al. (90) reported the endoscopic removal of mediastinal parathyroid tumors. Four patients with failed neck explorations were found to have mediastinal parathyroid glands on localization studies. Through three ports placed in left intercostal spaces, the glands were successfully removed.

In 1995 Wei et al. (91) reported the successful endoscopic removal of a 1.6 g adenoma in a patient who had three failed neck explorations and later had an anterior mediastinal gland located by Tc99m sestamibi radionuclide scan. Subxiphoid and suprasternal ports were used to dissect the thymus and pleura from the sternum; the heart and great vessels fell posteriorly, the adenoma was removed, and the patient became normocalcemic.

Gagner, who successfully treated a patient with familial hyperplasia in 1996, introduced endoscopic removal of parathyroid glands in the neck (92).

Although the indications for endoscopic parathyroidectomy have yet to been defined, it is hoped that the removal of mediastinal adenomas by mediastinoscopy and endoscopy will become the management of choice, sparing patients a sternal splitting incision.

19 FUTURE OF LIMITED ACCESS SURGERY

New techniques in localization and surgical approach are developing rapidly and are embraced with enthusiasm; further innovations can be expected. Time and experience will be required to evaluate and refine the benefits and limitations of these evolving methods and establish their place in parathyroid surgery (93).

A recent study of 80 patients with primary hyperparathyroidism and a single abnormal parathyroid gland (identified by sestamibi scans or ultrasound), compared bilateral and focal explorations. Although all patients became normocalcemic, those having bilateral explorations had a 15% higher rate of multiple parathyroid tumors, suggesting that some histologically abnormal parathyroid glands do not function or that there may be recurrences in the focal explorations (94).

Other concepts may develop. A new small molecule therapeutic (Cinacalcet), developed by Amgen, is in phase 3 clinical trials. This orally active compound specifically binds and modulates the calcium-sensing receptors on the surface of the parathyroid gland, decreasing secretion of parathormone. If successful, this may alter the approach to hyperparathyroidism, particularly to borderline disease and the hypercalcemia of end-stage renal disease (95).

REFERENCES

1. Cope O. The story of hyperparathyroidism at the Massachusetts General Hospital. N Engl J Med 1966; 274: 1174–1182.
2. Åkerström G, Malmeus J, Bergtröm R. Surgical anatomy of human parathyroid glands. Surgery 1984; 95:14–21.
3. Wang C-A. The anatomic basis of parathyroid surgery. Ann Surg 1976; 183:271–275.
4. Edis AJ, Purnell DC, van Heerden JA. The undescented "parathymus": an occasional cause of failed neck exploration for hyperparathyroidism. Ann Surg 1979; 190:64–68.
5. Albright F. A page out of the history of hyperparathyroidism. J Clin Endocrinol 1948; 8:637–657.
6. Halsted WS. Hypoparathyreosis, status parathyreoprivus, and transplantation of the parathyroid glands. Am J Med Sci 1907; 134:1–12.
7. Åkerström G, Grimelius L, Johansson H, Lundqvist H, Pertoft H, Bergström R. The parenchymal cell mass in normal human parathyroid glands. Acta Pathol Microbiol Immunol Scand (A) 1981; 89:367–375.
8. Ghandur-Mnaymneh L, Cassady J, Hajianpour MA, et al. The parathyroid glands in health and disease. Am J Pathol 1986; 125:292–299.
9. Grimelius L, Åkerström G, Bondeson L, Juhlin C, Johannson H, Ljunghall S, Rastad J. The role of the pathologist in diagnosis and surgical decision making in hyperparathyroidism. World J Surg 1991; 154:698–705.
10. Åkerström G, Bergström R, Grimelius L, Johansson H, Ljunghall S, Lundström B, Palmer M, Rastad J, Rudberg C. Relation between changes in clinical and histopathological features of primary hyperparathyroidism. World J Surg 1986; 10:696–702.
11. Rosenberg CL, Kim HG, Shows TB, et al. Rearrangement and overexpression of D11S287E, a candidate oncogene on chromosome 11q13 in benign parathyroid tumors. Oncogene 1991; 6(3):449–453.
12. Heppner C, Kester MB, Agarwal SK, et al. Somatic mutation of the MEN1 gene in parathyroid tumours. Nat Genet 1997; 16(4):375–378.
13. Purnell DC, Scholz DA, Beahrs OH. Hyperparathyroidism due to single gland enlargement. Arch Surg 1977; 112:369–372.
14. Black WC III, Utley JR. The differential diagnosis of parathyroid adenoma and chief cell hyperplasia. Am J Clin Parthol 1968; 49:761–775.
15. Bonjer HJ, Bruiningg HA, Scholz DA, Purnell DC, Edis AJ, et al. Primary hyperparathyroidism with multiple parathyroid gland enlargement. Review of 53 cases. Mayo Clin Proc 1978; 53:792–797.
16. Scholz DA, Purnell DC, Edis AJ, et al. Primary hyperparathyroidism with multiple parathyroid gland enlargement. Review of 53 cases. Mayo Clin Proc 1978; 53:792–797.
17. Baloch ZW, LiVolsi VA. Double adenoma of parathyroid gland: does the entity exist? Arch Pathol Lab Med 2001; 125(2):178–179.
18. Tezelman S, Shen W, Shaver JK, et al. Double parathyroid adenomas. Clinical and biochemical characteristics before and after parathyroidectomy. Ann Surg 1993; 218:300–309.
19. Ghandur-Mnaymneh L, Kimura N. The parathyroid adenoma. A histopathologic definition with a study of 172 cases of primary hyperparathyroidism. Am J Pathol 1884; 115:70–83.
20. Edis AJ, Beahrs OH, van Heerden JA, Akwari OE. "Conservative" versus "liberal" approach to parathyroid neck exploration. Surgery 1977; 82:466–473.
21. Dufour DR, Wilkerson SY. The normal parathyroid revisited: percentage of stromal fat. Human Pathol 1982; 13:717–721.
22. Roth SI, Gallagher MJ. The rapid identification of "normal" parathyroid glands by the presence of intracellular fat. Am J Pathol 1976; 84:521–528.
23. Bonjer HJ, Bruining HA, Birkenhager JC, et al. Single and multigland disease in primary hyperparathyroidism: clinical follow-up, histopathology, and flow cytometric DNA analysis. World J Surg 1992; 16:737–744.
24. Nishiyama RH. The intraoperative diagnosis of parathyroid lesions. Acta Chir Aust 1994; 112:8.
25. Nussbaum SR, Zahradnik RJ, Lavigne JR, et al. Highly sensitve two-site immunoradiometric assay of parathyrin, and its clinical utility in evaluating patients with hypercalcemia. Clin Chem 1987; 33:1364–1367.
26. Marx SJ, Spiegel AM, Levine MA, et al. Familial hypocalciuric hypercalcemia: the relation to primary parathyroid hyperplasia. N Engl J Med 1982; 307:416–426.
27. Scholtz DA, Purnell DC. Asymptomatic primary hyperparathyroidism: 10 year prospective study. Mayo Clin Proc 1981; 56:473–478.
28. Joborn C, Hetta J, Rastad J, Agren H, Åkerström G, Ljunghall S. Psychiatric symptoms and cerebrospinal fluid monoamine metabolites in primary hyperparathyroidism. Biol Psychiatry 1988; 23:149–158.
29. Shen W, Düren M, Morita E, Higgins C, Duh Q-Y, Siperstein A, Clark O. Reoperation for persistent or recurrent primary hyperparathyroidism. Arch Surg 1996; 131:861–869.

30. Chan AK, Duh QY, Katz MH, et al. J Clinical manifestations of primary hyperparathyroidism before and after parathyroidectomy: a case-control study. Ann Surg 1995; 222:402–412.
31. Eigelberger MS, Clark OH. Surgical approach to primary hyperparathyroidism. Endocrinol Metab Clin North Am 2000; 29:479–502.
32. Clark OH, Wilkes W, et al. Diagnosis and management of asymptomatic hyperparathyroidism: safety, efficacy, and deficiencies in our knowledge. J Bone Miner Res 1991; 6(suppl):135–142.
33. Silverberg S, Locker F, Bilezikian J. Vertebral osteopenia, a new indication for surgery in primary hyperparathyroidism. J Clin Endocrin Metab 1996; 81:4007–4012.
34. Palmer M, Adami H-O, Bergström R, et al. Survival and renal function in persons with untreated hypercalcemia: a population-based cohort study with 14 years of follow-up. Lancet 1987; 1:59–62.
35. Hedback G, Oden A, Tisell LE. The influence of surgery on the risk of death in patients with primary hyperparathyroidism. World J Surg 1991; 15:399–405.
36. Edis AJ. Hyperparathyroidsm: what does surgery have to offer? Med J Austr 1998; 168:148–149.
37. Van Heerden JA, Farley DR. Parathyroid. In: Schwartz SI, ed. Textbook of Surgery. New York: McGraw-Hill, 1999: 1694–1713.
38. Mitchell BK, Merrell RC, Kinder BK. Localization studies in patients with hyperparathyroidism. Surg Clin North Am 1995; 75:3,483–498.
39. Clark OH. Surgical treatment of primary hyperparathyroidism. Adv Endocrinol Metab 1995; 6:1–16.
40. NIH Conference. Diagnosis and management of asymptomatic primary hyperparathyroidism: consensus development conference statement. Ann Intern Med 1991; 114:593–597.
41. Kohri K, Ishikawa Y, Kodama S, et al. Comparison of imaging methods for localization of parathyroid tumors Am J Surg 1992; 164:140–145.
42. Jaskowiak NT, Sugg SL, Helke J, et al. Pitfalls of intraoperative quick parathyroid hormone monitoring and gamma probe localization in surgery for primary hyperparathyroidism. Arch Surg. 2002; 137:659–669.
43. Numerow LM, Morita ET, Clark OH, Higgins CB, et al. Persistent/recurrent hyperparathyroidism: a comparison of sestamibi scintigraphy, MRI, and ultrasonography. J Magn Reson Imaging 1995; 5:702–708.
44. Rodriguez JM, Tezelman S, Siperstein AE, et al. Localization procedures in patients with persistent or recurrent hyperparathyroidism. Arch Surg 1994; 129:870–875.
45. Wright AR, Goddard PR, Nicholson S, et al. Fat suppression magnetic resonance imaging in the preoperative localization of parathyroid adenomas. Clin Radiol 1992; 46:324–328.
46. Sofferman RA, Nathan MH, Fairbank JT, et al. Preoperative technetium Tc 99m sestamibi imaging: paving the way to minimal-access parathyroid surgery. Arch Otolaryngol Head Neck Surg 1996; 122:369–374.
47. Westrich R, Brandwein M, Bergman D, Mechanick J, Urken M. Preoperative parathyroid localization: correlating false negative technetium 99m sestamibi scans with parathyroid disease. Laryngoscope 2003; 113(3): 564–572.
48. Doppman JL, Krudy AG, Marx SJ, et al. Aspiration of enlarged parathyroid glands for parathyroid hormone assay. Radiology 1983; 148:31–35.
49. Miller DL. Preoperative localization and interventional treatment of parathyroid tumors: when and how? World J Surg 1991; 15:706–715.
50. Doherty GM, Doppman JL, Miller DL, et al. Results of a multidisciplinary strategy for management of mediastinal parathyroid adenoma as a cause of persistent primary hyperparathyroidism. Ann Surg 1992; 215:101–106.
51. Edis A. Invited commentary. World J Surg 1986; 10: 694.
52. Hellman P, Åkerström G, Ljunghall S, Rastad J. Surgical findings and results of subtotal and total parathyroidectomy in hypercalcemic patients with uremic hyperparathyroidism. Acta Chir Scand 1989; 155:573–582.
53. Baker LR, Oteino LS, Brown AL, et al. Pitfalls after total parathyroidectomy and parathyroid autotransplantation in chronic renal failure. Am J Nephrol 1991; 11:186–191.
54. Clark OH, Hunt TK, Way LW. Recurrent hyperparathyroidism. Ann Surg 1976; 184:391–402.
55. Huang S-M. Familial hyperparathyroidism. In: Clark OH, Duh Q-Y, eds. Textbook of Endocrine Surgery. Philadelphia: WB Saunders, 1997: 385–393.
56. Wells SA, Stirman JA, Bolman RM. Parathyroid transplantation. World J Surg 1977; 6:747–756.
57. Saxe AW, Brennan MF. Reoperative parathyroid surgery for primary; hyperparathyroidism caused by multiple-gland disease: total parathyroidectomy and autotransplantation with cryopreserved tissue. Surgery 1982; 91:616–621.
58. Feldman AL, Sharaf RN, Scarulis MC, et al. Results of heterotopic parathyroid autotransplantation: a 13-year experience. Surgery 1999; 126:1042–1048.
59. Goretzki PE, Dotzenrath C, Roeher HD. Management of primary hyperparathyroidism caused by multiple gland disease. World J Surg 1991; 15:693–697.
60. Saxe A, Spiegel AM, Marx SJ, et al. Deferred parathyroid autografts with cryopreserved tissue after reoperative surgery. Arch Surg 1982; 117:538–543.
61. Wells SA, Frandon JR, Dale JK, et al. Long term evaluation of patients with primary parathyroid hyperplasia managed by total parathyroidectomy heterotopic autotransplantation. Ann Surg 1980; 192:451–458.
62. Kraimps JL, Barbier J. Familial hyperparathyroidism

in multiple endocrine neoplasia syndromes. In: Clark OH, Duh, eds. Textbook of Endocrine Surgery. Philadelphia: WB Saunders, 1997: 381–384.
63. Niederle B. The technique of parathyroid cryopreservation and the results of delayed autotransplantation—a review. Acta Chir Austriaca 1996; 124:68–71.
64. Saxe AW, Baier R, Tesluk H, et al. The role of the pathologist in the surgical treatment of hyperparathyroidism. Surg Gynecol Obstet 1985; 161:101–105.
65. Edis AJ, Beahrs OH, van Heerden JK, Akwari OE. "Conservative" versus "liberal" approach to parathyroid neck exploration. Surgery 1977; 82:466–473.
66. Halsted WS, Evans HM. The parathyroid glandules: their blood supply and their preservation in operation upon the thyroid gland. Ann Surg 1907; 46:489–506.
67. Shen W, Düren M, Morita E, Higgins C, Duh Q-Y, Siperstein A, Clark O. Reoperation for persistent or recurrent primary hyperparathyroidism. Arch Surg 1996; 131:861–869.
68. Brennan MF, Doppman JL, Marx SJ, et al. Reoperative parathyroid surgery for persistent hyperparathyroidism. Surgery 1978; 83:669–776.
69. Carty SE, Norton JA. Management of patients with persistent or recurrent primary hyperparathyroidism. World J Surg 1991; 15:716–723.
70. van Heerden JA, Grant CS. Surgical treatment of primary hyperparathyroidism: an institutional perspective. World J Surg 1991; 15:688–692.
71. Moore FD Jr. Oral calcium supplements to enhance early hospital discharge after bilateral thyroid surgery or parathyroid exploration. J Am Coll Surg 1994; 178:11–16.
72. Habener JF, Potts JT Jr. Parathyroid physiology and primary hyperparathyroidism. In: Avoli LV, Krane SM, eds. Metabolic Bone Disease. Philadelphia: Saunders, 1990: 475–575.
73. Patow CA, Norton JA, Brennan MF. Vocal cord paralysis and reoperative parathyroidectomy. A prospective study. Ann Surg 1986; 203:282–285.
74. Nussbaum SR, Thompson AR, Hutcheson KA, Gaz RD, Wang C. Intraoperative measurement of parathyroid hormone in the surgical management of hyperparathyroidism. Surgery 1988; 104:1121–1127.
75. Irvin GL, Dembrow VD, Prudhomme DL. Clinical usefulness of an intraoperative "quick parathyroid hormone" assay. Surgery 1993; 114:1019–1023.
76. Davies C, Demeure MJ, St.John A, et al. Study of intact (1–84) parathyroid hormone secretion in patients undergoing parathyroidectomy. World J Surg 1990; 14:355–359.
77. Eigelberger MS, Clark OH. Surgical approach to primary hyperparathyroidism. Endocrinol Metab Clin North Amer 2000; 29:479–502.
78. Worsey MJ, Carty SE, Watson CG. Success of unilateral exploration for sporadic primary hyperparathyroidism. Surgery 1993; 114:1024–1030.
79. Mandl F. Attempt to treat generalized fibrous osteitis by extirpation of parathyroid tumor. Zentralbl F Chir 1926; 53:260–264.
80. Lo Gerfo P. Bilateral neck exploration for parathyroidectomy under local anesthesia: a viable technique for patients with coexisting thyroid disease with or without sestamibi scanning. Surgery 1999; 126:1011–1015.
81. Schwartz AE, Clark OH, Ituarte P, Lo Gerfo P. Therapeutic controversy, thyroid surgery—the choice. J Clin Endocrinol Metab 1998; 83:1097–1105.
82. van Heerden JA, Grant CS. Surgical treatment of primary hyperparathyroidism: an institutional perspective. World J Surg 1991; 15:688–692.
83. Arici C, Cheah WK, Ituarte PH, Morita E, Lynch TC, Siperstein AE, Duh Q-Y, Clark OH. Can localization studies be used to direct focused parathyroid operations?. Surgery 2001; 129:720–729.
84. Gauger PG, Reeve TS, Delbridge LW. Endoscopically-assisted minimally-invasive parathyroidectomy. Br J Surg 1999; 86:1566–1583.
85. Chaffanjon CJ, Brichon P-Y, Sarrazin R. Bilateral oblique approach to parathyroid glands. Ann Surg 2000; 231:25–30.
86. Proye C, Carnaille FB, Bizard JP, et al. Multiglandular disease in seemingly sporadic primary hyperparathyroidism revisited; where are we in the early 1990's? A plea against unilateral parathyroid exploration. Surgery 1992; 112:1118–1122.
87. Shen W, Sabanci U, Morita ET, Siperstein AE, Duh YU, Clark OH. Sestamibi scanning is inadequate for directing unilateral neck exploration for first time parathyroidectomy. Arch Surg 1997; 132:969–976.
88. Irvin GL III, Carnerio DM. "Limited" parathyroidectomy in geriatric patients. Ann Surg 2001; 233(5):612–616.
89. Moore FD, Mannting F, Tanasijevic M. Intrinsic limitations to unilateral parathyroid exploration. Ann Surg 1999; 230:382–391.
90. Prinz RA, Lonchyna V, Carnaille B, et al. Thoracoscopic excision of enlarged mediastinal parathyroid glands. Surgery 1994; 116:999–1004.
91. Wei JP, Gadacz TR, Weisner LF, et al. The subxiphoid laparoscopic approach for resection of mediastinal parathyroid adenoma after successful localization with Tc99m sestamibi radionuclide scan. Surg Laparosc Endosc 1995; 5:402–406.
92. Gagner M. Endoscopic subtotal parathyroidectomy in patients with primary hyperparathyroidism (lett). Br J Surg 1996; 83:875.
93. Wang C-A. Parathyroid re-exploration. A clinical and pathological study of 112 cases. Ann Surg 1977; 186:140–145.
94. Hudai G, Morita E, Ferrier ND, et al. Differing histologic findings after bilateral and focused parathyroidectomy. 2003; 196:535–540.
95. Nemeth EF. The search for calcium receptor antagonists (calcilytics). J Mol Endocrinol 2002; 29(1):15–21.

20

Reoperation for Primary Hyperparathyroidism

Daniel F. Roses

New York University School of Medicine and New York University Medical Center, New York, New York, U.S.A.

1 INTRODUCTION

The truism that the best opportunity to cure a patient with a surgical disease is at the initial operation is particularly self-evident in the treatment of primary hyperparathyroidism. The initial operative procedure in experienced hands is successful in at least 95% of cases and is associated with negligible potential morbidity and the great satisfaction of knowing that surgical cure will persist in the vast majority of instances (1). Reoperative surgery following a failed initial operation, or for recurrence following a more prolonged period of normocalcemia, presents far more formidable challenges for the surgeon. Indeed, the first patient treated surgically in the United States, Captain Charles Martell, a sea captain in the merchant marines with severe debilitating skeletal sequelae from primary hyperparathyroidism, had six unsuccessful cervical procedures that included excision of two normal parathyroid glands in search of a parathyroid adenoma beginning in 1926 (2). Finally, at the captain's urging, a sternotomy in 1933 allowed the successful identification of a mediastinal parathyroid adenoma.

The initial operation for primary hyperparathyroidism in the previously unoperated neck is performed through normal anatomical planes. In recent years efforts have been made to even further minimize the dissection and expedite the surgery through a variety of adjunctive preoperative and intraoperative measures. Advocates of such approaches employing preoperative scintigraphy, intraoperative gamma probe–guided surgery, and rapid parathormone assays emphasize the reduction in size of incisions and surgical fields, and the use of regional-local anesthesia with the patient often treated on an ambulatory basis. This certainly contrasts with more extensive reoperative procedures through expanding surgical fields, often following more extensive preoperative localization, in efforts to optimize the chance of success and minimize the greater potential morbidity. These technical challenges, increased logistical considerations and expense, and the greater risk of failure make it imperative that the first operation be performed with as much attention as possible to optimizing the chance of success. It must be appreciated however, that any attempt to limit the extent and expense of the primary procedure will be insignificant if there is persistent or recurrent disease and a subsequent, more challenging procedure is required. Even with the appropriate recognition of the importance of a successful initial surgical procedure, failures or recurrences will continue to occur as the frequency of diagnosing and surgically treating primary hyperparathyroidism increases.

2 REASONS FOR PERSISTENT OR RECURRENT PRIMARY HYPER-PARATHYROIDISM FOLLOWING SURGICAL TREATMENT

The distinction between persistent or recurrent hyperparathyroidism is not always clear. Unless the diagnosis of primary hyperparathyroidism is in error, persistent hypercalcemia must be viewed as a failure of primary surgery (3,4). Recurrence of hypercalcemia after a period of normocalcemia, often defined as 6 months or longer, is less clearly a result of failure of the initial operation than is persistent hypercalcemia (5,6). In some instances a period of normocalcemia may in fact mask persistent hyperparathyroidism due to postoperative ischemic changes being superimposed on retained abnormal parathyroid tissue. This may occur even after a pathological gland has been removed and the patient presumably cured as a result of ischemia to retained multiglandular disease. Nevertheless, persistent hypercalcemia is the most common presentation following failure of the initial procedure. The causes are more varied than those instances of recurrent hyperparathyroidism where abnormal parathyroid tissue has been removed, but after a period of time additional hyperplastic tissue may proliferate and lead to the further clinical and biochemical manifestations of excess parathyroid hormone production. A review of the potential causes for persistent or recurrent hypercalcemia is therefore essential in planning a reoperative surgical approach. The causes are listed in Table 1.

Inappropriate surgery because of an incorrect diagnosis of primary hyperparathyroidism should be eliminated by the increasing specificity of immunoradiometric assays of intact parathyroid hormone. Hypercalcemia due to other diseases (sarcoidosis, multiple myeloma, skeletal metastases, and paraneoplastic syndromes) as well as medications (hypervitaminosis D, thiazide diuretics, lithium) should not only be readily apparent by clinical criteria but certainly distinguishable by double antibody assays (7). These assays should also enable the accurate diagnosis of primary hyperparathyroidism in those rare instances when it coexists with other pathologic and therapeutic entities that cause hypercalcemia.

Benign familial hypocalciuric hypercalcemia is a rare disease that may present a legitimate diagnostic dilemma (8). The hypercalcemia is frequently seen early in life, and the disease is characterized by both hypercalcemia and hypocalciuria. While the parathyroid hormone level is usually normal, it has been reported as being elevated in several instances, leading to obvious confusion with primary hyperparathyroidism. When surgical failure for hyperparathyroidism results, this rare condition should be considered if family screening reveals other members with hypercalcemia, as the disease is an autosomal dominant disorder with a high degree of penetrance (9). If suspected, it should be carefully sought, as reoperation will obviously again be met with failure.

3 INDICATIONS FOR TREATMENT OF PERSISTENT OR RECURRENT PRIMARY HYPERPARATHYROIDISM

The challenges of reoperative parathyroid surgery make the need for establishing clear indications for embarking on another attempt particularly important. What might be a clear indication for initial surgery might be viewed as less compelling in the reoperative setting. In general, indications for reoperative surgery should be the same as for the initial operation, particularly if an analysis of the prior procedure, as well as localizing efforts, indicate a high possibility of success. However, borderline or mild hypercalcemia in a patient with no clear signs and symptoms following an ordered, extensive, and competent effort at initial surgery make the indications for surgery less secure, and surveillance may be more prudent. Indications for surgery that may have been a

Table 1 Reasons for Persistent or Recurrent Hypercalcemia Following Surgery for Primary Hyperparathyroidism

1. Diagnostic error leading to inappropriate surgery
2. Inexperience of the surgeon as evidenced by the the presence of an abnormal parathyroid gland or glands in predictable normal locations at reoperation
3. Failure to recognize multiple or supernumerary gland disease
4. Failure to identify ectopically located abnormal parathyroid glands
5. Failure to recognize the potential pitfalls of localization procedures, as well as intraoperative parathyroid hormone assays and frozen sections leading to inadequate reduction of abnormal parathyroid tissue
6. Scattering and retention of abnormal parathyroid tissue leading to parathyromatosis or recurrent growth of malignant parathyroid tissue following resection of parathyroid carcinoma

source of controversy before the primary operative treatment become even more so before a reoperative procedure. Morbidity that may have resulted from the initial procedure, such as recurrent laryngeal nerve injury and vocal cord paralysis, or the histologically confirmed ablation of remaining normal parathyroid glands, thereby raising the risk of permanent hypoparathyroidism, as well as medical comorbidities that present an anesthesia risk, may make the need for reoperation less compelling unless the biochemical and clinical indications are significant.

In the early period following an initial failed exploration, a trial of observation may be appropriate to allow any devascularization or transient ischemia to hypercellular parathyroid tissue to reverse or alternatively to determine whether it fails to revascularize, thereby resulting in a persistent state of normocalcemia (10). Furthermore, reassessment of the extent of hyperparathyroidism biochemically after several months can better enable the indications for reoperation to be assessed and provide a more reliable baseline if performed. While indications for the primary surgical treatment of hyperparathyroidism may be quite liberal for patients without overt clinical manifestations, several investigators have endorsed the monitoring of patients not meeting criteria that include calcium levels of 11.5 mg/dL or greater and reduced cortical bone density to demonstrate if there is stability of mild hypercalcemia and a benign clinical course over prolonged periods of observation (11). These considerations must also be evaluated along with an assessment of the thoroughness of the initial surgical procedure and whether attempts at localization yield positive findings before arriving at a decision for reoperation. Furthermore, an overzealous initial failed procedure, in which multiple normal parathyroid glands were excised or devascularized, may position the surgeon of the reoperative procedure to render a patient permanently hypoparathyroid if the offending single adenoma is successfully ablated.

4 ASSESSING THE INITIAL OPERATION

The success of the initial procedure may reflect the inexperience of the surgeon if a single adenoma was not found in a normal location. Inexperience may also be reflected by a failure to systematically map normal glands in normal locations in an effort to direct the initial exploration to the potential ectopic site of a single adenoma. However, despite efforts at preoperative localization prior to the primary surgical procedure, failures may occur even in experienced hands due to both a failure to detect abnormal glands in ectopic sites at the initial procedure, despite an ordered search, and the inadequacies of available localizing techniques to detect ectopic or multiglandular disease, as discussed in prior chapters. The common ectopic locations have been well described and documented. They are more common in the neck, particularly if one includes the upper mediastinum accessible from a cervical approach, than they are in thoracic locations that require a thoracic surgical approach. The most common sites of abnormal glands at reoperation in numerous reported series vary, but a majority of ectopic locations have been confirmed to be in the neck, particularly if the thymus, accessible from a cervical approach, is included. In addition to the thymic tongue, the cervical locations include the para- and retrotracheal and para- and retroesophageal spaces, subcapsular and intrathyroidal sites, sites within the carotid sheath, and those above the thyroid lobe, including those resulting from failure of descent of a parathyroid gland from its point of embryological origin. Mediastinal sites account for less than half of ectopically located glands with distributions in most series equally divided between anterior and superior-posterior locations (12–17).

The most common cause of a failed primary procedure after the undetected single adenoma is the inadequate appreciation and identification of multiglandular disease in patients with sporadic hyperparathyroidism as well as in those with familial disease and multiple endocrine neoplasias (18–22). Even with the identification of all parathyroid glands at surgery, asymmetrical enlargements may mislead the surgeon into presuming that the largest gland is the unifocal source of hyperparathyroidism. Slightly enlarged glands, however, even if smaller than a significantly enlarged one, may also be responsible for contributing to the patient's hyperparathyroidism and, if not ablated, may result in surgical failure. We reported on four patients with marked asymmetry of two enlarged glands in which failure to excise the smaller gland led to persistent or recurrent hyperparathyroidism cured by excision of the initially retained, slightly enlarged gland at reoperation (20). Double adenomas have been documented and are not uncommonly diagnosed at reoperation following the initial excision of a presumed single adenoma (23). Certainly the inadequacy of localizing procedures to identify multiglandular disease is well recognized, and this can further mislead the primary surgeon (17,22–25). The intraoperative quick parathyroid hormone assay may compensate for this by indicating that an enlarged gland, when excised, fails to result in a significant enough reduction in parathyroid hormone levels (generally > 50%) from baseline values. Four-gland hyperplasia as well may present with significant asymmetry leading to inadequate extirpation of hypercellular tissue. This may be particularly true in multiple endocrine neoplasia (MEN) patients and those with familial hyperparathyroidism (18). Another cause of failure may be the dispersion of parathyroid tissue at initial surgery leading to parathyromatosis, the hyperplastic implanted fragments becoming vascularized and viable in the initial surgical field (26). In addition, local recurrence is common with parathyroid carcinoma, leading to recurrent hyperparathyroidism (27). Furthermore, a rare hypercellular supernumerary gland may be the cause of persistent or recurrent hyperparathyroidism (28), even with thorough identification of four parathyroid glands and excision of a presumed single adenoma, as reported by the author (20) and by Harness and associates (19) in a review of patients with multiple adenomas.

Presently limited explorations augmented by either technetium 99m–sestamibi scintigraphy and guided gamma probe–directed dissections, as well as intraoperative quick parathyroid hormone assay monitoring to confirm the adequacy of resection, have replaced the more traditional bilateral exploration to identify all cervical parathyroid tissue in many centers. Conversely, in the face of multiglandular disease, bilateral exploration including the thymic tongue to detect supernumerary glands is advisable. An appreciation of the various pitfalls of primary surgery is therefore essential for a surgeon assessing a patient for reoperation. If the reoperative surgeon performed the initial unsuccessful procedure, these considerations can be evaluated more clearly than by the surgeon who is called upon to assess the first procedure that he or she did not perform. In such instances the surgeon most often has to rely on the description of the procedure as detailed in the operative report and by available pathology reports and slides. If no abnormal parathyroid tissue was removed, then a critical assessment of the adequacy of the initial procedure, paying attention to the usual locations of parathyroid tissue as well as any ectopic sites, must be evaluated. If a single large parathyroid gland was histologically confirmed to be hypercellular and consistent with an adenoma, then consideration must focus on the possibility that multiglandular disease was underappreciated (29). Here, too, a careful review of the extent of exploration, as well as any additional measures that were taken to augment the procedure, must be considered. Likewise, if parathyroid tissue was excised but not histologically hypercellular on subsequent review, then the responsible parathyroid gland or glands have been overlooked.

Questions that must be asked by the surgeon evaluating the patient with persistent or recurrent hyperparathyroidism vary depending on the circumstances, but most often include the following: Were all parathyroid glands identified? If no abnormal parathyroid gland was excised, how many normal glands were identified, and where were they located? If an abnormal gland was not identified, were all ectopic sites searched, including the intrathymic, retroesophageal, carotid sheath, intrathyroidal, and suprathyroid locations? It must be appreciated, however, that the reported identification of normal parathyroid glands may not be reliable and their misidentification attributable to lymph nodes or stained fat globules. Perhaps more importantly, if persistent or recurrent disease follows what is reportedly the removal of abnormal parathyroid tissue, the histology should be reviewed to optimally confirm if indeed the tissue removed was parathyroid and, if so, whether it was hypercellular or even malignant. Finally, a decision must be made as to the appropriateness and extent of localizing procedures. This may be a particularly important component of the fundamental decision regarding surgery and the subsequent surgical approach. Even without a clear decision as to the appropriateness of reoperative surgery, and faced with an understandable unwillingness of the patient to undergo a second attempt at surgical treatment after a failed initial attempt, successful localization may provide an appropriate incentive for the patient and a more confident strategy for the surgeon. Even if surgery is not pursued, non-operative attempts at parathyroid ablation may be pursued in selected cases if localization is successful. Most importantly, localization, if successful, can indicate whether the pathology should be sought in the neck or the mediastinum. If localization is to a cervical location, it can further direct the surgeon to the most expeditious approach through what may have been a previously explored and potentially scarred surgical field.

5 LOCALIZATION FOLLOWING FAILED INITIAL SURGERY

Traditional surgical doctrine tended to discount the value of preoperative localization for primary surgical procedures. Refinements in localizing techniques and recent interest in more limited approaches to surgery have led to a reassessment of the value of localization. When faced with the prospect of reoperation, however, there is a consensus that efforts at localization are clearly indicated (10,13,14,30–32). The presence of scar in the operative field from prior surgery, often a procedure that was more extensive and prolonged due to failure to locate the offending pathology, makes the ability to preoperatively localize the site of possible abnormal parathyroid tissue self-recommending. Furthermore, successful preoperative localization of an intrathoracic parathyroid adenoma is obviously invaluable. If successful, localization can help the surgeon navigate through difficult and scarred tissue planes, which may further decrease the risk of morbidity. Localization studies may also assist in indicating the potential for intraoperative adjuncts to surgery, including ultrasonography- and gamma probe–directed procedures, and may even offer the opportunity to use nonoperative approaches at parathyroid ablation. The available techniques include technetium 99m–sestamibi scanning, ultrasonography, magnetic resonance imaging (MRI), computed tomography (CT) scanning, selective venous catheterization for intact parathyroid hormone, and angiography.

6 NONINVASIVE LOCALIZING STUDIES

6.1 Technetium 99m–Sestamibi Scanning

Technetium 99m–sestamibi scintigraphy with single photon emission computed tomography (SPECT) imaging has emerged as the localizing procedure with the greatest sensitivity and specificity in the preoperative evaluation of the primary surgical procedure (33,34). However, there are pitfalls in the overutilization of this modality, most commonly due to false-negative studies in patients with multiple gland disease and false-positive studies in patients with nodular thyroid disease (17,24). In the reoperative setting a positive sestamibi scan, particularly if corroborated with sonography, and in conjunction with additional information from the primary procedure, may be of great usefulness in localizing the source of persistent or recurrent hyperparathyroidism. In addition, a positive scan offers the opportunity to utilize a gamma probe for intraoperative localization, an adjunct to surgery that may be particularly helpful in a scarred surgical field where the opportunities for dissection along traditional surgical planes may be limited (35). Certainly an advantage of technetium 99m–sestamibi scanning with SPECT imaging as reported from its use in primary procedures is the ability to image both anterior and lateral views, which may be particularly helpful in planning the operative approach (36–38). Technetium 99m–sestamibi scintigraphy also provides the possibility of identifying ectopic mediastinal tumors (15,33,39). In a report by Thompson and associates (17) on its efficacy in the reoperative setting, sensitivity and accuracy rates were reported as 82% and 67%, respectively, with higher doses of the radionuclide in the later cases increasing the sensitivity to 90%. Shen and associates (15) reported a sensitivity of 77% and, importantly, found it equally accurate for both tumors in normal as well as ectopic sites.

6.2 Ultrasonography

High-resolution (10 MHz) real-time ultrasonography represents the second common modality for preoperative localization and is complimentary to technetium 99m–sestamibi scintigraphy, corroborating positive studies, and often detecting missed, enlarged cervical parathyroid glands. It may also lead to the suspicion of an intrathyroidal parathyroid adenoma if a dominant finding is present in an otherwise normal thyroid gland, particularly with positive uptake on the sestamibi study (40–42). Thompson and associates (17) reported an accuracy rate of 65% and a sensitivity of 75% for ultrasonography in the reoperative setting. Shen and associates (15) reported a sensitivity of 57% in the reoperative setting, confirming the accuracy of ultrasonography for identifying enlarged glands adjacent to or within the thyroid as well as its limitations for ectopic and mediastinal lesions. Ultrasonography has particular utility within the soft tissues of the neck but is limited in its ability to detect parathyroid abnormalities behind the air-filled trachea, particularly in the retroesophageal midline location overlying the vertebra, and near or behind the upper sternum or clavicles (14,43–45). When there is concordance between the technetium 99m–sestamibi scan and the sonogram, there is a greater confidence in an accurate and precise localization of a missed abnormal parathyroid gland (14). Some investigators have advocated fine needle aspiration by sonographic guidance to confirm a preoperative diagnosis. The aspirate can be used for confirmatory cytology or for a bioassay for parathyroid hormone (PTH) (17,46–48).

6.3 Magnetic Resonance Imaging

MRI, like CT scanning, is most often reserved as a second echelon localizing procedure when technetium 99m–sestamibi scintigraphy and ultrasonography fail to identify an abnormal parathyroid gland or glands or when there is discordance between those studies (14,49,50) A positive sestamibi scan with increased uptake in locations where the accuracy of ultrasonography is limited, such as behind the trachea or close to bony structures, if corroborated with MRI, may provide greater confidence for a focused procedure that corroboration by ultrasonography might ordinarily provide in other locations. In the report of Shen and associates (15) on 23 patients having reoperative surgery for whom sestamibi scanning, ultrasonography, and MRI were utilized, all abnormal glands were identified in 87% of cases, leading to the recommendation that all three studies be used in evaluation prior to reoperative surgery.

6.4 Computed Tomography

CT scans, like MRI, are most often utilized when scintigraphy and ultrasonography fail to demonstrate an abnormal parathyroid gland, or where scintigraphy alone has been positive and the accuracy of sonography is compromised. The accuracy of the CT scan is comparable to that of MRI, but MRI has achieved a position of preference over CT scanning because of the lower rate of false-positive results reported in most series and a greater ability to image the infrathyroid region due to the shoulder artifact that may often be present with CT scanning (10,25,49).

7 INVASIVE LOCALIZING PROCEDURES

When technetium 99m–sestamibi scintigraphy, ultrasonography, MRI, and/or CT scanning fail to identify any abnormal parathyroid gland, or when the results of the localizing procedures are equivocal or discordant, more aggressive radiological localization attempts are justified. The differential diagnostic considerations for the surgeon remain even more compelling in the reoperative setting when noninvasive attempts at localization associated with sensitivity rates exceeding 50% have failed. These diagnostic issues remain not only single versus multiple gland disease, an ectopic versus a normal anatomical site or sites for the abnormal gland or glands, supernumerary gland disease, right versus left neck for single gland cervical disease, a cervical versus an intrathoracic location, but, perhaps most significantly, whether reoperative surgery is indicated when the chance of success is compromised or extensive dissection required. This last consideration hinges as well on a review of the previous procedure, as will be discussed, but can obviously be influenced significantly by a predictive localizing procedure. The two invasive radiological techniques are angiography and selective venous sampling for intact PTH.

It is reasonable to initiate the invasive radiological work-up with selective angiography of the vessels of the neck and mediastinum. Angiography is capable of demonstrating a vascular blush that is ovoid or spherical consistent with an adenoma (Fig. 1), but even in the absence of a definite parathyroid enlargement, abnormal venous drainage patterns can be appreciated on delayed angiographic views, particularly in the previously explored neck, that result in shifts or distortion of venous anatomy (25,50–56). Defining such changes can assist the radiologist in sampling venous drainage sites and identifying their specific locations. Angiographic examination includes selective catheterization of the thyrocervical trunks for glands in lower cervical sites, the carotid arteries and superior thyroid arteries for upper cervical sites, and the internal mammary arteries for thymic and anterior mediastinal sites. Accuracy rates of 60% have been reported, but the experiences in the reoperative setting are limited and highly selected (57).

Venous catheterization is performed through a femoral vein with sampling of the superior, middle, and inferior thyroid veins when present, and the internal jugular vein, which is of particular importance when smaller venous drainage sites have been disrupted by prior surgery. The thymic and vertebral veins, if possible, are sampled as well. Intact PTH assays are obtained

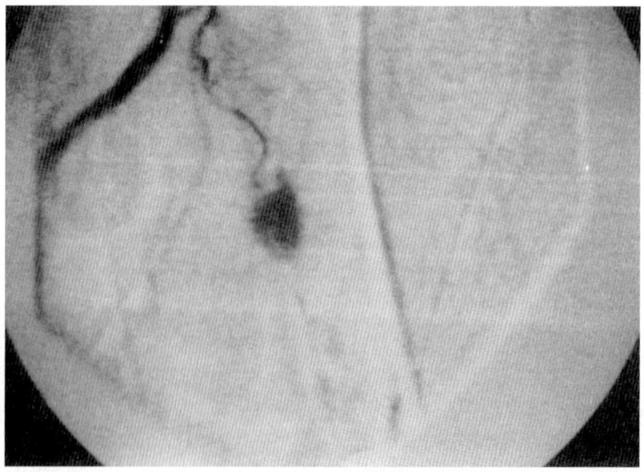

Figure 1 Selective angiogram of the left internal mammary (lateral view) demonstrating a hypervascular mass from a branch off the left internal mammary artery in a 37-year-old man with persistent hypercalcemia following excision of a cervical parathyroid adenoma and histological confirmation of three additional normal parathyroid glands. A median sternotomy revealed a second parathyroid adenoma in a supernumerary gland. Excision resulted in normocalcemia that has persisted for over 10 years following resection.

and then compared to a baseline value established from a femoral vein sample, and any gradients determined as they relate to the neck versus the chest or the right versus the left neck along with any greater degree of anatomic specificity that can be suggested. For example, an upper versus a lower neck gradient might be suggestive of an undescended parathyroid adenoma. In series of selected patients, selective (14,15,25,58,59) venous catheterization has shown variable success rates. A series of 86 patients from the National Insititutes of Health (NIH) having selective venous catheterization prior to surgery, as reported by Sugg and associates (56), demonstrated a sensitivity of 88%.

8 NONOPERATIVE APPROACHES TO PERSISTENT OR RECURRENT HYPERTHYROIDISM

The patient with a clearly localized single adenoma, particularly in the mediastinum, is faced with the choice of whether to have surgery to extirpate the gland or an attempt at nonoperative ablation. For most patients, the decision favors surgery. Surgical extirpation is definitive, histologically confirmed, and provides tissue for cryopreservation and autotransplantation in selected instances. However, in the high-risk patient with significant medical comorbidities, or in those unwilling to have reoperative surgery after failed attempts, two nonoperative techniques are available: embolization of an angiographically defined adenoma or alcohol injection of a sonographically defined adenoma in the neck. Experience with each of these techniques has been limited. Certainly angiographic ablation of a mediastinal adenoma that is not accessible through a cervical incision would be appealing to many patients. Even with the availability of thoroscopy, which may enable surgery to be more limited and acceptable to patients, angiographic ablation is an alternative for any patient at significant high risk for anesthesia or for those resistant to another surgical procedure. High-pressure delivery of ionic contrast material into the vessel supplying the angiographically identified adenoma is performed to destroy the gland. Successful ablation has been achieved in limited series in fewer than half of patients (39,60).

Alcohol ablation has been detailed by Harmon and associates (61) in a series of 36 patients whose indications included medical comorbidities, the technical risks from complications of previous procedures, or patient preference. Optimally, enlarged parathyroid glands are confirmed by fine needle aspiration with cytology and/or PTH assay. Ultrasound-guided injection (from one to three, depending on the estimated volume of the sonographically visualized gland) of 95% ethanol is performed. While 33% of patients remain normocalcemic, partial ablation was the goal in many who had been operated on previously for multigland disease and were left with a possible single intact enlarged gland, making the risk of hypoparathyroidism significant if complete ablation were achieved.

Nonoperative approaches must be carefully weighed against the advantages of surgery. This has limited the use of angiographic ablation or percutaneous sonographically controlled alcohol ablation to very high-risk patients and those insistent on a nonoperative attempt, particularly as results to date indicate a very real risk of recurrence following initial normocalcemia.

9 SURGERY FOR PERSISTENT OR RECURRENT HYPERPARATHYROIDISM

For the great majority of patients, surgery represents the treatment of choice for persistent or recurrent disease (17,62–66). The operative approaches are varied depending on a careful review of the previous operative report and the pathology, the success of preoperative localization, the likelihood of single versus multiglandular disease, the risk of anesthesia, and the availability of ancillary techniques including the intraoperative quick PTH assay, gamma probe–directed surgery for those patients with scintigraphically localized findings, and intraoperative ultrasonography for those patients with sonographically localized findings.

9.1 Patients for Whom Localization Procedures Indicate a Positive Unifocal Lateral Cervical Location

In patients in which two preoperative localizing procedures are concordant in demonstrating a unifocal enlarged parathyroid gland or a single localizing procedure is strongly positive for such a finding, particularly if review of previous operative and pathology reports indicate the removal or identification of parathyroid glands in other locations, a selective and focused laterocervical approach is appropriate (13,17,67). The previous cervical incision and subplatysmal planes are reentered and flaps elevated. Instead of attention being directed to the midline, the anterior border of the sternocleidomastoid muscle on the localized side of the neck lateral to the strap muscles is identified. The deeper structures are then approached by dissecting and entering the plane anterior to the sternocleidomastoid muscle and retracting the jugulo-carotid structures laterally. The omohyoid muscle may be retracted laterally and superiorly or divided to allow optimal exposure. Dissection may then be carried toward the thyroid gland through planes that may have developed little scarring from previous surgery. Entering this plane allows identification of the recurrent laryngeal nerve, exploration of the parathyroidal region adjacent to the trachea and esophagus, and excision of a gland localized on preoperative studies. The presence of an esophageal probe further facilitates orientation and enables careful and safe access to the retroesophageal region. This approach also allows access to the posterior superior mediastinum, which can be digitally explored along the prevertebral space, a site associated with a significant incidence of missed descended superior parathyroid adenomas. The posterior thyroid region may be explored, as can the extent of the carotid sheath. These are all areas in which preoperative localization studies suggested a laterally located enlarged parathyroid gland. If these maneuvers fail to reveal an enlarged gland, contralateral exploration may be carried out in a similar manner.

The use of preoperative technetium 99m–sestamibi scintigraphy with SPECT imaging has also created an opportunity for the use of gamma probe–directed surgery when the scan is positive (35,68,69). Gamma probe–directed surgery has been used extensively for sentinel lymphadenectomy for both malignant melanoma and breast cancer, and may be used to augment selective, limited surgical approaches to parathyroid adenomas. Technetium 99m–sestamibi is given at least 2 hours prior to surgery, which is facilitated by a handheld gamma probe equipped with a collimator for directed, shielded identification of radioactivity without background interference from intrathoracic structures. The role of gamma–probe directed surgery in the reoperative setting has not been evaluated extensively, but certainly is recommendable to augment surgical exploration, particularly where extensive scarring is predicted by assessment of previous surgery and a positive preoperative radionuclide localization study strongly suggests single gland disease.

9.2 Equivocal or Negative Localization and Review of Prior Surgery Suggestive of Failure to Identify any Parathyroid Tissue

When localizing studies have failed to identify an abnormal parathyroid gland but selective venous catheterization reveals a gradient favoring the neck, and one side in particular, exploration through an anterior cervical approach would seem prudent. The previous incision is extended laterally on both sides over the borders of the sternocleidomastoid muscle. If initial attempts at anterior midline mobilization of the strap muscles reveal extensive scarring, a lateral approach anterior to the sternocleidomastoid muscle can be performed as previously described on the side favored by the venous catheterization data or, in the absence of any lateralizing gradient, by the surgeon's preference. The midline approach does provide greater access to anterior dissection inferiorly towards the thymus, a common site for ectopically located glands and certainly a high priority when localizing procedures have not specifically identified the site of abnormal parathyroid tissue. Alternatively, if the plane anterior to the sternocleidomastoid muscles has been entered, the strap muscles may be divided inferior to the lower pole of the thyroid to allow access to the anterior-superior mediastinum. With both approaches, the thymus may be delivered by progressive dissection and careful upward traction. Laterally, dissection may be carried along the carotid sheath as high as the angle of the mandible, particularly when an undescended parathymic parathyroid gland is suspected (70–72). Thyroid lobectomy may be appropriate when other sites have failed, particularly if only a single unidentified parathyroid gland remains after bilateral exploration (73,74).

The routine use of intraoperative ultrasonography using a 10 mHz transducer has been particularly recommended for the identification of intrathyroidal parathyroid adenomas and may facilitate excision of the gland without a concomitant thyroid lobectomy. It has demonstrated utility as well in identifying glands in the intrathymic, paraesophageal, and carotid sheath locations (13,75).

9.3 Equivocal or Negative Localization Procedures with a Review of Previous Records Suggestive of Possible Multiple Gland Disease

In instances in which review of the previous operative reports and pathology indicates that a hypercellular parathyroid gland or glands have been removed, or when the surgeon for the reoperative procedure also performed the initial operation and can confirm this firsthand, the possibility of multiglandular disease must be considered. The extent of surgery will be dictated by previous findings, but reentering the previous transverse cervical incision and extending it laterally if needed on each side is appropriate. An exploration for all remaining parathyroid tissue as well as possible supernumerary parathyroid glands, particularly in the thymus, must be considered. In these situations as well, the use of the intraoperative quick PTH assay (QPTH) provides an appropriate adjunct and is particularly recommended (76–80). The QPTH may be performed in the operating room at the initiation of the procedure and then at appropriate intervals (generally every 10 minutes) after extirpation of abnormal parathyroid tissue. The assay has a 10-minute turnaround time, and a drop of 50% or greater has been reportedly associated with surgical cure, although several investigators have cautioned that a greater fall from baseline in the range of 70% is recommended for multiglandular disease. Data from Gauger and associates (81) on the use of intraoperative PTH monitoring in patients with double parathyroid adenoma had a false-positive rate of 55% if it relied on a 50% or greater fall below baseline value. For multiglandular disease, therefore, PTH monitoring must be used in the context of all available preoperative and localizing information.

When neck reexploration fails, the most significant issue is whether to follow through with a sternotomy at the same procedure. Indeed, this issue should be raised with the patient and appropriate consent obtained if this is planned should the cervical attempt fail. However, most investigators feel that a sternotomy should be limited only to those instances where localization procedures indicate a mediastinal enlarged parathyroid gland not retrievable through a cervical incision.

The patients with persistent or recurrent hyperparathyroidism with familial hyperparathyroidism or multiple endocrine neoplasia syndromes MENI or IIa present special challenges. Familial hyperparathyroidism in the absence of multiple endocrinopathy is rare, but hyperplasia of all parathyroid tissue in such instances is common (82). In patients with a MEN syndrome, the hyperparathyroidism is uniformly the result of hyperplasia but the gland size may be asymmetrical (83). Supernumerary glands that are hyperplastic at initial surgery, as well as ectopic parathyroid rests in cervical and mediastinal locations that become hyperplastic, have been reported (84–86). I have performed three procedures following an initial recurrence of hyperparathyroidism after a primary procedure by another surgeon over a 20-year period of time for recurrent hyperparathyroidism in a patient with familial hyperparathyroidism. In each instance the patient was rendered normocalcemic only to recur despite histologically confirmed extirpation to date of six hyperplastic parathyroid glands from normal locations as well as within the carotid sheath and thymus. The fourth procedure was performed with gamma probe–assisted localization of a scintigraphically identified gland within the carotid sheath. She is presently mildly hypercalcemic.

The role of cryopreservation and autotransplantation of hyperplastic parathyroid tissue is particularly relevant in patients with multiglandular disease having reoperative surgery. The extent of prior resection, or the degree to which other parathyroid glands may have been rendered ischemic, is often uncertain. If multigland disease is clearly at issue, cryopreservation of resected glands after histological confirmation using a fragment of each gland is appropriate (87). More controversial is the issue of immediate autotransplantation. The advantage over cryopreservation for potential subsequent autotransplantation is the more predictable success rate for immediately autografted tissue compared to cryopreserved tissue (83,88). However, the frequency of supernumerary glands and recurrent hyperparathyroidism compel many to follow a policy of biochemical observation. Cryopreservation of a portion of resected tissue is therefore appropriate in reoperative cases, and particularly so in the patient with multiglandular disease or in those instances where prior operative information indicates the resection of multiple glands, which may then place the patient at risk of hypoparathyroidism following resection of adenomas or hyperplastic glands at reoperation. In the reoperative setting and faced with possible multiglandular disease, the QPTH would appear to be a most useful adjunct to titrate biochemical response to parathyroid resection (89,90).

9.4 Preoperative Localization Suggestive of Mediastinal Parathyroid Adenoma

In those instances where preoperative localization indicates a mediastinal parathyroid adenoma, those in the upper mediastinum can be approached initially through a cervical incision (91–93). Where this is not likely, approaches include limited sternotomy, thorascopic excision, or anterior mediastinotomy (Chamberlain parasternal approach) (94,95) (Fig. 2). The appropriate approach will be dependent upon careful consideration of the localizing procedures and the depth of the lesion in the mediastinum. When precise localization has not been achieved, and only selective venous catheterization demonstrates a gradient strongly favoring an intrathoracic location, a limited sternal splitting procedure is indicated if an attempt at retrieval through the neck is unsuccessful. Partial sternotomy to a transverse inverted T incision at the third intercostal space allows excellent access of the superior anterior mediastinum. A total sternotomy may be required in selected instances. Precise localization, however, can allow a more limited

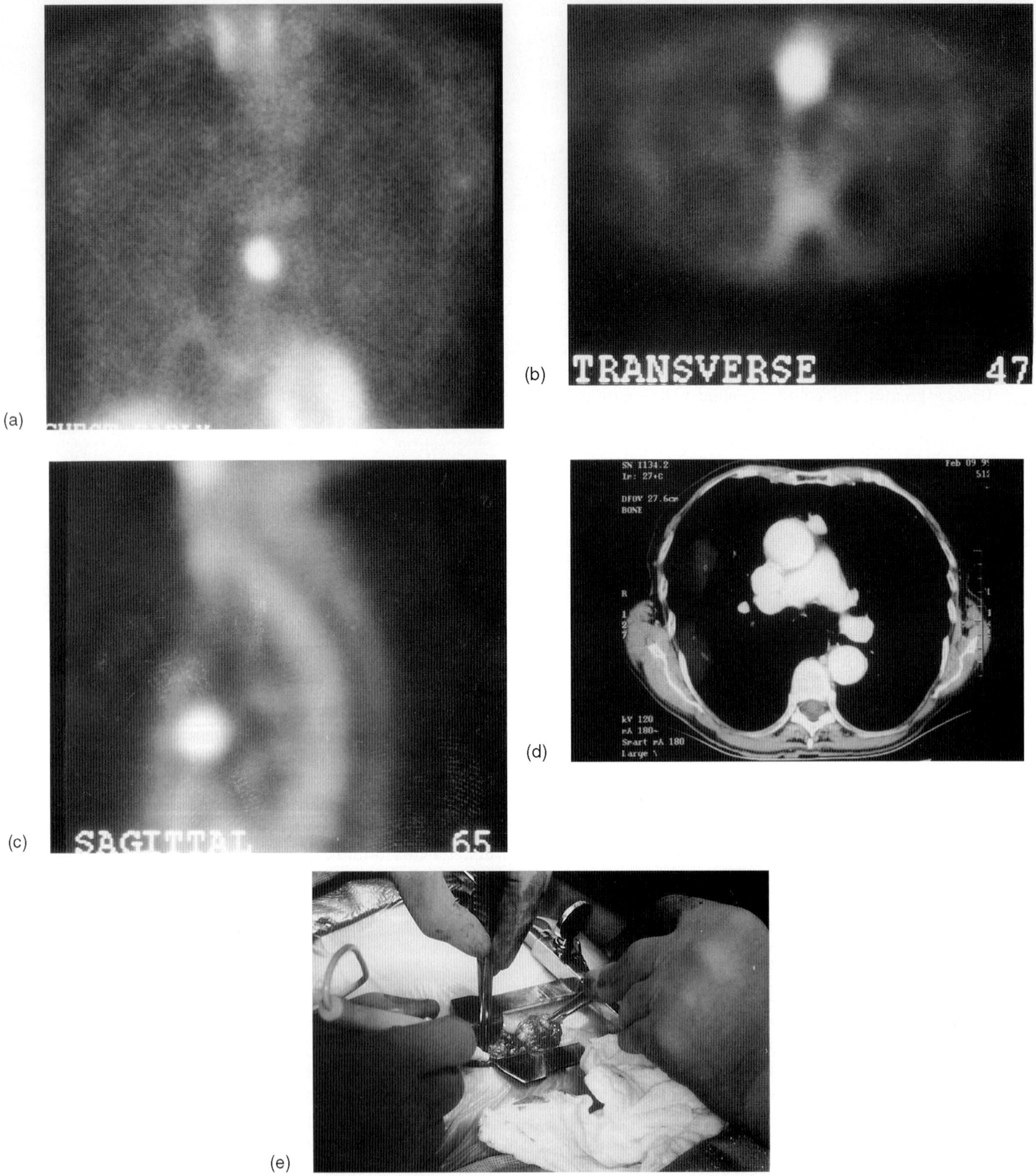

Figure 2 A technetium-99m–sestamibi scan demonstrated marked uptake in the chest in this 78-year-old woman with hyperparathyroidism on early chest (a), transverse (b), and sagittal (c) views. On CT scan (d) a nodule was noted adjacent to the aortic arch. A parathyroid adenoma was excised (e) through a limited anterior parasternal incision (Chamberlain approach).

Table 2 Results of Reoperations for Persistent or Recurrent Hyperparathyroidism

Author(s) (Ref.)	Year	No. of patients	% Cured
Wang (12)	1977	112	91
Brennan and Norton (29)	1985	175	90
Grant et al. (10)	1986	157	89
Levin (43)	1989	81	91
Cheung et al. (102)	1989	83	86
Rothmund et al. (100)	1990	70	96
Carty and Norton (13)	1991	206	95
Jarhult et al. (64)	1993	93	82
Rodriguez et al. (14)	1994	152	93
Shen et al. (15)	1996	102	95
Jaskowiak et al (16)	1996	222	97
Mariette et al. (65)	1998	38	92
Thompson et al. (17)	1999	124	88

parasternal approach. More recently, video-assisted thoracoscopy has successfully allowed excision of mediastinal parathyroid adenomas that were precisely localized preoperatively (96,97).

Special considerations apply to the patient treated for parathyroid cancer or likely to have parathyromatosis. Patients who had previous treatment for parathyroid carcinoma may develop recurrent disease in the neck. Localizing studies in patients with recurrent parathyroid carcinoma may be helpful but do not detect all foci of disease (27). In patients with familial histories of hyperparathyroidism as well as with MEN syndromes, prior procedures may lead to the implantation of hyperplastic parathyroid tissue in the surgical field. Meticulous assessment of the prior surgery, a more extensive use of localizing procedures, and more complete and thorough explorations may be required to ablate hyperplastic parathyroid tissue in this situation, and once again, the intraoperative QPTH may have particular efficacy.

10 SUCCESS AND MORBIDITY

Results of large series (Table 2) from centers that have acquired significant experiences with reoperative cases indicate a success rate in the 80–90% range. In the largest series of 222 patients from the NIH, as detailed by Jaskowiak and associates (16), a success rate of 97% was reported. A more significant rate of permanent hypoparathyroidism clearly resulted from these procedures than from primary operations. The NIH series reported a rate of 12%, Thompson and associates 13% (17), and Shen and associates 1% (15). Vocal cord paralysis rates in the 5% range have been reported, certainly higher than primary operations, where this complication is rare (98). Certainly the cost of reoperative surgery is more significant (99). All of these considerations make attention to detail especially important for reoperative cases. Most importantly, the challenges of reoperative cases provide compelling incentives for as thorough, expeditious, and successful an approach to the initial procedure as possible (100–102).

REFERENCES

1. van Heerden JA, Grant CS. Surgical treatment of primary hyperparathyroidism: an institutional perspective. World J Surg 1991; 15:688–692.
2. Bauer W, Federman DD. Hyperparathyroidism epitomized: case of Captain Charles E. Martell. Metabolism 1962; 11:21–30.
3. Martin JK, van Heerden JA, Edis AJ, Dahlin DC. Persistent postoperative hyperparathyroidism. Surg Gynecol Obstet 1980; 151:764–768.
4. McGarity WC, Goldman AL. Reoperation for primary hyperparathyroidism. Ann Surg 1981; 194:134–139.
5. Muller H. True recurrence of hyperparathyroidism: proposed criteria of recurrence. Br J Surg 1975; 62:556–559.
6. Rudberg C, Akerstrom G, Palmer M, et al. Late results of operation for primary hyperparathyroidism in 441 patients. Surgery 1986; 99:643–651.
7. Chan FKW, Koberle LMC, Thys-Jacobs S, Bilezikian JP. Differential diagnosis, causes and management of hypercalcemia. Curr Problems Surg 1997; 34:449–523.
8. Heath H III. Familial benign (hypocalciuric) hypercalcemia: a troublesome mimic of mild primary hyperparathyroidism. Endocrinol Metab Clin North Am 1989; 18:723–740.
9. Marx SJ, Stock JL, Attie MF, et al. Familial

hypocalciuric hypercalcemia: recognition among patients referred after unsuccessful parathyroid exploration. Ann Intern Med 1980; 92:351–356.
10. Grant CS, van Heerden JA, Charboneau JW, et al. Clinical management of persistent and/or recurrent primary hyperparathyroidism. World J Surg 1986; 10:555–565.
11. Consensus Development Conference Panel. Diagnosis and management of asymptomatic primary hyperparathyroidism: Consensus Development Conference Statement. Ann Intern Med 1991; 114:593–597.
12. Wang CA. Parathyroid re-exploration: a clinical and pathological study of 112 cases. Ann Surg 1977; 186: 140–145.
13. Carty SE, Norton JA. Management of patients with persistent or recurrent primary hyperparathyroidism. World J Surg 1991; 15:716–723.
14. Rodriguez JM, Tezelman S, Siperstein AE, et al. Localization procedures in patients with persistent or recurrent hyperparathyroidism. Arch Surg 1994; 129: 870–875.
15. Shen W, Duren M, Morita E, et al. Reoperation for persistent or recurrent hyperparathyroidism. Arch Surg 1996; 131:861–869.
16. Jaskowiak N, Norton JA, Alexander HR, et al. A prospective trial evaluating a standard approach to reoperation for missed parathyroid adenoma. Ann Surg 1996; 224:308–322.
17. Thompson GB, Grant CS, Perrier ND, et al. Reoperative parathyroid surgery in the era of sestamibi scanning and intraoperative parathyroid hormone monitoring. Arch Surg 1999; 134:699–704.
18. Marx SJ, Menczel J, Campbell G, Aurbach GD, Spiegel AM, Norton JA. Heterogeneous size of the parathyroid glands in familial multiple endocrine neoplasia type 1. Clin Endocrinol 1991; 35:521–526.
19. Harness JK, Ramsburg SR, Nishiyama RH, et al. Multiple adenomas of the parathyroids: do they exist? Arch Surg 1979; 114:468–474.
20. Roses DF, Karp NS, Sudarsky LA, et al. Primary hyperparathyroidism associated with two enlarged parathyroid glands. Arch Surg 1989; 121:1261–1265.
21. Verdonk CA, Edis AJ. Parathyroid double adenomas: fact or fiction? Surgery 1981; 90:523–526.
22. Attie JN, Bock G, Auguste L-J. Multiple parathyroid adenomas: report of thirty-three cases. Surgery 1990; 108:1014–1020.
23. Tezelman S, Shen W, Siperstein AE, Duh QY, Clark OH. Persistent or recurrent hyperparathyroidism in patients with double adenomas. Surgery 1995; 118: 1115–1124.
24. Kraimps J-L, Duh Q-Y, Demeure M, Clark OH. Hyperparathyroidism in multiple endocrine neoplasia syndrome. Surgery 1992; 112:1080–1088.
25. Clark OH, Way LW, Hunt TK. Recurrent hyperparathyroidism. Ann Surg 1976; 184:391–402.
26. Fitko R, Sanford IR, Hines JR, Roxe DM, Cahill E. Parathyromatosis in hyperthyroidism. Hum Pathol 1990; 21:234–237.
27. Kebekou E, Arici C, Duh Q-Y, Clark O. Localization and reoperation results for persistent and recurrent parathyroid carcinoma. Arch Surg 2001; 136:878–885.
28. Wang CA, Mahaffey, Axelrod L, Perlman JA. Hyperfunctioning supernumerary parathyroid glands. SGO 1979; 148:711–714.
29. Brennan MF, Norton JA. Reoperation for persistent and recurrent hyperparathyroidism. Ann Surg 1985; 201:40–44.
30. Brennan MF, Marx SJ, Doppman J, et al. Results of reoperation for persistent and recurrent hyperparathyroidism. Ann Surg 1981; 194:671–676.
31. Peeler BB, Martin WH, Sandler MP, Goldstein RE. Sestamibi parathyroid scanning and preoperative localization studies for patients with recurrent/persistent hyperparathyroidism or significant comorbid conditions: development of an optimal localization strategy. Am Surg 1997; 63:37–46.
32. Sarfati E, Billotey C, Halimi B, Fritsch S, Cattan P, Dubost C. Early localization and reoperation for persistent primary hyperparathyroidism. Br J Surg 1997; 84:98–100.
33. Weber CJ, Vansant J, Alazraki N, et al. Value of technetium 99m sestamibi iodine 123 imaging in reoperative parathyroid surgery. Surgery 1993; 114: 1011–1018.
34. Thompson GB, Mullen BP, Grant CS, et al. Parathyroid imaging with technetium-99m–sestamibi: an initial institutional experience. Surgery 1993; 116:966–973.
35. Norman J, Denham D. Minimally invasive radioguided parathyroidectomy in the reoperative neck. Surgery 1998; 124:1088–1093.
36. Sfakianakis GN, Irvin GL, Foss J, et al. Efficient parathyroidectomy guided by SPECT-MIBI and hormonal measurements. J Nucl Med 1996; 37:798–804.
37. Carty SE, Worsey MJ, Virgi MA, et al. Concise parathyroidectomy: the impact of preoperative SPECT 99mTc sestamibi scanning and intraoperative quick parathormone assay. Surgery 1997; 122:1107–1116.
38. Chen H, Sokoll LJ, Udelsman R. Outpatient minimally invasive parathyroidectomy: a combination of sestamibi-SPECT localization, cervical block anesthesia, and intraoperative parathyroid hormone assay. Surgery 1999; 126:1016–1022.
39. Doherty GM, Doppman JL, Miller DL, et al. Results of a multidisciplinary strategy for management of mediastinal parathyroid adenoma as a cause of persistent hyperparathyroidism. Ann Surg 1992; 215:101–106.
40. Kern KA, Shawker TH, Doppman JL, et al. The use of high-resolution ultrasound to locate parathyroid tumors during reoperations for primary hyperparathyroidism. World J Surg 1987; 111:579–585.
41. Krudy AG, Shawker TH, Doppman JL, et al. Ultrasonic parathyroid localization in previously operated patients. Clin Radiol 1984; 35:113–118.

42. Reading CC, Charboneau JW, James EM, et al. Postoperative parathyroid high-frequency sonography: evaluation of persistent or recurrent hyperparathyroidism. AJR 1985; 144:399–400.
43. Levin KE, Clark OH. The reasons for failure in parathyroid operations. Arch Surg 1989; 124:911–915.
44. Oertli D, Richter M, Kraenzlin M, et al. Parathyroidectomy in primary hyperthyroidism: preoperative localization and routine biopsy of unaltered glands are not necessary. Surgery 1994; 117:392–396.
45. Mitchell BK, Merrell RC, Kinder BK. Localization studies in patients with hyperparathyroidism. Surg Clin North Am 1995; 75:483–498.
46. Gooding GA, Clark OH, Stark DD, et al. Parathyroid aspiration biopsy under ultrasound guidance in the postoperative hyperparathyroid patient. Radiology 1985; 155:193.
47. Doppman JL, Krudy AG, Marx SJ, et al. Aspiration of enlarged parathyroid glands for parathyroid hormone assay. Radiology 1983; 148:31–35.
48. McFarland MP, Fraker DL, Shawker TH, et al. Use of preoperative fine-needle aspiration in patients undergoing reoperation for primary hyperparathyroidism. Surgery 1994; 116:959–964.
49. Auffermann W, Gooding GAW, Okerlund MD, et al. Diagnosis of recurrent hyperparathroidism: comparison of MR imaging and other imaging techniques. AJR 1988; 150:1027–1033.
50. Miller DL. Preoperative localization and interventional treatment of parathyroid tumors: when and how? World J Surg 1991; 15:706–715.
51. Fayet P, Hoeffel C, Fulla Y, et al. Technetium-99-m-sestamibi scintigraphy, magnetic resonance imaging and venous blood sampling in persistent and recurrent hyperparathyroidism. Br J Radiol 1997; 70:459–464.
52. Levy JM, Hessel SJ, Dioppe SE, et al. Digital subtraction angiography for localization of parathyroid lesions. Ann Intern Med 1982; 97:710–712.
53. Krudy AG, Doppman HL, Miller DL, et al. Abnormal parathyroid glands: comparison of nonselective arterial digital arteriography, selective parathyroid arteriography and venous digital arteriography as methods of detection. Radiology 1983; 148:23–29.
54. Obley DL, Winzelberg GG, Jarmmolowski CR, et al. Parathyroid adenomas studied by digital subtraction angiography. Radiology 1984; 153:449–451.
55. Krudy AG, Doppman JL, Miller DL, et al. Detection of mediastinal parathyroid glands by nonselective digital arteriography. AJR 1984; 142:693–695.
56. Sugg SL, Fraker DL, Alexander R, et al. Prospective evaluation of selective venous sampling for parathyroid hormone concentration in patients undergoing reoperations for primary hyperparathyroidism. Surgery 1993; 114:1004–1010.
57. Miller DL, Doppman JL, Krudy AG, et al. Localization of parathyroid adenomas in patients who have undergone surgery: Part II. Invasive procedures. Radiology 1987; 162:133–137.
58. Nilsson BE, Tisell LE, Jansson S, Zackrisson BF, Lindstedt G, Lundberg PA. Parathyroid localization by catheterization of large cervical and mediastinal veins to determine serum concentrations of intact parathyroid hormone. World J Surg 1994; 18:605–611.
59. Granberg PO, Hamberger B, Johanson G, et al. Selective venous sampling for localization of hyperfunctioning parathyroid glands. Br J Surg 1988; 73: 118–123.
60. Miller DL, Doppman JL, Chang R, et al. Angiographic ablation of parathyroid adenomas: lessons from a 10-year experience. Radiology 1987; 165:601–607.
61. Harmon CR, Grant CS, Hay ID, et al. Indications, technique and efficacy of alcohol injection of enlarged parathyroid glands in patients with primary hyperparathyroidism. Surgery 1998; 124:1011–1020.
62. Weber CJ, Sewell CW, McGarity WC. Persistent and recurrent sporadic primary hyperparathyroidism: histopathology, complications and results of operation. Surgery 1994; 116:991–998.
63. Wadstrom C, Zedenius J, Guinea A, Reeve TS, Delbridge L. Reoperative surgery for recurrent or persistent primary hyperparathyroidism. Aust NZ J Surg 1998; 68:103–107.
64. Jarhult J, Nordenstrom J, Perbeck L. Reoperation for suspected primary hyperparathyroidism. Br J Surg 1993; 80:453–456.
65. Mariette C, Pellissier L, Combemale F, Quivreuz JL, Carnaille B, Proye C. Reoperation for persistent or recurrent primary hyperparathyroidism. Langenbecks Arch Surg 1998; 383:174–179.
66. Block MA, Frame B, Keerekoper M, et al. Surgical management of persistence or recurrence after subtotal parathyroidectomy for primary hyperparathyroidism. Am J Surg 1979; 138:561–566.
67. Akerstrom G, Rudberg C, Grimelius L, et al. Causes of failed primary exploration and technical aspects of reoperation in primary hyperparathyroidism. World J Surg 1992; 16:562–568.
68. Norman J, Chheda H, Farrell C. Minimally invasive parathyroidectomy for primary hyperparathyroidism: decreasing operative time and potential complications while improving cosmetic results. Am Surg 1998; 64: 391–396.
69. Norman, Chheda H. Minimally invasive parathyroidectomy facilitated by intraoperative nuclear mapping. Surgery 1997; 122:998–1004.
70. Billingsley KG, Fraker DL, Doppman JL, et al. Localization and operative management of undescended parathyroid adenomas in patients with persistent primary hyperthyroidism. Surgery 1994; 116:982–990.
71. Edis AJ, Purnell DC, van Heerden JA. The undescended parathymus: an occasional cause of failed neck

exploration of hyperparathyroidism. Ann Surg 1979; 190:64–68.
72. Fraker DL, Doppman JL, Shawker TH, et al. Undescended parathyroid adenoma: an important etiology for failed operations for primary hyperparathyroidism. World J Surg 1990; 14:342–348.
73. Libutti SK, Bartlett DL, Jaskowiak NT, et al. The role of thyroid resection during reoperation for persistent or recurrent hyperparathyroidism. Surgery 1997; 122: 1183–1188.
74. Wang CA. Hyperfunctioning intrathyroid glands: a potential cause of failure in parathyroid surgery. J R Soc Med 1981; 74:49–51.
75. Norton JA, Shawker TH, Jones BL, et al. Intraoperative ultrasound and reoperative parathyroid surgery: an initial evaluation. World J Surg 1986; 10: 631–639.
76. Patel PC, Pellitteri PK, Patel NM, Fleetwood MK. Use of rapid intraoperative parathyroid hormone assay in the surgical management of parathyroid disease. Arch Otolaryngol Head Neck Surg 1998; 123: 559–562.
77. Irvin GL, Dembrow VD, Prudhomme DL. Clinical usefulness of an intraoperative "quick parathyroid hormone assay. Surgery 1993; 114:1019–1023.
78. Kao PC, van Heerden JA, Taylor RL. Intraoperative monitoring of parathyroid procedures by a 15-minute parathyroid hormone immunochemiluminometric assay. Mayo Clin Proc 1994; 69:532–537.
79. McHenry CR, Pollard A, Walfish PG, Rosen IB. Intraoperative parathormone level measurement in the management of hyperparathyroidism. Surgery 1990; 108:801–808.
80. Nussbaum SR, Thompson AR, Hutcheson KA, Gaz RD, Wang C-A. Intraoperative measurement of parathyroid hormone in the surgical management of hyperparathyroidism. Surgery 1988; 104:1121–1127.
81. Gauger PG, Agarwal G, England BG, et al. Intraoperative parathyroid hormone monitoring fails to detect double parathyroid adenoma: a 2-institution experience. Surgery 2001; 130:1005–1010.
82. Stevens LE, Bloomer A, Castleton KB. Familial hyperparathyroidism. Arch Surg 1967; 94:524–529.
83. Kivlen MH, Bartlett DL, Libutti SK, et al. Reoperation for hyperparathyroidism in multiple endocrine neoplasia type I. Surgery 2001; 130:991–998.
84. Gilmour JR. Some developmental abnormalities of the thymus and parathyroids. J Pathol 1941; 52:213–218.
85. Akerstrom G, Malmaeus J, Bergstrom R. Surgical anatomy of human parathyroid glands. Surgery 1984; 95:14–21.
86. Rizzoli R, Green J III, Marx SJ. Primary hyperparathyroidism is familial multiple endocrine neoplasia type I: long-term follow-up of serum calcium levels after parathyroidectomy. Am J Med 1985; 78:467–474.
87. Caccitolo JA, Farley DR, van Heerden JA, et al. The current role of parathyroid cryopreservation and autotransplantation in parathyroid surgery: an institutional experience. Surgery 1997; 122:1062–1067.
88. Demeter JG, DeJong SA, Lawrence AM, Paloyan E. Recurrent hyperparathyroidism due to parathyroid autografts: incidence presentation and management. Am Surg 1993; 59:178–181.
89. Gordon LL, Snyder WH, Wians F, Nwariaku F, Kim LT. The validity of quick intraoperative parathyroid hormone assay: an evaluation in 72 patients based on gross morphologic criteria. Surgery 1999; 126:1030–1035.
90. Nussbaum SR, Thompson AR, Hutcheson KA, Gaz RD, Wang CA. Intraoperative measurement of parathyroid hormone in the surgical management of hyperparathyroidism. Surgery 1988; 104:1121–1127.
91. Nathaniels EK, Nathaniels AM, Chiu an Wang. Mediastinal parathyroid tumors. A clinical and pathological study of 84 cases. Ann Surg 1970; 171:165–170.
92. Wang CA, Gaz RD, Moncure AC. Mediastinal parathyroid exploration: a clinical and pathological study of 47 cases. World J Surg 1986; 10:687–695.
93. Clark OH. Mediastinal parathyroid tumors. Arch Surg 1988; 123:1096–1099.
94. Russell CF, Edis AJ, Scholz DA, Sheedy PF, van Heerden JA. Mediastinal parathyroid tumors: experience with 38 tumors requiring mediastinostomy for removal. Ann Surg 1981; 193:805–809.
95. Norton JA, Schneider PD, Brennan MF. Mediastinal sternotomy in reoperations for primary hyperparathyroidism. World J Surg 1985; 9:807–813.
96. Prinz RA, Lonchyna V, Carnaille B, Wurtz A, Proye C. Thorascopic excision of enlarged mediastinal parathyroid glands. Surgery 1994; 116:999–1005.
97. Knight R, Ratzer ER, Fenoglio ME, Moore JT. Thorascopic excision of mediastinal parathyroid adenomas: a report of two cases and review of the literature. J Am Coll Surg 1997; 185:481–485.
98. Patow CA, Norton JA, Brennan MF. Vocal cord paralysis and reoperative parathyroidectomy. Ann Surg 1986; 203:282–285.
99. Doherty GM, Weber B, Norton JA. Cost of unsuccessful surgery for primary hyperparathyroidism. Surgery 1994; 116:954–958.
100. Rothmund M, Wagner PK, Seesko H, Zielke A. Lessons from reoperations in 55 patients with primary hyperparathyroidism. Dtsch Med Wochenschr 1990; 115:1579–1585.
101. Poole GV Jr, Albertson DA, Myers RT. Causes of the failed cervical exploration for primary hyperparathyroidism. Am Surg 1988; 54:553–557.
102. Cheung PSY, Borgstrom A, Thompson NW. Strategy in reoperative surgery for hyperparathyroidism. Arch Surg 1989; 124:676–680.

21

Parathyroid Carcinoma

John A. Olson, Jr.

Duke University Medical Center, Durham, North Carolina, U.S.A.

1 DEFINITION

Parathyroid carcinoma (PC) is a rare, malignant neoplasm of the parathyroid glands that causes parathyroid hormone–dependent hypercalcemia. The distinction between primary hyperparathyroidism due to the common parathyroid adenoma and the rare parathyroid carcinoma is rarely made on clinical grounds. Parathyroid carcinoma may be identified during surgery, but the diagnosis is made only after careful histopathological examination of the resected specimen or at recurrence months or years following resection. A diagnosis of parathyroid carcinoma is made with certainty by the demonstration of direct invasion of adjacent tissues, synchronous or metachronous cervical lymph node, or distant metastases.

2 EPIDEMIOLOGY

2.1 Incidence and Prevalence

Parathyroid carcinoma is rare; the true incidence of this disease in the general population is unknown. It represents 1% of cases of primary hyperparathyroidism in the United States and up to 5% of cases in published series from Japan and Italy (2–4). Fewer than 300 cases of parathyroid carcinoma were reported in the English literature prior to 1992, and an additional 100 cases have been reported in 16 published papers since 1992 (5). The largest series of parathyroid carcinoma published to date documents 286 cases of parathyroid cancer registered over a 10-year period in the National Cancer Data Base in the United States, representing 0.005% of all cases in this registry (Fig. 1) (6).

2.2 Demographic Features

The female-to-male ratio is 1:1 for parathyroid carcinoma. This is in sharp contrast to the female preponderence (3–4:1) observed in primary hyperparathyroidism due to sporadic benign parathyroid adenomas. The mean age of presentation of parathyroid carcinoma in most series is between 48 and 53 years, nearly a decade lower than the average age at presentation of benign parathyroid adenoma (Table 1). It has been reported in children less than 15 years of age (6–8). There is no racial predilection. It is unclear whether the higher incidence of parathyroid carcinoma in series of from Japan and Italy reflects true ethnic differences in disease susceptibility or differences in diagnostic criteria.

3 RISK FACTORS

3.1 Environmental

Environmental risk factors for parathyroid carcinoma are unknown. Reports of parathyroid carcinoma developing in patients with a history of head and neck irra-

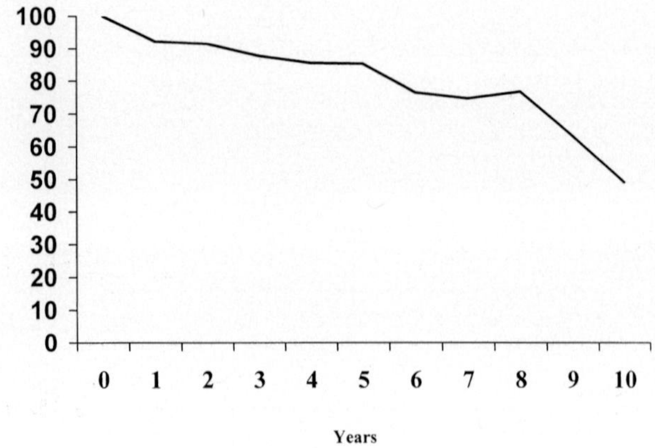

Figure 1 Overall percentage survival from parathyroid carcinoma over a 10-year period ($N = 134$). (Data from Ref. 6.)

diation support a role for ionizing radiation–induced genetic mutations in this disease (9,10).

3.2 Genetic

Parathyroid carcinoma has been reported as a feature of both familial isolated hyperparathyroidism (FIHP) and familial hyperparathyroidism–tumor jaw syndrome (FHPT-TJ). These inherited diseases are likely caused by the same gene, located on chromosome 1q25-31 (11–13). In these syndromes, hyperparathyroidism is inherited in an autosomal dominant fashion. Familial HPT can also occur in the context of several other diseases, including multiple endocrine neoplasia type 1 (MEN1) and type 2 (MEN2); however, parathyroid carcinoma is not a feature of the MEN syndromes.

Streeten et al. reported two cases of parathyroid carcinoma and two cases of atypical parathyroid adenomas in a family with primary hyperparathyroidism with apparent autosomal dominant transmission (14). Constitutional karyotypes were normal in all four patients, although three chromosomal abnormalities (a reciprocal translocation between chromosomes 3 and 4, trisomy 7, and a pericentric inversion in chromosome 9) were identified in cultured parathyroid carcinoma tissue from one patient. There was no evidence of ras gene mutations, PTH gene rearrangement, or allelic loss from the MEN1 locus on chromosome 11q13 in tumor DNA from one case of PC and one of atypical adenoma.

Wassif et al. described 19 members of a large four-generation family with autosomal dominant FIHP (15). DNA markers closely linked to the MEN1 and MEN2A loci and the prepro-PTH gene excluded linkage to these syndromes. In one individual a parathyroid carcinoma

Table 1 Selected Series of Parathyroid Carcinoma with 10 or More Patients

Author/institution (Ref.)	Year	Study type		Pathology review	Female:male ratio	Average age, yr (range)
Hundahl et al./ United States (6)	1985–1995	National registry	286	No	1:1	55 (14–88)
Sandelin et al./ Sweden (3)	1968–1990	International registry	95	Yes	1:1	55 (20–83)F 52 (24–78)M
Schantz and Castleman (8)	1930–1972	Single institution review	70	Yes	1:1	44 (13–84)
Shane et al./ Columbia (2)	1966–1982	Literature review	62	No	1:1	48 (18–73)
Holmes et al./NIH (7)	1933–1968	Literature review	50	No	1:1	44 (12–72)
Wang and Gaz/ MGH (29)	1948–1983	Single institution review	28	No	1:1	45 (28–72)
Wynne et al./ Mayo Clinic (31)	1920–1991	Single institution review	43	Yes	1:1	54 (29–78)
Favia et al./Padua	1980–1996	Single institution review	16	Yes	1:2	61 (30–78)
Levin et al./UCSF (39)	1966–1985	Single institution review	10	Yes	1:2	49 (23–68)
Anderson et al./ MDACC (48)	1968–1982	Single institution review	15	Yes	1:1	(27–61)
Chow et al./PMH, Toronto (47)	1958–1996	Single institution review	10	Yes	1:1	53 (14–72)

was found after recurrence of hypercalcemia, leading these investigators to conclude that FIHPT is a genetically and clinically distinct entity with an increased risk of malignant transformation of parathyroid tumors.

3.3 Secondary Hyperparathyroidism

Parathyroid carcinoma has been described in several patients with secondary hyperparathyroidism (sHPT) due to end-stage renal disease. This observation suggests that chronic stimulation of the parathyroid glands may lead to parathyroid carcinoma (16,17). The development of asymmetrical nodular parathyroid growth in hyperplastic glands in sHPT supports the notion that chronic parathyroid stimulation can lead to neoplastic transformation of parathyroid cells (18). Parathyromatosis, the implantation and growth of hyperplastic parathyroid glands following tumor spillage during para-thyroidectomy, is a well-recognized outcome following parathyroidectomy for benign sHPT (19). Whether this phenomenon represents parathyroid cancer in these patients with sHPT is unclear. The observation that benign parathyroid tissue may grow heterotopically and cause recurrent hyperparathyroidism supports the contention that not all parathyromatosis represents parathyroid carcinoma (40).

4 ETIOLOGY AND PATHOGENESIS

The cause of parathyroid carcinoma is unknown. An association of parathyroid carcinoma with FIHP suggests a genetic predisposition. The association with secondary HPT also suggests that chronic parathyroid stimulation or environmental factors are also important in the pathogenesis of parathyroid carcinoma. Isolated instances of synchronous parathyroid carcinoma and adenoma have been reported (20); however, the largest pathological review of parathyroid carcinoma reported no cases of parathyroid carcinoma developing in a preexisting parathyroid adenoma or hyperplasia (8).

Oncogenes implicated in the pathogenesis of parathyroid carcinoma include the cell cycle regulators, retinoblastoma (Rb) gene, and P53. Several investigators have reported somatic loss of the DNA at the Rb locus using polymorphic DNA markers (21–23) and decreased immunohistochemical staining of Rb protein in parathyroid carcinoma (21,24). However, other studies have failed to identify such loss, and mutations in this gene have not been reported (25). Loss of DNA in the region of P53 and abnormal P53 immunostaining have also been described in a small number of parathyroid carcinomas, although mutations in P53 have not been described (26). Mutations in PRAD1 (cyclin fused to PTH promoter in 5% of parathyroid adenomas), menin (MEN1), and ret (MEN2A), genes associated with benign parathyroid neoplasia have not been reported in parathyroid carcinoma.

5 CLINICAL PRESENTATION

5.1 Symptoms and Signs

Virtually all patients with parathyroid carcinoma are symptomatic at the time of diagnosis. Symptoms reflect marked hypercalcemia and significanty elevated parathyroroid hormone, rather than local effects of tumor growth (Table 2). These symptoms are similar to advanced hyperparathyroidism and most commonly include polyuria, polydypsia, weakness and fatigue, nausea and vomiting, dyspepsia and constipation (2). Depression and psychosis are also commonly described. Rare asymptomatic patients with nonfunctioning parathyroid carcinoma have been reported; such patients present with a neck mass without clinical or biochemical features of hyperparathyroidism (27,28).

Most patients with parathyroid cancer have severe renal and skeletal manifestations of hyperparathyroidism. This syndrome is again similar to the presentation of longstanding benign primary hyperparathyroidism, before the widespread use of the multichannel blood analyzer. Since most patients diagnosed today with hyperparathyroidism are asymptomatic, patients with severe symptoms and hypercalcemic crisis may be suspected of having parathyroid cancer (1). Up to 15% of

Table 2 Clinical Features of Parathyroid Carcinoma

Feature	Frequency (%)
Bone disease	46–73
Nephrolithiasis	30–64
Renal insufficiency	21,
Pancreatitis	10–15
Weakness	8
Nausea and vomiting	5
Peptic ulcer	8–18
Hypercalcemic crisis	14
Local recurrence	25–30
Lymphatic metastases	10–15
Distant metastases	25–30
Hypercalcemia (> 14 mg/dL)	40–70
Palpable neck mass	30–50
Vocal cord paralysis	15

Source: Refs. 7, 8, 29.

patients present in hypercalcemic crisis, with dehydration, mental status changes, and profoundly elevated serum calcium (> 14 mg/dL) (29). The clinical manifestations of severe hypercalcemia are variable and reflect altered central nervous system (CNS), cardiovascular, and gastrointestinal physiology (30). CNS dysfunction is characterized by confusion, impaired cognition, obtundation, and coma in severe cases. Cardiovascular effects include hypertension and a shortened QT interval on electrocardiogram. Gastrointestinal symptoms such as anorexia, nausea, vomiting, and occasionally pancreatitis can be present. A palpable neck mass is uncommon in benign parathyroid disease and its presence usually indicates the presence of a thyroid nodule. In contrast, a palpable neck mass is reported in 32–50% of patients with parathyroid carcinoma. This finding, in conjunction with very high PTH levels, should raise the suspicion of parathyroid cancer in hypercalcemic patients (29,31,32). Patients with parathyroid carcinoma may infrequently present with vocal cord paralysis, hoarsness, or dysphagia because of locally advanced disease involving the recurrent laryngeal nerve, esophagus, or trachea.

5.2 Laboratory Tests

Hypercalcemia is the hallmark feature of parathyroid carcinoma. Hypercalcemia in these cases is often severe; between 39 and 75% of patients with parathyroid carcinoma have a serum calcium concentration greater than 14 mg/dL (1). Patients with parathyroid carcinoma also have significant elevations of parathyroid hormone (5–70 times normal range) (2,20). Associated laboratory abnormalities include hypophosphatemia, elevated alkaline phosphatase, and hyperchloremic metabolic acidosis due to bicarbonate excretion in the urine.

5.3 Imaging

The routine use of preoperative localization studies in hyperparathyroid patients without a history of prior neck surgery is controversial. Until recently, imaging studies to preoperatively locate enlarged parathyroid glands were discouraged. However, recent data suggest that ^{99}Tc sestamibi identifies parathyroid adenomas with high sensitivity and may be used to select patients for directed parathyroidectomy with good success (32,33). Localization studies are clearly useful in reoperative parathyroidectomy, a small percentage of which is performed for recurrent parathyroid carcinoma. When parathyroid carcinoma is suspected on clinical grounds, preoperative imaging may be indicated to assess involvement of contiguous structures or to identify distant metastases. Effective noninvasive imaging studies to identify parathyroid tissue include ^{99}Tc sestamibi scanning, ultrasound, computed tomography (CT) scan, magnetic resonance (MR) imaging, and FDG-PET. In selected cases, invasive imaging with selective venous sampling for parathyroid hormone may be useful. Despite an abundance of literature regarding the effectiveness of these imaging modalities in benign parathyroid disease, the experience with various approaches to imaging parathyroid carcinoma is anecdotal.

Although frequently reported for localizing parathyroid adenomas, ^{99}Tc sestamibi has been reported in only a few cases of primary and recurrent parathyroid carcinoma. Aigner was one of the first to describe focal Tc-99m–MIBI uptake in parathyroid carcinoma (34). Subsequently, Al Sobhi reported a case of locally recurrent parathyroid carcinoma with involved lymph nodes that was localized by Tc-99m–sestamibi imaging and was confirmed surgically and pathologically (35) Neumann and colleagues also described a 65-year-old man with recurrent hyperparathyroidism after resection of parathyroid carcinoma. However, double-phase Tc-99m–sestamibi scintigraphy gave misleading localization and the location and extent of the parathyroid carcinoma were correctly detected by PET using 18F-fluorodeoxyglucose (36). More recently, Favia et al. reported true positive findings (93.7% sensitivity) for sestamibi in 15 of 16 patients with parathyroid carcinoma (4). This compared favorably to ultrasound (11 of 13 true positive, 85% sensitivity) and CT scan (4 of 4 true positive, 100% sensitivity) for localizing parathyroid carcinoma. Based on limited published experience, Tc-99m–sestamibi should be considered to localize suspected primary or recurrent parathyroid carcinoma.

High-frequency (10 MHz) ultrasonography has been reported for preoperative localization and for differentiating parathyroid carcinoma from adenoma (37). On ultrasound, parathyroid carcinomas are ovoid or round with a lobulated contour. They are predominantly hypoechoic relative to the adjacent thyroid but may contain both hypoechoic and hyperechoic regions and cystic spaces. Gross invasion of surrounding structures may be seen. In their series of over 70 parathyroid neoplasms imaged with ultrasound, Hara et al. reported that a depth-width ratio greater than or equal to 1 was identified in 15 (94%) of the 16 cases of carcinoma, whereas only 3 (5%) of the 61 adenomas had a similar ratio (38). Ultrasonographic features of parathyroid carcinoma include large, inhomogeneous, hypoechoic masses with lobulated contours. In contrast, parathy-

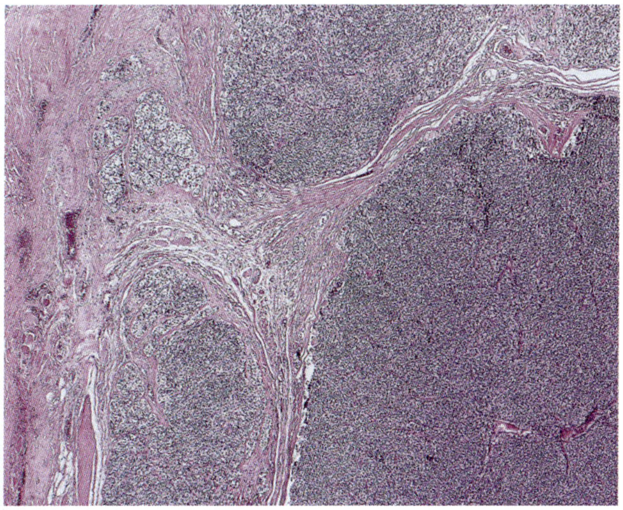

Figure 2 Parathyroid carcinomas are typically surrounded by a thick fibrous capsule, and invasion into or through the capsule is typical. (H&E × 10.) (Courtesy of John F. Madden, Duke University, Durham, NC.)

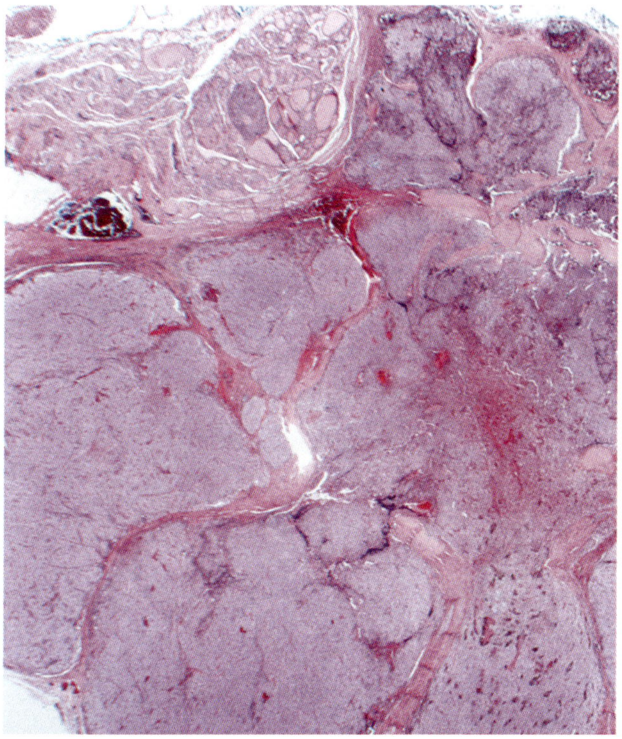

Figure 3 Fibrous bands divide the tumor into irregular lobules. Tumor is attached to thyroid at the upper left. Similar features may be seen in degenerative parathyroid adenomas, so evidence of vascular and capsular/extracapsular invasion is a crucial finding. (H&E) (Courtesy of John F. Madden, Duke University, Durham, NC.)

(a)

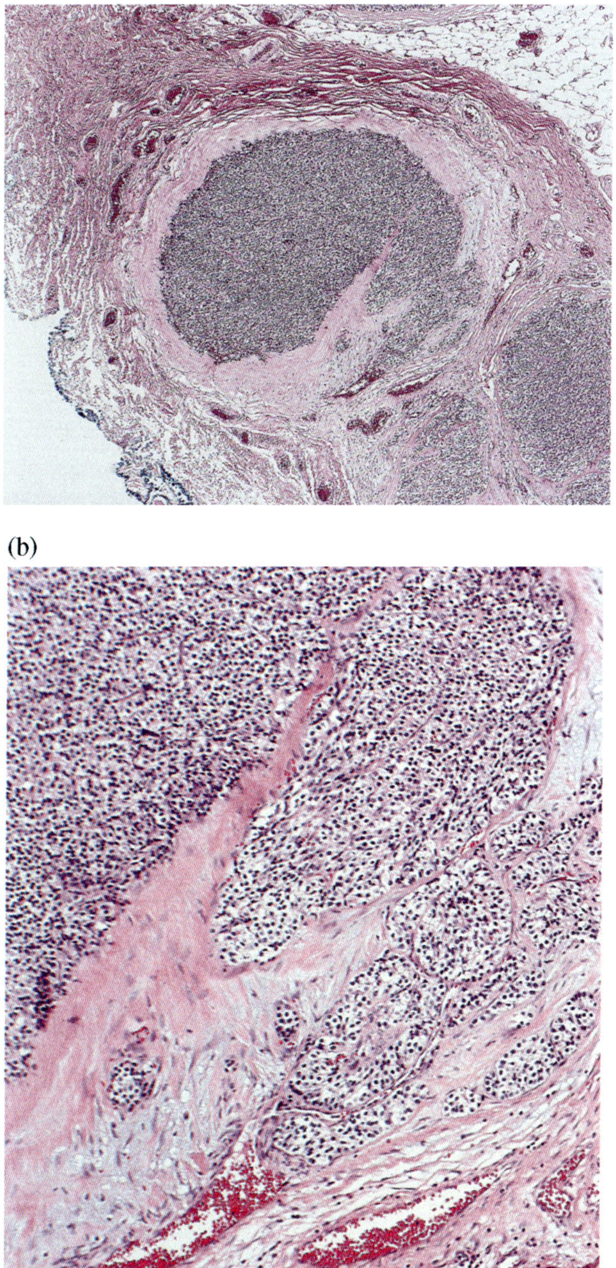

(b)

Figure 4 (a) The presence of invasive tumor nodules within the parathyroidal soft tissue is an unequivocal malignant feature. Note fat at the upper right. Irregular tongues of tumor infiltrate around the margins of the nodule. (H&E × 4.) (b) Invasion of blood vessels, usually in or around the capsule, indicates malignancy. In this field, in addition to vascular invasion there is marked stromal desmoplastic reaction (pale blue stroma). (H&E × 10.) (Courtesy of John F. Madden, Duke University, Durham, NC.)

roid adenomas appear as small, homogeneous, hypoechoic masses with smooth borders.

6 DIAGNOSIS

A high index of suspicion is required to prospectively identify malignant parathyroid disease (Table 3). A relative predisposition of males and younger patients to parathyroid cancer versus benign parathyroid disease has been noted; however, these trends are usually not helpful in assessing individual patients.

Parathyroid cancer should be suspected during parathyroidectomy when a firm, grey enlarged parathyroid gland is encountered. In these cases, the gland is fixed to surrounding structures and is difficult to dissect from adjacent tissues. This is in sharp contrast to benign parathyroid adenomas, which are the oval, soft, reddish-brown, and are easily dissected from the thyroid. Malignant parathyroid glands can be quite large, weighing up to 120 g. The discovery of pathological cervical adenopathy or frank invasion of nearby structures confirms the presence of parathyroid carcinoma. Despite these seemingly obvious criteria, a diagnosis of parathyroid carcinoma is rendered at the primary operation in only 15–80% of cases (3,6).

A pathological diagnosis of grossly unapparent parathyroid cancer can be quite difficult. The most commonly accepted criteria to differentiate parathyroid carcinoma from adenoma were initially proposed by Schantz and Castleman (8). Pathological features of parathyroid carcinoma include a trabecular cell pattern, mitotic figures, thick fibrous bands, and capsular and blood vessel invasion. (Figs. 2–4). However, parathyroid adenomas may also have some of these features, making them unreliable and the diagnosis of parathyroid carcinoma in these cases uncertain (39). Other parameters, including nuclear diameter, tumor aneuploidy, Rb and P53 gene expression, Ki-67 expression, and gelatinase mRNA expression, have been proposed as specific tests for parathyroid carcinoma, yet none has provided superior discriminating power over histopathology (1). The most certain method of diagnosis of a malignant tumor of the parathyroid is the identification of local tissue invasion or the presence of nodal or distant metastases. Consequently, a diagnosis of parathyroid carcinoma may be made following local or systemic recurrence of parathyroid carcinoma months to years following resection of a presumed benign parathyroid adenoma. Even then, local recurrence does not necessarily confirm the presence of carcinoma since autotransplanted benign parathyroid adenomas have been shown to proliferate ectopically (40).

Table 3 Clinical Features Suggestive of Parathyroid Carcinoma

Severe renal/bone manifestations
Hypercalcemic crisis
Calcium > 14 mg/dL
Intact PTH > 5 times normal
Palpable neck mass
Male sex

7 NATURAL HISTORY

Owing to the rarity of the disease, there have been few independent studies to define the natural history of this disease (29,41). Most published series reveal that parathyroid carcinoma is an indolent, yet tenacious malignancy. Parathyroid carcinoma is most prone to direct, local spread, with metastases to cervical lymph nodes occurring late in the disease. Distant metastasis to the lungs and liver and occasionally, bone, adrenals, and pancreas is usually a late event (29,42).

Untreated, parathyroid carcinoma proceeds slowly, and patients often experience progressive decline secondary to severe hyperparathyroidism. Morbidity and mortality are usually due to metabolic complications of hypercalcemia including uremia, arrhythmias, chronic wasting, hypercalcemic crisis, and pancreatitis (7). Morbidity due to mass effect of invasion of contiguous structures is less frequent.

8 TREATMENT

8.1 Surgery

Aggressive surgical resection is the treatment of choice for primary parathyroid carcinoma. The initial operation for localized disease includes en bloc removal of the parathyroid tumor, the ipsilateral thyroid lobe, and any adherent tissue. Long-term studies have shown that 50% or more of patients with parathyroid cancer will be cured by adequate surgical resection. The most important factor related to cure is en bloc surgical resection without rupture or tumor spillage (29). In a careful analysis of factors predicting survival, the extent of surgical resection (i.e., tumor excision vs. tumor excision with either thyroid lobectomy or total thyroidectomy) correlated significantly with overall survival from parathyroid cancer (3).

Fragmentation and piecemeal resection of parathyroid cancer is to be strictly avoided, but unfortunately is not uncommon. In most series, fragmentation of parathyroid cancer is reported up to 28–40% of the time (6,29). This error seems to occur as the surgeon attempts to dissect an expected benign adenoma, only to realize that "something isn't right" as the tenacious capsule is violated and tumor is spilled. This error often results in tumor spillage and implantation, leading to recurrence. In the largest series of parathyroid carcinoma, survival at 10 years was better in patients with measured and presumably nonfragmented primary tumors (6).

Occasionally, locally advanced parathyroid carcinoma involves the strap muscles, esophagus, or trachea, necessitating resection of these structures. In a review of 163 reported cases of parathyroid carcinoma, Obara and Fujimoto reported local invasion in 38 patients. In these patients, the thyroid gland was most commonly involved (63%), followed by the recurrent laryngeal nerve (16%), and the strap muscles, esophagus, and trachea (43). The most important principle in surgical resection of parathyroid carcinoma is recognition of the cancer and complete, en bloc resection of the tumor and involved structures.

The management of recurrent laryngeal nerve involvement is controversial. Some authors advocate resection of a functioning, involved nerve, while others advocate shaving the tumor from the nerve. Frozen section examination is not reliable for establishing a diagnosis in the absence of clear invasion of cervical structures (7). Given the difficulty in establishing the diagnosis during the primary operation, a conservative approach to a functioning recurrent nerve seems justified. Resection of an involved recurrent nerve is justifiable in repeat resections for cure of parathyroid carcinoma.

The indication for cervical lymphadenectomy during initial resection for recognized parathyroid carcinoma is controversial. Holmes et al. documented a 32% incidence of cervical metastases, leading them to conclude that a central and ipsilateral radical cervical lymphadenectomy should be performed (7). Hundahl et al. documented cervical lymph node involvement in up to 15% of cases of parathyroid carcinoma supporting this observation (6). In contrast, Sandelin et al. reported cervical lymph node involvement in less than 3% of patients at initial operation for parathyroid cancer (3). This observation is supported by Obara and Fujimoto, who identified only 7 patients with cervical metastases in their series of 163 patients (43). Ipsilateral central (level VI) and upper mediastinal (level VII) lymph nodes should be excised during the initial operation for parathyroid cancer. Elective lateral lymph node dissection is rarely indicated during initial surgery for parathyroid carcinoma. The fact that several series have shown that the inclusion of cervical lymphadenectomy had no impact on disease outcome (3,6) supports the recommendation that lateral neck dissection (levels II–IV) should be reserved for gross nodal metastases.

The association of parathyroid carcinoma with familial HPT suggests that patients with parathyroid carcinoma are at risk for multiple gland neoplasia. Hence, all patients with parathyroid carcinoma should have complete neck exploration with identification of all parathyroid glands. Indeed several reports have documented patients with concurrent benign and malignant parathyroid neoplasms (20). Sandelin et al. reported that multiple gland resection was performed in approximately 4% of cases of parathyroid carcinoma (3).

Surgical resection is also the treatment of choice for local recurrence and for low-volume distant metastases from parathyroid carcinoma (7,44). As with other endocrine tumors, symptoms reflect excess hormone production, rather than local tumor effects. Furthermore, most patients die of uncontrolled hypercalcemia rather than replacement of organs by tumor (8). Local recurrence in the neck should be suspected first, followed by metastases to distant sites, including lung, bone, liver, and adrenal. Localization of metastatic parathyroid can be difficult (42). Radiological studies including chest x-ray, cervical ultrasound, CT scans, and selective venous sampling may be used. Studies should be guided by local symptoms (e.g., bone pain). Resection of distant metastases has been reported to achieve sustained control of hypercalcemia in many cases (42,44,45). The chance for cure in this situation is low; however, significant palliation from the effects of severe hypercalcemia can be achieved. Obara et al. reported 7 patients with pulmonary metastases from parathyroid carcinoma and reviewed the reported outcome in an additional 22 cases from the literature (46). Six of their 7 patients underwent either unilateral or staged bilateral thoracotomies to resect up to 55 total lesions. In 4 patients, normocalcemia was achieved after multiple thoracotomies. Three patients had persistent hypercalcemia and all died; two had concurrent bone metastases. Their review of 22 published cases revealed that aggressive resection of pulmonary metastases can result in improvements in serum calcium and long-term (9–30 years) survival in up to 50% of patients with pulmonary metastases from parathyroid cancer. Patient selection for metastectomy is essential. Patients with concurrent multiple sites of metastases and those with a short (< 2 yr) disease-free interval after primary surgery are unlikely to benefit from metastectomy (8). Sandelin et al. also reported results in 6 patients with metastatic parathyroid carcinoma (42). Only one of these patients had normalization of calcium after repeat neck exploration. All patients with multiple site disease (pulmonary, bone, liver) had persistent, severe hypercalcemia or died of disease despite resection of both pulmonary and bone metastases.

8.2 Radiation Therapy

Parathyroid carcinoma is not a radiosensitive malignancy (7). However, series of adjuvant or palliative radiation have been reported. In the Princess Margaret Hospital experience, 9 of 10 patients received radiation therapy (47). In this series, indications for adjuvant radiation included close (< 2 mm) or positive resection margins. Six patients received electron beam adjuvant radiotherapy delivering 40–45 Gy in 15–25 daily fractions. No complications were reported, and all 6 patients are free of disease at a mean follow-up of 62 months (range 12–156 months). Three patients in this series had palliative radiotherapy for local and distant recurrence; two for progressive disease.

8.3 Chemotherapy

Chemotherapy is ineffective in parathyroid carcinoma. Anderson et al. reported that combination chemotherapy with doxorubicin, cyclophosphamide, and 5-fluorouracil was ineffective in two patients with unresectable metastases from parathyroid carcinoma (48). Three of 7 patients with metastatic parathyroid carcinoma reported by Obara et al. received chemotherapy with a variety of agents including dacarbazine, cyclophosphamide, 5-fluourouracil, and vincristine, none of which demonstrated response in terms of correcting hypercalcemia or impacting tumor burden (46). Wynne et al. showed no benefit of chemotherapy in terms of lowering calcium or prolonging life in 6 patients treated with combinations including mithramycin, 5-fluorouracil, and doxorubicin (31).

8.4 Hypercalcemic Crisis

Severe hypercalcemia is generally defined as an albumin-corrected serum calcium concentration greater than 14 mg/dL. Clinical manifestations of hypercalcemic crisis include mental status changes, hypertension, prolonged QT interval on the electrocardiogram, nausea and vomiting, and occasionally pancreatitis. Patients with hypercalcemia of this degree, as well as those who are symptomatic at lower degrees of hypercalcemia, should be treated. The management of acute, severe hypercalcemia due to parathyroid carcinoma is no different than that due to other causes. Goals of treatment are to restore intravascular volume, promote renal excretion of calcium, and inhibit osteoclast-mediated bone resorption.

Specific medical management can be broken down into measures that promote calcium excretion and those that inhibit osteoclast-mediated bone resorption. Initial measures aimed at promoting calcium excretion should include infusion of normal saline to reverse intravascular volume depletion and administration of loop diuretics to promote calciuresis. These measures alone are usually ineffective in hypercalcemia due to parathyroid carcinoma and must be complemented with other agents. Bisphosphonates (etidronate, pamidronate, and clodronate) are the drugs of choice in this setting (30). In particular, a single 24-hour infusion of up to 90 mg of pamidronate results in normalization of serum in 70–100% of patients (49,50). Other active agents include plicamycin, calcitonin and gallium nitrate, glucocorticoids, and sodium phosphate. Calcitonin 4 U per kg every 12 hours is first-line therapy when hypercalcemia is life threatening and rapid correction of serum calcium is necessary (30). The effect of calcitonin is short-lived, and additional treatment, usually with a bisphosphonate, is usually necessary.

9 PROGNOSIS

Even following adequate surgical resection, approximately one third to one half of patients with parathyroid carcinoma will experience recurrence (3,8). Prediction of outcome from parathyroid carcinoma is imprecise. Tumor size and lymph node status were not predictive of outcome in the largest series of parathyroid carcinoma published to date, making a TNM-type staging scheme unlikely to be useful (6). In contrast, extent of initial surgery (presence or absence of thyroidectomy), age of the patient at onset, and pathological confirmation of malignancy were most predictive of mortality from parathyroid carcinoma on univariate and multivariate analysis of 95 cases performed by Sandelin et al. (3).

Recurrences from parathyroid carcinoma most often develop within 3 years and are heralded by recurrent hypercalcemia (7). Recurrences within 2 years, in particular, are associated with poor outcome (8,48). Five-year disease-free and overall survival range from 30 to 80% and 45 to 85%, respectively (Table 4). Patients

Table 4 Outcome from Parathyroid Carcinoma

Author/institution (Ref.)	Pts	Follow-up (months)	Recurrence (%)	Median time to recurrence (months)	Survival at 5/10 years (%)	Median survival (months)
Hundahl et al./United States (6)	286	60	NR	NR	85.5/49.1	NR
Sandelin et al./Sweden (3)	95	84	42	33 (1–228)	85/70 43/43	28
Schantz and Castleman (8)	70	60	31	NR	69/NR	NR
Shane et al./Columbia (2)	62	NR	NR	36	50/35	NR
Wang and Gaz/MGH (29)	28	24–264	39	18	44/22	91
Holmes et al./NC (7)	46	NR	81	NR	50/13	60
Wynne et al./Mayo Clinic (31)	43	83(14–228)	67	28 (3–228)	69/56	36

with recurrence are infrequently cured, with death resulting from the complications of hypercalcemia rather than from organ invasion (2,8,29).

10 FOLLOW-UP

Patients with resected parathyroid carcinoma should be followed with serum calcium, physical examination, and chest x-ray. Since up to 50% of both local and distant recurrences occur within the first 2 years of resection, intensity of follow-up should be highest during this time. Long-term follow-up is indicated for all patients because recurrence has been documented up to 15 years following resection of parathyroid carcinoma (29).

11 SUMMARY POINTS

1. Parathyroid carcinoma represents 1% of hyperparathyroidism.
2. Clinical features of parathyroid carcinoma reflect severe hyperparathyroidism and are indistinguishable from those of longstanding, symptomatic benign parathyroid disease.
3. Severe hypercalcemia with very high PTH levels in a young male patient with a palpable neck mass are the classic "at-risk" signs to suggest parathyroid carcinoma.
4. At operation, parathyroid carcinoma appears as a gray to white, firm enlarged parathyroid with a thick fibrous capsule. Adherence to and invasion of surrounding structures is common.
5. Complete en bloc resection of parathyroid carcinoma with ipsilateral thyroid lobectomy and ipsilateral paratracheal lymphadenectomy is the best surgical procedure. Removal of adjacent structures, including strap muscles, esophagus, nerves, and vessels, is indicated when invasion is encountered. Piecemeal resection of parathyroid carcinoma is to be strictly avoided.
6. Disease-free survival of 20–70% and overall survival of 13–70% can be expected 10 years following resection of parathyroid carcinoma. Local recurrence develops in up to 50% of patients. Distant metastases to regional lymph nodes, lung, liver, and bone can be expected in 30% of patients. There are no reliable prognostic factors for parathyroid carcinoma.
7. Surgical resection of locoregional or isolated distant metastases can provide effective palliation for hypercalcemia resulting from recurrent parathyroid carcinoma. Disease-free survival less than 2 years and multiple site recurrence portends a poor outcome from surgical palliation. Chemotherapy and radiation therapy are ineffective in this disease.

REFERENCES

1. Fujimoto Y, Obara T. How to recognize and treat parathyroid carcinoma. Surg Clin North Am 1987; 67(2): 343–357.
2. Shane E, Bilezikian JP. Parathyroid carcinoma: a review of 62 patients. Endocr Rev 1982; 3(2):218–226.
3. Sandelin K, Auer G, Bondeson L, Grimelius L, Farnebo LO. Prognostic factors in parathyroid cancer: a review of 95 cases. World J Surg 1992; 16(4):724–731.
4. Favia G, Lumachi F, Polistina F, D'Amico DF. Parathyroid carcinoma: sixteen new cases and suggestions for correct management. World J Surg 1998; 22(12):1225–1230.
5. Shane E. Parathyroid carcinoma. In: Bilezikian JP, Marcus R, Levine MA, eds. The Parathyroids. San Diego: Academic Press, 2001:515–525.

6. Hundahl SA, Fleming ID, Fremgen AM, Menck HR. Two hundred eighty-six cases of parathyroid carcinoma treated in the US between 1985-1995: a National Cancer Data Base Report. The American College of Surgeons Commission on Cancer and the American Cancer Society. Cancer 1999; 86(3):538–544.
7. Holmes EC, Morton DL, Ketcham AS. Parathyroid carcinoma: a collective review. Ann Surg 1969; 169(4): 631–640.
8. Schantz A, Castleman B. Parathyroid carcinoma. A study of 70 cases. Cancer 1973; 31(3):600–605.
9. Mashburn MA, Chonkich GD, Chase DR, Petti GH Jr. Parathyroid carcinoma: two new cases—diagnosis, therapy, and treatment. Laryngoscope 1987; 97(2):215–218.
10. Ireland JP, Fleming SJ, Levison DA, Cattell WR, Baker LR. Parathyroid carcinoma associated with chronic renal failure and previous radiotherapy to the neck. J Clin Pathol 1985; 38(10):1114–1118.
11. Mendelian inheritance in man. OMIM (TM) Johns Hopkins University, 2002.
12. Fujikawa M, Okamura K, Sato K, Mizokami T, Tamaki K, Yanagida T, et al. Familial isolated hyperparathyroidism due to multiple adenomas associated with ossifying jaw fibroma and multiple uterine adenomyomatous polyps. Eur J Endocrinol 1998; 138(5):557–561.
13. Yoshimoto K, Endo H, Tsuyuguchi M, Tanaka C, Kimura T, Iwahana H, et al. Familial isolated primary hyperparathyroidism with parathyroid carcinomas: clinical and molecular features. Clin Endocrinol (Oxf) 1998; 48(1):67–72.
14. Streeten EA, Weinstein LS, Norton JA, Mulvihill JJ, White BJ, Friedman E, et al. Studies in a kindred with parathyroid carcinoma. J Clin Endocrinol Metab 1992; 75(2):362–366.
15. Wassif WS, Moniz CF, Friedman E, Wong S, Weber G, Nordenskjold M, et al. Familial isolated hyperparathyroidism: a distinct genetic entity with an increased risk of parathyroid cancer. J Clin Endocrinol Metab 1993; 77(6):1485–1489.
16. Miki H, Sumitomo M, Inoue H, Kita S, Monden Y. Parathyroid carcinoma in patients with chronic renal failure on maintenance hemodialysis. Surgery 1996; 120 (5):897–901.
17. Tominaga Y, Numano M, Uchida K, Sato K, Asano H, Haba T, et al. Lung metastasis from parathyroid carcinoma causing recurrent renal hyperparathyroidism in a hemodialysis patient: report of a case. Surg Today 1995; 25(11):984–986.
18. Tominaga Y, Takagi H. Molecular genetics of hyperparathyroid disease. Curr Opin Nephrol Hypertens 1996; 5(4):336–341.
19. Lee PC, Mateo RB, Clarke MR, Brown ML, Carty SE. Parathyromatosis: a cause for recurrent hyperparathyroidism. Endocr Pract 2001; 7(3):189–192.
20. Shapiro DM, Recant W, Hemmati M, Mazzone T, Evans RH. Synchronous occurrence of parathyroid carcinoma and adenoma in an elderly woman. Surgery 1989; 106(5):929–933.
21. Cryns VL, Thor A, Xu HJ, Hu SX, Wierman ME, Vickery AL Jr, et al. Loss of the retinoblastoma tumor-suppressor gene in parathyroid carcinoma. N Engl J Med 1994; 330(11):757–761.
22. Dotzenrath C, Teh BT, Farnebo F, Cupisti K, Svensson A, Toell A, et al. Allelic loss of the retinoblastoma tumor suppressor gene: a marker for aggressive parathyroid tumors? J Clin Endocrinol Metab 1996; 81(9): 3194–3196.
23. Pearce SH, Trump D, Wooding C, Sheppard MN, Clayton RN, Thakker RV. Loss of heterozygosity studies at the retinoblastoma and breast cancer susceptibility (BRCA2) loci in pituitary, parathyroid, pancreatic and carcinoid tumours. Clin Endocrinol (Oxf) 1996; 45(2): 195–200.
24. Subramaniam P, Wilkinson S, Shepherd JJ. Inactivation of retinoblastoma gene in malignant parathyroid growths: a candidate genetic trigger? Aust NZ J Surg 1995; 65(10):714–716.
25. Farnebo F, Auer G, Farnebo LO, Teh BT, Twigg S, Aspenblad U, et al. Evaluation of retinoblastoma and Ki-67 immunostaining as diagnostic markers of benign and malignant parathyroid disease. World J Surg 1999; 23(1):68–74.
26. Cryns VL, Rubio MP, Thor AD, Louis DN, Arnold A. p53 abnormalities in human parathyroid carcinoma. J Clin Endocrinol Metab 1994; 78(6):1320–1324.
27. Klink BK, Karulf RE, Maimon WN, Peoples JB. Nonfunctioning parathyroid carcinoma. Am Surg 1991; 57 (7): 463–467.
28. Aldinger KA, Hickey RC, Ibanez ML, Samaan NA. Parathyroid carcinoma: a clinical study of seven cases of functioning and two cases of nonfunctioning parathyroid cancer. Cancer 1982; 49(2):388–397.
29. Wang CA, Gaz RD. Natural history of parathyroid carcinoma. Diagnosis, treatment, and results. Am J Surg 1985; 149(4):522–527.
30. Bilezikian JP. Management of acute hypercalcemia. N Engl J Med 1992; 326(18):1196–1203.
31. Wynne AG, van Heerden J, Carney JA, Fitzpatrick LA. Parathyroid carcinoma: clinical and pathologic features in 43 patients. Medicine (Baltimore) 1992; 71(4):197–205.
32. Udelsman R, Donovan PI, Sokoll LJ. One hundred consecutive minimally invasive parathyroid explorations. Ann Surg 2000; 232(3):331–339.
33. Irvin GL III, Prudhomme DL, Deriso GT, Sfakianakis G, Chandarlapaty SK. A new approach to parathyroidectomy. Ann Surg 1994; 219(5):574–579.
34. Aigner RM, Fueger GF, Lax S. A case of parathyroid carcinoma visualized on Tc-99m-sestamibi scintigraphy. Nuklearmedizin 1997; 36(7):256–258.
35. Al Sobhi S, Ashari LH, Ingemansson S. Detection of metastatic parathyroid carcinoma with Tc-99m sestamibi imaging. Clin Nucl Med 1999; 24(1):21–23.

36. Neumann DR, Esselstyn CB, Kim EY. Recurrent postoperative parathyroid carcinoma: FDG-PET and sestamibi-SPECT findings. J Nucl Med 1996; 37(12):2000–2001.
37. Edmonson GR, Charboneau JW, James EM, Reading CC, Grant CS. Parathyroid carcinoma: high-frequency sonographic features. Radiology 1986; 161(1):65–67.
38. Hara H, Igarashi A, Yano Y, Yashiro T, Ueno E, Aiyoshi Y, et al. Ultrasonographic features of parathyroid carcinoma. Endocr J 2001; 48(2):213–217.
39. Levin KE, Galante M, Clark OH. Parathyroid carcinoma versus parathyroid adenoma in patients with profound hypercalcemia. Surgery 1987; 101(6):649–660.
40. Brennan MF, Brown EM, Marx SJ, Spiegel AM, Broadus AE, Doppman JL, et al. Recurrent hyperparathyroidism from an autotransplanted parathyroid adenoma. N Engl J Med 1978; 299(19):1057–1059.
41. Sandelin K, Tullgren O, Farnebo LO. Clinical course of metastatic parathyroid cancer. World J Surg 1994; 18(4):594–598.
42. Sandelin K, Thompson NW, Bondeson L. Metastatic parathyroid carcinoma: dilemmas in management. Surgery 1991; 110(6):978–986.
43. Obara T, Fujimoto Y. Diagnosis and treatment of patients with parathyroid carcinoma: an update and review. World J Surg 1991; 15(6):738–744.
44. Flye MW, Brennan MF. Surgical resection of metastatic parathyroid carcinoma. Ann Surg 1981; 193(4): 425–435.
45. Dubost C, Jehanno C, Lavergne A, Le Charpentier Y. Successful resection of intrathoracic metastases from two patients with parathyroid carcinoma. World J Surg 1984; 8(4):547–551.
46. Obara T, Okamoto T, Ito Y, Yamashita T, Kawano M, Nishi T, et al. Surgical and medical management of patients with pulmonary metastasis from parathyroid carcinoma. Surgery 1993; 114(6):1040–1048.
47. Chow E, Tsang RW, Brierley JD, Filice S. Parathyroid carcinoma—the Princess Margaret Hospital experience. Int J Radiat Oncol Biol Phys 1998; 41(3):569–572.
48. Anderson BJ, Samaan NA, Vassilopoulou-Sellin R, Ordonez NG, Hickey RC. Parathyroid carcinoma: features and difficulties in diagnosis and management. Surgery 1983; 94(6):906–915.
49. Thiebaud D, Jaeger P, Burckhardt P. Response to retreatment of malignant hypercalcemia with the bisphosphonate AHPrBP (APD): respective role of kidney and bone. J Bone Miner Res 1990; 5(3):221–226.
50. Gucalp R, Ritch P, Wiernik PH, Sarma PR, Keller A, Richman SP, et al. Comparative study of pamidronate disodium and etidronate disodium in the treatment of cancer-related hypercalcemia. J Clin Oncol 1992; 10(1): 134–142.

22

Endoscopic Parathyroidectomy

Michel Gagner

Mount Sinai School of Medicine, New York University, New York, New York, U.S.A.

Francesco Rubino

IRCAD–European Institute of Telesurgery, Strasbourg, France

1 INTRODUCTION

The first successful parathyroidectomy for primary hyperparathyroidism was performed in Vienna, Austria, in 1925. Since then, parathyroidectomy has been routinely performed in many specialized centers worldwide. Due to the fact that a subset of patients with primary hyperparathyroidism (PHPT) has a multiglandular disease caused by four-gland hyperplasia or multiple adenomas, most surgeons have recommended routine bilateral exploration and identification of all glands.

The advent of more reliable preoperative imaging techniques such as high-resolution ultrasonography and sestamibi scan and the development of an intraoperative assay to confirm normalization of parathyroid hormone (PTH) have allowed important changes in the treatment of primary hyperparathyroidism. More surgeons today are comfortable with unilateral exploration, which allows for smaller incisions, shorter operative times, and use of sedation instead of general anesthesia in some instances.

Laparoscopic procedures were initially limited to body areas with preexisting cavities; more recently, access to potential spaces has extended the spectrum of minimally invasive endoscopic surgery. Since the first report of an endoscopic parathyroidectomy in 1996 (1), video-assisted techniques have been applied to surgery of the neck, and several series have documented the feasibility of these approaches for parathyroid and thyroid diseases (2–5).

Three major techniques are currently utilized for the minimally invasive treatment of hyperparathyroidism:

1. *The endoscopic approach*: As originally described by Gagner, it includes constant gas insufflation and four trocars placed on the anterior aspect of the neck. Other authors have subsequently described technical variations such as using a combination of an external lift device and/or a modified hernia balloon to create a working space (6,7) or performing an axillary approach (8) with the aim to avoid scars in the neck area.
2. *Video-assisted parathyroidectomy*: Miccoli et al. (9) have described a video-assisted parathyroidectomy withouth gas insufflation. Their technique is performed through a 15 mm incision at the sternal notch, which is then held open with conventional retractors. The operation is performed using a 5 mm endoscope and 2 mm forceps and scissors passed through the incision at the sternal notch.
3. *Video-assisted parathyroidectomy by lateral approach*: This approach, described by Henry et al.

(10), is characterized by a 15 mm transversal skin incision on the anterior border of the sternocleidomastoid muscle (SCM), on the side of the supposed lesion. Dissection of the fascia connecting the lateral portion of the strap muscles and the thyroid lobe with the carotid sheath is then performed prior to introduce a 12 mm trocar through the incision and two 2.5 mm trocars on the line of the anterior border of the SCM, above and below the first trocar. Carbon dioxide is then used at 8 mmHg. Unilateral video-assisted parathyroid exploration can be therefore carried out using a 10 mm 0-degree endoscope.

In this chapter we will describe in detail the operative technique of endoscopic parathyroidectomy and its current indications and contraindications. We will also discuss the clinical outcomes and advantages of minimally invasive neck surgery in general and of the endoscopic technique in particular.

2 ENDOSCOPIC PARATHYROIDECTOMY

2.1 Indications

Indications for the procedure are as follows:

1. Laboratory evidence of primary hyperparathyroidism associated with solitary adenoma, being unequivocal at a single site documented by technetium Tc-99m–sestamibi and/or ultrasonographic scanning.
2. Availability of the quick PTH assay (QPTH).

Since the neck offers a limited working space for endoscopic maneuvering, the ideal candidate is a thin patient with a moderately enlarged gland (1–2 cm).

2.2 Contraindications

Relative contraindications are as follows:

1. Evidence of multiple gland disease
2. Likelihood of hyperplasia of the parathyroids or multiple gland disease
3. History of renal disease, family history of parathyroid disease, or suspected multiple endocrine neoplasia syndrome
4. Goiter
5. Previous neck surgery or irradiation of the neck
6. Lithium-associated PHPT
7. Abnormal neck structure (skeletal or soft tissue)
8. Obesity (a short, wide neck can limit maneuverability)

Absolute contraindications are preoperative evidence or suspicion of parathyroid carcinoma:

1. The endoscopic approach may lead to inadequate staging.
2. The removal of a parathyroid carcinoma through a small incision or through an endoscopic port or cannula provides a situation of risk for rupture with potential cell spillage, leading to disease recurrence.

3 THE TECHNIQUE OF ENDOSCOPIC PARATHYROIDECTOMY

3.1 Patient's Position

After inducing general endotracheal anesthesia, the patient is placed on the operating table in the supine position with the neck slightly extended and rotated to the contralateral side. A donut is used to stabilize the head.

3.2 Team Set-Up

The surgeon stands on the side of the patient contralateral to the affected parathyroid gland. The first assistant who maneuvers the camera stands on the surgeon's left. A second assistant, if available, may stand on the contralateral side of the table. The scrub nurse stands on the side of the table opposite the surgeon.

3.3 Equipment

One screen is placed slightly above the head of the patient, on the same side of the lesion, therefore being opposite to the surgeon and first assistant. A second screen is placed on the contralateral side and used by the third assistant. Laparoscopic and video units are usually placed behind the surgeon.

3.4 Instruments

Optical devices include a 0 degree 5 mm laparoscope, a 30 degree 5 mm laparoscope, and a 30 degree 3 mm laparoscope. Operating devices include 2–3 mm and 5 mm trocars and 2–3 mm dissectors, graspers, and scissors with a length of about 18–20 cm (Figs. 1–3).

3.5 Incision and Placement of Trocars

Anatomical landmarks are outlined with a marking pen, including the sternal notch, the midline, the anterior border of the sternocleidomastoid muscle, and the external jugular veins (Fig. 4). The head of the patient is slightly rotated on the opposite side of the lesion to maximize access to the ipsilateral neck.

A 0.5 cm skin incision is made at the sternal notch (Fig. 5). A blunt-tipped Kelly clamp is used to enter the subplatysmal space under direct vision. Blunt dissection is performed to develop a space along the anterior border of the ipsilateral SCM. A pursestring suture (2/0 silk) is placed around the incision in order to minimize gas leakage from this port site. The pursestring should be placed in the subcutaneous tissue, since placing it transcutaneously seems to increase the risk of keloids.

After insertion of the first trocar, carbon dioxide is insufflated to a pressure of 12 mmHg until an adequate working space is developed by gently advancing a 0 degree 5 mm endoscope along the avascular space of the anteromedial border of the ipsilateral SCM. Once the working space is developed, the insufflation pressure is decreased to 8–10 mmHg for the remainder of the procedure.

The 0 degree endoscope is then replaced by a 30 degree 5 mm endoscope, which is used for the remainder of the case. Three additional trocars are then inserted under direct vision: (1) one 2–3 mm trocar at the mid-portion of the ipsilateral SCM, (2) one 2–3 mm or one 5 mm trocar at the midline, and (3) one 2–3 mm trocar superolaterally, along the anterior border of the SCM (Fig. 6).

3.5.1 Dangers and Intraoperative Complications

Rarely, an external jugular vein or smaller venous vessels such as subplatysmal or subcutaneous veins or anterior cervical veins may be injured during trocar insertion. These types of vascular injuries may be concealed by the tamponade effect of insufflation or the trocar itself during the operation. Hence, these types of injuries may only be revealed at the end of the operation when the trocars are removed and the neck is desufflated.

3.5.2 Tips

Trocar insertion needs to be performed carefully. It is mandatory to have a clear view of the area where the trocar is being inserted. In order to minimize the risk of injury to vessels or to the trachea during trocar insertion, it is a good practice to direct the tip of the trocar toward the laparoscope. Care should be taken to avoid insertion of the trocars through the fibers of the sternocleidomastoid muscle to avoid injuring the jugular vein or the carotid artery. The first trocar must be inserted by an open technique, while other trocars are inserted under direct vision.

3.6 Dissection of the Operative Site and Mobilization of Structures

The carotid artery is identified and the space between the lateral border of the strap muscles and the medial edge of the carotid artery is developed (Fig. 7). Strap muscles are retracted antero-medially in order to visualize the lateral aspect of the thyroid lobe. The thyroid lobe is then gently retracted medially in order to provide further exposure of the area, exposing the loose connective tissue posterolateral to the thyroid lobe. If needed, the middle thyroid vein can be ligated using 5 mm clips or a 5 mm harmonic scalpel introduced through the trocar at the sternal notch. While performing this step, a 3 mm endoscope must be inserted through the superolateral trocar on the anterior border of the SCM. This maneuver allows safer medial retraction of the thyroid lobe and can facilitate exposure of the deeper tissue planes.

3.6.1 Dangers and Intraoperative Complications

Bleeding from a middle thyroid vein may significantly compromise view of structures and be difficult to manage endoscopically. The use of cautery is to be avoided since the small working space favors inadvertent contacts between endoscopic instruments with consequent possible spreading of energy and injury to nervous and vascular structures.

3.6.2 Tips

The combination of blunt dissection and gas insufflation allows easy separation of structures, minimizing the need for sharp dissection. This avoids annoying oozing from small vessels and helps maintain a clear endoscopic view. If the source of moderate bleeding is a small venous vessel, hemostasis can be effectively achieved by just crushing it with the tips of the grasper for approximately one minute. In addition to the advantage of reducing the risk of electrical injury, this method avoids the switching of instrumentation in and out of the neck, thereby decreasing the risk of traumatic injury to organs.

3.7 Anatomical Landmarks and Dissection of the Recurrent Laryngeal Nerve

Dissection directed medially on the posterolateral aspect of the thyroid will allow identification of the recurrent laryngeal nerve and parathyroid glands (Figs. 8,9). The inferior thyroid artery is a useful landmark for locating the recurrent laryngeal nerve. As the artery passes medially behind the thyroid gland, it crosses the recurrent laryngeal nerve in front, behind, or on both sides. The easiest site to identify the recurrent laryngeal nerve is near where the inferior thyroid artery crosses the lateral border of the lower pole of the thyroid gland. The nerve or one of its branches may pass behind, between, or in front of the branches of the artery. Another site to identify the nerve is more caudally, where it crosses behind the cranial and medial curves of the common carotid artery and can be identified dissecting along the medial surface of the artery. The superior parathyroid glands will be found most often at the level of the upper two thirds of the posterior thyroid capsule. The inferior thyroid artery or its branches leads in most cases to the inferior parathyroid glands.

3.7.1 Dangers and Intraoperative Complications

In approximately 1% of cases the right recurrent nerve is nonrecurrent and originates in a superior level of the vagus nerve, therefore having a lateral direction and being susceptible to injury.

3.7.2 Tips

To prevent injury of the nerve, coagulation or clip application in close proximity to the nerve or when the nerve is not yet identified should be minimized or avoided. The use of bipolar coagulation or ultrasonic energy for hemostasis is preferable due to limited lateral spread. The nerve should also be separated from the thyroid gland before the gland is retracted medially or manipulated to avoid stretching and axon damage.

Although the operative field during endoscopic thyroidectomy is limited, the magnification allowed by the laparoscope provides improved visualization of small anatomical details that might help decrease the risk of injury the nerve. The vasa nervorum running along the recurrent laryngeal nerve may in fact be easily recognized (Fig. 5) and help identification and preservation of the nerve.

3.8 Identification of Parathyroid Adenoma

When the plane between the thyroid and the carotid sheath is developed, using either an inferior view or a lateral view, and the recurrent laryngeal nerve and inferior thyroid artery are identified, the next step is the location of the parathyroid gland (Fig. 10). When parathyroid glands are not immediately visualized, classic anatomical landmarks should lead the dissection. The endoscopic approach makes it possible to locate glands located deeply in the tracheoesophageal groove or even downward in the superior mediastinum.

When performing dissection of the posterolateral aspect of the thyroid, a 3 mm endoscope should be placed through the superolateral trocar (the most cranial of the two trocars placed along the SCM), while a 5 mm endopeanut is introduced through the sternal port and used to retract the thyroid lobe medially. Positioning the endoscope in this position allows one to approach the recurrent laryngeal nerve and parathyroid glands frontally and assists in dissection of the base of the neck or superior mediastinum if ectopic parathyroid glands need to be located.

3.9 Freeing of the Parathyroid Adenoma

When the parathyroid gland/adenoma is identified, the parathyroid gland can be retracted bluntly by pushing the gland with the closed tip of a grasper forceps. While retracting maneuvers provide tension, a curved scissor or a curved dissector is used to dissect the gland away from surrounding structures and loose areolar tissue until complete mobilization is achieved and the vascular pedicle of the gland clearly identified.

When the parathyroid adenoma is completely freed and the vascular pedicle circonferentially dissected by using a curved dissector or a right-angled dissector, a 5 mm clip applier is introduced through the trocar at the sternal notch. After placing two 5 mm clips proximally and one distally, a 2–3 mm scissor is introduced through the trocar located at the midportion of the SCM in order to divide the pedicle between clips (Fig. 11).

Alternatively, a 5 mm harmonic scalpel can be passed through the trocar at the sternal notch and used to coagulate and divide the parathyroid vascular pedicle.

3.10 Extraction of the Specimen

A small sac fashioned by removing the thumb portion of a surgical glove and placing a pursestring on the opening is introduced through the 5 mm trocar. The specimen is then placed into the sac and the pursestring pulled to ensure tight closure of the opening during the extraction. The free tails of the pursestring are then grabbed and pulled through the trocar at the sternal notch by using a grasper forceps. The trocar is then removed and the sac extracted through the port site incision, which may need to be slightly enlarged to accommodate the specimen (Fig. 12).

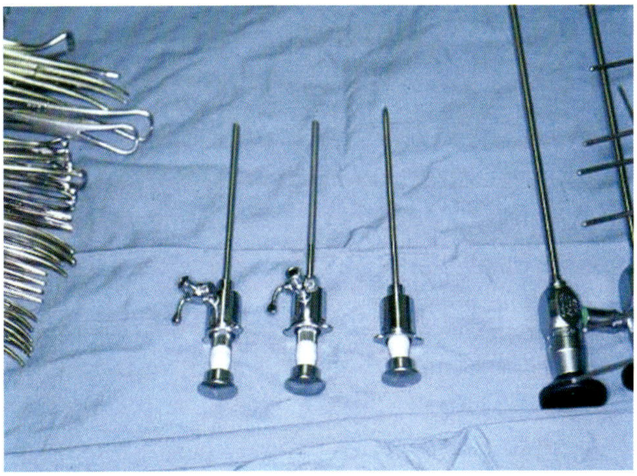

Figure 1 Trocars of 3 mm (Karl Storz Endoscopy of America, Culver City, CA).

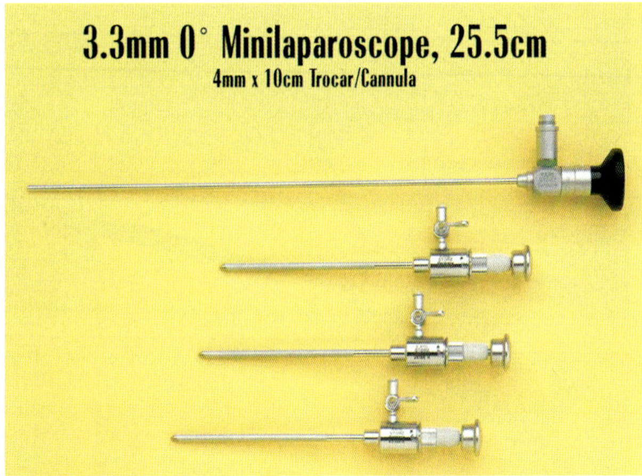

Figure 3 Endoscope of 3.3 mm (Karl Storz Endoscopy of America, Culver City, CA).

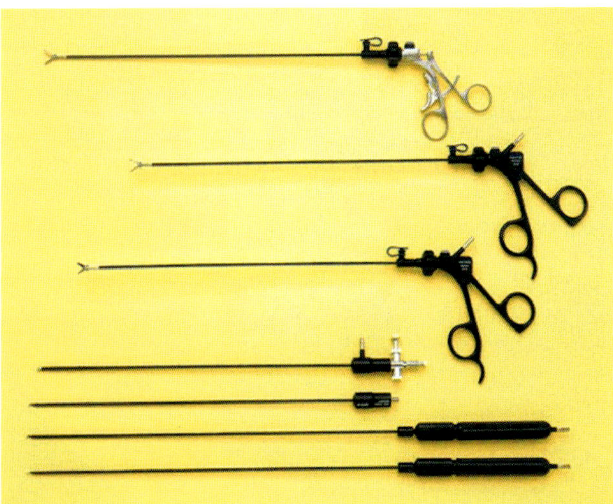

Figure 2 Instruments of 3 mm (Karl Storz Endoscopy of America, Culver City, CA).

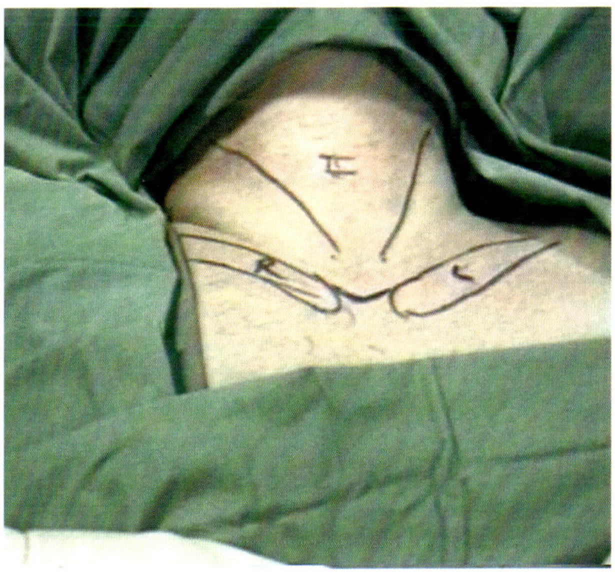

Figure 4 Neutral cervical position.

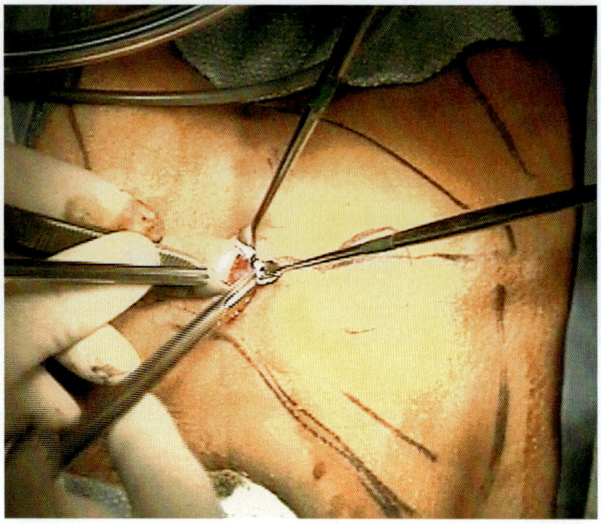

Figure 5 Small transverse incision for a lateral approach, anterior to the sternocleidomastoid muscle.

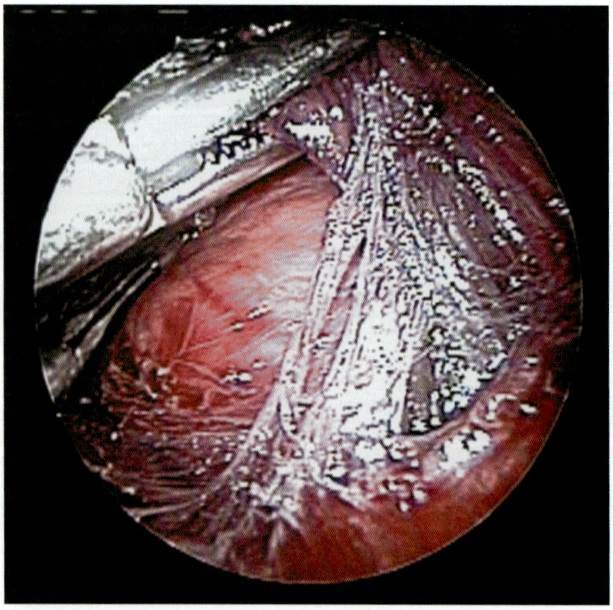

Figure 6 Creation of the space, deeper plane under the platysma muscle.

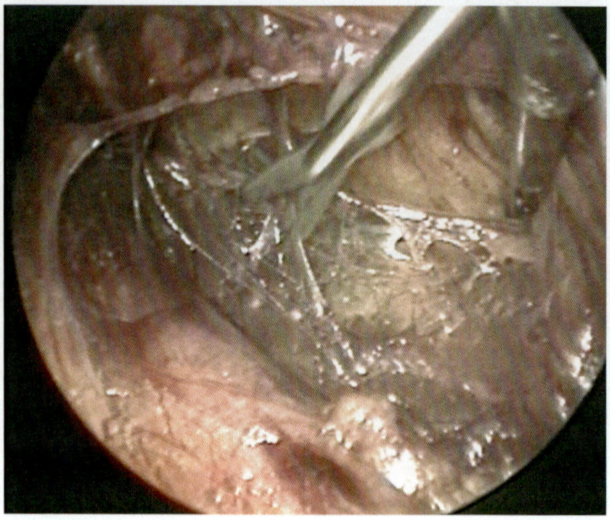

Figure 7 Dissection medial to the cartoid sheath, near the tracheo-esophageal groove.

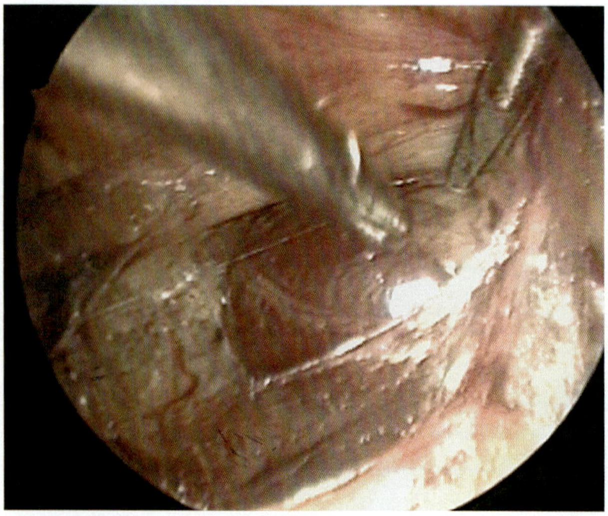

Figure 8 Dissection of a parathyroid adenoma by blunt dissection around the capsule.

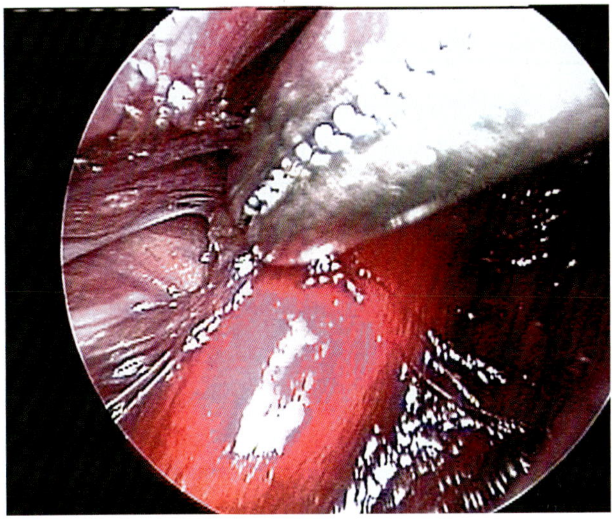

Figure 9 Identification of the recurrent laryngeal nerve on the right side.

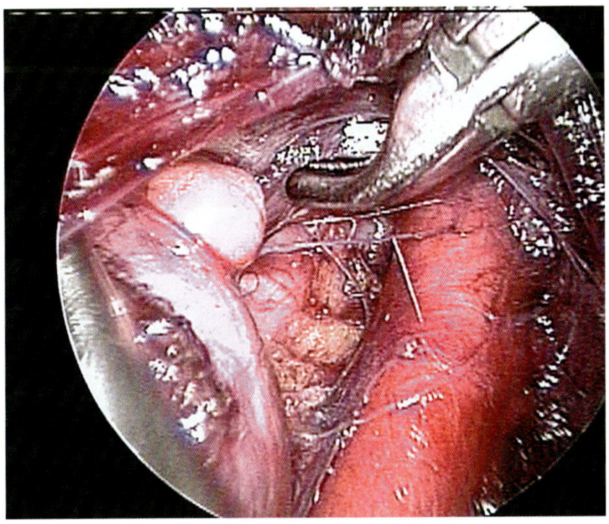

Figure 10 Identification of a normal ipsilateral parathyroid gland.

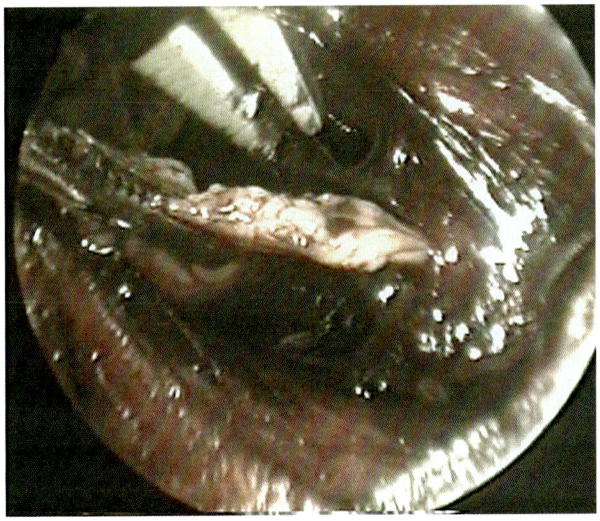

Figure 11 Ligating the blood supply, parathyroid artery and vein, with a 5 mm titanium clip.

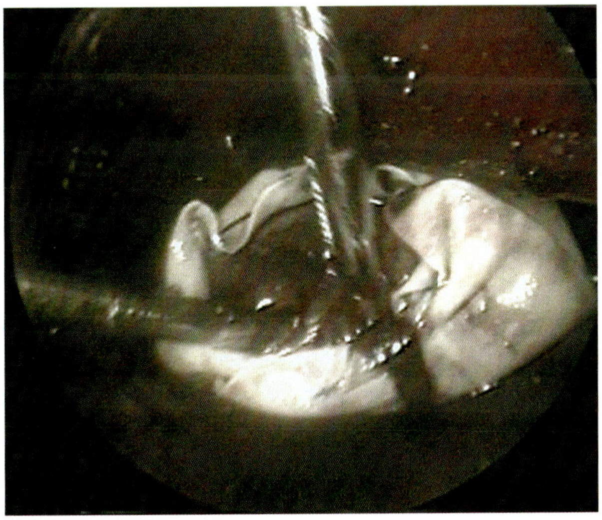

Figure 12 Extraction performed with a latex bag (tip of a glove with a polene pursestring.

3.11 End of the Procedure

After extraction of the specimen, the trocar is reinserted at the sternal notch and exploration of the working cavity is carefully performed to check hemostasis and integrity of other cervical structures. Routine use of drains is unnecessary. The neck is then desufflated and trocars removed (Fig. 12).

Two blood samples are obtained at 10 and 20 minutes from the ligature of the parathyroid peduncle and quick PTH assay (QPTH) performed to verify that at least a 50% decrease of preoperative hormonal levels is achieved. The specimen is submitted for frozen section analysis to confirm extraction of parathyroid adenomatous tissue.

If results of QPTH and frozen section are consistent with successful removal of parathyroid adenoma, the operation can be concluded and the skin incision closed. Steri-strips are used to close the incisions at the 2–3 mm port sites, while the incision of the 5 mm trocar can be closed either by steri-strips or by using a subcuticular 4/0 absorbable suture. The latter is recommended in case the incision is enlarged to accommodate the specimen during extraction.

4 POSTOPERATIVE MANAGEMENT

A test for possible bleeding at the conclusion of the parathyroidectomy should be performed. The head can be tilted down and the lungs hyperinflated by the anesthetist to increase intrathoracic pressure as well as blood pressure in the neck veins. Patients should be observed for several hours after surgery, with head and shoulders elevated 10–20 degrees, if necessary, to keep a negative pressure in the veins. Vocal cord dysfunction should be ruled out with laryngoscopy during extubation.

After extubation, the patient should be observed for a few hours to ensure that recovery from anesthesia is uneventful and to monitor other possible sequelae of neck carbon dioxide insufflation. Continuous end-tidal monitoring is suggested during the operation. Arterial blood gas determination could be necessary in the first few hours postoperatively in patients who develop hypercarbia intraoperatively, since it has been shown that increased values of Pa_{CO_2} may persist as long as 2 hours after desufflation.

Patients should have one determination of serum calcium and magnesium levels during the first 12 hours postoperatively and then once a day at least for the following 2–3 days to monitor for possible hypoparathyroidism.

5 CLINICAL OUTCOMES AND ADVANTAGES OF MINIMALLY INVASIVE NECK SURGERY

Despite the increasing interest in minimally invasive neck surgery over the last few years, published series are relatively small and do not allow firm conclusions to be drawn as to whether the minimally invasive approach results in significant improvements in clinical outcomes compared to open surgery. Nevertheless, several hundred patients have been reported to have undergone minimally invasive neck surgery over the last 3 years (11), and some conclusions can therefore be made about the feasibility, safety, reported and/or potential complications, as well as advantages and future developments.

5.1 Feasibility

Feasibility of a minimally invasive approach for surgery of the parathyroid and thyroid has been well demonstrated. The technical difficulty and endoscopic skills required for performance of these operations vary greatly depending on the technique utilized. Both unilateral and bilateral explorations have been showed to be feasible by both videoassisted (9) and pure endoscopic technique (12).

5.2 Safety and Complications

In general, the complication rate for minimally invasive parathyroidectomy seems to be as low as that of traditional surgery (13). Most reported series of minimally invasive neck surgery show a rate of recurrent nerve palsies of <1% (14,15), which compares favorably with the results of the most important series of conventional techniques reported over the last 10 years (16,17).

An important issue when dealing with parathyroid surgery for HPT is the risk of persistent and recurrent disease. Miccoli reported 1.6% persistent disease in a series of 200 patients undergoing videoassisted parathyroidectomy (13). Other series of endoscopic procedures also show overall cure rates comparable to standard bilateral open exploration (17,18), possibly due to the use of intraoperative use of PTH, which has been shown to minimize the number of persistent PHPT. Since persistence of disease is not increased by minimally invasive techniques, it seems reasonable to expect that long-term recurrences will not be increased either.

Postoperative hypocalcemia is a well-known risk of parathyroidectomy. Reported rates of postoperative symptomatic hypocalcemia after minimally invasive parathyroidectomy can be as low as 4–6% (13,18). This apparently lower risk of developing postoperative hypocalcemia after minimally invasive procedures may be due to the lesser extent of dissection or a less invasive approach to the parathyroid gland, avoiding any gland biopsy.

Sustained supraventricular tachycardia, subcutaneous emphysema, and increased levels of arterial CO_2 and acidosis have been regarded as specific complications of the pure endoscopic technique (19). Severe acidosis and hypercapnia may theoretically have a negative inotropic effect on myocardial cells (20) and produce a decrease in peripheral vascular resistance. Despite this potential risk, most recently published clinical series (21,22) have not reported these complications. The use of a lower CO_2 insufflation level with respect to the early reports may explain this. Our experiments in a large animal model suggest that insufflation of CO_2 at 15 and 20 mmHg may cause significant increase in central venous pressure as well as increased values of intracranial pressure. Insufflation pressure up to 10 mmHg does not cause significant changes in intracranial pressure levels or significant hemodynamic alterations (23,24).

Subcutaneous emphysema has been reported to follow gas insufflation for endoscopic neck surgery (19). In our experience, it seems to be caused by both high levels of insufflation pressure and the modality of initial dissection. It may also caused by the development of pneumomediastinum. Subcutaneous emphysema might play an important role in the mechanism of production of hypercarbia because it increases the total gas exchange area.

Reducing the level of insufflation pressure may reduce the passage of gas in the subcutaneous tissue. The creation of a working space below the strap muscle may also thicken the anatomical barrier to absorption of CO_2 in the subcutaneous tissue.

5.3 Advantages

Demonstrating the advantages of minimally invasive techniques for parathyroid surgery is not easy. Unlike abdominal operations, conventional procedures for surgery of the neck are generally associated with very low morbidity, almost zero mortality, and early discharge from the hospital, often allowing for "same-day surgery" or performance of surgery under local anesthesia. It is difficult to challenge these results with a new technique and more difficult to document that the new one is advantageous. Furthermore, most advantages of the minimally invasive neck approach consist of subjective aspects, such as satisfaction with the scar and level of postoperative distress, which are difficult to measure and use reliably as an endpoint in comparative studies.

Nevertheless, one prospective randomized study demonstrated that video-assisted parathyroidectomy results in significantly better cosmesis and decreased postoperative pain (25). Another randomized study reported similar results for video-assisted thyroidectomy (26). Pure endoscopic thyroidectomy has been also associated with earlier return to work (22).

Minimally invasive neck surgery has other potential advantages. The magnification provided by the endoscope improves visualization of anatomical details that may theoretically result in decreased incidence of injuries (27). However, due to the low incidence of morbidity with conventional techniques, this hypothesis needs much larger series to be tested and verified.

The pure endoscopic technique for parathyroidectomy seems to be more time consuming than either the conventional approach and the video-assisted gasless technique. The longer operative time represents, at present, the most important drawback of endoscopic parathyroidectomy. It is, however, reasonable to expect that, with more experience and dedicated surgical instruments, endoscopic parathyroidectomy may become easier and faster. Increased experience with endoscopic parathyroidectomy should make surgeons more confident about using this approach, and such confidence could extend beyond the performance of parathyroid and thyroid surgery. The endoscopic approach, in fact, allows a wider exposure of cervical structures than video-assisted gasless techniques, as these are more targeted on the parathyroid and thyroid gland. The insufflation of the neck with CO_2 creates a larger working cavity in which structures can be identified without distortion due to mechanic retraction. The lack of a fixed angle of view, as in the video-assisted techniques, also makes it possible to follow anatomical landmarks which can be dissected when needed. For this reason, the pure endoscopic approach lends itself better than other minimally invasive techniques to other operations, such as for cervical spine and carotid artery surgery, whose feasibility we have recently reported in an experimental model (28,29).

There is no doubt that future technological developments, in particular the availability of dedicated instruments of small diameter and appropriate length, can dramatically improve the technique of endoscopic parathyroidectomy.

6 CONCLUSIONS

The results of published experimental studies and clinical series provide evidence that endoscopic parathyroidectomy is feasible and safe. This minimally invasive approach has better cosmetic results and the potential to decrease morbidity and allow earlier return to work activity. Larger experience and comparative studies are needed to assess its specific role in the management of parathyroid diseases. Technical difficulties may be overcome as experience increases and specific instrumentation becomes available. Experience in preoperative management of hyperparathyroidism and detailed knowledge of cervical anatomy remain the key for successful treatment of primary hyperparathyroidism.

REFERENCES

1. Gagner M. Endoscopic subtotal parathyroidectomy in patients with primary hyperparathyroidism. Br J Surg 1996; 83(6):875.
2. Huscher CS, Recher A, Napolitano G, Chiodini S. Endoscopic right thyroid lobectomy. Surg Endosc 1997; 11:877.
3. Shimizu K, Akira S, Jasmi A Y, Kitamura Y, Kitagawa W, Akasu H, Tanaka S. Video-assisted neck surgery: endoscopic resection of thyroid tumors with a very minimal neck wound. J Am Coll Surg 1999; 188(6):697–703.
4. Video-assisted neck surgery: endoscopic resection of thyroid tumors with a very minimal neck wound. J Am Coll Surg 1999; 188(6):697–703.
5. Chowbey PK, Mann VI, Khullar R, Sharma A, Baijal M, Vashistha A. Endoscopic neck surgery: expanding horizons. J Laparoendosc Adv Surg Tech A 1999; 9(5):397–400.
6. Brunt LM, Jones DB, Wu JS, Quasebarth MA, Meininger T, Soper NJ. Experimental development of an endoscopic approach to neck exploration and parathyroidectomy. Surgery 1997; 122(5):893–901.
7. Okido M, Shimizu S, Kuroki S, Goto K, Yokohata K, Uchiyama A, Mizumoto K, Tanaka M. Video-assisted parathyroidectomy by a skin-lifting method for primary hyperparathyroidism. JSLS 2001; 5(2):197–200.
8. Ikeda Y, Takami H, Sasaki Y, Kan S, Niimi M. Endoscopic neck surgery by the axillary approach. J Am Coll Surg 2000; 191(3):336–340.
9. Miccoli P, Bendinelli C, Vignali E, Mazzeo S, Cecchini GM, Pinchera A, Marcocci C. Endoscopic parathyroidectomy: report of an initial experience. Surgery 1998; 124(6): 1077–1079.
10. Henry JF, Defechereux T, Gramatica L, de Boissezon C. Minimally invasive videoscopic parathyroidectomy by lateral approach. Langenbecks Arch Surg 1999; 384(3): 298–301.
11. Miccoli P, Monchik JM. Minimally invasive parathyroid surgery. Surg Endosc 2000; 14(11):987–990.
12. Cougard P, Goudet P, Bilosi M, Peschaud F. Videoendoscopic approach for parathyroid adenomas: results of a prospective study of 100 patients. Ann Chir 2001; 126(4): 314–319.
13. Miccoli P. Minimally invasive surgery for thyroid and parathyroid diseases. Surg Endosc Online publication, October 31, 2001.
14. Lorenz K, Nguyen-Thanh P, Dralle H. Unilateral open and minimally invasive procedures for primary hyperparathyroidism: a review of selective approaches. Langenbecks Arch Surg 2000; 385(2):106–117.
15. Miccoli P, Berti P, Conte M, Raffaelli M, Materazzi G. Minimally invasive video-assisted parathyroidectomy: lesson learned from 137 cases. J Am Coll Surg 2000; 191(6): 613–618.
16. Carty SE, Worsey J, Virji MA, Brown ML, Watson CG. Concise parathyroidectomy: the impact of preoperative SPECT 99mTc sestamibi scanning and intraoperative quick parathormone assay. Surgery 1997; 122(6):1107–1116.
17. Duh QY, Uden P, Clark OH. Unilateral neck exploration for primary hyperparathyroidism: analysis of a controversy using a mathematical model. World J Surg 1992; 16(4): 654–662.
18. Lorenz K, Miccoli P, Monchik JM, Duren M, Dralle H. Minimally invasive video-assisted parathyroidectomy: multiinstitutional study. World J Surg 2001; 25(6):704–707.
19. Gottlieb A, Sprung J, Zheng XM, Gagner M. Massive subcutaneous emphysema and severe hypercarbia in a patient during endoscopic transcervical parathyroidectomy using carbon dioxide insufflation. Anesth Analg 1997; 84(5): 1154–1156.
20. Van den Bos GC, Drake AJ, Noble MI. The effect of carbon dioxide upon myocardial contractile performance, blood flow and oxygen consumption. J Physiol 1979; 287: 149–161.
21. Ochiai R, Takeda J, Noguchi J, Ohgami M, Ishii S. Subcutaneous carbon dioxide insufflation does not cause hypercarbia during endoscopic thyroidectomy. Anesth Analg 2000; 90(3):760–762.
22. Gagner M, Inabnet WB III. Endoscopic thyroidectomy for solitary thyroid nodules. Thyroid 2001; 11(2):161–163.
23. Bellantone R, Lombardi CP, Rubino F, Perilli W, Sollazzi L, Mastroianni G, Gagner M. Arterial PCO_2 and cardiovascular function during endoscopic neck surgery with CO_2 insufflation. Arch Surg 2001; 136(7): 822–827.
24. Rubino F, Pamoukian VN, Zhu JF, Deutsch H, Inabnet WB, Gagner M. Endoscopic endocrine neck surgery with carbon dioxide insufflation: the effect on intracranial

pressure in a large animal model. Surgery 2000; 128(6): 1035–1042.
25. Miccoli P, Bendinelli C, Berti P, Vignali E, Pinchera A, Marcocci C. Video-assisted versus conventional parathyroidectomy in primary hyperparathyroidism: a prospective randomized study. Surgery 1999; 126(6):1117–1122.
26. Miccoli P, Berti P, Raffaelli M, Materazzi G, Baldacci S, Rossi G. Comparison between minimally invasive video-assisted thyroidectomy and conventional thyroidectomy: a prospective randomized study. Surgery 2001; 130(6): 1039–1043.
27. Naitoh T, Gagner M, Garcia-Ruiz A, Heniford BT. Endoscopic endocrine surgery in the neck. An initial report of endoscopic subtotal parathyroidectomy. Surg Endosc 1998; 12(3):202–206.
28. Rubino F, Deutsch H, Pamoukian V, Zhu JF, King WA, Gagner M. Minimally invasive spine surgery: an animal model for endoscopic approach to the anterior cervical and upper thoracic spine. J Laparoendosc Adv Surg Tech A 2000; 10(6):309–313.
29. Rubino F, Nahouraii R, Deutsch H, King WA, Inabnet WB, Gagner M. Endoscopic approach for carotid artery surgery. Surg Endosc 2002; 16(5):789–794.

23

Video-Assisted Parathyroidectomy in the Management of Patients with Primary Hyperparathyroidism

Jean François Henry and Frédéric Sebag

Hôpital de la Timone, Marseille, France

1 INTRODUCTION

In 1925, Felix Mandel of Vienna published the first successful case of parathyroidectomy (1). The following three decades have been marked by a rapid worldwide acceptance of this procedure by most surgeons, because specific steps of the procedure have been well described. Presently, during the first intervention for primary hyperparathyroidism, an endocrine surgeon can assure his or her patient of a successfull outcome in more than 95% of cases when all four glands are explored through a transverse cervicotomy (2). Failures have been observed in patients with multiglandular disease, supernumerary glands, major ectopia, or exceptionally a rare carcinoma. Not only can we expect no mortality and a very low morbidity from this surgery, but also a short hospital stay of less than 48 hours, with an excellent cosmetic outcome in most patients.

We have recently seen the appearance of several new techniques for parathyroidectomy: the unilateral approach (3–5), radioguided surgery (6,7), open minimally invasive techniques (mini-incision with or without local anesthesia) (8–10), and minimally invasive video-assisted or fully endoscopic (11–21). The common threads among these techniques are (a) they all have a limited incision when compared to classic open transverse cervical incision, and (b) the surgery is targeted on one specific parathyroid gland. In most cases the exploration of other glands is not performed or is limited. These conceivable minimally invasive interventions are successfuly performed for three main reasons. First, the available imaging techniques permit us to localize with precision most adenomas to be excised. Second, the use of rapid intraoperative parathyroid hormone (PTH) assay (rPTH) can confirm the succesful extirpation of the diseased gland, obviating exploring others. Finally, new instrumentation and miniaturized cameras have been adapted for this kind of surgery. Let us add also that parathyroidectomy performed with minimally invasive techniques is well suited because of the lack of elaborate surgical reconstruction, where suturing would be needed, whereas only simple removal of a small benign tumor is necessary. Also, patients reluctant to have a visible scar in the neck prefer this technique. Since 1998 we have proposed a video-assisted parathyroidectomy (VAP) technique to some of our patients with primary hyperparathyroidism.

2 PATIENTS AND METHODS

During a 5-year period (1998–2002) we operated on 528 patients with primary hyperparathyroidism in the division of endocrine surgery at Hopital de la Timone in Marseille. Major contraindications included the presence of a large goiter or previous thyroid/parathyroid surgery. All cases of sporadic primary hyperparathyroidism had a cervical ultrasonography and a MIBI scan performed preoperatively to confirm the solitary character of the lesion. Two video-assisted approaches were used: lateral (22) and central (23).

3 TECHNIQUE

For video-assisted parathyroidectomy using the lateral approach, the endoscopic instrumentation is as follows: one 10–12 mm trocars and two 2.5 mm trocars; a 2 mm guide stick on which the 2.5 mm trocars can be adapted; and various 2 mm instruments (grasper, dissector, scissors, palpator, canula for suction). These instruments measure 25 cm in length. Endoscopic visualization is performed with a 10 mm 0° endoscope (Fig. 1).

All three trocars are positioned on the line of the anterior border of the sternocleidomastoid muscle (SCM). The procedure is performed in three steps: the procedure starts open (Fig. 2). A 15 mm transverse skin incision is made on the anterior border of the SCM, just caudad to the cricoid cartilage. Dissection should start in the plane between the anterior border of the SCM and the posterior border of the strap muscles, just below the omohyoid muscle. Then the fascia connecting the posterior aspect of the thyroid lobe to the carotid sheath is gently divided with scissors far enough to visualize the prevertebral fascia. In order to enlarge the working area, one or two small humid swabs are stuffed, upward and downward, deeply into the initially created space. This blind maneuver allows a surprisingly quick, efficient, and bloodless exposure of the operative field.

The transparietal path of the 2.5 mm trocar is made through the incision, from the inside to the outside, using a guide stick. The pathway of the guide stick must follow the anterior border of the SCM. Then the 2.5 mm trocars are adapted to the guide stick, to be put into place in the initially created space (Fig. 3).

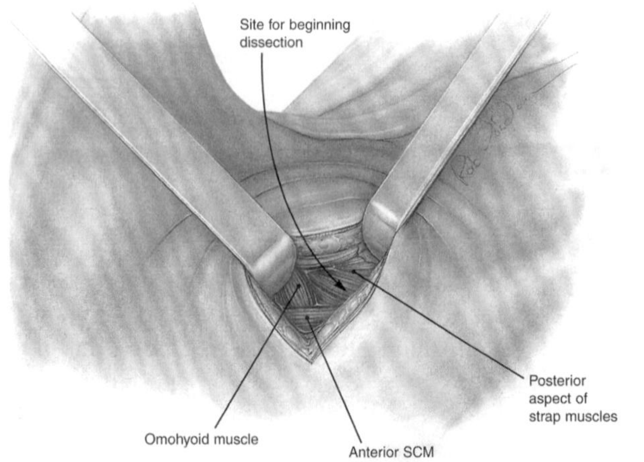

Figure 2 Space creation between the carotid sheath.

A purse-string suture is placed around the 15 mm transverse skin incision. It will prevent both gas leakage and the 10 mm trocar from slipping out of the wound. The purse-string suture is tightened around the trocar, into which is inserted a 10 mm 0° endoscopic camera. Carbon dioxide is insufflated to 8 mmHg. The assistant takes care of the endoscope and the surgeon works through the other two trocars (Fig. 4).

The second step of the operation is the endoscopic exploration. Immediately after introducing the endoscope and with a minimum of dissection, all anatomial structures can be easily identified. The recurrent laryngeal nerve should be searched for first (Fig. 5). If possible, the ipsilateral gland should also be checked (Fig. 6). During this endoscopic dissection, ligatures or clip applications are not necessary. The adenoma is progressively dissected from adjacent structures and more particularly from the recurrent laryngeal nerve (Fig. 7). When its pedicle is isolated, it is not necessary to continue the endoscopic dissection.

After removing the three trocars, the third step of the procedure is performed, again openly. Directly through the largest trocar site, the thyroid lobe is retracted medially and anteriorly. The adenoma is visualized and its pedicle can be ligated or clipped without any difficulty. The adenoma is extracted from the neck directly through the incision (Fig. 8). There is no need to place it in a sterile plasic bag. Draining is not necessary. This approach, initially proposed to all patients, has now been used principally for adenomas located behind the thyroid lobe.

The central approach is now reserved for adenomas localized much inferiorly near the thymus from a 15 mm transverse incision in the suprasternal notch. Through this incision, conventional instruments like retractors and dissectors are used to isolate the inferior parathyroid glands under the strap muscles, with video-assisted images of an endoscope (5 mm, 0° or 30°) in the incision. All maneuvers are therefore performed openly without the need of gas insufflation. This dissection is anterior to the trachea, mostly in the thymus and thyreothymic ligaments, and does not necessitate identification of the recurrent laryngeal nerve, which is posterior.

A rapid PTH assay was used to confirm a succesfull VAP on all patients. Blood was drawn at the time of intubation, first skin incision, adenoma extraction, and 5–15 minutes after extirpation. The highest pre-excision level of rPTH falling more than 50% was con-

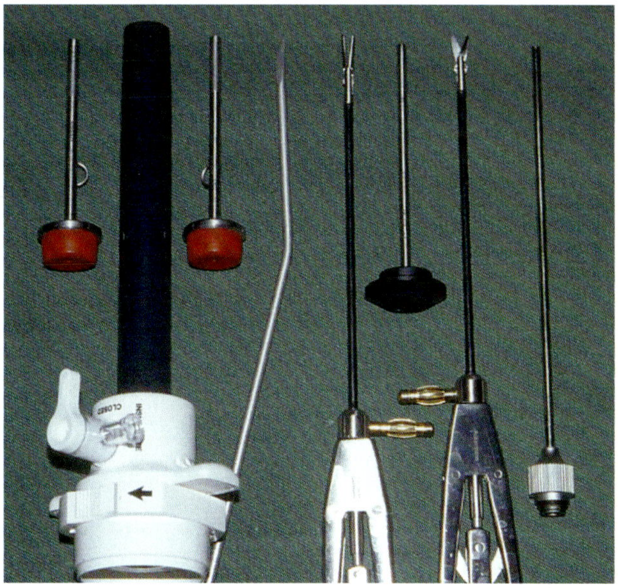

Figure 1 Instrumentation for video-assisted parathyroidectomy.

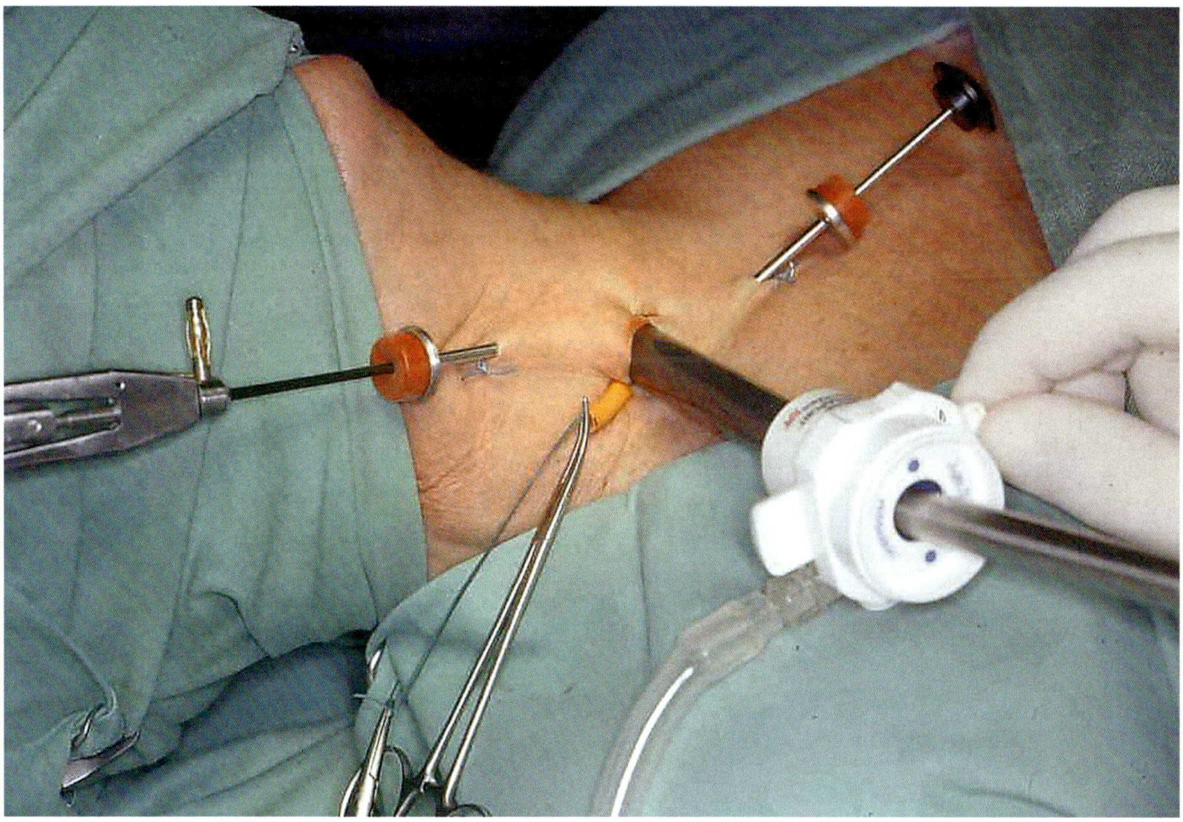

Figure 4 Trocar position for a lateral view.

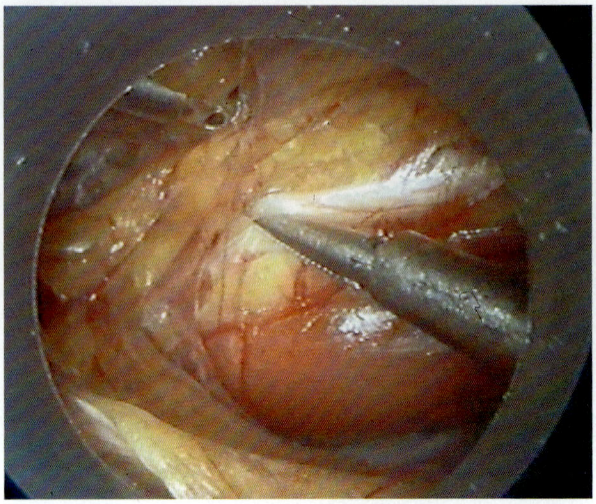

Figure 5 Identification of a recurrent laryngeal nerve.

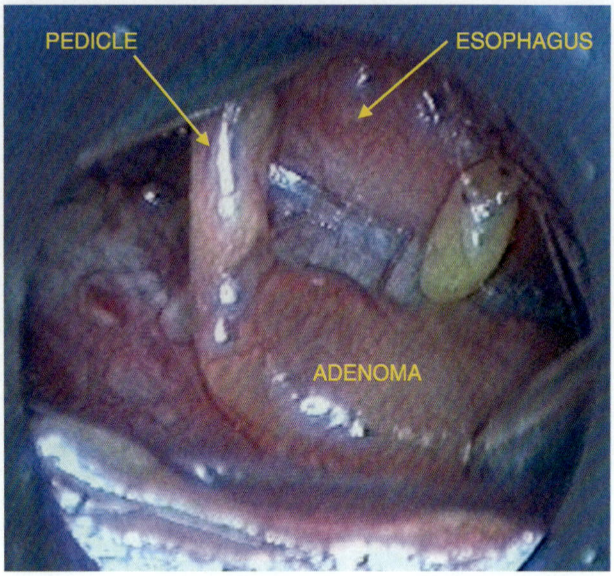

Figure 7 Dissection of a superior parathyroid adenoma.

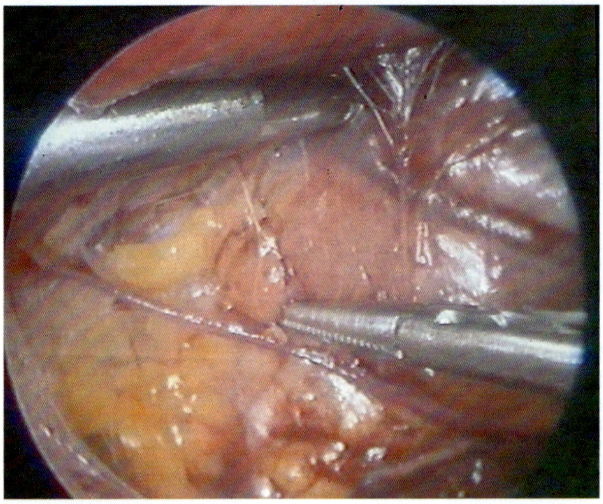

Figure 6 Identification of a normal left parathyroid gland.

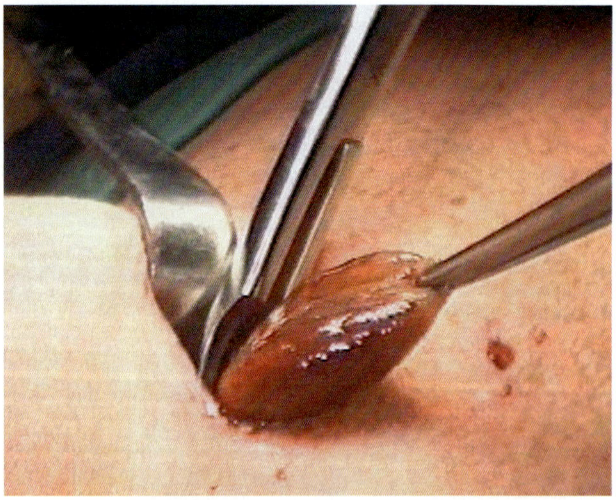

Figure 8 Extraction process.

(a)

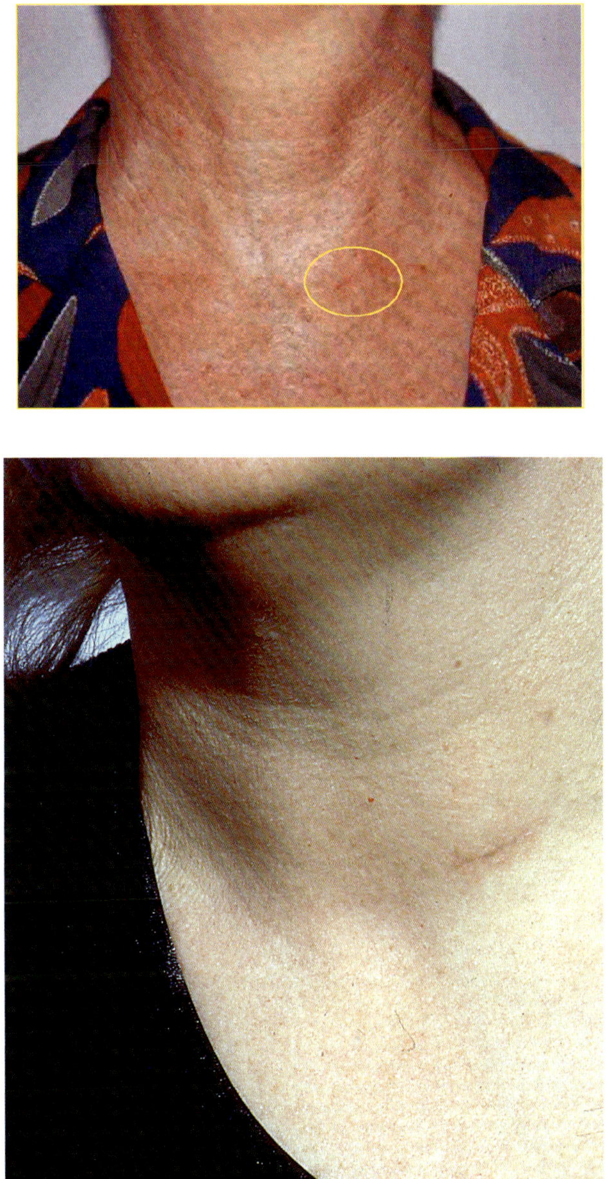

(b)

Figure 9 (a) Cervical scar after 1 week. (b) Cervical scar after 1 month.

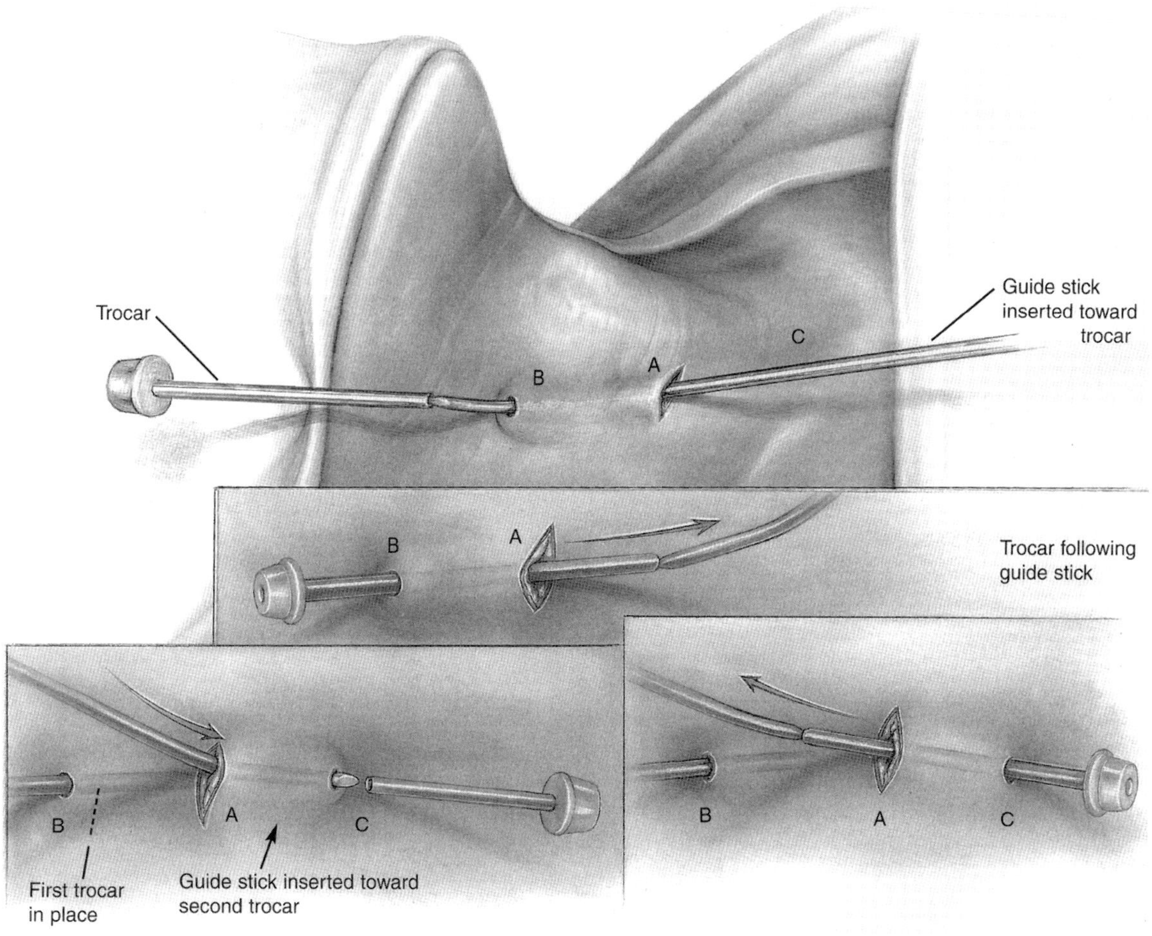

Figure 3 Trocar positions (2.5 mm).

sidered significant. Other biochemical tests performed included serum calcium, serum phosphorus, and serum PTH on the first postoperative day, 1 week, and 1 year later. Vocal cord mobility was also assessed pre- and postoperatively.

4 RESULTS

Of the 528 surgical patients, 228 (43%) had a conventional open approach and 300 (57%) a video-assisted technique. Patients who underwent an open approach had some contraindications to a minimally invasive approach: mostly a large multinodular goiter that needed an associated thyroidectomy in 99 cases, previous cervical surgery in 42 cases, suspicion of multiglandular disease in 25 cases, inconclusive localizing studies in 48 cases, and other reasons in 14 cases (Table 1).

VAP was performed in 300 patients (233 women and 67 men) with a median age of 60 years. All of these patients had a sporadic primary hyperparathyroidism,

Table 1 Contraindications to Video-Asssisted Parathyroidectomies in 228 Primary Hyperparathyroidisms

Associated multiglandular goiter	99
Previous cervical surgery	42
Inconclusive preop localization	48
Suspicion of multiglandular disease	25
Acute hyperparathyroidism	4
Too large lesion	4
Local anesthesia	3
Major ectopia	2
Cervical hematoma	1

removed by lateral approach most frequently in 282 cases or by a central approach in 17 cases. One interesting case was operated by thoracoscopy for a very lowly located adenoma in the anterior mediastinum, which we knew would be impossible to reach from a low transverse neck incision. Of the 17 patients who had a central approach, 2 had an associated lobar thyroidectomy.

The median operative time recorded was 50 minutes (20–130), which has been lowered to 41 minutes in the last 100 cases. Recurrent laryngeal nerves were identified in 94.6% of cases, as was the ipsilateral parathyroid gland in 63.8% of cases when a lateral approach was used. A bilateral approach was needed in 5 patients due to false-negative imaging studies (4 cases) or the presence of a double adenoma (1 case).

We were obliged to perform 10 conversions to open surgery (and one case converted to a bilateral video-assisted technique) due to multiglandular disease that was not detected by preoperative imaging (4 double adenomas and 7 hyperplasias). Among those 289 single lesions, the average weight recorded was 1087 mg (range : 100–7080 mg); 4 adenomas were atypical and 3 were malignant. Actually, the latest pathologies described needed conversions in 5 cases and reoperation by an open approach 3 months later in 1 case. Also, 42 patients (14%) had a conversion to open surgery (via a transverse cervicotomy) (Table 2). Causes for conversion included none found after 2-hour search (11 cases), large adenoma taking most of the working space (7 cases), false-positive imaging studies (11 cases), and inadequate fall of rapid PTH assay (13 cases). Interestingly, 10 of those 13 patients had a multiglandular disease during open conversion and 3 had a false-negative rapid PTH assay. Postoperative morbidity included permanent recurrent laryngeal nerve damage in one patient, two hematomas in the sternocleidomastoid muscle, and five capsular tears necessitating a conversion. These capsular disruptions are believed to occur in large and fragile adenomas weighing on average 4200 mg (range : 750–6800 mg). There was no mortality, and most patients are discharged without morbidity from the hospital the next day. Two patients were left with hypercalcemia—one after ablation of a 280 mg adenoma [calcium : 2.75 mmol/L (*N*: 2.20–2.60) and PTH: 12 pg/mL (*N*: 10–55)] and the other after ablation of a 450 mg adenoma (calcium: 2.78 mmol/L; PTH: 60 pg/mL). Persistent hyperparathyroidism is suspected in the first patient; another cause of hypercalcemia is likely in the second patient. With a median follow-up of 20.5 months, one of 150 patients had recurrent hypercalcemia (Calcium: 2.68 mmol/L; PTH: 64 pg/mL) after removal of a 600 mg adenoma, where for 15 months she had normal serum calcium levels.

Table 2 Causes for Conversions in 42 Cases from 300 Video-Assisted Parathyroidectomies

Adenomas not found	11
Difficult dissections	7
Multiglandular disease	10[a]
False-negative rPTH	3
False-positive MIBI	10
False-positive U/S	1

RPTH: rapid parathyroid hormone assay; MIBI: methyl-iodo-benzyl iguanine nuclear scan; U/S: cervical ultrasonography.
[a] Diagnosed by rPTH.

5 DISCUSSION

We find it appropriate to cluster all interventions of parathyroid glands where the surgeon is using an endoscope, either during the full intervention or part of it, under the term "endoscopic parathyroidectomy or video-assisted technique." The first application of the endoscope in parathyroid surgery was described for the removal of mediastinal parathyroid adenomas by thoracoscopy (24). In these rare cases of major ectopia, the advantages to the patient are irrefutable. However, the same advantages are more difficult to demonstrate for all cervical approaches. Two studies comparing conventional parathyroid surgery to endoscopic techniqes have clearly shown a diminution of postoperative pain and better cosmetic results with endoscopic techniques (25,26) (Fig. 9). Those results await confirmation by randomized studies, and their use in parathyroidectomy remains controversial.

From our own experience, we judge the use of endoscopic techniques superior because they provide a greater and better surgical image, with magnification of all anatomical structures normally encountered in conventional open surgery. It is probably more difficult to get an adequate view of structures through mini-incisions that do not use an endoscope, and it is our belief that optimal conditions for exploration are not met even if those surgeons use frontal lamps and surgical loops.

We found a permanent recurrent laryngeal nerve injury, which of course we deplore, and think is mechanism of injury was probably due to damage during the extraction process. As the nerve was properly identified during the earlier dissection surrounding the adenoma, but not the pedicle, the accident must have occurred during the open part of the operation through the mini-incision, where the pedicle is ligated.

According to our experience, not all patients presenting with primary hyperparathyroidism are candidates for this surgery. Contraindications are mainly due to a large goiter, previous surgery in the parathyroid vicinity, suspicious multiglandular disease, and equivocal preoperative localizating studies. Depending upon the operator's experience and according to the specific technique utilized, these contraindications can become relative. The central approach appears to be the best one for cases where a bilateral exploration is anticipated or if localization is uncertain. According to certain authors, more than 60% of patients with primary hyperparathyroidism are candidates for video-assisted parathyroidectomy (27,28).

Occasionally one can performed a video-assisted technique by lateral approach in patients who had a previous low transverse neck incision. In this series, 7 patients were operated without difficulties: 5 after previous thyroid operations on the contralateral side and 2 after previous tracheostomy. Large adenomas (>3 cm) should not be considered an absolute contraindication, especially if situated in the postero-superior mediastinum. The pedicle is easily dissected at the level of the inferior thyroid artery, and their shape is amenable to expeditious extraction. With limited experience, some surgeons can encounter major difficulties while dissecting voluminous adenomas, which may lead to a capsular rupture and local seeding of parathyroid adenomatous cells. When this happens, we suggest a conversion. In the five cases where this occurred, we have seen no signs of reccurence, and we continue to follow these patients closely for any signs.

Absolute contraindications remain the presence of a carcinomatous parathyroid gland and/or a voluminous goiter, no matter the experience of the surgeon or type of endoscopic technique employed.

The percentage of patients with a proper indication for VAP has not changed through the years: it was 56.7% for our first 166 cases (29), and is now 57%.

The lateral approach is the procedure of choice in most cases because it provides the best access to the posterior aspect of the ipsilateral thyroid lobe. The working space is easily created with minimal dissection and maintained with low CO_2 pressure at 8 mmHg. We have not seen subcutaneous emphysema or pneumomediastinum. The lateral approach also permits a complete exploration of all anatomical elements present in this retro-thyroidal area from the superior pedicle to the postero-superior mediastinum. It is therefore applicable in all cases where the parathyroid lesion is located posteriorly, meaning superior parathyroid glands, since their enlargement pushes them to migrate posteriorly and slides along the prevertebral plane next to the lateral esophageal border. The lateral approach is also ideal for inferior parathyroid glands located posterior to the inferior poles of the thyroid lobe. It is in these cases that they become intimate with the recurrent laryngeal nerve. The lateral view permits an easy identification of the nerve abutting the adenoma, and therefore allows a secure dissection.

However, for inferior peri-thymic locations, we tend to prefer the central approach. Because of their anterior locations, one can easlily reach them with a suprastrenal insicion, between the superficial muscles. Early in our experience, for glands situated near the thymus, we have experienced the lateral approach. In 6 out of 11 attempts we had to convert because we could not find the adenoma.

The surgeon is dependent upon the quality of preoperative imaging to make a judicious choice for a VAP. Once contraindications have been eliminated, all patients with sporadic primary hyperparathyroidism are considered candidates for this approach. The choices between approaches is dependent on the quality and adequate interpretation of preoperative imaging studies. For example, if the cervical ultrasonography and the nuclear scan do not correlate with a unique lesion at the same site, we recommend a traditional open cervical transverse incision. However, if the lesion is unique and confirmed by both studies, then depending on a posterior or anterior location and superior or inferior site, we will choose a central or lateral approach.

In this cohort of 300 patients with VAP, the sensitivity of cervical ultrasonography was determined to be 60.2% and for MIBI nuclear scan 89.3%. We know that ultrasonographic results are operator dependent and that MIBI scanning was a strong condition for a successful VAP and therefore could explain some skewed results from a predetermined process. When a global analysis of imaging is done, we find that 21 of 42 conversions were caused by erroneous imaging results: 10 multiglandular disease undetected, 10 false-positive MIBI scans, and 1 false-positive ultrasound (table 2). The risk of multiglandularity is nearly zero when both studies are positive for the same lesion site. This has been found to be 3.6% when only one exploration is positive versus 31.6% when both are negative. Even if the risk is low, we think that the use of intraoperative rPTH is justified. We had 11 cases of nonsuspected multiglandular disease which were correctly identified by an absence of the typical decrease in rPTH after one gland ablation. However, one of our patients has a persistent primary hyperparathyroidism, and we also suspect a recurrent disease in another case. In two cases we saw an adequate 50% fall in the rate of rPTH. We have found that interpretation of rPTH is not always evident, especially when one deals with moderate renal insufficiency. Three of our conversions have been in cases with a false-negative rate of rPTH, where normal glands were found on open exploration with normal recovering levels of PTH in the immediate postoperative period.

Unfortunately, we cannot compare results of those operated with an open technique with those of a VAP because they have been performed in different patients. However, we know that our results have been similar to our previous series of conventional traditional open pararthyroidectomies before the arrival of minimally invasive techniques (30). It is still too soon to evaluate the recurrence rate of these new techniques, which must be compared with an already very low, practically nonexistent rate of recurrent primary hyparparathyroidism following open surgery for a solitary lesion.

6 CONCLUSION

Contrary to open surgery, where the surgeon alone can be successful in more than 95% of cases, the video-assisted surgeon must depend on multiple technologies like special surgical instruments, rapid PTH assay intraoperatively, and preoperative specialized imaging. A cost analysis was not performed but must be part of a future prospective evaluation.

Among many minimally invasive techniques applied to parathyroidectomy, the video-assisted technique has the main advantage of offering a magnified view that permits a precise and careful dissection with minimal risks. In more than 50% of patients we are able to propose this new technique for primary hyperparathyroidism. In our experience, VAP and open surgery are complementary techniques.

If proper selection of patients is observed, the final results of video-assisted parathyroidectomy should equal those of conventional open surgery. A longer follow-up is needed before one can evaluate the real risk of recurrent or persistent hyperparathyroidism following video-assisted techniques.

ACKNOWLEDGMENTS

This manuscript was translated from French to English by Michel Gagner, M.D., Professor of Surgery at Mount Sinai School of Medicine, New York, NY.

REFERENCES

1. Mandl F. Therapeutischer Versuch bei Ostitis fribrosa generalisata mittels Extirpation eines Epithelkorpercher-tumors. Wien Klin Wschr 1925; 38:1343–1344.
2. Duh QY. Surgical approach to primary hyperparathyroidism: bilateral approach. In: Clark O, Duh QY, eds. Textbook of Endocrine Surgery. Philadelphia: Saunders, 1997:357–363.
3. Tibblin SA, Bondeson AG, Ljunberg O. Unilateral parathryoidectomy in hyperparathyroidism due to single adenoma. Ann Surg 1982; 195:245–252.
4. Russel CF, Laird JD, Fergusson WR. Scan-directed unilateral cervical exploration for parathyroid adenoma: a legitimate approach? World J Surg 1990; 14:406–409.
5. Chapuis Y, Richard B, Fulla Y, Bonnichon Ph, Tarla E, Icard Ph. Chirurgie de l'hyperparathyroïdie primaire par abord unilatéral sous anesthésie locale et dosage per opératoire de la PTH 1–84. Chirurgie 1993–1994; 119: 121–124.
6. Norman J, Chheda H. Minimally invasive parathyroidectomy facilitated by intraoperative nuclear mapping. Surgery 1997; 122:998–1004.
7. Burkey SH, Van Heerden JA, Farley DR, Thompson GB, Grant CS, Curlee KJ. Will directed parathyroidectomy utilizing the gamma probe or intraoperative parathyroid hormone assay replace bilateral cervical exploration as the preferred operation for primary hyperparathyroidism? World J Surg 2002; 26:914–920.
8. Udelsman R, Donovan PI, Sokoll LJ. One hundred consecutive minimally invasive parathyroid explorations. Ann Surg 2000; 232:331–339.
9. Inabnet WB, Biertho L. Chirurgie parathyroïdienne dirigée: une série de 100 patients consécutifs. Ann Chir 2002; 127:751–756.
10. Ikeda Y, Takami H, Tajima G, Sasaki Y, Takayama J, Kurihara H, et al. Direct mini-incision parathyroidectomy. Biomed Pharmacother 2002; 56(suppl 1):14s–17s.
11. Gagner M. Endoscopic parathyroidectomy. Br J Surg 1996; 83:875.
12. Miccoli P, Bendinelli C, Vignali E, Mazzeo S, Cecchini GM, Pinchera A, et al. Endoscopic parathyroidectomy: report of an initial experience. Surgery 1998; 124:1077–1080.
13. Henry JF, Defechereux T, Gramatica L, De Boissezon C. Parathyroïdectomie vidéo-assistée par abord latéro-cervical. Ann Chir 1999; 53:302–306.
14. Cougard P, Goudet P, Osmak L, Ferrand L, Letourneau B, Brun JM. La vidéo-cervicoscopie dans la chirurgie de l'hyperparathyroïdie primitive. Etude préliminaire portant sur 19 patients. Ann Chir 1998; 52:885–889.
15. Gauger PG, Reeve TS, Delbridge LW. Endoscopically-assisted minimally invasive parathyroidectomy. Br J Surg 1999; 86:1563–1566.
16. Duh QY. Videoscopic parathyroidectomy: rationales,

techniques, indications and contraindications. Acta Chir Austriaca 1999; 31:214–217.
17. Lorenz K, Nguyen-Thanh P, Dralle H. First experience with minimally invasive video-assisted parathyroidectomy. Acta Chir Austriaca 1999; 30:218–220.
18. Yeung GHC. Endoscopic surgery of the neck. A new frontier. Surg Laparosc Endosc 1998; 8:227–232.
19. Okido M, Shimizu S, Kuroki S, Yokohata K, Uchiyama A, Tanaka M. Video-assisted parathyroidectomy for primary hyperparathyroidism: an approach involving a skin-lifting method. Surg Endosc 2001; 15:1120–1123.
20. Ikeda Y, Takami H, Tajima G, Sasaki Y, Takayama J, Kurihara H, Niimi M. Total endoscopic parathyroidectomy. Biomed Pharmacother 2002; 56(suppl 1):22s–25s.
21. Suzuki S, Fukushima T, Ami H, Asahi S, Takenoshita S. Video-assisted parathyroidectomy. Biomed Pharmacother 2002; 56(suppl 1):18s–21s.
22. Henry JF. Endoscopic exploration. In: Van Heerden JA, Farley DR, eds. Operative Technique in General Surgery. Surgical Exploration for Hyperparathyroidism. Philadelphia: WB Saunders, 1999:49–61.
23. Miccoli P, Bendinelli C, Conte M. Endoscopic parathyroidectomy by a gasless approach. J Laparoendosc Adv Surg Tech A 1998; 8:189–194.
24. Prinz RA, Longhyna V, Carnaille B, Wurtz A, Proye C. Thoracoscopic excision of enlarged mediastinal parathyroid glands. Surgery 1994; 116:999–1004.
25. Miccoli P, Bendinelli C, Berti P, Vignali E, Pinchera A, Marcocci C. Video-assisted versus conventional parathyroidectomy in primary hyperparathyroidism: a prospective randomized study. Surgery 1999; 126:1117–1122.
26. Henry JF, Raffaelli M, Iacobone M, Volot F. Video-assisted parathyroidectomy via lateral approach versus conventional surgery in the treatment of sporadic primary hyperparathyroidism. Results of a case-control study. Surg Endosc 2001; 15:116–119.
27. Miccoli P, Berti P, Conte M, Raffaelli M, Materazzi G. Minimally invasive video-assisted parathyroidectomy: lesson learned from 137 cases. J Am Coll Surg 2000; 191: 613–618.
28. Cougard P, Goudet P, Bilosi M, Peschaud F. Exérèse vidéoendoscopique des adénomes parathyroïdiens: résultats à propos d'une série prospective de 100 patients. Ann Chirur 2001; 126:314–319.
29. Henry JF, Iacobone M, Mirallié E, Deveze A, Pili S. Indications and results of video-assisted parathyroidectomy by a lateral approach in patients with primary hyperparathyroïdism. Surgery 2001; 130:999–1004.
30. Henry JF, Denizot A, Porcelli A. Chirurgie de l'hyperparathyroïdisme primaire au début des années 1990. Rev Franç Endocrinol Clin 1993; 34:49–55.

24

Adrenocortical Function and Adrenal Insufficiency

J. Lester Gabrilove

Mount Sinai School of Medicine, New York University, New York, New York, U.S.A.

1 EMBRYOLOGY

The adrenal cortex and gonads arise in common from the urogenital ridge and share a common pathway to androgen and estrogen. Except in virilizing and feminizing disorders of the adrenal cortex, the androgen-estrogen pathway in the adrenal cortex plays a minor role compared to that in the ovary or testis. The dominant function of the adrenal cortex is the biosynthesis of cortisol and aldosterone.

2 HORMONE SYNTHESIS

The basic building block of adrenal steroid synthesis is cholesterol, which in large measure is brought to the adrenal via a hematogenous route. Following cleavage of the side chain of cholesterol, the steroid nucleus is available for the formation of the adrenal steroids. There are three pathways of hormone synthesis in the adrenal cortex: (1) to androgen and estrogen, (2) to cortisol, and (3) to aldosterone (1). The adrenal cortex possesses a unique ability to 21-hydroxylate the steroid nucleus, a prerequisite in the aldosterone and cortisol synthetic pathways. The cortisol pathway requires subsequent 17- and 11-β-hydroxylation, whereas the aldosterone pathway requires only 11-β-hydroxylation and the introduction of an aldehyde group at the C-18 position (Fig. 1).

3 HISTOLOGY

The adrenal cortex consists of three layers: (1) the zona glomerulosa, the site of aldosterone synthesis, (2) the zona fasciculata where cortisol is produced, and (3) the zona reticularis, the reserve area and probable site of formation of androgens and estrogens.

4 PHYSIOLOGY

The adrenal cortex is primarily regulated by the secretion of corticotropin (ACTH) from the adenohypophysis, and, in turn, the hypophyseal secretion of corticotropin is controlled by corticotropin-releasing hormone (CRH) from the hypothalamus. Excess secretion of ACTH results in hypertrophy of the zona fasciculata and induces an increase in the secretion of cortisol. This is accompanied by minor increases in the production of aldosterone and the sex hormones, the latter presumably from the overflow of precursor steroids in the cortisol pathway. In turn, the excessive production of cortisol by the adrenal cortex suppresses CRH and, secondarily, ACTH secretion and its consequent effect on the adrenal cortex.

The mechanism of control of androgen and estrogen secretion by the adrenal cortex is not well understood. However, androgen production by the adrenal is increased at the time of puberty (adrenarche) and is also increased in the presence of congenital adrenal hyperplasia associated with enzymatic defects in the steroid pathways. For example, 21-hydroxylase deficiency results in decreased cortisol secretion, which accelerates ACTH formation, resulting in excess steroid precursors driven mostly into the androgen pathway. In the presence of severe 21-hydroxylase blockade, the flow into the aldosterone pathway is also restricted.

Aldosterone secretion is primarily controlled by the renin-angiotensin system and the serum concentration of potassium.

4.1 Metabolic Effects of Adrenocortical Steroids

Excess cortisol acts as an antianabolic or catabolic agent. Protein wasting leads to a decrease in collagen production and to thinning of the skin. Decrease in osteoid formation results in osteoporosis and fractures. The excessive cortisol production also interferes with carbohydrate metabolism with ensuing impaired glucose tolerance or overt diabetes mellitus. Another significant effect of excessive cortisol production is suppression of immune function. Aldosterone regulates sodium-potassium homeostasis by the kidney. In the presence of sodium deprivation, renin is secreted by the juxtaglomerular apparatus of the kidney. It then cleaves angiotensinogen to produce angiotensin 1. The latter is in turn converted in the lung to angiotensin 2, and further cleavage results in angiotensin 3. Angiotensin 2 is the potent force driving aldosterone production by the adrenal cortex. Aldosterone acts on the distal convoluted tubule to retain sodium in exchange for potassium. This signals the juxtaglomerular apparatus to decrease renin production. Advantage is taken of this in the diagnosis of primary aldosteronism by the finding of a high serum aldosterone following a high-sodium diet and a low serum renin activity following a low-sodium diet. The ratio of plasma aldosterone to plasma renin activity is often employed in the diagnosis of primary aldosteronism, especially if it is greater than 50. The physiological effects of androgen and estrogen are well recognized and need not be detailed. They are manifested at puberty in the sexual development seen following secretion of these compounds by the ovary or testis. As mentioned, the adrenal elaboration of these hormones is ordinarily minimal, but it is significant in virilizing or feminizing tumors of the adrenal cortex or in congenital adrenal hyperplasia.

5 CLINICAL SYNDROMES

5.1 Hyperfunction

Hyperfunctioning syndromes of the adrenal cortex are seen in association with either tumor or hyperplasia. Overproduction of cortisol results in Cushing's syndrome. This is far more commonly the result of a corticotropin-secreting tumor of the adenohypophysis and less frequently due to an adrenal adenoma or carcinoma. Even more uncommon are ectopic ACTH-secreting tumors, which are usually carcinoids in the lung, pancreas, or thymus. On rare occasions an ectopic ACTH-secreting tumor is seen in association with a pheochromocytoma. Other less common causes of Cushing's syndrome are autonomous micronodular or macronodular hyperplasia. CRH secreting tumors are exceedingly rare.

Overproduction of aldosterone results from either a small adrenocortical tumor or hyperplasia. The primary cause of hyperplasia is unknown. The differentiation of tumor from hyperplasia is usually accomplished by computed tomography (CT), magnetic resonance imaging (MRI), or ultrasound imaging or less frequently by selective adrenal vein sampling or iodocholesterol nuclear scanning.

The virilizing and feminizing syndromes caused by adrenocortical tumors have been well described (2,3). Virilization and, far less frequently, feminization are also seen in congenital adrenocortical hyperplasia due to congenital enzymatic defects in the adrenal biosynthetic pathway to cortisol. In these latter disorders, particularly in 21-hydroxylase deficiency, concomitant excessive production of androgens ensues. Acquired nontumorous syndromes of adrenal virilism or feminism are rare.

5.2 Hypofunction

Unrecognized adrenocortical insufficiency is of particular importance to the surgeon, as failure of recognition in a patient undergoing surgery may lead to fatal shock. Adrenal insufficiency may be either of primary (Addison's disease) or secondary (pituitary) etiology. Primary adrenal insufficiency results from destruction or atrophy of the adrenal. In the past, Addison's disease was in large measure due to tuberculosis, but in more recent times autoimmune atrophy has become the most common cause. Other less common causes include human immunodeficiency virus (HIV) infection, amyloid, metastatic carcinoma, fungal infection,

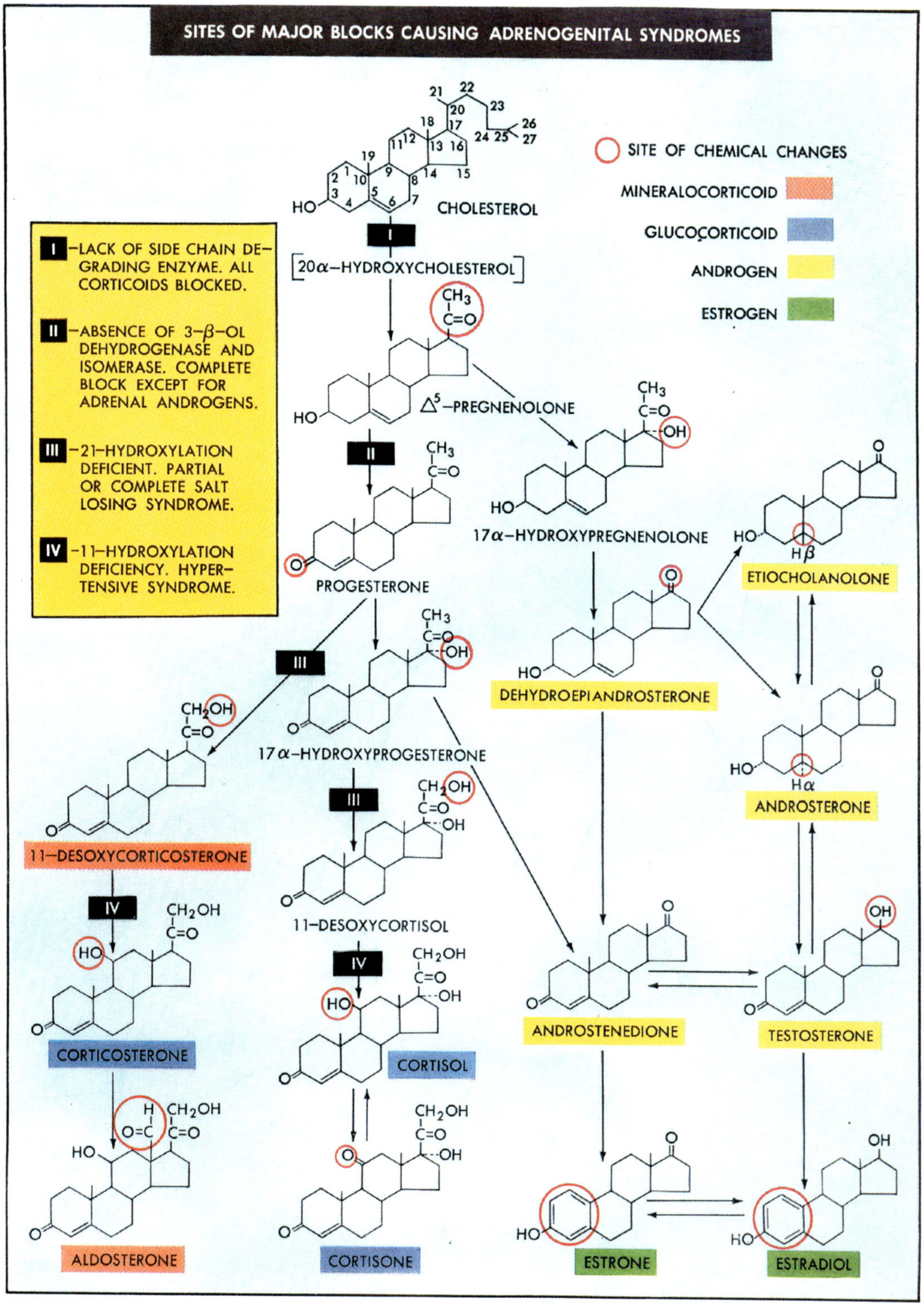

Figure 1 Adrenal biosynthetic pathways of steroids. Sites of major blocks causing adrenogenital syndromes.

meningitis, and hemorrhagic disorders resulting from shock or excessive anticoagulation. Adrenal cortical insufficiency is also encountered in the untreated patient with congenital adrenocortical hyperplasia, particularly of the 21-hydroxylase variety. Some less common forms of adrenal insufficiency, particularly in the pediatric age group, have been described (4).

5.2.1 Clinical Manifestations of Adrenocortical Insufficiency

The symptoms and signs of primary adrenal insufficiency include marked asthenia and fatigue, pigmentation of the skin, mucous membranes and scars, weight loss, gastrointestinal symptoms, and hypotension (Table 1). The serum sodium may be low, as sodium wasting is part of this disorder. However, the use of sodium withdrawal as a diagnostic test is no longer employed. The diagnosis is based on finding a low serum cortisol or, more definitively, a failure of the serum cortisol to rise significantly following the administration of the ACTH analog cosyntropin. Debate is still ongoing as to whether a low dose (1 μg) or a high dose (250 μg) is preferable. A normal response is a rise in the serum cortisol to above 20 μg/dL at the end of 30–60 minutes. The use of adrenal antibodies to establish the autoimmune etiology of the insufficiency may be employed as well. Other commonly employed diagnostic tools include a tine test to exclude tuberculosis and CT of the adrenals to delineate their size and characteristics.

Table 1 Clinical and Laboratory Findings in Primary Adrenal Insufficiency

Weakness
Fatigue
Pigmentation and vitiligo
Weight loss
Hypotension
Shock[a]
Nausea and vomiting[a]
Flank pain (due to hemorrhage)
Fever[a]
Psychiatric manifestations (e.g., anorexia)
Hyponatremia
Hyperkalemia
Azotemia
Low serum cortisol
Lack of response to ACTH

[a] In the presence of crisis.

5.2.2 Secondary Adrenal Insufficiency

Secondary adrenal insufficiency is seen in association with destructive lesions of the adenohypophysis such as pituitary tumors, craniopharyngiomas, and Sheehan's syndrome. This form of adrenal insufficiency is also encountered in patients with suppression of adrenal function secondary to long-term glucocorticoid administration or following the removal of a glucocorticoid-secreting adrenal adenoma or carcinoma. When the basic defect is in the hypothalamus and CRH is no longer produced, the term tertiary adrenal insufficiency may be used.

In patients with secondary adrenal insufficiency, there is a lack of pigmentation and the plasma ACTH concentration level is low. In contrast, a high serum level of ACTH is seen in primary adrenal insufficiency and is usually associated with abnormal pigmentation. The serum sodium is usually maintained in secondary adrenal insufficiency except in the face of marked salt deprivation. The adrenal usually responds to the administration of ACTH unless the pituitary hypofunction is of long duration.

The symptoms of adrenal insufficiency may be subtle, and the diagnosis may be first considered when a patient goes into shock following a surgical procedure or in the presence of minor or major infection. The shock is unresponsive to the usual methods of treatment and responds only to the administration of a glucocorticoid.

5.2.3 Treatment

In general, treatment of adrenal insufficiency consists of the administration both of a salt-retaining steroid and a glucocorticoid. If the patient is in adrenal crisis, usually provoked by surgery or infection, large doses of a glucocorticoid are given parenterally in dosages of up to 300 mg of cortisol a day. If infection is suspected, antibiotic therapy is also warranted. The patient is weaned from the cortisol to a maintenance dosage as the condition improves. In the maintenance phase, treatment consists of fludrocortisone in a dosage of 0.1–0.2 mg/day and cortisol in a dosage of 12.5–37.5 mg/day.

Doses of cortisol exceeding 15 mg/day provide sufficient sodium-retaining ability to obviate the need for fludrocortisone, whereas equivalent doses of dexamethasone and prednisone require the additional use of a salt-retaining hormone. The administration of intravenous isotonic saline is usually warranted depending on the state of hydration and sodium depletion (Fig. 1.).

REFERENCES

1. Gabrilove JL. A biologic concept of adrenocortical function. Acta Endocrinol 1961; 36:281–286.
2. Gabrilove JL, Seman AT, Sabet R, Mitty HA, Nicolis GL. Virilizing adrenal adenoma with studies on the steroid content of the adrenal venous effluent and a review of the literature. Endocrinol Rev 1981; 2:462–470.
3. Gabrilove JL, Sharma DC, Wotiz HH, Dorfman RI. Feminizing adrenocortical tumors in the male. A review of 52 cases. Medicine 1965; 44:37–79.
4. Ten S, New M, McLaren N. Clinical review 130: Addison's disease 2001. J Clin Endocrinol Metab 2001; 86:2909–2922.

25

The Sympathoadrenal System: Its Physiology and Function

Laura Bertani Dziedzic and Stanley Walter Dziedzic

Mount Sinai School of Medicine, New York University, New York, New York, U.S.A.

1 INTRODUCTION

Nowhere in the human body is the intimate relationship that exists between the nervous system and the endocrine system more apparent than in the connection between the sympathetic nervous system itself and the adrenal medulla (the sympathoadrenal system). This concept was postulated as early as Aristotle's time, with the term "neurohumor" (a word demonstrating the involvement of both systems) used to describe substances released by a system for use at a distant site. Even today this definition can be superficially used to describe the regulation of homeostasis by the catecholamine neurotransmitters (1). The sympathetic nervous system allows for rapid adjustment to change by elaboration of the transmitter, which acts quickly at the site of release. On the other hand, the substance secreted by the endocrine system acts more slowly and at distant sites. Classically, the three naturally occurring catecholamines in the human subject that function as neurotransmitters for major portions of the central and autonomic nervous systems are norepinephrine (NE, noradrenaline, levarterenol), epinephrine (E, adrenaline), and dopamine (DA). One would expect that these compounds would participate in the metabolic changes associated with innumerable pathophysiological situations. NE is the transmitter released from postganglionic axons of the sympathetic nervous system as well as from central nervous system noradrenergic neurons. It exerts a direct effect where it is released at the junctional cleft, while E elaborated from the adrenal medulla affects sites far distant from where it is secreted. Although it is postulated that a peripheral dopaminergic system exists, it has not been fully elucidated (2,3).

Since the chromaffin cells of the adrenal medulla and neuronal cells of the sympathetic nervous system develop together and are derived from the same neuroectodermal cells in the embryo, it is not surprising that their physiological functions, including the chemical structures of the hormones synthesized and stored in different organs, are similar. In response to cortisol, the precursor cells in the center of the gland differentiate. Further differentiation occurs in response to nerve growth factor producing sympathetic neurons. Sympathetic ganglia differ from the adrenal medulla in that in many species, including human beings, NE is secreted preferentially in response to stimulation in the sympathetic nervous system, whereas E is released in the medulla. The adrenal gland itself in many mammalian species is comprised of two distinct entities: the medulla, surrounded by the much larger cortex. Although the gland was first described in the sixteenth century, its function was not elucidated until Addison's research (4). Studies since that time have shown that aberrations in adrenal function are associated with many diseases (5–8).

The adrenal medulla and the sympathetic nervous system are innervated by pre-ganglionic sympathetic nerves. The major outer portion of the adrenal, the cortex, secretes steroid hormones, while the inner portion, the medulla, elaborates biologically active amines called catecholamines. The nomenclature of the compounds classified as catecholamines is derived from the "dihydroxy" modification of the aromatic phenyl ring in their structure (Fig. 1). The terminology "chromaffin" cells, which constitute the adrenal medullary tissue, is used because the catecholamines contained in these polyhedral structures can precipitate chromium salts.

The autonomic or involuntary nervous system is comprised of nerves, ganglia, and plexuses, which are widely distributed throughout the human body and provide innervation to the heart, blood vessels, and smooth muscles, where it regulates functions that occur without conscious control. The autonomic nervous system is divided into two parts: the sympathetic nervous system (thoracolumbar outflow) and the parasympathetic nervous system (craniosacral outflow). The sympathetic nervous system is widely distributed throughout the body, whereas parasympathetic distribution is limited to its proximate effector sites. Both systems appear to exhibit opposing effects, which contribute to the maintenance of homeostasis of the human organism. The operation of the sympathetic nervous system by its storage, release, and metabolism of NE permits fine adjustments to be made in order to maintain a steady state. The amount of activity varies from moment to moment in response to stresses placed on the organism. This chapter will focus primarily on the syn-

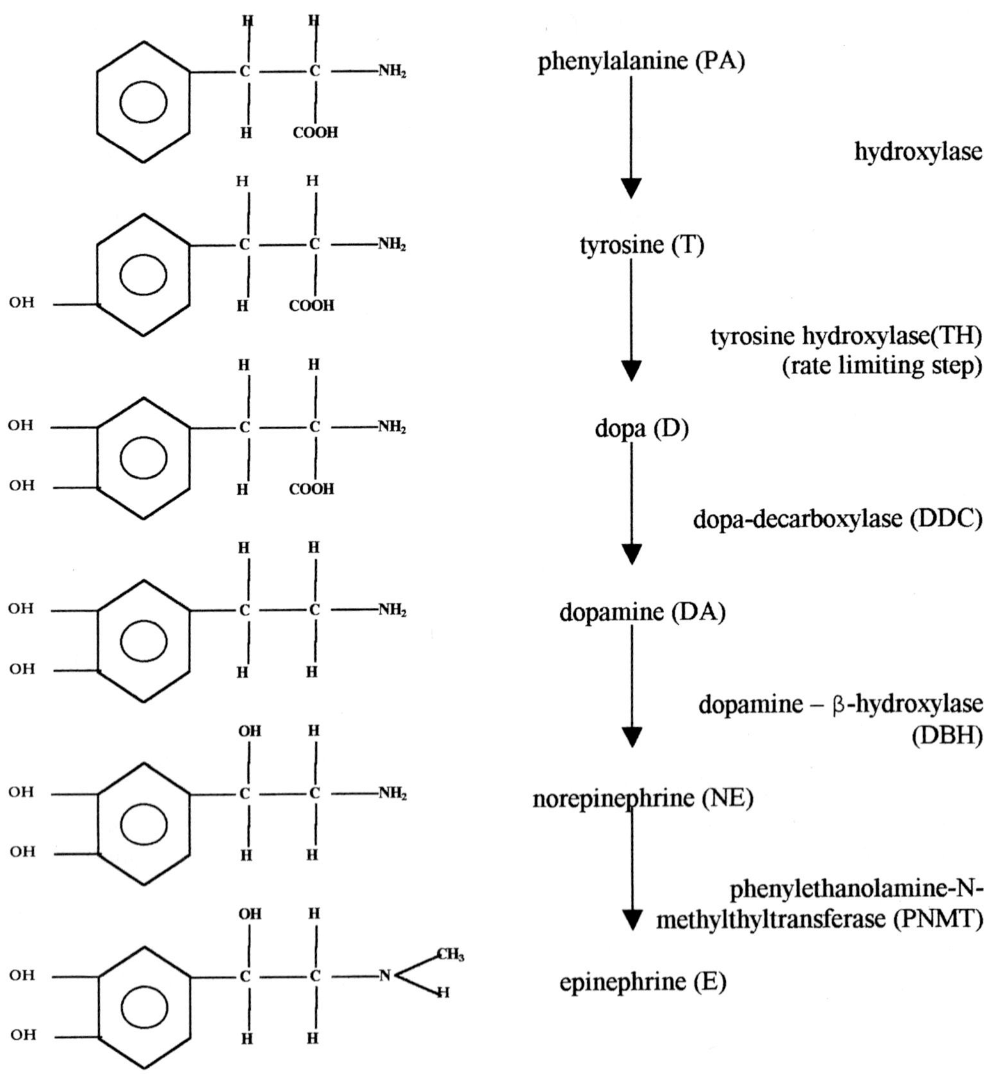

Figure 1 Biosynthesis of catecholamines.

thesis, actions, and degradation of the neurotransmitters of the aforementioned system.

2 NEUROTRANSMITTER BIOSYNTHESIS

Nerves transmit their impulses and elicit responses in target organs via the elaboration of specific chemical compounds. By the early twentieth century it had been conclusively established that catecholamines (sympathin) were the primary mediators in the sympathetic nervous system (9). Although the catecholamines are still considered the principal neurotransmitters, recent observations have suggested that synaptic transmission may be mediated by release of more than a single substance. These additional neurotransmitters may include peptides (e.g., enkephalin, substance P, neuropeptide Y, VIP, somatostatin), purines (e.g., ATP, adenosine) and small molecules (e.g., nitric oxide) (10,11). In general terms, when a nerve impulse arrives at the axonal terminal, it initiates a series of steps that transmit the impulse across the neuroeffector junction or junctional cleft. The neurotransmitter is released from synaptic storage vesicles and combined with postjunctional receptors, where an action potential is generated. After each impulse the transmitter itself is either destroyed or dissipated by reuptake or simple diffusion.

The three bioactive amines, NE, E, and DA, are derived from a common precursor, the dietary essential amino acid phenylalanine (PA). E originates almost entirely in the adrenal medulla, whereas NE is synthesized in the central nervous system (CNS) as well as the sympathetic postganglionic fibers. The function of DA, which acts as a transmitter in the CNS, has a less clearly defined role. The synthesis of the catecholamine transmitters involves five enzymatic steps (Fig. 1). The enzymes involved are localized in both the cytoplasm and the vesicles of neural and chromaffin cells (12). All the enzymes involved in this biosynthetic pathway have been cloned and characterized (13). The resultant synthesis of E or NE is dependent on the presence of phenylethanol-*N*-methyl transferase (PNMT). Initially, PA is hepatically converted into the neutral amino acid tyrosine (T), which can also be directly ingested from food. T is then hydroxylated further via tyrosine hydroxylase (TH) to 3,4-dihydroxyphenylalanine (DOPA). The enzyme TH is the product of a single, multiple exonic gene (14). The hydroxylation of the phenolic ring requires molecular oxygen, ferrous ion, and reduced pteridine as co-factors and is the rate-limiting step in this biosynthetic pathway (15). Other neurotransmitters, including acetylcholine, released from preganglionic neurons interact with receptors on the postganglionic neurons and play an important part in the regulation of this enzyme.

A subsequent enzymatic step promotes the conversion of DOPA to DA via cytosolic dopamine decarboxylase (DDC). Pyridoxal phosphate (vitamin B_6) is the cofactor required in this step. In the CNS, DA itself is the neurotransmitter, and in certain neurons this is the final biosynthetic step. This enzyme is expressed in monoamine-producing neuronal cells and in thymic, liver, and kidney cells. Approximately one half of the DA is actually transported to dopamine-β-hydroxylase (DBH)–containing storage vesicles, while the remainder is deaminated to 3,4-dihydroxyphenylacetic acid (DOPAC) and subsequently O-methylated to homovanillic acid (HVA). In the sympathetic neurons as well as in medullary cells, the next step that occurs involves the conversion of DA to NE via DBH (16), a copper containing enzyme. Molecular oxygen and ascorbic acid are needed for this reaction to occur. Many other phenylethylamines can serve as the substrate for this oxidase, which employs both ascorbic acid and molecular oxygen as proton donors. In sympathetic neurons and approximately 20% of chromaffin cells, NE is the final metabolic product. However, in the chromaffin cells of the adrenal medulla and in the organ of Zuckerkandl, the cytosolic enzyme (PNMT) converts NE to E. Smaller amounts of PNMT have also been isolated in some CNS adrenergic neurons and other extra-adrenal sources (17). Almost without exception, tumors that secrete E arise in these sites. PNMT requires S-adenosylmethionine (SAME) as a methyl donor and can utilize many other phenylethanolamine derivatives as substrates for this catalytic step.

3 STORAGE, RELEASE, AND METABOLISM OF CATECHOLAMINES

Synthesized catecholamines are sequestered from the cytosol and stored in osmophilic granules or vesicles associated with adenosine triphosphate (ATP). These membrane-limited organelles also contain DBH and chromogranin A. The granules, isolated from tissue from the adrenal medulla, splenic nerves, and CNS, contain a "reserve pool" of E in the adrenal medulla and NE in the adrenergic fibers. The uptake of catecholamines into these sites is mediated by vesicular monoamine transporters, wherein the energy required results from a proton (H^+) gradient maintained through a H^+-

ATPase system (18–20). The ratio of catecholamine to ATP is 4:1 in adrenal medullary granules and 6–8:1 in noradrenergic neuronal vesicles. Under physiological conditions in the granules, the cationic (positively charged) catecholamines react with the anionic (negatively charged) phosphate groups. For every catecholamine molecule taken up, two protons are released. The active transport mechanism is sodium dependent and can be blocked by a number of drugs, including cocaine and imipramine (21). This promotes the binding of the catecholamines to chromogranin A to some extent. It is in this way that the catecholamines are protected from degradation by metabolic enzymes . Thus, the catecholamines remain in a reserve pool until there is a stimulus to secrete them. A multipool system exists in the vesicles (or granules) wherein the large reserve pool exists in equilibrium with smaller mobile pools within the cytoplasm (22).

The compartmentalization of these pools is very significant for the regulation of the secretion of the catecholamines, which is principally mediated by acetylcholine. The storage of E and NE in their respective pools prevents their leakage outside the cell. Release of E in the adrenal medulla occurs by the liberation of acetylcholine by preganglionic fibers via nicotinic receptors, which causes a variation in the permeability for calcium and other ions. The entrance of calcium ion into the vesicle causes release of hormone. This secretion can also be stimulated by histamine receptors, potassium ion, bradykinin, and other neuromodulators (23,24). The regulation of catecholamine secretion (a process called "exocytosis") under physiological conditions is very tightly controlled. Although the mechanisms involved in exocytosis for the adrenergic system have not been fully elucidated, it is known that the processes of synthesis and reuptake allow NE output to be sustained during prolonged stimulation. A significant portion of the NE is released intraneuronally, ultimately arrives at the circulation, and is catabolized to the amine-oxidized byproducts vanillylmandelic acid (VMA) and 3-methoxy-4-hydroxyphenylethylglycol (MHPG) (Fig. 2). It is noteworthy that circulating catecholamines are rapidly cleared extrarenally and have a very short half-life (1–2 min). On the other hand, neural impulses result in the quantal release of NE into the junctional cleft, followed by receptor response and diffusion of the transmitter to distant sites, to the local intraneuronal storage granules (neuronal reuptake) or to the enzymatic mechanisms responsible for biochemical degradation of NE to its O-methylated congener normetanephrine (NM). Neuronal reuptake is characterized by its location at the pre-synaptic axonal membrane, dependence on extracellular sodium, and inhibition by pharmacological substances such as antidepressants and cocaine. In much the same manner, the adrenal medulla releases its humoral agent, E, into the general circulation in response to specific preganglionic stimulation or certain neurochemical phenomena such as hypoglycemia. The state of the art concerning information about storage of catecholamines has been obtained from adrenergically innervated organs and adrenal medullary tissue. Chromaffin granules are composed of 21% dry weight of catecholamines, ascorbic acid, ATP, chromogranins, DBH, and peptides (e.g., enkephalin and neuropeptide). In sympathetic nerve terminals there are two types of vesicles: large dense core (similar to chromaffin granules) and small dense core vesicles. In the sympathetic neurons, the enzymes that catalyze the synthesized NE are formed in the neuron cell body and transported along the neuron to the axon's terminal, while the hydroxylation of T and decarboxylation of DA occur in the cytoplasm. In the adrenal medulla there exist two distinct catecholamine-containing cell types: those with NE and those with E. In the latter cells, which contain NE as well as the enzyme PNMT, the synthesized NE diffuses out of the granules and is methylated in the cytoplasm to E. E then reenters the chromaffin granules, where it is stored until needed. Any persistent stress on the system mobilizes the secretion of both cortisol in the adrenal cortex and E from the adrenal medulla. Three pathways that terminate the actions of catecholamines govern their clearance from the circulation: (1) a specific reuptake mechanism by the sympathetic neurons, (2) dilution by diffusion out of the junctional cleft terminals and nonspecific reuptake at extraneuronal sites, and (3) degradation by peripheral tissues followed by urinary excretion.

Catecholamines are metabolized in liver and kidneys by two enzymes, monoamine oxidase (MAO) and catechol-O-methyltransferase (COMT), to produce inactive metabolites, which are renally cleared and measured in urine as free compounds or as conjugates of glucuronide or sulfate (Fig. 2). In addition, phenol sulfotransferases can metabolize catecholamines (25). However, a preeminent degradative pathway such as that which exists for acetylcholine is not present in the adrenergic nervous system. Neurotransmitters that are released within the nerve and terminated by entrance into the circulation are metabolized by MAO and COMT. Both enzymes are distributed widely in the human body, with the highest concentrations existing in the liver and kidneys. Interestingly, COMT is almost completely absent from adrenergic neurons. COMT is located primarily in cytoplasm, whereas MAO is prin-

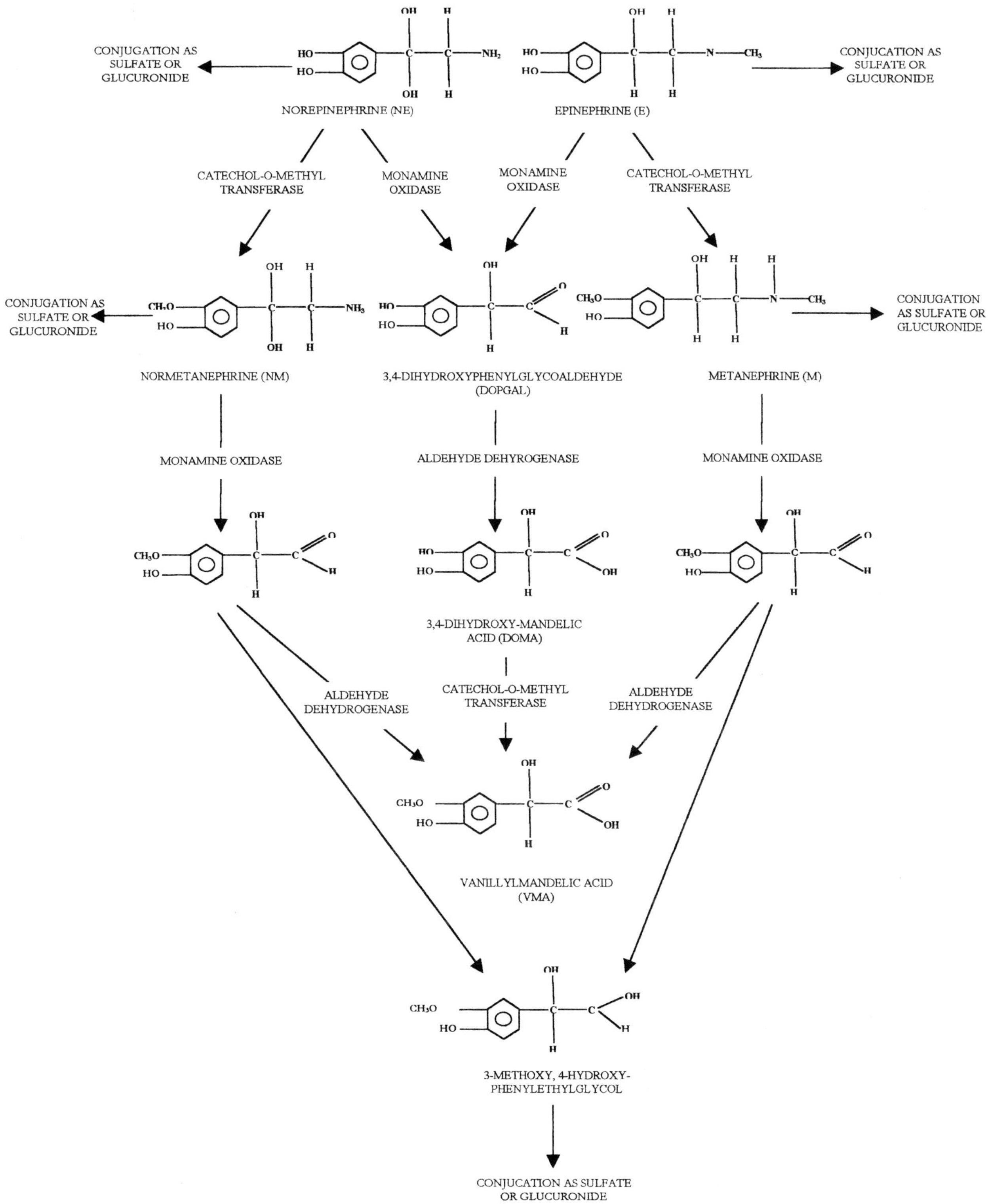

Figure 2 Metabolism of catecholamines.

cipally in found on the outer surface of the mitochondrion. Two isoenzymes, MAO-A and MAO-B, exist in widely varying portions within the cells and can be inhibited very selectively by a variety of specific drugs (26,27). As shown in Figure 2, the conjugation of catecholamine byproducts as glucuronides and sulfates is an important mode for inactivation of catecholamine metabolites. Over 50% of the NE and E in biological fluids is conjugated in this manner (28).

4 ADRENERGIC RECEPTORS

Essential to understanding the diverse physiological role of the catecholamines themselves is knowledge of the structure and function of receptors located in the effector cells. The differing physiological effects of NE and E led Ahlquist to propose the existence of more than one type of receptor (29). For smooth muscle, where processes such as excitation and relaxation were measured, the two types of structurally related receptors were designated as α or β, depending on whether catecholamines produced excitatory or inhibitory responses (30). The variety of hemodynamic and metabolic effects produced by catecholamines are the result of their occupancy of the adrenergic receptors on the surface membrane of the target cell and the events that cascade from this situation.

As more information was obtained, β receptors were subclassified into β_1, β_2, and β_3, dependent upon sensitivity to the transmitters (31). The heterogeneity of α receptors has also been appreciated. This group of adrenergic receptors has also been subdivided into α_1 and α_2 receptors, which have been further subclassified into α_{1A} and α_{1B}. Cloning has revealed further incompletely characterized subtypes of adrenergic receptors (32,33).

Although controlling different functions, all adrenoreceptors appear to be comprised of closely related proteins similar to receptors for other hormones that are coupled to G-proteins (guanine nucleotide regulatory proteins) (34). These proteins have characteristic features, including seven membrane-spanning hydrophobic regions containing 20–28 amino acids each. These domains are essential for determining ligand binding. In addition, the binding of ligands (usually antagonists) and the competition for these sites by agonists and antagonists "in vitro" determine the characteristics of the receptors. NE and E are mixed agonists interacting with both α and β receptors to different extents. E appears to be the more potent substance, which has a greater affinity for receptors.

5 PHYSIOLOGICAL EFFECTS OF CATECHOLAMINES

Different hemodynamic patterns emerge from the interaction of catecholamines with the heart and vasculature. NE produces increases in both systolic and diastolic blood pressure, which in turn limits the heart rate increase. The elevated blood pressure stimulates the carotid and aortic baroreceptors, producing reflex bradycardia that overrides the direct cardioacceleration and cardiac output per minute decreases. On the other hand, E increases heart rate and cardiac output while causing a rise in systolic but a decrease in diastolic blood pressure. NE and E also increase myocardial excitation, giving rise to extra systoles and occasionally to even more serious cardiac arrhythmias. NE causes vasoconstriction, whereas E dilates the blood vessels in the skeletal muscle and liver. E and NE, when injected, can cause changes to occur in potassium ion concentration and hence play a significant role in the regulation of intracellular and extracellular concentration of this ion.

The multiplicity of direct influences of the catecholamines on the major organ systems is dramatic. Profound effects on the cardiovascular system, metabolic rates (e.g., heat production), and fluid and electrolyte balance have been exhibited. In addition, indirect effects on the endocrine system have been demonstrated (35,36). Catecholamines play a preeminent role in response to stressors and are crucial in responses to perceived threats (37). The initial release of catecholamines is followed by an increase in the expression of genes that encode catecholamine-synthesizing enzymes. Although E and NE are equipotent in increasing alertness, E evokes more anxiety and fear in humans.

There is little doubt that we have witnessed during the last century tremendous growth in the role played by the catecholamines in both normal and disease states. Biochemical assays, gene cloning, and computer-derived models have begun to replace the pathologist's microscope in diagnosing illnesses arising from aberrations in catecholamine metabolism. It is therefore quite natural to experience excitement regarding the anticipated revelations of the new millennium.

REFERENCES

1. von Euler US. Historical perspective: growth and impact of the concept of chemical neurotransmission. In: Stjärne L, Hedquist P, Lagerkrantz H, Wennhalm A, eds. Chemical Neurotransmission—75 Years. London: Academic Press, 1981:3–12.

2. O'Connor DT. The adrenal medulla, catecholamines and pheochromocytoma. In: Goldman L Bennett JC, eds. Cecil Textbook of Medicine. 21st ed. New York: W.B. Saunders, 2000:1258–1259.
3. Lansberg LB, Young JB. The sympathetic nervous system and the adrenal medulla. In: Fauci AS, Braunwald E, Isselbacher KJ, Wilson JD, Martin JB, Kasper DL, Hauser SL, Longo DL, eds. Harrison's Principles of Internal Medicine. 14th ed. New York: McGraw-Hill, 1998:431–442.
4. Addison T. On the Constitutional and Local Effects of disease of the suprarenal capsules. London: Highly, 1885.
5. Walters W, Wilder RM, Kepler EJ. The suprarenal cortical syndrome with presentation of ten cases. Ann Surg 1934; 100:670–679.
6. Conn JW. Presidential address: (1) painting background; (2) primary aldosteronism. J Lab Clin Med 1955; 45:661.
7. DeChrecchio L. Sapra un caso di apparenzi virili in una donna. Morgagni 1865; 7:151.
8. Young WF. Pheochromocytoma and primary aldosteronism: diagnostic approaches. Endocrinal Metab Clin North Am 1997; 27:801–827.
9. Loewi O, Navratil E. Über humorale Übertragbarkeit der Herznervenwirkung. Mitteilung über das Schicksal des Vagustoff. Pflügers Arch. Gesamte Physiol 1926; 214: 678–688.
10. Bartfai T, Iverfeldt K, Fisone G, Serfozo P. Regulation of the release of coexisting neurotransmitters. Annu Rev Pharmacol Toxicol 1988; 28:285–310.
11. Lundberg JM. Pharmacology of cotransmission in the autonomic nervous system: integrative aspects on amines, neuropeptides, adenosine triphosphate, amino acids and nitric oxide. Pharmacol Rev 1996; 48: 113–178.
12. Blaschko H. The specific action of L-dopa decarboxylase. J Physiol Lond 1939; 96:50–51.
13. Nagatsu T. Genes for human catecholamine-synthesizing enzymes. Neurosci Res 1991; 12:315–345.
14. Sabban EL, Kvetňansky R. Stress-triggered activation of gene expression in catecholaminergic systems; dynamics of transcriptoral events. Trends Neurosci 2001; 24:91–98.
15. Zigmond RE, Schwartzchild MA, Rittenhouse AR. Acute regulation of tyrosine hydroxylase by nerve activity and by neurotransmitters via phosphorylation. Annu Rev Neurosci 1989; 12:415–461.
16. Winkler H. Membrane composition of adrenergic large and small dense cored vesicles and of synaptic vesicles, consequences for their biogenesis. Neurochem Res 1997; 22: 921–932.
17. Kennedy B, Ziegler MG. Cardiac epinephrine synthesis. Regulation by a glucocorticoid. Circulation 1991; 84: 891–895.
18. Schuldiner S. A molecular glimpse of vesicular monoamine transporters. J Neurochem 1994; 62:2067–2078.
19. Brownstein MJ, Hoffman BJ. Neurotransmitter transporters. Recent Prog Horm Res 1994; 49:27–42.
20. Varoqui H, Erickson JD. Vesicular neurotransmitter transporters. Potential site for regulation of synaptic function. Mol Neurobiol 1997; 15:165–191.
21. Iversen LL. Uptake processes for biogenic amines. In: Iversen LL, Iversen SD, Snyder SH, eds. Vol. 3. Handbook of Psychopharmacology. New York: Plenum Press, 1975:381–442.
22. De Robertis ED. Adrenergic endings and vesicles isolated from brain. Pharmacol Rev 1966; 18:413–424.
23. Aunis D. Exocytosis in chromoffin cells of the adrenal medulla. Int Rev Cytol 1998; 181:213–320.
24. Bowersox SS, Singh T, Nadsdi L, Zukowska-Grojec A, Valentino K, Hoffman BB. Cardiovascular effects of omega-conopeptides in conscious rats: mechanisms of action. J Cardiovasc Pharmacol 1992; 20:756–764.
25. Dooley TP. Cloning of the human phenol sulfotransferase gene family: three genes implicated in the metabolism of catecholamines, thyroid hormones and drugs. Chem Biol Interact 1998; 109:29–41.
26. Volz HP, Gleiter CH. Monoamine oxidase inhibitors. A perspective on their use on the elderly. Drugs Aging 1998; 13:341–355.
27. Wouters J. Structural aspects of monoamine oxidase and its reversible inhibition. Curr Med Chem 1998; 5:137–162.
28. Cryer PE. Pheochromocytoma. West J Med 1992; 156: 399–407.
29. Ahlquist RP. A study of the adrenotropic receptors. Am J Physiol 1948; 153:586–600.
30. Lefkowitz RJ, Kobilka BK, Benovic JL. Molecular Biology of Adrenergic Receptors Cold Spring Harbor Symposia on Quantative Biology. Vol. 53. Cold Spring Harbor, NY: Cold Spring Harbor Laboratories, 1988: 507–514.
31. Emorine LJ, Marullo S, Briend-Sutren MM. Molecular characterization of the human β_3-adrenergic receptor. Science 1989; 245:1118–1121.
32. Docherty JR. Subtypes of functional alpha1 and alpha2-adrenoreceptors. Eur J Pharmacol 1998; 361:1–5.
33. Starke K. Presynaptic α-autoreceptors. Rev Physiol Biochem Pharmacol 1987; 107:73–146.
34. Strader CD, Fong TM, Tota MR, Underwood D, Dixon RA. Structure and function of G protein-coupled receptors. Annu Rev Biochem 1994; 63:101–132.
35. Clutter WE, Rizza RA, Gerich JE, Cryer PE. Regulation of glucose metabolism by sympathochromaffin catecholamines. Diabetes Metab Rev 1988; 4:1–15.
36. Berk MA, Clutter WE, Skor DA. Enhanced glycemic responsiveness to epinephrine in insulin dependent diabetes mellitus is the result of the inability to secrete insulin. J Clin Invest 1985; 75:1842–1851.
37. Sabban EL, Kveňtansky R. Stress-triggered activation of gene expression in catecholaminergic systems: dynamics of transcriptional events. Trends Neurosci 2001; 24:91–98.

26

Surgical Pathology of the Adrenal Glands

Pamela Unger

Mount Sinai School of Medicine, New York University, New York, New York, U.S.A.

1 ADRENAL CORTICAL PATHOLOGY

1.1 Nonfunctioning Adrenal Cortical Nodule/Adenoma

The incidental finding of a cortical nodule/adenoma is not uncommon. Autopsy and clinical studies revealed an incidence of 1.4–3.0% and 0.6–1.3%, respectively. A higher incidence is noted in elderly, hypertensive, and diabetic patients. There are no established size criteria to differentiate a nodule from an adenoma, although measurements of less than 0.5–1.0 cm are usually accepted for a nodule. The average size from several studies is 2.5 cm, but larger lesions of 5–6 cm have been reported. In nonautopsy material, patients are most frequently women with an average age of 60 years. Grossly, these lesions are well circumscribed yellow masses (Fig. 1). On histology, the lesions are composed of cortical cells with variable lipid contents (1–5).

1.2 Functioning Adrenal Cortical Adenomas

1.2.1 Adrenal Cortical Adenoma with Cushing's Syndrome

Adrenal cortical adenomas with Cushing's syndrome are usually solitary unilateral lesions weighing less than 50 g, although tumors weighing over 100 g are rarely reported. Grossly, the lesions are sharply circumscribed and well demarcated from the nonneoplastic adrenal. The average size is approximately 4 cm. Typically the tumor tissue is solid and golden yellow in color, similar to the nonneoplastic cortex (Fig. 2). Areas of brown discoloration due to hemmorhage, lipid depletion, or lipofuscin deposition are frequently seen. In larger lesions, degenerative changes such as fibrosis and cystification may be present. Histology shows a well-demarcated mass (Fig. 3). The tumor cells are arranged in cords, nests, or trabeculae. The cytoplasm is usually pale staining due to the abundance of lipid droplets (Fig. 4). Occasional lipid-depleted cells will have a pink (eosinophilic) appearance. Lipofuscin deposits, if present, are brown droplets in the cytoplasm. The nuclei can vary from round and regular, similar to normal cortical nuclei, to enlarged and hyperchromatic. Focally there may be significant nuclear atypia; however, mitosis will be absent (Fig. 5). The remaining adrenal cortical tissue is usually atrophic. The gross and microscopic findings for any adrenal lesion have to be correlated with the clinical findings. There are no gross or mircroscopic findings (with rare exceptions) that indicate that an adrenal neoplasm is functional or what the hormonal product of the lesion is. Additional histological stains that may be useful are those that bring out the lipid content of the tumor. These include Sudan black on paraffin-embedded tissue and oil red O on fresh or frozen samples. Ultrastructural evaluation will show abundant lipid droplets in the cytoplasm. Mitochondria can be numerous and contain tubular and vesicular cristae. (Figs. 2–5) (6–9).

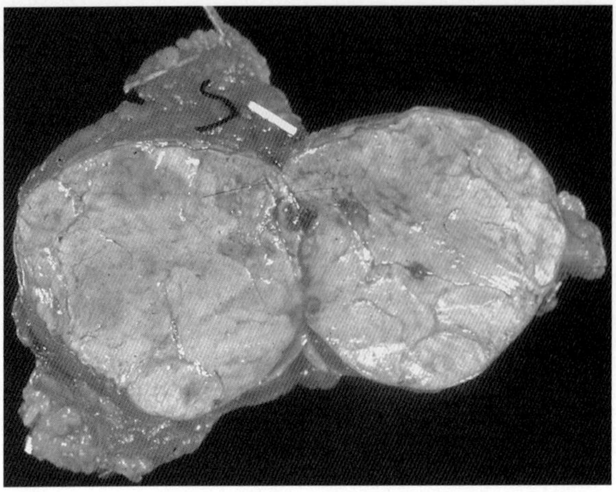

Figure 1 A nonfunctioning incidental adrenal cortical adenoma. The lesion is composed of uniform golden yellow tissue.

1.2.2 Adrenal Cortical Adenoma with Primary Hyperaldosteronism

An adrenal cortical adenoma associated with hypertension and hypokalemia was first described by Conn in 1955. Primary aldosteronism is estimated to occur in 2% of hypertensive patients, mostly in the third to fifth decades. These adenomas are usually small (2 cm in diameter), weigh less than 10 g, are sharply demarcated from the surrounding tissue, and their color is described as canary yellow (Fig. 6). Most tumors are unilateral and solitary.

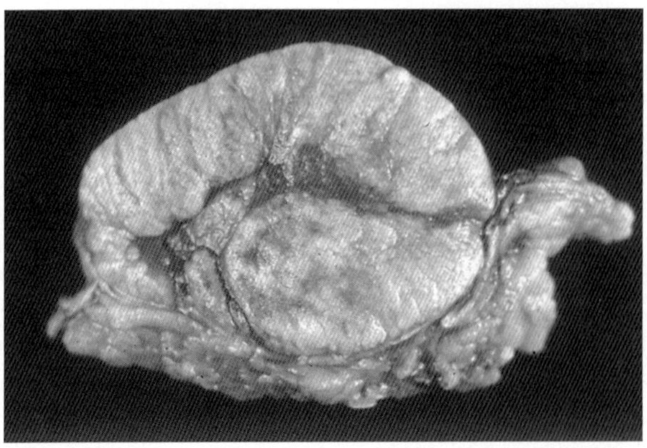

Figure 2 Adrenalectomy specimen with a cortical adenoma in a patient who clinically had Cushing's syndrome. The lesion is composed of uniform yellow tissue.

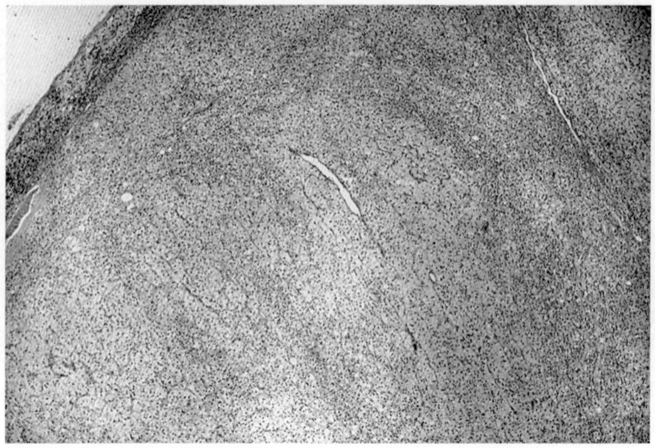

Figure 3 An adrenal cortical adenoma associated with Cushing's syndrome. There is compressed atrophic adrenal cortical tissue at the upper left. The lesion is composed of cords of clear cells (hemotoxylin/eosin ×4).

Microscopically, the adenoma is well demarcated from the nonneoplastic tissue. The tumor cells are arranged in nests or cords, with the neoplastic cells having abundant fine lipid droplets, but lipid-depleted cells are also present. The cell size may be similar to or smaller than seen in the nonneoplastic zona fasciculata and the normal zona glomerulosa. Eosinophilic intracytoplasmic inclusions which have a scroll-like appearance may be seen in neoplastic and nonneoplastic cortical cells (Fig. 7). These are termed spironolactone bodies because they develop in patients treated with the

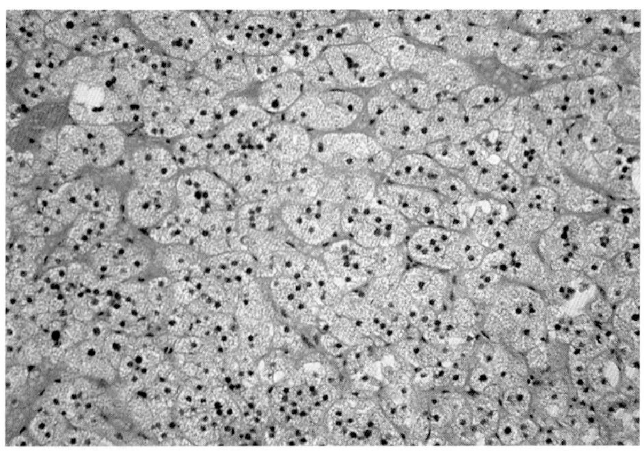

Figure 4 Adrenal cortical adenoma composed of nests of tumor cells separated by a delicate vascularity. The cells have bubbly, clear cytoplasm and uniform, round nuclei (hemotoxylin/eosin ×20).

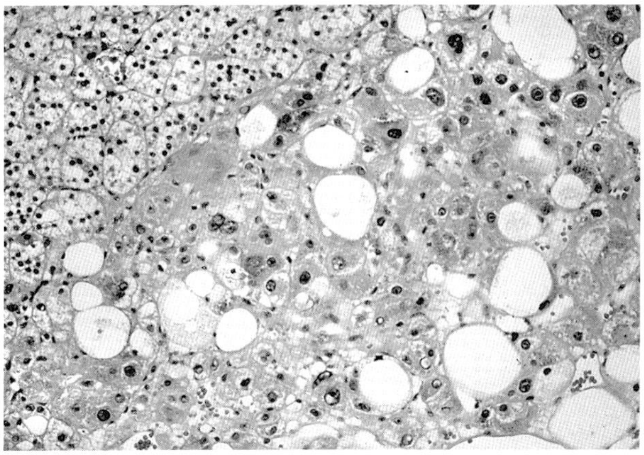

Figure 5 Adrenal cortical adenoma showing an area of nuclear pleomorphism and atypia. The cytoplasm is lipid depleted and is eosinophilic. At the upper left are cortical adenoma cells with clear cytoplasm and uniform nuclei (hemotoxylin/eosin ×40).

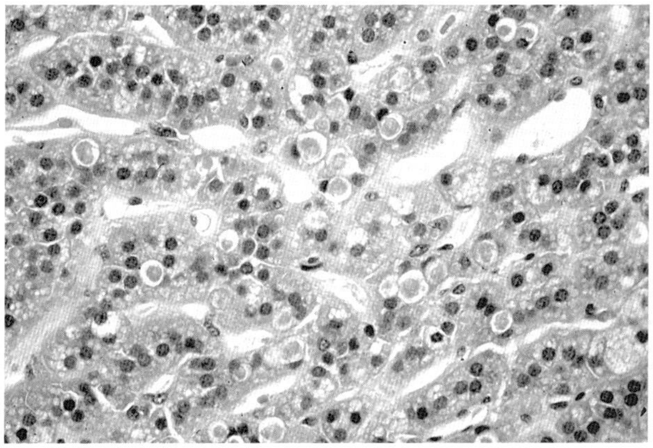

Figure 7 Histological section of an aldosterone-producing adenoma. The cells are arranged in cords with pale to clear cytoplasm. The cytoplasm contains pink scroll-like structures, which are the spironolactone bodies (hemotoxylin/eosin ×40).

aldosterone antagonist spironolactone. They range in size from 2 to 12 μm and are surrounded by a clear space. Immunohistochemistry demonstrates the presence of aldosterone in these inclusions. Nuclei of the adenomas are generally round and regular. The remaining cortex most often appears normal but may be atrophic or even hyperplastic. On ultrastructural examination, in addition to the lipid droplets, there is abundant endoplasmic reticulum and mitochondria, which may have normal or abnormal configurations with vesicular or lamellar cristae. The spironolactone bodies consist of electron dense material surrounded by endoplasmic reticulum (Fig. 6, 7) (10–16).

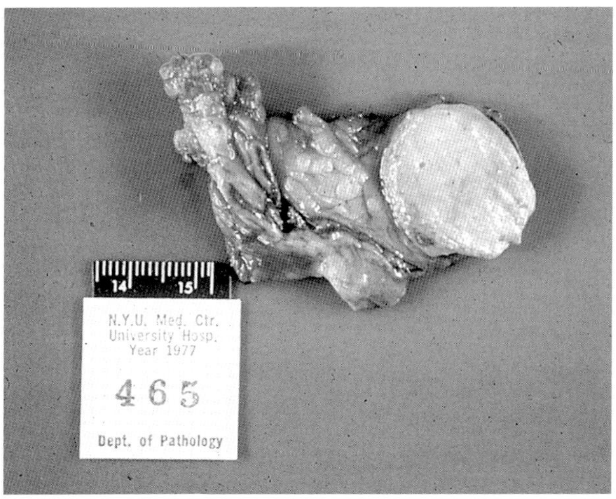

Figure 6 Adrenalectomy specimen with an aldosterone-producing adenoma. The lesion consists of uniform bright yellow (canary yellow) tissue. There is nonneoplastic adrenal tissue on the lower left of the specimen.

1.2.3 Adrenal Cortical Neoplasms with Virilization or Feminization

The majority of these cortical neoplasms have a malignant course. The feminizing tumors occur in adult patients in the second to fifth decades, while the virilizing tumors occur frequently in the pediatric population in addition to adults. In feminizing tumors—almost

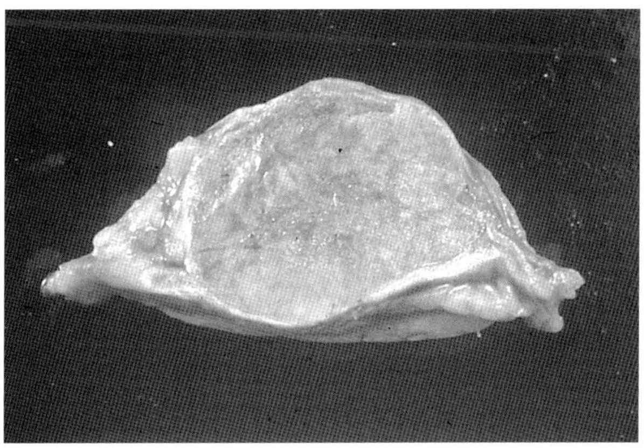

Figure 8 Adrenalectomy specimen with a tan yellow adenoma, which was clinically virilizing.

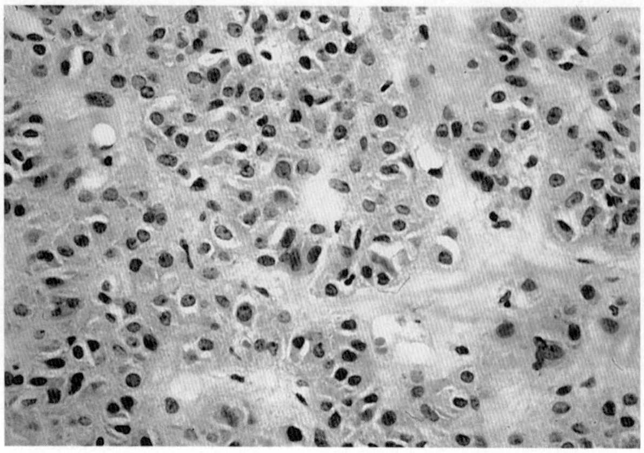

Figure 9 Histological section of a virlizing cortical adenoma. It is composed of cords of pale pink cells with uniform nuclei (hemotoxylin/eosin ×40).

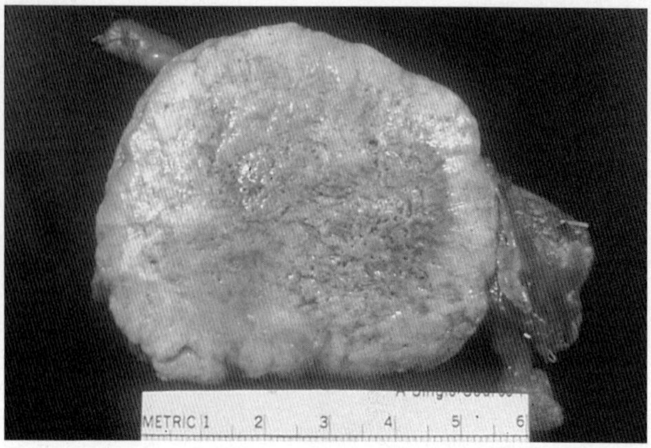

Figure 10 Adrenalectomy specimen of a cortical carcinoma. The carcinoma has a central zone of necrosis. Nonneoplastic adrenal tissue is seen on the right of the specimen.

always malignant—male adult patients present mostly with gynecomastia. Grossly, these tumors are of variable sizes, but most cases weigh over 100 g and they may be over 1000 g. The neoplasms are sharply circumscribed and usually have a tan or brown color (Fig. 8). Cells are arranged in cords or nests. Histologically, there is a predominance of lipid-depleted, eosinophilic, compact cells (Fig. 9). The remaining cortex, when visible is atrophic or normal in appearance.

Criteria for malignancy will be discussed in the next section (Figs. 8, 9) (17–19).

2 ADRENAL CORTICAL CARCINOMA

Adrenal cortical carcinoma (ACC) is a rare malignancy occurring predominantly in adults, but it can also affect the pediatric age group. Most large series show a slight female predilection, and the left adrenal is more often involved than the right. Metastases as an initial presentation occur in 15–25% of patients. At the clinical level these carcinomas may appear to be nonfunctional or hormonally active. Functional tumors are either monohormonal (i.e., Cushing's syndrome) or polyhormonal (i.e., Cushing's syndrome and virilization). The figures for patients presenting with hormonally inactive disease span a large range and may represent insensitivity in assessing steroid production. In several series the percentages of nonfunctional ACCs ranged from 25 to 75%. Overall, ACCs appear to be less efficient in hormone production than their benign counterparts because of deficiencies in enzymes essential for steroidogenesis. On gross examination these tumors are usually very large, weighing several hundred grams (Fig. 10). In general, adrenal cortical lesions weighing more than 100 g are suspect of being malignant, but definitive diagnosis of malignancy rests on characteristic histological findings. Additional gross features of ACC include fleshy, bulging tan nodules, which may have areas of necrosis and hemorrhage. Particularly large tumors may show gross evidence of infiltration into surrounding tissues. Histologically, the tumor cells are arranged in sheets, cords, or nests (Fig. 11), and broad areas of necrosis may be present. The vascularity of these tumors is less pronounced than that seen in adenomas. The predominant cell type, termed compact cell, is large and lipid

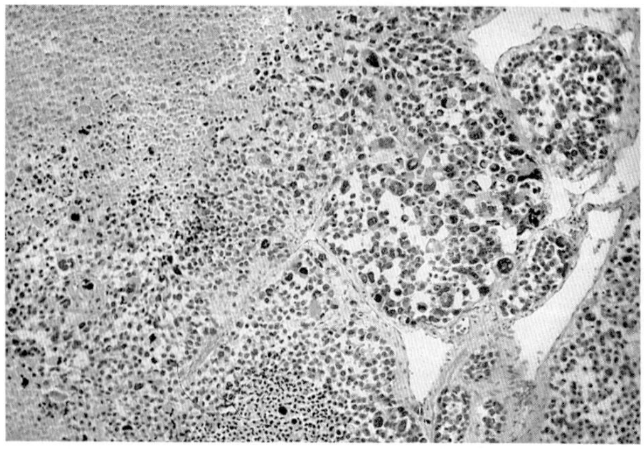

Figure 11 Histological section of a cortical carcinoma. The cells are in solid nests with areas of tumor necrosis on the left. The cells show nuclear pleomorphism and are lipid depleted (hemotoxylin/eosin ×10).

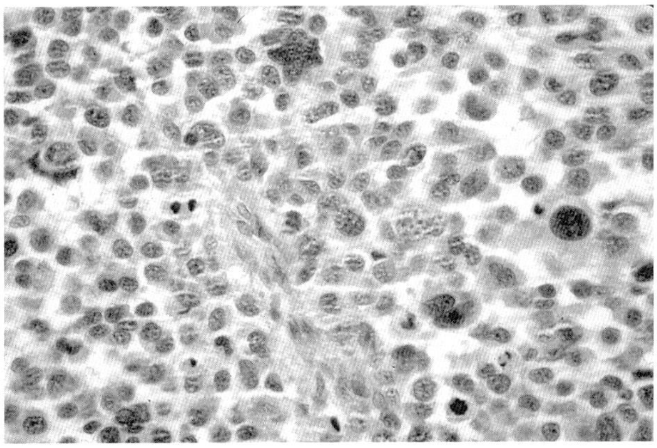

Figure 12 High magnification of an adrenal cortical carcinoma. The cells are in solid sheets and show marked nuclear pleomorphism with mitotic figures. The cells are lipid depleted and have eosinophilic cytoplasm (hemotoxylin/eosin ×40).

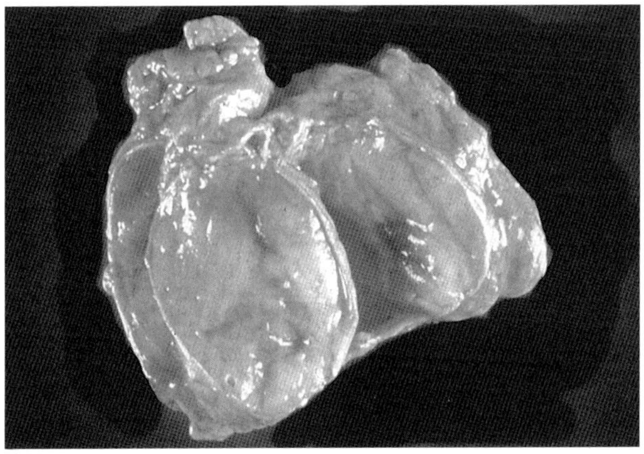

Figure 13 Adrenalectomy specimen of an adrenal pheochromocytoma. The tumor has a tan-red color, and there is a thin rim of adrenal cortical tissue at the periphery of the specimen.

depleted with adundant eosinophilic cytoplasm, but pale, lipid-rich cells may also be found. There is usually significant nuclear pleomorphism and atypia. Nuclear pseudoinclusions (cytoplasmic invaginations into the nucleus) can be seen. Mitotic figures are usually easily located, may be atypical in form (Fig. 12), and vascular/lymphatic invasion may be identified.

Immunohistochemistry is limited in this diagnosis. Unlike the majority of carcinomas, these carcinomas usually do not react with keratin antibodies but will react with the steroid marker inhibin, and vimentin is usually positive. Ultrastructural examination shows the lipid-depleted cells to contain abundant mitochondria and smooth endoplasmic reticulum. Rare cases may contain electron dense neuroendocrine-type cytoplasmic granules. Criteria established for the diagnosis of ACC in the absence of metastasis include vascular invasion, extensive capsular invasion, marked nuclear pleomorphism, and mitosis with atypical forms. In a study by Weiss (26), the only features associated with metastases were mitosis greater than 6 per 50 high-power fields and vascular invasion. There are a minority of cases where histology cannot definitively distinguish between a benign and malignant adrenal cortical tumor. These cases may be termed "adrenal cortical neoplasm of indeterminate malignant potential" (Figs. 10–12) (20–35).

3 ADRENAL PHEOCHROMOCYTOMA

Adrenal pheochromocytoma arises from the medullary chromaffin cells. This is the most common tumor of the adult adrenal medulla. The average age of patients is in the fifth decade. It is often termed the 10% tumor, with roughly 10% of the cases being malignant, bilateral, extra-adrenal, and occurring in childhood. These figures, however, have to be modified for sporadic and familial pheochromocytomas. Grossly, pheochromocytoma is a well-circumsrcibed red/brown mass (Fig. 13). The average size is approximately 4 cm. In smaller lesions, remnant adrenal medullary and overlying cortical tissue may be visualized and large lesions may show areas of cystification. The larger tumors may extend beyond the adrenal into adjacent structures, including the inferior vena cava. The classic histological pattern is a nested aggregation of cells termed Zellballen (Fig. 14).

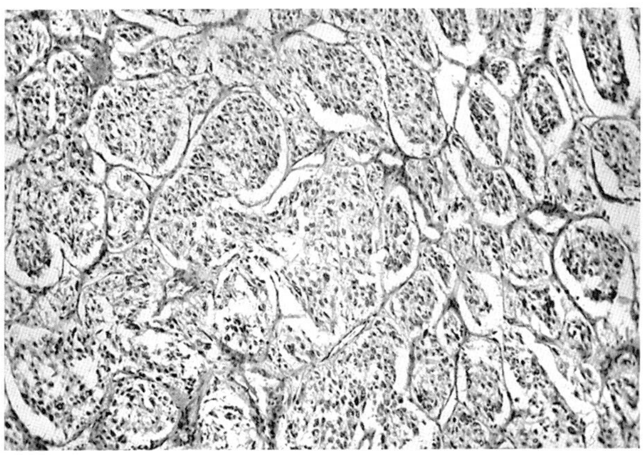

Figure 14 Adrenal pheochromocytoma showing the characteristic nested (Zellballen) arrangement of the tumor (hemotoxylin/eosin ×10).

Other patterns include trabecular and solid. An abundant capillary vasculature is found in all cases. The main cell population consists of chief cells, which have a round, polygonal, or spindle configuration. The cytoplasm is granular and may be eosinophilic, basophilic, or amphophilic. A rare degenerative change is the presence of cytoplasmic lipid droplets, which may cause confusion with a cortical tumor. Nuclei may vary greatly in size and shape (Fig. 15). Intranuclear pseudoinclusions as well as cytoplasmic hyalin globules may be seen and may be related to catecholamine production. Rare mitotic figures can be seen in benign cases. The stroma may show extensive sclerosis, and amyloid deposition can occur. Special histochemical stains can support the diagnosis of pheochromocytoma. A reticulin stain will enhance the Zellballen arrangement of the cells (Fig. 16). Silver stains such as grimelius will react with the catecholamine neurosecretory granules. Immunohistochemistry can also play a role in establishing the diagnosis in difficult cases. The chief cells will react with neuroendocrine markers such as chromogranin, synaptophysin, neuron-specific enolase, and Leu 7. The chief cells may also react with a variety of neuropeptides and hormones. A second population of cells, the sustentacular cells, which cannot be visualized with the routine hemotoxylin and eosin stain, will stain with the immunohistochemical marker S100 protein. The sustentacular cells are believed to play a supporting role in the tumor's composition. Ultrastructural examination is noteworthy for the presence of dense core neurosecretory granules. Two types of granules have been described, the epinephrine and the norepinephrine types. The epinephrine type has a uniform appearance, while the norepinephrine type is more variable and has a halo surrounding the granule. Correlation of ultrastructural findings with catecholamine production is, however, not reliable.Of historical interest is the chromaffin reaction, which aided the pathologist in establishing the diagnosis of pheochromocytoma. The reaction is the oxidation of the cathecholamines, which occurs following fixation of the tissue in solutions such as a dichromate fixative or, more commonly, formalin. The oxidation causes the fixative and the tissue to turn brown. Malignancy is uncommon and ranges from 3 to 14% of the adrenal pheochromocytomas (Fig. 17). Malignant cases tend to be larger, being several hundred grams in weight, show necrosis, vascular invasion, and have numerous mitotic figures. At present, however, there is no reliable morphological feature to distinguish

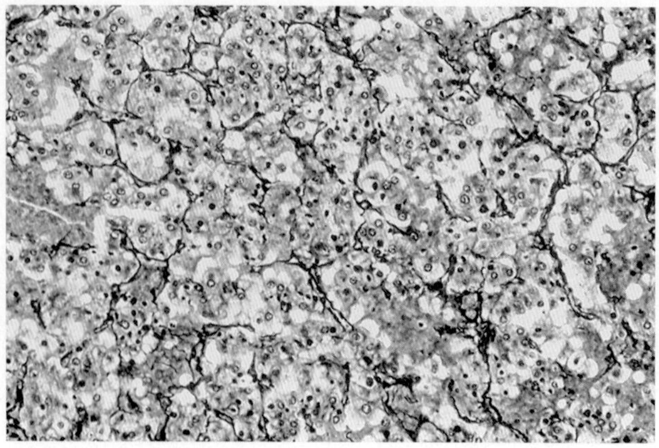

Figure 16 Reticulin stain highlighting the nested pattern of an adrenal pheochromocytoma (reticulin ×10).

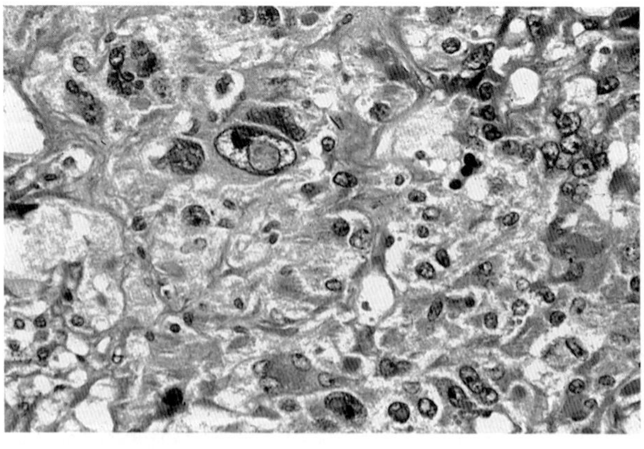

Figure 15 Adrenal pheochromocytoma showing nuclear atypia and an intranuclear inclusion. The cytoplasm is finely granular and basophilic (hemotoxylin/eosin ×40).

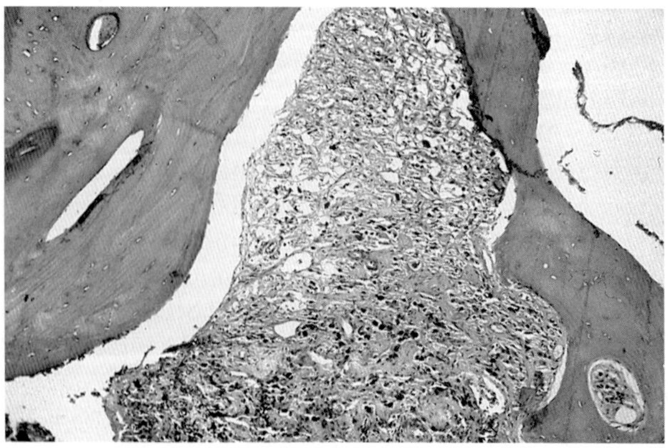

Figure 17 Metastatic pheochromocytoma in bone (hematoxylin/eosin ×10).

a benign from a malignant pheochromocytoma in the absence of mestastases (Figs. 13–17) (36–39).

4 NEUROBLASTOMA/ GANGLIONEUROBLASTOMA

Neuroblastoma/ganglioneuroblastoma (NB/GNB) is one of the most common childhood malignancies. The vast majority of these neoplasms arise in either the adrenal gland or the sympathetic ganglia. The gross appearance is usually a well-circumscribed nodule or group of nodules, which are tan and soft (Fig. 18). There may be areas of hemorrhage and necrosis, calcifications may be visible, and some tumors may have nodules of different appearance, corresponding to areas of varying maturation. Neuroblastoma is histologically composed of "round blue cells" with little appreciable cytoplasm in the most immature cells. Cells with some degree of maturation have more abundant cytoplasm and may have fibrillar material extending from the cells. These cells may be aggregated so that the fibrillar material protrudes centrally and forms what is termed a Homer-Wright pseudorosette (Fig. 19). The tumor cells can be arranged in sheets or in an organoid pattern. There is a prominent delicate background vascularity. GNBs will have a gross appearance similar to NB but will have a firmer consistency (Fig. 20). Histologically, cells show ganglionic differentiation with larger eccentric nuclei and have prominent nucleoli and abundant eosinophilic cytoplasm (Fig. 21). There is prominent fibrillar material in the background. Ultrastructural studies demonstrate a paucity of cytoplasmic organelles, rare electron dense neurosecretory granules, and neuritic cell pro-

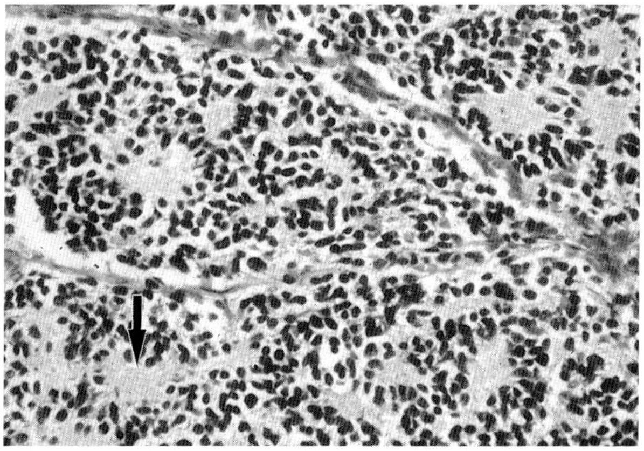

Figure 19 Neuroblastoma composed of small round blue cells, some forming Homer-Wright rosettes (arrow) with central neuropil fibrils (hemotoxylin/eosin ×40).

cesses. Immunohistochemical stains that are positive in these tumors include neuron-specific enolase (NSE), chromogranin, and synaptophysin. Tumors that have schwannian differentiation will react with S100 protein. There are several grading systems for these tumors, taking into consideration the degree of maturation in the lesion. The most universal system presently in use is the Shimada classification, which stratifies patients by age and tumor differentiation. Tumors are broadly divided into stroma-rich and stroma-poor groups. In the stroma-rich group, there are further subdivisions into tumors with abundant stroma and no nodules (the well-differentiated group and intermixed group), which is a favorable prognostic group, and those stroma-rich

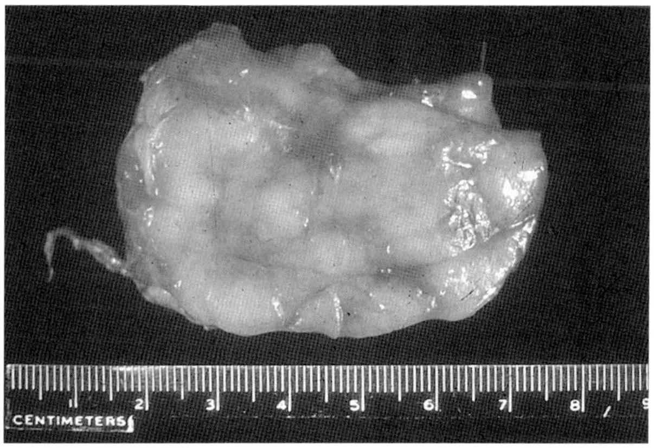

Figure 18 Adrenal neuroblastoma replacing the adrenal gland. The tumor is composed of fleshy tan tissue.

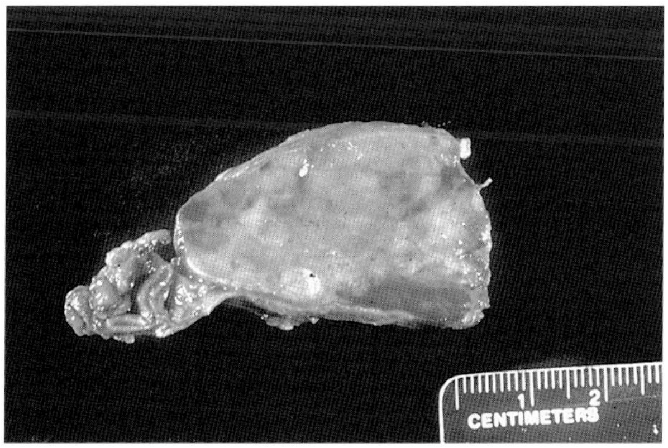

Figure 20 Adrenalectomy specimen with a ganglioneuroblastoma. There is attached nonneoplastic adrenal tissue on the left of the specimen.

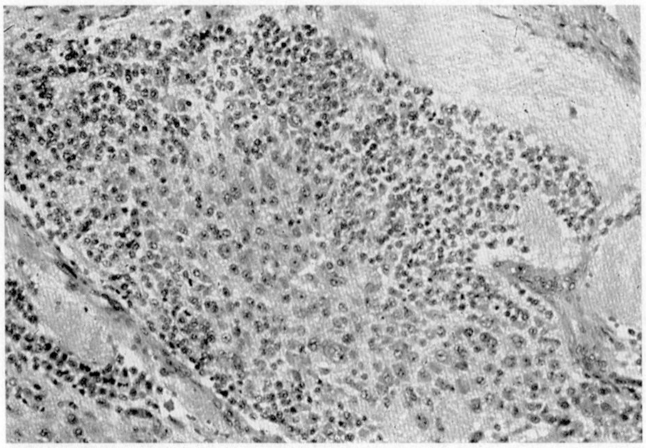

Figure 21 Ganglioneuroblastoma composed of larger more mature ganglionic cells which are surrounded by smaller undifferentied neuroblasts (hemotoxylin/eosin ×20).

cases with nodules showing different levels of maturation, i.e., neuroblastoma and ganglioneuroblastoma, in two grossly distinct nodules. This is considered an unfavorable prognosis. The stroma-poor group is stratified by age, tumor differentiation, and mitotic/karyorrhexis index (MKI). Stroma-poor tumors in patients less than 1.5 years of age and a MKI less than 200 fall into the favorable prognostic group. The other stroma-poor tumors are in patients less than 1.5 years of age with a MKI greater than 200, patients older than 5 years, and patients between 1.5 and 5 years with undifferentiated tumors. Patients 1.5–5 years of age with differentiated tumors and a MKI less than 100 fall in between the favorable and unfavorable groups. Overall adverse prognostic findings in NB/GNB include older age at diagnosis, advanced stage, N-myc oncogene amplification, and cytogenetic abnormalities of chromosome 1. These tumors will rarely spontaneously regress or mature into a ganglioneuroma. Metastatic spread occurs most often to the bone marrow, bone, lymph nodes, liver, skin, testis, and intracranial structures. (Figs. 18–21) (40–54).

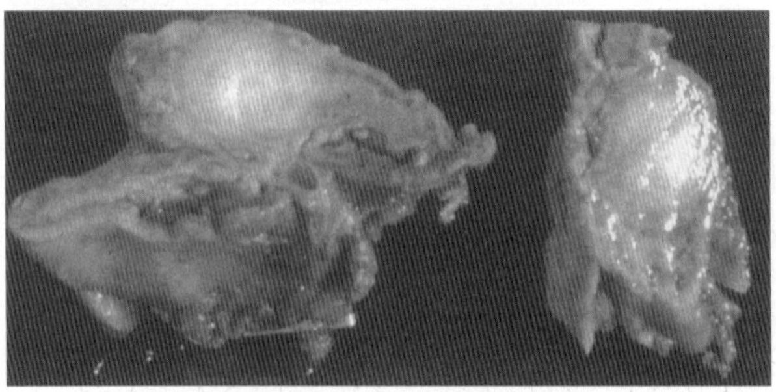

Figure 22 Adrenalectomy specimen with a ganglioneuroma. The lesion is well circumscribed and light tan in color.

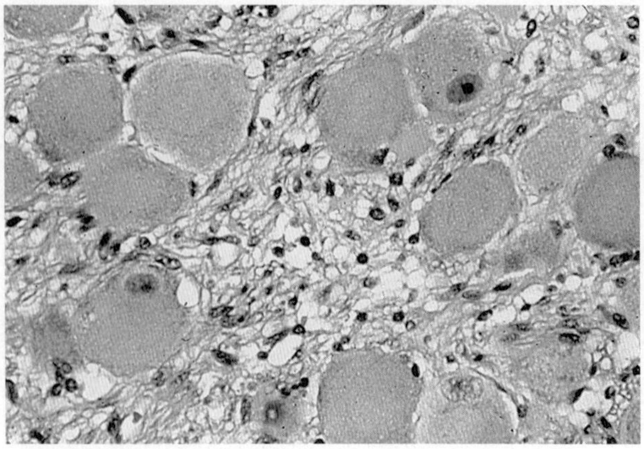

Figure 23 Histological section of a ganglioneuroma with mature ganglia (hemotoxylin/eosin ×40).

5 GANGLIONEUROMA

Ganglioneuroma is the mature neuroendocrine tumor occurring in the posterior mediastinum followed by the retroperitoneum and rarely in the adrenal medulla. Patients are usually older than the neuroblastoma group, and the tumor can occur in adults. Grossly, the tumors are well circumscribed, light, tan and firm (> Fig. 22). Calcifications may be felt on gross inspection. The adrenal tumors are usually smaller than those found in the more common locations. Histologically, there is a disorganized arrangement of mature ganglia and spindle Schwann cells (Fig. 23) (55–57).

REFERENCES

1. Commons RR, Callaway CP. Adenoma of the adrenal cortex. Arch Intern Med 1948; 81:37–41.
2. Kokko JP, Brown TC, Berman MM. Adrenal adenoma and hypertension. Lancet 1967; 1:468–470.
3. Shamma AH, Goddard JW, Sommers SC. A study of the adrenal status in hypertension. J Chron Dis 1958:587–595.
4. Abecassis M, Mc Loughlin MJ, Langer B, Kudlow JE. Serendipitous adrenal masses: prevalence, significance, and management. Am J Surg 1985; 49:783–788.
5. Prinz RA, Brooks MH, Churchill R, et al. Incidental asymptomatic adrenal masses detected by computed

tomographic scanning. Is operation required? JAMA 1982; 248:701–704.

6. Harrison JH, Mahoney EM, Bennett AH. Tumors of the adrenal cortex. Cancer 1973; 32:1227–1235.
7. Lack EE, Travis WD, Oretel LE. Adrenal cortical neoplasms. In: Lack EE, ed. Pathology of the adrenal glands. New York: Churchill Livingstone, 1990:115–171.
8. Neville AM, O'Hare MJ. Histopathology of the human adrenal cortex. Clin Endocrinol Metab 1985; 14:791–820.
9. Tannenbaum M. Ultrastructural pathology of the adrenal cortex. Pathol Annu 1973; 8:109–156.
10. Conn JW. Primary aldosteronism. J Lab and Clin Med 1955; 45:661–664.
11. Young WF Jr, Hogan MJ, Klee GG, Grant CS, van Heerden JA. Primary aldosteronism: diagnosis and treatment. Mayo Clin Proc 1990; 65:96–110.
12. Lack EE, Travis WD, Oertel JE. Adrenal cortical neoplasms. In: Lack EE, ed. Pathology of the Adrenal Glands. New York: Churchill Livingstone, 1990:115–171.
13. Eto T, Kumanoto K, Kawasaki T, Omae T, Masaki Z, Yamamoto T. Ultrastructural types of cells in adrenal cortical adenoma with primary aldosteronism. J Pathol 1979; 128:1–6.
14. Davis DA, Medline NM. Spironolactone (aldactone) bodies: concentric lamellar formations in the adrenal cortices of patients treated with spironolactone. Am J Clin Pathol 1970; 54:22–32.
15. Hsu SM, Raine L, Martin HF. Spironolactone bodies. An immunoperoxidase study with biochemical correlation. Am J Clin Pathol 1981; 75:92–95.
16. Kovacs K, Horvath E, Singer W. Fine structure and morphogenesis of spironolactone bodies in the zona glomerulosa of the human adrenal cortex. J Clin Pathol 1973; 26:949–957.
17. DelGaudio A, DelGaudio GA. Virilizing adrenocortical tumors in adult women. Report of 10 patients, 2 of whom each had a tumor secreting only testosterone. Cancer 1993; 72:1997–2003.
18. Gabrilove JL, Sharma DC, Wotiz HH, Dorfman RI. Feminizing adrenocortical tumors in the male. A review of 52 cases including a case report. Medicine 1965; 44:37–79.
19. Lee PD, Winter RJ, Green OC. Virilizing adrenocortical tumors in childhood: eight cases and a review of the literature. Pediatrics 1985; 76:437–444.
20. Cohn K, Gottesman L, Brennan M. Adrenocortical carcinoma. Surgery 1986; 100:1170–1177.
21. Wooten MD, King DK. Adrenal cortical carcinoma. Epidemiology and treatment with mitotane and a review of the literature. Cancer 1993; 72:3145–3155.
22. King DR, Lack EE. Adrenal cortical carcinoma. A clinical and pathological study of 49 cases. Cancer 1979; 44:239–244.
23. Van Slooten H, Schaberg A, Smeenk D, Moolenaar AJ. Morphologic characteristics of benign and malignant adrenocortical tumors. Cancer 1985; 55:766–773.
24. Lewinsky BS, Grigor KM, Symington T, Neville AM. The clinical and pathologic features of non-hormonal adrenocortical tumors. Report of twenty new cases and review of the literature. Cancer 1974; 33:778–790.
25. D'Agata R, Malozowski S, Barkan A, Cassorla F, Loriaux D. Steroid biosynthesis in human adrenal tumors. Horm Metabol Res 1987; 19:338–352.
26. Weiss LM. Comparative histologic study of 43 metastasizing and nonmetastasizing adrenocortical tumors. Am J Surg Pathol 1984; 8:163–169.
27. Tang CK, Gray GF. Adrenocortical neoplasms. Prognosis and morphology. Urology 1975; 5:691–695.
28. Mackay B, El-Naggar A, Ordonez NG. Ultrastructure of adrenal cortical carcinoma. Ultrastruct Pathol 1994; 18:181–190.
29. Miettinen M. Neuroendocrine differentiation in adrenocortical carcinoma. New immunohistochemical findings supported by electron microscopy. Lab Invest 1992 :169–174.
30. Gaffey MJ, Traweek ST, Mills SE, et al. Cytokeratin expression in adrenocortical neoplasia: an immunohistochemical and biochemical study with implications for the differential diagnosis of adrenocortical, hepatocellular and renal cell carcinoma. Hum Pathol 1992; 23:144–153.
31. Wick MR, Cherwitz DL, McGlennan RC, Dehner LP. Adrenocortical carcinoma. An immunohistochemical comparison with renal carcinoma. Am J Pathol 1986; 122:343–352.
32. Mc Cluggage WG, Burton J, Maxwell P, Sloan JM. Immunohistochemical staining of normal, hyperplastic and neoplastic adrenal cortex with a monoclonal antibody against alpha inhibin. J Clin Pathol 1998; 2:114–116.
33. Hough AJ, Hollifield JW, Page DL, Hartmann WH. Prognostic factors in adrenal cortical tumors. A mathematical analysis of clinical and morphologic data. Am J Clin Pathol 1979; 72:390–399.
34. O'Hare MJ, Monaghan P, Neville AM. The pathology of adrenocortical neoplasia: a correlated structural and functional approach to the diagnosis of malignant disease. Hum Pathol 1979; 10:137–154.
35. Lack EE, Travis WD, Ortel JE. Adrenal cortical neoplasms. In: Lack EE, ed. Pathology of the Adrenal Glands. New York: Churchill Livingstone, 1990:115–171.
36. Hume DM. Pheochromocytoma in the adult and in the child. Am J Surg 1960; 99:458–496.
37. Lack EE. Pathology of adrenal and extra adrenal paraganglia. In: Major Problems in Pathology. Vol. 29. Philadelphia: WB Saunders, 1994:229–272.
38. Stackpole RH, Melicow MM, Uson AC. Pheochromocytoma in children. Report of 9 cases and review of the first 100 published cases with follow up studies. J Pediatr 1963; 63:315–330.

39. Page DL, DeLellis RA, Hough AJ Jr. Tumors of the adrenal. In: Atlas of Tumor Pathology, 2nd Series, Fascicle 23. Washington, DC: Armed Forces Institute of Pathology, 1986:223–253.
40. Young JL Jr, Miller RW. Incidence of malignant tumors in US children. J Pediatr 1975; 86:254–258.
41. Young Jr, Ries LG, Silverberg E, Horm JW, Miller RW. Cancer incidence, survival and mortality for children younger than age 15 years. Cancer 1986; 58:598–602.
42. Lack EE. Pathology of adrenal and extra adrenal paraganglia. In: Major Problems in Pathology. Vol. 29. Philadelphia: WB Saunders, 1994:315–370.
43. Dehner LP. Pathologic anatomy of classic neuroblastoma:including prognostic features and differential diagnosis. In: Pochedly C, ed. Neuroblastoma: Tumor Biology and Therapy. Boca Raton, FL: CRC Press, 1990:111–143.
44. Lack EE, Kozakewich HP. Adrenal neuroblastoma, ganglioneuroblastoma, and related tumors. In: Lack EE, ed. Pathology of the Adrenal Glands. New York: Churchill Livingstone, 1990:277–309.
45. Shimada H, Chatten J, Newton WA Jr, et al. Histopathologic prognostic factors in neuroblastic tumors: definition of subtypes of ganglioneuroblastoma and age–linked classification of neuroblastoma. J Natl Cancer Inst 1984; 73,405–416.
46. Taxy JB. Electron microscopy in the diagnosis of neuroblastoma. Arch Pathol Lab Med 1980; 104:355–360.
47. Triche TJ. Differential diagnosis of neuroblastoma and related tumors. In: Lack EE, ed. Pathology of the Adrenal Glands. New York: Churchill Livingstone, 1990: 323–350.
48. Thomas P, Battifora H, Manderino GL, Patrick J. A monoclonal antibody against neuron-specific enolase. Immunohistochemical comparison with a polyclonal antiserum. Am J Clin Pathol 1987; 88:146–152.
49. Cooper MJ, Hutchins GM, Cohen PS, Helman LJ, Mennie RJ, Isreal MA. Human neuroblastoma tumor cell lines correspond to the arrested differention of chromaffin adrenal medullary neuroblasts. Cell Growth Diff 1990:149–159.
50. Misugi K, Aoki I, Kikyo S, Sasaki Y, Tsunoda A, Nakajima T. Immunohistochemical study of neuroblastoma and related tumors with anti-s-100 protein antibody. Pediatr Pathol 1985; 3:217–226.
51. Beckwith JB, Martin RF. Observations on the histopathology of neuroblastomas. J Pediatr Surg 1968; 3:106–110.
52. Brodeur GM, Azar C, Brother M, et al. Neuroblastoma. Effect of genetic factors on prognosis and treatment. Cancer 1992; 70:1685–1694.
53. Brodeur GM, Seeger RC, Schwab M, Varmus HE, Bishop JM. Amplification of N-myc in untreated human neuroblastomas correlates with advanced disease stage. Science 1984; 24:1121–1124.
54. Savilo E, Harnish D, Barr R, deSa D. A comparison of the prognostic significance of the Shimada classification and N-myc oncogene amplification in neuroblastoma and ganglioneuroblastoma: a prospective study. Mod Pathol 1994; 7:8P.
55. Hamilton JP, Koop CE. Ganglioneuromas in children. Surg Gynecol Obstet 1965; 121:803–812.
56. Stout AP. Ganglioneuroma of the sympathetic of the sympathetic nervous system. Surg Gynecol Obstet 1947; 84:101–110.
57. Lack EE. Pathology of Adrenal and Extraadrenal Paraganglia. Major Problems in Pathology. Vol. 29. Philadelphia: WB Saunders, 1994.

27

Ultrasonography of the Adrenal Gland

Hsu-Chong Yeh

Mount Sinai School of Medicine, New York University, New York, New York, U.S.A.

Ultrasonographic delineation of the adrenal glands and small adrenal lesions is usually more difficult than that of other abdominal organs because these small structures are located high and deep in the rib cage, especially the left adrenal gland, which may be obscured by bowel gas or lung. Successful scanning usually requires prior knowledge of detailed anatomy in the adrenal areas and a careful and appropriate scanning method. With the advent of many improvements in ultrasound equipment, e.g., well-focused beam profile, tissue harmonic imaging, and compound real-time scanning, adrenal lesions are becoming more readily visible by ultrasonography.

1 ULTRASOUND FEATURES OF NORMAL ADRENAL GLANDS

The adrenal glands are a pair of flat organs, triangular on the right and semilunar shaped on the left. They are about 4–6 cm in length and 2–3 cm in width. They are characteristically thin, only 2–6 mm thick, and in cross-sectional imaging with ultrasound, computed tomography (CT), and magnetic resonance (MR), the glands appear as variations of linear or curvilinear structures and not as triangular or semilunar configurations. The adrenal glands consist of an anteromedial ridge and two wings that open posterolaterally (1). The medial wing is larger superiorly and smaller or absent inferiorly, and vice versa for the lateral wing (2). On transverse scan, the superior section of the adrenal gland is a vertical linear or curvilinear structure consisting of only the anteromedial ridge and the medial wing. In the middle section, both wings are equally seen and an inverted "Y" (or inverted "V" when the anteromedial ridge is small)–shaped structure may be seen. The inferior section shows little or no medial wing, resulting in an "L" (left adrenal) or reverse "L" (right adrenal) shape. In longitudinal or coronal scan, the glands appear as a linear, curvilinear, or horizontal "Y" or "V" shape (2). Therefore, depending on the shape of the gland on image, the level of scanning plane can be determined on transverse scan.

The success rates of visualization of the right and left adrenal glands are 78% and 44%, respectively, by manual scanning (1), 92% and 71%, respectively, by real-time scanning (4). The medulla may sometimes be seen as a highly echogenic line sandwiched between two thin layers of hypoechoic cortex (5). This is more frequently seen in the newborn and in the hypertrophic adult gland.

2 SCANNING TECHNIQUE

The best scanning approach for the adrenal gland is transverse intercostal scanning from the upper lateral abdomen (1). The right adrenal gland is enclosed in a small area between the crus of diaphragm, liver, inferior vena cava, and the upper pole of the kidney. The left adrenal gland is located lateral to the aorta and crus of diaphragm, medial to the spleen, anteromedial to the

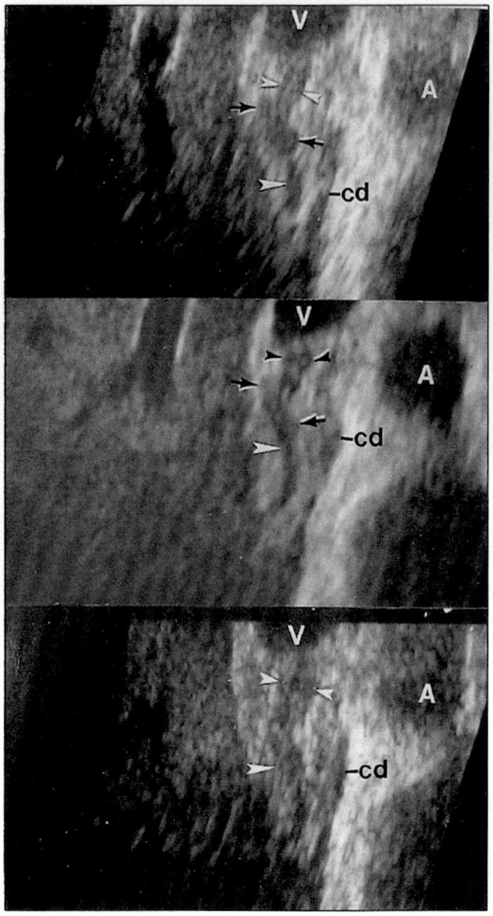

Figure 1 Nodular hyperplasia of adrenal glands. A series of three transverse sections of the superior aspect of the right adrenal gland are shown. There are only two parts of the gland in these sections: the antero-medial ridge and the medial wing forming a vertical curved band-like structure. The anterior part of the structure represents the antero-medial ridge, and the posterior part, which is curved, represents the medial wing. (Top) The uppermost section shows two small nodules (black arrows) at the junction between the antero-medial ridge (small white arrowheads) and the medial wing (large white arrowhead). Note the linear echogenic medulla running through the center of the antero-medial ridge. V = inferior vena cava; A = aorta; cd = crus of diaphragm. (Middle) Four nodules are seen: two tiny ones (black arrowheads) in the cortex of the antero-medial ridge where the echogenic medulla is again seen; two nodules (black arrows) at the junction between the antero-medial ridge and the medial wing, same as above. V = inferior vena cava; A = aorta; cd = crus of diaphragm. (Bottom) This section shows the thickest part of adrenal gland, 0.9 cm in thickness in the antero-medial ridge (between small white arrowheads). Large white arrowhead = medial wing; V = inferior vena cava; A = aorta; cd = crus of diaphragm.

upper pole of the left kidney, and posterior to the stomach and pancreas. The left adrenal gland is usually more difficult to scan than the right because it may be obscured by gastric or bowel gas. Therefore, the transducer position should be more posterior than for the right gland, usually at the posterior axillary line. A gentle sweeping motion of the transducer to scan from 3–4 cm above the upper pole of the kidney downward to the renal hilum level will allow the adrenal areas to be completely examined. Longitudinal (i.e., coronal) scan from the same transducer position may also show the adrenal areas.

3 SMALL ADRENAL MASSES

Small adrenal masses are usually hypoechoic and round or oval in shape, and they are thicker than the normal adrenal gland and easier to visualize than the normal gland. The incidence of visualization of a small mass is 97% by an experienced ultrasonographer (1). Therefore, when the adrenal area is thoroughly scanned and the area is not obscured by bowel gas and no mass is found, a mass can be practically excluded even though the normal adrenal gland is not visualized.

A mass of 1 cm or smaller can be seen by ultrasonography (5). Although a small mass frequently represents a benign adenoma, it cannot be differentiated from a metastatic malignant tumor or hyperplastic nodule (Fig. 1) by ultrasonography, and the latter may or may not be associated with an enlarged (thickened) adrenal gland. When differentiation between hyperplastic nodules and tumor is impossible with ultrasound, CT, or MR, adrenal venography with venous blood sampling or adrenal scintigraphy may be necessary.

Adrenal adenoma with a high lipid content such as aldosteronoma (Fig. 2) may present as a low-density lesion similar to a cyst even on enchanced CT (6). When the density is very low and blends with surrounding fat, it may become difficult to recognize on CT, but ultrasonography will clearly delineate it as a solid mass.

4 LARGE ADRENAL MASSES

Since the adrenal gland is located anteromedially to the upper pole of the kidney, a large adrenal mass usually displaces the upper pole of the kidney laterally (7). Some larger adrenal masses, however, may extend down anterior to the kidney without causing much displacement of the latter (8). A right adrenal mass may also

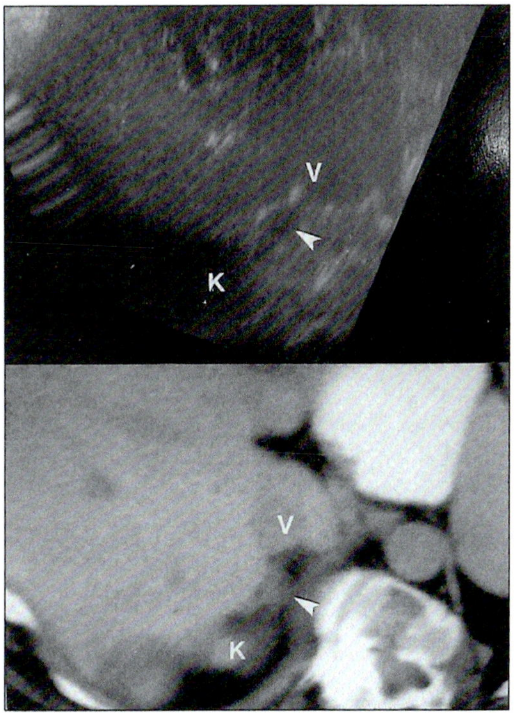

Figure 2 A 1.4 cm aldosteronoma in the right adrenal gland. (Top) Transverse scan shows a 1.4 cm mass (arrowhead) in the right adrenal gland. Note normal part of the adrenal gland anterior and posterior to the mass are also seen. The adrenal gland is located immediately posterior to inferior vena cava (V), which is not clearly seen in this section. K = upper pole of right kidney. (Bottom) Corresponding CT shows the small adrenal mass (arrowhead) and normal parts of the adrenal gland anteriorly and posteriorly. V = inferior vena cava; K = kidney. Note the medial part of the mass has low density due to high lipid content.

extend anteriorly between the inferior vena cava and aorta.

A large adrenal mass may markedly indent the kidney or liver so that the mass may appear to arise from either of the two organs. There are some ultrasonographic features that help to differentiate an adrenal from a renal or hepatic mass: (1) a highly echogenic demarcation line between the mass and the kidney or the liver may represent a thin layer of perirenal fat, therefore the mass is extrarenal or extrahepatic in origin; (2) a notch at the edge of demarcation; (3) a larger portion of the mass outside the kidney or the liver; (4) during deep inspiration, a relative motion can be seen between the mass and the kidney or the liver; (5) on color Doppler study, if intrarenal or intrahepatic vessels are seen to enter the mass, the mass is likely to be renal or hepatic.

5 DIFFUSE ENLARGEMENT OF THE ADRENAL GLAND

In diffuse enlargement of the adrenal gland, the most important ultrasonographic feature is thickening of the adrenal gland to more than 0.7 cm measured for each part of the gland (9) and not at the confluence of adrenal parts. The length and width of the entire gland are much less important. The enlargement or thickening may be more marked in one part than in others (Fig. 1), and the largest number is taken. When the confluent point is measured, the normal thickness can be up to 1 cm (10). When the adrenal gland is mildly (0.7–1.2 cm thick) to moderately (1.3–2.5 cm thick) enlarged, the basic form of the normal adrenal gland is still easily recognizable in each scanning plane except that the gland appears thicker or fatter (11). The enlargement of the gland may be asymmetrical. This is best observed in the middle-scanning plane in which both wings are equally visualized. One wing may be thicker than the other. When the gland is markedly enlarged, i.e., more than 2.6 cm thick, the features are more distorted. In the upper transverse section it may be a vertical oval or pear shaped. In the middle section, it may be a fat inverted "V" shape, triangular shaped, inverted heart shaped, or pentagonal shaped with rounded-off corners. A small notch at the base of the inverted heart shape represents the residual space between the two wings. In the lower section, it may appear as a fat "L" or reverse "L" shape, a wedge, a rhomboid shape, or a horizontally elongated oval shape. When the gland is extremely enlarged, it may appear nodular or irregular in contour even though the gross appearance of the basic feature is preserved. On coronal scan, a characteristic horn shape is seen. If one does not have prior knowledge of the features of a markedly enlarged adrenal gland on serial sections or if one does not systemically study the entire series of sections, one can easily mistake it as focal mass lesion (11). Recognition of a diffusely enlarged adrenal gland is important because this will narrow down the differential diagnoses to the following (9):

1. Bilateral hyperplasia: since there is no infiltration, destruction, or invasion of the gland by inflammatory or neoplastic process, the medulla is usually preserved (Fig. 1) and easier to see than

a normal gland. In marked enlargement of the gland, which usually is due to ectopic ACTH syndrome, the medulla may appear as a thin echogenic line in a very "fat" gland, and careful examination is necessary to find the medulla. The presence of medulla in a large gland is characteristic of hyperplasia (9,11).

2. Infiltrating neoplastic disease: the most common tumor is lymphoma, mostly non-Hodgkin's lymphoma (9) (Fig. 3). Diffuse involvement of the adrenal glands by lymphoma is usually bilateral. It is frequently associated with retroperitoneal lymphadenopathy but can be primary adrenal involvement. Massive enlargement of adrenal glands is not uncommonly seen and the enlarged adrenal glands may have homogeneous or somewhat nodular echotexture. Metastatic lesions may also cause diffuse enlargement of the adrenal gland (8), most commonly from lung (Fig. 4), but may also from stomach, breast, uterus, kidney, and pancreas primaries.

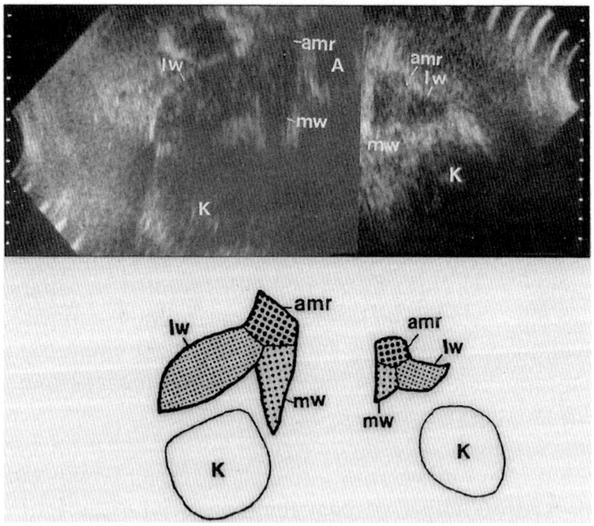

Figure 3 Bilateral diffusely enlarged adrenal glands due to primary adrenal lymphoma. (Top) A composite image of transverse scans of the right and left adrenal glands. Both glands show inverted thick "Y"-shaped structures representing the middle section of the glands. No medulla was detected on scanning. amr = artero-medial ridge; lw = lateral wing; mw = medial wing; K = kidney; A = aorta. (Bottom) Drawing shows three parts of the enlarged adrenal gland corresponding to the above images.

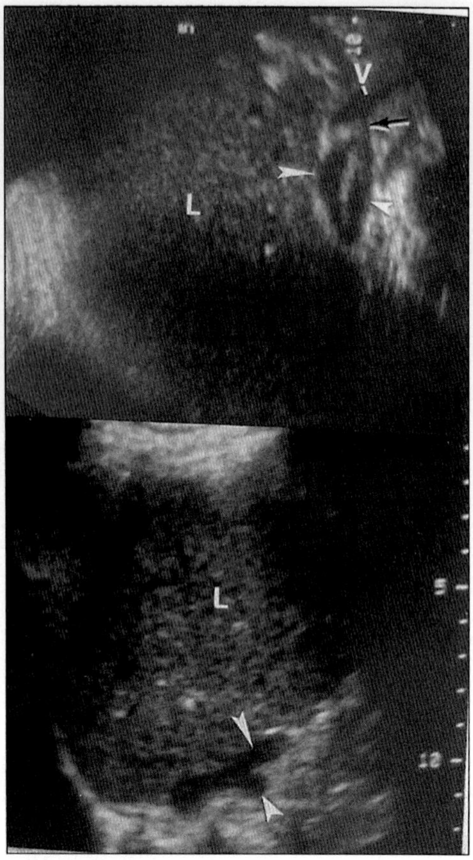

Figure 4 Diffuse involvement of the right adrenal gland by lung cancer. (Top) Transverse scan from the right upper flank region shows diffusely enlarged right adrenal gland medial to the liver (L) posterior to inferior vena cava (V). The image is rotated 90° counterclockwise to show the same orientation as a transaxial CT scan. This is section of the midportion of the gland, and both lateral (long arrowhead) and medial (short arrowhead) wings are equally seen. The lateral wing is the largest, 1 cm in thickness. The antero-medial ridge (arrow) is only slightly enlarged. (Bottom) Coronal scan shows the diffusely enlarged right adrenal gland with lateral (long arrowhead) and medial (short arrowhead) wings. L = liver. Ultrasound-guided transhepatic fine needle biopsy of the right adrenal gland proved metastatic lung cancer.

3. Adrenal hemorrhage: may be focal or generally diffuse, diffuse cortical or diffuse medullary.
4. Infectious disease, e.g., tuberculosis, histoplasmosis, blastomycosis, cryptococcus.
5. Congenital metabolic deficiency: lipoid adrenal hyperplasia, cholesterol desmolase deficiency. There is accumulation of lipids and cholesterol in the adrenal cortex.

6 ADRENAL HEMORRHAGE

A focal adrenal hemorrhage is usually round or oval in shape. It may be echo-free (12,13) but may contain echoes due to blood clots. The echoes may disappear in a few days due to lysis of clots. The hematoma usually decreases in size in 4–5 weeks, and internal echoes reappear due to organization of the hematoma. The hematoma may further shrink down and may calcify in 4–9 months (14), seen by ultrasonography as a small highly echogenic lesion with acoustic shadow.

In diffuse hemorrhage, the adrenal gland is diffusely enlarged. moderately echogenic, similar to infiltrating tumor (9). CT without intravenous injection of contrast material may show high-density areas in the gland representing blood clots.

7 ADRENAL CALCIFICATIONS

Adrenal calcifications usually result from hemorrhage but may also be from tumors (neuroblastoma, carcinoma, pheochromocytoma, adenoma, myelolipoma) or infection such as tuberculosis (15). They are usually small, irregular-shaped highly echogenic lesions with acoustic shadow but may also appear as thin peripheral calcification. Calcification in adrenal cystic wall may appear as a curvilinear echogenic structure with shadowing. Adrenal cysts have a high incidence of wall calcification, and a calcified adrenal cyst does not have the same ominous significance as indicating a tumor as does a renal cyst (15).

8 ADRENAL TUMORS

8.1 Cortical Adenomas

Nonfunctioning (nonhyperfunctioning) adenomas are usually small, ranging up to 2.5 cm (15) in diameter, rarely exceeding 5 cm, being found in 2% of postmortem examinations. They are usually found incidentally during examination for other purposes. On ultrasonography, they cannot be differentiated from a small primary or metastatic tumor or functioning tumor except that the latter causes abnormal clinical endocrinological manifestations. Low density on unenhanced CT will differentiate adenoma from nonadenoma (16), which is the advantage of CT over ultrasonography.

Functioning adenomas may cause Cushing's syndrome, primary aldosteronism, or virilization. Ultrasonographically, functioning adenomas cannot be differentiated from nonfunctioning adenomas.

8.2 Carcinomas

Carcinomas may also be functioning or nonfunctioning. The tumors are large, sometimes exceeding 20 cm in diameter (15). They frequently have hemorrhagic, cystic, or necrotic changes. The hemorrhage and necrosis may result in hyperechoic or hypoechoic areas, depending on the age of the clot, amount of debris, edema, and liquefication of clot or necrotic tissue (8). Therefore, a tumor may appear heterogeneous. The contour of a tumor may be smooth or irregular (8,6,16). A small carcinoma cannot be differentiated from an adenoma (17).

8.3 Pheochromocytoma

This is an uncommon tumor, mostly arising in chromaffin cells of the adrenal medulla, but 10% arise in the autonomic nervous system, usually in the organ of Zuckerkandl in the para-aortic areas. Multiple pheochromocytomas, unilateral or bilateral, are frequently associated with various hereditary syndromes. Although it is reported that the pheochromocytomas are usually large when discovered (18), small masses less than 3 cm are not uncommonly seen (20% in the author's experience) (5). The tumor may be homogeneous in echo texture but hemorrhage and necrosis are frequently seen, even in a small tumor. This may result in heterogeneity with hyperechoic (Fig. 5) or hypoechoic or echo-free areas. Total hemorrhage may result in a cystic appearance that may occur even in a small tumor (e.g., 2 × 3 cm) (8).

8.4 Myelolipoma

This tumor arises from the adrenal cortex and is composed of fat and bone marrow elements in varying proportions. It is endocrinologically nonfunctioning, although bilateral large tumors may cause endocrine disturbance. There is no malignant potential. Ultrasonographically, the tumor is diffusely highly echogenic (19,20), usually homogeneous. It is quite similar to angiomyolipoma of the kidney, and therefore, when the mass indents on the kidney, angiomyolipoma should also be considered. When a large amount of myeloid element or hemorrhage and/or necrosis is present, the tumor may appear heterogeneous. Some other tumors, e.g., carcinoma or pheochromocytoma, should also be

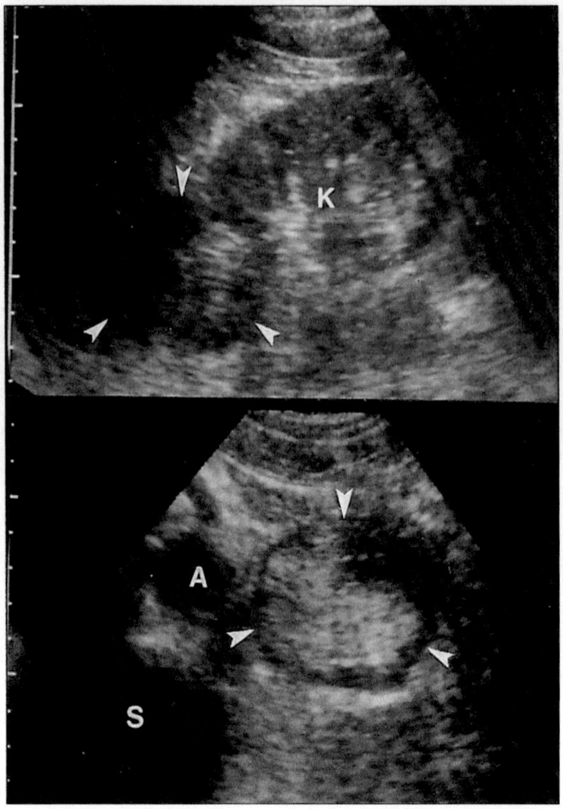

Figure 5 A necrotic pheochromocytoma in the left adrenal gland. (Top) Coronal scan of left kidney (K) shows a mass (arrowheads) antero-medial to the upper pole of the kidney. (Bottom) Transverse scan showed the mass to be highly echogenic in most part. A = aorta; S = vertebral body. Pathological examination shows extensive necrosis and hemorrhage in the mass. High echogenicity was due to debris and blood clot.

considered in such an instance. During needle biopsy, if only fatty tissue is obtained one may not be certain if the specimen is from perirenal fat or from a myelolipoma. Repeat biopsy should be done in different areas to obtain myeloid tissue in order to confirm the diagnosis.

9 METASTATIC MASSES OF THE ADRENAL GLAND

The adrenal glands are the fourth most common site in the body for metastases, after the lungs, the liver, and the bones. Adrenal metastases were found in 27% in a series of 1000 autopsied patients with malignancies (21). The most common primary sites are lung (75.6%) and breast (53.9%) (21). Others include the gastrointestinal tract, kidney, and ovary. Therefore, scanning of both adrenal areas should be done for patients known to have primary malignancy to detect adrenal masses. Most adrenal metastases are round or oval and poorly echogenic (22), but a large metastasis may be irregular in shape (6). Ultrasonography, including color Doppler scanning, usually cannot differentiate between a metastasis and a benign adenoma (23) except that if the mass is large (>5 cm) and/or irregular in shape, metastasis rather than adenoma is more likely.

REFERENCES

1. Yeh HC. Ultrasonography of normal adrenal gland and small adrenal masses. Am J Roentgenol 1980; 1135: 1167–1177.
2. Yeh HC. Ultrasonography of the adrenal gland. In: Resnick MI, Sanders RC, eds. Ultrasound in Urology. Baltimore: Williams and Wilkins, 1984:285–306.
3. Marchal G, Gelin J, Verbeken E, Baert A, Lauwerins J. High-resolution real time sonography of the adrenal glands: a routine examination? J Ultrasound M 1986; 5:65–68.
4. Oppenheimer DA, Carroll BA, Yousem S. Sonography of the normal neonatal adrenal gland. Radiology 1983; 146:157–160.
5. Yeh HC. Adrenal gland and nonrenal retroperitoneum. Urol Radiol 1987; 9:127–140.
6. Yeh HC. Ultrasonography of the adrenal glands. In: Resnick MI, Rifkin MD, eds. Ultrasonography of the Urinary Tract. 3d ed. Baltimore: Williams and Wilkins, 1991.
7. Yeh HC, Mitty HA, Rose JS, Wolf BS, Gabrilove LL. Ultrasonography of adrenal masses, usual manifestations. Radiology 1978; 127:467–474.
8. Yeh HC, Mitty HA, Rose JS, Wolf BS, Gabrilove LL. Ultrasonography of adrenal masses, unusual manifestations. Radiology 1978; 127:475–483.
9. Yeh HC. US and CT evaluation of diffusely enlarged adrenal gland. Crit Rev Diagn Imaging 1992; 33(5):437–460.
10. Montagne JP, Kressel HY, Korobkin M, Moss AA. Computed tomography of the normal adrenal gland. Am J Roentgenol 1978; 130:963–966.
11. Yeh HC, Bhardwaji S, Gabrillove JL, Cuttner J. Imaging of diffusely enlarged adrenal glands. Hospimedica 1991; 9:37–42.
12. Mittlestaedt CA, Volberg FM, Merten DF, Brill PW. The sonographic diagnosis of neonatal adrenal hemorrhage. Radiology 1979; 131:453–457.
13. Mineau DE, Koehler PR. Ultrasound diagnosis of neonatal adrenal hemorrhage. Am J Roentgenol 1979; 132:443–444.
14. Pery M, Kaftori JK, Bar-Maor JA. Sonography for

diagnosis and follow-up of neonatal adrenal hemorrhage. J Clin Ultrasound 1981; 9:397–401.
15. Mitty HA, Yeh HC. Radiology of the Adrenals with Sonography and CT. Philadelphia: WB Saunders, 1982.
16. Korobkin M, Brodeur FJ, Yutzy GG, Francis IR, Quint LE, Dunnick NR, Kazerooni EA. Differentiation of adrenal adenomas from nonadenomas using CT attenuation values. Am J Roentgenol 1996; 166:531–536.
17. Hamper UM, Fishman EK, Hartman DS, Roberts DS, Sanders RC. Primary adrenocortical carcinoma: sonographic evaluation with clinical and pathologic correlation in 26 patients. Am J Roentgenol 1987; 148:915–919.
18. Bowerman RA, Silver TM, Jaffe MH, Stuck KJ, Hinerman DL. Sonography of adrenal pheochromocytomas. Am J Roentgenol 1981; 137:1227–1231.
19. Musante F, Derchi LE, Zappasodi F, Bazzocchi M, Riviezzo GC, Banderali A, Ciccio GR. Myelolipoma of the adrenal gland: sonographic and CT features. Am J Roentgenol 1988; 151:961–964.
20. Vick CW, Zeman RK, Mannes E, Cronan JJ, Walsh JW. Adrenal myelolipoma: CT and ultrasound findings. Urol Radiol 1984; 6:7–13.
21. Abrams HL, Spiro R, Goldstein N. Metastases in carcinoma. Cancer 1950; 3:74–85.
22. Forsythe JR, Gosink BB, Leopold GR. Ultrasound in the evaluation of adrenal metastases. J Clin Ultrasound 1977; 5:31–34.
23. Ghiatas AA, Chopra S, Schnitker JB. Is sonographic flow imaging useful in the differential diagnosis of adrenal masses? Br J Radiol 1996; 69:1005–1008.

28

Computed Tomography of the Adrenal Glands

David S. Mendelson and William L. Simpson, Jr.

Mount Sinai School of Medicine, New York University, New York, New York, U.S.A.

1 TECHNOLOGY

Computed tomography (CT) is often regarded as a mature technology. In fact, it is a constantly evolving technology much different in its current implementation than it was at its inception 25 years ago. While the basic premise, the delivery of a cross-sectional image, remains the same, the scope of what can be delivered is currently much greater than when it entered the marketplace during the late 1970s.

Currently, imaging of the abdomen can be performed in a single breath-hold, with a z-axis (craniocaudad) resolution of less than 1 mm, utilizing a technology known as multidetector CT (MDCT) (1,2). This technology is enabled by exposing multiple rows of CT detectors simultaneously, rather than the conventional single row. At the time of this writing, four-detector-row CT devices are common, and instrumentation with up to 32 detector rows is being introduced. In the most simplistic scheme, the presence of four rows reduces the imaging time by a factor of four. Other advances have further reduced scanning time, including faster rotation of the x-ray tube around the patient (0.5 sec), and faster transit of the patient through the CT gantry.

What have these advances in engineering attained from a clinical perspective? Combined with the gains in affordable computer processing, we have a host of tools directed at volumetric imaging. Isotropic data sets are obtained; that is, the voxels that comprise the CT image are close to equal in all three dimensions. The end result is that we can look at the CT data as representing a volume, rather than a plane, and reconstruct images along any axis we wish, maintaining a high image quality. We can deliberately select a viewing plane that emphasizes the anatomy of interest (Fig. 1). Images can be presented in a three-dimensional (3-D) mode, enhancing our ability to appreciate spatial relationships. We have made great strides to graphically present human anatomy in a realistic fashion.

These technological advances have also allowed the enhancement of more conventional CT diagnostic techniques. The improved spatial resolution permits the performance of thin sections (< 1 mm). Smaller structures, both normal and abnormal, can be delineated. Whereas we have long utilized iodinated contrast media to simply identify vascular structures, we now routinely speak of CT angiography. In many clinical settings CT angiography has replaced conventional angiography.

2 CT ANATOMY OF THE NORMAL ADRENAL

The adrenal glands are thin, inverted V- or Y-shaped structures, adjacent to the upper poles of the kidneys (Fig. 1A,B). They are of soft tissue density, measuring approximately 40–50 Hounsfield units (HU). Though anatomically composed of a medulla and cortex, these components are not distinguishable on CT. On the right

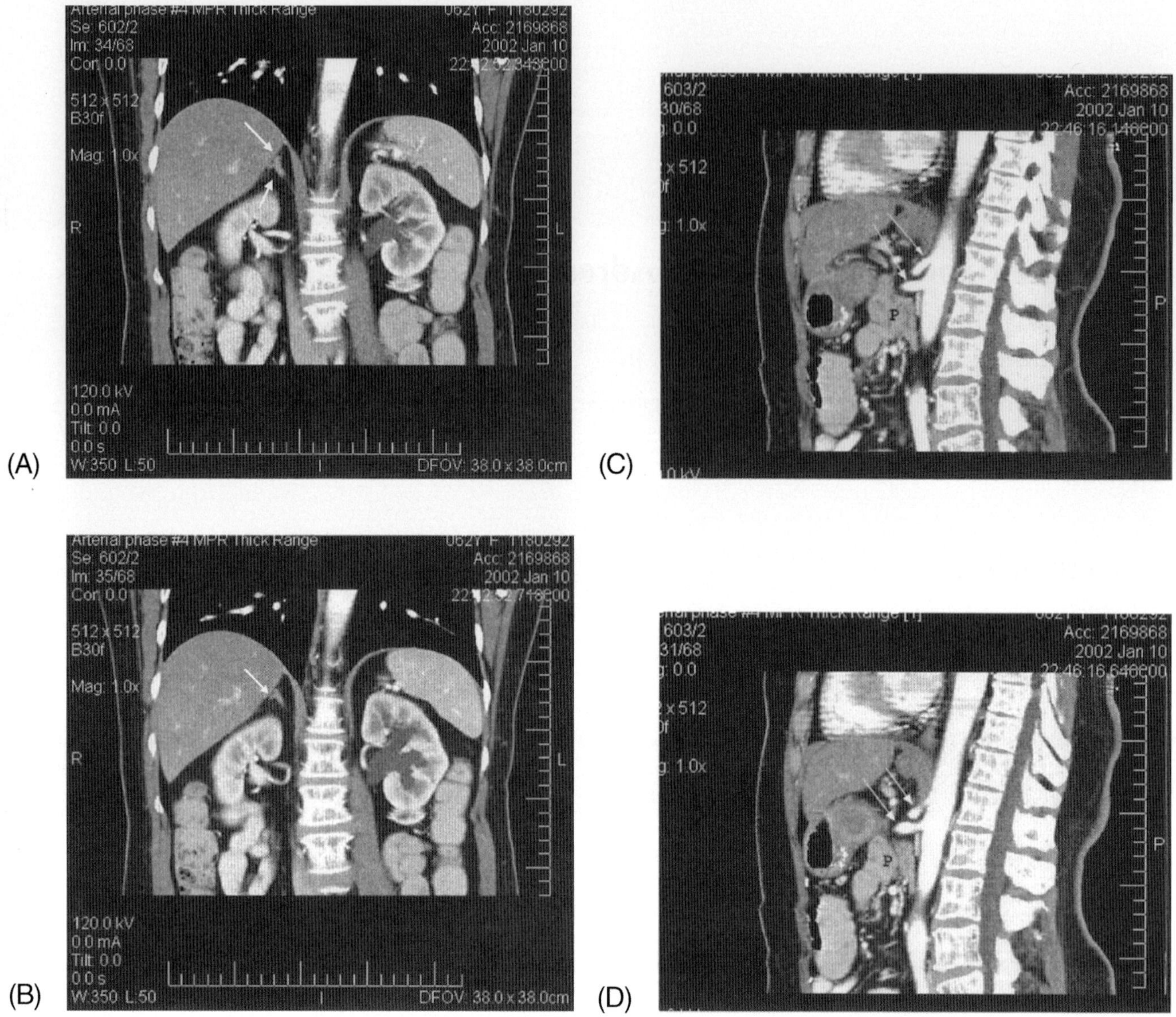

Figure 1 Normal anatomy of the adrenals and pancreas depicted in multiple planes. (A,B) Two views in the coronal plane of the normal right adrenal, seen as a thin inverted V, easily demonstrate its relationship to the upper pole of the right kidney. (C,D) Two saggital views demonstrate a portion of the pancreatic head (P), and importantly the origins of the celiac (superior arrow) and superior mesenteric (lower arrow) arteries. When a pancreatic tumor is present, the status of these vessels is important in performing surgical planning; these are best visualized in this plane.

side, the junction of the medial and lateral limbs usually resides just dorsal to the inferior vena cava (IVC), between the liver and kidney. The junction is slightly thickened compared to each of the limbs, which are draped around the upper pole of the kidney. Usually there is a substantial plane of fat separating all these soft tissue density structures. The fat is relatively lucent, and the lucency provides contrast, making identification of the various organs easy.

The left adrenal is similar to the right but is sometimes slightly more difficult to identify, given the absence of the larger landmarks and the presence of several similar caliber vascular structures running nearby. It is not unusual for a novice observer to mistake a portion of the splenic vein or some branch vessel for the adrenal gland.

A good rule of thumb during a quick visual assessment of the adrenals is that the limbs of the adrenal should be no thicker than the nearby crura of the diaphragms. While there is no strict measurement distinguishing the normal from abnormal adrenal, the thickness is usually on the order of several millimeters.

On closer inspection further detail can be resolved. Often one can identify the vascular supply of each adrenal, with the attendant variations in the origin of the vessels. These vascular landmarks can become useful in the patient with congenital anomalies in whom the site of an adrenal gland is in question. In a difficult case, one may first identify one of these vessels and trace their way back to the adrenal.

3 CT EVALUATION OF THE ADRENAL NODULE

3.1 Identification

An adrenal mass may be identified on a CT exam either deliberately, that is, the CT was performed specifically to detect such a mass, or as an incidental finding as part of a CT performed for some other reason. There are several reasons that a CT may be performed with attention directed at the adrenal (3,4). In a patient with an endocrinological syndrome with evidence suggesting that the adrenal may be involved, CT is the first-line radiological examination. The adrenal is easily identified, and CT can quickly establish in most patients whether or not the gland is morphologically normal. It is a rare patient who has a syndrome for which the adrenal glands are the source who does not have some morphological abnormality. This applies to syndromes including both hyperactive and hypoactive states.

The other reason to assess the adrenals with CT is in the staging of patients with a neoplasm. The adrenals are a common site of metastases, particularly in lung cancer. At the time of death, up to 33% of patients with lung cancer will have adrenal metastases.

Once an adrenal mass is identified, there is generally an attempt to further chararacterize it. Size alone, while not specific, can still yield some useful information. Almost all lesions 4 cm and greater are malignant, whether primary or metastatic. Lesions under 2 cm are quite common and statistically often benign, thus known as "incidentalomas."

3.2 Technique

The adrenal is optimally evaluated with sections on the order of 3–5 mm in thickness as a preliminary examination. On occasion there may be a need for thinner sections, dictated by the findings on the preliminary examination. The use of intravenous contrast is optional and often dependent on the clinical situation. One may obtain excellent images of the adrenal glands without iodinated contrast. Below we discuss CT densitometry and the role of IV contrast in this setting.

4 ANALYSIS OF AN ADRENAL NODULE

The CT approach to analyzing an adrenal nodule will vary depending on whether or not the presence of the nodule was anticipated prior to the performance of the CT. There are many variations of abdominal CT, utilizing intravenous and oral contrast, which may suffice to establish whether or not an adrenal nodule is present, particularly when the CT is performed for an indication other than adrenal assessment. However, these techniques are not optimized for fully assessing an adrenal nodule. When an examination is targeted specifically at assessing an adrenal nodule, thin section techniques should be employed and performance of CT densitometry should be considered.

5 CT DENSITOMETRY

CT densitometry offers a good deal of information that can help in the management of the patient with an adrenal nodule. There is a growing literature that supports the utilization of CT to characterize adrenal masses. We regard a section thickness of 3 mm or thinner as optimal for CT densitometry.

Initially a contrast minus (C-) examination should be performed. The value of this exam lies in the observation that most benign adrenal adenomas contain a large amount of lipid. Fat has a lower CT value, i.e., generally in the −40 to −100 HU range, than soft tissue, usually +40 HU or above. The presence of fat in the adenoma often results in an average CT number near 10 HU, much lower than the typical soft tissue mass, 40–50 HU.

Several studies have corroborated this finding in practice (5–7). Different authors have set various thresholds, between 0 and 18 HU, and measured the sensitivity and specificity of a C- CT for the prediction of a benign adenoma. In a meta-analysis of this body of work, Boland et al. (6) noted that a threshold of 10 HU had a sensitivity of 71% and a specificity of 98% for distinguishing benign from malignant tumors.

The C- examination may be followed by an examination with intravenous contrast. Several authors have demonstrated that the use of CT density washout measurements is an accurate means of identifying adrenal adenomas (8–13). While both benign adenomas and malignant neoplasms enhance, there is a rapid washout of contrast in the group of benign adenomas. This can be measured with the following technique.

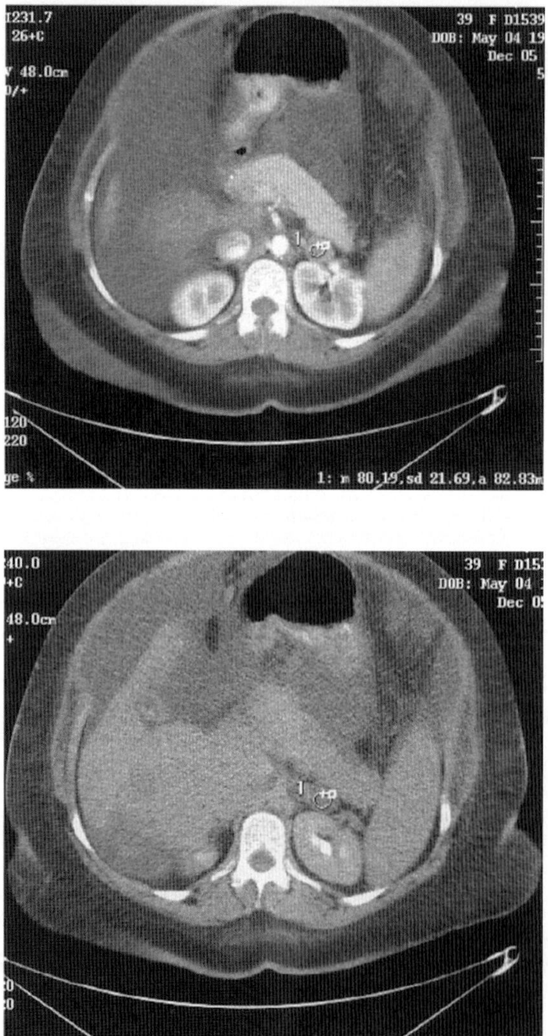

(A)

(B)

Figure 2 This patient demonstrates a 2.2 × 2.0 cm left adrenal mass that initially enhanced to 80 HU (A) and subsequently diminished to 14 HU (B) on a 15-minute delayed study. By both a raw threshold of 24 HU and a relative washout percentage of 84%, this pattern suggests an adenoma.

Percentage washout = {(Peak CT # - Delayed CT number) / (Peak CT # - C- CT #) }X 100

Figure 3 Formula for calculating percentage washout.

After a C- CT, a C+ exam is conducted in two phases; the first is performed approximately 70 seconds after intravenous contrast injection has commenced, usually at a rate of 2–3 cc/sec, with sections 3–5 mm in thickness. This is followed by similar thickness imaging 15 minutes later, selectively through the adrenals. Measurements are taken of the adrenal mass at each time (Fig. 2). A percentage of washout (Fig. 3)—a measure of the diminution from peak enhancement—of 60% or greater is typical of benign adenomas. Other neoplasms remain enhanced to a greater degree at the 15-minute interval and thus demonstrate a smaller percentage of washout.

A variant of this technique has been described which accounts for the common situation in which only a C+ CT was performed (9,10). A value, the relative percentage of washout, is calculated (Fig. 4), which takes into account only the initial enhancement (peak CT number) and the 15-minute delay value, since a C- exam for baseline comparison was not performed.

These techniques have been repeatedly demonstrated to have sensitivities on the order of 88% and specificities of 95%. There have been modifications of the technique and the thresholds, but all variants have had similar results. While the one described above is generally considered the standard practice at this time, some authors have suggested that rather than calculate a percentage or relative percentage washout at 15 minutes, one can simply set a CT measurement threshold of 24 HU or less on a C+ exam at 15 minutes and attain a specificity and sensitivity of 96% (12,13). Conceptually these authors are measuring the same thing, CT enhancement, utilizing a slightly different technique.

Relative Percentage enhancement washout = {(Peak CT # - Delayed CT number) / Peak value}X 100

Figure 4 Formula for calculating relative percentage washout.

6 CT FINDINGS IN SPECIFIC ADRENAL SYNDROMES AND NEOPLASMS

6.1 Pheochromocytoma

Pheochromocytoma is a neoplasm arising in the adrenal medulla which secretes catecholamines. Identification of a pheochromocytoma on CT is often easy, at least in the patient in whom it occurs spontaneously, as they are relatively large tumors, often several centimeters in size (Fig. 5). The exception to this rule is the patient with a familial syndrome in whom pheochromocytoma is simply one manifestation of a multiorgan disease. Pheochromocytoma may be discovered when significantly smaller in size in these patients, whether or not they are symptomatic. This observation particularly includes the MEN syndromes. Whereas a small adrenal nodule un-

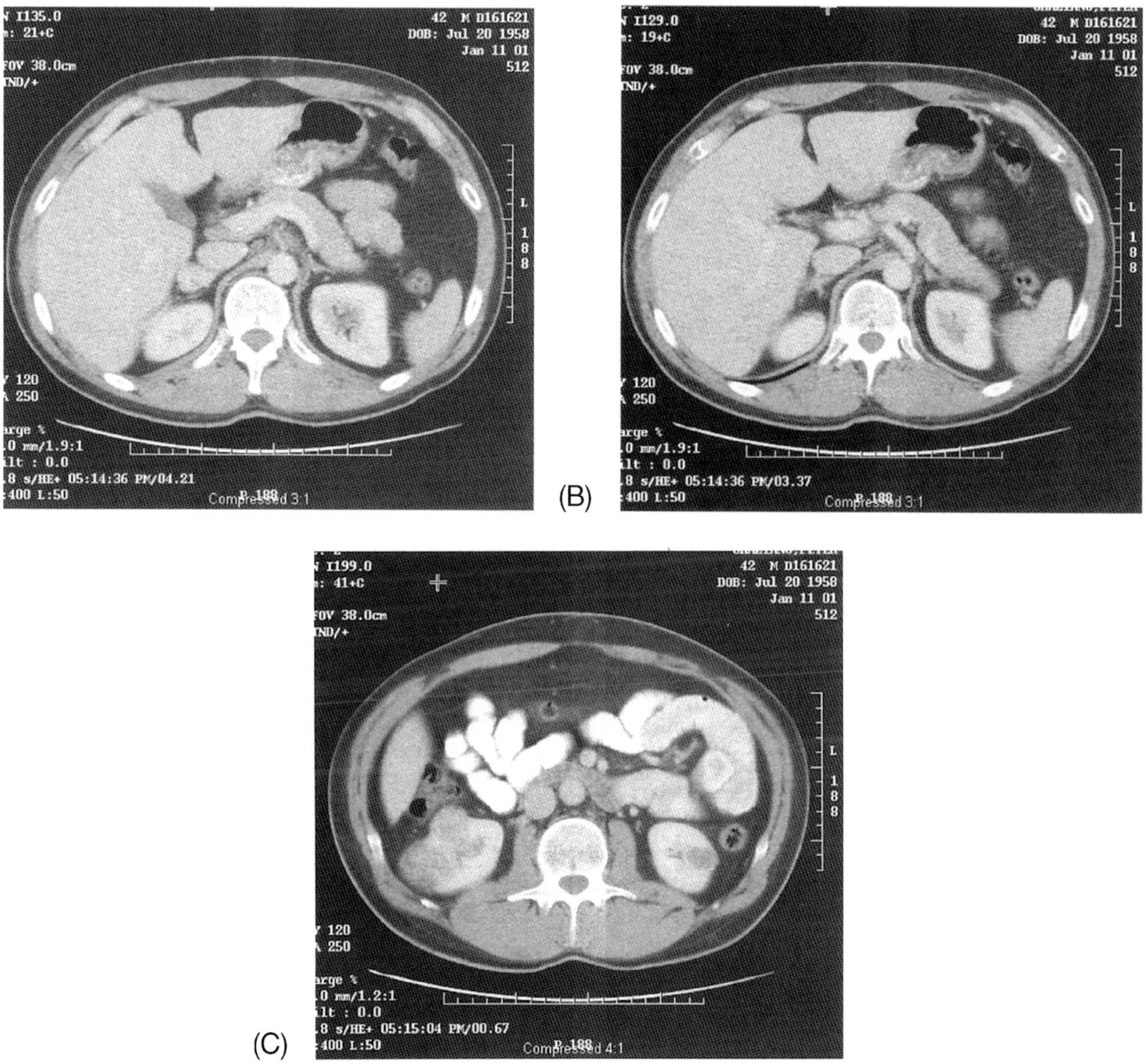

(A) (B) (C)

Figure 5 This patient with Von Hippel Lindau syndrome demonstrates a mass at the right adrenal, which proved to be a pheochromocytoma (A). There is an additional subcentimeter nodule noted at the left adrenal, which proved to be a second pheochromocytoma (B). This latter lesion is unusual in that it is small. Generally these tumors first come to attention when several centimeters in size. However, in the event of a familial syndrome, when deliberately searched for they can be discovered when quite small. One can also see several solid renal masses, consistent with hypernephromas (C), also a part of this syndrome.

der 1–2 cm in size, the incidentaloma, may simply be followed in an otherwise normal host, all such nodules must be regarded as suspicious for pheochromocytoma in the patient with a familial syndrome.

Its origin from the adrenal medulla is not discernible on CT, even with thin sections. Thus, when identified in an asymptomatic patient, CT does not provide many clues to distinguish this tumor from other neoplasms.

Intravenous contrast must be employed judiciously in a patient with a pheochromocytoma (4,14,15). The utilization of contrast is contraindicated in patients with this tumor if they are not pharmacologically blocked with alpha and beta antagonists, as an adrenergic crisis may be induced. There is some evidence that this reaction is less likely to occur with the newer nonionic contrast agents (15).

A significant number of pheochromocytomas, up to 10%, arise in an extra-adrenal location. While they may occur almost anywhere in the body, the sympathetic chain is a common site. Thus, CT has the advantage of providing good visualization of most of the sites at which this tumor may occur. Given the relatively high frequency of occurrence along the sympathetic chain, attention to the paraspinal region is warranted.

6.2 Cushing's Syndrome

The status of the adrenals will vary depending on the underlying etiology of the patient's Cushing's syndrome (16). The most straightforward finding is in the 20% of patients in whom the cause of Cushing's syndrome is an isolated adrenal cortical adenoma secreting cortisol. Such functioning adenomas are often over 2 cm in diameter and easily discerned on CT. The more common etiology of Cushing's syndrome is Cushing's disease, in which there is an ACTH-secreting pituitary tumor. In this situation both of the adrenals may vary in appearance from normal to thickened.

6.3 Conn's Syndrome—Hyperaldosteronism

Hyperaldosteronism is caused by a benign adrenal adenoma in up to 65–80% of cases (3,17). The remainder of the cases usually have bilateral adrenal hyperplasia. This diagnosis may be suspected when a patient is undergoing an evaluation for hypertension and hypokalemia is detected. The adenomas causing this syndrome are usually small, measuring less than 1 cm (18). However, given the current state of CT, they are easily detectable. If fact, the challenge is to distinguish these small tumors from normal variants and/or bilateral hyperplasia. In one study, Doppman et al. (19), found that the most common error was to interpret thickened adrenals with multiple small nodules as bilateral hyperplasia, when in fact there was a small adenoma present; their conclusion was that one may be confident of a diagnosis of adenoma on CT but must be wary of a diagnosis of hyperplasia. The therapies are different: surgical in the case of the adenoma and medical for hyperplasia.

6.4 Myelolipoma

Myelolipoma is an unusual tumor of the adrenal. It is composed of mixed elements, including myeloid, erythroid, and fatty elements. They have a typical appearance on CT examination; that is, they can be seen to contain a significant amount of discrete fat (20). The demonstration of islands of fat in a small to moderate-sized lesion is considered diagnostic. Sometimes this requires measuring CT numbers. Note that as opposed to benign adenomas in which the fat is histologically intermixed throughout the tumor, the fat in a myelolipoma is in well-delineated and bounded collections.

6.5 Adrenal Carcinoma

Adrenal carcinoma is usually a large neoplasm arising from the adrenal cortex. They are often larger than 4 cm in size, and they on occasion may be bilateral. Approximately one half of these tumors are functioning with some secondary syndrome related to the production of hormones. Their large size is recognized on CT, where they are usually noted to be heterogeneous and occasionally demonstrate flecks of calcium. They are indistinguishable from large metastasis.

6.6 Adrenal Hemorrhage

A variety of etiologies can cause adrenal hemorrhage, including trauma, stress, shock, postpartum necrosis, and coagulopathy. These may all result in hypofunction of the glands, particularly when bilateral. Acute hemorrhage is characterized on CT by enlargement of the gland, which may or may not maintain its shape, and an increase in the density of the gland. The region of hemorrhage usually diminishes in both size and density over time and may ultimately calcify.

6.7 Adrenal Calcifications

Adrenal calcification may be noted in several conditions, some neoplastic and some not. In the context of endocrine disease it is simply a sign that some pathological process has occurred in the adrenals and may be an etiology of an endocrinological syndrome. They can be seen at the site of old granulomatous infections and prior hemorrhage. They can also be seen as part of neoplastic processes, including adrenal carcinoma. Hence, the presence of a calcification in a mass does not exclude the possibility of a tumor, even a malignant one.

REFERENCES

1. Hu H. Multi-slice helical CT: scan and reconstruction. Med Phys 1999; 26:5–18.
2. Klingenbeck-Regn K, Schaller S, Flohr T, Ohnesorge B, Kopp AF, Baum U. Subsecond multi-slice computed tomography: basics and applications. EurJ Radiol 1999; 31:110–124.
3. Mayo-Smith WW, Boland GW, Noto RB, Lee ML. State of the art adrenal imaging. RadioGraphics 2001; 21:995–1012.
4. Lockhart ME, Smith JK, Kenney PJ. Imaging of adrenal masses. Eur J Radiol 2002; 41(2):95–112.
5. Lee MJ, Hahn PF, Papanicolaou N, et al. Benign and malignant adrenal masses: CT distinction with attenuation coefficients, size, and observer analysis. Radiology 1991; 179:415–418.
6. Boland GW, Lee MJ, Gazelle GS, Halpern EF, McNicholas MM, Mueller PR. Characterization of adrenal masses using unenhanced CT: an analysis of the CT literature. Am J Roentgenol 1998; 171:201–204.
7. Korobkin M, Brodeur FJ, Yutzy GG, et al. Differentiation of adrenal adenomas from nonadenomas using CT attenuation values. Am J Roentgenol 1996; 166:531–536.
8. Korobkin M, Brodeur FJ, Francis IR, Quint LE, Dunnick NR, Goodsitt M. Delayed enhanced CT for differentiation of benign from malignant adrenal masses. Radiology 1996; 200:737–742.
9. Szolar DH, Kammerhuber FH. Adrenal adenomas and nonadenomas: assessment of washout at delayed contrast-enhanced CT. Radiology 1998; 207:369–375.
10. Caoili EM, Korobkin M, Francis IR, Cohan RH, Dunnick NR. Delayed enhanced CT of lipid poor adrenal adenomas. Am J Roentgenol 2000; 175:1411–1415.
11. Szolar DH, Kammerhuber FH. Quantitative CT evaluation of adrenal gland masses: a step forward in the differentiation between adenomas and nonadenomas? Radiology 1997; 202:517–521.
12. Boland GW, Hahn PF, Pena C, Mueller PR. Adrenal masses: characterization with delayed contrast-enhanced CT. Radiology 1997; 202:693–696.
13. Korobkin M, Brodeur FJ, Francis IR, Quint LE, Dunnick NR, Londy F. CT time-attenuation washout curves of adrenal adenomas and nonadenomas. Am J Roentgenol 1998; 170:747–752.
14. Raisanen J, Shapiro B, Glazer GM, Desai S, Sisson JC. Plasma catecholamines in pheochromocytoma: effect of urographic contrast media. Am J Roentgenol 1984; 143:43–46.
15. Mukherjee JJ, Peppercorn PD, Reznek RH, Patel V, Kaltsas G, Besser M, Grossman AB. Pheochromocytoma: effect of nonionic contrast medium in CT on circulating catecholamine levels. Radiology 1997; 202:227–231.
16. Sohaib SA, Hanson JA, Newell-Price JDC, et al. CT appearance of the adrenal glands in adrenocorticotrophic hormone-dependent Cushing's syndrome. Am J Roentgenol 1999; 172:997–1002.
17. Blevins LS Jr, Wand GS. Primary aldosteronism: an endocrine perspective. Radiology 1992; 184:599–600.
18. Dunnick NR, Leight GS, Robidoux MA, Leder RA, Paulson E, Kurylo L. CT in the diagnosis of primary aldosteronism: sensitivity in 29 patients. Am J Roentgenol 1993; 160:321–324.
19. Doppman JL, Gill JR Jr, Miller DL, Chang R, Gupta R, et al. Distinction between hyperaldosteronism due to bilateral hyperplasia and unilateral aldosteronoma: reliability of CT. Radiology 1992; 184(3):667–682.
20. McNicholas MM, Lee MJ, Mayo-Smith WW, Kenney PJ, Wagner BJ, Rao P, Heffess CS. Myelolipoma: CT and pathologic features. Radiology 1998; 208:87–95.

29

Magnetic Resonance Imaging of Endocrine Adrenal Tumors

Angela R. Berning and Jeffrey P. Goldman

Mount Sinai School of Medicine, New York University, New York, New York, U.S.A.

1 INTRODUCTION

Endocrine tumors of the adrenal arise from either the cortex or the medulla. Magnetic resonance imaging (MRI) is most commonly used to investigate a clinical syndrome caused by hormonal hypersecretion or to study an adrenal mass detected on some other imaging test. Functional tumors are usually smaller and more difficult to detect than nonfunctional tumors, which usually present at a later stage with local complications of a mass or metastatic disease. Less commonly, patients with a known primary malignancy are evaluated for possible adrenal metastasis (1–4).

2 MR IMAGING

Particularly useful in the imaging of the adrenals is a variation on the T1 sequence called the chemical shift (CS) technique, which utilizes the principle of the differences in motion or rotational frequencies of water and lipid protons. Two T1-weighted gradient echo sequences are performed with different echo times. The first is called an "in-phase" sequence, where water and fat are at the same point in their cycle and so their signals are additive. Second, an "out-of-phase" sequence is performed in which fat and water are at opposite points in their cycle and so their contributions to the MR signal are destructive and cancel out. Observation of a relative loss of signal intensity on opposed-phase images compared with that on in-phase images indicates the presence of relatively small amounts of intracellular lipid in tissues (15). This finding has been shown to correlate well with density measurements in computed tomography (CT) (16) and histological findings (17). Adrenal adenomas are homogeneous with low signal intensity on T2-weighted images.

For many years CT was the imaging method of choice (18–21) in evaluating a possible adrenal mass. Means of differentiating benign from malignant lesions include evaluation of attenuation values or "density" and contrast enhancement patterns (22,23). There is no doubt that MR is playing an ever-increasing role in the evaluation of adrenal lesions.

3 MR IMAGING OF THE NORMAL ADRENAL GLAND

The normal adrenal gland is hypo-intense or dark in relation to the liver and renal cortex but more intense or bright than adjacent vascular structures on T1- and T2-weighted images (Fig. 1). Some authors purport to being able to differentiate between two regions of different signal intensity thought to represent cortex and medulla differentiation, with the medulla being brighter than the cortex (27). The normal gland enhances homogeneously with the maximal signal intensity

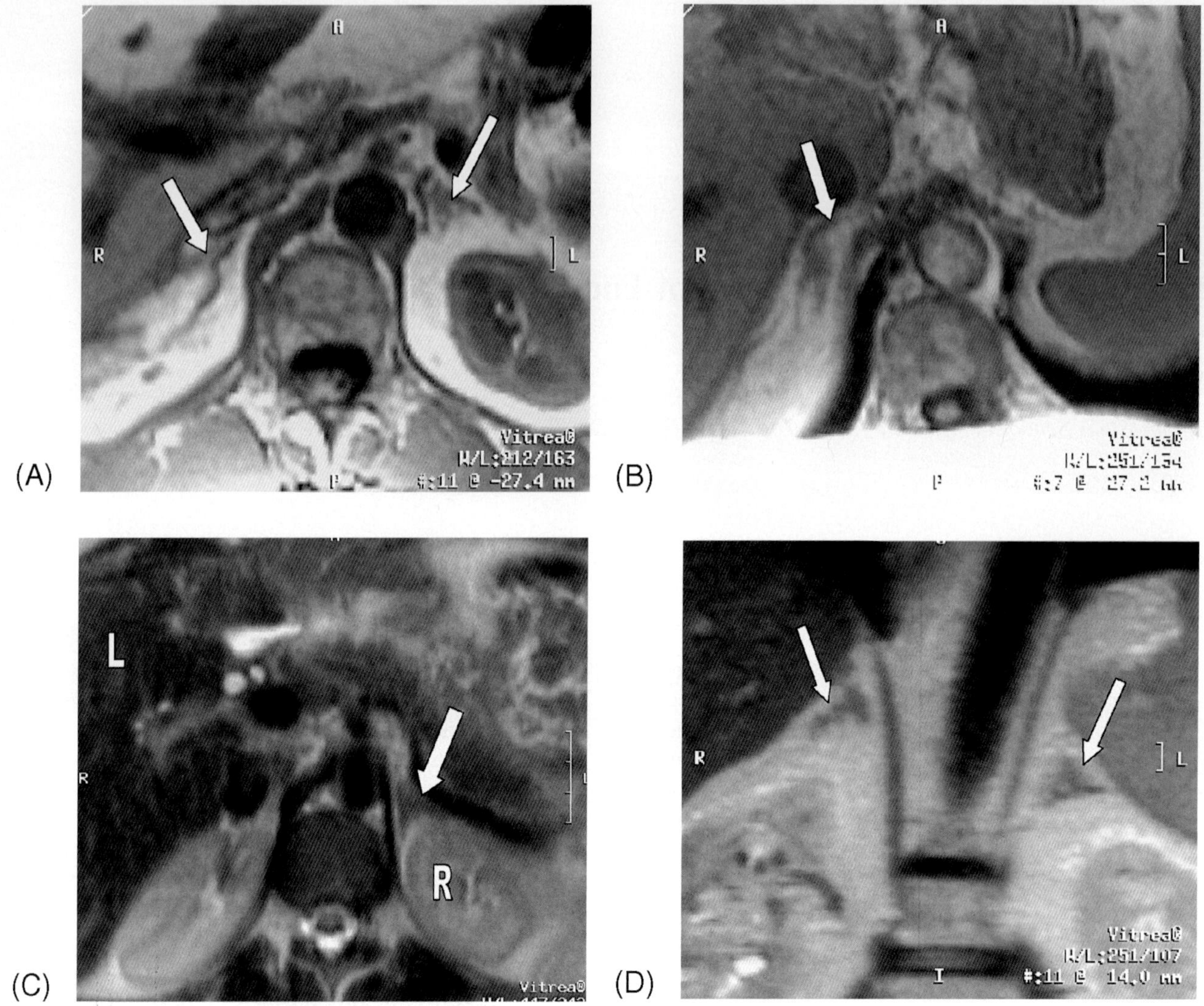

Figure 1 Axial T1 (A and B), axial T2 (C), and coronal T2 (D) MR images of normal adrenal.

observed at approximately 2.5 minutes after injection of contrast (28). This remains elevated to at least 50% of maximal intensity for up to 20 minutes (29) (Fig. 2).

When the adrenals are inspected either qualitatively or quantitatively with the chemical shift technique, the signal intensity of the adrenal is compared to that of an adjacent organ in both the in-phase and out-of-phase sequences. Although traditionally the liver was used as the comparative organ, the adrenal: spleen ratio has been found to be the most accurate (35) (Fig. 3). The singnal intensity measurements of these organs are applied to a formula to assess whether or not there is signal loss and, therefore, the presence of intracellular lipid (Fig. 4). A number of studies have compared the value of qualitative and quantitative assessment of the adrenals (35–38), with most concluding that experienced observers were able to differentiate adenomas from metastases just as well as quantitative measures.

A study of the adrenal gland should, therefore, include high-resolution images through both glands. Slice thickness should be 4 mm or less. A standard examination of the adrenal should include the following: T1 in- and out-of-phase gradient echo images and a T2 sequence. Optional sequences include postcontrast (41).

(A) (B)

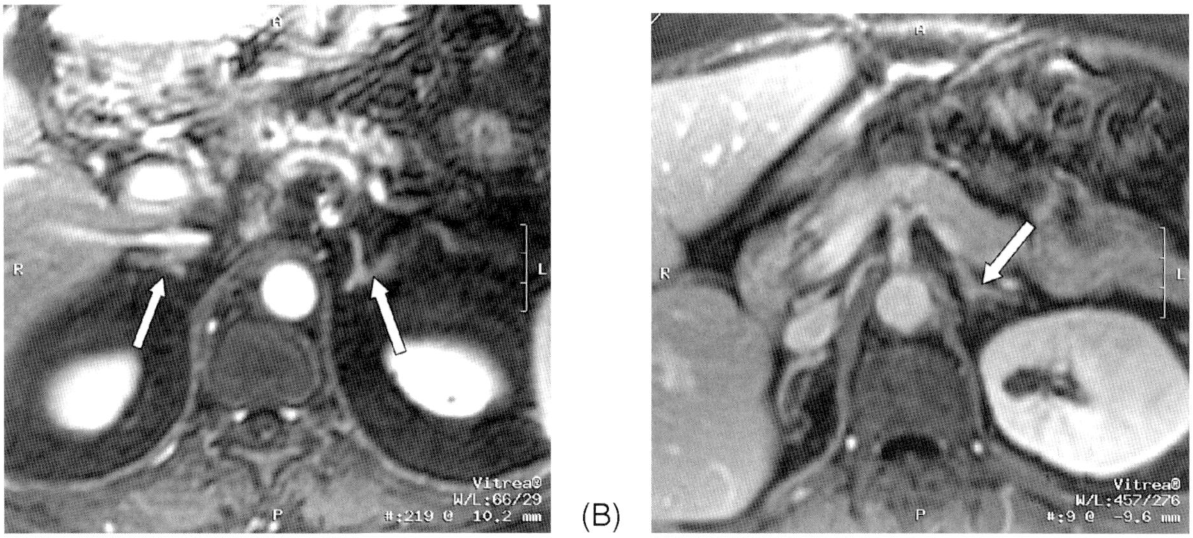

Figure 2 Axial T1 MR images with fat suppression of normal adrenal glands (arrows) shows some mild early enhancement following the injection of gadolinium (A), which washes out on glands (arrows) in different patients. In all sequences the adrenals are relatively low in signal intensity in relation to the liver (L) and renal cortex (R) delayed postcontrast images (B).

(A) (B)

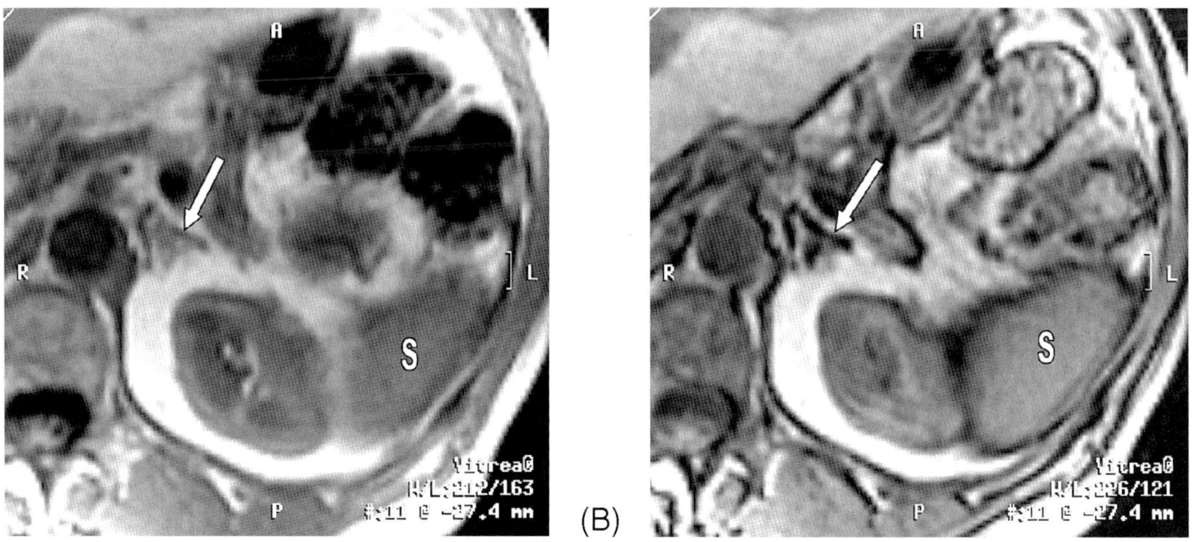

Figure 3 Axial T1 MR images of a normal left adrenal gland both in (A) and out of phase (B) (arrows). Due to the small size of the adrenals, comparison with the spleen (S) is difficult. Note the India ink or chemical shift artifact at the junction between the adrenal and the surrounding fat seen on the out-of-phase images (B).

(A) (B)

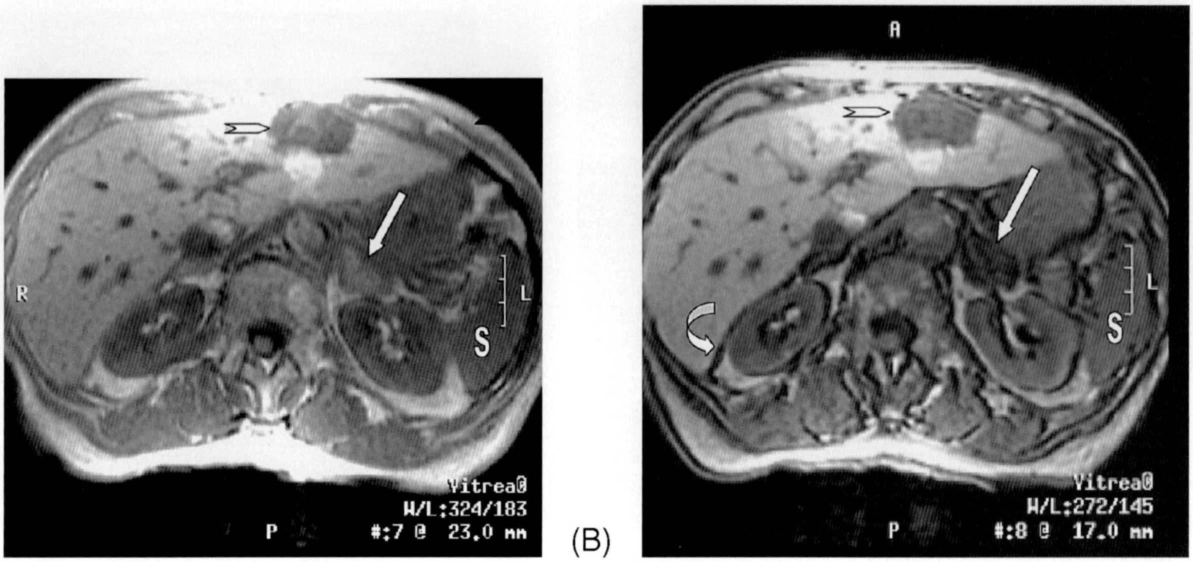

Figure 4 Axial T1 MR images demonstrating a loss of signal of the left adrenal gland (arrows) in relation to the spleen (S) on the out-of-phase images (B) compared to the in-phase images (A). This indicates the presence of intracellular lipid and is in keeping with an adenoma. Incidentally there is a left lobe hepatic hemangioma (arrowhead). Note again that the out-of-phase sequence (B) can be identified by the chemical shift or India ink artifact outlining organs at the fat/fluid interfaces (curved arrow).

4 MR IMAGING OF ADRENAL TUMORS

The use of MR in the investigation of the adrenal gland in neuroendocrine disease is well documented in the literature (1,42–44). Adenomas usually are low in signal intensity and are iso-intense to liver on T1 and T2 sequences (39), similar in appearance to the normal gland (45) (Figs. 4A, 5–7). Adrenal carcinomas may be iso-intense or hypo-intense to liver on T1 but are usually hyper-intense on T2 and heterogeneous on T2-weighted images (46) (Figs. 8 and 9A). Metastases are also often heterogeneous and high in signal intensity on the T2-weighted sequences (30).

Numerous studies have established the superiority of the chemical shift technique in differentiating adenomas from malignant lesions when compared to other sequences (15,38,47–49). Adrenal adenomas are derived from cells of the adrenal cortex that contain intracellular lipid, and so they characteristically lose signal on the out-of-phase sequence using the chemical shift technique (Figs. 4, 7A,C). Malignant lesions and metastases have very little if any intracytoplasmic lipid and so do not lose signal (Fig. 8). The larger the percentage of lipid, the more definitively one is able to differentiate adenomatous from nonadenomatous lesions.

The majority of adenomas show a homogeneous capillary blush on immediate postcontrast images with rapid washout (50,51) (Fig. 7D). Some studies describe a central spot of hyperintensity (39,52). Malignant lesions do not demonstrate the capillary blush and usually show marked enhancement on delayed images (13,34), but overlap in appearances does exist (13,37, 51,53–55) (Fig. 9B–D).

The most comprehensive study to date compared over 100 patients with adrenal masses with histopathological results using a combination of chemical shift and dynamic gadolinium-enhanced images confirming that MR can be used to characterize adrenal lesions with a high degree of specificity and sensitivity (18). Sensitivities, specificities, and accuracies of 91, 94, and 93%, respectively, were achieved. While a number of other studies have proposed a combination of chemical shift and gadolinium techniques (24,37,48,56,57), the use of contrast enhancement patterns to differentiate adrenal lesions still remains an optional and complementary technique (50). Chemical shift remains the single preferred method of evaluating the adrenals in most institutions.

The problem, however, still remains of delineation of indeterminate lesions (30,31,58,59). This is due to the

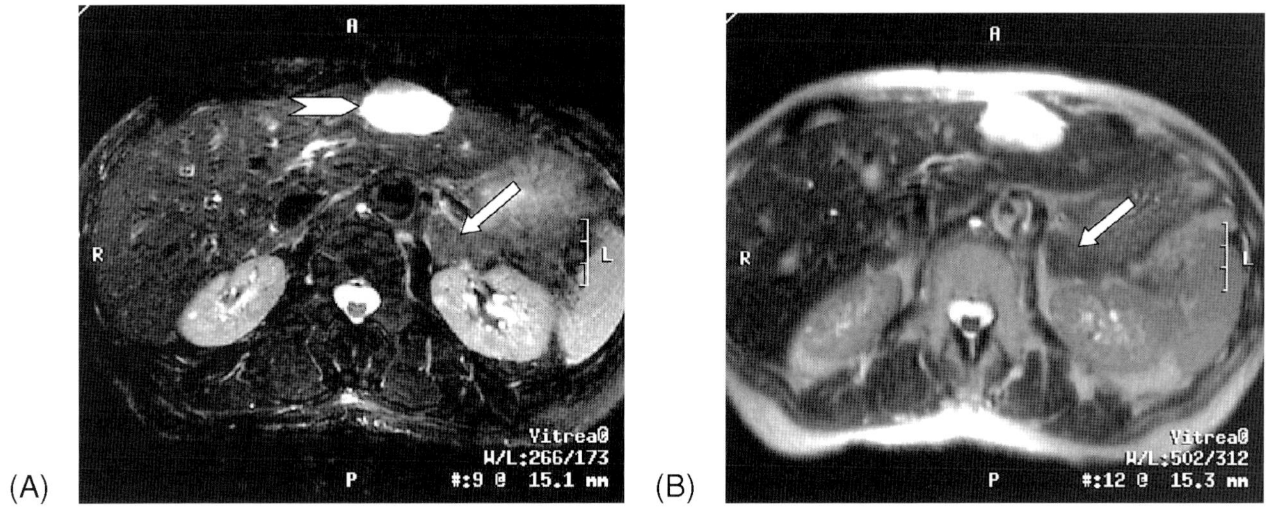

Figure 5 Axial T2 FSE (A) and single-shot (B) images of the same patient. In A the image is fat-suppressed, which increases the conspicuity of the adrenal lesion (arrow). The hepatic hemangioma is bright on both sequences (arrowheads).

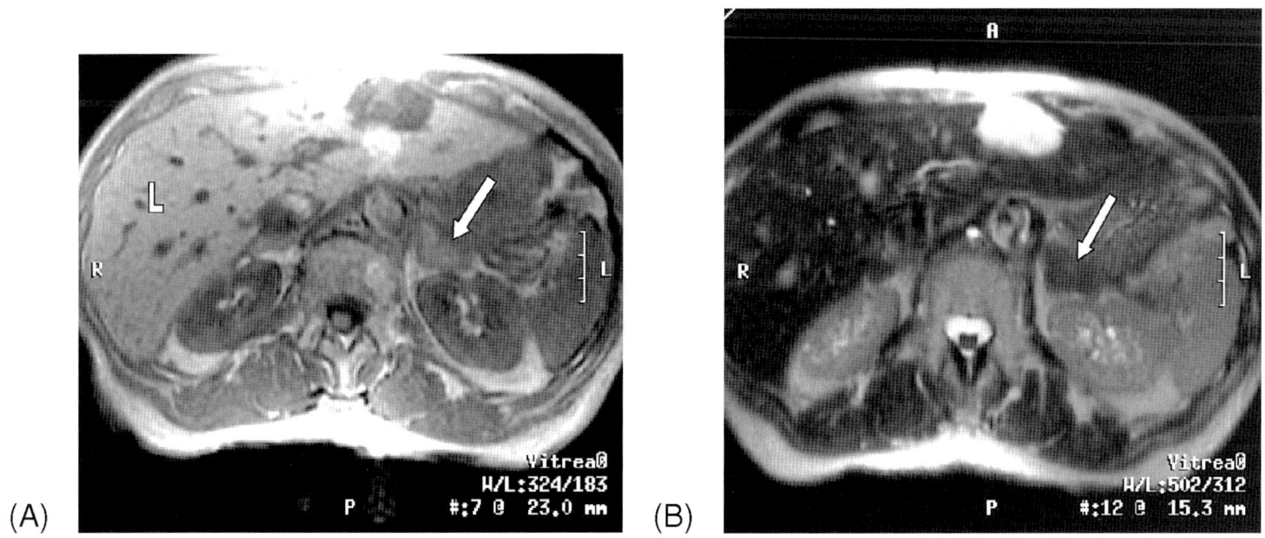

Figure 6 Axial T1 in-phase (A) and single-shot T2 (B) MR images of a left adrenal adenoma (arrow) seen in Figures 4 and 5, which is iso-intense on both sequences when compared to the liver (L).

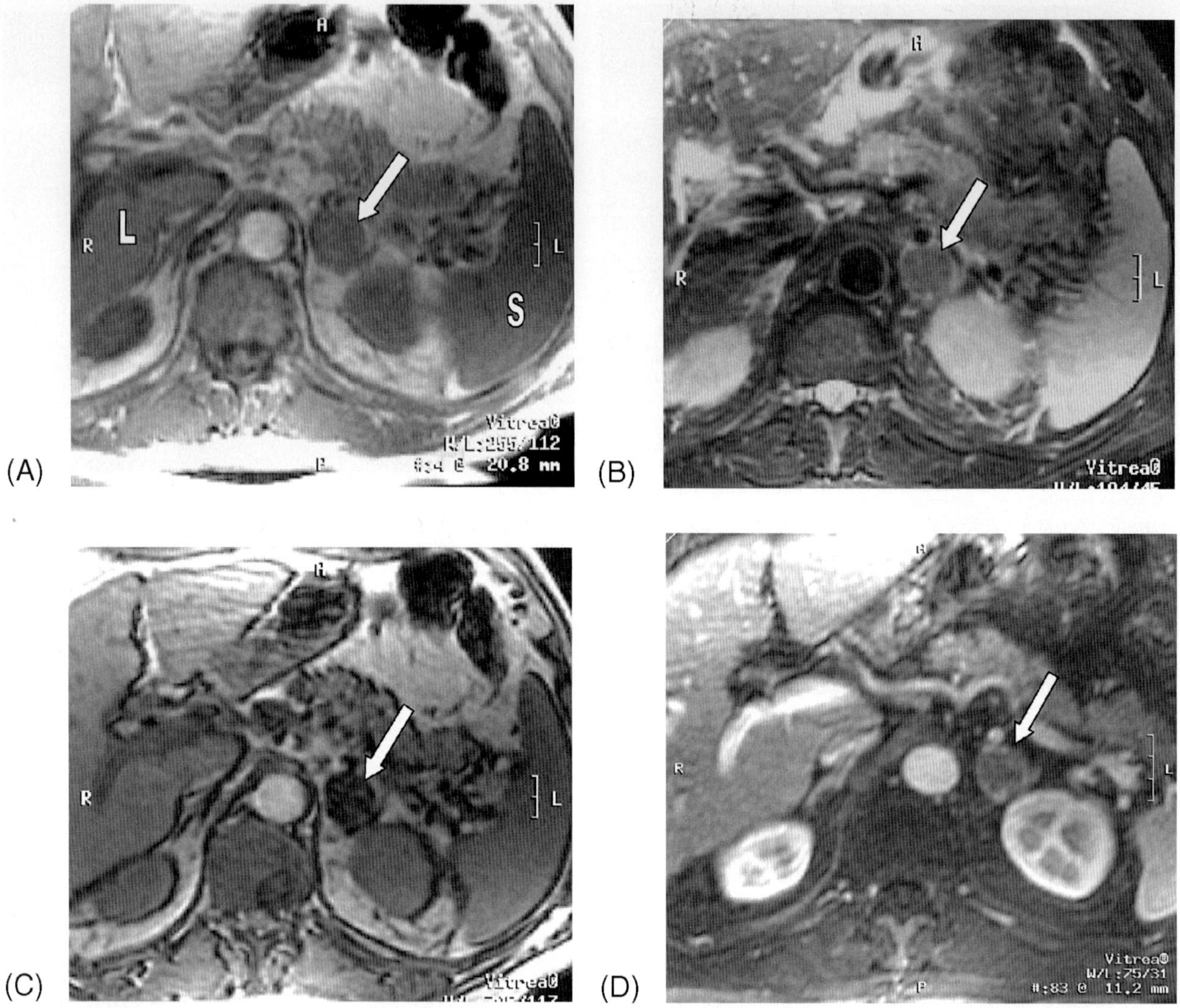

Figure 7 Axial T1 in-phase (A) and single-shot T2 (B) MR images of a left adrenal mass (arrow) in a different patient which is also relatively iso-intense on both sequences when compared to the liver (L). In (A) the intensity of the adrenal is similar to that of the spleen (S). On the out-of-phase image (C), the adenoma loses signal in relation to the spleen, indicating the presence of intracellular lipid and, therefore, in keeping with an adenoma. Axial T1 with fat suppresion immediate postgadolinium image (D) shows minimal enhancement.

wide variation in histological characteristics of both benign and malignant lesions (60–62), which contributes to a wide range of T1 and T2 values as well as varying appearances on chemical shift techniques. In particular, larger adenomas, which may contain foci of calcification, cystic change, degeneration, and hemorrhage, may be impossible to differentiate from carcinomas (63). Two other entities complicate the differentiation: collision tumors where benign and malignant tumors coexist, and a zonal phenomenon where adjacent lipid-rich and lipid-poor regions abut one another (60,62).

5 SPECIFIC SYNDROMES

5.1 Cushing's Syndrome

Most patients with Cushing's syndrome do not have a primary neoplasm of the adrenal cortex but have increased corticotrophin production by the pituitary

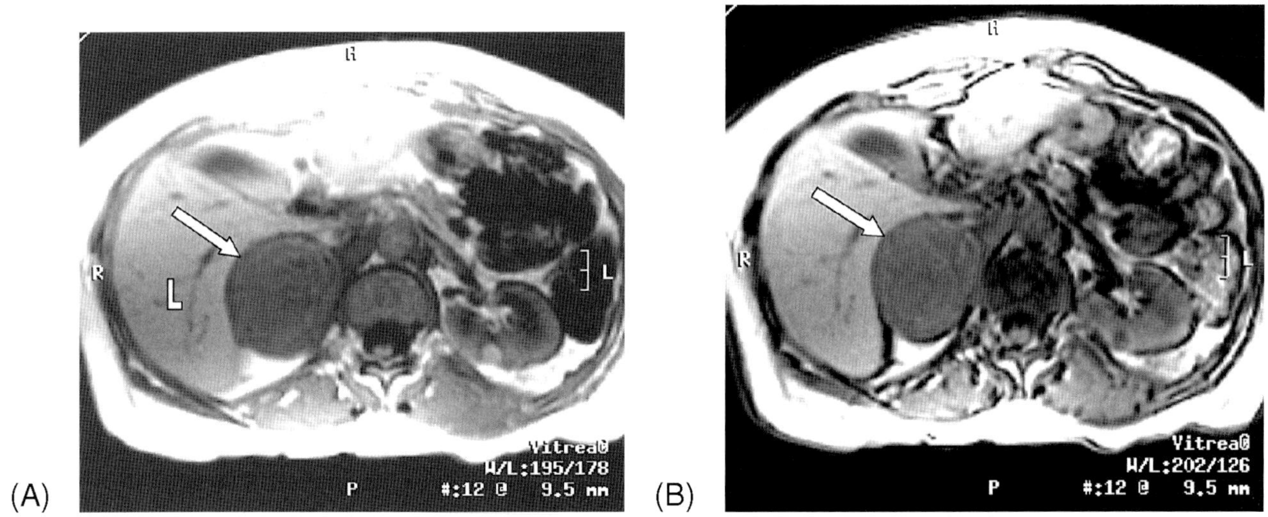

Figure 8 Axial T1 MR images demonstrating a moderate-to-large sized right adrenal mass (arrow), which is hypo-intense when compared to the liver (L) and shows no loss of signal on out of phase images (A) when compared to the in-phase images (B). Unfortunately, the patient has no spleen for comparison, so the liver is used instead.

gland (70–90%). Such patients may demonstrate hyperplasia of both glands (64,65), which have the same signal characteristics as the normal adrenal gland. The other 10–30% of Cushing's patients have a demonstrated focal mass, of which about 70% are adenomas (Fig. 10). Characteristically adenomas are intermediate in size (mean 3.3 cm) and are accompanied by atrophy of the nonneoplastic adrenal tissue. Other causes of Cushing's syndrome include carcinoma or unilateral adrenal hyperplasia (66). Carcinomas are larger, with a mean size of 8.6 cm. The first line of investigation in Cushing's syndrome, therefore, should be MR of the pituitary gland. If this examination is negative, then evaluation of the adrenals with MR may be performed to locate a possible adrenal mass.

5.2 Conn's Syndrome

Approximately two thirds of cases of Conn's syndrome demonstrate an adrenal adenoma which is characteristically small (<2 cm) and homogeneous in appearance with the typical signal intensities described for adenomas (25,67). Alternatively, hormone hypersecretion may be due to unilateral adrenal hyperplasia or bilateral hyperplasia with no true adenoma (68,69). Adrenal vein sampling remains the gold standard for lateralization of function and cure by unilateral adrenalectomy. Fewer than 1% of cases are due to carcinoma. One study demonstrated decreased intracellular lipid in some adenomas, but this has not been shown to affect the signal intensity on chemical shift techniques.

5.3 Pheochromocytoma

Pheochromocytoma arises from the adrenal medulla, can appear brighter than the adrenal cortex, but iso- or hypo-intense to liver on T1 (Fig. 12) and markedly hyper-intense or bright on T2 (Fig. 13A). These tumors are hypervascular and show significant enhancement with gadolinium with a variable homogeneous/heterogeneous pattern (70,71)(Fig. 13B). They may be complicated by hemorrhage, cystic degeneration, or necrosis, which can alter the imaging findings. Adrenal medullary hyperplasia, which may occur as a precursor to frank pheochromocytoma, has similar imaging, appearance (72,73).

Pheochromocytomas may be associated with a multiple endocrine neoplasia (MEN), a neuroectodermal disorder, or with other inherited neoplastic syndromes. Extra-adrenal pheochromocytoma can occur anywhere along the sympathetic chain from the neck to the sacrum (74). However, because 98% of tumors are subdiaphragmatic and 85–90% arise within the adrenal medulla, imaging the upper abdomen and adrenal area is usually adequate.

Ten percent of pheochromocytomas are malignant, with the diagnosis usually made clinically based on the

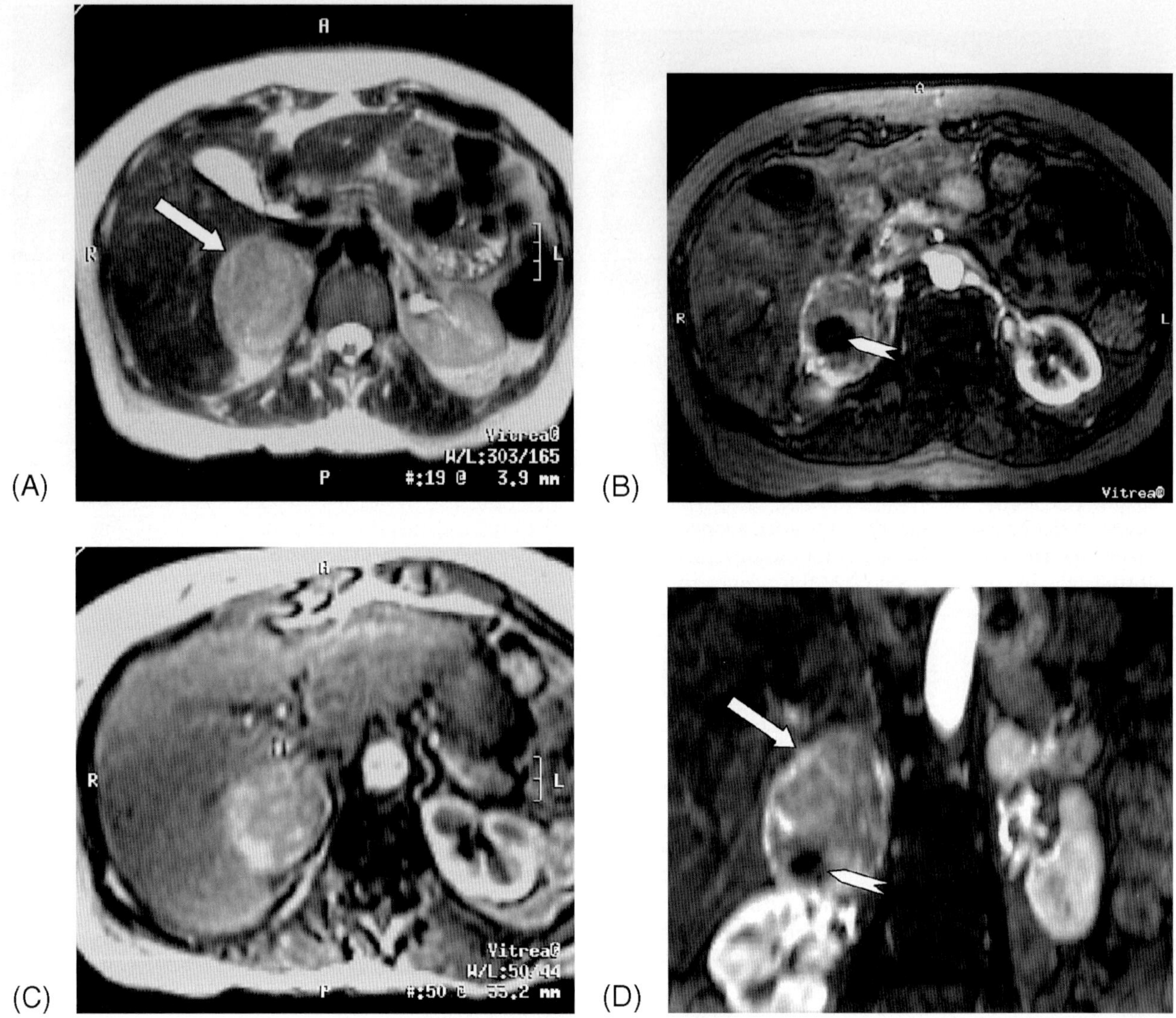

Figure 9 On the axial T2 MR images (A) the mass (arrow) is only mildly hyper-intense but shows quite significant enhancement with contrast (B–D). There is a central area of decreased intensity in keeping with hemorrhage or necrosis (arrowhead). This was histologically proven to be an adreno-cortical carcinoma.

presence of extensive local invasion or, more reliably, metastatic disease. Although nuclear pleomorphism and other findings suggestive of malignancy are present in some tumors, they do not correlate with malignant behavior. Metastases may occur in liver, bone, lymph nodes, brain, and lung and may be hormonally active. Metastases must be distinguished from multifocal tumors occurring elsewhere in areas of neural crest tissue (75), which occur in about 10% of cases. Although scintigraphy with iodine-labeled meta-iodobenzylguanidine (MIBG) offers the greatest specificity, it is not as sensitive as MR imaging, failing to visualize some tumors. In a recent study of 282 patients in which MR imaging, CT, and MIBG were compared, MR imaging was the most sensitive study for localizing adrenal and extra-adrenal pheochromocytomas (76).

5.4 Adrenocortical Carcinoma

Adrenocortical carcinoma is rare. Thirty-eighty percent are functional lesions, usually small in size, most commonly resulting in Cushing's syndrome. Nonfunction-

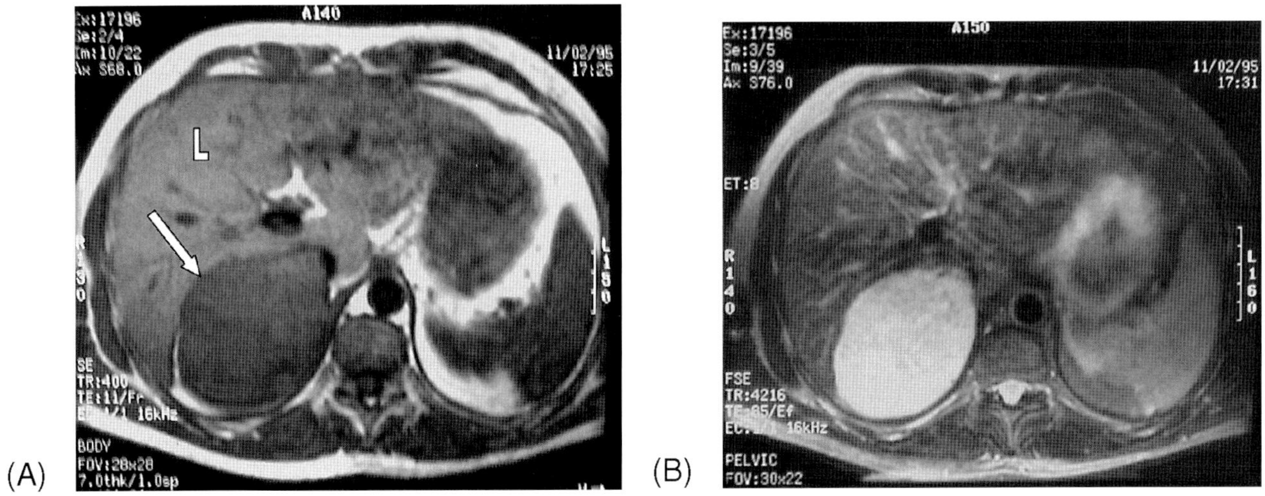

Figure 10 Axial T1 in phase (A) and T2 fat-suppressed (B) MR images of a right adrenal mass (arrow) in a patient with increased cortisol production. The mass is relatively low signal on T1 and high signal on T2 in relation to the liver (L). Despite its large size and discrepant features, this proved to be a benign cortisol-secreting adenoma.

ing lesions are usually large (12–16 cm), show heterogeneous enhancement, intermediate to high signal intensity on T2 and possibly high signal intensity on T1 if there is complicating hemorrhage. They do not lose signal on out-of-phase imaging and show progressive enhancement on delayed images (Figs. 8, 9). Local and distant metastatic spread may occur. Local invasion may involve the adrenal veins, IVC, and right atrium. Metastatic deposits occur in the liver, lungs, bone, and regional lymph nodes.

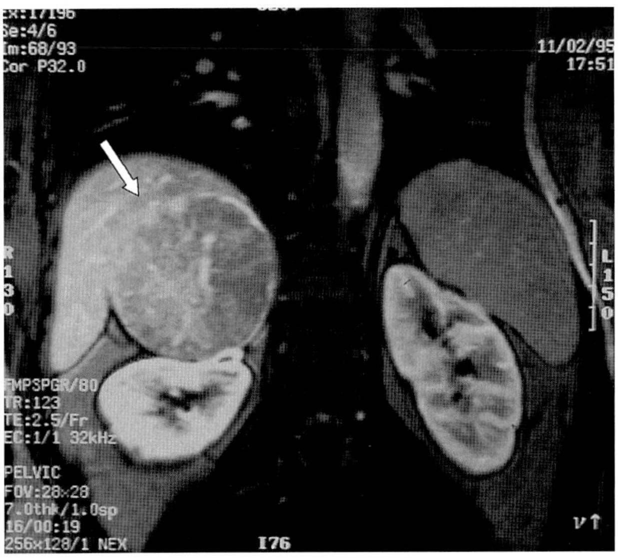

Figure 11 Axial T1 fat-suppressed postcontrast MR image of the same patient demonstrates minimal enhancement (arrow).

5.5 Differential Diagnoses

5.5.1 Metastases

Adrenal metastatic masses may occur with a known or unknown primary source and may or may not be associated with a hormonal clinical syndrome. The lesions are characteristically intermediate in size (mean size 4 cm), show rapid growth, have ill-defined margins, and show heterogeneous signal intensity and variable enhancement.

5.5.2 Adrenal Myelolipoma

These lesions demonstrate increased signal intensity relative to liver on T1 and T2 sequences, but appearances vary depending on the amount of fat they contain and the predominance of other tissue (77,78) (Fig. 14).

5.5.3 Hematoma (Adrenal Pseudocyst)

Variation in appearance depending on the stage of hemoglobin degradation is seen in hematomas (79,80). Serial imaging, however, usually demonstrates an evolving lesion that changes in signal intensity and may shrink or totally disappear over time (Fig. 15). There usually is minimal rim enhancement.

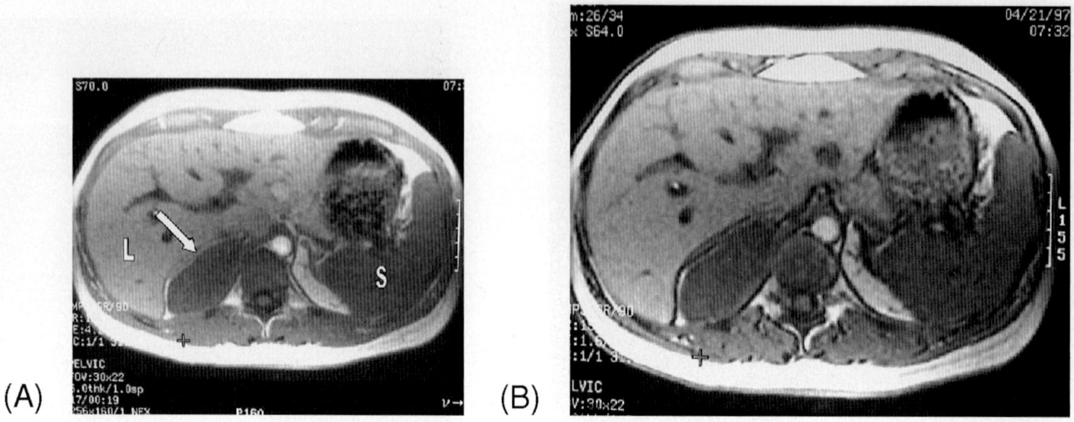

Figure 12 Axial T1 in- (A) and out-of-phase (B) MR images of a moderate-sized right adrenal mass (arrow), which is relatively hypo-intense to the liver (L) and shows no signal loss in relation to the spleen (S) on the out-of-phase images.

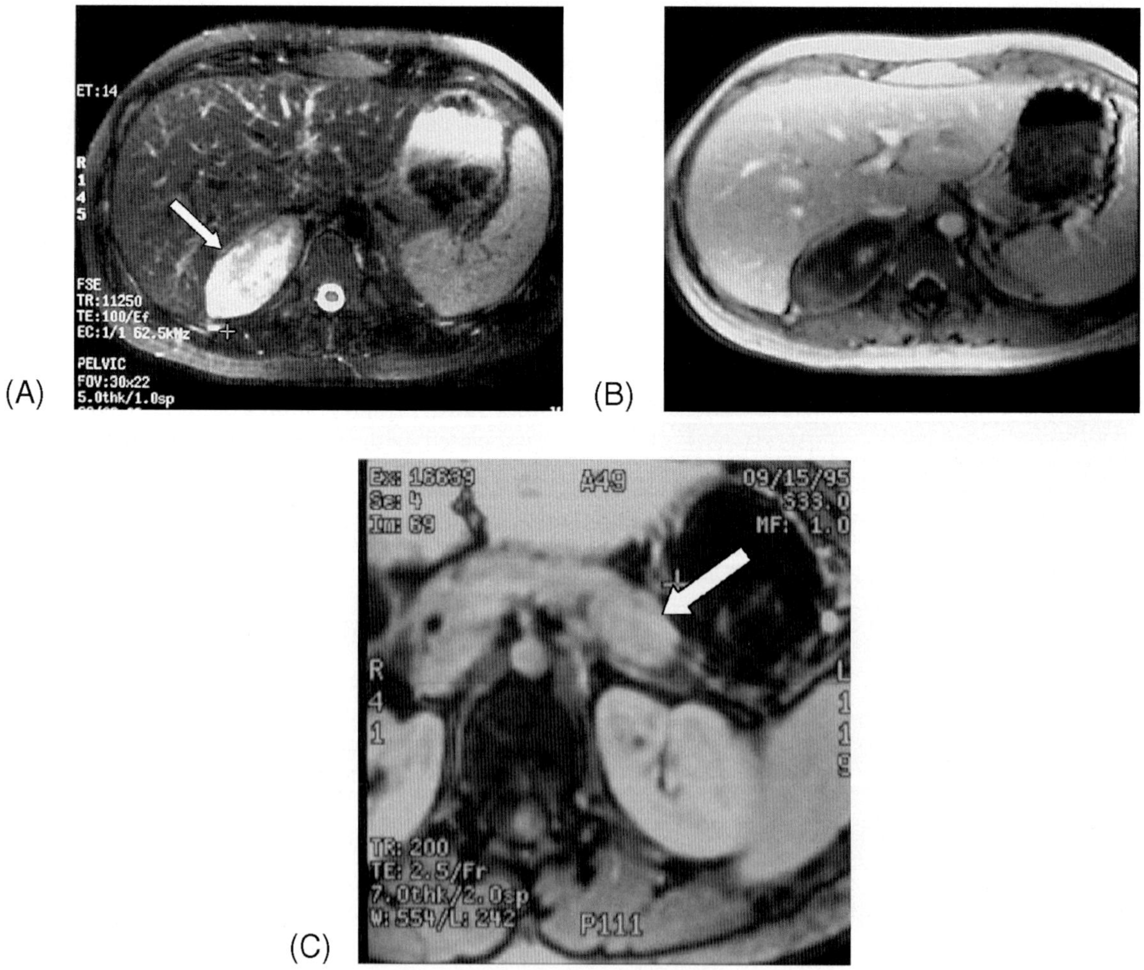

Figure 13 Axial T2 fat-suppressed (A) MR image demonstrates marked hyper-intensity of the adrenal mass (arrow), which is typical for a pheochromocytoma. The axial T1 postgadolinium (B) MR image shows minimal enhancement.

5.5.4 Lymphoma and Adenomatoid Tumor

Both of these may produce nonspecific findings approximating those of carcinoma or metastases (59,81).

5.5.5 Retroperitoneal Bronchogenic Cyst

This lesion is rare but may present as a retroperitoneal lesion which is bright on T2 sequences and, therefore, may be mistaken for pheochromocytoma (82).

5.5.6 Congenital Adrenal Hyperplasia and Ectopic Adrenal Cortex

Adrenals may be hyperplastic or ectopic but usually display signal intensities of normal adrenals (83,84).

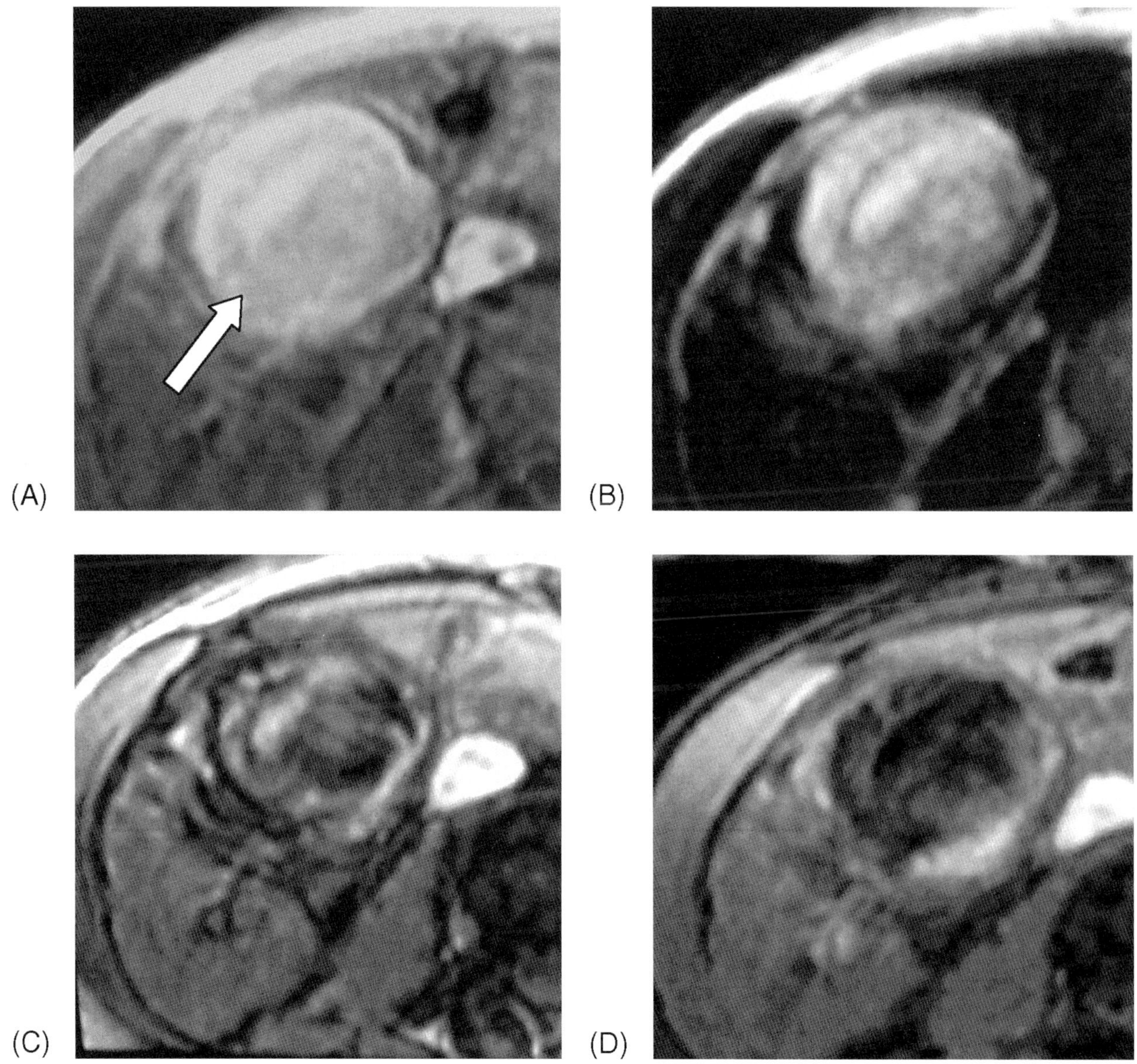

Figure 14 Axial T1 (A), single-shot T2 (B) and fat-suppressed postgadolinium MR images (C and D) of a right adrenal angiomyelolipoma (arrow). In A and B it is bright but loses signal on the fat-suppressed postgadolinium images, indicating the presence of fat.

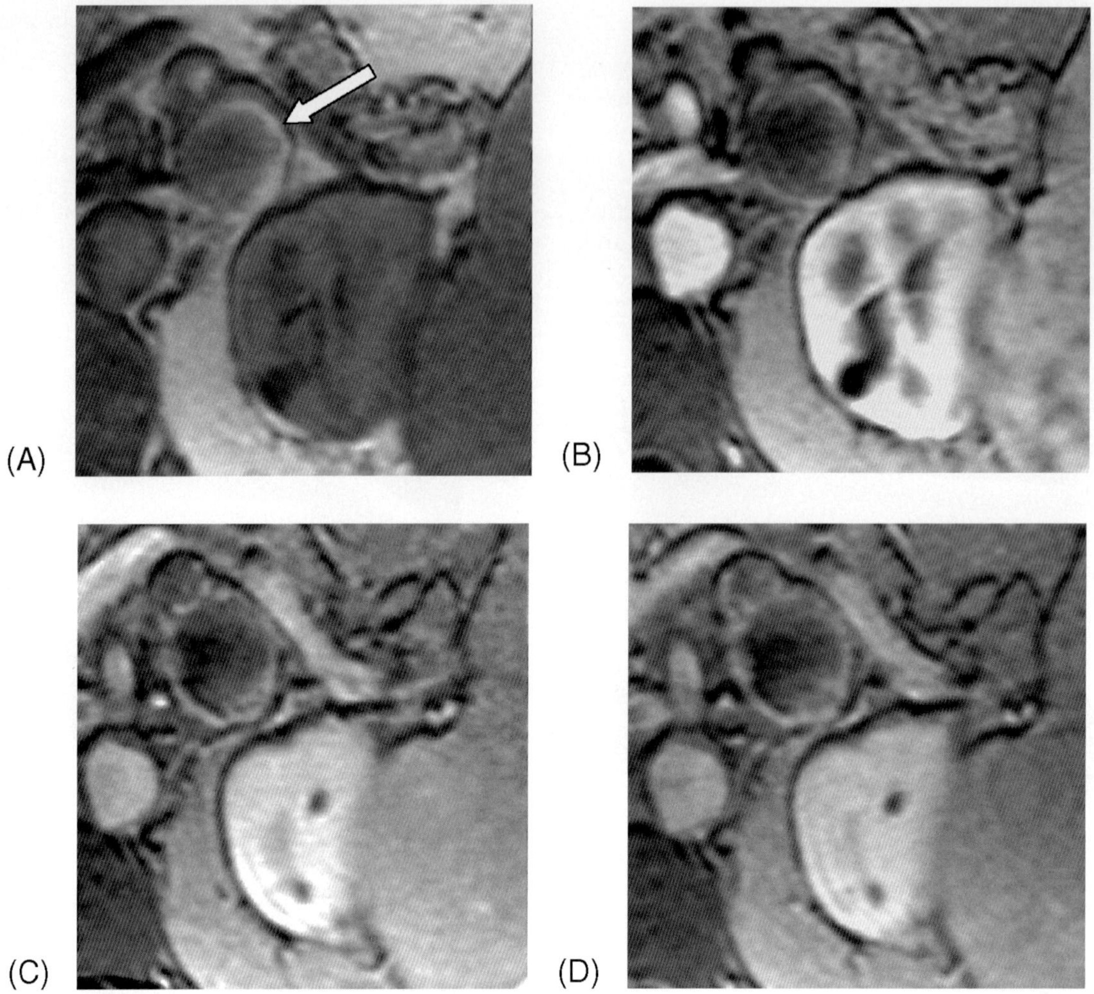

Figure 15 Axial T1 pre- (A) and postgadolinium (B–D) MR images demonstrate a left adrenal mass (arrow), which is bright peripherally on T1 and shows no enhancement with contrast. This mass disappeared over a period of 3 months, in keeping with a resolving hematoma.

6 CONCLUSION

The choice of preoperative imaging will depend very much on the specific clinical problem, the local expertise, and the availability of imaging techniques. The chemical shift technique is undoubtedly extremely useful in identifying benign adrenal lesions, but the problem still remains of classifying indeterminate lesions. MR, however, should be the examination of choice in patients with renal disease and compromised renal function.

ACKNOWLEDGMENT

The authors would like to thank Dr. Emil Cohen for his assistance with presenting the images.

REFERENCES

1. Krebs TL, Wagner BJ. MR imaging of the adrenal gland: radiologic-pathologic correlation. Radiographics 1998; 18(6):1425–1440.
2. Francis IR, Korobkin M. Incidentally discovered adrenal masses. Magn Reson Imaging Clin North Am 1997; 5(1): 147–164.
3. Gilfeather M, Woodward PJ. MR imaging of the adrenal glands and kidneys. Semin Ultrasound CT MR 1998; 19(1):53–66.
4. Korobkin M, et al. The incidental adrenal mass. Radiol Clin North Am 1996; 34(5):1037–1054.
5. Megibow AJ, Lavelle MT, Rofsky NM. MR imaging of the pancreas. Surg Clin North Am 2001; 81(2):307–320, ix-x.
6. Prince MR, Arnoldus C, Frisoli JK. Nephrotoxicity of

high-dose gadolinium compared with iodinated contrast. J Magn Reson Imaging 1996; 6(1):162–166.
7. Murphy KJ, Brunberg JA, Cohan RH. Adverse reactions to gadolinium contrast media: a review of 36 cases. Am J Roentgenol 1996; 167(4):847–849.
8. Dwamena BA, et al. Diagnostic evaluation of the adrenal incidentaloma: decision and cost-effectiveness analyses. J Nucl Med 1998; 39(4):707–712.
9. Semelka RC. Pancreatic disease: prospective comparison of CT,ERCP,and 1.5T MR imaging with dynamic gadolinium enhancement and fat suppression. Radiology 1991; 181: 785–791.
10. Siegelman ES, et al. Fat suppression by saturation/opposed-phase hybrid technique: spin echo versus gradient echo imaging. Magn Reson Imaging 1995; 13(4):545–548.
11. Ichikawa T, et al. Depiction of the normal adrenal gland evaluation with 0.5 tesla MRI. Nippon Igaku Hoshasen Gakkai Zasshi 1991; 51(8):906–911.
12. Siegelman ES. MR imaging of the adrenal neoplasms. Magn Reson Imaging Clin North Am 2000; 8(4):769–786.
13. Semelka RC, et al. Evaluation of adrenal masses with gadolinium enhancement and fat-suppressed MR imaging. J Magn Reson Imaging 1993; 3(2):337–343.
14. Bilal MM, Brown JJ. MR imaging of renal and adrenal masses in children. Magn Reson Imaging Clin North Am 1997; 5(1):179–917.
15. Tsushima Y, Ishizaka H, Matsumoto M. Adrenal masses: differentiation with chemical shift, fast low-angle shot MR imaging. Radiology 1993; 186(3):705–709.
16. Outwater EK, et al. Adrenal masses: correlation between CT attenuation value and chemical shift ratio at MR imaging with in-phase and opposed-phase sequences. Radiology 1996; 200(3):749–752.
17. Korobkin M, et al. Adrenal adenomas: relationship between histologic lipid and CT and MR findings. Radiology 1996; 200(3):743–747.
18. Heinz-Peer G, et al. Characterization of adrenal masses using MR imaging with histopathologic correlation. Am J Roentgenol 1999; 173(1):15–22.
19. Francis IR, et al. Integrated imaging of adrenal disease. Radiology 1992; 184(1):1–13.
20. Dunnick NR. Hanson lecture. Adrenal imaging: current status. Am J Roentgenol 1990; 154(5):927–936.
21. Dunnick NR. CT and MRI of adrenal lesions. Urol Radiol 1988; 10(1):12–16.
22. Berland LL, et al. Differentiation between small benign and malignant adrenal masses with dynamic incremented CT. Am J Roentgenol 1988; 151(1):95–101.
23. Szolar DH, Kammerhuber F. Quantitative CT evaluation of adrenal gland masses: a step forward in the differentiation between adenomas and nonadenomas? Radiology 1997; 202(2):517–521.
24. Slapa RZ, Jakubowski W, Szopinski K. Magnetic resonance techniques used in the differentiation of adrenal tumors. Pol Merkuriusz Lek 2000; 8(48):436–440.
25. Wang JH, et al. High resolution MRI of adrenal glands in patients with primary aldosteronism. Zhonghua Yi Xue Za Zhi (Taipei) 2000; 63(6):475–481.
26. Rossi GP, et al. Identification of the etiology of primary aldosteronism with adrenal vein sampling in patients with equivocal computed tomography and magnetic resonance findings: results in 104 consecutive cases. J Clin Endocrinol Metab 2001; 86(3):1083–1090.
27. Schultz CL, et al. Magnetic resonance imaging of the adrenal glands: a comparison with computed tomography. Am J Roentgenol 1984; 143(6):1235–1240.
28. Small WC, Bernardino ME. Gd-DTPA adrenal gland enhancement at 1.5 T. Magn Reson Imaging 1991; 9(3): 309–312.
29. Huch-Boni RA, Debatin JF, Krestin GP. Contrast-enhanced MR imaging of the kidneys and adrenal glands. Magn Reson Imaging Clin North Am 1996; 4(1):101–131.
30. Reinig JW, et al. MRI of indeterminate adrenal masses. Am J Roentgenol 1986; 147(3):493–496.
31. Chezmar JL, et al. Adrenal masses: characterization with T1-weighted MR imaging. Radiology 1988; 166(2):357–359.
32. Chang A, et al. Adrenal gland: MR imaging. Radiology 1987; 163(1):123–128.
33. Leroy Willig A, et al. In vitro adrenal cortex lesions characterization by NMR spectroscopy. Magn Reson Imaging 1987; 5(5):339–344.
34. Mitchell DG, et al. Benign adrenocortical masses: diagnosis with chemical shift MR imaging. Radiology 1992; 185(2): 345–351.
35. Mayo-Smith WW, et al. Characterization of adrenal masses (< 5 cm) by use of chemical shift MR imaging: observer performance versus quantitative measures. Am J Roentgenol 1995; 165(1):91–95.
36. Namimoto T, et al. Adrenal masses: quantification of fat content with double-echo chemical shift in-phase and opposed-phase FLASH MR images for differentiation of adrenal adenomas. Radiology 2001; 218(3):642–646.
37. Korobkin M, et al. Characterization of adrenal masses with chemical shift and gadolinium- enhanced MR imaging. Radiology 1995; 197(2):411–418.
38. Outwater EK, et al. Distinction between benign and malignant adrenal masses: value of T1-weighted chemical-shift MR imaging. Am J Roentgenol 1995; 165(3): 579–583.
39. Boraschi P, et al. Diagnosis of adrenal adenoma: value of central spot of high-intensity hyperintense rim sign and homogeneous isointensity to liver on gadolinium-enhanced fat-suppressed spin-echo MR images. J Magn Reson Imaging 1999; 9(2):304–310.
40. Outwater EK, et al. Detection of lipid in abdominal tissues with opposed-phase gradient- echo images at 1.5 T: techniques and diagnostic importance. Radiographics 1998; 18(6):1465–1480.
41. Mitchell DG, et al. Fatty tissue on opposed-phase MR images: paradoxical suppression of signal intensity by

paramagnetic contrast agents. Radiology 1996; 198(2): 351–357.
42. Teeger S, Papanicolaou N, Vaughan ED Jr. Current concepts in imaging of adrenal masses. World J Urol 1999; 17(1):3–8.
43. Weishaupt D, Debatin JF. Magnetic resonance: evaluation of adrenal lesions. Curr Opin Urol 1999; 9(2):153–163.
44. Mantero F, Arnaldi G. Investigation protocol: adrenal enlargement. Clin Endocrinol (Oxf) 1999; 50(2):141–146.
45. Ogita M, et al. Magnetic resonance imaging of the adrenal gland. Nippon Igaku Hoshasen Gakkai Zasshi 1991; 51(12):1431–1441.
46. Dunnick NR, Korobkin M, Francis I. Adrenal radiology: distinguishing benign from malignant adrenal masses. Am J Roentgenol 1996; 167(4):861–867.
47. Bilbey JH, et al. MR imaging of adrenal masses: value of chemical-shift imaging for distinguishing adenomas from other tumors. Am J Roentgenol 1995; 164(3): 637–642.
48. Peppercorn PD, Reznek RH. State-of-the-art CT and MRI of the adrenal gland. Eur Radiol 1997; 7(6):822–836.
49. Outwater EK, Mitchell DG. Differentiation of adrenal masses with chemical shift MR imaging. Radiology 1994; 193(3):877–878.
50. Chung JJ, Semelka RC, Martin DR. Adrenal adenomas: characteristic postgadolinium capillary blush on dynamic MR imaging. J Magn Reson Imaging 2001; 13(2):242–248.
51. Krestin GP, Steinbrich W, Friedmann G. Adrenal masses: evaluation with fast gradient-echo MR imaging and Gd-DTPA-enhanced dynamic studies. Radiology 1989; 171(3):675–680.
52. Ichikawa T, et al. Adrenal adenomas: characteristic hyperintense rim sign on fat-saturated spin-echo MR images. Radiology 1994; 193(1):247–250.
53. Krestin GP, et al. Evaluation of adrenal masses in oncologic patients: dynamic contrast- enhanced MR vs CT. J Comput Assist Tomogr 1991; 15(1):104–110.
54. Krestin GP, Lorenz R, Steinbrich W. Magnetic resonance tomography of adrenal gland tumors. Detection and differentiation using fast gradient echo sequences and dynamic contrast media studies. Radiology 1990; 30(5):228–234.
55. Reinig JW, et al. Differentiation of adrenal masses with MR imaging: comparison of techniques. Radiology 1994; 192(1):41–46.
56. Schwartz LH, et al. Comparison of two algorithms and their associated charges when evaluating adrenal masses in patients with malignancies. Am J Roentgenol 1997; 168(6):1575–1578.
57. Zimmermann GG, Debatin JF, Krestin GP. The differentiation of adrenal gland tumors: an improvement in accuracy by a combination of fat-sensitive, T2-weighted and contrast-enhanced MR sequences. Rofo Fortschr Geb Rontgenstr Neuen Bildgeb Verfahr 1997; 167(2): 153–159.
58. Korobkin M, et al. Differentiation of adrenal adenomas from nonadenomas using CT attenuation values. Am J Roentgenol 1996; 166(3):531–536.
59. Rodrigo Gasque C, et al. MR imaging of a case of adenomatoid tumor of the adrenal gland. Eur Radiol 1999; 9(3):552–554.
60. Ramsay JA, et al. Lipid degeneration in pheochromocytomas mimicking adrenal cortical tumors. Am J Surg Pathol 1987; 11(6):480–486.
61. Cotran RS, Kumar V, Robbins SL, eds. Robbins Pathological Basis of Disease. Philadelphia: WB Saunders.
62. Custodio CM, et al. Adrenal neuroblastoma in an adult with tumor thrombus in the inferior vena cava. J Magn Reson Imaging 1999; 9(4):621–623.
63. Newhouse JH, et al. Large degenerated adrenal adenomas: radiologic-pathologic correlation. Radiology 1999; 210(2): 385–391.
64. Miyajima A, et al. ACTH-independent bilateral macronodular adrenocortical hyperplasia caused Cushing's syndrome. Urol Int 1997; 58(4):259–261.
65. Doppman JL, et al. Adrenocorticotropin-independent macronodular adrenal hyperplasia: an uncommon cause of primary adrenal hypercortisolism. Radiology 2000; 216(3): 797–802.
66. Otsuka F, et al. Cushing's syndrome due to unilateral adrenocortical hyperplasia. Intern Med 1998; 37(4):385–390.
67. Sohaib SA, et al. Primary hyperaldosteronism (Conn syndrome): MR imaging findings. Radiology 2000; 214(2): 527–531.
68. Haenel LCt., Hermayer KL. A case of unilateral adrenal hyperplasia: the diagnostic dilemma of hyperaldosteronism. Endocr Pract 2000; 6(2):153–158.
69. Otsuka F, et al. Hormonal characteristics of primary aldosteronism due to unilateral adrenal hyperplasia. J Endocrinol Invest 1998; 21(8):531–536.
70. Garritano A, et al. Pheochromocytoma. A case report. Minerva Chir 1999; 54(4):283–286.
71. Neumann K, Langer R. Imaging methods in diagnosis of pheochromocytoma. Zentralbl Chir 1997; 122(6):438–442.
72. Yung BC, et al. Sporadic bilateral adrenal medullary hyperplasia: apparent false positive MIBG scan and expected MRI findings. Eur J Radiol 2000; 36(1):28–31.
73. Fink IJ, et al. MR imaging of pheochromocytomas. J Comput Assist Tomogr 1985; 9(3):454–458.
74. Dahnert WF. Dahnert's Radiology Review Manual. 4th ed. Williams and Wilkins, 1999.
75. Walther MM, Keiser HR, Linehan WM. Pheochromocytoma: evaluation, diagnosis, and treatment. World J Urol 1999; 17(1):35–39.
76. Jalil ND, et al. Effectiveness and limits of preoperative imaging studies for the localisation of pheochromocytomas and paragangliomas: a review of 282 cases. French Association of Surgery (AFC), and The French Associ-

ation of Endocrine Surgeons (AFCE). Eur J Surg 1998; 164(1):23–28.
77. Huang SP, et al. Adrenal myelolipoma—report of two cases. Kaohsiung J Med Sci 2000; 16(10):542–547.
78. Boraschi P, et al. Adrenal myelolipomas: their magnetic resonance assessment. Clin Ter 1996; 147(11): 549–557.
79. Prokesch RW, et al. Adrenal hemorrhage after orthotopic liver transplantation: MR appearance. Eur Radiol 2001; 11(12):2484–2487.
80. Sakamoto T, et al. Idiopathic adrenal hemorrhage: a case report. Hinyokika Kiyo 1998; 44(11):805–807.
81. Li JK, et al. Adrenal and hypophyseal non-Hodgkin's lymphoma presenting with panhypopituitarism. Int J Clin Pract 1998; 52(7):513–514.
82. Doggett RS, Carty SE, Clarke MR. Retroperitoneal bronchogenic cyst masquerading clinically and radiologically as a phaeochromocytoma. Virchows Arch 1997; 431(1): 73–76.
83. Giacaglia LR, et al. Adrenal nodules in patients with congenital adrenal hyperplasia due to 21-hydroxylase deficiency: regression after adequate hormonal control. J Pediatr Endocrinol Metab 2001; 14(4):415–419.
84. Souverijns G, et al. Ectopic localisation of adrenal cortex. Eur Radiol 2000; 10(7):1165–1168.
85. Beckmann N, et al. Non-invasive, quantitative assessment of the anatomical phenotype of corticotropin-releasing factor-overexpressing mice by MRI. NMR Biomed 2001; 14(3):210–216.

30

Scintigraphic Imaging of the Adrenal Cortex

Neeta Pandit-Taskar

Memorial Sloan–Kettering Cancer Institute, New York, New York, U.S.A.

Samuel D. J. Yeh

Memorial Sloan–Kettering Cancer Institute and Cornell University, New York, New York, U.S.A.

1 INTRODUCTION

Almost 70 years ago, George Hevesy initiated the use of radioactive tracers to map metabolic processes (1,2). In the mid-1930s, studies in human subjects were accomplished primarily in the thyroid gland using radioactive iodine (I-131). For many decades, I-131 remained the only specific radionuclide for the diagnosis and treatment of thyroid diseases (3–7). Subsequently, phosphorus (P-32) was used for treatment of patients with bone tumors, leukemia, polycythemia vera, and bony metastases from cancer of the breast and prostate. Prior to the development of computed tomography (CT) scanning and magnetic resonance imaging (MRI), abdominal ultrasound, plain radiographs, and pyelography were the means of initial evaluation of the adrenal masses. Definitive diagnosis was made by invasive procedures like arteriography, venography, and adrenal venous sampling.

The development of scintigraphy as a noninvasive means of studying the adrenal cortex relied on several discoveries. It was known that labeled cholesterol is concentrated in the adrenal cortex and is the precursor for synthesis of adrenal corticosteroids. Later, it was found that carbon (C-14)-labeled cholesterol was avidly taken up by the adrenals in many species of animals (8). C-14 cholesterol cannot be used for imaging, but this observation led to imaging of the adrenal glands in vivo by noninvasive methods using labeled cholesterol analogues with other isotopes. Endocrine imaging using specific radiopharmaceuticals has been quite successful in answering many important functional and biochemical questions related to specific clinical problems raised by clinicians and basic scientists. Subsequent improvement in the anatomical imaging techniques using high-resolution CT scan and MRI have given better anatomical diagnosis, but the unique physiological information provided by scintigraphic imaging remains clinically important.

2 ANATOMY

The adrenal glands are inverted V-shaped, triangular structures located along the upper medial pole of the kidneys at the level of the 11th thoracic vertebra on the left and first lumbar vertebra on the right. The average weight of a single gland is about 5 g, measuring 5 cm in length, 2.5 cm in width, and 0.6 cm in thickness. The adrenal cortex forms about 80–90% of the entire gland. The outermost layer of the cortex, the zona glomerulosa, represents about 15% of the total mass and is the primary site for aldosterone secretion. The next layer, the zona fasciculata, represents 75% of the adrenal cortex and is the main site for cortisol secretion, while the innermost layer, the zona reticularis, represents about 10% of the adrenal cortex and is the primary site for androgen and estrogen production (9).

3 ROLE OF IMAGING

Tumors of the adrenal glands are relatively uncommon. With improvement of imaging modalities, clinically unimportant nodular changes caused by fibrosis, hemorrhage, and cyst formation can be detected (10–12). Three percent of normotensive individuals may show such changes with this percentage increasing with advanced age. These nodules may measure up to 3 cm and are more frequently seen in hypertensive and diabetic patients. Moreover, during routine abdominal examination with CT scan, many benign masses less than 1 cm may be detected. MRI and sonogram can detect slightly larger lesions. Patterns in MRI may differentiate benign from malignant tumors and identify specific tumor types, especially when chemical shift, fast low-angle shot MR (FLASH) imaging is used (13–16). Radionuclide studies, however, are simple, noninvasive, and probably the most cost-effective procedures to elucidate functional abnormalities in the adrenal cortex.

3.1 Tracers

Various radiopharmaceuticals used for adrenal cortical imaging are shown in Table 1. In 1971, it was found that C-14–labeled cholesterol is avidly taken up by the adrenals in many species of animals and is the precursor for synthesis of adrenal corticosteroids (8). C-14 has no gamma emission and is therefore not suitable for imaging. Many attempts to label cholesterol with I-131 were unsuccessful until 19-iodocholesterol was synthesized (Fig. 1a). After 8 days of injection, the adrenal-to-liver ratio of 19-iodocholesterol was 200:1, and uptake in tissues other than adrenal was largely cleared (17,18). Later, the contaminant from 19-iodocholesterol synthesis, 6-β-iodomethyl-19-norcholesterol (NP-59) (Fig. 1b) was found to have 5–10 times higher uptake than 19-iodocholesterol in the adrenals (19). Attempts to synthesize even more avid compounds for adrenal localization such as 6-iodocholesterol, side chain modifications, or labeling various esters or stigmasterol were not successful. In the United States, NP-59 can be obtained from the radiopharmacy of the University of Michigan as an investigating radiopharmaceutical requiring individual IND from the FDA. In Europe, selenium (Se-75) methyl-selenocholest-5(6)en-3-β-ol and (Se-75) 6-β-methyl-selenomethyl-19-norcholest-5(10)en-3-β-ol, which has a biodistribution similar to I-131 NP 59, is also available (20). Due to the longer physical half-life of Se-75 and better photon contribution for imaging, Se-75 methyl-cholesterol, which is available from Amersham as Scintadren, is preferable. In China, cholesterol labeled at the 7 position was found to be more stable, and its synthesis is much simpler than labeling at the 19 position (21).

Table 1 Radiopharmaceuticals for Adrenal Cortical Imaging

19-Iodocholesterol
6-β-Iodomethyl-19-norcholesterol (NP-59)
6-Iodocholesterol
Se-75 methyl-selenocholest-5(6)en-3-beta-ol
Se-75 6-β-methyl-selenomethyl-19-norcholest-5(10)en-3-β-ol
Se-75 methyl-cholesterol
I-131 norcholesterol
F18 FDG
C-11 metomidate

3.2 Pharmacokinetics

Following intravenous injection, I-131 NP-59 is carried in low-density lipoprotein (LDL), red blood cells, and other lipoproteins and is stored within the lipid pool at the LDL receptors of adrenocortical cells. Unlike C-14 cholesterol, NP-59 is not utilized for steroid synthesis. The uptake in the normal adrenal in humans is about 0.16% (0.073–0.26%). The uptake of Se-75 methyl-norcholesterol is 0.19% (0.09–0.30%) (20). The dosimetry of radiocholesterol is shown in Table 2 (22–24). Once inside the adrenocortical cells, the radiocholesterol is esterified, without any further metabolism of the 6-β-norcholesterol. The enterohepatic circulation may cause some background intestinal activity and visualization of gallbladder. Medications that affect tracer uptake include steroids, loop diuretics, aminoglutethemide, mitotane, and spironolactone. Adrenal secretagogues adrenocorticotropic hormone (ACTH) and angiotensin II have significant effects on accumulation of labeled cholesterols and may increase adrenal uptake of the tracer. Adrenal uptake of NP-59 is inversely related to cholesterol pool size. Low uptake may be seen in patients with serum cholesterol above 300 mg/dL or after administration of potent corticosteroids. Dexamethasone may suppress uptake to about 50% of normal.

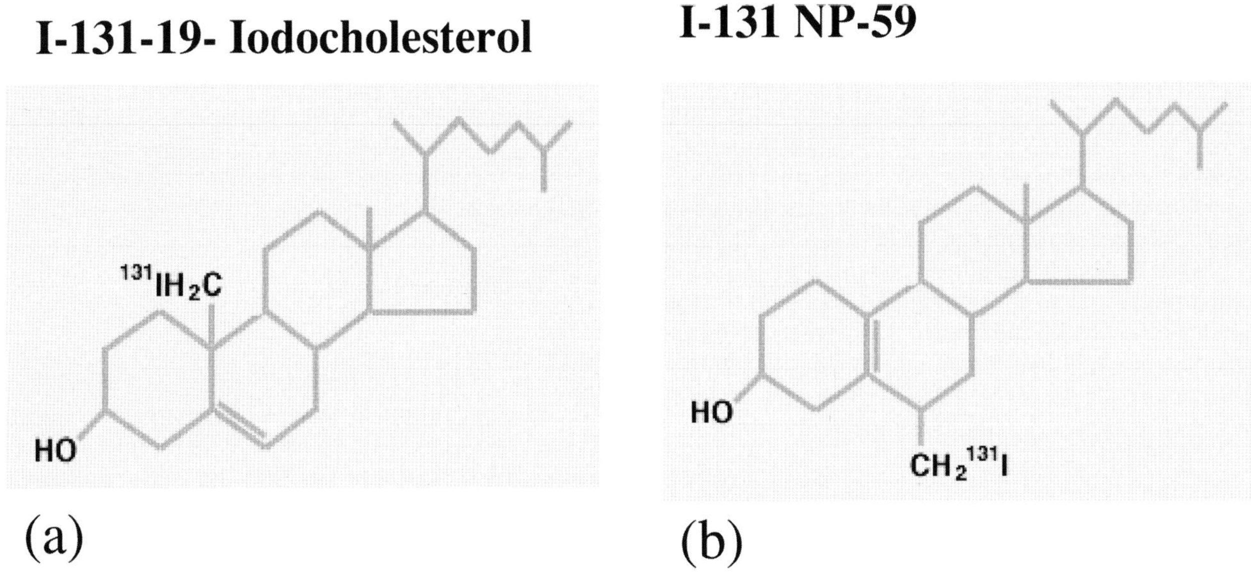

Figure 1 (a, b) Chemical structures of adrenal cortical imaging agents.

3.3 Scintigraphy Technique

Prior preparation for scanning with supersaturated potassium iodide (SSKI), using 5–7 drops for adults and 2 drops for children, is started 2 days prior to the day of the scan and continued for the entire period of the study, blocking uptake by the thyroid. Dexamethasone is given at a dose of 1 mg orally every 6 hours starting one week prior to the initiation of the scan and continued during the period of scanning. The activity of normal cortical cells is suppressed by this dosing, while functioning neoplastic cortical lesions are not. Laxatives may be used to decrease the bowel activity and are given in the evening prior to imaging. Intravenous injection of 0.5–1 mCi of labeled NP-59 is given slowly with the patient in supine position in an attempt to minimize side effects (25). Some patients may complain of dizziness, shortness of breath, chest tightness, palpitation, or nausea, and hypotension may also occur. At Memorial Sloan Kettering Cancer Center (MSKCC), more than 80 patients have been studied without any side effects. Thirty-minute posterior images of the lumbar area, including the kidneys, are obtained on days 3 and 5, and reimaging may be done on day 7. If needed, anterior and lateral or oblique images are obtained as well. SPECT imaging may also be performed with good target-to-nontarget ratio (26,27) using a 360 degree acquisition with 64 30-second steps.

Table 2 Radiation Dosimetry for Radiotracers

	I-131 NP-59 (rad/mCi)	Se-75 methyl-norcholesterol (rad/mCi)
Total body	1.8	1.4
Adrenals	26	6.1
Ovaries	8	1.9
Testes	2.3	—
Liver	2.4	3.5

4 CLINICAL APPLICATIONS

Silent adrenal masses are due to a number of causes, such as cysts, lipomas, nonfunctioning adenomas, or primary or metastatic carcinoma (12). Lymphoma may involve the adrenal, causing diffuse rather than nodular disease, occurring more often in non-Hodgkin's lymphoma than in Hodgkin's disease. It is present in about 4% of in lymphomatous patients on abdominal CT scan but rarely causes impairment of adrenal functions. Hemangioma is rare. Adrenal metastases may originate from malignant melanoma, small-cell lung carcinoma (found in 21–38%), renal cell carcinoma, breast, gastrointestinal, or ovarian primary (33).

Adrenal carcinoma is extremely rare and represents 0.05–0.2% of neoplastic disease (33). The mass is usually quite large at the time of diagnosis. Twenty to 40% present with a mass of about 1000–5000 g, rarely less than 100 g. Local nodal invasion and hematogenous spread to lung and liver is common. Analysis of data at Memorial Sloan Kettering Cancer Center from January 1980 to December 1991 showed that 44 of 73 patients had functioning tumors with excessive corticosteroid but normal aldosterone secretion, and that 29 tumors were nonfunctioning. One third of the patients had tumors larger than 4 cm, one third had local invasion with positive lymph node involvement, and 35% had distant metastases to liver, lung, and bone (34). In 156 patients analyzed by the French Association of Endocrine Surgery, half had functioning tumors (35) with a mean tumor weight of 714 g (12–4750 g). Twenty-two patients had metastases at presentation.

5 SCINTIGRAPHIC FINDINGS

5.1 Normal Scan Findings

Uptake can be seen in normal adrenals on or after the fifth day. There is usually mild asymmetrical adrenal uptake with the left lower, more posterior, and more intense than the right. There may be a 20–30% difference in counts, and this normal pattern should be recognized (25,28).

Dexamethasone suppression can be used to distinguish the differential cortical uptake, and the duration of the dexamethasone administration helps distinguish the pattern (25,29,30). ACTH has been used to improve the visualization of the suppressed adrenals (31,32). Forty units of ACTH by intramuscular injection 2 days prior to and 1 day after the tracer administration facilitates visualization of the suppressed glands as in cases of Cushing's adenoma and autoimmune adrenal dysfunction (30).

5.2 Cushing's Syndrome

In patients with Cushing's syndrome subjected to adrenal scintigraphy, one third may show normal looking adrenals, one third may show ACTH-dependent hyperplasia, and about one third may show one or more distinct focal masses in the diffusely enlarged, normal, or atrophic gland. Cholesterol imaging may show symmetrical or asymmetrical increase of NP-59 or selenomethylcholesterol uptake in the adrenals or concentration in one adrenal with nonvisualization of the other, depending on the functional status and degree of suppressibility of circulating steroid hormones (29,36,37). Bilateral symmetrical uptake is seen in Cushing's disease from pituitary, hypothalamic pituitary or ectopic ACTH hypersecretion. Bilateral uptake that is asymmetrical is seen in ACTH-independent conditions like cortical nodular hyperplasia, while bilateral nonvisualization is usually seen in adrenal carcinoma. Unilateral uptake is due to adenoma. Cholesterol imaging is also

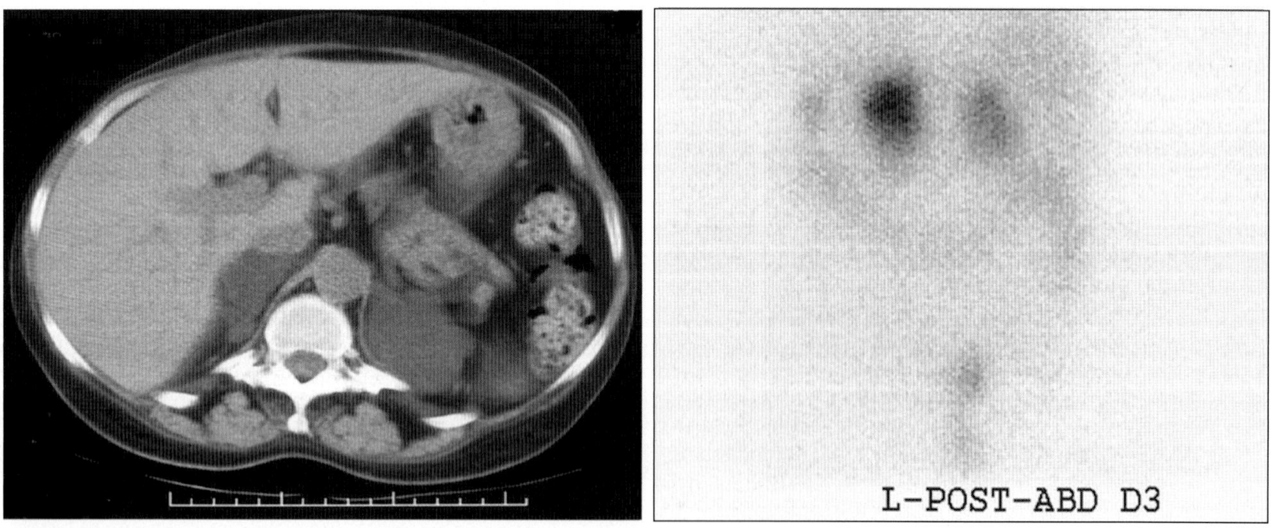

Figure 2 53-year-old female with diabetes and refractory hypertension. Cushing features and hirsutism were present. There was elevated serum and urinary free cortisol and suppressed ACTH level. A left adrenal mass and right adrenal hyperplasia was seen on CT scan. NP-59 scan shows bilateral but asymmetrical uptake with more intense activity in left adrenal gland, consistent with bilateral hyperplasia.

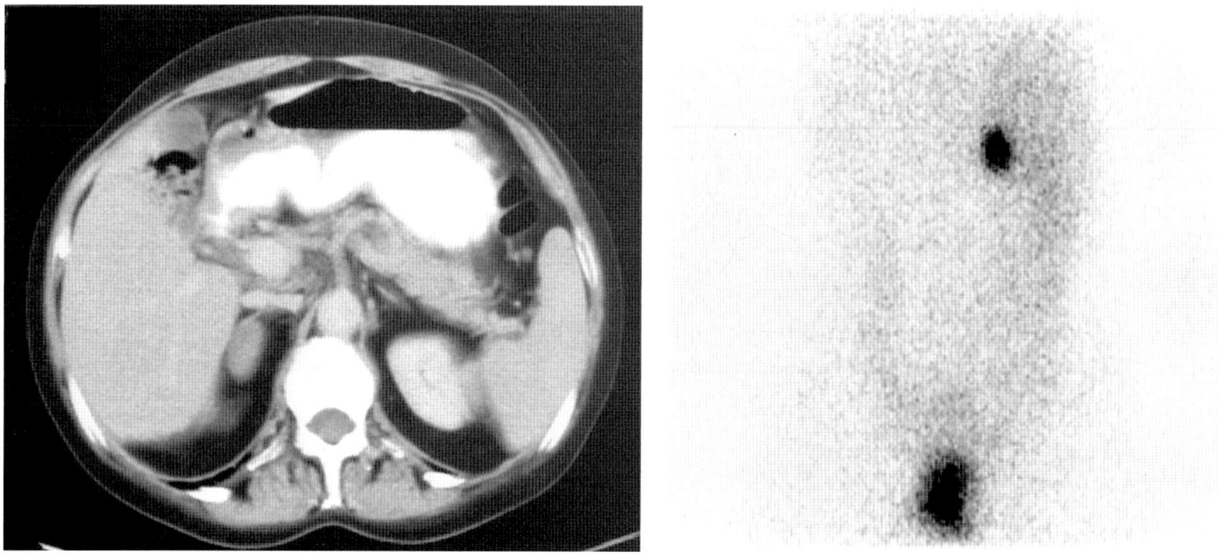

Figure 3 51-year-old female with hypertension, increased serum and urinary free cortisol, low ACTH, and right adrenal mass on CT scan. NP-59 scan without dexamethasone suppression shows unilateral adrenal uptake consistent with adenoma.

often performed to assess the suppressibility of an adrenal mass by a more potent corticosteroid such as dexamethasone or to search for residual functioning adrenal tissue following bilateral adrenalectomy (25).

Figure 2 shows a scan of a middle-aged woman with Cushing's manifestations, high plasma and urinary cortisol, bilateral enlargement of the adrenals on CT, with nodular appearance in the left. There was early and persistent bilateral increase of uptake of NP-59 with particularly high uptake in the left adrenal. Eventually this patient had bilateral adrenalectomy for hyperplasia. At surgery, the left adrenal gland measured 55 g and right adrenal gland measured 86.4 g, consistent with bilateral hyperplasia.

Figure 3 shows unilateral uptake in a woman with Cushing's adenoma. Adrenal scintigraphy can also be helpful in localizing recurrent disease (Fig. 4).

5.3 Hyperfunctioning Adrenal Carcinoma

In general, adrenal carcinoma and metastatic lesions do not take up I-131 NP-59. Some data are available that suggest that certain carcinomas may show increased I-131 NP-59 or Se-75 methylcholesterol uptake (38–41),

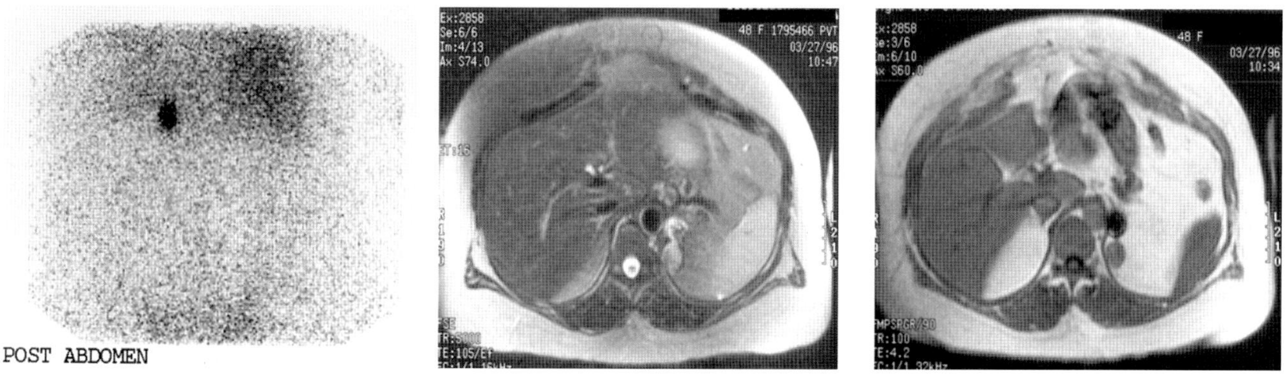

Figure 4 49-year-old female had left adrenalectomy in 1970 for cortisol-producing tumor. She had recurrence of symptoms. NP 59 scan showed uptake in left adrenal bed. At surgery, 2.5 × 1.8 cm tumor was removed. In 1996, patient had recurrent symptoms and NP-59 scan again showed left adrenal uptake, consistent with recurrence.

possibly due to more well-differentiated histology. Studies have shown that CT scan and MRI may be more informative and show typical appearance of a large adrenal tumor with central attenuation and calcification in 30% of patients, with evidence of extension into the left renal vein or inferior vena cava and presence of tumor thrombi or local nodal involvement and visceral metastases. Overall, radionuclide imaging with cholesterol analogues does not play a very important role in assessment of the functional status of these tumors. F-18 flurodeoxyglucose PET imaging has been found to be useful and shows hypermetabolic areas of primary or metastatic disease of adrenal glands.

5.4 Primary Aldosteronism

Adrenal imaging is important in assessing adrenal adenoma in patients with hyperaldosteronism (42–45). Patients with Conn's syndrome may show high plasma aldosterone and low renin levels. This occurs in about 0.1–0.5% of hypertensive patients. About 70% of these patients may have aldosterone-producing adenomas and 15–30% have bilateral hyperplasia.

Hypo functioning or nonfunctioning adenomas may take up I-131 NP-59 or Se-75 methylcholesterol. There may be bilateral symmetrical or asymmetrical uptake. Administration of dexamethasone 1 mg every 6 hours for 7 days may suppress the normal adrenal completely but not the hyperfunctioning adrenal adenoma. The appearance of unilateral adrenal uptake under dexamethasone suppression before the fifth day indicates the presence of an aldosterone-producing adenoma. Bilateral early visualization before the fifth day, under dexamethasone suppression, suggests the presence of bilateral adrenal hyperplasia, which should be treated medically. Bilateral late visualization of the adrenals is nondiagnostic. SPECT imaging has also been used for distinction between hyperplasia and adenoma (46).

About 12–20% of aldosteronomas are less than 1 cm and may be difficult to localize on CT scans. Also, diffuse hyperplasia of both glands may not produce visible distortions on anatomical imaging. Scintigraphy may help in such situations. NP-59 imaging with dexamethasone suppression is the most important tool for identifying surgically curable hypertension due to aldosterone-producing adenoma.

Figure 5 shows adrenal uptake of NP-59 at 72 hours after injection and 7 days after dexamethasone . Surgical removal of such tumor may cure the elevated blood pressure, correct electrolyte abnormalities, and abolish abnormal aldosterone secretion in two thirds of patients. The results of Se-75 methylcholesterol and I-131 NP-59 are comparable. The failure of blood pressure control after removal of aldosterone-producing adenomas is usually due to coexisting macronodules in the contralateral gland. Figure 6 shows bilateral uptake in glands of a patient with hyperaldosteronism consistent with bilateral hyperplasia.

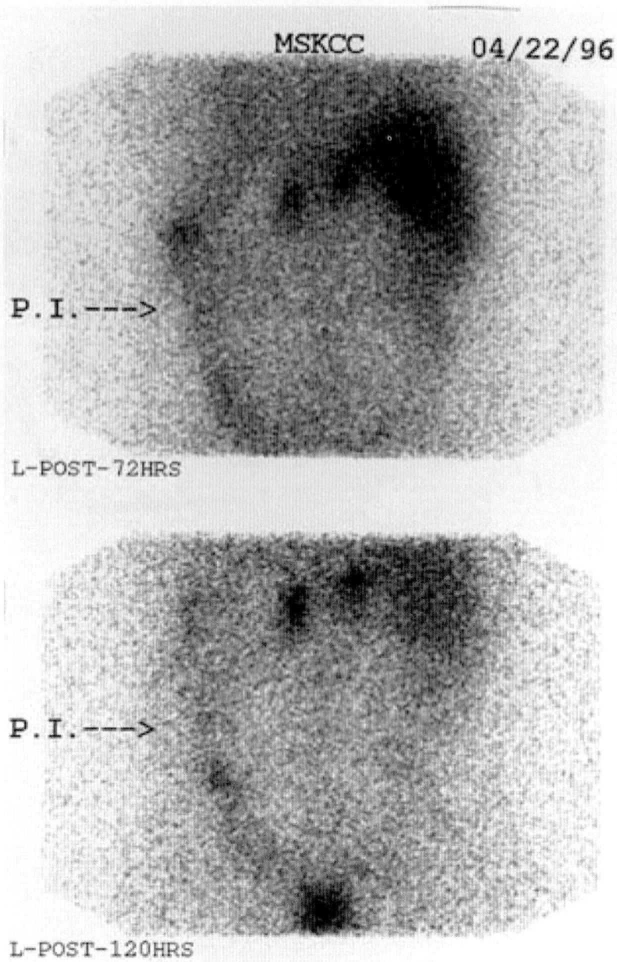

Figure 5 50-year-old male with low plasma renin activity, high serum aldosterone, and hypokalemia. NP-59 study showed bilateral adrenal uptake with dexamethasone suppression, consistent with bilateral adrenal hyperplasia.

5.5 Adrenal Hyperandrogenism

Cholesterol imaging can be also used to detect the source for hyperandrogenism in patients with virilism and excessive secretion of adrenal androgens (30,47). Bilateral early visualization is seen in bilateral hyperplasia, while androgen-secreting adenomas are seen as unilateral focal uptake on the dexamethasone suppres-

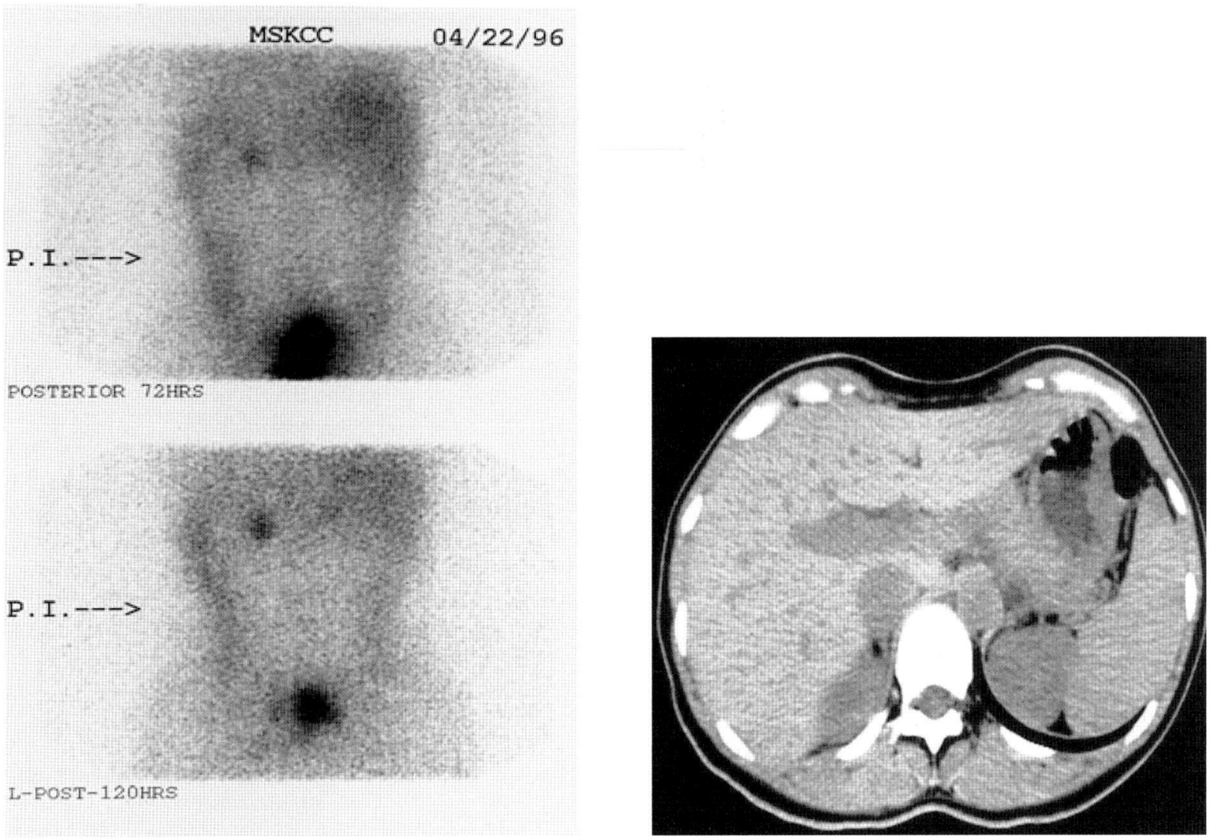

Figure 6 35-year-old female with hypertension for 10 years which was not well controlled. There was low plasma renin activity, high serum aldosterone, and low serum potassium level. CT scan showed a left adrenal mass, and high aldosterone levels were found in the left adrenal vein. NP-59 study showed left adrenal uptake. At surgery, there was 2.5 × 1.5 cm tumor and a 1 cm nodule in the left adrenal gland. After surgery the blood pressure and serum potassium levels returned to normal.

sion scan (29). Functional tumorous and nontumorous ovarian disease has been evaluated by scintigraphy (48). Bilateral late visualization is seen in the polycystic ovarian disease and congenital adrenal hyperplasia. Early nonvisualization may be seen in ovarian and peripheral hyperandrogenism. Late bilateral visualization may mean a normal pattern versus peripheral hypersensitivity to androgens.

6 INCIDENTALOMAS OR ASYMPTOMATIC ADRENAL MASSES

Scintigraphy using I-131 NP-59 has been shown to be useful for evaluation of incidentalomas. When compared with CT scanning, adenomas will show uptake at the site of the lesion (concordant imaging) and carcinoma or metastatic lesions will show no uptake at the site of CT masses (discordant imaging) (39,49). The sensitivity is reported to be about 30–70%, while specificity may be close to 100%. For lesions greater than 2 cm, the sensitivity is 100%. The sensitivity for lesions less than 2 cm is 30% (50).

7 PET IMAGING

Positron emission tomography has been used for the evaluation of many tumors, and its use in adrenal masses has been studied (51–53). The sensitivity and specificity of PET FDG imaging was about 100% and 94–97%, respectively. It was found to be very useful in initial staging and follow-up of patients. Another tracer that has been used is the 11-β-hydroxylase inhibitor carbon (C-11) metomidate. This inhibits the synthesis of cortisol and aldosterone within the adrenal cortex. It shows high uptake in adrenal cortical tumors, with low uptake in other organs (53).

REFERENCES

1. Hevesy G. The absorption and translocation of lead by plants. Biochem J 1923; 17:439.
2. Hevesy G. Adventures in Radioisotope Research: The Collected Papers of George Hevesy. New York: Pergamon, 1962.
3. Schoenheimer R, Rittenberg D. Isotopes in Biology: Dynamic State of Body Constituents. Cambridge: Harvard University Press, 1962.
4. Hertz S, Roberts A, Evans RD. Radioactive iodine as an indicator in the study of thyroid physiology. Proc Soc Exp Biol Med 1938; 38:510–513.
5. Werner SC, Quimby EH, Schmidt C. Clinical experience in the diagnosis and treatment of thyroid disorders with radioactive iodine (eight day half life). Radiology 1948; 51:564–578.
6. Fitzgerald PJ, Foote FW Jr, Hill RF. Concentration of I^{131} in thyroid cancer shown by radioautography. Cancer 1950; 3:86–105.
7. Seidlin SM, Marinelli LD, Oshry E. Radioactive iodine therapy, effect on functioning metastases of adenocarcinoma of thyroid. JAMA 1946; 132:838–847.
8. Applegren LE. Sites of steroid hormone formation: autoradiographic studies using labeled precursors. Acta Physiol Scand 1967; 301(suppl):1.
9. Fauci AS, Braunwald E, Isselbacher KJ, Wilson JD, Martin JB, Kasper DL, Hauser SL, Longlo DI. Harrison's Principles of Internal Medicine. 14th ed. New York: McGraw-Hill, 1998:2035–2056.
10. Krestin GP, Friedmann G, Fischbach R, Neufang KFR, Allolio B. Evaluation of adrenal masses in oncologic patients: dynamic contrast-enhanced MR Vs CT. J Comput Assist Tomog 1991; 15:104–110.
11. Dunnick NR. Adrenal imaging: current status. AJR 1990; 154:927–936.
12. Gajrag H, Young AE. Adrenal incidentaloma. Br J Surg 1993; 80:422–426.
13. Reinig JW, Doppman JL, Dwyer AJ, Johnson AR, Knop RH. Adrenal masses differentiated by MR. Radiology 1986; 158:81–84.
14. Mitchell DG, Crovello M, Matteucci T, Petersen RO, Miettinen MM. Benign adrenocortical masses: diagnosis with chemical shift MR imaging. Radiology 1992; 185: 345–351.
15. Tsushima T, Ishizaka H, Matsumoto M. Adrenal masses; differentiation with chemical shift, fast low-angle shot MR Imaging. Radiology 1993; 186:705–709.
16. Reinig JW. MR imaging differentiation of adrenal masses: has the time finally come. Radiology 1992; 185: 339–340.
17. Counsell RE, Ranade VV, Blair RJ, Beierwaltes WH, Weinhold PA. Tumor localizing agents IV Radioiodinated cholesterol. Steroid 1970; 15:3127–3128.
18. Beierwaltes WH, Lieberman LM, Ansari AN, Nishiyama H. Visualization of human adrenal glands in vivo by scintillation scanning. JAMA 1971; 216:275–277.
19. Sarkar SD, Beierwaltes WH, Ice RD, Basmadijian GP, Hetzel KR, Kennedy WP, Mason MM. A new and superior adrenal scanning agent, NP 59. J Nucl Med 1975; 16: 1038–1042.
20. Sarkar SD, Ice RD, Beierwaltes WR, Gill SP, Balachandran S, Basmadijian GP. Selenium-75-19-seleno cholesterol-a new adrenal scanning agent with high concentration in the adrenal medulla. J Nucl Med 1976; 17:212–217.
21. Ma JX, Zhu RS. ^{131}I-6-iodocholesterol, an agent for imaging the adrenal gland. Chin Med J 1979; 92:237–246.
22. Thrall JH, Freitas JE, Beierwaltes WH. Adrenal scintigraphy. J Nucl Med 1978; 8:23–41.
23. Blau M. Radiation dosimetry of ^{131}-I-iodocholesterol: the pitfalls of using tissue concentration data. J Nucl Med 1975; 16:247–249.
24. Kirschner AS, Ice RD, Beierwaltes WH. Radiation dosimetry of ^{131}I-19-iodocholesterol. J Nucl Med 1973; 14:713–717.
25. Gross MD, Shapiro B. Scintigraphic studies in adrenal hypertension. Sem Nucl Med 1989; 19:122–143.
26. Britton KE, Shapiro B, Hawkins LA. Emission tomography for adrenal imaging. Nucl Med Commun 1980; 1:20–23.
27. Ishimura J, Kawanaka M, Fukuchi M. Clinical application of SPECT on adrenal imaging with iodine 131-6 beta-iodomethyl-19 norcholesterol. Clin Nucl Med 1989; 14:278–281.
28. Freitas JE, Thrall JH, Swanson DP, Rifai A, Beierwaltes WH. Normal adrenal asymmetry: explanation and interpretation. J Nucl Med 1979; 19:149–154.
29. Gross MD, Freitas JE, Swanson DP, Brady T, Beurwaltes WH. The normal dexamethasone suppression adrenal scintiscan. J Nucl Med 1979; 20:1131–1135.
30. Gross MD, Shapiro B, Freitas JE, Ayers J, Swanson DP, Woodbury MC, Schteingart DE, Beierwaltes WH. The relationship of I-131 6 beta-iodomethyl-19-norcholesterol(NP-59) adrenal cortical uptake to indices of androgen secretion in women with hyperandrogenism. Clin Nucl Med 1984; 9:264–270.
31. Gross MD, Valk TW, Swanson DP, et al. The relationship of adrenal iodomethylnorcholesterol uptake to indices of adrenal cortical function in Cushing's syndrome. J Clin Endocrinol Metab 1981; 52:1062–1066.
32. Nakajo M, Sakata H, Shirona K, Shimabukuro K, Onohara S. Application of ACTH stimulation to adrenal imaging with radiocholoesterol. Clin Nucl Med 1983; 8:112–120.
33. Page DL, DeLellis RA, Hough AJ. Tumors of the Adrenal. Washington, DC: Armed Forces Institute of Pathology, 1986:45–46.
34. Pommier RF, Brennan MF. An eleven-year experience with adrenocrotical carcinoma. Surgery 1992; 112:963–971.

35. Icard P, Chapuis Y, Andreassian B, Bernard A, Proye C. Adrenocrotical carcinoma in surgically treated patients: a retrospective study on 156 cases by the French Association of Endocrine Surgery. Surgery 1992; 112:972–980.
36. Ney RI, Shianzes N, Nicholson WE, Island DP, Liddle G. Correlation of plasma ACTH concentration with adrenocortical response in normal human subjects, surgical patients and patients with Cushing's disease. J Clin Invest 1963; 42:1669–1677.
37. Barbarino A, Demarinis L, Liberace I, Menini E. Evaluation of steroid laboratory tests and adrenal gland imaging with radiocholesterol in the etiological diagnosis of Cushing's syndrome. Clin Endocrinol 1979; 10:107–121.
38. Gross MD, Wilson GP, Shapiro B, Cho K, Samuels BI, Bouffard JA, Glazer G, Grekin RJ, Brady T. Functional and scintigraphic evaluation of the silent adrenal mass. J Nucl Med 1987; 28:1401–1407.
39. Gross MD, Shapiro B, Bouffard JA, Glazer GM, Francis IR, Wilson GP, Khafagy F, Sonda LR. Distinguishing benign from malignant adrenal masses. Ann Int Med 1988; 109:613–618.
40. Shapiro B, Britton KE, Hawkins LA, Edwards CRW. Clinical experience with ^{75}Se selenomethylcholesterol adrenal imaging. Clin Endocrinol 1981; 15:19–27.
41. Reschini E, Catania A. Clinical experience with the adrenal scanning agents iodine 131-19-iodocholesterol and selenium 75-6-selenomethylcholesterol. Eur J Nucl Med 1991; 18:817–823.
42. Young WF, Klee GG. Primary aldosteronism: diagnostic evaluation. Endocrinol Metab Clin North Am 1988; 17:367–395.
43. Lim RC, Nakayama DK, Biglieri EG, Schambelan M, Hunt TK. Primary aldosteronism: changing concepts in diagnosis and management. Am J Surg 1986; 152:116–121.
44. Grant CS, Carpenter P, van Heerden JA, Hamberger B. Primary aldosteronism. Clinical management. Surgery 1984; 119:585–589.
45. Obara T, Ito Y, Okamoto T, Kanaji Y, Yamashita T, Aiba M, Fujimoto Y. Risk factors associated with postoperative persistent hypertension in patients with primary aldosteronism. Surgery 1992; 112:987–993.
46. Ishimura J, Fukuchi M. High diagnostic accuracy of qualitative adrenal SPECT imaging without dexamethasone suppression in primary aldosteronism [abstr]. J Nucl Med 1992; 33:384.
47. Freitas JE, Beierwaltes WH, Nishiyama RH. Adrenal hyperandrogenism: detection by adrenal scintigraphy. J Endocrinol Invest 1978; 1:59–64.
48. Mountz JM, Gross MD, Shapiro B, Barkan AL, Woodbury MC, Schteingart DE, Ayers JWT. Scintigraphic localization of ovarian dysfunction. J Nucl Med 1988; 29: 1644–1650.
49. Gross MD, Shapiro B, Francis IR, Gldzer GM, Bree RL, Arcumano MA, Schteingart DE, McLeod MK, Sanfield JA, Thompson NW. Scintigraphic evaluation of clinically silent adrenal masses. J Nucl Med 1994; 35:1145–1152.
50. Kloos RT, Gross MD, Shapiro B, Francis TR, Korobki M, Thompson NW. Diagnostic dilemma of small incidentally discovered adrenal masses: role for I-131 6 beta iodomethyl norcholesterol scintigraphy. World J Surg 1997; 21:36–40.
51. Yun M, Kim W, Alnafisi N, Lacorte L, Jang S, Alavi A. F-18 FDG PET in characterizing adrenal lesions detected on CT or MRI. J Nucl Med 2001; 42:1795–1799.
52. Becherer A, Vierhapper H, Potzi C, Karanikas G, Kutaran A, Schmaljohann J, Standenhertz A, Dudezak R, Kletter K. FDG PET in adrenocortical carcinoma. Cancer Biother Radiopharm 2001; 16(4):289–295.
53. Rastad J, Akerstrom G, Langstrom B. PET imaging of adrenal cortical tumors with the 11 beta hydroxylase tracer C-11 metomidate. J Nucl Med 2000; 41:275–282.

31

Radionuclide Imaging of Adrenal Medullary Tumors

Chun Ki Kim, Borys R. Krynyckyi, and Josef Machac

Mount Sinai School of Medicine and Mount Sinai Medical Center, New York, New York, U.S.A.

1 INTRODUCTION

Iodine-131 (or iodine-123) *meta*-iodobenzylguanidine (MIBG), a norepinephrine analogue, and indium-111 octreotide, a somatostatin analogue, are the two most common radiotracers used for imaging adrenal medullary tumors. Fluorine-18 fluorodeoxyglucose (FDG), a positron-emitting radiotracer, has been utilized in selected cases of these tumors. This chapter discusses the diagnostic role of these radiotracers in the evaluation of adrenal medullary tumors. Therapeutic applications of iodine-131 MIBG will not be discussed.

2 RADIOTRACERS AND TECHNIQUES

2.1 Radioiodinated MIBG

Radioiodinated-MIBG, a structural analog of guanethidine and norepinephrine, was developed in 1980. It demonstrated concentration in the adrenal medulla (1). This compound is concentrated in tumors of sympathoadrenal lineage as well as a variety of neuroendocrine tumors (2–4).

The localization of MIBG occurs primarily through the type 1 amine uptake mechanism, with entry of the agent into catecholamine storage vesicles of adrenergic nerve endings and the cells of the adrenal medulla (5). There is evidence that MIBG uptake is proportional to the quantity of neurosecretory granules in the tumor. Drugs known to or expected to interfere with MIBG uptake include tricyclic antidepressants, cocaine, labetalol, reserpine, imipramine, calcium antagonists, and amphetamine-like drugs (6–9). Therefore, these drugs should be withdrawn before an MIBG study is performed.

MIBG labeled with either iodine-131 (I-131) or iodine-123 (I-123) can be used for imaging. While the latter provides images of a higher quality due to better physical characteristics of I-123, the former has a longer half-life, which enables delayed imaging. Only I-131 MIBG has been approved by the U.S. Food and Drug Administration (FDA). Because free radioiodine accumulates in the thyroid (Fig. 1), the patient should be pretreated with Lugol's solution (3 drops orally twice a day for a week, starting 1–2 days before injection of MIBG) in order to avoid excessive radiation exposure to the thyroid.

An MIBG scan shows varying levels of physiological activity in the salivary glands, myocardium, liver, spleen, and urinary bladder (Fig. 1). Activity in the colon is noted on delayed images in some patients. Normal adrenal glands, kidneys and renal pelvis, nasal mucosa and lacrimal glands may be visualized, particularly on I-123 MIBG images, due to the higher image quality compared to I-131 MIBG. Detailed information regarding the MIBG imaging technique has been described (10,11). Obtaining additional images after administration of renal radiotracer can be helpful in confirming retention of radioactivity in the renal pelvis (Fig. 2).

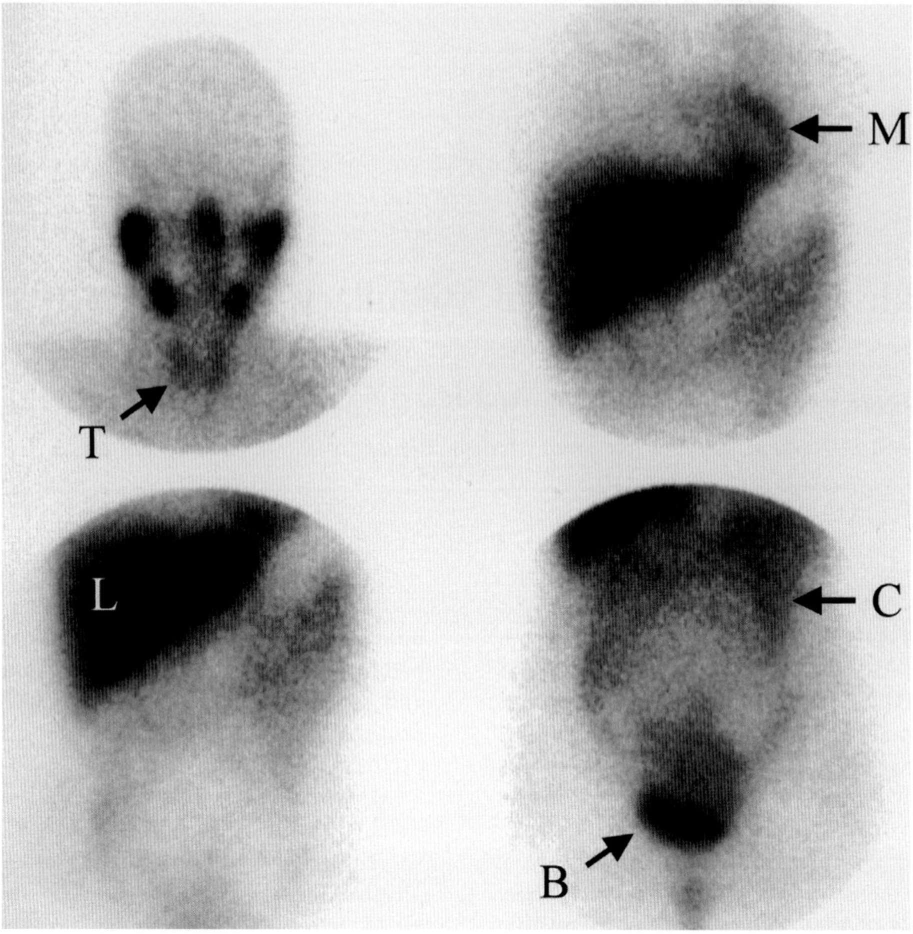

Figure 1 A normal I-123 MIBG scan showing physiological activity in the salivary glands, myocardium (M), liver (L), colon (C), and urinary bladder (B). Note that the thyroid gland (T) is also visualized, probably due to the presence of free iodine not bound to MIBG.

2.2 Indium-111 Octreotide

Indium-111 octreotide is a somatostatin analogue. Background information on this tracer is discussed in detail in Chapter 44.

2.3 Fluorine-18 Fluorodeoxyglucose

Since Warburg discovered more than a half century ago that cancer cells have increased glycolysis as compared to benign cells (12), various mechanisms have also been proposed for the accelerated glucose utilization by malignant cells. These include enhanced rates of glucose uptake by activation of glucose transporters, especially glucose transporter-1 (Glut-1) (13,14), increased concentration of hexokinase (15), and decreased rates of glucose-6-phosphatase–mediated dephosphorylation (16).

FDG is a glucose analogue. Aggressive and proliferative growth of tumors is typically associated with increased FDG uptake. FDG uptake may also be seen in active inflammatory/infectious lesions due to uptake by inflammatory cells. Thus, FDG uptake is not completely specific for malignancy. However, in general, the higher the uptake value, the more likely it is that malignant tissue is present. A negative study is very useful in excluding the presence of malignant tissue. Although FDG positron-emission tomography (PET) is currently a widely accepted technique for general tumor imaging, its utility in neuroendocrine tumors has not been fully established.

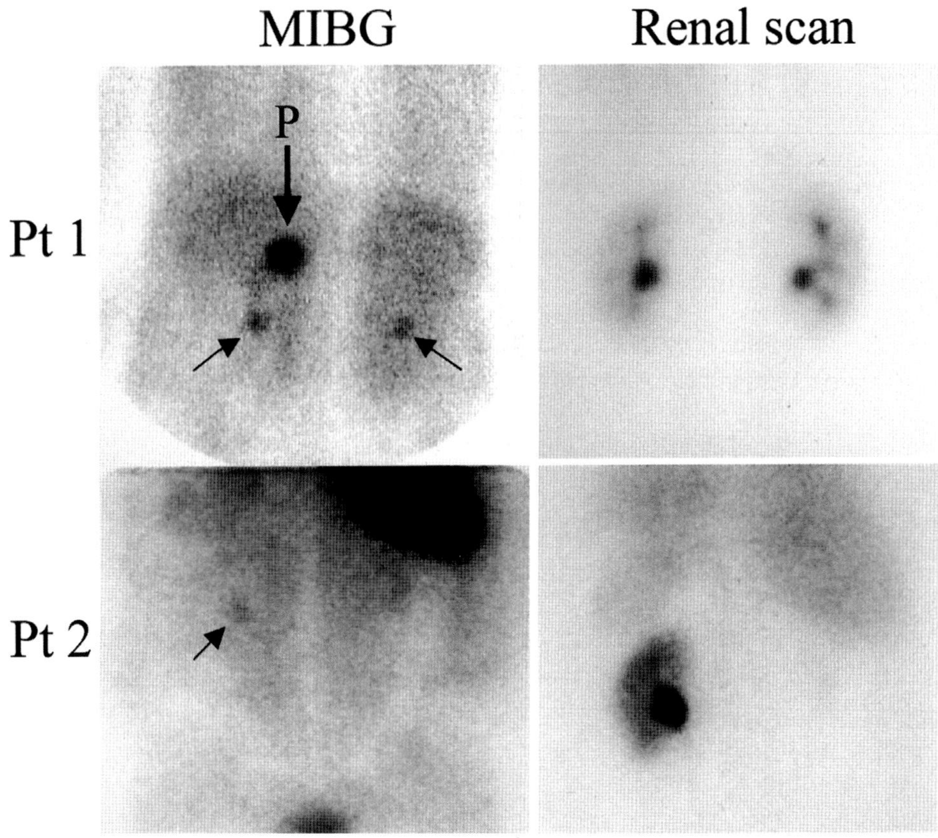

Figure 2 I-123 MIBG scintigraphy shows pheochromocytoma (P) in the left adrenal gland in Patient 1. Two additional small foci (short thin arrows) are noted, which correspond to urine activity retained in the renal pelvis of both kidneys. I-123 MIBG scintigraphy performed on Patient 2 shows a solitary focus of mildly increased activity, which also turned out to be urine retained in the left renal pelvis. The patient is status post–right nephrectomy.

3 PHEOCHROMOCYTOMA

3.1 Diagnostic Accuracy of Radionuclide Imaging

The initial experience in 400 patients at the University of Michigan (17) with MIBG scanning yielded a sensitivity of 78.4% for the detection of primary, sporadic pheochromocytoma (PCC), 92.4% in malignant PCC, and 94.3% in familial PCC, giving an overall sensitivity of 87.4%. The overall specificity was 99%. These authors found essentially identical overall sensitivity and specificity in a larger series (927 patients) that was probably expanded from their early series (18). Sensitivity and specificity reported by other investigators in review articles range from 79 to 95% and 88 to 99%, respectively (10,19), while a small series reported an exceptionally poor specificity (17%) of MIBG scintigraphy in 17 patients with multiple endocrine neoplasia (MEN) type II–related PCC (20).

For imaging of adrenal PCCs, somatostatin receptor scintigraphy (SRS) is less accurate than MIBG scintigraphy, which seems particularly true in benign PCC. This is probably because the majority of benign lesions do not express a sufficient amount of somatostatin receptors to be visualized. Another possible reason is intense renal uptake, which could potentially interfere with visualization of the adrenal gland. While the majority of malignant PCCs showed increased uptake on SRS with In-111 octreotide, only 20–25% of benign PCCs were visualized (21,22). However, while metastases were visualized with I-123 MIBG in 8 of 14 cases, with In-111 octreotide, 7 of 8 cases were visualized, including three I-123 MIBG–negative cases (22).

The overall accuracy of FDG PET for detecting PCCs as well as delineation of the tumor is somewhat inferior to those with MIBG scintigraphy. However, some aggressive tumors (MIBG-negative cases) show intense FDG uptake (23).

Overall, MIBG scanning has a high diagnostic accuracy in detecting PCC. False-positive studies are rare. MIBG scanning is particularly valuable in the localization of tumors located outside the adrenal gland and in determining the extent of disease (Fig. 3) (24). It appears reasonably safe to conclude, based on data in the literature, that MIBG scintigraphy is the radionuclide imaging of choice, and that while SRS and FDG PET are not as sensitive for detecting benign PCCs, they can add further information in malignant, MIBG-negative PCCs.

3.2 Radionuclide Imaging Versus Anatomical Imaging

Investigators have reported that computed tomography (CT) and magnetic resonance imaging (MRI) have a significantly higher diagnostic sensitivity compared to I-131 MIBG imaging during the initial evaluation, but I-131 MIBG imaging and MRI has slightly better sensitivity compared to CT when performed after surgery. I-131 MIBG has a higher specificity than CT/MRI both before and after surgery. These authors concluded that

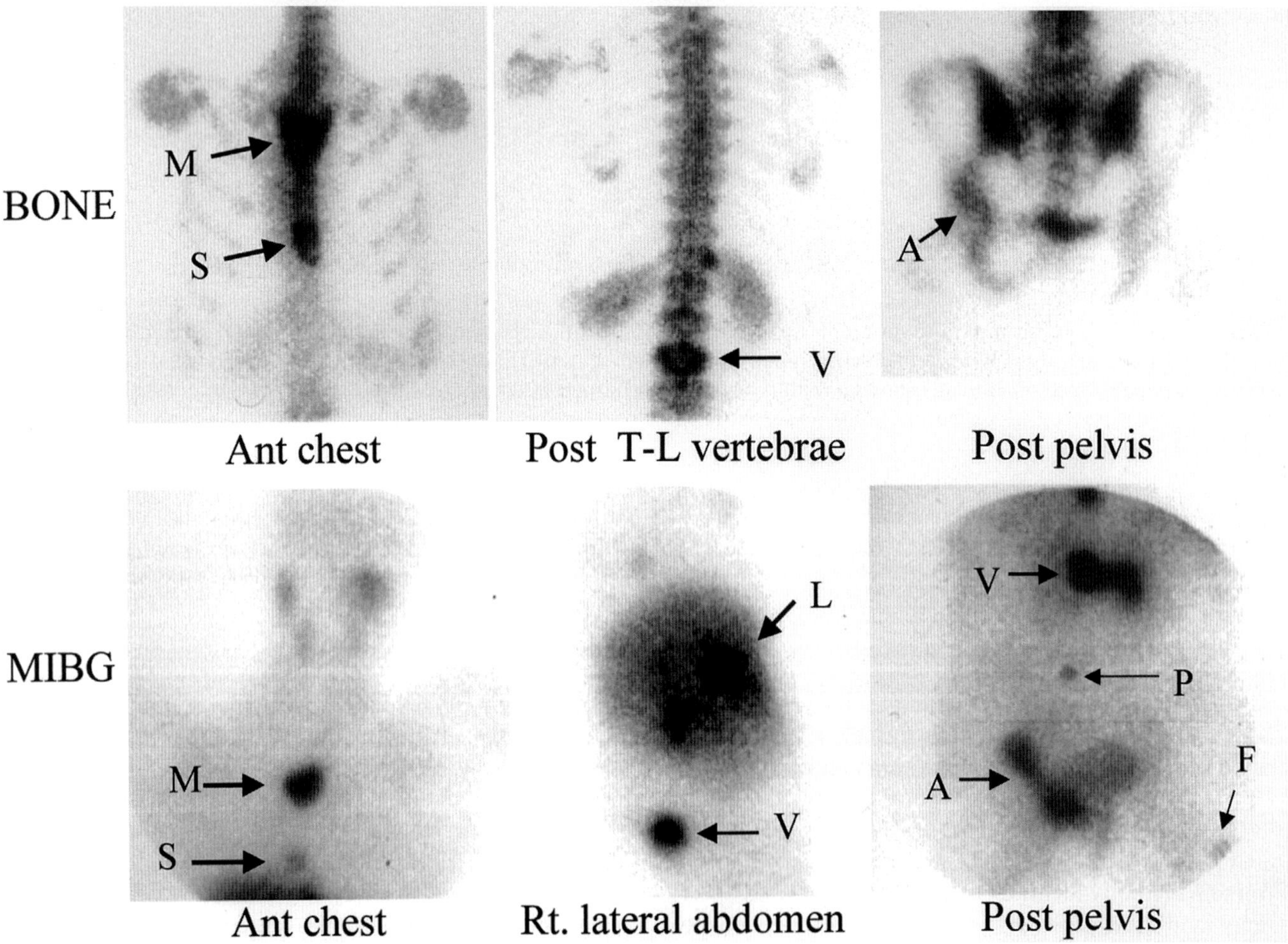

Figure 3 Metastatic pheochromocytoma. Bone scintigraphy demonstrating foci of increased activity in the manubrium (M), lower sternum (S), third lumbar vertebra (V), and right acetabular region (A), all of which are seen on the I-123 MIBG scan. The MIBG scan additionally shows a liver lesion (L), and small pelvic (P) and right proximal femoral lesions (F). The acetabular and vertebral lesions appear to be more extensive on the MIBG scan.

CT and MRI are useful in the initial evaluation of patients with suspected paragangliomas, but that MIBG should be recommended during the postsurgical follow-up (25).

While I-131 MIBG studies clearly have a lower sensitivity but a higher specificity compared to CT/MRI, investigators have reported that the sensitivity of I-123 MIBG imaging is similar to that of CT/MRI (11). This is supported by a study of 120 patients with I-123 MIBG, which suggested that I-123 MIBG imaging might be the most sensitive screening test available for diagnosing PCC (24).

In addition, MIBG scintigraphy can particularly be valuable in patients with inconclusive laboratory results and CT (26). Besides, whole body imaging can be performed with radionuclide studies as a single examination, which helps detect extra-adrenal neoplastic sites.

Radionuclide imaging was found to be useful in the characterization of nonhypersecreting unilateral adrenal tumors that had been originally detected on CT or MRI (27). In that series, norcholesterol imaging, MIBG imaging, and FDG PET imaging had a high PPV and NPV for adenoma, PCC, and a malignant tumor, respectively. Therefore, adrenal scintigraphy is recommended for tumor diagnosis and, hence, for appropriate treatment planning, particularly when CT or MRI findings are inconclusive for lesion characterization. Norcholesterol imaging and its role in management of adrenal tumors is discussed in another section of this book.

3.3 Treatment Planning

When I-131-MIBG therapy is considered, MIBG imaging should be performed before administering the ther-

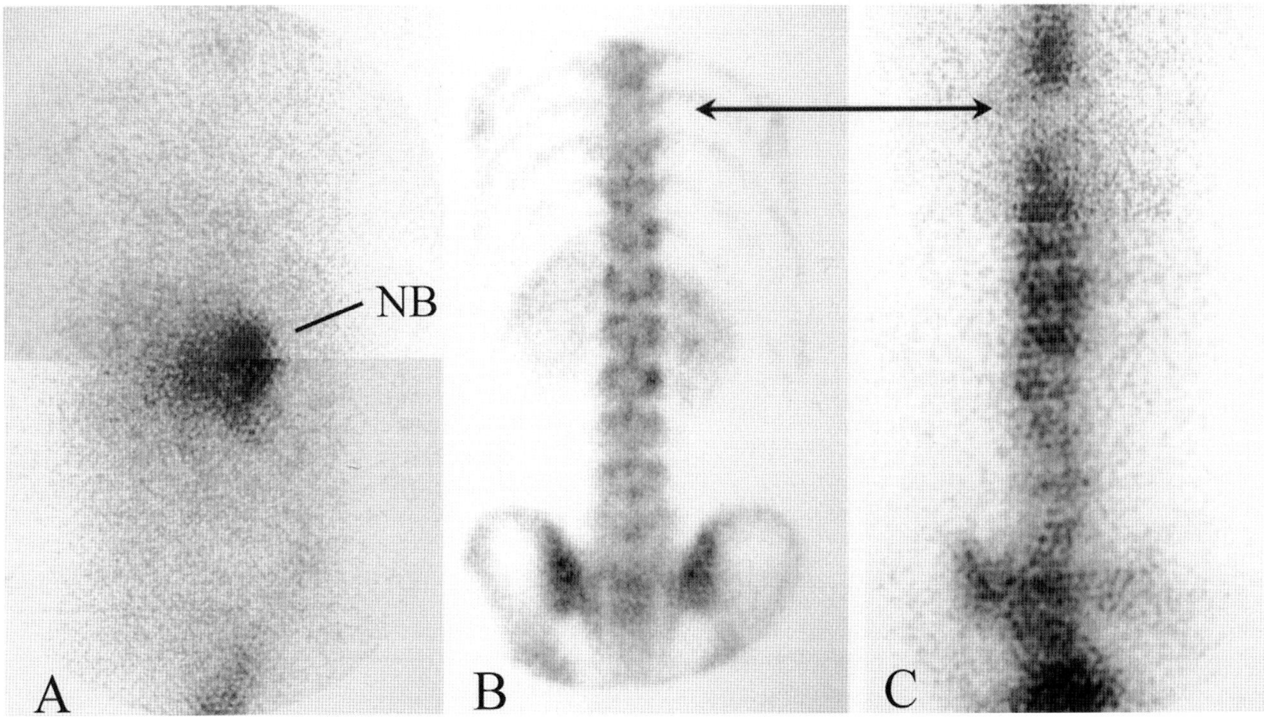

Figure 4 (A) I-131 MIBG scan in an 18-month-old child. Anterior view of the chest and abdomen shows a large focus of increased activity (NB) in the left upper quadrant of the abdomen consistent with neuroblastoma. (B) A follow-up bone scan. The patient is status post–resection of primary tumor. Posterior images show a somewhat heterogeneous distribution of tracer in the spine, but no discrete abnormalities. Initially, the bone scan was read as possibly demonstrating areas of decreased activity (arrow), which could represent aggressive lytic metastatic lesions. (C) MIBG scintigraphy performed subsequently demonstrates no uptake (which is normal) in the region of "relatively decreased" uptake on the bone scan. Actually, areas of "relatively normal" uptake on the bone scan correspond to areas of increased MIBG uptake that involves nearly the entire spine and pelvis. The patient was found to have diffuse marrow infiltration.

apy dose in order to assess tumor uptake and the biodistribution of the compound in the body.

4 NEUROBLASTOMA

4.1 MIBG Imaging

Neuroblastomas (NB) in neonates and infants are usually detected initially by ultrasonography. An accurate assessment of the disease extent and staging is essential for clinical management decision and prognostication. MIBG imaging is a well-established procedure in the evaluation of NB with a cumulative accuracy of ~90% (11). The highest sensitivity is shown in the detection of skeletal metastases (Fig. 4). MIBG imaging is reported to detect 10–40% more lesions than bone scintigraphy, although the latter remains the alternative modality in MIBG-negative cases (11).

A multicenter study has also found MIBG scintigraphy highly specific. Only 4 of 100 nonsympathomedullary tumors (non-PCC and nonneuroblastoma) in childhood showed MIBG uptake, of which only two were of non–neural crest origin (28).

4.2 Prognostic Value of Octreotide Imaging

Octreotide imaging, although not as sensitive for the detection of NB as MIBG imaging, does provide prognostic information. Several groups of investigators have reported that the absence of octreotide uptake in NB is associated with a poorer clinical outcome (29–31). While MIBG imaging remains the best scintigraphic method for detecting neuroblastoma tumor tissue, SRS can provide significant additional prognostic information.

4.3 Assessment of Therapeutic Response and Follow-Up

It has been reported that, in the presence of complete normalization of the MIBG scan after chemotherapy, the persistence of an abnormal signal in the bone marrow on MRI does not necessarily indicate persistence of disease and that attention must be paid to the delay of signal normalization on MRI in order to avoid false-positive interpretation (32).

4.4 Intraoperative Probe Localization

Injection of radiolabeled MIBG before surgery can be helpful for intraoperative detection of neuroblastoma (33,34). This technique can be particularly sensitive in the detection of early recurrence after treatment and may be used in children undergoing relaparotomy (33). Compared with I-123, I-125 labeling seems to have a similar sensitivity but a higher specificity (34). The method is reported to be useful to improve the quality of macroscopic resection in widespread neuroblastoma with nodal involvement, in sites with difficult access, and in operations for relapse.

5 CONCLUSION

MIBG scintigraphy is a valuable, highly specific and, if I-123 is used for labeling, fairly sensitive technique for imaging pheochromocytoma and neuroblastoma. It plays an important role in the diagnosis, staging, restaging, monitoring of the therapeutic response and follow-up, intraoperative radioguided surgery, and evaluation of biodistribution before I-131 MIBG therapy. In-111 octreotide imaging has a role in prognostication of patients with neuroblastoma. PET with FDG also provides some diagnostic and prognostic information, but further studies will be necessary to define its role more clearly.

REFERENCES

1. Wieland DM, Wu J, Brown LE, Mangner TJ, Swanson DP, Beierwaltes WH. Radiolabeled adrenergic neuron-blocking agents: adrenomedullary imaging with [131I]-iodobenzylguanidine. J Nucl Med 1980; 21:349–353.
2. Beierwaltes WH. Endocrine imaging: parathyroid, adrenal cortex and medulla, and other endocrine tumors. Part II. J Nucl Med 1991; 32:1627–1639.
3. McEwan AJ, Shapiro B, Sisson JC, Beierwaltes WH, Ackery DM. Radio-iodobenzylguanidine for the scintigraphic location and therapy of adrenergic tumors. Semin Nucl Med 1985; 15:132–153.
4. Slooter GD, Mearadji A, Breeman WA, Quet RL, de-Jong M, Krenning EP, van Eijck CH. Somatostatin receptor imaging, therapy and new strategies in patients with neuroendocrine tumours. Br J Surg 2001; 88:31–40.
5. Shapiro B, Wieland DM, Brown LE, Kline RC, Nakajo M, Sisson JC, Beierwaltes WH. 131I-Meta-iodobenzylguanidine (MIBG) adrenal medullary scintigraphy: interventional studies. In: Spencer RP, ed. Interventional Nuclear Medicine. New York: Grune & Stratton, 1983: 451–481.
6. Guilloteau D, Baulieu JL, Huguet F, Viel C, Chambon

C, Valat C, Baulieu F, Itti R, Pourcelot L, Narcisse G, et al. Meta-iodobenzylguanidine adrenal medulla localization: autoradiographic and pharmacologic studies. Eur J Nucl Med 1984; 9:278–281.
7. Tobes MC, Jaques S Jr, Wieland DM, Sisson JC. Effect of uptake-one inhibitors on the uptake of norepinephrine and metaiodobenzylguanidine. J Nucl Med 1985; 26:897–907.
8. Khafagi FA, Shapiro B, Fig LM, Mallette S, Sisson JC. Labetalol reduces iodine-131 MIBG uptake by pheochromocytoma and normal tissues. J Nucl Med 1989; 30:481–489.
9. Solanki KK, Bomanji J, Moyes J, Mather SJ, Trainer PJ, Britton KE. A pharmacological guide to medicines which interfere with the biodistribution of radiolabeled meta-iodobenzylguanidine (MIBG). Nucl Med Commun 1992; 13:513–521.
10. Hoefnagel CA. Metaiodobenzylguanidine and somatostatin in oncology: role in the management of neural crest tumours. Eur J Nucl Med 1994; 21:561–581.
11. Troncone L, Rufini V. Radiolabeled metaiodobenzylguanidine in the diagnosis of neural crest tumours. In: Murray IPC, Ell PJ, eds. Nuclear Medicine in Clinical Diagnosis and Treatment. Edinburgh: Churchill Livingstone 1998:843–857.
12. Warburg O. The Metabolism of Tumors. New York: Smith RR Inc., 1931:129–169
13. Merrall NW, Plevin R, Gould GW. Growth factors, mitogens, oncogenes and the regulation of glucose transport. Cell Signal 1993; 5:667–675.
14. Brown RS, Leung JY, Fisher SJ, Frey KA, Ethier SP, Wahl RL. Intratumoral distribution of tritiated-FDG in breast carcinoma: correlation between Glut-1 expression and FDG uptake. J Nucl Med 1996; 37:1042–1047.
15. Torizuka T, Tamaki N, Inokuma T, Magata Y, Sasayama S, Yonekura Y, Tanaka A, Yamaoka Y, Yamamoto K, Konishi J. In vivo assessment of glucose metabolism in hepatocellular carcinoma with FDG-PET. J Nucl Med 1995; 36: 1811–1817.
16. Graham MM, Spence AM, Muzi M, Abbott GL, Deoxyglucose kinetics in a rat brain tumor. J Cereb Blood Flow Metab 1989; 9:315–322.
17. Shapiro B, Copp JE, Sisson JC, Eyre PL, Wallis J, Beierwaltes WH. 131-Iodine-metaiodobenzylguanidine for the locating of suspected phaeochromocytoma: experience in 400 cases. J Nucl Med 1985; 26:576–585.
18. Shapiro B, Sisson JC, Sympatho-adrenal imaging with radio-iodinated meta-iodobenzylguanidine. In: Van Nostrand D, Baum S, eds. Atlas of Nuclear Medicine. Philadelphia: Lippincott, 1988:72–114.
19. Seregni E, Chiti A, Bombardieri E. Radionuclide imaging of neuroendocrine tumours: biological basis and diagnostic results. Eur J Nucl Med 1998; 25:639–658.
20. De Graaf JS, Dullaart RP, Kok T, Piers DA, Zwierstra RP. Limited role of meta-iodobenzylguanidine scintigraphy in imaging phaeochromocytoma in patients with multiple endocrine neoplasia type II. Eur J Surg 2000; 166:289–292.
21. Maurea S, Lastoria S, Caraco C, Klain M, Varrella P, Acampa W, Muto P, Salvatore M. The role of radiolabeled somatostatin analogs in adrenal imaging. Nucl Med Biol 1996; 23, 677–680.
22. van der Harst E, de Herder WW, Bruining HA, Bonjer HJ, de Krijger RR, Lamberts SW, van de Meiracker AH, Boomsma F, Stijnen T, Krenning EP, Bosman FT, Kwekkeboom DJ. [(123)I]Meta-iodobenzylguanidine and [(111)In]octreotide uptake in begnign and malignant pheochromocytomas. J Clin Endocrinol Metab 2001; 86:685–693.
23. Shulkin BL, Thompson NW, Shapiro B, Francis IR, Sisson JC. Pheochromocytomas: imaging with 2-[fluorine-18]fluoro-2-deoxy-D-glucose PET. Radiology 1999; 212:35–41.
24. Mozley PD, Kim CK, Mohsin J, Jatlow A, Gosfield E III, Alavi A, The efficacy of iodine-123-MIBG as a screening test for pheochromocytoma. J Nucl Med 1994; 35:1138–1144.
25. Maurea S, Cuocolo A, Reynolds JC, Neumann RD, Salvatore M. Diagnostic imaging in patients with paragangliomas. Computed tomography, magnetic resonance and MIBG scintigraphy comparison. Q J Nucl Med 1996; 40:365–371.
26. Berglund AS, Hulthen UL, Manhem P, Thorsson O, Wollmer P, Tornquist C. Metaiodobenzylguanidine (MIBG) scintigraphy and computed tomography (CT) in clinical practice. Primary and secondary evaluation for localization of phaeochromocytomas. J Intern Med 2001; 249:247–251.
27. Maurea S, Klain M, Mainolfi C, Ziviello M, Salvatore M. The diagnostic role of radionuclide imaging in evaluation of patients with nonhypersecreting adrenal masses. J Nucl Med 2001; 42:884–892.
28. Leung A, Shapiro B, Hattner R, Kim E, de Kraker J, Ghazzar N, Hartmann O, Hoefnagel CA, Jamadar DA, Kloos R, Lizotte P, Lumbroso J, Rufini V, Shulkin BL, Sisson JC, Thein A, Troncone L. Specificity of radioiodinated MIBG for neural crest tumors in childhood. J Nucl Med 1997; 38:1352–1357.
29. Kropp J, Hofmann M, Bihl H. Comparison of MIBG and pentetreotide scintigraphy in children with neuroblastoma. Is the expression of somatostatin receptors a prognostic factor? Anticancer Res 1997; 17(3B):1583–1588.
30. Schilling FH, Bihl H, Jacobsson H, Ambros PF, Tinsson T, Borgstrom P, Schwarz K, Ambros IM, Treuner J, Kogner P. Combined (111)In-pentetreotide scintigraphy and (123)I-mIBG scintigraphy in neuroblastoma provides prognostic information. Med Pediatr Oncol 2000; 35:688–691.
31. Orlando C, Raggi CC, Bagnoni L, Sestini R, Briganti V, La Cava G, Bernini G, Tonini GP, Pazzagli M, Serio M,

Maggi M. Somatostatin receptor type 2 gene expression in neuroblastoma, measured by competitive RT-PCR, is related to patient survival and to somatostatin receptor imaging by indium-111-pentetreotide. Med Pediatr Oncol 2001; 36:224–226.

32. Lebtahi N, Gudinchet F, Nenadov-Beck M, Beck D, Bischof Delaloye A. Evaluating bone marrow metastasis of neuroblastoma with iodine-123-MIBG scintigraphy and MRI. J Nucl Med 1997; 38:389–1392.
33. Heij HA, Rutgers EJ, de Kraker J, Vos A. Intraoperative search for neuroblastoma by MIBG and radioguided surgery with the gamma detector. Med Pediatr Oncol 1997; 28:171–174.
34. Martelli H, Ricard M, Larroquet M, Wioland M, Paraf F, Fabre M, Josset P, Helardot PG, Gauthier F, Terrier-Lacombe MJ, Michon J, Hartmann O, Tabone MD, Patte C, Lumbroso J, Gruner M. Intraoperative localization of neuroblastoma in children with 123I- or 125I-radiolabeled metaiodobenzylguanidine. Surgery 1998; 123:51–57.

32

Adrenal Vein Sampling

Harold A. Mitty

Mount Sinai School of Medicine, New York University, New York, New York, U.S.A.

1 INTRODUCTION

Adrenal venography has essentially been replaced by computed tomography (CT) and magnetic resonance (MR) as a method for detecting most adrenal masses. Nevertheless, catheterization of the adrenal veins remains a vital tool for obtaining blood for the localization of small aldosterone-producing adenomas. In addition, adrenal venous sampling is often necessary in patients with hyperaldosteronism to differentiate adenomas, bilateral hyperplasia, and automomous nodules in patients with bilateral findings (1). Finally, unilateral hyperplasia is a rare surgically correctable cause of hyperaldosteronism that may require adrenal venous sampling for accurate diagnosis (2).

2 TECHNIQUE

Adrenal venous sampling can be performed on ambulatory or hospitalized patients who have been off of steroids for one week. The common femoral vein is punctured and a 5 French vascular sheath is inserted. The right adrenal vein is generally more difficult to catheterize than the left as it enters the posterior aspect of the vena cava at the T-11 level in most patients. Recently, our greatest success in entering this vein has been with a Mickaelsson catheter, although a Cobra (C2) or Simmons 1 catheter may be successful in some patients. A blood sample is obtained by allowing the blood to drip from the catheter directly into the collection tube. One cannot aspirate blood from the gland with a syringe as it will collapse the tenuous venous system.

After the right-sided sample is collected, the catheter is withdrawn and a vena caval sample from below the renal veins is obtained. The right adrenal catheter is then exchanged for a left adrenal catheter and the left adrenal vein is entered. This is generally easier than the right side as the left adrenal vein has a fairly constant site of drainage into the superior aspect of the left renal vein at a point over the left pedicle of the corresponding lumbar vertebrae. Anomalies of the left renal vein such as circumaortic and retroaortic configurations will alter the site of left adrenal vein entry into the renal vein (3).

Once a blood sample is obtained from the left adrenal, we repeat the process in reverse after the slow administration of cosyntropin (Cortrosyn) 0.25 mg IV followed by an additional 0.25 mg mixed in 50 mL of saline, infused over 20 minutes. This agent will accentuate the differences between glands. The blood samples that are collected are assayed for aldosterone and cortisol so that a ratio can be generated that will take into account the dilution of adrenal blood by non-adrenal blood from collaterals, confluent branches, and the vena cava (4,5). Venography may be performed once adequate samples are obtained. The risk of damage

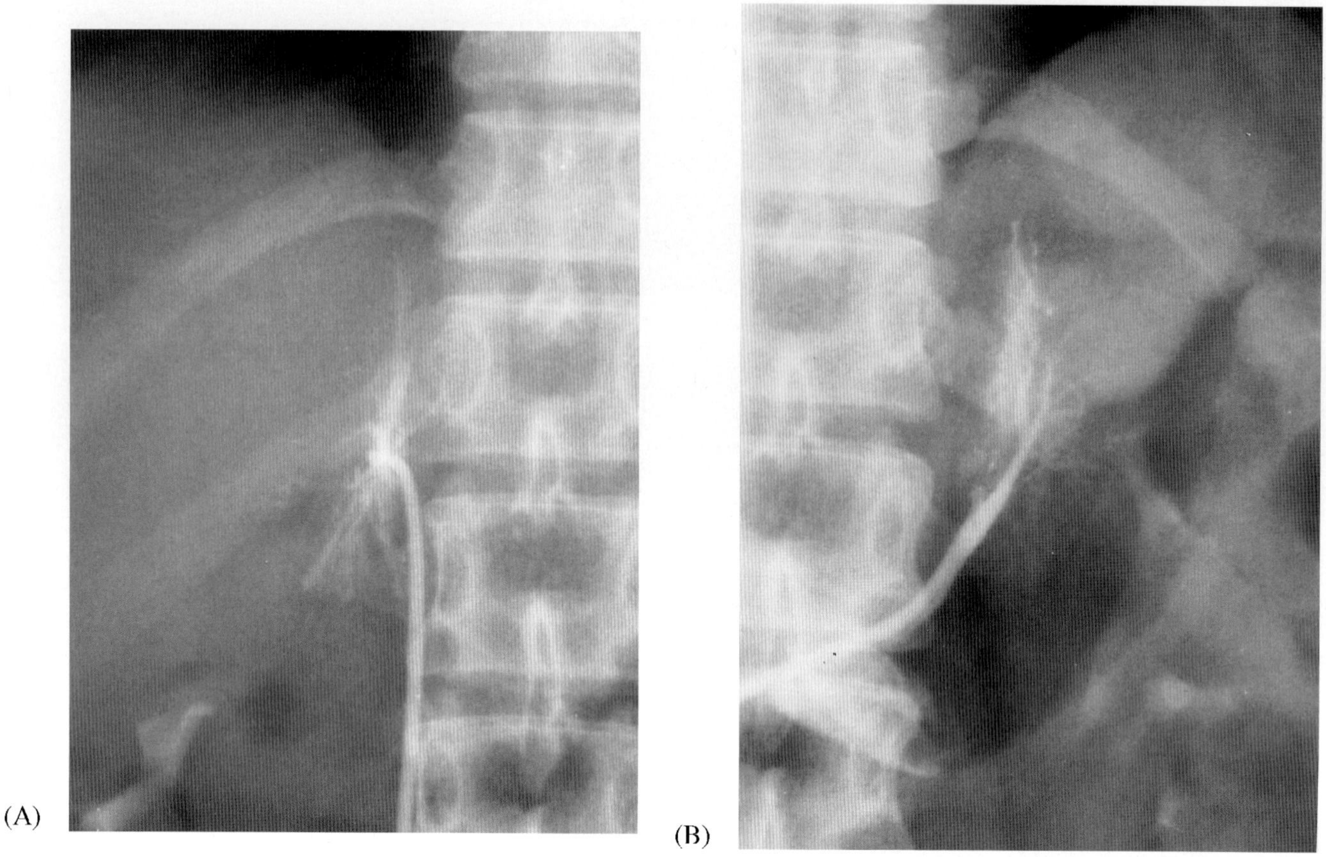

Figure 1 Normal adrenal venograms. (A) Right adrenal: note the triangular configuration with slightly concave boarders. (B) Left adrenal: triangular configuration maintained as gland extends towards left renal vein.

to the adrenal vein and gland by retrograde venography should be weighed against the potential benefit of additional information from this final venogram. Venograms may be of some value in documenting the site of the catheter at the time of sampling if assay results prove questionable.

Examples of venograms in patients with normal glands (Fig. 1), hyperplastic glands (Fig. 2), and a gland with a left adenoma (Fig. 3) are presented.

3 EVIDENCE SUPPORTING ADRENAL VEIN SAMPLING

The current role of adrenal venous sampling is essentially limited to the evaluation of functioning masses that are not successfully imaged on CT or MR. The problem of the small nonfunctioning adrenal adenoma may further confuse the significance of CT or MR findings (6).

A recent paper by Magill et al. comparing adrenal vein sampling and CT in 38 patients with aldosteronism gave the following results: 15 patients with aldosterone-producing adenomas proven by adrenal vein sampling were analyzed; 8 had concordant findings with CT, 4 had discordant findings, and 3 had normal CT studies (7). In a similar study in 34 patients by Young et al. (8), 4 of 9 patients with bilateral masses had a unilateral source of aldosterone production. Six of 15 with normal or minimal adrenal limb thickening had a unilateral source of aldosterone. Doppman et al. (1), in a study of 24 patients with primary aldosteronism, confirmed that the most common error in diagnosis was to conclude that the presence of bilateral nodules was consistent with hyperplasia. In 6 of 7 patients with such a diag-

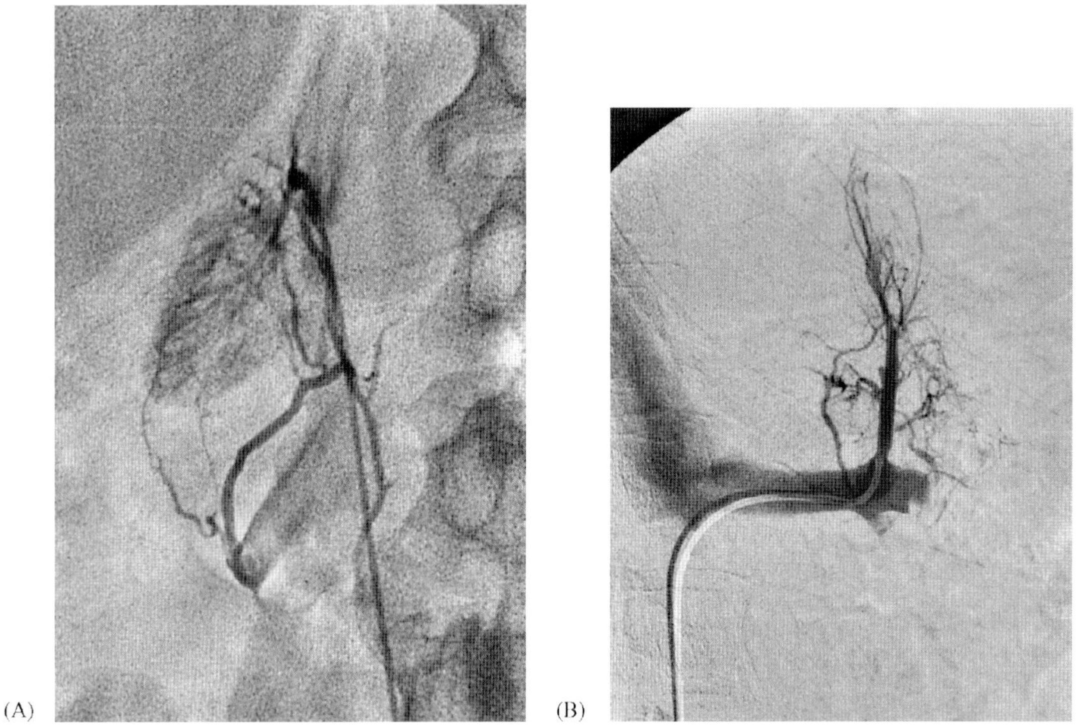

Figure 2 Hyperplasia. (A) Right: note the convex contour of the gland. (B) Left: contour less well-defined; venous system somewhat obscured by collateral vessels.

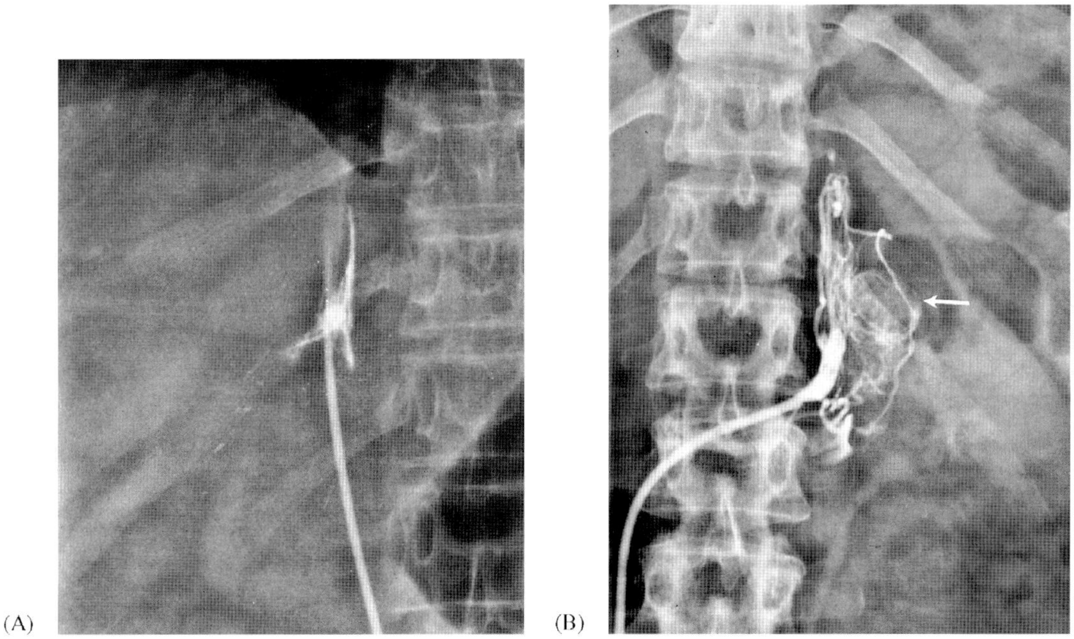

Figure 3 Aldosteronoma (Conn's tumor). (A) Normal right adrenal venogram. (B) Left adenoma (arrow).

nosis, sampling and surgery demonstrated a unilateral adenoma. The authors concluded that in a patient with bilateral nodules, CT cannot distinguish between adenoma and hyperplasia.

Thus, adrenal venous sampling combined with imaging studies offers the best means of demonstrating the source of hyperaldosteronism (9).

REFERENCES

1. Doppman JL, Gill JR Jr, Milker DL, et al. Distinction between hyperaldosteronism due to bilateral hyperplasia and unilateral aldosteronoma: reliability of CT. Radiology 1992; 184:677–682.
2. Morioka M, Kobayaski T, Sone A, et al. Primary aldosteronism due to unilateral adrenal hyperplasia: report of two cases and review of the literature. Endocr J 2000; 47:443–449.
3. Mitty HA, Yeh H-C. Radiology of the Adrenals. Philadelphia: W. B. Saunders and Co., 1982:49–58.
4. Rossi GP, Sacchatto A, Chiesura-Corona M, et al. Identification of the etiology of primary aldosteronism with adrenal vein sampling in patients with equivical CT and MR findings: results in 104 consecutive cases. J Clin Endocrinol Metab 2001; 86:1083–1090.
5. Doppman JL, Gill JR Jr. Hyperaldosteronism: sampling the adrenal veins. Radiology 1996; 198:309–312.
6. McAlister FA, Lewanczuk RZ. Primary hyperaldosteronism and adrenal incidentaloma: an argument for physiologic testing before adrenalectomy. Can J Surg 1998; 41:299–305.
7. Magill SB, Raff H, Shaker JL, et al. Comparison of adrenal vein sampling and computed tomography in the differentiation of primary aldosteronism. J Clin Endocrnol Metab 2001; 86(3):1066–1071.
8. Young WF Jr, Stanson AW, Grant CS, Thompson GB, van Heerden JA. Primary aldosteronism: adrenal venous sampling. Surgery 1996; 120:913–919.
9. Phillips JL, Walther MM, Pezzullo JC, et al. Predictive value of preoperative tests in discriminating bilateral adrenal hyperplasia from an aldosterone–producing adrenal adenoma. J Clin Endocrinol Metab 2000; 85:4526–4533.

33

Cushing's Syndromes, Adrenocortical Carcinoma, and Estrogen- and Androgen-Secreting Tumors

Moritz Wente

University of Heidelberg, Heidelberg, Germany

Guido Eibl and Oscar J. Hines

David Geffen School of Medicine at UCLA, Los Angeles, California, U.S.A.

1 CUSHING'S SYNDROMES

Cushing's syndrome is a symptom complex initially described by Harvey Cushing in 1932 as "pituitary basophilism" with a constellation of obesity, diabetes, arterial hypertension, muscular weakness, and adrenal hyperplasia (1). Whereas the term Cushing's syndrome is used for hypercortisolism of various etiologies, Cushing's disease, the most frequent form of the homonymous syndrome, is caused by excess pituitary adrenocorticotropic hormone (ACTH) from microadenoma. All symptoms of Cushing's syndrome result from long-term exposure of tissues to glucocorticoid excess. Although the entity is rare and difficult to diagnose, it should always be considered as the putative cause of many diverse and nonspecific clinical manifestations (2).

1.1 Epidemiology

There are limited epidemiological data about Cushing's syndrome. The annual incidence of pituitary-dependent Cushing's disease is in the range of 1–10 cases, and the prevalence is about 39 per million people (3,4). The female-to-male ratio in Cushing's syndrome ranges from 3 to 15:1 (3–5).

The most common cause of hypercortisolism is the exogenous use of glucocorticoids for treatment of other diseases. Eighty-five percent of endogenous Cushing's syndromes are caused by excess ACTH, mostly from autonomous pituitary adenomas (Table 1). Ectopic secretion of ACTH from endocrine tumors of the lung, thymus, or pancreas represents about 10% of the ACTH-dependent Cushing's syndromes (3,6,7). Adrenal adenomas and carcinomas comprise up to 25% of all cases of hypercortisolism and suppress pituitary ACTH production. Pseudo-Cushing's syndrome is caused by major depressive disorders or alcoholism resulting in hypercortisolism and clinical and biochemical features of Cushing's syndrome, which disappear with remission of the disorders (7) (Table 1).

1.2 Clinical Features

The most common and universal symptoms are weight gain leading to central obesity, diabetes mellitus type 2, and arterial hypertension, which are also prevalent in the general population and therefore nonspecific. Clinical manifestations more specific to Cushing's syndrome are facial rounding ("moon facies"), caused by thickening of facial fat, and a "buffalo hump," caused by increased fat in the dorsal neck and supra-

Table 1 Various Types of Cushing's Syndromes

Diagnosis	Frequency (%)		
	Study 1[a] ($n=302$)	Study 2[b] ($n=306$)	Study 3[c] ($n=630$)
ACTH-dependent Cushing's syndrome			
Cushing's disease	66.0	68.3	68
Ectopic ACTH syndrome	7.1	10.5	12
Ectopic CRH syndrome	>1	n.a.	<1
Unknown source of ACTH	n.a.	5.2	n.a.
ACTH-independent Cushing's syndrome			
Adrenal adenoma	18.0	7.8	10
Adrenal carcinoma	6.2	6.5	8
Nodular adrenal hyperplasia	2	1.6	1
Pseudo-Cushing's syndrome			
Major depressive disorder	n.a.	n.a.	1
Alcoholism	n.a.	n.a.	<1

[a] From Ref. 18.
[b] From Ref. 16.
[c] From Ref. 7.

clavicular areas combined with kyphosis induced by osteoporosis. Furthermore, patients may show signs of proximal muscular weakness with thin extremities and facial plethora or hirsutism. A relatively specific clinical finding is the appearance of multiple wide purple striae on the abdomen (wider than 1 cm), and virilization is often seen in adrenal carcinoma (3,7) (Table 2). In the early stage of the disease when the signs and symptoms are less clear, the diagnosis of Cushing's syndrome is difficult.

1.3 Diagnosis of Cushing's Syndrome

The first test in the diagnosis of Cushing's syndrome should be simple to perform, noninvasive, and should have a high sensitivity. Later, the definitive diagnosis should be confirmed using tests with high specificity (Fig. 1).

1.3.1 Urinary Free Cortisol

The measurement of urinary free cortisol (UFC) is the established and most widely used screening test for patients with clinical signs and symptoms of Cushing's syndrome. The normal range for UFC by radioimmunoassay (RIA) is 80–120 μg/24 h. Values greater than 400 μg/24 h are indicative of Cushing's syndrome (8). Assays of UFC in an outpatient setting offer a sensitivity of up to 100% and a specificity of 98% (9). Assay of urinary creatinine is needed to minimize pitfalls from incomplete collection and to ensure accurate results (7). It has been shown that up to 11% of patients with Cushing's syndrome may have normal values in one of four UFC assays. Therefore, the UFC should be performed in two or three consecutive 24-hour periods to increase the sensitivity and to avoid single test results with normal values (10). False-positive test results in UFC assays have been found in up to 50% of women with polycystic ovaries and in up to 40% of patients with major depression (11,12). Therefore, assays of UFC cannot be used to distinguish between true Cushing's and pseudo-Cushing's syndromes, but it is possible to exclude true Cushing's syndrome after obtaining several results in the normal range.

1.3.2 Low-Dose Dexamethasone Suppression Test

Another screening method is the oral low-dose dexamethasone suppression test (LDDST). Dexamethasone suppresses pituitary ACTH secretion through a negative-feedback mechanism without cross-reactivity in the RIA of cortisol. In healthy patients, full suppression of ACTH and cortisol production can be attained, whereas autonomous cortisol production cannot be inhibited. Two different tests are widely used: the 2-day test introduced by Liddle in 1960 and the overnight test introduced by Nugent in 1965. In the 2-day test (administration of 0.5 mg dexamethasone every 6 hours), a UFC value greater than 10 μg/24 h or a serum cortisol concentration higher than 50 nmol/L confirms the

Table 2 Clinical Manifestations of Hypercortisolism

Sign/symptom	Frequency (%)	
	Study 1[a]	Study 2[b]
Truncal obesity	96	95
Facial fullness ("moon facies")	n.a.	90
Hypertension	68	85
Facial plethora	82	80
Impaired glucose tolerance/ diabetes mellitus	80	80
Menstrual irregularities/gonadal dysfunctions	74	80
Hirsutism	72	70
Striae	n.a.	70
Muscle weakness	64	65
Osteoporosis	38	55
Bruising	62	55
Impaired wound healing	n.a.	55
Psychiatric disturbances/mood disorders	68	50
Headache	n.a.	40
Edema	18	40
Hypocalemic alkalosis	n.a.	40
Fractures	n.a.	35
Polydipsia	10	30
Fungal infections	6	n.a.

[a] From Ref. 13.
[b] From Ref. 39.

diagnosis of Cushing's syndrome with a sensitivity of 97–100% (5,13,14). In the overnight LDDST (administration of 1 mg dexamethasone at 11 p.m. or at midnight), a plasma cortisol level obtained at 8 am on the following day that is lower than 5 μg% or 138 nmol/L effectively rules out Cushing's syndrome (15). A lower cut-off value of serum cortisol less than 50 nmol/L reflects negative result and enhances the sensitivity up to 98% (16). Both tests have a specificity of 87.5–100% (13,17). The absorption and metabolism of dexamethasone, however, is influenced by various factors (18). Interactions with drugs accelerating the metabolism (e.g., phenytoin, rifampin) can induce increased hepatic clearance of dexamethasone and lead to a higher rate of false-positive results. Therefore, parallel measurements of cortisol and dexamethasone plasma levels should be taken into consideration to ensure adequate plasma concentrations (19). In conclusion, LDDST is a good screening test for Cushing's syndrome, and negative results of the UFC assays and use of low cut-off value for serum cortisol definitively exclude the diagnosis of Cushing's syndrome (5,20).

1.3.3 Differentiation Between ACTH-Dependent and ACTH-Independent Cushing's Syndrome

After establishing the diagnosis of Cushing's syndrome, studies should be performed to distinguish between ACTH-dependent and ACTH-independent forms of Cushing's syndrome. As shown in Table 1, the great majority of cases are ACTH-dependent, i.e., the cause is hypersecretion of pituitary or ectopic ACTH. In up to 25% of patients, the cause is primary adrenal and therefore ACTH-independent.

1.3.4 ACTH Assay

The most effective method of distinguishing between ACTH-independent and ACTH-dependent forms of Cushing's syndrome is a plasma ACTH assay (21, 22). Whereas in ACTH-independent cases the plasma ACTH levels are suppressed, the values for ACTH-dependent cases are normal or elevated. The best time to determine the plasma ACTH concentration is between midnight and 2 a.m., the period of physiologically lowest concentrations of cortisol and ACTH (23). Undetectable ACTH or levels < 5 pg/mL (normal basal ACTH levels 10–100 pg/mL) and a plasma cortisol > 15 μg/dL are typical for ACTH-independent Cushing's syndrome caused by primary adrenocortical source. This assay should be performed two or three times because of pulsatile ACTH and cortisol secretion in patients with Cushing's syndrome. Values of plasma ACTH > 35 pg/mL are strong indicators of an ACTH-dependent Cushing's syndrome. The higher the value, the more likely is an ectopic source of ACTH, mostly from small-cell lung cancer (7). Whereas the diagnosis of ACTH-independent Cushing's syndrome should lead to imaging of the adrenal glands, the differentiation among the various causes of ACTH-dependent Cushing's syndrome needs further diagnostic evaluation (Fig. 1).

1.3.5 High-Dose Dexamethasone Suppression Test

Whereas corticotroph cells in Cushing's disease retain partial responsiveness to negative feedback regulation, ectopic ACTH-secreting tumors generally resist feedback inhibition (5). The high-dose dexamethasone suppression test (HDDST) is most effective in distinguishing between Cushing's disease and ectopic ACTH syndrome. Nonsuppression or markedly elevated levels of ACTH reflect an ectopic source, whereas suppression of plasma ACTH and UFC indicates a pituitary adenoma. The standard procedure for the HDDST is a 2-day test with oral administration of 2 mg dexametha-

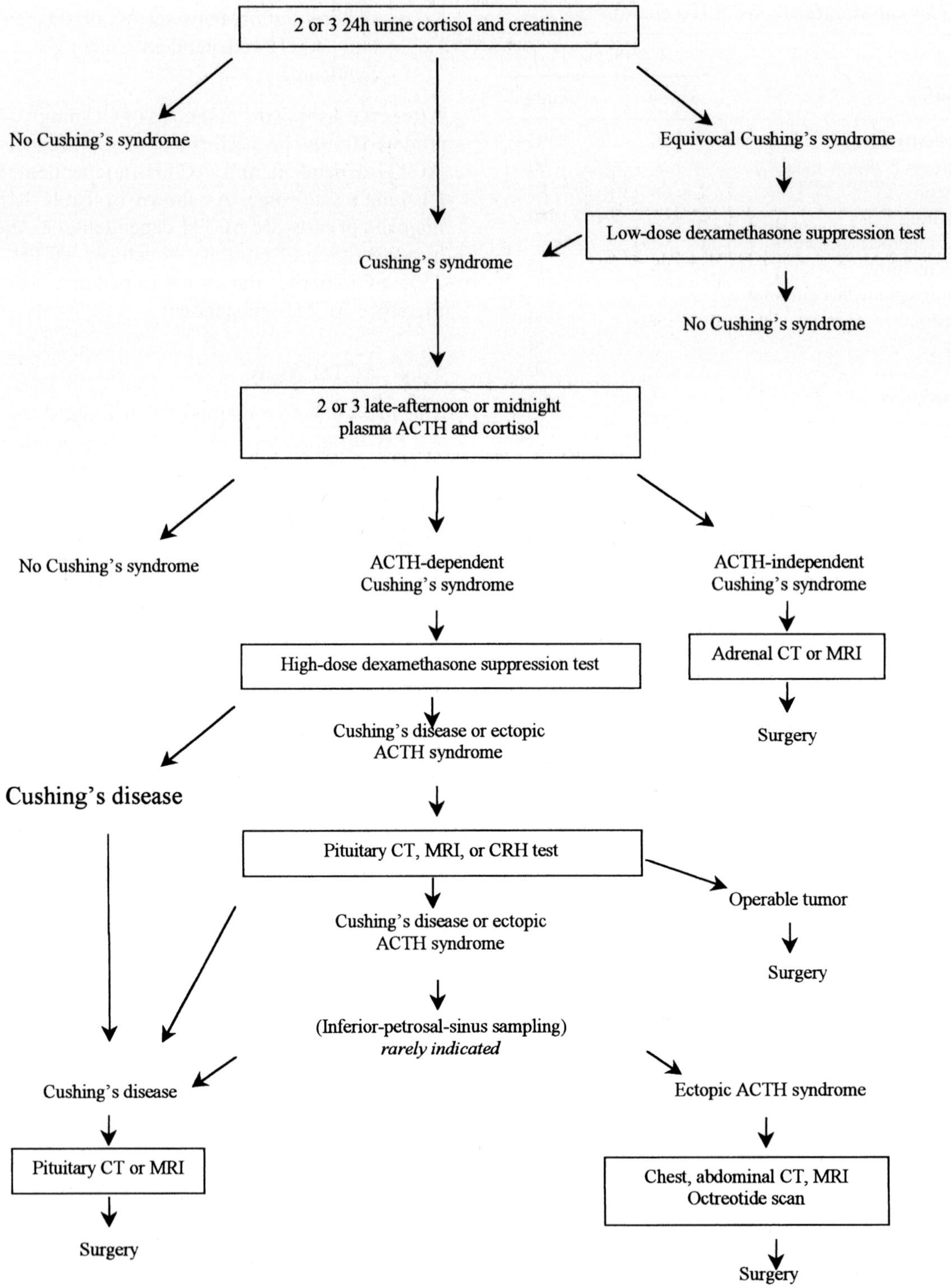

Figure 1 Flow chart diagnosis of Cushing's syndrome.

sone every 6 hours and determination of the 24-hour excretion of UFC on day 2 (14). Its efficacy has been tested repeatedly (24,25), and a suppression of more than 90% of the UFC on day 2 has a sensitivity of 69% and specificity of 100% in verifying hypercortisolism from an ACTH-secreting pituitary adenoma (26). Problems of the standard HDDST are similar to the pitfalls of the LDDST mentioned above, with inadequate dexamethasone levels caused by diminished absorption or increased clearance. Therefore, a modified test with intravenous administration of dexamethasone over a short period of time (1 mg/h for 7 h) has been recommended by some authors (27,28).

1.3.6 Corticotropin-Releasing Hormone Stimulation Test

Corticotropin-releasing hormone (CRH) induces an exaggerated ACTH and cortisol response in pituitary adenomas, but not in cases of ectopic ACTH secretion (29–31), because the former, but not the latter, express CRH receptors (32). Intravenous bolus of ovine CRH (1 μg/kg) is given and plasma ACTH and cortisol are measured before and 15, 30, 60, 90, and 120 minutes after CRH injection. An increase of plasma ACTH by at least 35% of the mean basal values 15 and 30 minutes after CRH injection has a sensitivity of up to 95% with a specificity of up to 100% (33). Meta-analysis of published series about the CRH stimulation test established criteria for a positive response to be an increase of more than 50% of plasma ACTH or greater than 20% of plasma cortisol. Using these criteria, sensitivities of 86% and 91% and specificities of 95% and 95% for ACTH and cortisol levels, respectively, were identified (34). Driven by the concerns of possible antigenic effects of the ovine CRH, the use of synthetic human CRH as the stimulatory agent has been analyzed (35,36). A comparison between ovine and human CRH revealed similar responses in patients with Cushing's disease, nevertheless ovine CRH caused a greater response (37,38). To date, no large studies using synthetic human CRH have been published. Some rare reports have shown a positive response in ectopic ACTH from CRH stimulation (39,40), but generally a combination of the CRH stimulation and HDDST will lead to correct differentiation between pituitary and ectopic ACTH hypersecretion.

1.3.7 Bilateral Inferior Petrosal Sinus Sampling

The simultaneous bilateral inferior petrosal sinus sampling (BIPSS) has been described as the most accurate and reliable method of distinguishing a pituitary from ectopic source of ACTH production (41,42). After placing catheters via the ipsilateral femoral vein into each inferior petrosal sinus, peripheral and petrosal sinus ACTH and cortisol are simultaneously measured before and after stimulation with CRH (1 μg/kg) at 3, 5, and 10 minutes (41,42). A >2 basal ratio of central: peripheral venous plasma ACTH and a threefold or higher ratio after CRH stimulation yields a sensitivity and specificity between 80 and 100% (21,43). In an overall analysis of 21 published studies, a basal ratio of >2 and a ratio of >3 after stimulation showed a sensitivity of 96% and 100%, respectively (5). Accurate BIPPS may also help to exactly localize the possible pituitary adenoma as there is limited mixing of intracavernous bloods from the two lobes of the pituitary gland. A gradient between the left and right greater than 1.4 may predict lateralization with an accuracy up to 80% (18,44,45). An analysis of 19 published reports showed an overall accuracy of 78% (range 50–100%) (5). A single study has shown that BIPPS might even have a higher diagnostic accuracy for the localization in patients with Cushing's disease than imaging using magnetic resonance imaging (MRI) (46). Furthermore, in at least 40–50% of cases of Cushing's disease, no abnormalities are detected by imaging (5). Although this invasive procedure results in low morbidity in the hands of experienced teams, it is not indicated as a routine procedure (7,3,47). Complications range from inguinal hematoma to serious neurological morbidities (48,49). Indications for BIPPS are patients with clinical Cushing's disease but negative or equivocal pituitary MRI, or patients with positive pituitary MRI but equivocal stimulation and suppression tests (3).

Typical results leading to the diagnosis of Cushing's disease are clinical symptoms of hypercortisolism with no suppression of cortisol and ACTH in the LDDST, but suppression in the HDDST with exaggerated cortisol and ACTH response with CRH stimulation test (Fig. 1).

1.4 Localization by Imaging

1.4.1 Pituitary Gland

In patients diagnosed with ACTH-dependent Cushing's syndrome, imaging should be used to identify and localize a microadenoma in the pituitary gland. Either computed tomography (CT) or MRI can be useful (2). The CT scan in patients with Cushing's disease caused by a pituitary microadenoma usually shows a hypodense lesion with no enhancement after contrast administration (50). The sensitivity and specificity for the detection of microadenomas is only 47% and 74%, respectively (34). The introduction of the gadolinium-enhanced MRI of the sella turcica established only a modest improvement with a sensitivity of 50–60% (51,52). In the majority of cases a positive MRI shows a hypodense signal, which usually fails to enhance after administration of gadolinium. In up to 5% of cases the microadenomas show an uptake of gadolinium, therefore imaging of the precontrast phase is essential to increase the sensitivity (53). Unfortunately, incidental tumors of the pituitary gland without clinical or biochemical signs of hypercortisolism are identified by MR in up to 10% of the population and are seen in 27% of autopsies. Thus, a positive scan does not absolutely con-firm the diagnosis (51,54). Furthermore, the localization of microadenomas on CT or MRI correlates with as little as 52% of intraoperative surgical findings (55,56). Therefore, all imaging results should always be correlated with clinical symptoms and biochemical tests (7).

1.4.2 Adrenal Glands

Imaging is especially important in patients with ACTH-independent Cushing's syndrome caused by an adrenal adenoma or adenocarcinoma. Both thin-slice CT (Fig. 2) and MRI of the adrenal glands have a sensitivity greater than 95%. The distinction between adenoma and adenocarcinoma has been shown to have an accuracy of up to 100% (57,58). MRI appears to be especially useful for differentiating between benign and malignant disease.

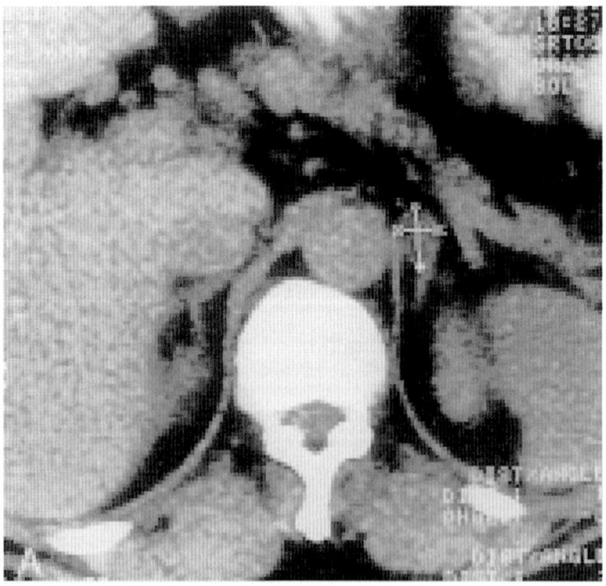

Figure 2 CT scan of the adrenals demonstrating a 1.5 cm nodule in the left adrenal gland and a normal right adrenal gland.

1.4.3 Ectopic Sources of Cushing's Syndrome

If clinical signs and biochemical tests reveal an ACTH-dependent hypercortisolism with negative results in the dexamethasone suppression tests, the search for a possible source of ectopic ACTH production should be performed using CT or MRI of the chest. A bronchial carcinoid or small-cell carcinoma of the lung is the most likely etiology (59–61). In cases of negative results following imaging of the chest, an abdominal CT or MRI may reveal rare sources of ectopic ACTH production, such as pancreatic islet tumors or intestinal carcinoid (62).

1.5 Surgical Treatment of Cushing's Syndromes

Depending on the cause of the hypercortisolism, the primary treatment of choice for the various types of Cushing's syndrome should be a surgical approach to the pituitary gland, the adrenal glands, or possible ectopic sources. Surgery is successful in more than 80% of cases.

1.5.1 Transsphenoidal Adenomectomy

In patients with Cushing's disease caused by a circumscribed microadenoma, surgery using trans-sphenoidal selective adenomectomy is the first-line treatment of choice (3). Otherwise, the neurosurgeon should resect 85–90% of the anterior pituitary gland (7). Total remission rates after transsphenoidal surgery are up to 80–90% in expert centers (63–65), but a recent large multicenter trial reported a remission rate of 69% (21). The main criterion of cure after transsphenoidal surgery for patients with Cushing's disease is an undetectable postoperative plasma cortisol level (66). Until recovery of normal hypothalamic-pituitary-adrenal function, patients require replacement therapy with oral hydrocortisone, 20–30 mg/day, for as long as 4–12 months after surgery (7). A relapse after initial surgery is defined as the recurrence of clinical and biochemical signs of Cushing's syndrome more than 6 months after surgery. The success rate for a reoperation is less than that of the initial surgical therapy, ranging between 22 and 64% (67,68). Therefore, only patients with clear signs of pituitary tumor on imaging should be considered for reoperation. More commonly the procedure of choice as second-line treatment for recurrent Cushing's disease after transsphenoidal surgery is irradiation, with a remission rate of 83% (69). Used as first-line treatment for patients with high surgical risk, irradiation will lead to remission in about 45–55% of adult patients (64). Because of the high remission rate of 85% in children, irradiation should be considered as the first-line treatment in children with Cushing's disease (7,70).

1.5.2 Laparoscopic Adrenalectomy

A bilateral adrenalectomy is a reasonable treatment for patients without cure after transsphenoidal surgery and irradiation of the pituitary (3). It is the procedure of choice delivering a definitive cure for hypercortisolism but requires a life-long substitution of glucocorticoids and mineralocorticoids. Furthermore, 10–25% of patients following bilateral adrenalectomy will develop Nelson's syndrome with the symptom triad of high ACTH levels, a pituitary tumor, and dark pigmentation of the skin (64). The surgical technique for the bilateral adrenalectomy, as for all benign adrenal diseases in general, should be the laparoscopic approach. This is a safe procedure with shorter hospital stay and lower complication rates than the traditional open approach (71–73).

Cushing's syndrome, as a primary adrenal disease caused by micro- or macronodular adrenal hyperplasia, also requires a bilateral adrenalectomy. On the other hand, in cases of ACTH-independent Cushing's syndrome caused by an adrenal adenoma or carcinoma, unilateral adrenalectomy is the treatment of choice (7). After unilateral adrenalectomy, replacement therapy of glucocorticoids should be administered until recovery of the hypothalamic-pituitary-adrenal axis (74).

1.5.3 Surgery for Ectopic ACTH Syndromes

As described above, the sources of ectopic ACTH syndromes are most likely bronchial carcinoids or small-cell lung carcinomas, which require a lung lobectomy for cure (75). If the tumors are non-resectable (metastatic, occult), control of hypercortisolism by bilateral adrenalectomy or treatment with enzyme inhibitors should be performed.

1.6 Medical Treatment of Cushing's Syndromes

Although a variety of different medical approaches have been established, the pharmacological therapy of patients with Cushing's syndrome should be considered as an alternative approach to addressing the underlying pathology. Possible targets for a medical approach are the hypothalamic-pituitary axis, corticoid production by the adrenal glands, or ACTH receptors directly.

1.6.1 Hypothalamic-Pituitary Axis

Drugs such as bromocriptine, cyproheptadine, ritanserine, ketanserine, and valproic acid have been shown to work only occasionally and are not definitively effective in the treatment of hypercortisolism (76–80). A trial of treatment with these drugs should cover at least 2 weeks with frequent measurements of ACTH and urinary free cortisol (UFC) to check for possible response to a specific drug or combination therapy (3,81).

1.6.2 Adrenal Glands

Various inhibitors of the steroid biosynthesis in the adrenal glands are already in clinical use. Examples are metapyrone, mitotane, and ketoconazole. These medications unfortunately interfere with a variety of reactions controlled by cytochrome P450. Therefore, extraadrenal effects are likely to occur (81). Metapyrone has been used for all kinds of Cushing's syndrome and as a result of androgen excess has side effects such as hirsutism and acne (82). The most widely used enzyme inhibitor is mitotane, which seems to have multifactorial effects on the regulation of the plasma cortisol level. Beside the direct inhibition of steroid synthesis, mitotane plays a role in the regulation of peripheral corticoid metabolism (3,83). Ketoconazole can be administered in lower doses than the other biosynthesis inhibitors (84,85). Treatment with 600–800 mg/d may keep the UFC values within upper normal levels, but in some cases results in hepatotoxicity (86). Ketoconazole treatment results in normalization of UFC in 43% of patients and a reduction of UFC in an additional 42% of patients, as reported in a recent multicenter study (21).

1.6.3 ACTH Receptor Level

The first clinical available antagonist with affinity to ACTH receptors in the adrenal glands is mifepristone. So far, the experience with this drug for the treatment of hypercortisolism is limited to a small number of patients, and the results have been mixed (87–89).

In summary, established medical therapy for the treatment of hypercortisolism is useful only as an adjunctive therapy in patients with mild disease or after surgery or pituitary irradiation. It may also be important for palliative treatment of hypercortisolism in malignant ectopic ACTH syndromes or adrenocarcinomas (7).

2 CORTICAL CARCINOMA

Adrenocortical carcinoma is a rare disease with a reported incidence in the United States of up to 2.0 cases per million persons per year and accounts for 0.2% of cancer deaths in the United States annually (90–94). Most published series demonstrate a bimodal distribution in the incidence of adrenal carcinoma peaking in the first and fourth decades (95,96). The bimodal age distribution is significant since several studies have found that children with localized adrenocortical carcinoma have a better prognosis after surgery compared to adults (97,98). The occurrence of adrenocortical cancer in adults seems to be associated with a more aggressive phenotype and poorer prognosis (99–101). Some studies demonstrate an equal gender distribution (102,103), while others show a predominance in female (95, 104,105) or male patients (106). Female patients, however, are more likely to harbor a hormonally active tumor with symptoms of hypercortisolism or hyperandrogenism. Very few data are available on the ethnic distribution of patients with adrenocortical carcinoma. Some studies suggest a predominance of Caucasians over patients with African and Asian ancestry (95, 107,108).

The etiology of adrenocortical carcinoma is unknown. Some believe that, like colon cancer, adrenocortical carcinoma develops from hyperplastic nodules in the adrenal gland, which form adenomas that later transform to a malignant phenotype. In support of this, some patients have abnormal adrenal steroid production preceding the development of adrenocortical carcinoma by over 10 years (109,110). Cytogenetic analysis suggests that loss of heterozygosity on chromosomes 11p, 13q, or 17p may be important in the pathogenesis (111,112). Several more recent studies have implicated p53 tumor suppressor gene in the pathogenesis of sporadic adrenocortical carcinoma (113–115).

2.1 Clinical Features

Patients' symptoms are first determined by the functional status of the tumor. Adrenocortical carcinomas are considered functional when they secrete significant amounts of hormones leading to clinical symptoms. Secretion of corticosteroids leads to Cushing's syndrome, secretion of sex hormones to virilization or feminization syndromes, and secretion of both hormones is associated with a mixed Cushing-virilizing/feminization syndrome. Isolated secretion of mineralocorticoids is rarely seen in patients with adrenocortical carcinoma (95,116,117). Tumors are considered nonfunctional when they do not produce significant quantities of hormones leading to clinical consequences. Tumors secreting large amounts of hormones (e.g., large quantities of estrogens in woman) that do not lead to clinical symptoms should be considered nonfunctional. Additionally, nonfunctional tumors can be transformed into functional adrenal tumors with significant clinical symptomatology.

Memorial Sloan-Kettering has reported that 60% of patients presented with clinically evident functional tumors and 40% presented with clinically nonfunctional tumors (118). Based on large epidemiological studies, most nonfunctional tumors arise in adult males, whereas functional tumors are more common in the younger population (< 30 years) and found more often in women (95,96).

Nonfunctional adrenocortical carcinomas are quite rare in children (97,98). Children who present with functional adrenocortical carcinomas most commonly have symptoms of virilization, and this is followed by a mixed Cushing-virilization phenotype (95). Isolated hypersecretion of corticosteroids leading to Cushing's syndromes is very rare in children (119).

In adults with functional adrenocortical carcinomas, the most common presentation is the mixed Cushing-virilization syndrome, followed by isolated virilization (99,102,105). Wajchenberg et al. found that 63% of the patients with mixed hormonal syndromes and 100% of the patients with Cushing's syndrome were adults, whereas 76% of the patients with virilization syndrome were children (95). Hypertension is a common symptom in patients with functional adrenal tumors. This may be related to the direct hormonal effect of glucocorticoids and/or mineralocorticoids or to the local tumor effect compressing the renal vasculature with subsequent activation of the renin-angiotensin system (103,107). An infrequent symptom for some patients may be fasting or postabsorptive hypoglycemia, resulting from production of insulin-like growth factor (120,121).

Other clinical manifestations of adrenocortical carcinoma include abdominal pain with palpable abdominal mass, weight loss, weakness, anorexia, nausea, emesis, and myalgias (102,105,108,122–125). Rare manifestations include hematuria (124,126), Budd-Chiari syndrome (127), urinary obstruction, and paraplegia (104). In the series of Kendrick et al., 48% of all patients with adrenocortical carcinoma presented with abdominal pain and 47% with various manifestations of endocrine syndromes (128).

2.2 Staging and Prognosis

According to MacFarlane (131) and Sullivan et al. (132), stage I and II adrenocortical carcinoma is con-

Table 3 Staging of Adrenocortical Carcinoma

Stage	TNM staging criteria
TNM	
T1	Tumor ≤ 5 cm, no invasion
T2	Tumor > 5 cm, no invasion
T3	Tumor any size, locally invading to, but not involving adjacent organs
T4	Tumor any size, locally invading adjacent organs
N0	No regional positive nodes
N1	Positive regional nodes
M0	No distant metastatic disease
M1	Distant metastatic disease
Tumor	
I	T1 N0 M0
II	T2 N0 M0
III	T1 N1 M0, T2 N1 M0, T3 N0 M0
IV	Tx Nx M1, T3 N1 T4

fined to the adrenal gland without local invasion or distant metastases and with a greatest tumor diameter of <5 cm (stage I) or >5 cm (stage II) (Table 3). Surgical excision is considered to be the treatment of choice in these patients. Complete resection of the adrenocortical carcinoma is associated with an improved outcome (138). Stage III adrenocortical carcinoma is defined by the presence of local tumor invasion that does not involve adjacent organs or regional lymph nodes. Distant metastases or local invasion into adjacent organs plus regional lymph nodes is considered stage IV (Table 3). In pooled data from multiple institutions, 2% of patients present as stage I, 19% as stage II, 18% as stage III, and 61% as stage IV (Table 4) (133). In most patients primary diagnosis is made at an advanced tumor stage of the disease (101–103,120,122,123,139). In a review by Wooten and King (96), 49% of all patients were diagnosed with stage IV disease. The overall 5-year survival in patients with adrenocortical carcinoma ranged from 16 to 35% in large series (Table 4) (115,134).

Although some authors suggested a better prognosis in patients with functional adrenocortical carcinoma (123,142), most studies have found no relation of prognosis to functional status (105,107,108,122,139). Wajchenberg et al. found in their series that patients with functional tumors presenting with virilization syndrome had a better prognosis (81% of whom were children) than patients presenting with a mixed Cushing-virilization phenotype (63% of whom were adults) (95). The occurrence of adrenocortical carcinomas is sometimes associated with secondary tumors, which apparently has an influence on the natural course of the disease. In a series published by Venkatesh et al. the most frequent secondary tumors arise within the breast, thyroid, and skin (melanoma) (102). The occurrence of adrenocortical carcinomas in families with histories of malignant tumors has also been described (130).

2.3 Diagnosis of Cortical Carcinoma

Ultrasonography, CT, and MRI are the main imaging techniques employed in the diagnosis and classification of adrenal tumors, although some scintigraphy may be used in specific cases. Each of the main diagnostic modalities will be discussed separately.

2.3.1 Ultrasonography

Ultrasonography is in most cases the initial diagnostic modality and has been shown to be effective in identification of adrenal tumors as small as 1.3 cm (135). However, this technique is very operator-dependent, and reliable diagnosis requires great experience. Adrenal tumors usually appear as smooth, rounded, solid masses, which replace the usual triangular shaped adrenal gland. In addition to detecting the adrenal tumor, ultrasonography is also able to show effects of local tumor growth, e.g., displacement of adjacent organs. Unfortunately, ultrasonography cannot reliably differentiate benign from malignant tumors. However, in some cases local infiltration into the inferior vena

Table 4 Survival Rates of Patients with Adrenocortical Carcinoma

			5-year survival (%)		
Authors (ref.)	Year	Patients (n)	Overall	Complete resection	Incomplete resection
Soreide et al. (106)	1991	99	16	62	0
Icard et al. (100)	1992	156	34	42	0
Zografos et al. (103)	1994	53	19	38	0
Haak et al. (171)	1995	96	27	49	9
Crucitti et al. (176)	1996	129	35	48	7

cava as a sign of malignancy can be identified by ultrasonography.

2.3.2 Computed Tomography

Computed tomography is generally considered to be the gold standard in the radiodiagnostic evaluation of adrenal tumors. Using conventional CT, tumors of 1 cm can be reliably identified. Smaller tumors of 0.5 cm can be detected with more advanced CT scanning techniques (136–138). However, using conventional CT it is difficult to differentiate between benign and malignant adrenal tumors. This has become a major issue with the more widespread use of CT and the detection of more adrenal incidentalomas. Radiological series show the prevalence of incidentalomas of the adrenal gland to be in the range of 1–2% (149). In the evaluation of an incidentaloma, the possibility of metastatic disease must be considered and excluded. Some authors suggest that lesions <3 cm in diameter are probably benign, whereas masses >5 cm are most likely to be malignant (140,141). However, the differentiation between benign and malignant lesions can not be based on tumor size alone, because tumor size is a function of duration. Therefore, other radiological features, such as tumor tissue heterogeneity and contrast enhancement, have been considered to be more reliable parameters for the differentiation between benign and malignant adrenal masses (Fig. 3) (136–138). Malignant tumors appear to be larger in diameter, present with blurred margins and irregular shape, and are more often found to have an inhomogeneous contrast enhancement, whereas benign masses tend to be smaller, have sharp borders, and exhibit a more homogeneous contrast enhancement (95,136,137,142,143).

2.3.3 Magnetic Resonance Imaging

MRI improves adrenal imaging through the specific tissue characteristics of adrenal tissue on T1- and T2-weighted images (144) (Fig. 4). Adrenal tissue appears darker than surrounding adipose tissue on both T1 and T2 images. Although MRI offers information to help tissue-specific diagnosis among adrenal lesions, it is also limited in differenting benign from malignant masses. However, MRI is sometimes able to discriminate between the different types of adrenal tumors on the basis of T1- and T2-weighted signal intensities (145,146). Adrenocortical carcinomas characteristically have signal intensities that are isointense with the liver on T1-weighted images and hyperintense on T2-weighted images. The accuracy in detecting malignant tumors is improved by using intravenous gadolinium with gradient echo magnetic resonance imaging. Using this technique, adenomas show mild enhancement of the paramagnetic contrast medium with a quick washout, whereas malignant tumors have a stronger enhancement and slower washout (147–153).

2.3.4 Adrenal Cortical Scintigraphy

Whereas CT and MRI are effective in identifying adrenal masses, adrenal cortical scintigraphy using radiocholesterol can complement the biochemical and radiologic imaging data to identify abnormal adrenal function in adenomas and can suggest the presence of adrenal carcinoma or delineate the functional status of adrenal masses identified with CT or MRI (154,155).

2.3.5 Imaging of Local Invasion and Distant Metastasis

The invasion of the inferior vena cava by adrenocortical carcinoma is not uncommon. Precise and detailed

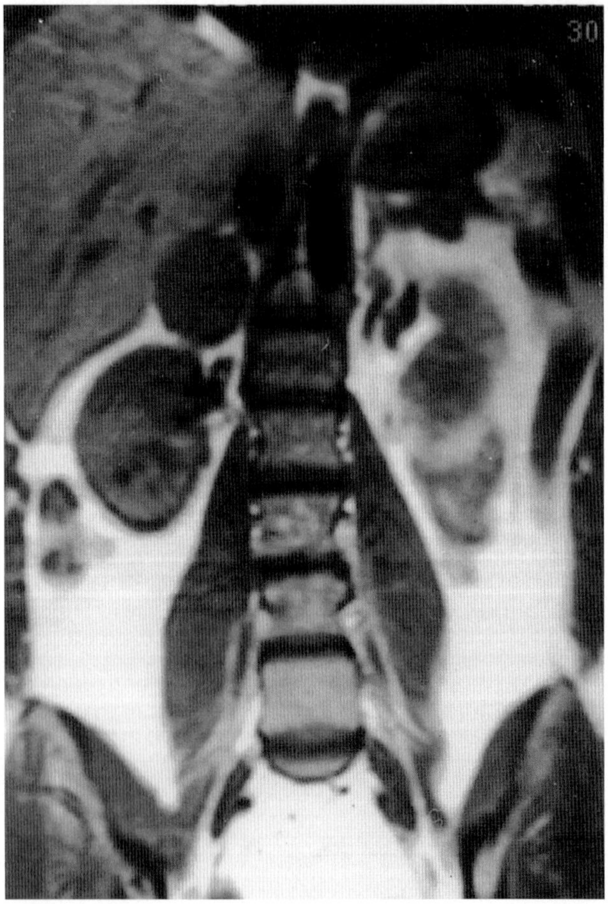

Figure 3 A CT scan of the abdomen demonstrates a large left-sided adrenal tumor which is heterogeneous and calcified, suggesting an adrenal carcinoma.

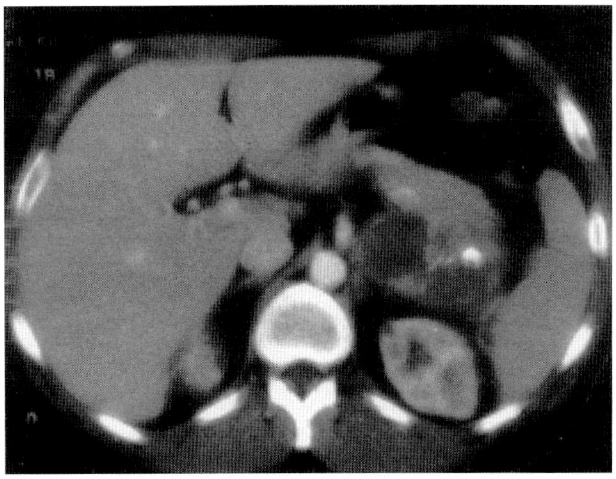

Figure 4 An axial MRI demonstrates a right adrenal lesion just above the right kidney.

information about the involvement and extent of inferior vena caval infiltration is essential for planning surgery. Adrenocortical carcinomas that involve the inferior vena cava tend to arise from the right side (83%) and tend to be large (156). Large lesions on the left commonly involve the left renal vein. Ultrasonography reliably demonstrates vena caval extension, and the cranial extension of the tumor thrombus is usually seen well (157). CT and, moreso, MRI have been proven very helpful in identifying inferior vena caval involvement, especially in patients who are difficult to examine with ultrasonography (158). In the series of Wajchenberg et al. (95) MRI was superior to CT and ultrasonography in identifying inferior vena caval involvement.

Adrenocortical carcinoma preferentially metastasizes to the liver (85%), followed by lung (60%), bone (10%), and lymph nodes (10%) (95). The presence of liver metastases can be best evaluated by CT, in which metastatic lesions appear as usually homogeneous, rounded, and hypodense masses with variable sizes (95). CT is usually considered the imaging technique of choice for identifying lung metastases.

2.4 Pathology of Cortical Carcinoma

Except for patients with distant metastasis and local invasion in whom malignancy is obvious, it may be difficult histologically to differentiate between benign and malignant tumors. Early proposed criteria for malignancy included capsular and vascular invasion, mitotic activity, necrosis, hemorrhage, calcification, and nuclear polymorphism (159,160). Weiss et al. (161) proposed nine histological criteria associated with adrenocortical carcinoma: (1) high nuclear grade, (2) mitotic rate >5 per 50 high-power fields, (3) atypical mitotic figures, (4) eosinophilic tumor cell cytoplasm (>75% of tumor cells), (5) diffuse architecture present in ≥33% of the tumor, (6) necrosis, (7) invasion of venous structures, (8) invasion of sinusoidal structures, and (9) capsular invasion. Adrenal tumors with three or more of the above criteria were considered to be malignant (162). In the Memorial Sloan-Kettering experience the mean size of the carcinomas at presentation was 16 cm (range 6–40 cm) and the mean weight was 1190 g (range 320–2600 g) (163). In a series from France with 156 cases, the mean size of the carcinomas at presentation was 12 cm (range 3–30 cm) and the mean weight was 714 g (range 12–4750 g) (164).

More recently, immunohistochemical markers have been evaluated for identification of adrenocortical carcinomas. Wajchenberg et al. (95) found that the most common immunoprofile for an adrenocortical carcinoma was positive staining for vimentin. The proportions of the other markers tested including cytokeratin 8/18, the monoclonal antibody D11 that has been reported to be specific for adrenocortical tissue, and p53 was not striking. Other laboratories similarly failed to find a specific immunohistochemical marker for adrenocortical carcinoma (165–169). Cell DNA content and cell proliferation measurements, including determination of DNA ploidy, S-phase fraction, mitotic counting, AgNOR counting, and immunohistochemical detection of nuclear proteins, are interesting research topics but are still controversial in assessing adrenal neoplasms (170–172).

2.5 Treatment of Cortical Carcinoma

Determination of optimal treatment of patients with adrenocortical carcinoma is difficult given the low incidence of the disease. Large randomized prospective studies are lacking. The mainstay of treatment in less advanced stages of adrenocortical carcinoma remains surgical resection. Surgery has been shown to improve survival. In order to improve outcome many different chemotherapeutic agents have been tested, of which o,p'-DDD (mitotane) is the most commonly used. However, whether mitotane significantly improves survival has yet to be determined. In an attempt to overcome the lack of prospective data, the American College of Surgeons Oncology Group is currently in the process of preparing an international, prospective, randomized trial evaluating the role of adjuvant mitotane in adrenocortical carcinoma. Patients with stage I and II disease will be randomized to receive adjuvant mitotane or placebo. Patients with stage III or IV disease will be randomized to receive either mitotane or standard chemotherapy (cisplatin/etoposide).

2.5.1 Surgery

Complete surgical excision is the treatment of choice in patients with stage I and II tumors and in children. In case of a tumor thrombus in the inferior vena cava, an aggressive surgical approach should be used to extract the tumor thrombus (173). In patients who have biochemically active tumors that secrete corticosteroids and who have suppressed the contralateral gland, careful attention must be given to corticosteroid replacement. In patients with stage III and IV, the indication for surgical therapy is more controversial. Some studies suggest a maximal tumor debulking when complete excision is not possible (174,175). Other series clearly demonstrated that palliative surgery has no influence on patients survival (135,136,139). The 5-year survival rate of patients with adrenocortical carcinomas who undergo surgical excision is 15–30%. In one study, the median survival of patients with complete resection was 50.6 months compared to 7.6 months in patients with incomplete resection (128). In other series complete resection of all disease yielded a 5-year survival of 38–62%. Incomplete resection offered a 5-year survival of 0–9% (118,134,164,176–178) (Table 4). Recurrence often occurred even in patients in whom resection was considered complete. Kendrick et al. saw a 73% recurrence rate with a median time to recurrence of 17 months (138). Patients who underwent resection of recurrent disease had an improved survival over patients who did not, with a median survival of 29 months vs. 11 months, respectively (138). Similar findings were reported by Schulick and Brennan (179). However, whether surgical re-resection of recurrent disease should be offered to any patient with recurrent adrenocortical carcinoma is still not certain. When metastatic disease was present at diagnosis, patients generally did not survive more than 1 year (103,105, 122,123,175). In most patients in whom surgical resection is indicated, an ipsilateral adrenalectomy is performed. Depending on the local tumor growth, adrenalectomy is performed together with nephrectomy and/or splenectomy. Wajchenberg et al. (95) operated on 46 patients with adrenocortical carcinoma and performed an ipsilateral adrenalectomy alone in 50%, an adrenalectomy and nephrectomy in 39%, and an adrenalectomy, nephrectomy, and splenectomy in the remaining patients.

Many centers prefer open surgery with either a subcostal, thoracoabdominal, or abdominal midline incision depending on the size and extent of the adrenal mass as defined by radiological imaging. In a review of Schulick et al. (179), the authors preferred a bilateral subcostal incision for adrenocortical carcinoma less than 10 cm in size, allowing adequate access to the liver, omentum, peritoneum, and periaortic nodes (common sites of metastasis). For larger lesions (>10 cm) a thoracoabdominal approach was recommended for better access. With the rise of laparoscopic adrenalectomy for benign disorders, the question has a risen whether laparoscopic resection of malignant adrenal tumors is appropriate (180). When CT or MRI demonstrates a small adrenal tumor with no invasion or infiltration of adjacent structures suggesting malignancy, the laparoscopic approach seems to be justified (181).

2.5.2 Medical Therapy

Of the pharmacological agents known to suppress adrenal function, mitotane has gained widespread use in the past for the nonoperative treatment with advanced adrenocortical carcinoma. Mitotane inhibits corticoid biosynthesis and causes mitochondrial and cell death (182,183). In doses less than 3 g per day, mitotane primarily suppresses adrenal corticoid secretion, whereas doses exceeding 3 g per day have been shown to have an adrenocidal effect. Mitotane has been proven effective in patients with metastatic or unresectable adrenocortical carcinoma (102,105,122,139,175). Although mitotane has been shown to lead to tumor regression, a beneficial effect of patients' survival is questionable (128,184,185). Generally mitotane treatment is associated with frequent side effects, e.g., nausea, vomiting, anorexia, diarrhea, lethargy, somnolence, skin rash, and dose-dependent hepatotoxicity. These frequent, often intolerable, side effects of mitotane which lead to noncompliance in patients are the reasons why adequate large prospective studies are missing. More recently, evaluation of a "low-dose" mitotane has surfaced with greater patient compliance (186,187). In large series including adults and children with adrenocortical carcinoma, the response to mitotane was not influenced by the age of the patient (184,188,189). Because survival appears to depend on the size of the primary lesion and the extent of local and distant tumor growth, it has been suggested that mitotane should be administered as an early adjuvant therapy after surgical resection of the primary tumor. Some studies employing this approach demonstrated encouraging results (188–190), while others failed to prove any beneficial effect (101,191).

2.5.3 Chemotherapy

In patients in whom surgery is not an option and mitotane treatment can no longer be administered, other chemotherapeutic agents have been suggested. Among the various agents, cisplatin, cyclophosphamide, doxorubicin, and 5-fluorouracil or different combinations have lead to partial responses or disease stabilization (96,120,192). Suramin, which decreases cortisol secretion and inhibits serum-induced proliferation of cultured adrenocortical cells, has been tested in patients with advanced adrenocortical carcinomas and led to partial, however transient, tumor responses (193, 194). Patients treated with suramin suffered from serious side effects, including coagulopathy, thrombocytopenia, polyneuropathy, and allergic skin reactions (193). Another promising chemotherapeutic agent for patients with metastatic adrenocortical carcinoma is gossypol, a biphenolic derivative extracted from cottonweeds. Some patients who were resistant to other chemotherapeutic regimens have been treated with gossypol with very few side effects and had partial responses that lasted several months (195).

2.5.4 Radiotherapy

Anecdotal studies have reported occasional control of nonresectable adrenocortical carcinomas with external radiotherapy. However, the majority of studies indicate that external radiotherapy is ineffective in the treatment of patients with adrenocortical carcinoma and should be considered only as a palliative measure in patients with severe pain from bone metastases (95, 123,129,190).

3 ESTROGEN- AND ANDROGEN-SECRETING TUMORS

3.1 Androgen-Secreting Tumors

Androgen-producing tumors of the adrenal gland cause the symptomatolgy of sex steroid excess. Prepubertal males present with isosexual precocious puberty leading to penile enlargement, hair development, and secondary sexual characteristics. The clinical manifestations in adult males are minimal and may include early hair loss and acne. For prepubertal females, virilization leads to the inappropriate manifestation of acne, hirsutism, and clitoromegaly. The adult female usually presents with arrest of menarche and virilization.

Diagnosis of an adrenal tumor in these patients includes the measurement of plasma DHEA, DHEAS, androstenedione, testosterone, and urinary 17-ketosteroids. Since patients can have a combined presentation of androgen excess and corticosteroid excess, they should be evaluated for Cushing's syndrome as outlined above. The adrenal androgens will not suppress with dexamethasone if an adrenal tumor is the etiology (196). In prepubertal patients it is important to rule out benign premature adrenarche. Differential diagnosis includes androgen-secreting tumors of the ovaries, polycystic ovarian disease, endocrine tumors of the testicle, and congenital adrenogenital syndrome. The adrenals may be imaged by ultrasound, CT, or MRI. These tumors are usually small, unilateral, and have no enhancement on T2-weighted MR images. Cortical carcinomas may also secrete virilizing hormones in combination with glucocorticoids and mineralocorticoid activity. These tumors are more likely to be larger than benign androgen-secreting tumors and enhance on T2 images.

As with all primary tumors of the adrenal gland, surgical excision is the mainstay of treatment for benign and malignant disease. For patients with malignant androgen-secreting tumors, the medical therapy as outlined above for cortical carcinoma is appropriate. For patients with metastatic disease, steroid synthesis inhibitors and androgen antagonists may help address symptoms.

3.2 Estrogen-Secreting Tumors

Estrogen-secreting tumors of the adrenal gland are often associated with carcinoma. In the female patient, menstrual irregularity is often the only clinical manifestation and in males a loss of libido, gynecomastia, and female distribution of the hair. As with androgen-secreting tumors of the adrenal gland, urinary 17-ketosteroids are often elevated and do not suppress with dexamethasone. In addition, estrone, 11-deoxycortisol, and androstenedione levels help to confirm the diagnosis. Imaging may include those studies listed above. To rule out an ovarian source of steroid excess, some physicians utilize a NP-59 nuclear medicine study to confirm the accumulation of this tracer by a functional tumor of the adrenal gland. Treatment is surgical excision of the tumor.

REFERENCES

1. Cushing H. The basophil adenomas of the pituitary body and their clinical manifestations (pituitary basophilism). Bull Johns Hopkins Hosp 1932; 50:137–195.
2. Perry LA, Grossman AB. The role of the laboratory in

the diagnosis of Cushing's syndrome. Ann Clin Biochem 1997; 34(pt 4):345–359.
3. Boscaro M, Barzon L, Fallo F, Sonino N. Cushing's syndrome. Lancet 2001; 357:783–791.
4. Etxabe J, Vazquez JA. Morbidity and mortality in Cushing's disease: an epidemiological approach. Clin Endocrinol (Oxf) 1994; 40:479–484.
5. Newell-Price J, Trainer P, Besser M, Grossman A. The diagnosis and differential diagnosis of Cushing's syndrome and pseudo-Cushing's states. Endocr Rev 1998; 19:647–672.
6. Becker M, Aron DC. Ectopic ACTH syndrome and CRH-mediated Cushing's syndrome. Endocrinol Metab Clin North Am 1994; 23:585–606.
7. Orth DN. Cushing's syndrome. N Engl J Med 1995; 332:791–803.
8. Nieman LK. Cushing's syndrome. In: de Groot LJ, Jameson JL, eds. Endocrinology. 4th ed. Philadelphia: WB Saunders, 2001:1691–1713.
9. Mengden T, Hubmann P, Muller J, Greminger P, Vetter W. Urinary free cortisol versus 17-hydroxycorticosteroids: a comparative study of their diagnostic value in Cushing's syndrome. Clin Investig 1992; 70: 545–548.
10. LK Nieman, GB Cutler Jr. The sensitivity of the urine free cortisol measurement as a screening test for Cushing's syndrome. 72nd Annual Meeting of The Endocrine Society, Atlanta, GA, 1990:822.
11. Carroll BJ, Curtis GC, Davies BM, Mendels J, Sugerman AA. Urinary free cortisol excretion in depression. Psychol Med 1976; 6:43–50.
12. Cizza G, Nieman LK, Doppman JL, Passaro MD, Czerwiec FS, Chrousos GP, Cutler GB Jr. Factitious Cushing syndrome. J Clin Endocrinol Metab 1996; 81: 3573–3577.
13. Kennedy L, Atkinson AB, Johnston H, Sheridan B, Hadden DR. Serum cortisol concentrations during low dose dexamethasone suppression test to screen for Cushing's syndrome. Br Med J 1984; 289:1188–1191.
14. Liddle GW. Tests of pituitary-adrenal suppressibility in the diagnosis of Cushing's syndrome. J Clin Endocrinol Metab, 1539–1560.
15. Nugent CA, Nichols T, Tyler FH. Diagnosis of Cushing's syndrome—single dose dexamethasone. Arch Intern Med 1965; 116:172–176.
16. Newell-Price J, Trainer P, Perry L, Wass J, Grossman A, Besser M. A single sleeping midnight cortisol has 100% sensitivity for the diagnosis of Cushing's syndrome. Clin Endocrinol (Oxf) 1995; 43:545–550.
17. Cronin C, Igoe D, Duffy MJ, Cunningham SK, McKenna TJ. The overnight dexamethasone test is a worthwhile screening procedure. Clin Endocrinol (Oxf) 1990; 33:27–33.
18. Boscaro M, Barzon L, Sonino N. The diagnosis of Cushing's syndrome: atypical presentations and laboratory shortcomings. Arch Intern Med 2000; 160: 3045–3053.
19. Meikle AW. Dexamethasone suppression tests: usefulness of simultaneous measurement of plasma cortisol and dexamethasone. Clin Endocrinol (Oxf) 1982; 16:401–408.
20. Wood PJ, Barth JH, Freedman DB, Perry L, Sheridan B. Evidence for the low dose dexamethasone suppression test to screen for Cushing's syndrome—recommendations for a protocol for biochemistry laboratories. Ann Clin Biochem 1997; 34(pt 3):222–229.
21. Invitti C, Giraldi FP, de Martin M, Cavagnini F. Diagnosis and management of Cushing's syndrome: results of an Italian multicentre study. Study Group of the Italian Society of Endocrinology on the Pathophysiology of the Hypothalamic-Pituitary-Adrenal Axis. J Clin Endocrinol Metab 1999; 84:440–448.
22. Meier CA, Biller BM. Clinical and biochemical evaluation of Cushing's syndrome. Endocrinol Metab Clin North Am 1997; 26:741–762.
23. Weitzman ED, Fukushima D, Nogeire C, Roffwarg H, Gallagher TF, Hellman L. Twenty-four hour pattern of the episodic secretion of cortisol in normal subjects. J Clin Endocrinol Metab 1971; 33:14–22.
24. Dichek HL, Nieman LK, Oldfield EH, Pass HI, Malley JD, Cutler GB Jr. A comparison of the standard high dose dexamethasone suppression test and the overnight 8-mg dexamethasone suppression test for the differential diagnosis of adrenocorticotropin-dependent Cushing's syndrome. J Clin Endocrinol Metab 1994; 78:418–422.
25. Nieman LK, Chrousos GP, Oldfield EH, Avgerinos PC, Cutler GB Jr, Loriaux DL. The ovine corticotropin-releasing hormone stimulation test and the dexamethasone suppression test in the differential diagnosis of Cushing's syndrome. Ann Intern Med 1986; 105:862–867.
26. Flack MR, Oldfield EH, Cutler GB Jr, Zweig MH, Malley JD, Chrousos GP, Loriaux DL, Nieman LK. Urine free cortisol in the high-dose dexamethasone suppression test for the differential diagnosis of the Cushing syndrome. Ann Intern Med 1992; 116:211–217.
27. Biemond P, de Jong FH, Lamberts SW. Continuous dexamethasone infusion for seven hours in patients with the Cushing syndrome. A superior differential diagnostic test. Ann Intern Med 1990; 112:738–742.
28. Croughs RJ, Docter R, de Jong FH. Comparison of oral and intravenous dexamethasone suppression tests in the differential diagnosis of Cushing's syndrome. Acta Endocrinol (Copenh) 1973; 72:54–62.
29. Gold PW, Loriaux DL, Roy A, Kling MA, Calabrese JR, Kellner CH, Nieman LK, Post RM, Pickar D, Gallucci W. Responses to corticotropin-releasing hormone in the hypercortisolism of depression and Cushing's disease. Pathophysiologic and diagnostic implications. N Engl J Med 1986; 314:1329–1335.
30. Lytras N, Grossman A, Perry L, Tomlin S, Wass JA,

Coy DH, Schally AV, Rees LH, Besser GM. Corticotrophin releasing factor: responses in normal subjects and patients with disorders of the hypothalamus and pituitary. Clin Endocrinol (Oxf) 1984; 20:71–84.
31. Orth DN, DeBold CR, DeCherney GS, Jackson RV, Alexander AN, Rivier J, Rivier C, Spiess J, Vale W. Pituitary microadenomas causing Cushing's disease respond to corticotropin-releasing factor. J Clin Endocrinol Metab 1982; 55:1017–1019.
32. Chrousos GP, Schuermeyer TH, Doppman J, Oldfield EH, Schulte HM, Gold PW, Loriaux DL. NIH conference. Clinical applications of corticotropin-releasing factor. Ann Intern Med 1985; 102:344–358.
33. Nieman LK, Oldfield EH, Wesley R, Chrousos GP, Loriaux DL, Cutler GB Jr. A simplified morning ovine corticotropin-releasing hormone stimulation test for the differential diagnosis of adrenocorticotropin-dependent Cushing's syndrome. J Clin Endocrinol Metab 1993; 77:1308–1312.
34. Kaye TB, Crapo L. The Cushing syndrome: an update on diagnostic tests. Ann Intern Med 1990; 112:434–444.
35. Fukata J, Shimizu N, Imura H, Hibi I, Tanaka K, Tanaka T, Nakagawa S, Takebe K, Kimura K, Yoshinaga K. Human corticotropin-releasing hormone test in patients with hypothalamo-pituitary-adrenocortical disorders. Endocr J 1993; 40:597–606.
36. Tanaka K, Shimizu N, Imura H, Fukata J, Hibi I, Tanaka T, Nakagawa S, Fujieda K, Takebe K, Yoshinaga K. Human corticotropin-releasing hormone (hCRH) test: sex and age differences in plasma ACTH and cortisol responses and their reproducibility in healthy adults. Endocr J 1993; 40:571–579.
37. Doppman JL, Nieman L, Miller DL, Pass HI, Chang R, Cutler GB Jr, Schaaf M, Chrousos GP, Norton JA, Ziessman HA. Ectopic adrenocorticotropic hormone syndrome: localization studies in 28 patients. Radiology 1989; 172:115–124.
38. Trainer PJ, Faria M, Newell-Price J, Browne P, Kopelman P, Coy DH, Besser GM, Grossman AB. A comparison of the effects of human and ovine corticotropin-releasing hormone on the pituitary-adrenal axis. J Clin Endocrinol Metab 1995; 80:412–417.
39. Loriaux DL, Nieman L. Corticotropin-releasing hormone testing in pituitary disease. Endocrinol Metab Clin North Am 1991; 20:363–369.
40. Malchoff CD, Orth DN, Abboud C, Carney JA, Pairolero PC, Carey RM. Ectopic ACTH syndrome caused by a bronchial carcinoid tumor responsive to dexamethasone, metyrapone, and corticotropin-releasing factor. Am J Med 1988; 84:760–764.
41. Findling JW, Kehoe ME, Shaker JL, Raff H. Routine inferior petrosal sinus sampling in the differential diagnosis of adrenocorticotropin (ACTH)-dependent Cushing's syndrome: early recognition of the occult ectopic ACTH syndrome. J Clin Endocrinol Metab 1991; 73:408–413.
42. Oldfield EH, Doppman JL, Nieman LK, Chrousos GP, Miller DL, Katz DA, Cutler GB Jr, Loriaux DL. Petrosal sinus sampling with and without corticotropin-releasing hormone for the differential diagnosis of Cushing's syndrome. N Engl J Med 1991; 325:897–905.
43. Kaltsas GA, Giannulis MG, Newell-Price JD, Dacie JE, Thakkar C, Afshar F, Monson JP, Grossman AB, Besser GM, Trainer PJ. A critical analysis of the value of simultaneous inferior petrosal sinus sampling in Cushing's disease and the occult ectopic adrenocorticotropin syndrome. J Clin Endocrinol Metab 1999; 84:487–492.
44. McCance DR, McIlrath E, McNeill A, Gordon DS, Hadden DR, Kennedy L, Sheridan B, Atkinson AB. Bilateral inferior petrosal sinus sampling as a routine procedure in ACTH-dependent Cushing's syndrome. Clin Endocrinol (Oxf) 1989; 30:157–166.
45. Tabarin A, Greselle JF, San Galli F, Leprat F. Usefulness of the corticotropin-releasing hormone test during bilateral inferior petrosal sinus sampling for the diagnosis of Cushing's disease. J Clin Endocrinol Metab 1991; 73:53–59.
46. Booth GL, Redelmeier DA, Grosman H, Kovacs K, Smyth HS, Ezzat S. Improved diagnostic accuracy of inferior petrosal sinus sampling over imaging for localizing pituitary pathology in patients with Cushing's disease. J Clin Endocrinol Metab 1998; 83:2291–2295.
47. Kaltsas GA, Newell-Price JD, Trainer PJ, Besser GM, Grossman AB. Complications of inferior petrosal sinus sampling. J Clin Endocrinol Metab 85:1741–2000.
48. Miller DL, Doppman JL, Peterman SB, Nieman LK, Oldfield EH, Chang R. Neurologic complications of petrosal sinus sampling. Radiology 1992; 185:143–147.
49. Sturrock ND, Jeffcoate WJ. A neurological complication of inferior petrosal sinus sampling during investigation for Cushing's disease: a case report. J Neurol Neurosurg Psychiatry 1997; 62:527–528.
50. Marcovitz S, Wee R, Chan J, Hardy J. The diagnostic accuracy of preoperative CT scanning in the evaluation of pituitary ACTH-secreting adenomas. AJR Am J Roentgenol 1987; 149:803–806.
51. Hall WA, Luciano MG, Doppman JL, Patronas NJ, Oldfield EH. Pituitary magnetic resonance imaging in normal human volunteers: occult adenomas in the general population. Ann Intern Med 1994; 120:817–820.
52. Newton DR, Dillon WP, Norman D, Newton TH, Wilson CB. Gd-DTPA-enhanced MR imaging of pituitary adenomas. AJNR Am J Neuroradiol 1989; 10:949–954.
53. Findling JW, Doppman JL. Biochemical and radiologic diagnosis of Cushing's syndrome. Endocrinol Metab Clin North Am 1994; 23:511–537.
54. Burrow GN, Wortzman G, Rewcastle NB, Holgate RC, Kovacs K. Microadenomas of the pituitary and

abnormal sellar tomograms in an unselected autopsy series. N Engl J Med 1981; 304:156–158.
55. Buchfelder M, Nistor R, Fahlbusch R, Huk WJ. The accuracy of CT and MR evaluation of the sella turcica for detection of adrenocorticotropic hormone-secreting adenomas in Cushing disease. AJNR Am J Neuroradiol 1993; 14:1183–1190.
56. de Herder WW, Uitterlinden P, Pieterman H, Tanghe HL, Kwekkeboom DJ, Pols HA, Singh R, van de Berge JH, Lamberts SW. Pituitary tumour localization in patients with Cushing's disease by magnetic resonance imaging. Is there a place for petrosal sinus sampling? Clin Endocrinol (Oxf) 1994; 40:87–92.
57. Fig LM, Gross MD, Shapiro B, Ehrmann DA, Freitas JE, Schteingart DE, Glazer GM, Francis IR. Adrenal localization in the adrenocorticotropic hormone-independent Cushing syndrome. Ann Intern Med 1988; 109:547–553.
58. Dunnick NR, Schaner EG, Doppman JL, Strott CA, Gil JR, Javadpour N. Computed tomography in adrenal tumors. AJR Am J Roentgenol 1979; 132:43–46.
59. Newell-Price J, Grossman A. Diagnosis and management of Cushing's syndrome. Lancet 1999; 353:2087–2088.
60. Cederna P, Eckhauser FE, Kealey GP. Cushing's syndrome secondary to bronchial carcinoid secretion of ACTH: a review. Am Surg 1993; 59:438–442.
61. Hofland J, Schneider AJ, Cuesta MA, Meijer S. Bronchopulmonary carcinoids associated with Cushing's syndrome—report of a case and an overview of the literature. Acta Oncol 1993; 32:571–573.
62. Vincent JM, Trainer PJ, Reznek RH, Marcus AJ, Dacie JE, Armstrong P, Besser GM. The radiological investigation of occult ectopic ACTH-dependent Cushing's syndrome. Clin Radiol 1993; 48:11–17.
63. Mampalam TJ, Tyrrell JB, Wilson CB. Transsphenoidal microsurgery for Cushing disease. A report of 216 cases. Ann Intern Med 1988; 109:487–493.
64. Sonino N, Zielezny M, Fava GA, Fallo F, Boscaro M. Risk factors and long-term outcome in pituitary-dependent Cushing's disease. J Clin Endocrinol Metab 1996; 81:2647–2652.
65. Swearingen B, Biller BM, Barker FG, Katznelson L, Grinspoon S, Klibanski A, Zervas NT. Long-term mortality after transsphenoidal surgery for Cushing disease. Ann Intern Med 1999; 130:821–824.
66. Estrada J, Garcia-Uria J, Lamas C, Alfaro J, Lucas T, Diez S, Salto L, Barcelo B. The complete normalization of the adrenocortical function as the criterion of cure after transsphenoidal surgery for Cushing's disease. J Clin Endocrinol Metab 2001; 86:5695–5699.
67. Ludecke DK. Transnasal microsurgery of Cushing's disease 1990. Overview including personal experiences with 256 patients. Pathol Res Pract 1991; 187:608–612.
68. Ram Z, Nieman LK, Cutler GB Jr, Chrousos GP, Doppman JL, Oldfield EH. Early repeat surgery for persistent Cushing's disease. J Neurosurg 1994; 80:37–45.
69. Estrada J, Boronat M, Mielgo M, Magallon R, Millan I, Diez S, Lucas T, Barcelo B. The long-term outcome of pituitary irradiation after unsuccessful transsphenoidal surgery in Cushing's disease. N Engl J Med 1997; 336:172–177.
70. Jennings AS, Liddle GW, Orth DN. Results of treating childhood Cushing's disease with pituitary irradiation. N Engl J Med 1977; 297:957–962.
71. Henry JF, Defechereux T, Raffaelli M, Lubrano D, Gramatica L. Complications of laparoscopic adrenalectomy: results of 169 consecutive procedures. World J Surg 2000; 24:1342–1346.
72. Lanzi R, Montorsi F, Losa M, Centemero A, Manzoni MF, Rigatti P, Cornaggia G, Pontiroli AE, Guazzoni G. Laparoscopic bilateral adrenalectomy for persistent Cushing's disease after transsphenoidal surgery. Surgery 1998; 123:144–150.
73. Smith CD, Weber CJ, Amerson JR. Laparoscopic adrenalectomy: new gold standard. World J Surg 1999; 23:389–396.
74. Doherty GM, Nieman LK, Cutler GB Jr, Chrousos GP, Norton JA. Time to recovery of the hypothalamic-pituitary-adrenal axis after curative resection of adrenal tumors in patients with Cushing's syndrome. Surgery 1990; 108:1085–1090.
75. Pass HI, Doppman JL, Nieman L, Stovroff M, Vetto J, Norton JA, Travis W, Chrousos GP, Oldfield EH, Cutler GB Jr. Management of the ectopic ACTH syndrome due to thoracic carcinoids. Ann Thorac Surg 1990; 50:52–57.
76. Invitti C, de Martin M, Danesi L, Cavagnini F. Effect of injectable bromocriptine in patients with Cushing's disease. Exp Clin Endocrinol Diabetes 1995; 103:266–271.
77. Waveren Hogervorst CO, Koppeschaar HP, Zelissen PM, Lips CJ, Garcia BM. Cortisol secretory patterns in Cushing's disease and response to cyproheptadine treatment. J Clin Endocrinol Metab 1996; 81:652–655.
78. Sonino N, Fava GA, Fallo F, Franceschetto A, Belluardo P, Boscaro M. Effect of the serotonin antagonists ritanserin and ketanserin in Cushing's disease. Pituitary 2000; 3:55–59.
79. Beckers A, Stevenaert A, Pirens G, Flandroy P, Sulon J, Hennen G. Cyclical Cushing's disease and its successful control under sodium valproate. J Endocrinol Invest 1990; 13:923–929.
80. Colao A, Pivonello R, Tripodi FS, Orio F Jr, Ferone D, Cerbone G, Di Somma C, Merola B, Lombardi G. Failure of long-term therapy with sodium valproate in Cushing's disease. J Endocrinol Invest 1997; 20:387–392.
81. Sonino N, Boscaro M. Medical therapy for Cushing's disease. Endocrinol Metab Clin North Am 1999; 28:211–222.

82. Verhelst JA, Trainer PJ, Howlett TA, Perry L, Rees LH, Grossman AB, Wass JA, Besser GM. Short and long-term responses to metyrapone in the medical management of 91 patients with Cushing's syndrome. Clin Endocrinol (Oxf) 1991; 35:169–178.
83. Luton JP, Mahoudeau JA, Bouchard P, Thieblot P, Hautecouverture M, Simon D, Laudat MH, Touitou Y, Bricaire H. Treatment of Cushing's disease by o,p'DDD. Survey of 62 cases. N Engl J Med 1979; 300:459–464.
84. Chou SC, Lin JD. Long-term effects of ketoconazole in the treatment of residual or recurrent Cushing's disease. Endocr J 2000; 47:401–406.
85. Sonino N, Boscaro M, Paoletta A, Mantero F, Ziliotto D. Ketoconazole treatment in Cushing's syndrome: experience in 34 patients. Clin Endocrinol (Oxf) 1991; 35:347–352.
86. Sonino N. The use of ketoconazole as an inhibitor of steroid production. N Engl J Med 1987; 317:812–818.
87. Bertagna X, Bertagna C, Laudat MH, Husson JM, Girard F, Luton JP. Pituitary-adrenal response to the antiglucocorticoid action of RU 486 in Cushing's syndrome. J Clin Endocrinol Metab 1986; 63:639–643.
88. Sartor O, Cutler GB Jr. Mifepristone: treatment of Cushing's syndrome. Clin Obstet Gynecol 1996; 39: 506–510.
89. Norton JA, Li M, Gillary J, Le HN. Cushing's syndrome. Curr Probl Surg 2001; 38:488–545.
90. Brennan MF. Adrenocortical carcinoma. CA Cancer J Clin 1987; 37:348–365.
91. Javadpour N, Woltering EA, Brennan MF. Adrenal neoplasms. Curr Probl Surg 1980; 17:1–52.
92. Plager JE. Carcinoma of the adrenal cortex: clinical description, diagnosis, and treatment. Int Adv Surg Oncol 1984; 7:329–353.
93. National Cancer Institute, Third National Cancer Survey: Incidence Data. Bethesda, MD: National Cancer Institute, 1975:785–787.
94. Steiner PE. Cancer: Race and Geography: Some Etiological, Environmental, Ethnological, Epidemiological, and Statistical Aspects in Caucasoids, Mongoloids, Negroids and Mexicans. Baltimore: Williams and Wilkins, 1954:25.
95. Wajchenberg BL, Albergaria Pereira MA, Medonca BB, Latronico AC, Campos CP, Ferreira AV, Zerbini MC, Liberman B, Carlos GG, Kirschner MA. Adrenocortical carcinoma: clinical and laboratory observations. Cancer 2000; 88:711–736.
96. Wooten MD, King DK. Adrenal cortical carcinoma. Epidemiology and treatment with mitotane and a review of the literature. Cancer 1993; 72:3145–3155.
97. Mendonca BB, Lucon AM, Menezes CA, Saldanha LB, Latronico AC, Zerbini C, Madureira G, Domenice S, Albergaria MA, Camargo MH. Clinical, hormonal and pathological findings in a comparative study of adrenocortical neoplasms in childhood and adulthood. J Urol 1995; 154:2004–2009.
98. Sabbaga CC, Avilla SG, Schulz C, Garbers JC, Blucher D. Adrenocortical carcinoma in children: clinical aspects and prognosis. J Pediatr Surg 1993; 28:841–843.
99. Cohn K, Gottesman L, Brennan M. Adrenocortical carcinoma. Surgery 1986; 100:1170–1177.
100. Icard P, Louvel A, Chapuis Y. Survival rates and prognostic factors in adrenocortical carcinoma. World J Surg 1992; 16:753–758.
101. Pommier RF, Brennan MF. An eleven-year experience with adrenocortical carcinoma. Surgery 1992; 112: 963–970.
102. Venkatesh S, Hickey RC, Sellin RV, Fernandez JF, Samaan NA. Adrenal cortical carcinoma. Cancer 1989; 64:765–769.
103. Zografos GC, Driscoll DL, Karakousis CP, Huben RP. Adrenal adenocarcinoma: a review of 53 cases. J Surg Oncol 1994; 55:160–164.
104. Bertagna C, Orth DN. Clinical and laboratory findings and results of therapy in 58 patients with adrenocortical tumors admitted to a single medical center (1951 to 1978). Am J Med 1981; 71:855–875.
105. Luton JP, Cerdas S, Billaud L, Thomas G, Guilhaume B, Bertagna X, Laudat MH, Louvel A, Chapuis Y, Blondeau P. Clinical features of adrenocortical carcinoma, prognostic factors, and the effect of mitotane therapy. N Engl J Med 1990; 322:1195–1201.
106. Soreide JA, Brabrand K, Thoresen SO. Adrenal cortical carcinoma in Norway, 1970-1984. World J Surg 1992; 16:663–667.
107. Hutter AM Jr, Kayhoe DE. Adrenal cortical carcinoma. Clinical features of 138 patients. Am J Med 1966; 41:572–580.
108. King DR, Lack EE. Adrenal cortical carcinoma: a clinical and pathologic study of 49 cases. Cancer 1979; 44:239–244.
109. Hamwi GJ, Serbin RA, Kruger FA. Does adrenocortical hyperplasia result in adrenocortical carcinoma? N Engl J Med 1957; 257:1153–1157.
110. Plager JE. Carcinoma of the adrenal cortex: clinical description, diagnosis, and treatment. Int Adv Surg Oncol 1984; 7:329–353.
111. Henry I, Grandjouan S, Couillin P, Barichard F, Huerre-Jeanpierre C, Glaser T, Philip T, Lenoir G, Chaussain JL, Junien C. Tumor-specific loss of 11p15.5 alleles in del11p13 Wilms tumor and in familial adrenocortical carcinoma. Proc Natl Acad Sci USA 1989; 86:3247–3251.
112. Yano T, Linehan M, Anglard P, Lerman MI, Daniel LN, Stein CA, Robertson CN, LaRocca R, Zbar B. Genetic changes in human adrenocortical carcinomas. J Natl Cancer Inst 1989; 81:518–523.
113. McNicol AM, Nolan CE, Struthers AJ, Farquharson MA, Hermans J, Haak HR. Expression of p53 in

adrenocortical tumours: clinicopathological correlations. J Pathol 1997; 181:146–152.
114. Ohgaki H, Kleihues P, Heitz PU. p53 mutations in sporadic adrenocortical tumors. Int J Cancer 1993; 54:408–410.
115. Reincke M, Karl M, Travis WH, Mastorakos G, Allolio B, Linehan HM, Chrousos GP. p53 mutations in human adrenocortical neoplasms: immunohistochemical and molecular studies. J Clin Endocrinol Metab 1994; 78:790–794.
116. Brooks RV, Felix-Davies D, Lee MR, Robertson PW. Hyperaldosteronism from adrenal carcinoma. Br Med J 1972; 1:220–221.
117. Hyodo T, Megyesi K, Kahn CR, McLean JP, Friesen HG. Adrenocortical carcinoma and hypoglycemia: evidence for production of nonsuppressible insulin-like activity by the tumor. J Clin Endocrinol Metab 1977; 44:1175–1184.
118. Pommier RF, Brennan MF. An eleven-year experience with adrenocortical carcinoma. Surgery 1992; 112:963–970.
119. Holcombe JH, Physher TJ, Kirkland RT. Functioning adrenocortical tumors in childhood. In: Humphrey GB, Grindey GB, Dehner LP, Acton RT, Pysker TJ, eds. Adrenal and Endocrine Tumors in Children. Boston: Martinus Nijhoff Publishers, 1983:277–290.
120. Kasperlik-Zaluska AA, Migdalska BM, Zgliczynski S, Makowska AM. Adrenocortical carcinoma. A clinical study and treatment results of 52 patients. Cancer 1995; 75:2587–2591.
121. Zapf J, Futo E, Peter M, Froesch ER. Can "big" insulin-like growth factor II in serum of tumor patients account for the development of extrapancreatic tumor hypoglycemia? J Clin Invest 1992; 90:2574–2584.
122. Henley DJ, van Heerden JA, Grant CS, Carney JA, Carpenter PC. Adrenal cortical carcinoma—a continuing challenge. Surgery 1983; 94:926–931.
123. Hogan TF, Gilchrist KW, Westring DW, Citrin DL. A clinical and pathological study of adrenocortical carcinoma: therapeutic implications. Cancer 1980; 45: 2880–2883.
124. Karakousis CP, Rao U, Moore R. Adrenal adenocarcinomas: histologic grading and survival. J Surg Oncol 1985; 29:105–111.
125. Prinz RA, Brooks MH, Churchill R, Graner JL, Lawrence AM, Paloyan E, Sparagana M. Incidental asymptomatic adrenal masses detected by computed tomographic scanning. Is operation required? JAMA 1982; 248:701–704.
126. Lewinsky BS, Grigor KM, Symington T, Neville AM. The clinical and pathologic features of "non-hormonal" adrenocortical tumors. Report of twenty new cases and review of the literature. Cancer 1974; 33: 778–790.
127. Carbonnel F, Valla D, Menu Y, Lecompte Y, Belghiti J, Rueff B, Benhamou JP. Acute Budd-Chiari syndrome as first manifestation of adrenocortical carcinoma. J Clin Gastroenterol 1988; 10:441–444.
128. Kendrick ML, Lloyd R, Erickson L, Farley DR, Grant CS, Thompson GB, Rowland C, Young WF Jr, van Heerden JA. Adrenocortical carcinoma: surgical progress or status quo? Arch Surg 2001; 136:543–549.
129. Bodie B, Novick AC, Pontes JE, Straffon RA, Montie JE, Babiak T, Sheeler L, Schumacher P. The Cleveland Clinic experience with adrenal cortical carcinoma. J Urol 1989; 141:257–260.
130. Lynch HT, Mulcahy GM, Harris RE, Guirgis HA, Lynch JF. Genetic and pathologic findings in a kindred with hereditary sarcoma, breast cancer, brain tumors, leukemia, lung, laryngeal, and adrenal cortical carcinoma. Cancer 1978; 41:2055–2064.
131. MacFarlane DA. Cancer of the adrenal cortex, The natural history, prognosis and treatment in a study of fifty-five cases. Ann R Coll Surg Engl 1958; 23:155–186.
132. Sullivan M, Boileau M, Hodges CV. Adrenal cortical carcinoma. J Urol 1978; 120:660–665.
133. Jaques DP, Brennan MF. Tumors of the adrenal cortex. In: Cameron JL, ed. Current Surgical Therapy. Toronto: BC Decker, 1989:435–444.
134. Soreide JA, Brabrand K, Thoresen SO. Adrenal cortical carcinoma in Norway, 1970–1984. World J Surg 1992; 16:663–667.
135. Ferrucci JT Jr. Body ultrasonography. N Engl J Med 1979; 300:590–602.
136. Edelman RR, Hesselink JR. Adrenal glands. Clinical Magnetic Resonance Imaging. Philadelphia: WB Saunders Co, 1990:888–894.
137. Lee JK, Sagel SS, Stanley RJ. Adrenal glands. Computed Body Tomography with MRI Correlation. 2d ed. New York: Raven Press, 1989:827–849.
138. Schultz CL, Haaga JR, Fletcher BD, Alfidi RJ, Schultz MA. Magnetic resonance imaging of the adrenal glands: a comparison with computed tomography. AJR Am J Roentgenol 1984; 143:1235–1240.
139. Li BD, Douglass HO. Management of the incidentally discovered adrenal mass or "incidentaloma." J La State Med Soc 1997; 149:291–299.
140. Falke TH, te SL, Shaff MI, Sandler MP, Kulkarni MV, Partain CL, Nieuwenhuizen-Kruseman AC, James AE Jr. MR imaging of the adrenals: correlation with computed tomography. J Comput Assist Tomogr 1986; 10:242–253.
141. McLoughlin RF, Bilbey JH. Tumors of the adrenal gland: findings on CT and MR imaging. AJR Am J Roentgenol 1994; 163:1413–1418.
142. Davis PL, Hricak H, Bradley WG Jr. Magnetic resonance imaging of the adrenal glands. Radiol Clin North Am 1984; 22:891–895.
143. Krestin GP, Freidmann G, Fishbach R, Neufang KF, Allolio B. Evaluation of adrenal masses in oncologic

patients: dynamic contrast-enhanced MR vs CT. J Comput Assist Tomogr 1991; 15:104–110.
144. Chang A, Glazer HS, Lee JK, Ling D, Heiken JP. Adrenal gland: MR imaging. Radiology 1987; 163: 123–128.
145. Egglin TK, Hahn PF, Stark DD. MRI of the adrenal glands. Semin Roentgenol 1988; 23:280–287.
146. Peppercorn PD, Reznek RH. State-of-the-art CT and MRI of the adrenal gland. Eur Radiol 1997; 7:822–836.
147. Baker ME, Blinder R, Spritzer C, Leight GS, Herfkens RJ, Dunnick NR. MR evaluation of adrenal masses at 1.5 T. AJR Am J Roentgenol 1989; 153:307–312.
148. Doppman JL, Reinig JW, Dwyer AJ, Frank JP, Norton J, Loriaux DL, Keiser H. Differentiation of adrenal masses by magnetic resonance imaging. Surgery 1987; 102:1018–1026.
149. Glazer GM, Woolsey EJ, Borrello J, Francis IR, Aisen AM, Bookstein F, Amendola MA, Gross MD, Bree RL, Martel W. Adrenal tissue characterization using MR imaging. Radiology 1986; 158:73–79.
150. Korobkin M, Lombardi TJ, Aisen AM, Francis IR, Quint LE, Dunnick NR, Londy F, Shapiro B, Gross MD, Thompson NW. Characterization of adrenal masses with chemical shift and gadolinium-enhanced MR imaging. Radiology 1995; 197:411–418.
151. Outwater EK, Siegelman ES, Radecki PD, Piccoli CW, Mitchell DG. Distinction between benign and malignant adrenal masses: value of T1-weighted chemical-shift MR imaging. AJR Am J Roentgenol 1995; 165: 579–583.
152. Reinig JW, Stutley JE, Leonhardt CM, Spicer KM, Margolis M, Caldwell CB. Differentiation of adrenal masses with MR imaging: comparison of techniques. Radiology 1994; 192:41–46.
153. Schwartz LH, Panicek DM, Koutcher JA, Heelan RT, Bains MS, Burt M. Echoplanar MR imaging for characterization of adrenal masses in patients with malignant neoplasms: preliminary evaluation of calculated T2 relaxation values. AJR Am J Roentgenol 1995; 164:911–915.
154. Fig LM, Gross MD, Shapiro B, Ehrmann DA, Freitas JE, Schteingart DE, Glazer GM, Francis IR. Adrenal localization in the adrenocorticotropic hormone-independent Cushing syndrome. Ann Intern Med 1988; 109:547–553.
155. Thrall JH, Freitas JE, Beierwaltes WH. Adrenal scintigraphy. Semin Nucl Med 1978; 8:23–41.
156. Hedican SP, Marshall FF. Adrenocortical carcinoma with intracaval extension. J Urol 1997; 158:2056–2061.
157. Didier D, Racle A, Etievent JP, Weill F. Tumor thrombus of the inferior vena cava secondary to malignant abdominal neoplasms: US and CT evaluation. Radiology 1987; 162:83–89.
158. Goldfarb DA, Novick AC, Lorig R, Bretan PN, Montie JE, Pontes JE, Streem SB, Siegel SW. Magnetic resonance imaging for assessment of vena caval tumor thrombi: a comparative study with venacavography and computerized tomography scanning. J Urol 1990; 144:1100–1103.
159. Heinbecker P, O'Neil LW, Ackerman LV. Functional and nonfunctional adrenal cortical tumor. Surg Gynecol Obstet 1957; 105:21–33.
160. Schteingart DE, Oberman HA, Friedman BA, Conn JW. Adrenal cortical neoplasms producing Cushing's syndrome. A clinicopathologic study. Cancer 1968; 22:1005–1013.
161. Weiss LM. Comparative histologic study of 43 metastasizing and nonmetastasizing adrenocortical tumors. Am J Surg Pathol 1984; 8:163–169.
162. Weiss LM, Medeiros LJ, Vickery AL Jr. Pathologic features of prognostic significance in adrenocortical carcinoma. Am J Surg Pathol 1989; 13:202–206.
163. Cohn K, Gottesman L, Brennan M. Adrenocortical carcinoma. Surgery 1986; 100:1170–1177.
164. Icard P, Louvel A, Chapuis Y. Survival rates and prognostic factors in adrenocortical carcinoma. World J Surg 1992; 16:753–758.
165. Cote RJ, Cordon-Cardo C, Reuter VE, Rosen PP. Immunopathology of adrenal and renal cortical tumors. Coordinated change in antigen expression is associated with neoplastic conversion in the adrenal cortex. Am J Pathol 1990; 136:1077–1084.
166. Gaffey MJ, Traweek ST, Mills SE, Travis WD, Lack EE, Medeiros LJ, Weiss LM. Cytokeratin expression in adrenocortical neoplasia: an immunohistochemical and biochemical study with implications for the differential diagnosis of adrenocortical, hepatocellular, and renal cell carcinoma. Hum Pathol 1992; 23:144–153.
167. Henzen-Logmans SC, Stel HV, van Muijen GN, Mullink H, Meijer CJ. Expression of intermediate filament proteins in adrenal cortex and related tumours. Histopathology 1988; 12:359–372.
168. Komminoth P, Roth J, Schroder S, Saremaslani P, Heitz PU. Overlapping expression of immunohistochemical markers and synaptophysin mRNA in pheochromocytomas and adrenocortical carcinomas. Implications for the differential diagnosis of adrenal gland tumors. Lab Invest 1995; 72:424–431.
169. Schroder S, Padberg BC, Achilles E, Holl K, Dralle H, Kloppel G. Immunocytochemistry in adrenocortical tumours: a clinicomorphological study of 72 neoplasms. Virchows Arch A Pathol Anat Histopathol 1992; 420:65–70.
170. Cibas ES, Medeiros LJ, Weinberg DS, Gelb AB, Weiss LM. Cellular DNA profiles of benign and malignant adrenocortical tumors. Am J Surg Pathol 1990; 14: 948–955.
171. Haak HR, Cornelisse CJ, Hermans J, Cobben L, Fleuren GJ. Nuclear DNA content and morphological characteristics in the prognosis of adrenocortical carcinoma. Br J Cancer 1993; 68:151–155.
172. Sasano H, Imatani A, Shizawa S, Suzuki T, Nagura H.

Cell proliferation and apoptosis in normal and pathologic human adrenal. Mod Pathol 1995; 8:11–17.
173. Geelhoed GW, Dunnick NR, Doppman JL. Management of intravenous extensions of endocrine tumors and prognosis after surgical treatment. Am J Surg 1980; 139:844–848.
174. Grondal S, Cedermark B, Eriksson B, Grimelius L, Harach R, Kristoffersson A, Rastad J, Uden P, Akerstrom G. Adrenocortical carcinoma. A retrospective study of a rare tumor with a poor prognosis. Eur J Surg Oncol 1990; 16:500–506.
175. Thompson NW, Cheung PS. Diagnosis and treatment of functioning and nonfunctioning adrenocortical neoplasms including incidentalomas. Surg Clin North Am 1987; 67:423–436.
176. Crucitti F, Bellantone R, Ferrante A, Boscherini M, Crucitti P. The Italian Registry for Adrenal Cortical Carcinoma: analysis of a multiinstitutional series of 129 patients. The ACC Italian Registry Study Group. Surgery 1996; 119:161–170.
177. Haak HR, Hermans J, van de Velde CJ, Lentjes EG, Goslings BM, Fleuren GJ, Krans HM. Optimal treatment of adrenocortical carcinoma with mitotane: results in a consecutive series of 96 patients. Br J Cancer 1994; 69:947–951.
178. Zografos GC, Driscoll DL, Karakousis CP, Huben RP. Adrenal adenocarcinoma: a review of 53 cases. J Surg Oncol 1994; 55:160–164.
179. Schulick RD, Brennan MF. Long-term survival after complete resection and repeat resection in patients with adrenocortical carcinoma. Ann Surg Oncol 1999; 6:719–726.
180. Smith CD, Weber CJ, Amerson JR. Laparoscopic adrenalectomy: new gold standard. World J Surg 1999; 23:389–396.
181. Heniford BT, Arca MJ, Walsh RM, Gill IS. Laparoscopic adrenalectomy for cancer. Semin Surg Oncol 1999; 16:293–306.
182. Luton JP, Mahoudeau JA, Bouchard P, Thieblot P, Hautecouverture M, Simon D, Laudat MH, Touitou Y, Bricaire H. Treatment of Cushing's disease by o,p'DDD. Survey of 62 cases. N Engl J Med 1979; 300:459–464.
183. Schteingart DE. Cushing's syndrome. Endocrinol Metab Clin North Am 1989; 18:311–338.
184. Hutter AM Jr, Kayhoe DE. Adrenal cortical carcinoma. Results of treatment with o,p'DDD in 138 patients. Am J Med 1966; 41:581–592.
185. Lubitz JA, Freeman L, Okun R. Mitotane use in inoperable adrenal cortical carcinoma. JAMA 1973; 223:1109–1112.
186. Dickstein G, Shechner C, Arad E, Best LA, Nativ O. Is there a role for low doses of mitotane (o,p'-DDD) as adjuvant therapy in adrenocortical carcinoma? J Clin Endocrinol Metab 1998; 83:3100–3103.
187. Terzolo M, Pia A, Berruti A, Osella G, Ali A, Carbone V, Testa E, Dogliotti L, Angeli A. Low-dose monitored mitotane treatment achieves the therapeutic range with manageable side effects in patients with adrenocortical cancer. J Clin Endocrinol Metab 2000; 85:2234–2238.
188. Haak HR, Hermans J, van de Velde CJ, Lentjes EG, Goslings BM, Fleuren GJ, Krans HM. Optimal treatment of adrenocortical carcinoma with mitotane: results in a consecutive series of 96 patients. Br J Cancer 1994; 69:947–951.
189. Kasperlik-Zaluska AA, Migdalska B, Makowska A. Impact of adjuvant mitotane on the clinical course of patients with adrenocortical cancer. Cancer 1994; 73:1533–1535.
190. Schteingart DE, Motazedi A, Noonan RA, Thompson NW. Treatment of adrenal carcinomas. Arch Surg 1982; 117:1142–1146.
191. Vassilopoulou-Sellin R, Guinee VF, Klein MJ, Taylor SH, Hess KR, Schultz PN, Samaan NA. Impact of adjuvant mitotane on the clinical course of patients with adrenocortical cancer. Cancer 1993; 71:3119–3123.
192. Schlumberger M, Ostronoff M, Bellaiche M, Rougier P, Droz JP, Parmentier C. 5-Fluorouracil, doxorubicin, and cisplatin regimen in adrenal cortical carcinoma. Cancer 1988; 61:1492–1494.
193. Arlt W, Reincke M, Siekmann L, Winkelmann W, Allolio B. Suramin in adrenocortical cancer: limited efficacy and serious toxicity. Clin Endocrinol (Oxf) 1994; 41:299–307.
194. Dorfinger K, Niederle B, Vierhapper H, Astrid W, Czernin S, Nowotny P, Waldhausl W, Grubeck-Loebenstein B. Suramin and the human adrenocortex: results of experimental and clinical studies. Surgery 1991; 110:1100–1105.
195. Flack MR, Pyle RG, Mullen NM, Lorenzo B, Wu YW, Knazek RA, Nisula BC, Reidenberg MM. Oral gossypol in the treatment of metastatic adrenal cancer. J Clin Endocrinol Metab 1993; 76:1019–1024.
196. Kamilaris TC, Chrousos GP. Adrenal diseases. In: Moore WT, Eastman RC, eds. Diagnositic Endocrinology. Philadelphia: Decker, 1990:79–109.

34

Primary Aldosteronism: Pathophysiology, Diagnosis and Management

Sotirios G. Stergiopoulos, David J. Torpy*, and Constantine A. Stratakis

National Institute of Health, Bethesda, Maryland, U.S.A.

1 INTRODUCTION

Aldosterone, the major circulating mineralocorticoid, is a steroid hormone produced exclusively in the zona glomerulosa. The major regulators of aldosterone biosynthesis and secretion are the renin-angiotensin system and potasssium ion concentrations. Minor regulators include adrenocorticotropic hormone (ACTH) from the pituitary, atrial natriuretic peptide from the heart, and dopamine secreted locally in the adrenal. A number of aldosterone precursors, including deoxycorticosterone and 18-hydroxycorticosterone, have mineralocorticoid activity, and their hypersecretion in various pathological states may produce or exacerbate features typical of mineralocorticoid hypertension. Aldosterone acts mainly on the distal nephron, although several other sites of sodium reabsorption exist.

Hyperaldosteronism is characterized by excessive secretion of aldosterone with consequent increased sodium reabsorption and potassium and hydrogen ion loss. Clinical features include hypertension, hypokalemia, and metabolic alkalosis. It represents a subset of disorders causing mineralocorticoid hypertension, where the features of hypertension and hypokalemia can be produced by aldosterone, endogenous mineralocorticoid precursors, or intrinsic defects modulating aldosterone effects on its target tissues.

We have provided elsewhere a survey of familial hyperaldosteronism (1) and of other disorders of excess aldosterone secretion and action (2). This chapter focuses on primary hyperaldosteronism, although differential diagnosis is also discussed. Table 1 includes all disorders that should be considered in the hypertensive patient with real or apparent hyperaldosteronism.

*Current affiliation: Dept. of Medicine, University of Queensland, Greenslopes Hospital, Queensland, Australia.

2 PHYSIOLOGICAL MECHANISMS OF ALDOSTERONE SECRETION

2.1 Control of Aldosterone Secretion

Aldosterone participates in blood volume and serum potassium homeostasis, which, in turn, regulates aldosterone secretion by the zona glomerulosa of the adrenal cortex (2). Blood volume depletion or an increase in serum potassium concentration stimulates aldosterone secretion, whereas hypervolemia and hypokalemia suppress it. The mechanisms by which the homeostatic regulation of aldosterone secretion is accomplished are complex and involve the adrenal zona glomerulosa, the juxtaglomerular apparatus of the kidneys, the cardiovascular system, the autonomic nervous system, the lungs, and the liver.

Table 1 Causes of Hyperaldosteronism and Related Conditions with Diagnostic Laboratory Findings

Etiology	Laboratory and imaging findings
Primary aldosteronism	High aldosterone/low PRA**
Aldosterone-producing adenoma	Unilateral adrenocortical adenoma
Idiopathic hyperaldosteronism hyperplasia	Responds to posture/bilateral adrenal
Primary adrenal hyperplasia	Responds to posture/unilateral adrenal
Glucocorticoid-remediable aldosteronism (familial hyperaldosteronism type I)	Sustained suppression of aldosterone (<4 ng/dL) to dexamethasone/bilateral adrenal hyperplasia
Familial hyperaldosteronism type II	Familial (autosomal dominant) with lack of response to dexamethasone/bilateral adrenal hyperplasia with occasional adenoma(s)
Secondary hyperaldosteronism (>2 ng/mL)	High aldosterone/nonsuppressible PRA
Edema disorders, e.g., cardiac failure	
Renovascular hypertension	
Renin-producing tumors	
Pregnancy	
Aldosterone excess–like disorders	Low aldosterone/low PRA
Congenital adrenal hyperplasia (11-β-hydroxylase, 17-α-hydroxylase deficiencies)	Elevated steroid intermediaries
Primary glucocorticoid resistance	High glucocorticoid secretion unsuppressed by dexamethasone
DOC-secreting tumors upon imaging*	Elevated DOC levels/adrenal tumors
Apparent mineralocorticoid excess	Autosomal recessive/elevated urine cortisol(F)/cortisone (E) ratio
Liddle's syndrome	Autosomal dominant
Licorice ingestion	
Carbenoxolone	

* Deoxycorticosterone.
** Plasma-renin activity.

At the level of the zona glomerulosa, the major stimulatory influences are angiotensin II and serum potassium concentration (3,4). ACTH stimulates aldosterone secretion in an acute and transient fashion, but it is questionable whether ACTH plays a significant role in the chronic regulation of mineralocorticoid secretion (2). The major inhibitory influences affecting the zona glomerulosa are exerted by circulating atrial natriuretic peptide (ANP) and, locally, by dopamine (5). Although ANP levels are clearly increased in hyperaldosteronism, neither ANP nor dopamine has been implicated as a primary cause of clinically significant defects in aldosterone secretion. Metoclopramide increases aldosterone secretion, suggesting dopamine may inhibit aldosterone release (6–8). The physiological roles of adrenomedullin and vasoactive intestinal peptide (VIP) on aldosterone secretion remain to be clarified; it appears that both these neuropeptides are produced in the rat zona glomerulosa (9,10).

The major regulation of angiotensin II production occurs at the juxtaglomerular apparatus. The synthesis of prorenin, its conversion to renin, and the secretion of renin into the circulation are processes that are stimulated by blood volume contraction (stretch receptors), by the sympathetic nervous system (via α-adrenergic stimulation), and by prostaglandins (11–15). These processes are inhibited by volume expansion and ANP. Renin converts angiotensinogen, a liver protein, into the decapeptide angiotensin I. Angiotensin I is then converted into angiotensin II by angiotensin-converting enzyme, a protease that is active in the lungs. Angiotensin II, an octapeptide with both aldosterone-stimulating and vasopressor activities, is metabolized to angiotensin III, a heptapeptide characterized primarily by aldosterone-stimulating activity (13).

Prostaglandin synthesis and secretion of renin depend upon adequate amounts of intracellular ionized calcium (15). In addition, stretch sensor function may also depend on ionized calcium (13) Angiotensin II appears to stimulate renal prostaglandin secretion, as do catecholamines (13,14). Because of all these interrelationships, there are several points in this series of steps at which aldosterone secretion may be affected. Although this makes the diagnosis of hyperaldosteronism relatively complicated, especially in the elderly hypertensive patient who receives numerous medications, it also provides the opportunity for medical treatment at multiple levels.

2.2 Aldosterone Biosynthesis

Aldosterone is synthesized from cholesterol in a series of six biosynthetic steps (16). The first four steps are also involved in the synthesis of cortisol, whereas the last two pertain only to aldosterone (17). The product of the *CYP11B2* gene is capable of catalyzing both the 11-β-hydroxylase and 18-hydroxylase and 18-hydroxydehydrogenase steps in aldosterone biosynthesis (17–19). The CYP11B2 gene is located on human chromosome 8q24.3-tel (20).

2.3 Aldosterone Receptors

Aldosterone acts on its target tissues (distal renal tubule, sweat glands, salivary glands, large intestinal epithelium) via its own specific mineralocorticoid receptors (21). Mineralocorticoid receptors exhibit equal affinity for aldosterone and glucocorticoids (22), but distal renal tubular receptors are protected from the effects of cortisol by 11-β-hydroxysteroid dehydrogenase, which converts cortisol to inactive cortisone (23). More recently, non–steroid receptor effects of aldosterone have been described, although their pathophysiological relevance for primary aldosteronism is currently unknown (24).

2.4 Increased Mineralocorticoid Dependency in Childhood

The mineralocorticoid dependency of sodium reabsorption is increased in infancy and childhood, with its peak in the neonatal period; it progressively decreases with advancing age. There are several reasons for this fact, including changes in 11-β-hydroxysteroid dehydrogenase activity (25) and zona glomerulosa sensitivity to ACTH (26). In addition, proximal tubular sodium and water resorption is least efficient in early life, resulting in an increased sodium and water load at the level of the distal renal tubule (27). Because sodium and water resorption from the distal tubule is mediated by the renin-angiotensin-aldosterone axis, the plasma renin activity (PRA) of a newborn infant is approximately 10- to 20-fold higher than that of an adult. This results in increased aldosterone production (>300 μg/m^2/day in a newborn infant vs. 50 μg/m^2/day in an adult) and plasma aldosterone concentrations, in the neonate (80 vs. 16 pg/dL, respectively).

3 CLASSIFICATION AND MANAGEMENT OF HYPERALDOSTERONISM

Hyperaldosteronism is characterized by hypokalemia, which may produce neuromuscular symptoms such as weakness or paralysis and polyuria and polydipsia due to an associated renal concentrating defect. Hypokalemia also impairs insulin secretion and can promote the development of diabetes mellitus. The major causes and laboratory findings in hyperaldosteronism are listed in Table 1.

Hyperaldosteronism may be primary, representing a disorder of the zona glomerulosa, or may be secondary to factors beyond the mineralocorticoid axis, such as reduced effective circulating blood volume, where disorders such as hypovolemia, cardiac failure, or diuretic use can activate the renin-angiotensin system and stimulate aldosterone secretion (28). Primary and secondary aldosteronism can be differentiated with the aldosterone/PRA ratio; higher ratios are seen in primary aldosteronism (29). It is important to recognize that the features of aldosteronism can be produced without aldosterone hypersecretion resulting in non–aldosterone-mediated mineralocorticoid excess (Table 1). These include two causes of congenital adrenal hyperplasia (11-β-hydroxylase deficiency and 17-α-hydroxylase deficiency), the syndrome of apparent mineralocorticoid excess (AME) due to 11- β-hydroxysteroid dehydrogenase (11-β-HSD) deficiency, primary glucocorticoid resistance, Liddle's syndrome, and exogenous sources of mineralocorticoid such as licorice or drugs such as carbenoxolone (2). The features of mineralocorticoid excess are also often seen in Cushing's syndrome, particularly in patients with ectopic ACTH-producing tumors (2,3). In these cases it is postulated that excessive glucocorticoid levels overwhelm the ability of the 11-β-HSD enzyme to inactivate cortisol at the kidney mineralocorticoid receptor level.

3.1 Primary Aldosteronism

3.1.1 Prevalence

Primary aldosteronism was originally described by J. W. Conn (31) as a syndrome of hypertension associated with hypokalemia and postulated hypersecretion of an endogenous mineralocorticoid. Early cases were due to an aldosterone-producing adrenocortical adenoma, removal of which led to some of the earliest cures of hypertension (32). Primary aldosteronism is most frequently diagnosed in middle-aged adults, is more common in women, and is rare in children.

Earlier reliance on plasma potassium as a screening test, as advocated by some authorities (33), may have led to underrecognition of the contribution of primary aldosteronism to hypertension. An early study, using saline infusion as a screening test for primary aldosteronism reported a frequency of 2.2% of primary aldosteronism among 1036 unselected hypertensives, but a smaller study using the ratio of aldosterone to PRA concentrations in plasma suggested that primary aldosteronism may account for an even greater proportion of hypertension (33–35). The issue of whether we underdiagnose (36) or overdiagnose (37) primary aldosteronism is still highly controversial. There is little question, however, that the current incidence of this disease does not appear to be what was commonly accepted 10–20 years ago- the widely accepted incidence of 1–2% of all hypertensive adults may be closer to 5–10%. This corresponds to the increasing incidence of adrenal incidentalomas; in fact, it appears that a substantial number of patients with normokalemic hypertension have small, aldosterone-producing adrenocortical adenomas (38).

3.1.2 Classification of Aldosteronism

Primary aldosteronism has been traditionally classified on the basis of the presence or absence of an adrenal tumor and responses of aldosterone secretion to posture (34,35). In addition, glucocorticoid-remediable aldosteronism has been diagnosed on the basis of finding that aldosterone hypersecretion could be controlled with the adminstration of dexamethasone in physiological doses and the presence of a family history of hyperaldosteronism (39,40). In approximately 60% of cases, primary aldosteronism is due to an aldosterone-producing adenoma (APA) which is generally unresponsive to posture or angiotensin II infusion, indicating autonomous aldosterone secretion (41) (Fig. 1). At the other end of the spectrum, bilateral nonautonomous overproduction of aldosterone occurs in idiopathic hyperaldosteronism (IHA) (Fig. 2), where aldosterone secretion can be shown to increase in response to upright posture or angiotensin II infusion. This disease (as also shown in Fig. 2) is frequently associated with renal cysts (42). Rarer variants include primary adrenal hyperplasia (PAH), where unilateral autonomous aldosterone secretion occurs without a discrete tumor on gland resection. Also, angiotensin II–responsive aldosterone-producing adenoma represents a significant subset of APA (34,35,41).

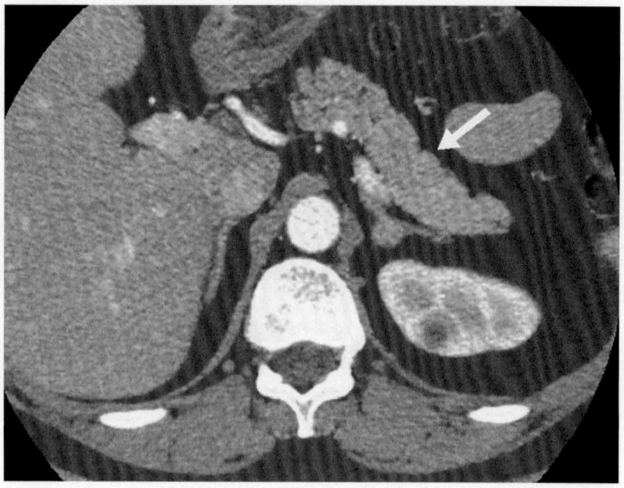

Figure 1 Left-sided adrenocortical adenoma (arrow) in a 49-year-old male patient with primary aldosteronism; unilateral adrenalectomy in this patient led to cure of his hypertension.

3.1.3 Familial Hyperaldosteronism

In 1966, the first familial cases of hypertension due to hyperaldosteronism were reported (39); this autosomal dominant disease came to be known as glucocorticoid-

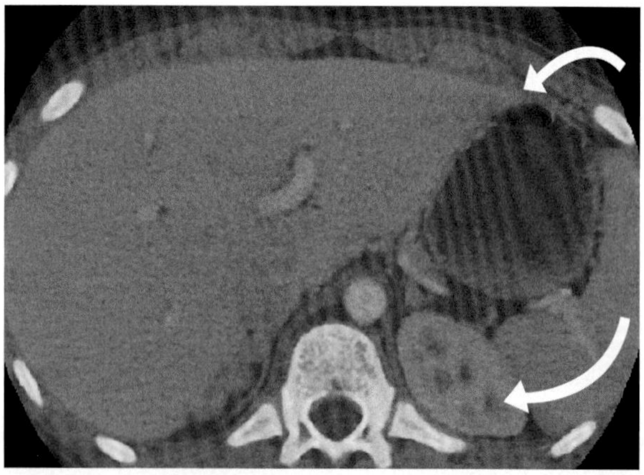

Figure 2 Bilateral adrenocortical hyperplasia (short arrow) in a 12-year-old patient with idiopathic primary aldosteronism; despite the apparent increased nodularity on the left side, adrenal venous sampling showed no ratio between the two glands. This patient is treated medically; he is currently normotensive 5 years after his original diagnosis. Renal cysts (long arrow) commonly associated with primary aldosteronism, are also seen in both kidneys.

remediable aldosteronism (GRA) or familial hyperaldosteronism type I (FH-I) (2,33). This disease is characterized by bilateral adrenal hyperplasia or, rarely, adrenal adenoma (40). GRA accounts for approximately 1% of cases of primary hyperaldosteronism. The genetic locus for this disorder was established by genetic linkage analysis, and the causative mutation was subsequently identified (43). The defect involves a crossover of genetic material between the gene that codes for the enzyme 11-β-hydroxylase (*CYP11B1*) (which catalyzes the last step in cortisol biosynthesis) and the gene for aldosterone synthesis (*CYP11B2*) (43,44). The *CYP11B1* and *CYP11B2* genes are closely located on chromosome 8, and the mutation involves a fusion of a portion of the regulatory region of *CYP11B1*, the ACTH-responsive promoter, with the coding region of the *CYP11B2* gene. Hence, aldosterone synthesis is directed by ACTH, resulting in pathologically high levels of aldosterone and extreme suppressibility of aldosterone by exogenous glucocorticoid administration. Elucidation of this mutation readily explained the cardinal pathophysiological features of the disorder. The synthesis of "hybrid" steroids such as 18-oxocortisol require the action of 17-α-hydroxylase on aldosterone, an enzyme expressed only in the zona fasciculata, suggesting that aldosterone is synthesized in the zona fasciculata in this disorder. Higher blood pressure in the offspring of affected mothers rather than affected fathers has been attributed to the effects of high maternal aldosterone on the fetus rather than imprinting (45,46). Importantly, not all individuals with the GRA mutation have hypertension, and ongoing studies of the physiological and genetic bases of their counterbalancing hypotensive systems are in progress (43–46). The lack of hypokalemia in many subjects with GRA has been related to a blunted aldosterone response to potassium, which may reduce the severity of hyperaldosteronism (47).

Familial hyperaldosteronism type II as a distinct entity was recognized by R. D. Gordon (48,49), although other familial cases of non–dexamethasone-suppressible hyperaldosteronism have also been reported (50,51). To date, 14 families (41 individuals) with FH-II have been identified by the Gordon group (52). The first occurrence of two cases of FH-II in a single family was identified serendipitously, but subsequent cases have been identified by application of the aldosterone: renin ratio screening test and confirmed by full diagnostic testing, and surgery, if indicated. In one large family, with seven affected members, exclusion of involvement of the angiotensin II type I (*AT1*) receptor gene and the *CYP11B2* locus has been performed with genetic linkage analysis (52,53). More recently, a genetic locus on chromosome 7 (7p) for the largest among the families was identified by our group (54); the responsible gene, however, remains elusive.

It should be also be noted also that hyperaldosteronism is also rarely seen in multiple endocrine neoplasia type-1 (MEN 1) (55), and thus the recently identified MEN 1 gene (*menin*) may indeed play some role in *zona glomerulosa* tumorigenesis.

Other familial cases of primary aldosteronism have also been reported, and they are reviewed elsewhere (56).

3.1.4 Diagnosis

The decision to screen for hyperaldosteronism is often prompted by the finding of hypokalemia in a hypertensive patient; whether hypokalemia is spontaneous or thiazide-associated, it is suspicious for hyperaldosteronism and should be investigated. The coexistence of both hypertension and hypokalemia predicts primary aldosteronism in 50% of cases (2,57,58). Hypertension and hypokalemia in the remaining cases indicate renovascular hypertension due to fibromuscular hyperplasia in the younger patient or atherosclerotic disease in older individuals. Although the hypertension in these cases is aldosterone-mediated, PRA is not suppressed. Other causes of hypertension and hypokalemia are presented in Table 1. Among the other endocrine causes of hypertension, screening for the presence of pheochromocytoma should comprise a search for symptoms such as headaches, palpitations, and sweating and measurement of plasma and urinary catecholamines and their metabolites, especially metanephrines (see chapter on Pheochromocytoma).

Screening for primary aldosteronism can be performed with the aldosterone:renin ratio, obtained under random conditions with respect to sodium intake (2,34,35). Values obtained in the upright position (standing for 2h) have greater sensitivity than supine tests. It should be noted that patients should be normokalemic, because low potassium can suppress aldosterone secretion. A ratio of plasma aldosterone (ng/dL) to plasma renin activity (ng/mL/h) of >20 with a plasma aldosterone >15 ng/dL is highly suggestive of primary aldosteronism.

The ratio of plasma aldosterone to PRA (ARR) was first described as a screening test for primary aldosteronism in 1981, and recent studies have confirmed its diagnostic accuracy (2,57,58). The principle is that, as aldosterone secretion rises, PRA, a measure of the rate of production of angiotensin I from endogenous angiotensinogen in ex vivo testing should fall because of sodium retention. This negative feedback response should occur when the aldosterone is supraphysiological for that individual patient, and hence PRA may fall well before plasma aldosterone is clearly increased.

The most important factors that interfere with the diagnostic reliability of the ARR test are drugs and renal impairment. Although a recent study suggested that discontinuation of antihypertensive medications may not be necessary prior to the work-up for primary aldosteronism (59), a wider investigation of this proposal is needed prior to its general application in all patients with this disease and hypertension. This is because β-blockers can reduce PRA levels leading to a falsely elevated ratio; dihydropyridine calcium antagonists can reduce aldosterone levels tending to lead to a falsely normal ratio in some patients with primary aldosteronism; diuretics tend to induce secondary aldosteronism; and, finally, spironolactone, an aldosterone receptor antagonist, can raise plasma renin levels.

We generally recommend that spironolactone and diuretics should be witheld for 6 weeks before testing (this may not be necessary or applicable in all patients; other centers recommend a much shorter, if any, washout time), and β-blockers and dihydropyridine calcium antagonists should be witheld for several days. We then usually control the patients' blood pressure with diltiazem during testing. It should also be noted that renal impairment can lead to a high aldosterone/renin ratio in patients without primary aldosteronism as fluid retention suppresses PRA and hyperkalemia stimulates aldosterone secretion.

After a positive screening test, subsequent testing is directed at (1) confirming aldosterone secretory autonomy and (2) determining if the patient is likely to have an APA, which can be treated surgically, or IHA, in which case medical treatment is indicated. The possibility of GRA, which accounts for approximately 1% of primary aldosteronism, should be kept in mind.

3.1.5 Confirmatory Tests for the Diagnosis of Primary Aldosteronism

Autonomous aldosterone secretion can be confirmed by the saline infusion test (60,61). Other tests described include the measurment of urine aldosterone excretion during oral salt loading or the fludrocortisone suppresion test (62). All tests rely on the principle that a lack of suppression of aldosterone excretion with intravascular expansion is indicative of autonomous aldosterone production. The saline infusion test is performed by infusing 2 L of isotonic saline over 4 hours. Plasma aldosterone and cortisol are measured before and at the end of infusion. A fall in plasma aldosterone to <10 ng/dL occurs in those without primary aldosteronism. Plasma aldosterone values of >10 ng/dL confirm primary aldosteronism. For several patients with other evidence supportive of primary aldosteronism, a response between 5 and 10 ng/dL may not be considered negative, and the test may be repeated. Cortisol levels are taken to exclude an ACTH-related rise in aldosterone. Consideration should be given to the risks of fluid expansion or hypokalemia in susceptible patients.

The oral salt loading test consists of administering 12 g sodium chloride tablets and ad libitum diet for 3 days followed by a 24-hour urinary aldosterone measurement (60,61). Values above 10–14 μg/day with urine sodium excretion >250 nmol/day are considered diagnostic of primary aldosteronism. The fludrocortisone suppression test utilizes fludrocortisone (0.1 mg q6h) and salt loading (63); this test is less frequently used today.

The captopril test, which is based on the principle that inhibition of angiotensin II production should not affect autonomous secretion of aldosterone in primary aldosteronism, has also been used for screening (64,65). Application of the 60-minute aldosterone/renin ratio after 25 mg oral captopril yielded a sensitivity of 100% and specificity of 83% for diagnosis of primary aldosteronism, but the test was only marginally better than baseline values (64). Somewhat lower sensitivity was noted in a larger study using aldosterone and PRA 90 minutes after a 50 mg dose of captopril (65).

3.1.6 Differential Diagnosis Between Adenoma and Other Forms of Primary Aldosteronism

The unique steroid production profile of an APA is used for its identification (66). The following tests are useful to differentiate between an APA and other forms of primary aldosteronism: postural testing, serum 18-hydroxycorticosterone, adrenal CT, and adrenal venous sampling.

Postural testing is best performed after overnight recumbency. An intravenous catheter is inserted at 7 a.m. and baseline aldosterone, cortisol, and PRA are obtained at 8 a.m. After 2 hours of ambulation, repeat aldosterone, cortisol, and PRA are obtained. Typically APAs are angiotensin II-unresponsive, and a fall in aldosterone over 2 hours parallels the reduction of circadian ACTH and cortisol release. A rise (or no significant change) in aldosterone is seen in IHA. Cortisol levels are used to validate the test, since a rise in cortisol release suggests an ACTH surge, which invalidates the test. Diagnostic accuracy of 85% is reported (66).

Levels of 18-hydroxycorticosterone are elevated (>100 ng/dL) in APA and lower than this value in IHA. Although a diagnostic accuracy of 82% is reported (66), it has been noted that 18-hydroxycorticosterone levels parallel the severity of aldosteronism: levels of aldosterone and clinical severity are greater in APA than IHA.

Adrenal computed tomography (CT) is 70% sensitive in detecting APAs (67). Mean APA size was 1.8 cm in one large series; however 19% of these tumors were smaller than 1 cm (67,68). As adrenal incidentalomas are also common in older adults, adrenal CT is adjunctive and cannot be used to direct adrenalectomy without other confirmatory data (67). This also true for magnetic resonance imaging (MRI) of the adrenal glands; use of MRI may also be complicated by motion in the retroperitoneal area.

Adrenal venous sampling requires considerable skill; the right adrenal vein drains directly into the inferior cava and can be difficult to catheterize (67). This test can, however, be performed on an outpatient basis. Infusion of ACTH into a peripheral vein (50 μg/h, starting 30 min before sampling) masks the effects of confounding ACTH peaks during sampling. Venography is avoided to reduce the risk of adrenal hemorrhage. Comparison of aldosterone/cortisol ratios in the adrenal veins and the inferior vena cava allows detection of unilateral or bilateral sources of aldosterone hypersecretion. The cut-off for lateralization is controversial; both 5:1 and 10:1 have been advocated (67,68); everything >10:1 is consistent with unilateral secretion. Thus, adrenal venous sampling is the gold standard for differential diagnosis for primary aldosteronism.

Adrenal scintigraphy has insufficient diagnostic accuracy for routine use (68).

Other causes of primary aldosteronism that have been identified include adrenal carcinoma (69) and extra-adrenal aldosterone secretion such as from ovarian and renal tumors. The rapid changes of an adrenocortical mass upon serial imaging and/or additional hormonal steroid secretion should prompt investigation for cancer and or tumors in other organs.

3.1.7 Variants of Primary Aldosteronism

Two forms of unilateral aldosterone hypersecretion are recognized: angiotensin II–responsive APA and primary adrenal hyperplasia. Angiotensin II–responsive APA exhibits a rise in aldosterone with upright posture but lateralizes with adrenal vein sampling. Primary adrenal hyperplasia does not respond to upright posture but lateralizes on adrenal vein sampling, and pathological changes of micronodular or macronodular hyperplasia are seen (34,35,68).

In cases of bilateral aldosterone secretion, or when the diagnosis is suspected on the basis of family history, GRA can be excluded with a 4-day dexamethasone suppression test (0.5 mg q6h). The aldosterone and renin levels can be measured before, at 2 days, and 4 days of suppression testing. The typical response in patients without GRA is for the aldosterone levels to fall by approximately 50% and return to normal levels by the end of testing, but persistent suppression of aldosterone levels to <4 ng/dL are also reported in GRA. The test achieves a sensitivity of 92% and specificity of 100% for the diagnosis of GRA compared to direct genetic testing (70). Biochemically unique markedly elevated levels of 18-oxo-cortisol and 18-hydroxy-cortisol (>100 nmol/dL) are also observed in GRA (70). Today, the hybrid gene mutation that causes GRA can be identified by Southern blotting or a long-PCR technique (71,72).

3.1.8 Treatment

All patients need to have blood pressure and potassium levels controlled pre-operatively (72). Assuming proper preparation for surgery, the procedure becomes less and less of an issue: today, surgical treatment of an APA may be done laparoscopically (73–76), a procedure that can be performed on an outpatient basis (77). Transcatheter arterial ablation with high-concentration ethanol injection of APA in 18 patients has also been reported (78).

What is clearly an issue is the effectiveness of surgical therapy. Removal of an adrenal lesion by adrenalectomy often does not result in normotension, although it improves blood pressure control and restores normokalemia in most patients (79,80). Transient postoperative hypoaldosteronism is common; however, immediate post-operative declines in blood pressure may not be sustained. In a recent study of 93 patients with primary aldosteronism who underwent adrenalectomy, normotension without the use of any medications was achieved in only 33% of the patients. Negative family history and easier control of the hypertension preoperatively were the two most important factors that predicted cure after surgery. Other such factors included young age and short duration of the disease (79). On the other hand, changes in heart and kidney function and/or cardiac and renal vasculature were predictors of pure response of blood pressure to surgery. Thus, persistent hypertension despite control of hyperaldosteronism may be due to preexistent essential hypertension and/or long-term secondary vascular effects of hyperaldosteronism. Finally, occasionally another cause of secondary hypertension may be present: both pheochromocytoma (81,82) and renal artery stenosis (83) have been reported to coexist with an APA.

Control of hypertension in GRA can be achieved by treatment with physiological doses of dexamethasone (48,49,72). GRA is associated with intracranial aneurysm and hemorrhagic stroke, and screening for intracranial aneurysm in patients with proven GRA has been recommended (49). Normalization of urinary steroid levels and abolition of ACTH-dependent aldosterone production is not necessary in patients with GRA; doses of 0.125 to 0.25 mg of dexamethasone/day are usually adequate for hypertension control and do not lead to Cushinoid features (84).

Medical therapy for primary aldosteronism may be the preferred mode of treatment for IHA. Control of hypokalemia and hypertension in IHA can be achieved with spironolactone (100–400 mg/d) or amiloride (5–30 mg/d), but additional antihypertensives are often needed in this patient group (72,85).

REFERENCES

1. Jackson RV, Laffery A, Torpy DJ, Stratakis CA. New genetic insights in familial hyperaldosteronism. Ann NY Head Sci 2002; 970:77–88.
2. Torpy DJ, Stratakis CA, Chrousos GP. Hyper- and hypoaldosteronism. Vitam Horm 1999; 57:177–216.
3. McKenna TJ, Island DP, Nicholson WE, Liddle GW. The effect of potassium on early and late steps in aldosterone biosynthesis in cells of the zona glomerulosa. Endocrinology 1978; 141:103.
4. Clyne CD, Zhang Y, Slutsker L, Mathis JM, White PC, Rainey WE. Angiotensin II and potassium regulate human CYP11B2 transcription through common cis-elements. Mol Endocrinol 1997; 11:638–649.
5. Brown JJ, Davies DL, Lever AF. Variations in plasma renin concentration in several physiological and pathological states. Can Med Assoc J 1964; 90:201–205.
6. Blair-West JR, Coughlin JP, Denton DA. A dose response comparison of the actions of angiotensin II and III in sheep. J Endocrinol 1980; 87:409.
7. Kono T, Oseko F, Ikeda F, et al. Biological activity of des-asp ileu^8-angiotensin II (ileu^8-angiotensin 3) in man. J Clin Endocrinol Metab 1976; 43:940.
8. Carey RM. Acute dopaminergic inhibition of aldosterone secretion is independent of angiotensin II and adrenocorticotropin. J Clin Endocrinol Metab 1982; 54: 463–469.
9. Kapas S, Hinson JP. Adrenomedullin in the adrenal. Microsc Res Tech 2002; 57:91–97.
10. Hinson JP, Puddefoot JR, Kapas S. Actions of vasoactive intestinal peptide on the rat adrenal zona glomerulosa. J Endocrinol 1999; 161:51–57.
11. Cantin M, Genest J. The heart and artrial natriuretic factor. Endocrinol Rev 1985; 6:107.
12. McKenna TJ, Island DP, Nicholson WE, Liddle GW. Dopamine inhibits angiotensin stimulated aldosterone biosynthesis in bovine adrenal cells. J Clin Invest 1979; 64: 247.
13. David JO, Freeman RH. Mechanisms regulating renin release. Physiol Rev 1976; 56:1.
14. Gordon RD, Kuchel O, Liddle GW, Island DP. Role of the sympathetic nervous system in regulating renin and aldosterone production. J Clin Invest 1967; 46:598.
15. Whorton AR, Lazar JD, Smigel MD, Oates JA. Prostaglandins and renin release: III. Effects of PGE1, E2 F2 alpha and D2 on renin release from rabbit renal cortical slices. Prostaglandins 1981; 22:455–468.
16. Muller J, Lauber M. Regulation of aldosterone biosynthesis: a continual challenge. Am J Hypertens 1991; 4: 280–282.
17. Muller J. Final steps of aldosterone biosynthesis: molecular solution of a physiological problem. J Steroid Biochem Mol Biol 1993; 45:153–159.
18. Curnow KM, Tusie-Luna MT, Pascoe L, Natarajan R, Gu JL, Nadler JL, White PC. The product of the CYP11B2 gene is required for aldosterone biosynthesis in the human adrenal cortex. Mol Endocrinol 1991; 5: 1513–1522.
19. Russell DW, White PC. Four is not more than two. Am J Hum Genet 1995; 57:1002–1005.
20. Taymans SE, Pack S, Pak E, Torpy DJ, Zhuang Z, Stratakis CA. Human CYP11B2 (aldosterone synthase) maps to chromosome 8q243. J Clin Endocrinol Metab 1998; 83:1033–1036.
21. Funder JW. Aldosterone and mineralocorticoid receptors: orphan questions. Kidney Int 2000; 57:1358–1363.
22. Sheppard KE, Funder JW. Equivalent affinity of aldosterone and corticosterone for type I receptors in kidney and hippocampus: direct binding studies. J Steroid Biochem 1987; 28:737–742.
23. Funder JW. Apparent mineralocorticoid excess. Endocrinol Metab Clin North Am 1995; 24:613–621.
24. Losel RM, Feuring M, Falkenstein E, Wehling M. Nongenomic effects of aldosterone: cellular aspects and clinical implications. Steroids 2002; 67:493–498.
25. Dotsch J, Hohenberger I, Peter M, Sippell W, Dorr HG. Evidence for change of 11beta-hydroxysteroid dehydrogenase activity during infancy and childhood. Pediatr Res 2000; 48:697–700.
26. Lashansky G, Saenger P, Dimartino-Nardi J, Gautier T, Mayes D, Berg G, Reiter E. Normative data for the steroidogenic response of mineralocorticoids and their precursors to adrenocorticotropin in a healthy pediatric population. J Clin Endocrinol Metab 1992; 75:1491–1496.
27. Gaunt R. Action of adrenal steroids on electrolyte and

water metabolism. In: Christy NP, ed. The Human Adrenal Cortex. New York: Harper & Row, 1971:373.
28. McKenna TJ, Sequeira SJ, Heffernan A, Chambers J, Cunningham S. Diagnosis under random conditions of all disorders of the renin-angiotensin-aldosterone axis, including primary hyperaldosteronism. J Clin Endocrinol Metab 1991; 73:952–957.
29. Lim PO, Jung RT, MacDonald TM. Is aldosterone the missing link in refractory hypertension?: aldosterone-to-renin ratio as a marker of inappropriate aldosterone activity. J Hum Hypertens 2002; 16:153–158.
30. Moneva MH, Gomez-Sanchez CE. Pathophysiology of adrenal hypertension. Semin Nephrol 2002; 22:44–53.
31. Conn JW. Primary aldosteronism, a new clinical syndrome. J Lab Clin Med 1955; 45:3–17.
32. Conn JW, Knopf RF, Nesbit RM. Clinical characteristics of primary aldosteronism from an analysis of 145 cases. Am J Surg 1964; 107:159–172.
33. Gordon RD, Stowasser M, Tunny TJ, Klemm SA, Rutherford JC. High incidence of primary hyperaldosteronism in 199 patients referred with hypertension. Clin Exp Pharmacol Physiol 1994; 21:315–418.
34. Biglieri EG. Primary aldosteronism. Curr Ther Endocrinol Metab 1997; 6:170–172.
35. Young WF Jr. Primary hyperaldosteronism: update on diagnosis and treatment. Endocrinologist 1997; 7:213–221.
36. Gordon RD, Stowasser M, Rutherford JC. Primary aldosteronism: are we diagnosing and operating on too few patients? World J Surg 2001; 25:941–947.
37. Padfield PL. Primary aldosteronism, a common entity? The myth persists. J Hum Hypertens 2002; 16:159–162.
38. Bernini G, Moretti A, Argenio G, Salvetti A. Primary aldosteronism in normokalemic patients with adrenal incidentalomas. Eur J Endocrinol 2002; 146:523–529.
39. Sutherland DJA, Ruse JC, Laidlaw JC. Hypertension increased aldosterone secretion and low plasma renin activity relieved by dexamethasone. J Can Med Assoc 1966; 95:1109–1119.
40. Pascoe L, Jeunemaitre X, Lebrethon MC, Curnow KM, Gomez-Sanchez CE, Gasc JM, Saez JM, Corvol P. Glucocorticoid-suppressible hyperaldosteronism and adrenal tumors occurring in a single French pedigree. J Clin Invest 1995; 96:2236–2246.
41. Melby JC. Diagnosis of hyperaldosteronism. Endocrinol Metab Clin North Am 1991; 20:247–255.
42. Torres VE, Young WF Jr, Offord KP, Hattery RR. Association of hypokalemia, aldosteronism, and renal cysts. N Engl J Med 1990; 322:345–351.
43. Lifton RP, Dluhy RG, Powers M, Rich GM, Cook S, Ulick S, Lalouel JM. A chimaeric 11-hydroxylase/aldosterone synthase gene causes glucocorticoid-remediable aldosteronism and human hypertension. Nature 1992; 355:262–265.
44. White PC. Abnormalities of aldosterone synthesis and action in children. Curr Opin Pediatr 1997; 9:424–430.
45. Jamieson A, Slutsker L, Inglis GC, Fraser R, White PC, Connell JM. Glucocorticoid suppressible hyperaldosteronism: effects of cross-over site and parental origin of chimaeric gene on phenotypic expression. Clin Sci 1995; 88: 563–570.
46. Gates LJ, MacConnachie AA, Lifton RP, Hartes NE, Benjamin N. Variation of phenotype in patients with GRA. J Med Genet 1996; 33:25–28.
47. Litchfield WR, Coolidge C, Silva P. Impaired potassium-stimulated aldosterone production: a possible explanation for normokalemic glucocorticoid-remediable aldosteronism. J Clin Endocrinol Metab 1997; 82:1507–1510.
48. Stowasser M, Gordon RD, Tunny TJ, Klemm SA, Finn WL, Krek AL. Familial hyperaldosteronism type II: five families with a new variety of primary hyperaldosteronism. Clin Exp Pharmacol Physiol 1992; 19:319–322.
49. Gordon RD, Stowasser M, Klemm SA, Tunny TJ. Primary aldosteronism—some genetic, morphological, and biochemical aspects of subtypes. Steroids 1995; 60:35–41.
50. London N, Swales J, Hollinrake K, Bell P, Heagerty A. Familial Conn's syndrome. Postgrad Med J 1992; 68: 976–977.
51. Greco RG, Carroll JE, Morris DJ, Grekin RJ, Melby JC. Familial hyperaldosteronism, not suppressed by dexamethasone. J Clin Endocrinol Metab 1982; 55: 1013–1016.
52. Torpy DJ, Gordon RD, Lin JP, Huggard PR, Taymans SE, Stowasser M, Chrousos GP, Stratakis CA. Familial hyperaldosteronism type-II: description of a large kindred and exclusion of the aldosterone synthase (CYP11B2) gene. J Clin Endocrinol Metab 1998; 83: 3214–3218.
53. Torpy DJ, Gordon RD, Stratakis CA. Linkage analysis of familial hyperaldosteronism type II—absence of linkage to the gene encoding the angiotensin II receptor type 1. J Clin Endocrinol Metab 1998; 83:1046–1047.
54. Lafferty AR, Torpy DJ, Stowasser M, Taymans SE, Lin JP, Huggard P, Gordon RD, Stratakis CA. A novel genetic locus for low renin hypertension: familial hyperaldosteronism type II maps to chromosome 7 (7p22). J Med Genet 2000; 37:831–835.
55. Beckers A, Abs R, Willems PJ. Aldosterone secreting adenomas as part of multiple endocrine neoplasia type 1 (MEN 1): loss of heterozygosity for polymorphic chromosome 11 deoxyribonucleic acid markers, including the MEN 1 locus. J Clin Endocrinol Metab 1992; 75: 564–570.
56. Stowasser M, Gordon RD. Familial hyperaldosteronism. J Steroid Biochem Mol Biol 2001; 78:215–229.
57. Hiramatsu K, Yamada T, Yukimura Y, Komiya I, Ichikawa K, Ishihara M, Nagata H, Izumiyama T. A screeening test to identify aldosterone-producing adenoma by measuring plasma renin activity. Results in hypertensive patients. Arch Intern Med 1981; 141:1589–1593.

58. Ignatowska-Switalska H, Chodakowska J, Januszewicz W, Feltynowski T, Adamczyk M, Lewandowski J. Evaluation of plasma aldosterone to plasma renin activity ratio in patients with primary aldosteronism. J Hum Hypertens 1997; 11:373–378.
59. Gallay BJ, Ahmad S, Xu L, Toivola B, Davidson RC. Screening for primary aldosteronism without discontinuing hypertensive medications: plasma aldosterone-renin ratio. Am J Kidney Dis 2001; 37:699–705.
60. Holland OB, Brown H, Kuhnert L, et al. Further evaluation of saline for the diagnosis of primary aldosteronism. Hypertension 1984; 6:717–723.
61. Kem DC, Weinberger MH, Mayes DM, Nugent CA. Saline suppression of plasma aldosterone in hypertension. Arch Intern Med 1971; 128:380–386.
62. Young WF Jr, Klee GG. Primary aldosteronism: diagnostic evaluation. Endocrinol Metab Clin North Am 1988; 17:367–395.
63. Lund JO, Nielsen MD. Fludrocortisone suppression test in normal subjects, in patients with essential hypertension and in patients with various forms of aldosteronism. Acta Endocrinol (Copenh) 1980; 93:100–107.
64. Hambling C, Jung RT, Gunn A, Browning MC, Bartlett WA. Re-evaluation of the captopril test for the diagnosis of primary hyperaldosteronism. Clin Endocrinol (Oxf) 1992; 36:499–503.
65. Iwaoka T, Umeda T, Naomi S, Inoue J, Sasaki M, Yamauchi J, Sato T. The usefulness of the captopril test as a simultaneous screening for primary aldosteronism and renovascular hypertension. Am J Hypertens 1993; 6:899–906.
66. Ulick S, Blumenfield JD, Atlas SA, Wang JZ, Vaughan ED Jr. The unique steroidogenesis of the aldosteronoma in the differential diagnosis of primary aldosteronism. J Clin Endocrinol Metab 1993; 76:873–878.
67. Doppman JL, Gill JR Jr. Hyperaldosteronism: sampling the adrenal veins. Radiology 1996; 198:309–312.
68. Litchfield WR, Dluhy RG. Primary aldosteronism. Endocrinol Metab Clin North Am 1995; 24:593–612.
69. Dixon AN, Bing RF. Two cases of adrenocortical carcinoma presenting as Conn's syndrome. J Hum Hypertens 2001; 15:75–79.
70. Litchfield WR, New MI, Coolidge C, Lifton RP, Dluhy RG. Evaluation of the dexamethasone suppression test for the diagnosis of glucocorticoid-remediable aldosteronism. J Clin Endocrinol Metab 1997; 82:3570–3573.
71. Jonsson JR, Klemm SA, Tunny TJ, Stowasser M, Gordon RD. A new genetic test for familial hyperaldosteronism type 1 aids in the detection of curable hypertension. Biochem Biophys Res Comm 1995; 207: 565–571.
72. Blumenfield JD, Sealy JE, Schlussel Y, et al. Diagnosis and treatment of primary aldosteronism. Ann Intern Med 1994; 121:877–885.
73. Weisnagel SJ, Gagner M, Breton G, Pomp A, Pharand D, Lacroix A. Laparoscopic adrenalectomy. Endocrinologist 1996; 6:169–178.
74. Rutherford JC, Stowasser M, Tunny TJ, Klemm SA, Gordon RD. Laparoscopic adrenalectomy. World J Surg 1996; 20:758–760.
75. Gill IS. The case for laparoscopic adrenalectomy. J Urol 2001; 166:429–436.
76. Naya Y, Nagata M, Ichikawa T, Amakasu M, Omura M, Nishikawa T, Yamaguchi K, Ito H. Laparoscopic adrenalectomy: comparison of transperitoneal and retroperitoneal approaches. BJU Int 2002; 90:199–204.
77. Edwin B, Raeder I, Trondsen E, Kaaresen R, Buanes T. Outpatient laparoscopic adrenalectomy in patients with Conn's syndrome. Surg Endosc 2001; 15:589–591.
78. Inoue H, Nakajo M, Miyazono N, Nishida H, Ueno K, Hokotate H. Transcatheter arterial ablation of aldosteronomas with high-concentration ethanol: preliminary and long-term results. Am J Roentgenol 1997; 168:1241–1245.
79. Sawka AM, Young WF, Thompson GB, Grant CS, Farley DR, Leibson C, van Heerden JA. Primary aldosteronism: factors associated with normalization of blood pressure after surgery. Ann Intern Med 2001; 25(135):258–261.
80. Fukudome Y, Fujii K, Arima H, Ohya Y, Tsuchihashi T, Abe I, Fujishima M. Discriminating factors for recurrent hypertension in patients with primary aldosteronism after adrenalectomy. Hypertens Res 2002; 25:11–18.
81. Gordon RD, Bachmann AW, Klemm SA, et al. An association of primary aldosteronism and adrenaline-secreting pheochromocytoma. Clin Exp Pharmacol Physiol 1994; 21:219–222.
82. Nguyen HLT, Luong KVQ. Coexistence of primary aldosteronism and pheochromocytoma in a Vietnamese patient. Endocrinologist 1996; 6:490–493.
83. Stowasser M, Gordon RD, Klemm SA, Tunny TJ. Renin-aldosterone response to dexamethasone in glucocorticoid-suppressible hyperaldosteronism is altered by coexistent renal artery stenosis. J Clin Endocrinol Metab 1993; 77: 800–804.
84. Stowasser M, Buchmann AW, Huggard PR, Rossetti TR, Gordon RD. Treatment of familial hyperaldosteronism type I: only partial suppression of ACTH required to corect hypertension. J Clin Endocrinol Metab 2000; 85:3313–3318.
85. Lim PO, Young WF, MacDonald TM. A review on the medical treatment of primary aldosteronism. J Hypertens 2001; 19:353–361.

35

Adrenal Incidentalomas

David C. Aron

Case Western Reserve University School of Medicine and Louis Stokes Department of Veterans Affairs Medical Center, Cleveland, Ohio, U.S.A.

Job Kievit

Leiden University Medical Center, Leiden, The Netherlands

1 INTRODUCTION

The discovery of an adrenal mass in the course of abdominal imaging performed for other reasons, "adrenal incidentaloma," is a common clinical problem that poses a challenging management dilemma (1). This dilemma arises because while most incidentalomas will be clinically insignificant benign and hormonally inactive adenomas that neither pose a risk to a patient's health nor warrant the risks of further diagnosis and treatment, there may be some lesions that do pose a significant risk, either because of their hormonal activity or because of their malignant histology. The challenge is to recognize and treat these few, while leaving the others alone. As imaging techniques improve and their use becomes more widespread, we can expect to encounter this challenge more frequently. Over the years a myriad of approaches has been recommended: strategies for hormonal screening, radiological testing, and histopathological examination. However, even after a commissioned systematic review of the literature and a consensus conference sponsored by the National Institutes of Health, controversies remain and the medical decisions are laced with uncertainty (2,3).

2 THE MAGNITUDE OF THE PROBLEM

What is the magnitude of this management dilemma? The question is difficult to answer, in part due to lack of standard definitions, and in part due to variability in methods and circumstances of detection; incidentaloma is not so much a disease entity as it is a finding that may or may not represent disease (2). Different authors have varied in strictness as to what constitutes an adrenal incidentaloma. Most agree on the fact that it is a mass discovered by imaging done for reasons other than suspected adrenal pathology. Differences of opinion do exist about exclusion criteria, such as the known presence of extra-adrenal cancer, or the fact that the complaints setting off the diagnostic imaging later turn out to be caused by the adrenal mass after all. The prevalence of incidentaloma, however defined, will vary depending upon the circumstances under which these lesions are detected—both the methods of detection and the reasons for the imaging study. For example, the prevalence of clinically inapparent adrenal masses found at autopsy is about 2.1%, but "clinically inapparent" is in the eye of the beholder. Prevalence estimates range from about 0.1% for general health screening with ultrasound, to 0.4–1.9% among patients evaluated for nonendocrinologic complaints, to more than 4% among patients who have a previous cancer diagnosis (2). The prevalence of adrenal incidentalomas, increases with age.

The differential diagnosis of an incidentally discovered mass is extensive (Table 1), but most are nonsecreting cortical adenomas. In the recent systematic review that combined studies using the broadest definitions, adenomas accounted for 41%, metastases 19%, adrenocortical carcinoma 10%, myelolipoma 9%, and pheochromocytoma 8%, with other, mostly benign lesions comprising the remainder (2). Self-evidently, such percentages will change as other inclusion and exclusion criteria are applied, i.e., metastases becoming far less common if patients with known extra-adrenal cancer are excluded. The distribution of etiologies varies by size of the lesion; larger tumors are more likely to be malignant than smaller ones. Among lesions larger than 6 cm, adrenal carcinomas comprised 25% and metastases 18%, while adenomas accounted for only 18% (2). When bilateral adrenal masses are found, which occurs in about 10–15% of cases, several diagnoses are more likely. These include metastatic disease, congenital adrenal hyperplasia, lymphoma, infection (e.g., tuberculosis, fungal), hemorrhage, adrenocorticotropic hormone (ACTH)-dependent Cushing's syndrome, pheochromocytoma, amyloidosis, and infiltrative disease of the adrenal glands.

Table 1 Differential Diagnosis of an Incidentally Discovered Adrenal Mass

Adrenal cortical tumors
Adenoma[a]
Carcinoma[a]
Nodular hyperplasia[a]
Adrenal medullary tumors
Pheochromocytoma[a]
Ganglioneuroma/neuroblastoma[a]
Other adrenal tumors
Myelolipoma
Metastases
Miscellaneous, e.g., hamartoma, teratoma, lipoma, hemangioma
Infections, granulomas, infiltrations
Abscess
Amyloidosis
Fungal infection, e.g., histoplasmosis, coccidiomycosis, blastomycosis, tuberculosis
Sarcoidosis
Cytomegalovirus
Cysts and pseudocysts
Parasitic
Endothelial
Degenerative adenomas
Congenital adrenal hyperplasia[a]
Hemorrhage
Pseudoadrenal masses
Splenic, pancreatic, renal lesions
Vascular lesions (especially aneurysms and tortuous splenic veins)
Technical artifacts

[a] Potentially functional.

3 DEMOGRAPHICS AND GENETIC RISK FACTORS

The prevalence of adrenal incidentalomas identified at autopsy increases from <1% among individuals less than 30 years of age to about 7% in those 70 years of age or older (2). There appear to be no gender differences in prevalence from autopsy studies or general health exams. Patients with clinical features associated with functioning adrenal lesions (e.g., primary hyperaldosteronism, pheochromocytoma, Cushing's syndrome, and virilization) are more likely to have adrenal tumors. Although in many cases these features are subtle and do not prompt early diagnosis, whether one should consider these lesions to be "incidental" is controversial.

Although the molecular pathogenesis of adrenal tumors has not been elucidated, these mechanisms are under active investigation (4). A variety of rare genetic syndromes predispose to adrenocortical tumors: Beckwith-Wiedemann, Li-Fraumeni, multiple endocrine neoplasia (MEN) 1, Carney complex, and McCune-Albright syndromes. Similarly some syndromes predispose to adrenomedullary tumors: multiple endocrine neoplasia 2, von Hippel-Lindau disease, and neurofibromatosis type 1. Because of their rarity and obvious clinical characteristics, they are not diagnosed after the finding of an incidentaloma. Nevertheless, some of the molecular targets for these syndromes have been isolated. Understanding these targets may be relevant to the more typical sporadic adrenal incidentaloma and lead to better diagnostic, therapeutic, and preventive measures (4). For example, overexpression of the insulin-like growth factor II (IGF II) gene has been associated with the tumors of the Beckwith-Wiedemann syndrome. Germline mutations in the p53 tumor suppressor gene contribute to the high cancer risk (breast carcinoma, soft tissue and bone sarcoma, brain tumor, leukemia, and adrenocortical carcinoma) in the autosomal dominant Li-Fraumeni syndrome. Adrenal cancer is a very unusual presentation of this unusual syndrome. Abnormalities in the RET-2 proto-oncogene have been associated with pheochromocytoma in MEN 2. However, at the end of the day, while the risks for harboring an adrenal mass remain to be elucidated, the major risk factor for being diagnosed with adrenal incidentaloma is clear: undergoing an imaging procedure that includes the abdomen.

4 CLINICAL FEATURES—CLASSIC AND SUBTLE PHENOTYPIC EXPRESSIONS

A patient with an incidental adrenal mass is susceptible to three types of adverse outcomes: endocrinological or oncological morbidity, mortality, and anxiety from knowing about a tumor that might cause problems in the future (1,5). Hypersecretion of glucocorticoids, mineralocorticoids, sex steroids, or catecholamines produces clinical syndromes, each associated with morbidity and premature mortality. The clinical features associated with Cushing's syndrome, primary hyperaldosteronism, virilization, and pheochromocytoma are addressed in other chapters in this volume and elsewhere. More germane to the management of patients with adrenal incidentalomas is the potential morbidity and mortality of subclinical autonomous cortisol secretion and "silent" pheochromocytoma.

Subclinical autonomous glucocorticoid hypersecretion, sometimes misleadingly termed subclinical Cushing's syndrome, has been found in 5–20% of patients with adrenal incidentalomas (6–11). This autonomous hypersecretion is subtle and may be transient. Differences in prevalence relate to, among other things, lack of standardized criteria for the diagnosis (2). Yet, although by definition overt Cushing's syndrome must be absent, these patients have a high prevalence of obesity, hypertension, and diabetes and insulin resistance. Abnormalities in bone turnover and bone mass have been reported (12–17). Tauchmanova et al. (18) used the criteria of the National Italian Group on Adrenal Tumors. In addition to the absence of clinical signs of cortisol excess these include two abnormalities in the regulation of the hypothalamic-pituitary-adrenal axis: failure to suppress serum cortisol to less than 83 nmol/L (3 μg/dL) by a 2 mg dexamethasone suppression test and the combination of a low-ACTH, high–urinary free cortisol, and diminished response to corticotropin-releasing hormone. This study involved 28 consecutive patients and 100 age-, and sex-, and body mass index–matched controls. They found that systolic and diastolic blood pressures were higher in patients, as were fasting glucose, insulin, total cholesterol, and triglycerides. In addition to elevated insulin resistance, the patients had increased waist-to-hip ratios and high frequencies of hypertension (61%), lipid abnormalities (71%), and impaired glucose tolerance or diabetes (64%); 85% had multiple cardiovascular risk factors. Evidence of cardiovascular disease was present in a high proportion of patients based on clinical evidence, electrocardiogram, or carotid ultrasound examination. Whether these findings will have impact on long-term morbidity of patients with subclinical autonomous cortisol hypersecretion remains to be determined. However, these metabolic abnormalities may improve after removal of the adrenal incidentaloma. In the continuum from normal cortisol-ACTH feedback to autonomous cortisol production, the stage at which cortisol autonomy results in clinical morbidity is not clear. Tsagarakis et al. (19) performed dexamethasone suppression tests in 61 patients with incidentally detected adrenal masses. In a post hoc analysis patients were divided into three groups: patients with a post dexamethasone level of cortisol of >70 nmol/L (group A, $n = 19$), 30–70 nmol/L (group B, $n=27$), and <30 nmol/L (group C, $n = 15$) (19). Group A patients had significantly higher cholesterol and triglyceride concentrations than group C patients. In addition, the natural history of patients with subclinical Cushing's syndrome and, specifically, the risk of progression to overt Cushing's syndrome is unclear. Barzon et al. found that among 130 nonoperated patients with a follow-up ≥1 year, there were 8 patients who had subclinical autonomous cortisol secretion at diagnosis and 4 who developed overt Cushing's syndrome after 1–3 years (10,20–22). One of these had autonomous cortisol secretion at first diagnosis. The estimated cumulative risk for a non-secreting adrenal incidentaloma to develop subclinical hyperfunction was 3.8% after 1 year and 6.6% after 5 years and for patients with masses with subclinical autonomous glucocorticoid overproduction, estimated cumulative risk to develop overt Cushing's syndrome was 11% after 1 year and 26% after 5 years.

Although the classic features of pheochromocytoma are well known, many patients lack those features and the diagnosis is readily missed. Among patients with adrenal incidentalomas, about 8% prove to have pheochromocytomas. Among patients referred to the Mayo Clinic for management of adrenal pheochromocytoma, 10% were discovered in the course of evaluation for adrenal incidentalomas (23). These "silent" pheochromocytomas may also be lethal. The most feared diagnostic possibility for an adrenal incidentaloma is adrenal cancer, which has a mean survival of approximately 18 months and 5-year survival of approximately 16% (2,24,25). The clinical manifestations of this disorder are addressed in other chapters in this volume and elsewhere (2). Mercifully, clinically diagnosed cases are rare; the prevalence of adrenal carcinoma in general is approximately 12/1,000,000 (26). However, the relative frequency of adrenal cancer varies considerably among adrenal incidentaloma series: 4.2% in the whole National Italian Study Group (AI-SIE) series, but 25% in another study (27,28). The unknown is also a concern. Anxiety for both patient and physician from knowing about the presence of a mass is also not a trivial concern. All these findings suggest a benefit of presymptomatic diagnosis. However, at the population level the health risk posed by adrenal incidentaloma, though real, is small because of the low prevalence of clinically significant tumors with hormonal activity or malignant potential, and the presence of a nonfunctional adrenal incidentaloma is relatively common.

The adrenal glands are highly vascular organs and therefore common sites of metastases from extra-adrenal malignancy. In patients with a history of malignant disease, metastases are the most common cause of an incidental adrenal mass, regardless of size, accounting for 48% of all incidentalomas in these patients. Carcinomas of the lung, breast, kidney, and gastrointestinal tract and melanoma or lymphoma constitute the most common sources of adrenal metastases (2). In fact, of those who die of epithelial malignancies, adrenal metastases are found in 25–75%. The source of the primary malignancy usually is known when an adrenal incidentaloma is discovered; metastatic cancer presenting as an isolated true adrenal incidentaloma is distinctly unusual. Although adrenal metastases are generally bilateral and larger than 3 cm, they may be unilateral and small.

5 BIOCHEMICAL DIAGNOSIS

Established algorithms exist for the diagnosis of hormonally active adrenal lesions. When patients present with signs or symptoms of these disorders, diagnostic evaluation can proceed apace. However, when patients have few or no signs of a particular disorder, the evaluation is more challenging. Diagnostic test performance characteristics in such patients in actual practice are not known, but they will be less accurate than in patients with clinically apparent disease. Test sensitivity is likely to be lower than in the study population from which the original characteristics were derived (spectrum bias); test specificity is also likely to be lower. Moreover, the absence of gold standards for the diagnosis makes assessment of test characteristics problematic. Finally, predictive value is dependent upon the prevalence of disease. Even a test with high sensitivity and specificity will, when used to detect a rare condition, falsely identify many nonaffected individuals as having the disease. Notwithstanding these limitations, a few studies have evaluated test performance (2). For example, two studies have used unilateral uptake on NP-59 (radio-iodinated cholesterol) scintigraphy as the indicator of autonomous activity of the incidentaloma (29). No single test was found to discriminate well between unilateral and bilateral uptake on scintigraphy. Bardet et al. (29) found that low 8 a.m. dehydro-epiandrosterone sulfate, low 8 a.m. ACTH, basal urinary free cortisol, unsuppressed 8 a.m. serum cortisol after overnight 1 mg dexamethasone suppression, unsuppressed day 2 serum cortisol, and unsuppressed day 2 urinary free cortisol after low-dose dexamethasone suppression had low sensitivity (0–50%) and moderate specificity (79–94%) to differentiate unilateral from bilateral scintigraphy uptake. In contrast, Valli et al. found that unsuppressed 8 a.m. cortisol after overnight dexamethasone suppression had 100% sensitivity and 67% specificity to predict unilateral uptake (30). Studies of diagnosis of catecholamine excess and primary hyperaldosteronism reveal similar problems in sensitivity and specificity. The optimal strategy for biochemical evaluation of a patient with an incidentally discovered adrenal mass is unclear and remains controversial (see below). Regardless of the approach used, it should be tailored to what is available; tests should be chosen based on their performance characteristics in the laboratories actually used.

6 SERUM MOLECULAR MARKERS

A variety of tissue molecular markers have been used to distinguish malignant from benign adrenal tumors and determine prognosis. These include mutant p53, the proliferation-associated antigen Ki67 protein, loss of heterozygosity at the 17p13 and 11p15 loci, and overexpression of the insulin-like growth factor (IGF) II gene and other IGF system products such as IGF-binding protein 2 (4,31). Serum levels of IGF-binding protein 2 have been assessed as a tumor marker (32). Boulle et al. found no significant difference in plasma IGFBP-2 concentration between healthy controls and patients with complete remission or localized tumors (32). In contrast, patients with metastatic disease had significantly higher IGFBP-2 plasma levels than the control group ($p < 0.001$). IGFBP-2 levels in patients with metastatic disease were inversely correlated with survival ($R^2 = 0.308$; $p = 0.0026$). However, the overall sensitivity and specificity of this test were low; five patients (17.8%) with metastatic tumors had normal IGFBP-2 levels, and two patients (13.3%) in complete remission had high plasma IGFBP-2 levels, limiting its value in diagnosis and follow-up of adrenocortical carcinoma. In one small study, serum levels of vascular endothelial growth factor (VEGF) were significantly higher in patients with malignant incidentalomas than in those with benign ones, and they decreased after surgery (33).

7 IMAGING FOR ADRENAL INCIDENTALOMA

Various imaging methods have been used and advocated for the assessment of adrenal incidentaloma (34). They can be subdivided into purely morphological methods on the one hand and function-based imaging methods on the other. Examples of the first category are ultrasonography, computerized tomographic (CT) scanning, and magnetic resonance imaging (MRI), while the MIBG and NP59 scanning are well-known examples of the latter. The relevance of ultrasonography for adrenal incidentaloma is mainly in its role for detection. As ultrasound scanning is widely used for the assessment of gallbladder pathology, most ultrasound-detected incidentalomas are located in the right adrenal gland. For the diagnostic evaluation of adrenal incidentaloma, ultrasound is of limited use (35). It provides little information about the malignant or benign nature of a mass, and none about its functional status. However, ultrasound data may provide indirect evidence for or against malignancy. Large diameter (as opposed to small), solidity (as opposed to cystic nature), and rapid diameter increase (as opposed to slow growth) can be assessed by ultrasound and may be used as indicators of malignancy (36). However, both CT and MRI outperform ultrasound in their ability to diagnose malignancy.

CT has been used in the assessment of adrenal incidentaloma both to detect malignancy (i.e., to identify those incidentalomas that should be treated) and to identify adenoma (i.e., to identify those insignificant incidentalomas where treatment is not necessary). Large size, irregular shapes, vague contour, invasion into surrounding structures, and high signal intensity have all been used to identify malignancy (9,87). High signal intensity can be expressed in either so-called Hounsfield units (with an intensity higher than 10 or 20 units being used as diagnostic threshold) or in signal-lesion to signal-fat ratio (with SL/SF above 1.5 suggesting malignancy). The threshold used determines the sensitivity and specificity of the test. At low threshold, sensitivity for malignancy is around 0.9 and specificity around 0.4 (38). Higher thresholds lead to better specificity (around 0.9), but at the cost of lower sensitivity (0.55). More recently, excellent results have been claimed for the identification of adenomas by delayed enhanced CT, with sensitivity and specificity of 98% and 92%, respectively (for an overall accuracy of 96%) (39). Further research is needed to corroborate these promising results. A particular application of CT is CT-guided adrenal biopsy (40). Provided that pheochromocytoma has been excluded beforehand, such biopsy may provide a safe and reliable method for assessing the histology of an adrenal incidentaloma. Both cytology and histology provide better results for the detection of metastasis of extra-adrenal malignancy than for the recognition of primary adrenocortical cancer (40–42).

MRI may be used both to differentiate between benign or malignant tumors and to diagnose pheochromocytoma. Accuracy with respect to the first purpose is essentially no better than for CT scan. However, with respect to pheochromocytoma, MRI outperformed CT scanning. High signal intensity on T2-weighted MRI is suggestive for pheochromocytoma, with accuracy originally having been claimed as close to 100% (43,44). However, later studies have corrected this overoptimistic perspective (45). By combining the data of several studies, we estimated the sensitivity and specificity of T2-weighted MRI for pheochromocytoma at around 92% and 88%, respectively (38). If such accuracy were indeed true, this would make T2-weighted MRI more accurate for diagnosing pheochromocytoma than urine-VMA assessment. Examples of CT and MR imaging of adrenal incidentalomas are shown in Figures 1–5.

Of the function-based isotope imaging studies, the two most frequently used are ^{131}I- or ^{123}I-labeled metaiodobenzylguanidine (MIBG) and ^{131}betaiodomethylnorcholesterol (NP-59) (46). MIBG is mainly used to detect pheochromocytoma, while NP-59 has claimed to assess adrenal hormonal function as well as to differentiate between benign and malignant adrenal tumors. MIBG has the advantage over CT or MRI that it provides a whole-body image with the administration of one tracer dose. As pheochromocytoma may occur bilaterally and its occurrence is not confined to the periadrenal region (especially in case of malignant pheochromocytoma with metastases), MIBG may be used for whole-body screening on pheochromocytoma. For pheochromocytoma detection MIBG has sensitivity and specificity of around 87% and 95%, respectively (38). Positive and negative MIBG results therefore change the prior probability of pheochromocytoma in adrenal incidentaloma from 3.5% to around 40% and 0.5%, respectively. Scanning with NP-59 has been advocated as a means to assess adrenal masses (46–50). On the basis of concordant or discordant imaging activity, NP-59 has been claimed to help in the identification of adrenocortical cancer or in identifying hormonally active benign adenomas. The limited available evidence precludes a definitive conclusion about the

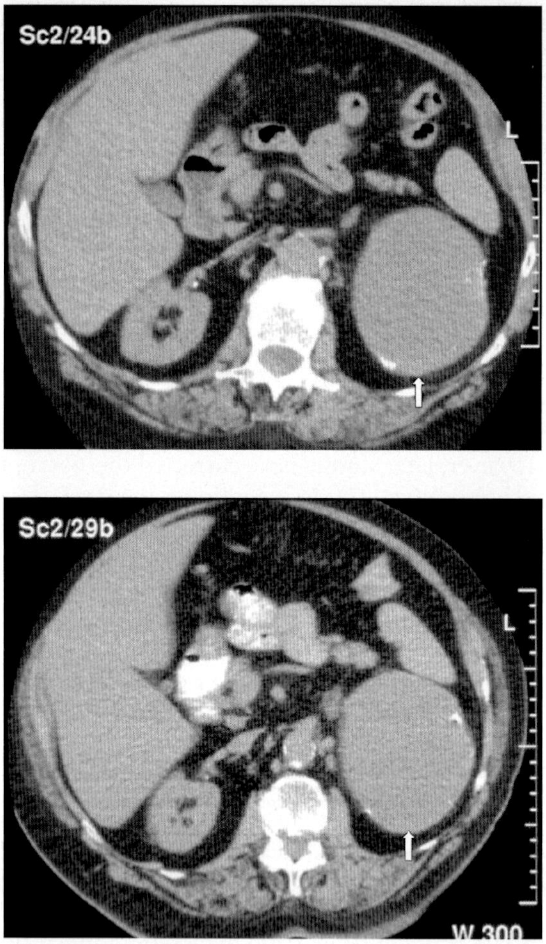

(A)

(B)

Figure 1 Patient B, female, 79 years old with large mass in left adrenal region (11 cm cystic incidentaloma), first seen at ultrasound examination for suspected gallstones. Because of the low suspicion of malignancy and no hormonal activity, physician and patient agreed on follow-up without surgery. The mass was stable over a 2-year period. (A) CT scan showing cystic incidentaloma 11 × 10 × 9.5 cm. (B) CT 2 years later: mass stable at 10.5 × 9 cm.

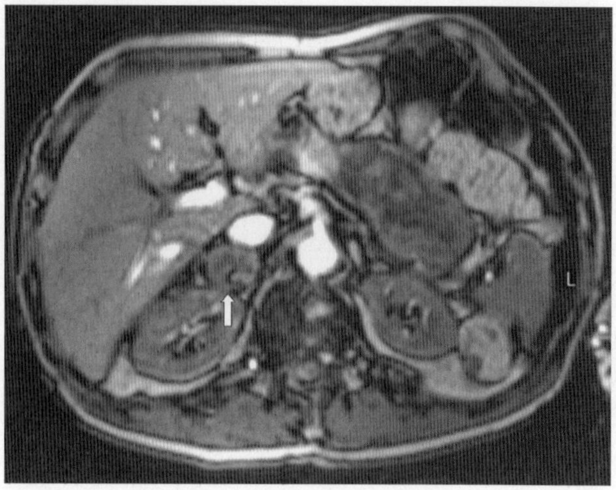

Figure 2 Patient K, male, 75 years old with multiple sclerosis and a 3 cm adrenal mass first seen at imaging for neurological assessment. He was normotensive and urinary catecholamines were not increased. MRI shows a 3 cm mass in right adrenal gland (see arrow), with fluid level, possibly necrosis, not typical for pheochromocytoma, but cystic pheochromocytoma cannot be excluded. A 5 × 3 cm pheochromocytoma was removed laparoscopically. Blood pressure was 150/80 without medication. Final diagnosis: asymptomatic pheochromocytoma.

usefulness of NP-59 in the assessment of adrenal incidentaloma. Apart from these four imaging techniques, others have been described. However, in the absence of convincing evidence for their added value, there is little or no reason to use other tests than the four described above, of which CT scan and MRI are the most commonly used and best documented.

8 DIAGNOSTIC THERAPEUTIC STRATEGIES FOR ADRENAL INCIDENTALOMA

Adrenal incidentaloma is a typical illustration of the fact that incidental findings by their nature pose a considerable threat of overdiagnosis and overtreatment (51). However, some adrenal incidentalomas are clinically significant, and inadvertently leaving them alone might damage the patient's health, not to mention the doctor's professional status. Therefore, detection of an incidentaloma creates a situation where a decision concerning its management has to be taken. Such a decision may range from a most conservative "leave alone" to a most aggressive "take the adrenal gland out right

(A)
(B)
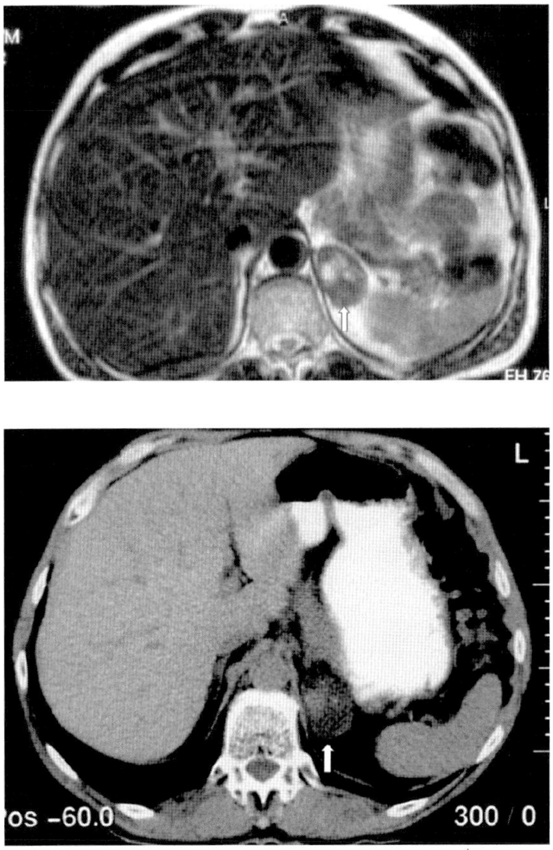

Figure 3 Patient D, male, 48 years old, with hypertension and marginally elevated 24-hour urinary cortisol excretion. (A) MRI: 4 × 3 cm adrenal mass (arrow), no specific characteristics, but consistent with an adenoma. (B) CT one year later: 3 × 4.5 cm mass (arrow). At laparoscopic adrenalectomy, an adenoma 8 × 5 × 2 cm was removed. Conclusion: probable subclinical autonomous cortisol hypersecretion.

away," preceded or not by additional biochemical or radiological assessment. Ideally, this decision is based on a careful weighing of the risks and benefits of each diagnostic and therapeutic step (38).

Many different strategies have been devised to deal with adrenal incidentaloma. Most of them are guided by the aim to elucidate at least two concerns: (1) assessment of function: Could the incidentaloma, in spite of its not being detected on the basis of clinical signs and symptoms, still be hormonally active and thereby pose a threat to the patients health?; and (2) assessment of histological nature: Could the incidentaloma mass itself be a malignant tumor, which, if left alone, will continue to grow and metastasize? The first concern is the reason that all strategies have some form of hormone assessment, focused on either the adrenal medulla (searching for pheochromocytoma), the adrenal cortex (searching for "subclinical Cushing," aldosteronoma, or sex hormone hyperactivity), or both. The second concern is less easily dealt with, as cytology is notoriously less reliable in the differentiation between benign or malignant primary adrenal tumors than for the detection of metastases from extra-adrenal origin in oncology patients (41,42,52). Below we will summarize some of the strategies that have been advocated and briefly assess their similarities and differences.

9 SPECIFIC STRATEGIES

We have translated four well-known strategies into simplified flowcharts and a table (Table 2) (which, by necessity, do not do justice to the complexity and nuances of the approaches) (26). Copeland's approach is among the best known and has been around the longest (Fig. 6) (3,26,53,54). Copeland first addresses diameter as the most easily available information item and one that has a close relationship to the chance of an incidentaloma being malignant. In addition, he proposes extensive hormonal screening. Ross and Aron focused on the hormonal evaluation of the patient with adrenal incidentaloma and clinical features consistent with hormonal hypersecretion rather than on diameter and/or imaging characteristics (Fig. 7) (53). Later advice not only specified diagnostic and therapeutic steps that should be taken at the time of discovery of an adrenal incidentaloma, but also took into account the fact that incidentalomas originally considered clinically insignificant may later turn out to be, or change into, significant disorders (21,22,55). Follow-up could then be used as a means to monitor change in functional activity or as a way to differentiate between malignant and benign lesions on the basis of increase in diameter over time. The strategy proposed by Young is an example of such an approach (Fig. 8) (23). More recently, in 2002, an NIH state-of-the-science conference summarized presently available evidence and issued a statement that advocates another, albeit similar approach (Fig. 9) (3).

10 ASSESSMENT OF STRATEGIES

Each of these strategies is based on the two concerns (potential hormonal activity and malignancy) described

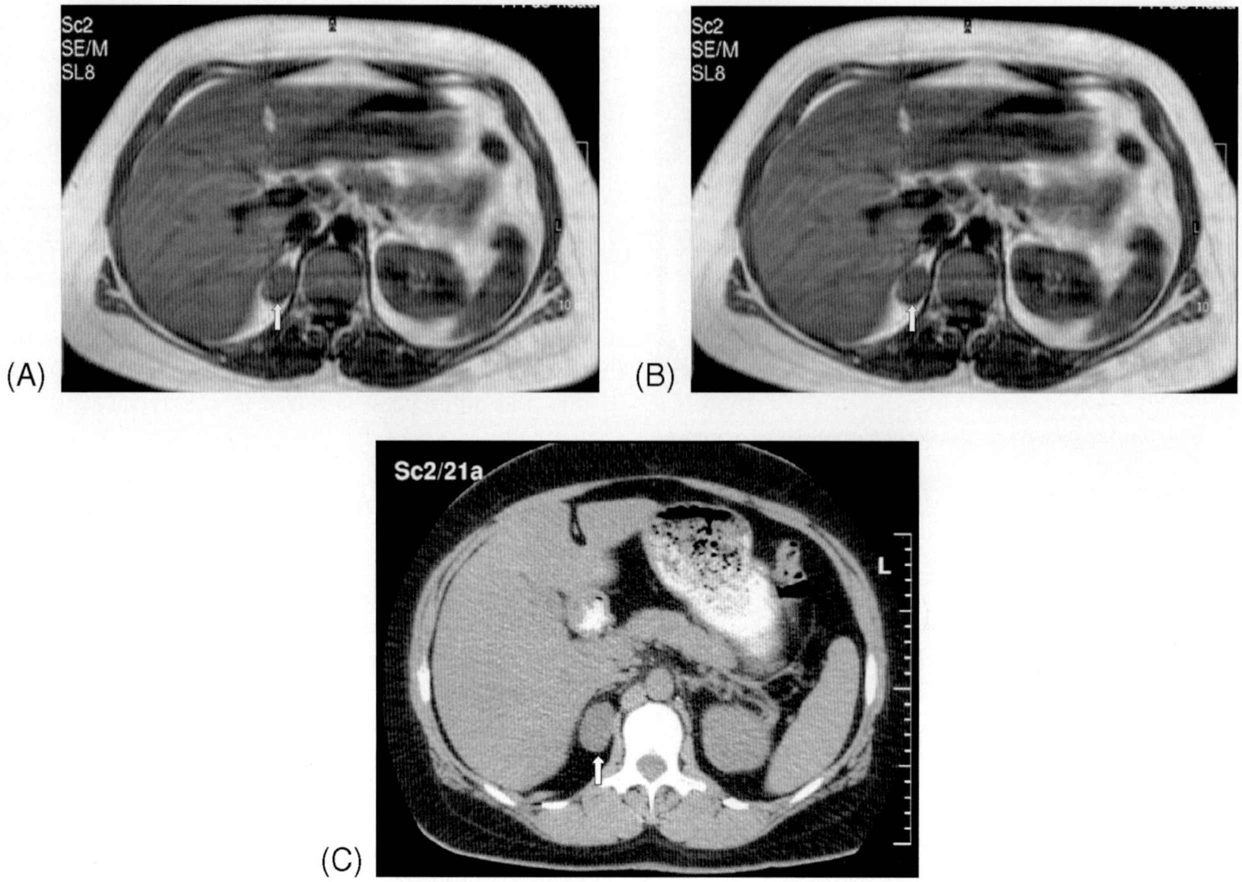

Figure 4 Patient S, female, 37 years old with hypertension and adrenal mass first seen at ultrasound imaging for dyspepsia. (A) MRI: 3 cm mass in right adrenal gland (arrow)—T1-weighted imaging. (B) MRI: 3 cm mass in right adrenal gland (arrow)—T2-weighted imaging; no elevated signal intensity. (C) CT: 3.3 × 2.5 cm mass (arrow), Houndsfield 17–20 U, possible cortical adenoma. Laboratory data showed marginally elevated urinary norepinephrine and dopamine, normal VMA, and marginally elevated cortisol excretion. Dexamethasone suppression test showed inadequate suppression. At laparoscopic adrenalectomy, a radical excision of an adenoma was performed. Final diagnosis: subclinical autonomous cortisol hypersecretion.

earlier. However, they use different instruments and cut-off points to get where they want to go. Assessment of function is done by hormonal analysis in all three strategies. However, they differ in the importance they lend to this step and in the focus they give to cortical and medullary hyperfunction, respectively. Finally, they differ in the specific tests they advise with respect to the function to be performed. Differences between strategies can be traced to three causes: (1) differences in the use of empirical data to assess the probability of different disorders being present; (2) differences in assumptions about diagnostic and therapeutic effectiveness, again traceable to available empirical evidence; and (3) differences in weight that are, either implicitly or explicitly, being attributed to various outcomes.

The first two causes relate to the quality and validity of the information used. Therefore, differences may be reduced or eliminated by using methods from evidence-based medicine to identify the correct underlying information. The third cause is not so easily solved, as it relates to judgment, not evidence. Examples of judgmental issues are the weight that is assigned to missing a relevant disorder, to short- or long-term morbidity and mortality, to life expectancy, quality of life, etc. Even the term "relevant" may be defined in different ways, pertaining to either "posing a severe risk to the patient" or to "where outcome can be affected by diagnosis and

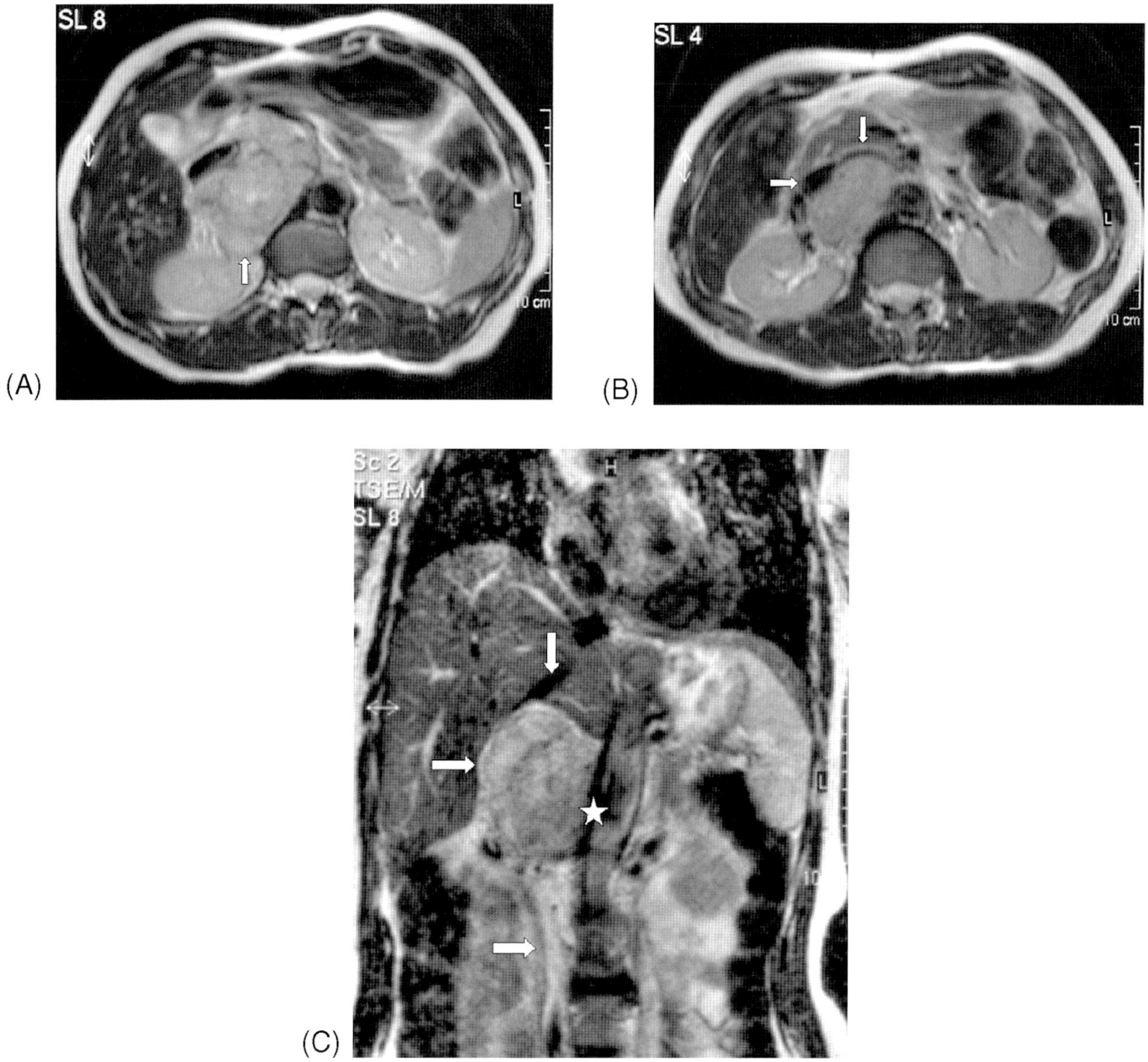

Figure 5 Pat T, female, 52 years old with hypertension (180/110), nonspecific chest pain, and upper abdominal discomfort, for which imaging was performed. (A) MRI (T2-weighted imaging): large 11 × 8 mass in right (peri-)adrenal region (arrow) with low signal intensity. No intravascular growth or other signs of malignancy. (B) MRI (T2-weighted imaging)—: arrows indicate the close relationship between the mass and the left renal vein and inferior vena cava. (C) MRI reconstruction in frontal plane. Arrows indicate relationship with inferior vena cava. The star indicates the aorta. Urinary catecholamines were elevated. Attempt at surgery, introduction of anesthesia has to be terminated because of uncontrollably elevated blood pressure. Two weeks later: successful extended transabdominal adrenalectomy, 12 × 8 × 5 cm pheochromocytoma with local perineural and intravascular growth. Final diagnosis: pheochromocytoma, malignancy cannot be excluded, but patient in excellent health 2 years after surgery.

Table 2 Simplified Summary of the Main Strategies Proposed to Deal with Adrenal Incidentalomas

	Functional assessment		Assessment of benign/malignant nature			
Author (Ref.)	Cortical function	Medullary function	Diameter threshold	Imaging characteristics	Isotope scanning	Fine needle aspiration cytology
Copeland, 1983 (26)	Urinary steroids (various) and 2-day low-dose dexamethasone suppression test	24-hr urinary vanillylmandelic acid, metanephrines, and catecholamines	6 cm	Solid versus cystic	—	Clear vs. bloody
Ross and Aron, 1990 (53)	–	24-hr urinary vanillylmandelic acid, metanephrines, and catecholamines	6 cm	–	–	–
Young, 2000 (54)	Overnight 1 mg dexamethasone suppression test	24-hr urinary vanillylmandelic acid, metanephrines, and catecholamines	4 cm	–	–	For suspected metastases or infection
NIH, 2002 (3)	Overnight 1 mg dexamethasone suppression test	Plasma-free metanephrines	4,6 cm	–	–	For suspected metastases

treatment." An adrenal metastasis is "relevant" in the first sense, but may be considered less relevant or even irrelevant in the second sense because of the impossibility to influence the bad prognosis. For such judgmental differences there are no universal right or wrong answers. The rise of evidence-based medicine is fostering transparency and accountability about the information we use in clinical practice. It is equally valuable to reveal how choices are guided by value judgments concerning process and outcome (38). The combination of best evidence and careful patient-centered value judgment is the key to good clinical practice for adrenal incidentaloma.

11 SURGERY FOR ADRENAL INCIDENTALOMA

Surgery offers the most direct solution to the diagnostic-therapeutic dilemma of an adrenal incidentaloma: tak-

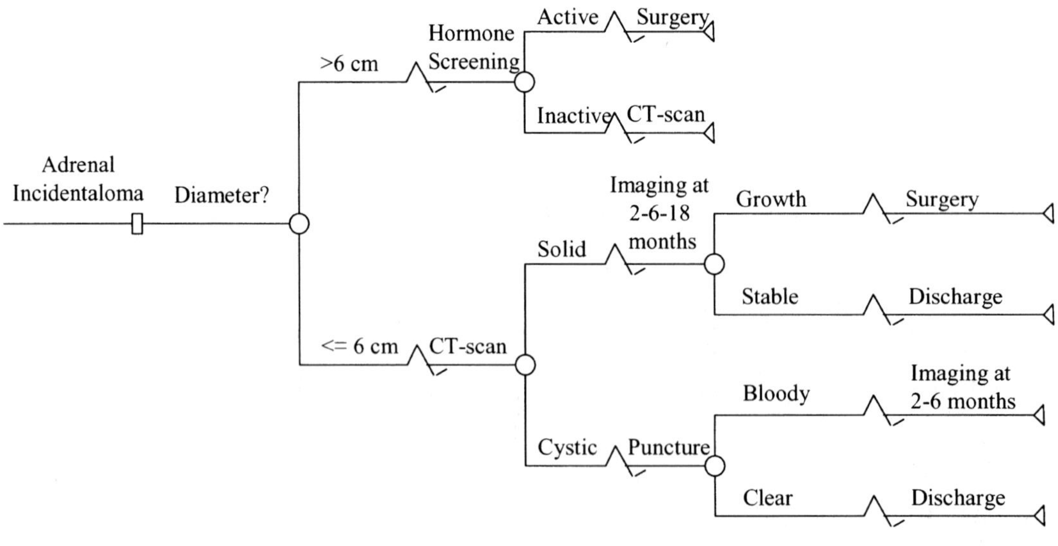

Figure 6 Strategic approach using a size criterion as the initial branch point. Translated into a simplified flowchart from the 1986 paper by Copeland (26).

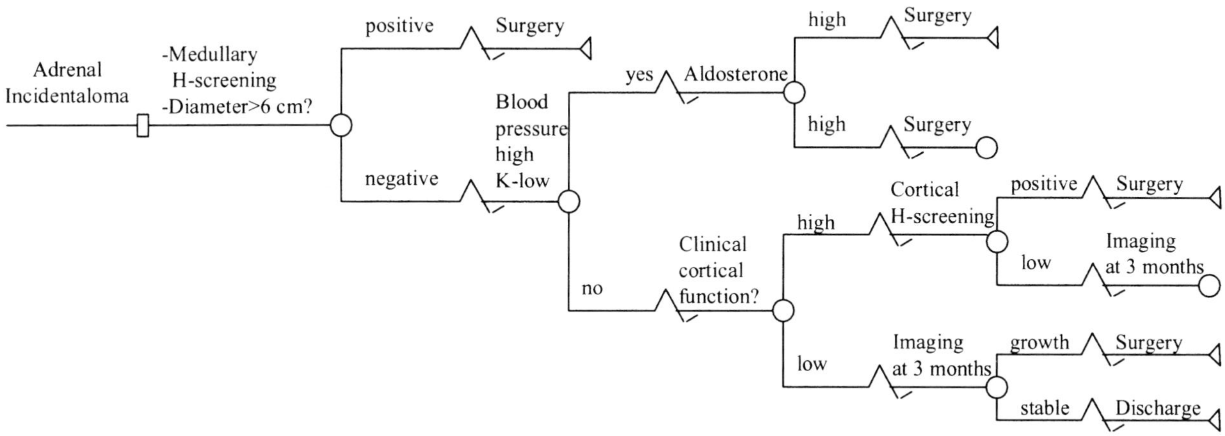

Figure 7 Strategic approach using a size criterion plus biochemical screening for pheochromocytoma as the initial branch point. Translated into a simplified flowchart from the 1990 paper by Ross and Aron (53).

ing out the mass and the adrenal gland both answers the diagnostic question and may offer cure for a disorder that needed treatment. The fact that diagnosis may be uncertain at the time of actual treatment makes surgery for adrenal incidentaloma different from surgery for a nonincidentaloma adrenal mass. Therefore, before surgery is undertaken, careful planning is needed with respect to preoperative, intraoperative, and postoperative management. Preoperative management issues include decisions about hormonal blocking of a suspected pheochromocytoma or of adrenocortical hyperfunction. Concerning intraoperative care, a choice must be taken for a laparoscopic or open surgical approach, depending on both the size and the suspected nature of the incidentaloma. In addition, both surgeon and anesthetist may have to deal with a pheochromocytoma or with a large ingrowing or intravascular growing cancer. Postoperative management includes anticipating upon the consequences of the reduction in stress hormone levels that follows pheochromocytoma-extirpation or the consequences of hormone withdrawal in case of clinical or subclinical autonomous cortisol hypersecretion.

12 PREOPERATIVE MANAGEMENT

Preoperative management ideally achieves maximum certainty concerning the absence or presence of adrenocortical or adrenomedullary hyperfunction. Pheochromocytoma presence, especially if unnoticed and not managed adequately by blockage of the adrenergic system, may increase perioperative risk (56–60). Certainly about pheochromocytoma status is not always easily obtained. Even if careful history taking reveals no pheochromocytoma triad (headache, palpitations, and diaphoresis) and if physical examination demonstrates normotension, this clinical information is insufficient proof of pheochromocytoma absence (61). Positive and negative likelihood ratios are 40 and 0.36, respectively, increasing the probability of a pheochromocytoma

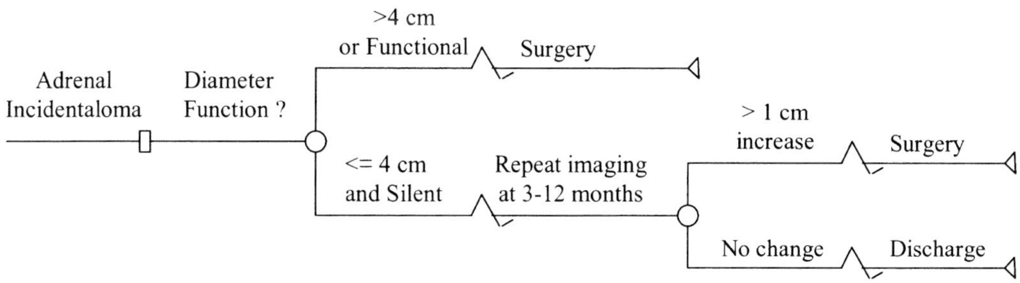

Figure 8 Strategic approach using a size criterion plus hormonal screening for pheochromocytoma, Cushing's syndrome, and hyperaldosteronism as the initial branch point. Translated into a simplified flowchart from the 2000 paper by Young (54).

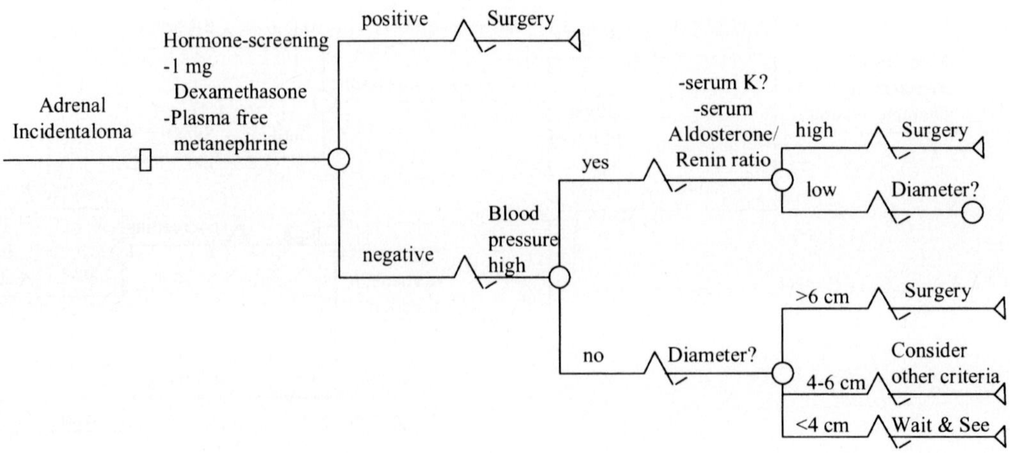

Figure 9 Strategic approach using a size criterion plus hormonal screening for pheochromocytoma, Cushing's syndrome, and hyperaldosteronism as the initial branch point. Translated into a simple flowchart from the 2002 NIH Consensus Panel (3).

from a prior 3.5% to around 60% in case of a positive triad, and reducing it to 1% in case of its absence (and changing from a prior probability of 8% as reported by Lau et al. to either 78% or 3%) (38). Hypertension provides even less reliable information, with positive and negative likelihood ratios of 2 and 0.6 changing the probability of a pheochromocytoma to 7% or 2% in the presence or absence of hypertension (or, again, from 8% to 15% and 5%, respectively). Various diagnostic tests are available to further reduce any clinical uncertainty about pheochromocytoma. High sensitivity maximizes the reliability of a negative test result, while high test specificity maximizes the reliability of a positive test. Hormonal testing for urinary or plasma metanephrines counts among the most reliable tests, with both sensitivity and specificity of around 95% (62,63). Testing for urinary catecholamines or vanillylmandelic acid (VMA) testing is notoriously unreliable, with dangerously low test sensitivities of 80–85% (64). Imaging techniques may be helpful; T2-weighted MRI may be used to demonstrate or exclude pheochromocytoma presence, although the high accuracy of 90–100% that was originally claimed has been challenged by more recent work that found a sensitivity of no more than 65% (44,45). A practical approach for ruling out pheochromocytoma would be a negative plasma or, if such testing were not available, urine metanephrine test, or the combination of a negative 24-hour urine testing for VMA in combination with negative T2-weighted MRI or positive testing for cortical hormonal hyperactivity. Ruling out cortical hyperfunction is likewise important, as hyperfunction of the involved gland (i.e., clinical or subclinical autonomous cortisol hypersecretion), apart from the long-term risks it may pose, might suppress the contralateral adrenal gland and thereby expose the patient to the risk of addisonian crisis after adrenalectomy (6,65). Diagnostic assessment of adrenocortical function is more easily resolved than that of adrenomedullary function, with dexamethasone suppression test being the standard workup for clinical or subclinical autonomous cortisol hypersecretion (66).

13 INTRAOPERATIVE CARE

Surgery for adrenal incidentaloma may pose challenges to both surgeon and anesthetist. Adrenal surgery requires careful tissue handling because of the friability of the adrenal gland and its tendency to easily and persistently bleed. Ideally a no-touch technique is used, "removing the patient from around the adrenal gland" instead of vice versa. Surgery for adrenal incidentaloma is further complicated by diagnostic uncertainty concerning pheochromocytoma or malignancy, making a no-touch technique even more important.

Even without randomized trials, laparoscopic adrenalectomy has rapidly become the standard for all adrenal masses where this approach is technically and medically feasible (67–74). This includes at least all those patients with small and medium-sized (up to 6 cm or more) incidentaloma, where no serious suspicion of malignancy exists. Laparoscopy eliminates the trauma associated with other approaches such as the dorsal lumbar approach or the median laparotomy. The laparoscopic approach may be less ideal for large or (potentially) malignant tumors, or for tumors that are highly vascular and/or have a close relationship to the aorta and/or the vena cava. Different views exist on whether laparoscopy should preferably be performed using a transabdominal or a lateral approach (75,76). The transperitoneal route enables the surgeon to take care of adrenal gland vessels before manipulation of the gland itself starts. However, traversing the abdominal cavity adds the risk of intraoperative intestinal trauma and potential morbidity in the form of postoperative paralytic ileus. A lateral extraperitoneal approach reduces these risks, but may be technically more difficult.

As adrenal tumors may remain asymptomatic for a long time, they may grow to considerable size and may extensively invade adjacent structures such as liver, diaphragm, kidneys, or abdominal wall. In addition, hypervascularity or intravascular growth in (ad)renal vein or vena cava may add to surgical technical complexity. If open surgery is deemed necessary because of size and/or malignant nature of the incidentaloma, several approaches are available (77). For large tumors with suspected ingrowth into surrounding structures such as diaphragm, spleen, or kidney, the thoraco-abdominal flank approach offers maximum access. While a retroperitoneal approach is ideally suited, intraoperative findings may necessitate switching to a transperitoneal approach. Large tumors located on the right side, in particular those that have a close relationship to the vena cava or the aorta, may alternatively be approached using a midline laparotomy. If this is combined with an extended Kocher's maneuver, wide access can be gained to the tumor, the adrenal vessels, as well as the vena cava and aorta (see Fig. 10), with less surgical trauma than with the thoraco-abdominal approach. In rare cases where extensive cardiac involvement is present, sternotomy and extracorporeal circulation may be used as a last resort (78). The dorsal lumbar approach, which was originally used for small to medium-sized benign tumors, has in almost all cases been replaced by laparoscopic adrenalectomy.

Anesthesia for adrenal incidentaloma surgery may likewise be a challenging endeavor. Although adrenalectomy generally can be performed with little or no blood loss, large hypervascular or intravascular growing tumors may create situations where the judicious use of blood (products) aims to prevent the vicious circle of blood loss, clotting disturbances, and additional blood loss. If adrenal tumors invade the vena cava or the right atrium, intraoperative variations in venous return may add to hemodynamic instability. In case of pheochromocytoma, the judicious and responsive intraoperative use of α- or β-adrenergic blockers is a prerequisite for adequate hemodynamic control. All such intraoperative situations can only be handled adequately through close cooperation between surgeon and anesthetist, who are aware of each other's specific needs and problems. Rapid-response reactions from either partner may be needed, with actions on the part of the surgeon being suspended or continued depending on anesthetic need and vice versa. In this sense, adrenal surgery, perhaps more than any other surgery, should be the product of close cooperation between surgeon, anesthetist, and referring internist/endocrinologist.

14 POSTOPERATIVE CARE

In most cases removal of an adrenal incidentaloma is not associated with specific postoperative problems. As with any major operation, general problems may arise such as bleeding, wound infection, or respiratory problems. Typically postoperative bleeding may occur as a retroperitoneal hematoma on the second or third postoperative day, after an essentially bloodless adrenalectomy. In patients with (sub)clinical Cushing, wound complications are more likely to occur than in those without. Specific problems, related to the nature of the adrenal incidentaloma, may arise in hormonally active disorders, being either cortical or medullary tumors. After removal of pheochromocytoma, chronically present vasoconstriction will give way to relative vasodilatation and thus will cause hypotension or overt hypovolemic shock. Replacement of intravascular volume should be performed under the guide of central venous pressure and urine production in an intensive or intermediate care setting. In most cases fluid balance and hemodynamic stability can be restored within 24 hours, with no need for further specific support or monitoring. Steroid-producing tumors (in case of either subclinical or clinical Cushing's syndrome) present a different picture. Removal of the hyperactive ipsilateral gland will leave only the suppressed contralateral adrenal gland to take care of cortical adrenal function. To prevent an addisonian crisis from occurring in such situations, intra- and postoperative substitution is necessary and should be continued for as long as it may take the other gland to fully restore adrenal cortical function. This may take up to a year or more in many cases.

15 PROGNOSIS

The natural history of adrenal incidentalomas is not well established, and observations vary depending on the composition of the study population and the size and pathological classification of the adrenal mass. Follow-up of patients with nonfunctioning adrenal masses suggests that 5–25% of masses increase in size by at least 1 cm and 3–4% decrease in size (2,21,22,55, 79–82). The threshold for clinically significant increase in size is unknown, particularly since the reproducibility of size determination by imaging procedures is unknown. The risk of malignancy is about 1/1000. Up to 20% of patients develop hormone overproduction. Little is known about whether early treatment is beneficial for these conditions before they cause significant symptoms, although the unpredictable lethality of pheochromocytoma and the insidious nature of the impact of the high cardiovascular risk associated with subclinical autonomous cortisol hypersecretion strongly suggest that early treatment would be beneficial. Masses greater than or equal to 3 cm are more likely to develop hyperfunction compared to smaller tumors.

The long-term prognosis of surgically treated benign adenomas causing catecholamine, cortisol or aldosterone excess appears to be reasonably good. Of note is the improvement in cardiovascular risk factors such as hypertension, hyperglycemia, and hypercholesterolemia after removal of an adrenal incidentaloma associated with subclinical autonomous cortisol hypersecretion. However, the immediate outcomes depend upon the quality of the operative and perioperative care. Especially relevant are the issues of the learning curve and the relationship between volume of procedures and outcome (83,84). For example, Fahlenkamp et al. described the experience with laparoscopic urological surgery (including but not limited to adrenalectomy) at four German centers (85). There were a total of 2407 such procedures. For the first 100 procedures, the complication rate was 13.3%, but for subsequent procedures the rate was 3.6%. Similarly, Catarci et al. reported on 1006 cases and found a complication rate of 6% for the first 50 cases and 1.9% for the rest (86). The existence of a learning curve for these complex procedures should not be surprising, and the poor initial outcomes from laparoscopic cholecystectomy should serve as a cautionary tale.

For those patients found to have adrenal gland metastases, prognosis is defined by the primary tumor—histology, grade, stage, and site. Approximately 25% of masses greater than 6 cm in diameter are adrenal cortical carcinomas, and these patients have very poor clinical outcomes. Among a large series of studies of adrenal cancer (usually not presenting as incidentalomas), 5-year survival ranged from 19 to 62% with a median of 34% (2). There is some evidence suggests that surgical extirpation of adrenal cancer at stage 1 or 2 may improve the survival rate.

16 SUMMARY AND CONCLUSIONS

The optimal strategy for evaluation of a patient with an incidentally discovered adrenal mass remains controversial. The quality of the data upon which such decisions are made remains imperfect, to say the least. We lack the randomized (or even nonrandomized) trials that would go a long way toward resolving the controversies. Even in the unlikely event that such trials were carried out, they would take years to yield results. Moreover, individual preferences are likely to be critical in such decision making. Review of the literature supports the view that such patients are at somewhat increased risk of morbidity and mortality, and this implies a benefit of early diagnosis for at least for some of the disorders. Our ability to accurately determine clinically those at increased risk among the vast majority who are not at increased risk is poor. We therefore rely on biochemical and radiological diagnostic tests, which have their own limitations. Subjecting patients to unnecessary testing and treatment carries its own set of risks. The diagnostic process itself may contribute considerable anxiety, expense, and, if invasive, cause pain and other morbidity. The harm that occurs as false-positive results are pursued has been termed the "cascade effect." We must avoid the pitfalls of overestimation of disease prevalence while taking advantage of the benefits of therapy resulting from advances in diagnostic imaging. In the meantime, we must use our best clinical judgment based upon the best available evidence to ensure that we maximize the benefit to those patients with adrenal incidentalomas who have clinically significant adrenal disorders and minimize the harm to those who do not.

REFERENCES

1. Aron DC. Endocrine incidentalomas. Endocrinol Metab Clin North Am 2002; 29:1–238.
2. Lau J, Balk E, Rothberg M, Ioannidid JPA, DeVine D, Chew P, Kupelnick B, Miller K. Management of Clinically Inapparent Adrenal Mass. AHRQ Publication No. 02-E014. Rockville, MD: Agency for Healthcare Research and Quality. Evidence Report/Technology Assessment, Number 56.
3. NIH Consensus Panel. NIH State of the Science Conference on the Management of the Clinically Inapparent Adrenal Mass, 2002.
4. Koch CA, Pacak K, Chrousos GP. The molecular

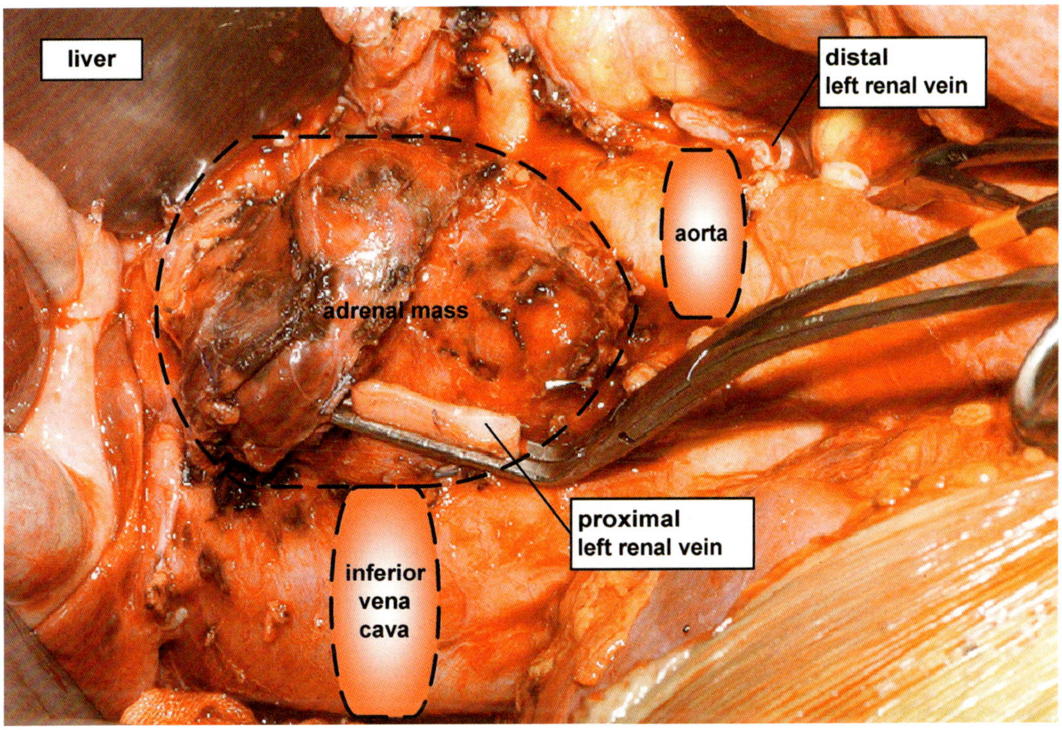

Figure 10 Intraoperative view (as seen from the right ventral side) of a large adrenal incidentaloma extending from the right adrenal gland behind the inferior vena. The tumor has its maximum diameter between the aorta and the inferior vena cava, pressing these two apart and thereby stretching the left adrenal vein and artery. To gain better access to the tumor, the right colon was mobilized upward, and the left adrenal vein was divided between clamps (with reanastomosis at the end of the operation). Histology demonstrated a pheochromocytoma with angioinvasive and perineural growth.

pathogenesis of hereditary and sporadic adrenocortical and adrenomedullary tumors. J Clin Endocrinol Metab 2002; 87:5367–5384.

5. Aron DC. The adrenal incidentaloma: disease of modern technology and public health problem. Rev Endocr Metab Disord 2001; 2:335–342.
6. Reincke M. Subclinical Cushing's syndrome. Endocrinol Metab Clin North Am 2000; 29:43–56.
7. Reincke M, Nieke J, Krestin GP, Saeger W, Allolio B, Winkelmann W. Preclinical Cushing's syndrome in adrenal "incidentalomas": comparison with adrenal Cushing's syndrome. J Clin Endocrinol Metab 1992; 75:826–832.
8. Terzolo M, Osella G, Ali A, Borreta G, Cesario F, Paccotti P, Angeli A. Subclinical Cushing's syndrome in adrenal incidentaloma. Clin Endocrinol (Oxf) 1998; 48:89–97.
9. Angeli A, Osella G, Ali A, Terzolo M. Adrenal incidentaloma: an overview of clinical and epidemiological data from the National Italian Study Group. Horm Res 1997; 47:279–283.
10. Barzon L, Boscaro M. Diagnosis and management of adrenal incidentalomas. J Urol 2000; 163:398–407.
11. Rossi R, Tauchmanova L, Luciano A, Di Martino M, Battista C, Del Viscovo L, Nuzzo V, Lombardi G. Subclinical Cushing's syndrome in patients with adrenal incidentaloma: clinical and biochemical features. J Clin Endocrinol Metab 2000; 85:1440–1448.
12. Tauchmanova L, Rossi R, Nuzzo V, del Puente A, Esposito-del Puente A, Pizzi C, Fonderico F, Lupoli G, Lombardi G. Bone loss determined by quantitative ultrasonometry correlates inversely with disease activity in patients with endogenous glucocorticoid excess due to adrenal mass. Eur J Endocrinol 2001; 145:241–247.
13. Torlontano M, Chiodini I, Pileri M, Guglielmi G, Cammisa M, Modoni S, Carnevale V, Trischitta V, Scillitani A. Altered bone mass and turnover in female patients with adrenal incidentaloma: the effect of subclinical hypercortisolism. J Clin Endocrinol Metab 1999; 84:2381–2385.
14. Midorikawa S, Sanada H, Hashimoto S, Suzuki T, Watanabe T. The improvement of insulin resistance in patients with adrenal incidentaloma by surgical resection. Clin Endocrinol (Oxf) 2001; 54:797–804.
15. Terzolo M, Pia A, Ali A, Osella G, Reimondo G, Bovio S, Daffara F, Procopio M, Paccotti P, Borretta G, Angeli A. Adrenal incidentaloma: a new cause of the metabolic syndrome? J Clin Endocrinol Metab 2002; 87:998–1003.
16. Chiodini I, Tauchmanova L, Torlontano M, Battista C, Guglielmi G, Cammisa M, Colao A, Carnevale V, Rossi R, Di Lembo S, Trischitta V, Scillitani A. Bone involvement in eugonadal male patients with adrenal incidentaloma an dsubclinical hypercortisolism. J Clin Endocrinol Metab 2002; 87:5491–5494.
17. Francucci CM, Pantanetti P, Garrapa GG, Massi F, Arnaldi G, Mantero F. Bone metabolism and mass in women with Cushing's syndrome and adrenal incidentaloma. Clin Endocrinol (Oxf) 2002; 57:587–593.
18. Tauchmanova L, Rossi R, Biondi B, Pulcrano M, Nuzzo V, Palmieri E-A, Fazio S, Lonbardi G. Patients with subclinical Cushing's syndrome due to adrenal adenoma have increased cardiovascular risk. J Clin Endocrinol Metab 2002; 87:4872–4878.
19. Tsagarakis S, Roboti C, Kokkoris P, Vasiliou V, Alevizaki C, Thalassinos N. Elevated post-dexamethasone suppression cortisol concentrations correlate with hormonal alterations of the hypothalamo-pituitary adrenal axis in patients with adrenal incidentalomas. Clin Endocrinol 1998; 49:165–171.
20. Barzon L, Scaroni C, Sonino N, Fallo F, Gregianin M, Macri C, Boscaro M. Incidentally discovered adrenal tumors: endocrine and scintigraphic correlates. J Clin Endocrinol Metab 1998; 83:55–62.
21. Barzon L, Scaroni C, Sonino N, Fallo F, Paoletta A, Boscaro M. Risk factors and long-term follow-up of adrenal incidentalomas. J Clin Endocrinol Metab 1999; 84:520–526.
22. Barzon L, Fallo F, Sonino N, Boscaro M. Development of overt Cushing's syndrome in patients with adrenal incidentaloma. Eur J Endocrinol 2002; 146:61–66.
23. Young WF Jr. Management approaches to adrenal incidentalomas. A view from Rochester, Minnesota. Endocrinol Metab Clin North Am 2000; 29:159–185, x.
24. Boscaro M, Fallo F, Barzon L, et al. Adrenocortical carcinoma: epidemiology and natural history. Minerva Endocrinol 1995; 20:89–94.
25. Icard P, Chapuis Y, Andreis M, et al. Adrenocortical carcinoma in surgically treated patients: a retrspective study on 156 cases by the French Association of Endocrine Surgery. Surgery 1992; 112:972–979.
26. Copeland PM. The incidentally discovered adrenal mass. Ann Intern Med 1983; 98:940–945.
27. Mantero F, Terzolo M, Arnaldi G, Osella G, Masini AM, Ali A, Giovagnetti M, Opocher G, Angeli A. A survey on adrenal incidentaloma in Italy. Study Group on Adrenal Tumors of the Italian Society of Endocrinology. J Clin Endocrinol Metab 2000; 85:637–644.
28. Terzolo M, Ali A, Osella G, Mazza E. Prevalence of adrenal carcinoma among incidentally discovered adrenal masses. A retrospective study from 1989 to 1994. Gruppo Piemontese Incidentalomi Surrenalici. Arch Surg 1997; 132:914–919.
29. Bardet S, Rohmer V, Murat A, Guillemot C, Marechaud R, Chupin M, Lecomte P, Simon D, Delemer B, Schneebelli S, Beutter D, Jacquin V, Peltier P, Charbonnel B. 1311-6 Beta-iodomethylnorcholesterol scintigraphy: an assessment of its role in the investigation of adrenocortical incidentalomas. Clin Endocrinol (Oxf) 1996; 44:587–596.
30. Valli N, Catargi B, Ronci N, Vergnot V, Leccia F, Ferriere JM, Chene G, Grenier N, Laurent F, Tabarin A. Biochemical screening for subclinical cortisol-secreting

adenomas amongst adrenal incidentalomas. Eur J Endocrinol 2001; 144:401–408.
31. Gicquel C, Bertagna X, Gaston V, Coste J, Louvel A, Baudin E, Bertherat J, Chapuis Y, Duclos JM, Schlumberger M, Plouin PF, Luton JP, Le Bouc Y. Molecular markers and long-term recurrences in a large cohort of patients with sporadic adrenocortical tumors. Cancer Res 2001; 61:6762–6767.
32. Boulle N, Baudin E, Gicquel C, Logie A, Bertherat J, Penfomis A, Bertagna X, Luton JP, Schlumberger M, Le Bouc Y. Evaluation of plasma insulin-like growth factor binding protein-2 as a marker for adrenocortical tumors. Eur J Endocrinol 2002; 144:29–36.
33. Kolomecki K, Stepien H, Bartos M, Kuzdak K. Usefulness of VEGF, MMP-2, MMP-3 and TIMP-2 serum level evaluation in patients with adrenal tumours. Endocr Regul 2001; 35:9–16.
34. Dunnick NR, Korobkin M. Imaging of adrenal incidentalomas: current status. AJR Am J Roentgenol 2002; 179:559–568.
35. Suzuki Y, Sasagawa, Suzuki H, Izumi T, Kaneko H, Nakada T. The role of ultrasonography in the detection of adrenal masses: comparison with computed tomography and magnetic resonance imaging. Int Urol Nephrol 2001; 32:303–306.
36. Fontana D, Porpiglia F, Destefanis P, Fiori C, Ali A, Terzolo M, Osella G, Angeli A. What is the role of ultrasonography in the follow-up of adrenal incidentalomas? The Gruppo Piemontese Incidentalomi Surrenalici. Urology 1999; 54:612–616.
37. Lumachi F, Zucchetta P, Marzola MC, Bui F, Casarrubea G, Angelini F, Favia G. Usefulness of CT scan, MRI and radiocholesterol scintigraphy for adrenal imaging in Cushing's syndrome. Nucl Med Commun 2002; 23:469–473.
38. Kievit J, Haak HR. Diagnosis and treatment of adrenal incidentaloma. A cost-effectiveness analysis. Endocrinol Metab Clin North Am 2000; 29:–69ix.
39. Caoili EM, Korobkin M, Francis IR, Cohan RH, Platt JF, Dunnick NR, Raghupathi KI. Adrenal masses: characterization with combined unenhanced and delayed enhanced CT. Radiology 2002; 222:629–633.
40. Mesurolle B, Ariche-Cohen M, Tardivon A, Gilles R, Couanet D, Vanel D. Retrospective analysis of 44 adrenal puncture biopsies under x-ray computed tomographic guidance. J Radiol 1996; 77:17–21.
41. Heaston DK, Handel DB, Ashton PR, Korobkin M. Narrow gauge needle aspiration of solid adrenal masses. AJR Am J Roentgenol 1982; 138:1143–1148.
42. Montali G, Solbiati L, Bossi MC, De Pra L, Di Donna A, Ravetto C. Sonographically guided fine-needle aspiration biopsy of adrenal masses. AJR Am J Roentgenol 1984; 143:1081–1084.
43. van Erkel AR, van Gils AP, Lequin M, Kruitwagen C, Bloem JL, Falke TH. CT and MR distinction of adenomas and nonadenomas of the adrenal gland. J Comput Assist Tomogr 1994; 18:432–438.
44. van Gils AP, Falke TH, van Erkel AR, Arndt JW, Sandler MP, van der Mey AG, Hoogma RP. MR imaging and MIBG scintigraphy of pheochromocytomas and extraadrenal functioning paragangliomas. Radiographics 1991; 11:37–57.
45. Varghese JC, Hahn PF, Papanicolaou N, Mayo-Smith WW, Gaa JA, Lee MJ. MR differentiation of phaeochromocytoma from other adrenal lesions based on qualitative analysis of T2 relaxation times. Clin Radiol 1997; 52:603–606.
46. Kurtaran A, Traub T, Shapiro B. Scintigraphic imaging of the adrenal glands. Eur J Radiol 2002; 41:123–130.
47. Francis IR, Smid A, Gross MD, Shapiro B, Naylor B, Glazer GM. Adrenal masses in oncologic patients: functional and morphologic evaluation. Radiology 1988; 166: 353–356.
48. Gross MD, Shapiro B, Shreve P. Radionuclide imaging of the adrenal cortex. Q J Nucl Med 1999; 43:224–232.
49. Kao CH, Liao SQ, Wang SJ, Lin MS, Hsu CY, Lin WY. I-131 NP-59 adrenal cortical scintigraphy in suspected primary aldosteronism. Gaoxiong Yi Xue Ke Xue Za Zhi 1992; 8:213–218.
50. Kloos RT, Gross MD, Shapiro B, Francis IR, Korobkin M, Thompson NW. Diagnostic dilemma of small incidentally discovered adrenal masses: role for 131I-6beta-iodomethyl-norcholesterol scintigraphy. World J Surg 1997; 21:36–40.
51. Pauker SG, Kopelman RI. Trapped by an incidental finding. N Engl J Med 1992; 326:40–43.
52. Harisinghani MG, Maher MM, Hahn PF, Gervais DA, Jhaveri K, Varghese J, Mueller PR. Predictive value of benign percutaneous adrenal biopsies in oncology patients. Clin Radiol 2002; 57:898–901.
53. Ross NS, Aron DC. Hormonal evaluation of the patient with an incidentally discovered adrenal mass. N Engl J Med 1990; 323:1401–1405.
54. Young WF Jr. Management approaches to adrenal incidentalomas. A view from Rochester, Minnesota. Endo Metab Clin North Am 2000; 29:159–185.
55. Siren J, Tervahartiala P, Sivula A, Haapiainen R. Natural course of adrenal incidentalomas: seven-year follow-up study. World J Surg 2000; 24:579–582.
56. Gotoh M, Ono Y, Hattori R, Kinukawa T, Ohshima S. Laparoscopic adrenalectomy for pheochromocytoma: morbidity compared with adrenalectomy for tumors of other pathology. J Endourol 2002; 16:245–249.
57. Kercher KW, Park A, Matthews BD, Rolband G, Sing RF, Heniford BT. Laparoscopic adrenalectomy for pheochromocytoma. Surg Endosc 2002; 16:100–102.
58. Orchard T, Grant CS, van Heerden JA, Weaver A. Pheochromocytoma—continuing evolution of surgical therapy. Surgery 1993; 114:1153–1158.
59. ReMine WH, Chong GC, van Heerden JA, Sheps SG, Harrison EG Jr. Current management of pheochromocytoma. Ann Surg 1974; 179:740–748.

60. Smith CD, Weber CJ, Amerson JR. Laparoscopic adrenalectomy: new gold standard. World J Surg 1999; 23: 389–396.
61. Neumann K, Langer R. Imaging methods in diagnosis of pheochromocytoma. Zentralbl Chir 1997; 122:438–442.
62. Lenders JW, Pacak K, Walther MM, Linehan WM, Mannelli M, Friberg P, Keiser HR, Goldstein DS, Eisenhofer G. Biochemical diagnosis of pheochromocytoma: which test is best? JAMA 2002; 287:1427–1434.
63. Lenders JW, Pacak K, Eisenhofer G. New advances in the biochemical diagnosis of pheochromocytoma: moving beyond catecholamines. Ann NY Acad Sci 2002; 970:29–40.
64. Mantero F, Masini AM, Opocher G, Giovagnetti M, Arnaldi G. Adrenal incidentaloma: an overview of hormonal data from the National Italian Study Group. Horm Res 1997; 47:284–289.
65. Reincke M, Nieke J, Krestin GP, Saeger W, Allolio B, Winkelmann W. Preclinical Cushing's syndrome in adrenal "incidentalomas": comparison with adrenal Cushing's syndrome. J Clin Endocrinol Metab 1992; 75:826–832.
66. Terzolo M, Osella G, Ali A, Borretta G, Cesario F, Paccotti P, Angeli A. Subclinical Cushing's syndrome in adrenal incidentaloma. Clin Endocrinol (Oxf) 1998; 48:89–97.
67. Gill IS, Soble JJ, Sung GT, Winfield HN, Bravo EL, Novick AC. Needlescopic adrenalectomy—the initial series: comparison with conventional laparoscopic adrenalectomy. Urology 1998; 52:180–186.
68. Gill IS. The case of laparoscopic adrenalectomy. J Urol 2001; 166:429–436.
69. Henry JF, Defechereux T, Gramatica L, Raffaelli M. Should laparoscopic approach be proposed for large and/or potentially malignant adrenal tumors? Langenbecks Arch Surg 1999; 384:366–369.
70. Henry JF, Defechereux T, Raffaelli M, Lubrano D, Gramatica L. Complications of laparoscopic adrenalectomy: results of 169 consecutive procedures. World J Surg 2000; 24:1342–1346.
71. Henry JF. Minimally invasive adrenal surgery. Best Pract Res Clin Endocrinol Metab 2001; 15:149–160.
72. Ortega J, Sala C, Garcia S, Lledo S. Cost-effectiveness of laparoscopic vs open adrenalectomy: small savings in an expensive process. J Laparoendosc Adv Surg Tech A 2002; 12:1–5.
73. Schell SR, Talamini MA, Udelsman R. Laparoscopic adrenalectomy for nonmalignant disease: improved safety, morbidity, and cost-effectiveness. Surg Endosc 1999; 13:30–34.
74. Valeri A, Borrelli A, Presenti L, Lucchese M, Manca G, Tonelli P, Bergamini C, Borrelli D, Palli M, Saieva C. The influence of new technologies on laparoscopic adrenalectomy: our personal experience with 91 patients. Surg Endosc 2002; 16:1274–1279.
75. Hsu TH, Gill IS. Bilateral laparoscopic adrenalectomy: retroperitoneal and transperitoneal approaches. Urology 2002; 59:184–189.
76. Naya Y, Nagata M, Ichikawa T, Amakasu M, Omura M, Nishikawa T, Yamaguchi K, Ito H. Laparoscopic adrenalectomy: comparison of transperitoneal and retroperitoneal approaches. BJU Int 2002; 90:199–204.
77. Nagesser SK, Kievit J, Hermans J, Krans HM, van de Velde CJ. The surgical approach to the adrenal gland: a comparison of the retroperitoneal and the transabdominal routes in 326 operations on 284 patients. Jpn J Clin Oncol 2000; 30:68–74.
78. Hartgrink HH, Roelfsema F, Tollenaar RA, Hiddema PA, Pijl ME, van de Velde CJ. Primary pheochromocytoma extending into the right atrium: report of a case and review of the literature. Eur J Surg Oncol 2001; 27:115–119.
79. Jockenhovel F, Kuck W, Hauffa B, Reinhardt W, Benker G, Lederbogen S, Olbricht T, Reinwein D. Conservative and surgical management of incidentally discovered adrenal tumors (incidentalomas). J Endocrinol Invest 1992; 15:331–337.
80. Kasperlik-Zeluska AA, Roslonowska E, Slowinska-Srzednicka J, Migdalska B, Jeske W, Makowska A, Snochowska H. Incidentally discovered adrenal mass (incidentaloma): investigation and management of 208 patients. Clin Endocrinol (Oxf) 1997; 46:29–37.
81. Grossrubatscher E, Vignati F, Possa M, Lohi P. The natural history of incidentally discovered adrenocortical adenomas: a retrospective evaluation. J Endocrinol Invest 2001; 24:846–855.
82. Libe R, Dall'Asta C, Barbetta L, Baccarelli A, Beck-Peccoz P. Long-term follow-up study of patients with adrenal incidentalomas. Eur J Endocrinol 2002; 147: 489–494.
83. Best MA, Slavin LP, Aron DC. To regionalize or not to regionalize: that is the question. Part II. Volume-outcome relationships-endocrine disorders and their treatment. Endocrinologist 2000; 10:265–269.
84. Slavin LP, Best MA, Aron DC. To regionalize or not to regionalize: that is the question. Part I. Volume-outcome relationships—conceptual framework. Endocrinologist 2000; 10:205–210.
85. Fahlenkamp D, Rassweiler J, Fornara P, Freda T, Loening SA. Complications of laparoscopic procedures in urology: experience with 2,407 procedures at 4 German centers. J Urology 2002; 162:770.
86. Catarci M, Zaraca F, Mulieri G, Di Paola M, Montemurro L, Filippoussis P, Greco E, Gossetti F, Carboni M. Surgical technique and results of 1006 consecutive cases of open laparoscopy. Chirurg Ital 2002; 51:151–158.

36

Pheochromocytoma: Diagnosis and Treatment

David S. Pertsemlidis and Demetrius Pertsemlidis

Mount Sinai School of Medicine, New York University, New York, New York, U.S.A.

1 INTRODUCTION

Pheochromocytoma is a neuroendocrine tumor, embryologically derived from the neural crest and located principally in the abdomen. The anatomical distribution conforms to that of the sympatho-adrenal system with predominant origin from the adrenal medulla in approximately 90% of cases. Most of the abdominal extra-adrenal tumors are clustered around the adrenals and the remaining small fraction originates from sympathetic neurons along the para-aortic, iliac, and pelvic regions. Extra-abdominal tumors, mainly in the mediastinum and rarely in the neck, comprise approximately 2% of all pheochromocytomas (1).

Until the early 1950s, about two thirds of all pheochromocytomas were discovered at autopsy (2). The absence of physical stigmata in sporadic pheochromocytoma and the nonspecific clinical manifestations precluded easy recognition of the syndrome. Greater awareness of endocrine etiologies of hypertension, advances in the assays of the metabolites and parent catecholamines in the urine and plasma, the evolution of imaging for localization, and the development of genetic testing have led to identification of the disease and its inherited associations with unprecedented speed and accuracy (3–8).

Surgery for pheochromocytoma has now attained a level of safety and efficacy that permits resection of benign or malignant tumors with minimal morbidity and rare mortality. For the endocrine surgeon, familiarity with the accuracy and limitations of biochemical diagnosis, localization by conventional and isotopic imaging, and perioperative pharmacological and surgical management are the only guarantees of successful outcome (9).

Differences in biological behavior, patterns of inheritance, association with other neoplastic syndromes, and distinction between benign and malignant disease dictate separate description and management of four categories: sporadic, inherited, extra-adrenal, and malignant tumors.

This chapter will also address the associations of pheochromocytoma with other cancer syndromes and clarify common misconceptions about the disease and its management. Genetic linkage to other endocrinopathies is well known, but the components of the associated hereditary neurocutaneous and other syndromes have not been sufficiently emphasized. Most clinicians are unaware of the risk of pancreatic neuroendocrine tumors in von Hippel-Lindau disease (10,11) or of the rare coexistence of pheochromocytoma with pulmonary chondroma and gastric leiomyosarcoma, a syndrome of unknown mendelian inheritance described by Carney et al. in 1977 (12).

Distorted impressions about the syndrome of pheochromocytoma and the appropriate treatment need to be demystified. These misconceptions are related to the source of excess catecholamines causing paroxysmal symptoms during physical or emotional stress, the presumed need for preoperative expansion of the blood volume, and the suggestion that early ligation of the main adrenal vein offers an advantage. Confusion persists regarding the fear of catecholamine release by the tumor with pneumoperitoneum, the choice of inhalation anesthetics and muscle relaxants, and the use of long-acting adrenergic blockers before and during surgery.

2 HISTORICAL LANDMARKS

In 1886, Felix Fraenkel was the first to give a pathological description of pheochromocytoma, and in 1912, Pick introduced the name to describe a tumor that stained brown when exposed to chromium salts (13,14). The three components of the name were derived from the Greek φαιόσ meaning brown, χρώμα, for color, and κύττωμα, for tumor. In 1926, the first successful surgical resections by César Roux in Switzerland and Charles Mayo were reported (13). Among the numerous biochemical discoveries that made the recognition of pheochromocytoma possible, several stand out as cornerstones. In 1946, Ulf Svante von Euler made a pioneering contribution to the field, which led to the pathophysiological characterization of pheochromocytoma. His discovery that norepinephrine is the neurotransmitter of the sympathetic nervous system earned him a share of the 1970 Nobel Prize in Physiology (13). The isolation of two catecholamine metabolites in the urine, vanillylmandelic acid (VMA) by Armstrong in 1956 (15) and metanephrines by Axelrod in 1957, were landmarks in biochemical diagnosis (16). Gitlow and coworkers from our institution contributed immensely to the perfection of biochemical diagnostic methods and their correlation with the clinical syndrome of pheochromocytoma (17–19).

Recent work done at the National Institutes of Health by Lenders et al. (3) and Eisenhofer and colleagues (4) have added new diagnostic dimensions. The two teams have shown that measurements of plasma free (unconjugated) metanephrines offer greater sensitivity and specificity than assays of the parent catecholamines and their urinary metabolites.

Historical observations of pathological and clinical associations with other entities ultimately led to genetic linkage of pheochromocytoma to multiple endocrine neoplasia Type 2 (MEN 2), neurocutaneous syndromes, especially von Hippel-Lindau disease (VHL) and neurofibromatosis Type 1 (NF 1), and the familial paraganglioma syndrome (13,20–24).

3 PREVALENCE AND DISTRIBUTION

The prevalence is less than 0.5% in hypertensive adults, but higher in hypertensive adolescents and children because of greater likelihood of inherited disease (1,5). In von Recklinghausen neurofibromatosis Type 1 and von Hippel-Lindau disease, pheochromocytoma occurs in up to 2 and 20% of such patients, respectively (22,23,25,26). However, patients with NF 1 and coexisting hypertension (27) or duodenal carcinoids (28) have a substantially greater prevalence of pheochromocytoma. Close to 40% of patients with MEN 2 harbor a pheochromocytoma (29).

Pheochromocytoma is neither gender nor race specific and can occur at any age. Sporadic tumors commonly present in the third and fourth decades of life, while familial disease is manifested one decade earlier. In sporadic cases, a single tumor arises from the adrenal medulla, almost never coexisting with extra-adrenal tumors. In the inherited syndromes, however, bilateral adrenal disease or multiple extra-adrenal tumors are often found, and medullary hyperplasia (diffuse or nodular) or multiple tumors are commonly identified within the involved ipsilateral and normal appearing contralateral glands. Finally, extra-adrenal tumors rarely, if ever, coexist with adrenal pheochromocytomas and have a predisposition to malignancy.

4 CLINICAL MANIFESTATIONS

Pheochromocytoma is a capricious neoplasm with nonspecific phenotypic manifestations and can therefore be difficult to diagnose clinically. Hypertension is almost always present and may be constant, rather than paroxysmal, in one third to one half of patients. Paroxysmal hypertensive crises may be so fleeting that they frequently escape detection. In a small minority of MEN 2 patients and those with predominantly epinephrine-secreting tumors, paroxysmal cardiac arrhythmia may be the presenting symptom.

Excess catecholamines affect a plurality of target organs, thus inducing a wide spectrum of symptoms which are often inseparable from those of a variety of common illnesses. In the broad constellation of symptoms, the triad of paroxysmal headaches, palpitations, and excess sweating is the most common expression in adults. In children, profuse sweating is a common manifestation, often ignored due to the infrequent use of blood pressure measurements. Some unusual clinical features are transient ischemic attacks, stroke, grand mal seizures, cardiomyopathy, gastrointestinal crises, and diabetes mellitus or insipidus. Severe constipation or pseudo-obstruction may be the initial manifestation (30) and secretory diarrhea from elaboration of vasoactive intestinal polypeptide or calcitonin by pheochromocytoma has been reported (31–34).

Paroxysmal events are usually precipitated by physical or emotional stress, which induces a flux of catecholamines from the expanded storage in the neurosecretory granules of the sympathetic neurons and adrenal medulla. Despite common misconceptions, stress-induced neural stimulation does not cause release of catecholamines directly from the tumor as no pathways of innervation exist. In fact, only direct mechanical pressure by blunt abdominal trauma, deep abdominal palpation, certain body postures, vigorous application of the ultrasound probe, retrograde adrenal venography, and intraoperative manipulation can cause sudden release of catecholamine by the tumor. An analogy to the compression-induced flux of catecholamines is the induction of symptoms during micturition in pheochromocytomas located in the wall of the urinary bladder.

Physical stigmata, seen mostly in inherited syndromes associated with pheochromocytoma, facilitate the recognition of the disease. Cutaneous neurofibromatosis Type 1 (Fig. 1), café-au-lait pigmentations, and Lisch nodules of the eye, especially with coexisting hypertension, should raise strong suspicion of pheochromocytoma. Visible neuromas of the oral mucosa, tongue, and conjunctiva (Fig. 2) and marfanoid habitus are indicative of MEN 2B. Loss of vision or of an eye from retinal angiomas or angioblastomas should alert the physician to possible existence of von Hippel-Lindau disease.

Family history is a reliable source of information that may lead to discovery of pheochromocytoma or coexisting but silent cancer syndromes. Sudden death of a parent or sibling at a young age, premature myocardial infarction or cardiomyopathy (35), endocrine surgery, and colorectal operation for Hirschsprung's disease, ganglioneuromatosis, or megacolon (30) are important leads in directing diagnostic investigations.

Offspring of parents harboring germline mutations of the autosomal dominant RET proto-oncogene mapped to chromosome 10 (10q11.2), the von Hippel-Lindau tumor suppressor gene mapped to chromosome 3 (3p25-26), or the neurofibromatosis Type 1 (NF 1) gene mapped to chromosome 17 (17q11.2) are at high risk for developing pheochromocytoma and other components of the neoplastic syndromes. About 20% of all pheochromocytomas are discovered by screening families with MEN 2 or neurocutaneous syndromes, especially VHL and NF 1. Phenotypic and genetic screening and surveillance are important because pheochromocytoma may be the first expression in about one third to one half of affected kindred in MEN 2 and VHL families (36). Family history of surgery for carotid body tumor, glomus jugulare, or other paraganglioma should initiate the search for extra-adrenal pheochromocytoma and screening for the presence of mutations of the genes for succinate dehydrogenase subunits D and B (SDHD and SDHB), which encode mitochondrial enzymes involved in oxidative phosphorylation (8).

A history of gastric leiomyosarcoma and pulmonary chondroma should alert the physician to possible coexistence of extra-adrenal pheochromocytoma. This syndrome described by Carney et al. (12) has no established etiology and no known mendelian inheritance. Other neurocutaneous syndromes which may be associated with pheochromocytoma are tuberous sclerosis and the Sturge-Weber syndrome. In tuberous sclerosis, visible angiofibromas distributed in a butterfly pattern on the cheeks, chin, and forehead coexist with malformations or tumors of the central nervous system. In the Sturge-Weber encephalo-trigeminal angiomatosis, there are visible cavernous hemangiomas along the distribution of the trigeminal nerve in association with hemangiomas of the leptomeninges.

5 BIOCHEMICAL DIAGNOSIS

Once clinical suspicion of pheochromocytoma is raised, treatment with oral long-acting α- and, if needed, β-adrenergic blockers should be started, and testing should be initiated under standardized, unstressed conditions. Physical or emotional stress, comatose state from subarachnoid hemorrhage or cerebral tumors, and congestive heart failure will raise the concentrations of catecholamines and their metabolites in the plasma and urine (17,18,37).

All medications should be screened, and those known to falsely elevate or suppress the catecholamines or their metabolite concentrations in the plasma or urine should be stopped for at least one week. Phenoxybenzamine and tricyclic antidepressants are major causes of false positive elevation of norepinephrine and its metabolites (38). Labetalol, one of the frequently used antihypertensive drugs, interferes with catecholamine and metanephrine assays and should be stopped one week before sampling of plasma or urine (39). Acetaminophen interferes with the analytical method of plasma normetanephrine assay and should be stopped several days before blood is collected (39). α-Methyl-DOPA, monoamino oxidase (MAO) inhibitors, amphetamine, cocaine, and calcium antagonists may interfere with assays of the parent catecholamines and metanephrines in the plasma and urine (39). Dietary caffeic acid, a catechol ingredient in natural and decaffeinated coffee, and its metabolite dihydrocaffeic acid interfere with assays of plasma catecholamines (39).

Provocative tests with histamine, glucagon, or phentolamine may cause severe paroxysmal rise or fall of the arterial pressure, resulting in stroke, myocardial infarction, or even death. Given the precision of current biochemical testing, these unnecessary provocative manipulations are strictly contraindicated. Patients should be fasting and resting in a quiet environment, and collection of blood should not be started until 10–15 minutes after venipuncture. Random samples of urine, preferably 50 mL of the first concentrated morning specimen, are sufficient, as the results are expressed in micrograms of the catecholamine metabolite per milligram of urinary creatinine. The assays of these stable urinary metabolites are valid even in the presence of renal dysfunction (17,18). Twenty-four hour urine collections, a cumbersome undertaking, are no longer necessary.

The diagnostic accuracy of measurements of urinary total metanephrines and VMA in two separate samples, approaches 98% (17–19,37). In healthy adults, the normal concentrations of urinary total metanephrines range from 0.05 to 1.2 (mean 0.61), and those of VMA from 0.25 to 3.5 (mean 1.4) μg/mg creatinine. In children the range of normal values is higher and should be interpreted with caution. The younger the child, the higher the normal concentration of metanephrines and VMA (40). Urinary homovanillic acid (HVA), a metabolite of dopamine, is always elevated in children with neuroblastomas and in some adults with ganglioneuromas or malignant pheochromocytoma. Normal urinary concentrations of HVA in adults range from 0.25 to 2.5 μg/mg urinary creatinine (17–19).

Assays of plasma catecholamines and their metabolites, especially norepinephrine and normetanephrine, are needed if the urinary test results are equivocal. The sensitivity and specificity of plasma free metanephrines has been reported to be 99 and 89%, respectively (38). In adults, the upper reference limits for plasma norepinephrine and epinephrine are 2.9 and 0.5 nmol/L, respectively, and for normetanephrine and metanephrine 0.6 and 0.3 nmol/L, respectively (38). Age-related scales of plasma catecholamines and metabolites have not been published.

Should both urine and plasma test results prove equivocal, the clonidine suppression test offers distinction between pheochromocytoma and essential hypertension. Nonsuppression of plasma norepinephrine by clonidine implies pheochromocytoma, whereas more than 50% suppression is indicative of essential hypertension (41). It should be noted that some pheochromocytomas elaborate the enzyme catechol-O-methyl transferase, resulting in intracellular conversion of catecholamines to the O-methylated compounds and elevation of metanephrines in the plasma and urine with normal concentrations of the parent catecholamines (38,39).

6 LOCALIZATION THROUGH IMAGING

Biochemical confirmation of pheochromocytoma is now followed routinely by efforts at localization. Current imaging technology permits anatomical and functional localization of tumors with unprecedented accuracy, far beyond the surgeon's visual and tactile skills. Prior to development of direct imaging of the adrenals and extra-adrenal sites, the surgical practice was to explore the abdomen after exclusion of a mediastinal tumor by conventional chest x-rays. Displacement of the right or left kidney on intravenous pyelography or the inferior vena cava on selective venography offered indirect evidence for the presence of a tumor. Selective arterial or venous angiography improved direct visualization of pheochromocytomas arising from the adrenals or the organ of Zuckerkandl (Fig. 3); however, the stress of invasive instrumentation and the sudden release of catecholamines by the tumor during retrograde venous injection of contrast proved risky. Pharmacological protection with adrenergic blockade was needed to prevent induction of hypertensive crises or cardiac arrhythmia during these now abandoned procedures.

Ultrasound examination has improved the direct imaging of adrenal tumors, but may be limited by the interposition of gastric and colonic gas. Small adrenal tumors measuring 1 cm or less can be detected by an experienced ultrasonographer (42). Patients with suspected pheochromocytoma should be protected with adequate adrenergic blockade to avoid induction of hypertensive crisis or cardiac arrhythmia from compression of the tumor by the ultrasound probe.

Computed tomography (CT) revolutionized the direct imaging of adrenal and extra-adrenal pheochromocytomas in the neck, mediastinum, abdomen, and pelvis (see Chapter 28). The resolution power of CT has permitted localization of tumors as small as 5 mm with a sensitivity and specificity of 88 and 95%, respectively. CT imaging also permits distinction between benign and

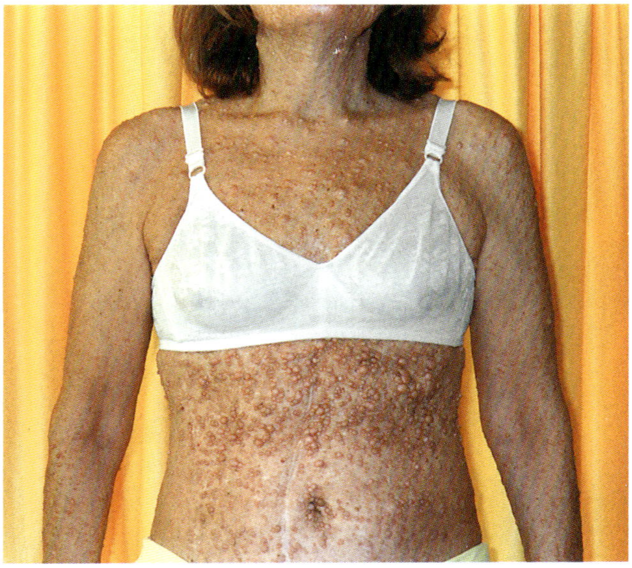

Figure 1 Inherited Type 1 neurofibromatosis with coexisting pheochromocytoma of the right adrenal, resected through open transperitoneal approach at age 27. The patient returned 21 years later with a gastrinoma, which was treated with distal pancreatectomy. Her father died following resection of a unilateral adrenal pheochromocytoma elsewhere, and autopsy revealed medullary hyperplasia of the remaining adrenal.

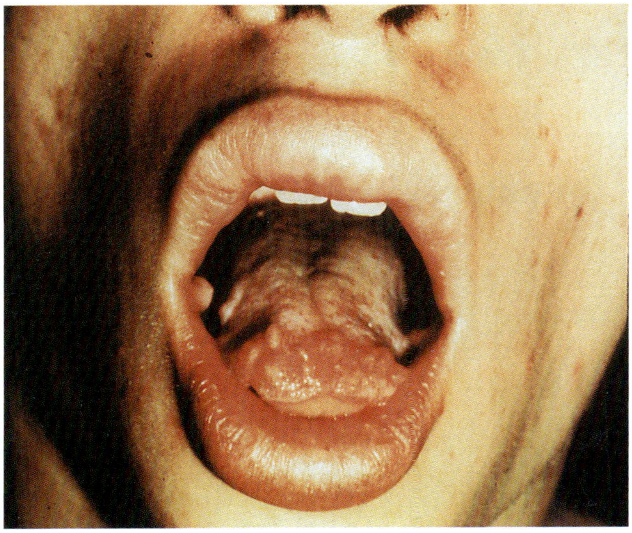

Figure 2 Oral and lingual mucosal neuromas in a patient with MEN 2B. (Courtesy of Dr. Donald Bergman, The Mount Sinai Hospital of New York.)

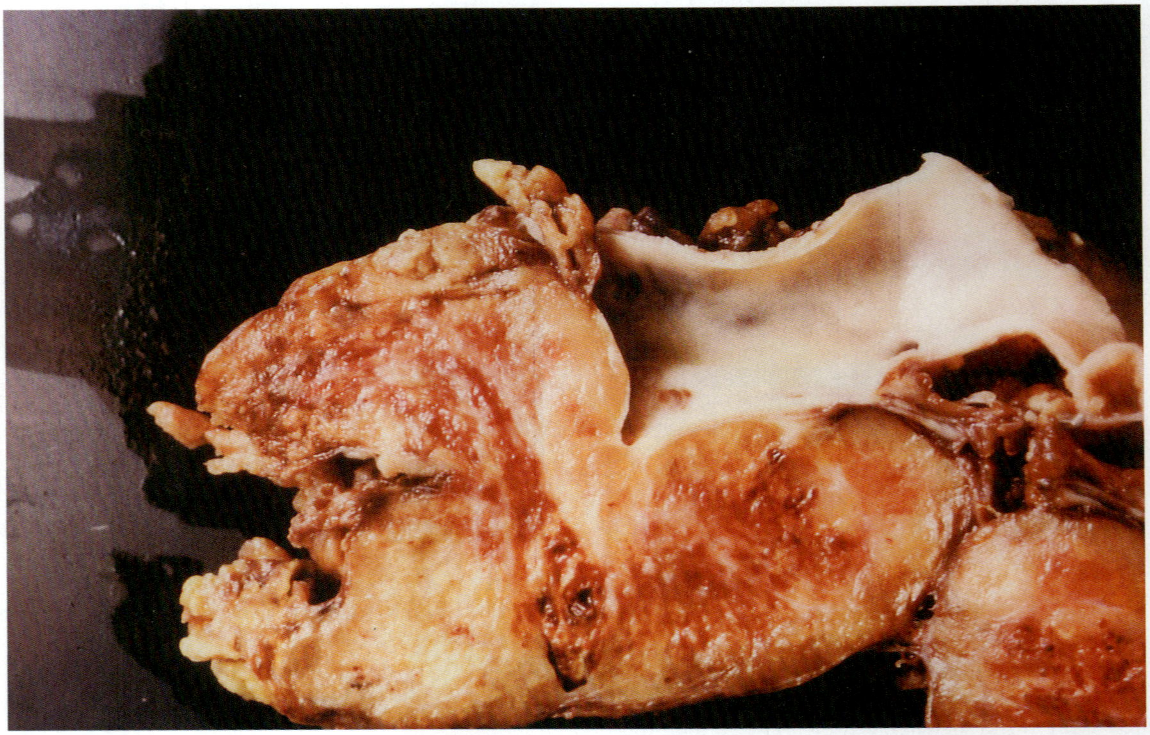

Figure 7 Malignant extra-adrenal para-aortic tumor invading the inferior vena cava. The patient had three operations for removal of extra-adrenal pheochromocytomas, the first at age 13. The involved infrarenal cava was resected and interposition vein graft was used. The patient died at the age of 39 from metastatic and locally recurrent disease.

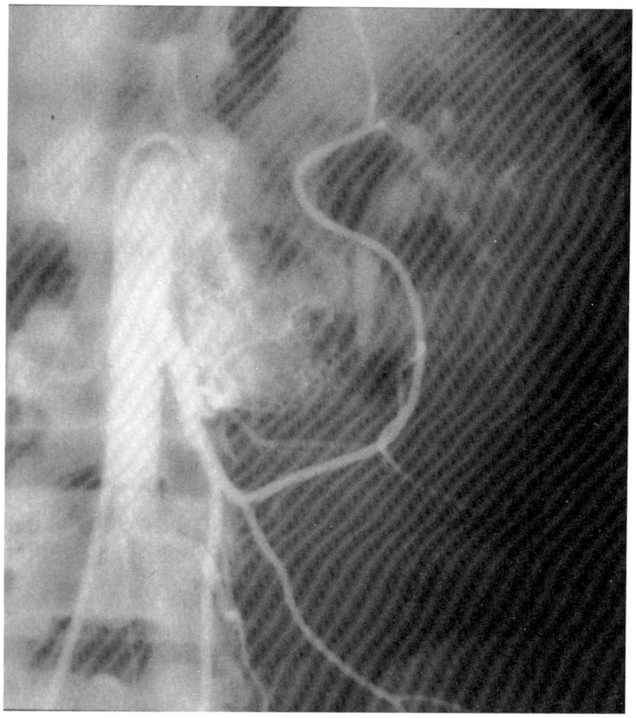

Figure 3 Arteriographic demonstration of a pheochromocytoma arising from the organ of Zuckerkandl adjacent to the inferior mesenteric artery.

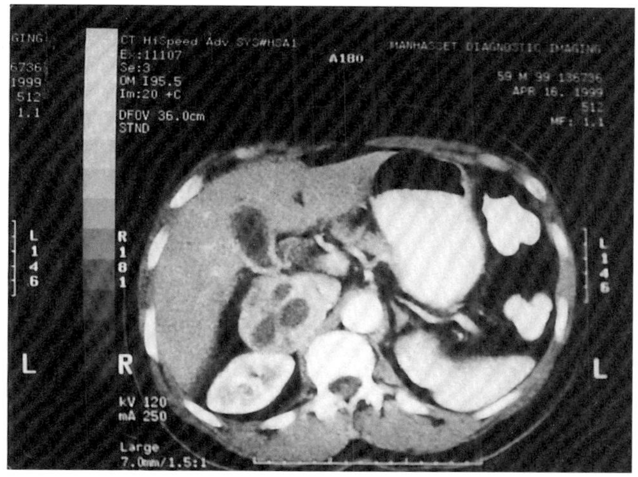

Figure 4 Large right adrenal pheochromocytoma with central necrosis raising suspicion of malignancy. Pathological examination revealed invasion of the capsule indicative of a malignant tumor.

malignant tumors (43). Large size, confluent necrosis, invasion of the capsule or adjacent organs, and large periadrenal nodes constitute features of malignancy (Fig. 4). All patients undergoing CT imaging for localization should be protected with adrenergic blockade to avoid induction of a crisis with ionic or nonionic contrast media (44,45).

The introduction of magnetic resonance imaging (MRI) has offered the additional feature of specificity through enhancement of signals on the T2-weighted images (Fig. 5A,B). Although this imaging property is also common in adrenocortical tumors and therefore not pathognomonic for pheochromocytoma, correlation with clinical and biochemical information offers an additional major diagnostic dimension.

Despite the high resolution of CT and MRI, these imaging modalities fail to screen the entire body and offer no definitive information on the functional status of the tumor. Scintigraphic studies, on the other hand, permit examination of the entire body and define the physiological properties of neoplasms. Scintigraphy with meta-iodobenzylguanidine (MIBG), an analogue of norepinephrine, labeled with iodine-123 (I-123) or iodine-131 (I-131), and indium-111–labeled octreotide, a somatostatin analogue, permits not only anatomical localization but also determination of function with the highest sensitivity and specificity. Selective uptake of MIBG by the sympatho-adrenal cells is dependent on the adequacy of neurosecretory granules in the tumor (see Chapter 31). Aside from anatomic and functional specificity, MIBG scintigraphy is superior in detecting small extra-adrenal tumors and metastases from malignant pheochromocytoma. The sensitivity and specificity of I-131 MIBG are 87 and 94%, respectively (46), with more recent studies reporting even higher percentages (47,48).

Indium-111–labeled octreotide scanning relies on the affinity of membrane receptors to somatostatin, present in most neuroendocrine tumors. The sensitivity of octreotide scintigraphy for pheochromocytoma ranges from 60 to 90%. Positron emission tomography (PET) after intravenous administration of fluorine-18–labeled deoxyglucose (FDG) is the most recent scintigraphic imaging method oriented toward anatomical localization and determination of the metabolic activity of adrenal and extra-adrenal pheochromocytoma. FDG uptake in pheochromocytoma does not depend on catecholamine uptake or abundance of neurosecretory granules in the tumor, but reflects proliferative activity and the number of viable tumor cells (see Chapter 31).

These isotopic studies should be used in a complementary fashion in cases of equivocal diagnostic results. Scintigraphy should not be used on pregnant women

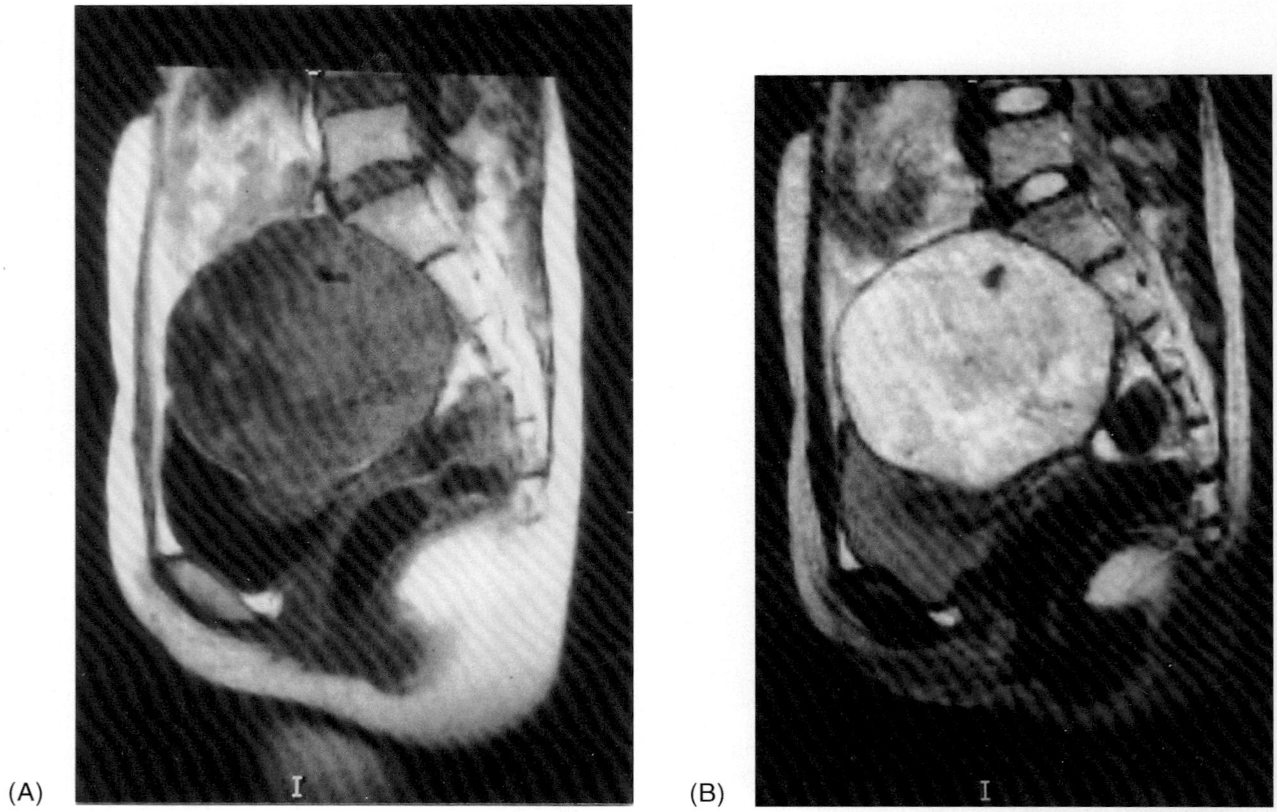

Figure 5 (A,B), Large pelvic pheochromocytoma with change of signal intensity from T1 to T2 MRI images. These imaging features are strongly suggestive but not pathognomonic for pheochromocytoma.

and should be used cautiously on women of childbearing age. MIBG and octreotide scintigraphy offer not only diagnostic localization, but also the ability to use the selective uptake of the isotope for therapy in the treatment of inoperable primary malignant and metastatic pheochromocytoma.

Angiographic selective sampling of blood from adrenal veins or extra-adrenal venous tributaries has not proven useful in localizing small pheochromocytomas because of the rapid turnover of catecholamines. Furthermore, the stress induced by invasive angiography results in variable flux of catecholamines from the expanded pool in the neurosecretory granules of the sympathetic neurons and adrenal medulla, rendering the assays virtually invalid.

The temptation to perform percutaneous CT-guided needle biopsy in suspected, but not proven, pheochromocytoma should be avoided due to the risk of inducing a crisis. In exceptional cases, such as patients with prohibitive surgical risk and equivocal diagnostic test results, percutaneous fine needle aspiration should only be performed under adequate adrenergic blockade.

The plurality of available conventional noninvasive and isotopic imaging methods has improved the precision of anatomical localization and the definition of physiological status of both benign and malignant tumors.

7 PERIOPERATIVE MANAGEMENT

7.1 Ambulatory Preoperative Care

Once the diagnosis of pheochromocytoma is established by biochemical parameters, α-adrenergic blockade should be initiated. Only after this blockade has established normotension can β-adrenergic inhibition be used to treat compensatory tachycardia. This sequence should never be reversed as β-adrenergic blockade alone inhibits β-receptor–mediated vasodilatation, allowing unopposed α-receptor stimulation and potentially inducing a hypertensive crisis. In the majority of patients, noncompetitive or selective α blockade alone is sufficient, reserving β antagonism for patients who develop significant tachycardia. Recent studies argue for the use of oral calcium channel blockade alone for the preoperative management of pheochromocytoma (49), but this regimen has not been widely adopted.

Phenoxybenzamine, a long-acting, nonselective oral α-blocker, is the drug of choice for outpatient management. An initial dose of 10 mg twice daily is used with progressive increases until normotension is achieved and paroxysmal symptoms are eliminated or minimized. Usually 30–40 mg/day, divided in 3 or 4 doses, are sufficient, although higher doses may be necessary. Prazocin, a selective α-receptor inhibitor with shorter duration of action than phenoxybenzamine, can be used at doses of 1–2 mg 3 times daily (50). Oral phentolamine, a short-acting α-receptor antagonist, has a variable absorption and is therefore unsuitable for therapy in the ambulatory setting. Similarly, the use of tyrosine hydroxylase inhibition with metyrosine is not useful in the management of benign pheochromocytoma as parkinsonian symptoms may occur. Oral β-receptor inhibition or calcium channel blockade can be achieved with a variety of selective and nonselective medications. Small doses of propranolol or atenolol usually provide adequate restoration of eurhythmia.

The debate over the need for expansion of the circulating blood volume in the preoperative phase is plagued by basic misconceptions. The notion that patients with pheochromocytoma are hypovolemic (51) is not valid. Measurements of plasma and red cell volumes in these patients have proven to be within the normal range (52) and, in fact, pheochromocytoma patients are hypervolemic relative to the capacity of the constricted vascular system. Attempts to expand the circulating volume with prolonged preoperative adrenergic blockade does not prevent intraoperative cardiovascular crises and the hypotension that follows tumor removal (53). The proposed 4- to 6- week delay for volume expansion serves only to increase the time period during which these patients are at continued risk from stress-induced paroxysmal crises. The surgical treatment of pheochromocytoma must be expeditious and should be performed immediately after diagnosis and localization. The appropriate timing of volume restoration is immediately after tumor removal.

7.2 In-Hospital Preoperative Preparation

In an era when the practice of surgery has, by necessity, shifted from the inpatient to the outpatient setting, the safest site for immediate preoperative management of a pheochromocytoma patient remains the critical care unit. The highest priority is optimal control of the arterial pressure and heart rate in a monitored setting. The choice of drugs for adrenergic inhibition is a matter of personal preference and institutional idiosyncrasy rather than scientific reasoning. The spectrum of pharmacological management includes α blockade, combined α and β blockade, short- or long-acting antagonists, and powerful vasodilating agents whose action is not mediated through adrenergic receptors.

The selection of the short-acting α-blocker phentolamine, alone or combined with the β-receptor antagonist esmolol, permits easy minute-to-minute titration of the doses needed to attain normotension and cardiac eurhythmia. The short half-life and virtual absence of toxicity renders these two medications highly desirable. The required infusion rates of these drugs are proportional to the levels of excess catecholamines in the plasma and tissues and the sensitivity of adrenergic receptors. The preoperative requirements of α- and β-blockers permit an estimate of the amounts needed during induction of anesthesia, endotracheal intubation, and intraoperative manipulation of the tumor (54).

Continuous intravenous infusion of phentolamine should be started at 10 mg/hour with incremental rates every 5–10 minutes until normotension is achieved. Usually, an average infusion rate of 35 mg/hr is sufficient, but the requirements may range from 10 to 100 mg/hr. Aside from normotension, the two other criteria for sufficiency of α blockade are a mild compensatory sinus tachycardia and nasal stuffiness. The solutions should be freshly prepared and contain 1.0 mg/mL of phentolamine in glucose/water. The concentration for intraoperative use should be two- to threefold higher to rapidly control intraoperative hypertensive events (9).

Continuous intravenous infusion of esmolol is started after the development of sinus tachycardia from adequate α-receptor blockade. The esmolol solution should contain 10 mg/mL of esmolol in glucose/water. The infusion rate should be started at 25 mg/hr with incremental titration until normal sinus rhythm is attained. The average infusion rate is 150 mg/hr. Labetalol, with combined long-acting β and intermediate α activity at a ratio of 7:1, offers the advantage of a single drug that can be used orally or intravenously (9). Despite this 7:1 ratio of β to α activity, the rapid onset of α blockade makes labetalol a useful drug in the perioperative period. Nitroprusside, a potent vasodilator and smooth muscle relaxant, should always be available in the perioperative setting for limited use during episodes when adrenergic blockade proves ineffective (50). Prolonged infusion rates greater than 2 μg/kg/min generate cyanide faster than the body can dispose, leading to toxicity and potential fatality (55).

The advantages of continuous intravenous use of short-acting adrenergic blockers are easy titration, rapid onset of action, negligible toxicity, and the restoration of physiological hemodynamic and cardiac parameters within minutes after stopping the drugs (9). Bolus injections of α- or β-receptor blockers may produce extreme fluctuations of arterial pressure and heart rate and should be avoided. Although the titration of intravenous infusion rates of short-acting antiadrenergic medications requires greater effort and subtlety, the ultimate benefits, especially during surgery, are superior to the "simplicity" of drugs with sustained action. The rapid control of intraoperative hypertensive or arrhythmic episodes, the quick return of physiological indices and the surgeon's ability to judge the completeness of tumor removal are powerful reasons for the preferential use of the continuous intravenous infusion of short-acting catecholamine antagonists.

Invasive instrumentation for monitoring of the peripheral and pulmonary arterial pressures should never be done without complete pharmacological protection with α-receptor blockade. Peripheral arterial and central venous catheters are necessary for monitoring of the respective pressures and pulmonary artery catheters are indicated in patients with previous myocardial infarction, arrhythmia, or cardiomyopathy.

7.3 Intraoperative Management

Patients should arrive in the operating room after a day's preparation in the critical care unit with appropriate monitors and well-controlled arterial pressure and heart rate with intravenous phentolamine and esmolol. All of the needed solutions must be freshly prepared and available in the operating room for immediate infusion through dedicated venous access. Delay in the control of a crisis, even for a few moments, may cause serious morbidity or death.

Phentolamine and esmolol solutions with concentrations of 2 mg/mL and 10 mg/mL in glucose/water, respectively, should be continuously infused at an appropriate rate. Sodium nitroprusside solution of 0.2 mg/mL (50 mg in 250 mL) of glucose/water should be available for brief use only to control paroxysmal hypertension that is not responsive to intravenous phentolamine. The solution should be protected from light using aluminum foil or other opaque material, but there is no need to cover the infusion chamber or tubing. Norepinephrine solution of 16 μg/mL (8 mg in 500 mL) of glucose/water should be ready for infusion in case of hypotension that is unresponsive to discontinuation of phentolamine and rapid volume infusion.

Surgery should not commence until adrenergic steady state is attained. Anesthetic induction and endotracheal intubation should be performed under optimal pharmacological protection to minimize induction of hypertension or arrhythmia. Continuous intravenous infusion of phentolamine and esmolol should be adjusted, when needed, to control hypertensive or arrhythmic events during unavoidable tumor manipulation in the course of mobilization and resection of the tumor.

The choice of inhalational anesthetic and muscle relaxant is no longer an issue of debate. Our experience and that of others (50) have demonstrated no correlation between the agent used and the incidence of cardiovascular events. The primary determinants of the safe conduct of anesthesia and of successful surgical outcome are the adequacy of adrenoreceptor blockade and the maintenance of sufficient anesthetic depth.

7.4 Surgical Approaches

Imaging-directed surgical approaches have totally eliminated the need for routine exploration of both adrenals, retroperitoneum, and pelvis by open laparotomy, which was practiced before the advent of ultrasound and other modern imaging methods. The choice between minimally invasive and traditional open surgery is a matter of the surgeon's experience and the limitations imposed by tumor size, suspicion of malignancy, adequacy of exposure, and comorbidities. Patients with recent cardiac failure or intracranial hemorrhage may be at greater surgical risk with minimally invasive surgery, compared to open techniques, because pneumoperitoneum lowers venous return to the heart and increases intracranial pressure (56). Small, benign, adrenal pheochromocytomas can be safely resected by endoscopic transperitoneal or retroperitoneal approaches, while tumors larger than 7 cm and with imaging features suggestive of malignancy should be accessed by open techniques. The open transperitoneal anterior approach offers excellent exposure for complete exploration, easier control of bleeding, and resection of large invasive tumors or multiple extra-adrenal pheochromocytomas. Minimally invasive techniques offer quick recovery, less adhesion formation, and superior cosmetic results.

The concern that the pressure of pneumoperitoneum may induce flux of catecholamines by the tumor has been dispelled by clinical observations and assays of plasma catecholamines during minimally invasive adrenalectomy for pheochromocytoma.

Experience with bilateral synchronous endoscopic adrenalectomy is still limited, and the safety of minimally invasive approaches for potentially malignant pheochromocytomas has not been yet established.

The approach to extra-adrenal abdominal pheochromocytomas depends on anatomical location, size, and multiplicity of the tumors. The deep retroperitoneal location, proximity to the aorta, cava, iliac vessels, or ureters and the potential malignancy dictate caution in employing an endoscopic approach.

Patients with left adrenal pheochromocytomas, especially large ones, should have preoperative antipneumococcal and antimeningococcal vaccinations because of the small likelihood of incidental splenectomy (1–2%). Knowledge of bilateral renal function with contrast-enhanced CT is essential because large or malignant pheochromocytomas may be difficult to resect completely without nephrectomy due to inseparable blood supply or direct invasion of the kidney. Informed consent should also be obtained from patients with large, vascular, invasive tumors, where nephrectomy may become necessary for oncological or vascular anatomical reasons. Cleansing of the colon is desirable but not necessary, but antibiotic prophylaxis against *Staphylococcus aureus* should be routine. Stress doses of cortisol are needed if bilateral synchronous adrenalectomy is planned, with or without orthotopic preservation or heterotopic autotransplantation of cortical tissue.

Early ligation of the main adrenal vein has been proposed to minimize hypertensive and arrhythmic events during dissection around the tumor. This concept ignores the presence of numerous emissary veins connecting the central vein with the pericapsular venous plexus and renal capsular veins. This alternate pathway for venous outflow is accelerated during stress and protects the gland from hemorrhage (57,58). Easier exposure, isolation, and ligation of the main adrenal veins, especially the short right, are facilitated greatly by dissection along the less vascular lateral, posterior, and apical planes first. Access to the planes along the renal vein on the left and inferior vena cava on the right is made easier with gentle retraction of the mobilized gland. A complete discussion of the techniques for minimally invasive and open adrenalectomy are described elsewhere in this volume.

Complete removal of the tumor is followed by a fall of systolic arterial pressure to less than 90 mmHg. This hypotension can be corrected within minutes by stopping the short-acting α-receptor blocker (phentolamine) and rapidly infusing 2–3 L of crystalloid. Infusion of norepinephrine to restore normotension should be avoided, as it prolongs undesirable vasoconstriction.

8 HEREDITARY PHEOCHROMOCYTOMA

Pheochromocytoma is often linked genetically to other neoplastic syndromes, inherited mostly by autosomal dominance. Associations with MEN 2, neurocutaneous syndromes, especially VHL and von Recklinghausen neurofibromatosis and the familial paraganglioma syndrome, have been documented (8,10,11,21–30).

Inherited pheochromocytoma occurs one decade earlier than sporadic in part because of earlier detection through screening of families. About 20% of all pheochromocytomas are discovered by prospective screening of families. In MEN 2A and VHL families the incidence of bilateral adrenal pheochromocytomas (synchronous or metachronous) is 90 and 60%, respectively (36). The multiplicity of tumors in each gland reflects evolution from medullary hyperplasia.

Familial pheochromocytoma alone has yet to be defined by genetic testing.

In a recent retrospective genetic study of 271 patients labeled as nonsyndromic (sporadic) pheochromocytoma, 66 (24%) were found to have mutations. Of those, 30 had mutations of the VHL gene, 13 of the RET proto-oncogene, 12 of SDHB, and 11 of SDHD genes. Patients with multifocal extra-adrenal pheochromocytomas presenting at age 18 or younger are more likely to have mutations of the SDHB and SDHD genes (8). This innovative study indicates that the prevalence of inherited pheochromocytoma is perhaps far greater than once thought.

8.1 Multiple Endocrine Neoplasia Type 2

MEN 2 is a cancer syndrome affecting organs derived from the neuroectoderm. The previous narrow definition of MEN 2A, which included medullary thyroid carcinoma (MTC) or thyroid C-cell hyperplasia, pheochromocytoma, and hyperparathyroidism has been broadened by the international RET Mutation Consortium (21). The MEN 2B phenotype was defined as the constellation of MTC with or without pheochromocytoma, usually without parathyroid disease, and characteristic clinical abnormalities (mucosal neuromas, marfanoid constitution and intestinal ganglioneuromatosis). The susceptibility gene for MEN 2 has been traced to chromosome 10 (10q11.2) (21).

In MEN syndromes, the full expression of the phenotype occurs sequentially, rather than simultaneously. In MEN 2A, only 20% of patients will present with clinical manifestation of all components. Prospective screening and long-term surveillance are therefore imperative to detect asymptomatic family members and the clinical or biochemical development of latent, subclinical components.

The prevalence of pheochromocytoma in MEN 2 families is about 40% (8). It usually originates from the adrenals, is bilateral (synchronous or metachronous) in 90% of MEN 2A families (9), and is rarely malignant (36). Multiple tumors or medullary hyperplasia (diffuse or nodular) are commonly present in the ipsilateral involved and contralateral adrenal, which appears normal on imaging.

The alarming report by Carney et al. in 1976 (59) that MEN 2 patients are at higher risk for malignancy proved incorrect. Subsequent larger series of MEN 2 and VHL patients did not verify the high risk for malignant pheochromocytoma in such families (29,36,60). As a result, the recommendation for prophylactic removal of the contralateral normal-appearing gland to prevent malignancy is no longer tenable.

Intestinal manifestations of MEN 2 include Hirschsprung's disease and ganglioneuromatosis. Familial Hirschsprung's disease can be autosomal dominant or recessive. Linkage to the chromosomal region containing the RET proto-oncogene has been documented (21). A recent study revealed that some patients with MEN 2A develop Hirschsprung's disease and kindred with MEN 2B develop intestinal neuromas and megacolon (30). Six of eight patients with Hirschsprung's disease among 83 MEN 2A families had surgery for aganglionosis 2–23 years prior to the diagnosis of MEN 2A. Almost all 28 patients with MEN 2B had gastrointestinal symptoms, but only one third had surgery (colectomy, colostomy or pull-through) 1–30 years prior to the MEN 2B diagnosis (30). Although this study was conducted with questionnaires and had only a 59% response, it has promoted awareness of the expanding spectrum of MEN manifestations and the need of prospective screening for MEN in children with intestinal manifestations.

8.2 Association with Neurocutaneous Syndromes

Pheochromocytoma can be genetically linked to neurocutaneous syndromes, also known as phacomatoses, which are inherited by autosomal dominance. In von Hippel-Lindau disease, pheochromocytoma occurs in about 20% of family members (23,26,60). Genetic linkage analysis showed that the gene responsible for VHL is located on the short arm of chromosome 3, within the region of 3p25-3p26 (61). The incidence of VHL is approximately 1:36,000. The spectrum of VHL-associated neoplasms also includes hemangioblastoma of the central nervous system and retina, renal cell carcinoma (usually bilateral), renal and pancreatic cysts, cystic or solid lesions of the liver, spleen, epididymis and ovary, and pancreatic neuroendocrine tumors (23,60,62). Of 256 VHL patients screened by history, physical examination, genotyping, and imaging studies, 30 (12%) had a pancreatic neuroendocrine tumor (11).

The incidence of type 1 neurofibromatosis (NF 1) is 1:3000, and pheochromocytoma is found in up to 2% of those patients and more frequently in those with coexisting hypertension or duodenal carcinoids (22,27, 28,63). The NF 1 gene has been localized on chromosome 17 (17q11.2) (63).

Pheochromocytoma is rarely associated with the Sturge-Weber syndrome and tuberous sclerosis. The former is also known as encephalo-trigeminal syndrome and is characterized by cavernous hemangioma along the facial distribution of the trigeminal nerve and venous hemangiomas of the leptomeninges. The syndrome of tuberous sclerosis comprises hypopigmented skin lesions, angiofibromas distributed in a butterfly configuration over the cheeks, chin, and forehead, and tumors of the central venous system.

8.3 Familial Paraganglioma Syndrome

The genotype of the familial paraganglioma syndrome has been recently defined through discovery of mutations in the genes of succinate dehydrogenase subunit D (SDHD) and succinate dehydrogenase subunit B (SDHB) encoding mitochondrial enzymes involved in oxidative phosphorylation (8,24). The syndrome comprises extra-adrenal pheochromocytoma and tumors of the carotid body, aortic arch, and jugulo-tympanic region. The mendelian inheritance of the syndrome is unknown.

9 EXTRA-ADRENAL PHEOCHROMOCYTOMA

The term functioning paraganglioma is synonymous with extra-adrenal pheochromocytoma. These tumors originate from the system of paraganglia, which extends from the base of the skull to the pelvis and includes the jugulotympanic, vagal, carotid body, laryngeal, aortico-pulmonary, and viscero-autonomic regions (65). The incidence of extra-adrenal tumors is 15–22% of all pheochromocytomas (66,67), with anatomical predilection to the peri-adrenal regions. Extra-adrenal pheochromocytomas rarely co-exist with primary adrenal tumors, sporadic or familial. Eighty-five percent of extra-adrenal pheochromocytomas are located in the abdomen (68) in anatomical regions defined as superior para-aortic, inferior para-aortic, and pelvic (69). The superior para-aortic region includes the peri-adrenal and peri-hilar sites, and the inferior para-aortic includes the inferior perinephric and iliac artery regions. The urinary bladder paragangliomas are classified separately because of their characteristic symptomatology (70). Multicentricity is high, ranging between 15 and 24% overall, and is higher in children (1,5,66–69). Extra-adrenal pheochromocytomas secrete exclusively norepinephrine, because they lack the cortisol-sensitive enzyme phenylethanolamine-*N*-methyltransferase, which catalyzes norepinephrine to epinephrine. Tumors arising from the organ of Zuckerkandl are the exception, as they do produce epinephrine. Localization and surgical treatment of extra-adrenal tumors is more difficult than primary adrenal pheochromocytomas. The small size and multiplicity are often difficult to detect, and confusion with enlarged lymph nodes is not unusual. The best imaging modality is the I-131 MIBG scintigraphy, which offers total body scanning and detection of metastatic disease.

Extra-adrenal pheochromocytomas are the most aggressive of the adult sympatho-adrenal tumors, should be considered malignant, and approached accordingly, whether in the abdomen, chest, or neck (Figs. 6,7). Multifocal disease does not have a higher rate for malignancy than solitary tumors. The reported incidence of malignancy in tumors arising from the organ of Zuckerkandl is 22% (70) and up to 15% in those originating from the urinary bladder (71).The deep retroperitoneal location, often between the cava

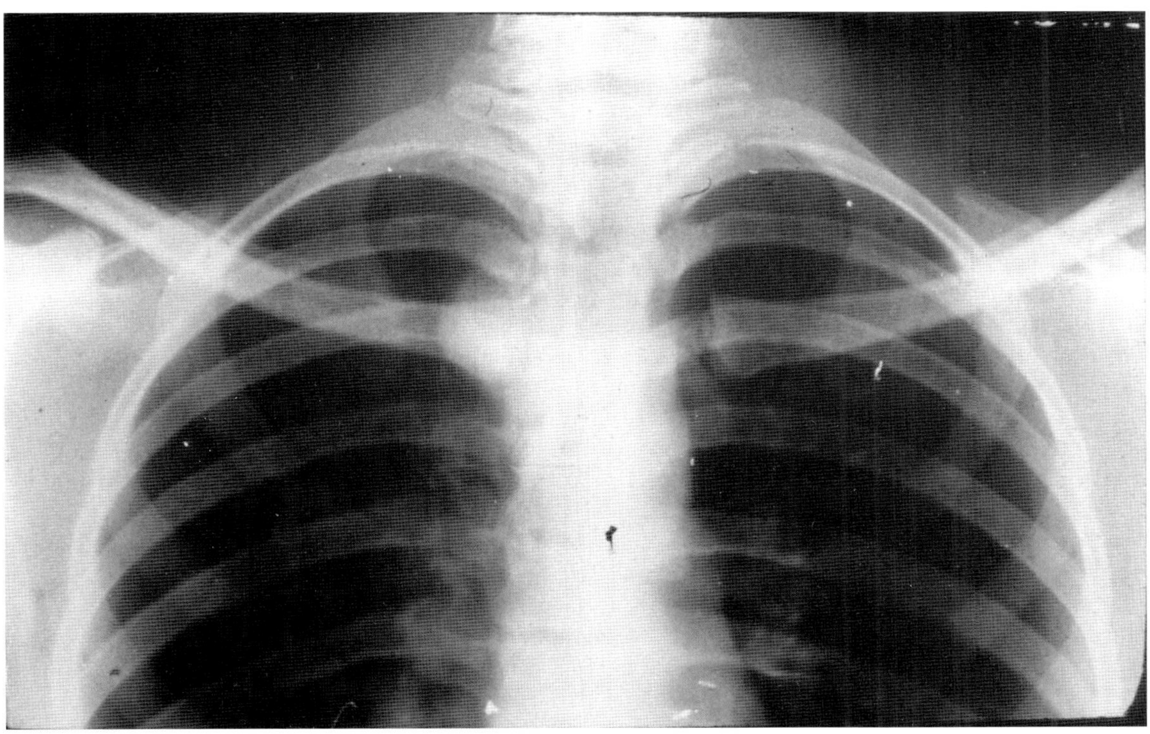

Figure 6 Pheochromocytoma of the superior mediastinum in a 13-year-old associated with one pharyngeal and 13 abdominal extra-adrenal pheochromocytomas. Ten were para-aortic, 2 in the urinary bladder and 1 in the vagina. The mediastinal and 5 para-aortic tumors were resected successfully. The patient died at age 19 from carotid bleeding following resection of the pharyngeal tumor by a different surgical team. Autopsy revealed 5 para-aortic tumors, 2 in the urinary bladder and 1 in the vagina. The adrenal glands were normal.

and aorta, the close proximity to the origin of the inferior mesenteric vessels in Zuckerkandl tumors and the malignant propensity dictate caution in approaching these tumors with endoscopic methods.

10 MALIGNANT PHEOCHROMOCYTOMA

Primary adrenal pheochromocytoma, whether sporadic or familial, carries a risk of malignancy of about 5%, whereas extra-adrenal origin is associated with 5- to 10-fold higher risk (36,68,72,73). In our experience and that of others, one half of all malignant pheochromocytomas arise from extra-adrenal sites (9,68,73,75,76). Patients with malignant tumors, irrespective of origin, typically present in their mid-forties, one decade later than those with benign pheochromocytoma and two decades later than those with familial disease. Other than extra-adrenal origin, there is no identifiable risk factor in the genesis of malignancy.

Markedly elevated serum chromogranin A and high excretion of urinary homovanillic acid are suggestive of malignant pheochromocytoma. Large size with confluent necrosis, local invasion, and distant metastases are the hallmarks of malignant disease as well. The histology of the primary tumor by light microscopy does not permit distinction between benign and malignant tumors. The natural history of malignant pheochromocytoma cannot be predicted by morphological or histochemical features of the primary or metastatic tumors. The typically slow growth of malignant pheochromocytomas favors aggressive surgical debulking and management with antihypertensive and antiarrhythmic medications. Overall, a 50% survival with advanced disease has been reported (9,68,72,75–79).

Reduction in tumor size, serum markers, catecholamine synthesis, and clinical improvement have been difficult to achieve with chemotherapy and conventional or isotope-based radiotherapy.

In a small sample of 14 patients, combination chemotherapy with cyclophosphamide, vincristine, and dacarbazine yielded complete and partial biochemical and clinical response in 79 and 57%, respectively, with a median duration of 21–22 months (80).

A larger experience using isotope-based radiotherapy has been recently reported. Meta-iodobenzylguanidine labeled with I-131 (I-131 MIBG) is taken up and concentrated by 85–90% of pheochromocytomas and metastases enabling delivery of selective therapeutic radiation (81). More than 100 patients have been treated with I-131 MIBG at several medical centers with doses ranging from 100 to more than 500 mCi in single or multiple sessions (82). The radionuclide is also concentrated in the sympathetic neurons and adrenal medulla, but there were no adverse effects on the sympathoadrenal system. Partial remission was reflected in reduction of tumor size and function in one third of the patients. Complete remissions were rare, and recurrence or progression were observed within 2 years. The only serious side effect was transient bone marrow depression.

11 PHEOCHROMOCYTOMA AND PREGNANCY

Hypertension and preeclampsia, common during gestation, the limitations in biochemical diagnosis and localization because of the stress of pregnancy and risk of exposure to ionizing radiation, and the unknown effects of adrenergic blockade on the fetus during the first two trimesters have magnified the challenges in the management of this problem.

Prior to the 1970s unrecognized pheochromocytoma before or during pregnancy, during delivery, and in the early postpartum recovery carried a mortality rate of about 50% for the fetus and the mother (83,84). More recently, improved recognition, localization, and management have resulted in drastic reduction of maternal mortality to 17% overall and to 1% if the diagnosis was made antepartum (85). In a review of 139 patients by Harper et al. (85) the correct diagnosis was made before delivery only in about one half of the cases.

The normal concentrations of catecholamines and their metabolites in the plasma and urine during pregnancy have not been adequately studied even though Freier and Thompson (86) found that they are not affected by pregnancy. Imaging of the abdomen is limited to ultrasonography and MRI as I-131 MIBG and CT are contraindicated because of unknown consequences to the fetus.

The surgical strategies are determined by the obstetrician, the endocrine physician and surgeon, and by the mother. Uncontrolled hypertension at any stage is an indication for immediate surgical intervention. After completion of organogenesis at about 24 weeks, adrenergic blockade is no longer contraindicated and pregnancy can be continued with adequate pharmacological control. In the second trimester, the risk of spontaneous abortion is low and laparoscopic or open surgery is apparently safe (87).

The safest surgical option remains synchronous Cesarian delivery and resection of the pheochromocytoma. Some reports have suggested vaginal delivery followed either by immediate or staged tumor resection as a viable option, provided that postpartum care is given in a monitored setting with strict pharmacological control.

12 PERSONAL EXPERIENCE

From September 1968 to September 2002, 181 operations were performed in 161 patients with pheochromocytoma by the senior author at the Mount Sinai Hospital in New York City. Hospital and office records were reviewed for demographic information, presenting symptoms, associated conditions and family history, laboratory evaluation, tumor localization, operative and pathological findings, and postoperative course. Follow-up information was obtained from charts, personal interviews and correspondence.

12.1 Demographics

There were 161 patients, 66 male and 95 female. There were 127 sporadic cases, 34 familial, 26 extra-adrenal, and 15 with malignant disease. The ages in years expressed in mean $\pm$ SD (range) were 42 $\pm$ 19 (5–86) overall, 45 $\pm$ 19 (5–86) for sporadic, 28 $\pm$ 11 (7–55) for familial, 37 $\pm$ 20 (7–83) for extra-adrenal, and 44 $\pm$ 20 (7–68) for malignant disease. Twenty-four of 26 extra-adrenal tumors and 14 of 15 malignant tumors were in patients diagnosed with sporadic disease, and 9 of the 15 malignancies were found in extra-adrenal locations.

Of the 34 patients with familial disease (17 males and 17 females), 16 were diagnosed with MEN 2A, 11 with von Hippel-Lindau disease, 4 with neurofibromatosis (NF 1), 2 with familial pheochromocytoma, and 1 with familial paraganglioma (PGLI) syndrome. At the time of presentation, 26 patients had a parent, 26 had a sibling, 11 had a second-degree relative, and 1 patient had a child with the same diagnosis. Bilateral tumors were found either synchronously or metachronously in 26 of 34 patients. Fourteen of 16 MEN 2A patients underwent thyroidectomy for medullary cancer, and only 2 were diagnosed with parathyroid disease. Of 11 patients with VHL, 7 developed retinal or CNS hemangiomas, 4 developed renal cell carcinoma, and 2 had pancreatic islet cell tumors. One of 4 with neurofibromatosis had a pancreatic gastrinoma. The 1 patient diagnosed with the newly described PGLI syndrome presented after resection of bilateral carotid body tumors with coexisting extra-adrenal pheochromocytoma and paraganglioma of the aortic arch.

12.2 Symptoms

In the sporadic group, the most common presenting symptoms were headache in 75 (59%), palpitations in 70 (55%), sweating in 60 (47%), dizziness in 18 (14%), nausea in 17 (13%), and blurred vision in 9 (7%). Twenty (16%) patients were asymptomatic on presentation.

The most common presenting symptoms in the familial group were palpitations in 17 (50%), headache in 15 (44%), sweating in 12 (35%), dizziness in 9 (26%), nausea in 6 (18%), and blurred vision in 2 (6%). Nine (26%) patients were asymptomatic on presentation. In both groups, less common complaints included flushing, abdominal pain, fatigue, and panic attacks.

12.3 Hypertension and Cardiac Disease

In the sporadic group, sustained hypertension was present in 78 (61%), paroxysmal hypertension was present in 58 (46%), arrhythmias in 26 (19%), and significant congestive heart failure, cardiomegaly, or cardiomyopathy was found in 3%.

In the familial cases, sustained hypertension was present only in 10 (29%), paroxysmal hypertension in 7 (21%), and an arrhythmia was found in 1 (3%) patient.

12.4 Laboratory Evaluation

Biochemical confirmation of the diagnosis was made by assays of urinary total metanephrines, VMA, and HVA in two separate random sample collections of about 1–2 fluid ounces, in the absence of stress. The results were expressed in μg of the metabolite per mg of urinary creatinine. In cases of equivocal urine assays, plasma catecholamines and metanephrine concentrations with or without clonidine suppression were used. Pharmacological provocative tests were never used because of the risk of serious morbidity caused by the sudden rise or decline in arterial pressure. With the use of combined urinary and serum assays and repeated sampling in borderline cases, a diagnostic accuracy of 98% was attained.

12.5 Localization

Prior to the availability of high-resolution imaging, our surgical approach consisted of open laparotomy with exploration of both adrenals, and the para-aortic, iliac, and uretero-vesical regions, after exclusion of mediastinal tumor by conventional x-ray. Current imaging techniques permit exploration of the abdomen and localization of pheochromocytomas with precision that surpasses the surgeon's tactile and visual sensitivity.

Abdominal ultrasound imaging was the first method of localization used in our series and was the first, and sometimes the only, radiographic study in 42 cases (33%). Ultrasonography proved valuable in large tumors, but had serious limitations in small tumors because of the interposition of gas between the ultrasonic probe and the retroperitoneal target. It has proved unhelpful in the detection of extra-adrenal pheochromocytomas.

Angiography and IVP were employed in 13 (10%) and 22 (17%), respectively, almost exclusively prior to the advent of CT scanning. The potential risk of invasive methods, especially retrograde venography, necessitated pharmacological protection with adrenergic blockers during the procedure to prevent paroxysmal hypertension and/or arrhythmia.

In our series, CT imaging was obtained in 89 patients (70%) and MRI was used in 39 (31%). These methods, used singly or combined, have proven highly successful in the localization of tumors as small as 1 cm.

MIBG and octreotide scintigraphies, which offer localization and high degree of specificity, were used only in 15 cases (12%). The former offers a sensitivity of 85–100% and specificity of 99%, and the latter a sensitivity of 60–90%. One case was diagnosed by PET scan.

12.6 Preoperative and Intraoperative Management

Intravenous continuous infusion of phentolamine at an average rate of 35 (range 5–100) mg/hr was used in all but 11 cases for the control of arterial pressure, and esmolol at an average rate of 154 (20–400) mg/hr for the control of heart rate in all but 20 cases. The two short-acting adrenergic blockers were started 12–24 hours preoperatively after insertion of arterial line and cardiac monitoring in the intensive care unit. Labetalol, a combined α- and β-receptor blocker, was used as a single agent in 11 cases.

12.7 Operative Procedures and Findings

Prior to 1993, an upper midline incision was used almost exclusively in resecting bilateral or unilateral adrenal and extra-adrenal pheochromocytomas. The laparoscopic transperitoneal lateral approach has now been used in 35 unilateral adrenalectomies with conversion to open laparotomy in 3 patients. Two mediastinal tumors were resected through postero-lateral thoracotomy in collaboration with the thoracic surgical service. With one exception, malignant pheochromocytomas were resected by conventional laparotomy.

Unilateral tumors were found in 98 (77%) of sporadic cases, equally divided between right and left. Bilateral pheochromocytomas were found in 5 (4%) patients: 4 synchronous and 1 metachronous. The latter case was that of a 5-year-old girl who had a 168-month interval between adrenalectomies. Autotransplantation of the adrenal cortex was performed twice without success. Extra-adrenal tumors were found in 24 (19%) and resected by open methods.

Unilateral tumors were found in 6 (18%) of familial cases, equally divided between right and left, and extra-adrenal tumors were found in 2 (6%) patients. Bilateral pheochromocytomas were found in 26 (76%) patients: 16 synchronous and 10 metachronous. In the metachronous cases, the average interval between adrenalectomies was 74 months with a range of 9–156 months. Autotransplantation of the adrenal cortex was performed in 16 patients, with success in 6. Three children with VHL disease and bilateral pheochromocytomas had orthotopic preservation of portions of one adrenal to avoid dependence on exogenous steroids during adolescence. All developed recurrence necessitating completion adrenalectomy at intervals of 1–13 years. A 15-year-old female with MEN 2A who had partial bilateral adrenalectomies elsewhere developed recurrence in both glands and underwent bilateral completion adrenalectomies here 3 years later.

In the malignant group, 7 of 15 patients had resection of the primary tumor elsewhere. The intervals between resection of the primary tumor and recurrence ranged from 2 to 19 years. Seven patients had more than one operation with an aggregate of 26 operations in 15 patients.

12.8 Pathology

The anatomical distribution of tumors in the 161 patients is shown in Table 1. Average tumor size in the sporadic group was nearly 7 cm in greatest diameter and was nearly 5 cm in the familial cases. Fourteen (11%) sporadic and 1 familial case had histological evidence of malignancy.

12.9 Postoperative Course

Mean hospital stay overall was 9.4 ± 7.6 days (2 – 55) in the sporadic group and 9.9 ± 5.4 (4 – 20) in the familial

Table 1 Anatomical Distribution of Tumors in (6) Patients

Location	Percentage
Adrenal	
Left	33
Right	32
Bilateral	19
Extra-adrenal Tumors	
Periadrenal/para-aortic	11
Organ of Zuckerkandl	5
Extra-abdominal (mediastinal)	1

group. Those patients who underwent laparoscopic resection had a mean hospital stay of 4.0 ± 2.1, while those undergoing open approaches had a mean stay of 10.8 ± 6.8 days.

12.10 Complications

The demographics and operative data for a case control group of 35 open and 35 laparoscopic cases are presented in Table 2, and the morbidities are presented in Table 3. The overall complications for the entire series are detailed in Table 4. Most notable in the laparoscopic era are a distal pancreatectomy during difficult left adrenal dissection and rupture of a large cystic tumor with subsequent development of multiple peritoneal implants. There was no operative mortality in our 181 operations.

12.11 Outcome

In the sporadic group, mean follow-up was 25 ± 49 months (0 – 328), and residual hypertension was found in 22 (17%), predominantly in patients with malignant disease. As would be expected, mean follow-up in the familial cases was significantly longer, 95 ± 111 months (1 – 336), and residual hypertension was found in 2 (6%). Of the 15 malignant cases, 2 were lost to follow-up and death from metastatic pheochromocytoma occurred in 5 patients after a mean survival of 132 months.

12.12 Discussion

There is no specific constellation of symptoms indicative of pheochromocytoma, but the triad of paroxysmal headaches, palpitations, and sweating should raise suspicion of the syndrome. New-onset hypertension, especially in the young and in families with MEN 2, neurocutaneous, and paraganglioma syndromes, should be promptly investigated. Rare initial presentations include stroke, seizures, diabetes mellitus and insipidus, or cardiomyopathy. Unrecognized pheochromocytoma still carries unacceptable serious morbidity and mortality in the settings of childbirth, unrelated surgery, trauma, and other physical or emotional stress. Two members of families under our care for MEN 2 and von Recklinghausen's disease died at other hospitals, one immediately postpartum and the other 3 days after left adrenalectomy for pheochromocytoma. Autopsy revealed medullary hyperplasia of the remaining adrenal. At our institution, a 47-year-old male underwent resection of a left adrenal pheochromocytoma one month after heart transplant for what was thought to be irreversible cardiomyopathy. Had the tumor been detected and treated, the transplant might have been unnecessary.

Biochemical diagnosis under standardized and unstressed conditions with urinary and, if needed, plasma catecholamines and their metabolites, with or

Table 2 Comparison of Laparoscopic and Open Experience

	Open (n = 35)	Laparoscopic (n = 35)
Female gender (%)	70	71
Age (mean)	44	46
Left side (%)	64	48
Tumor size (cm)	5.2	4.9
Phentolamine required (mg/hr)	32	26
Esmolol required (mg/hr)	208	118
Blood loss (mL)	410	135
Hospital stay (days)	10	4

Table 3 Operative Complications (Case-Control Study)

	Open (n = 35)	Laparoscopic (n = 35)
Pneumonia	2	0
Pneumothorax	1	1
Pleural effusion	1	0
Bleeding requiring reexploration	1	0
SBO requiring reexploration	1	0
Splenectomy	1	0
Distal pancreatectomy	0	1
Tumor rupture/seeding	0	1
Mortality	0	0

without clonidine suppression, approaches 100% accuracy. Provocative tests have no place in this disease because of the risk of morbidity and mortality. Pheochromocytomas can be localized using CT, MRI, and MIBG scintigraphy, alone or in combination, with a precision approaching 100%. Abdominal ultrasound and octreotide scanning offer a lower sensitivity. The accuracy with which noninvasive imaging techniques explore the abdomen have made routine surgical exposure of both adrenals and para-aortic and pelvic regions unnecessary. The open lumbar and laparoscopic approaches which limit access to one adrenal are now fully justified. Our current approach to diagnosis, localization, and treatment is depicted in the algorithm shown in Figure 8.

Continuous intravenous phentolamine and, if needed, esmolol offer the unique advantages of short half-life, no toxicity, and efficient regulation of arterial pressure and heart rate. The moment-to-moment adjustment of the infusion rates and the immediate cardiovascular response are critical to the safe conduct of the operation. The rapid restoration of physiological hemodynamic and cardiac indices after discontinuing adrenergic blockade permits accurate judgment regard-

Table 4 Operative Complications (Overall)

	Open (n = 146)	Laparoscopic (n = 35)
Pneumonia	5	0
Pneumothorax	1	1
Pleural effusion	3	0
Bleeding requiring reexploration	1	0
SBO requiring reexploration	2	0
Splenectomy	5	0
Splenorrhaphy	3	0
Distal pancreatectomy	0	1
Tumor rupture/seeding	1	1
Renal artery injury/repair	1	0
Unilateral loss of renal function	1	0
Incisional hernia	3	1
Perioperative CVA	2	0
Deep vein thrombosis	1	0
Pulmonary embolism	1	0
Infectious colitis	1	0
Mortality	0	0

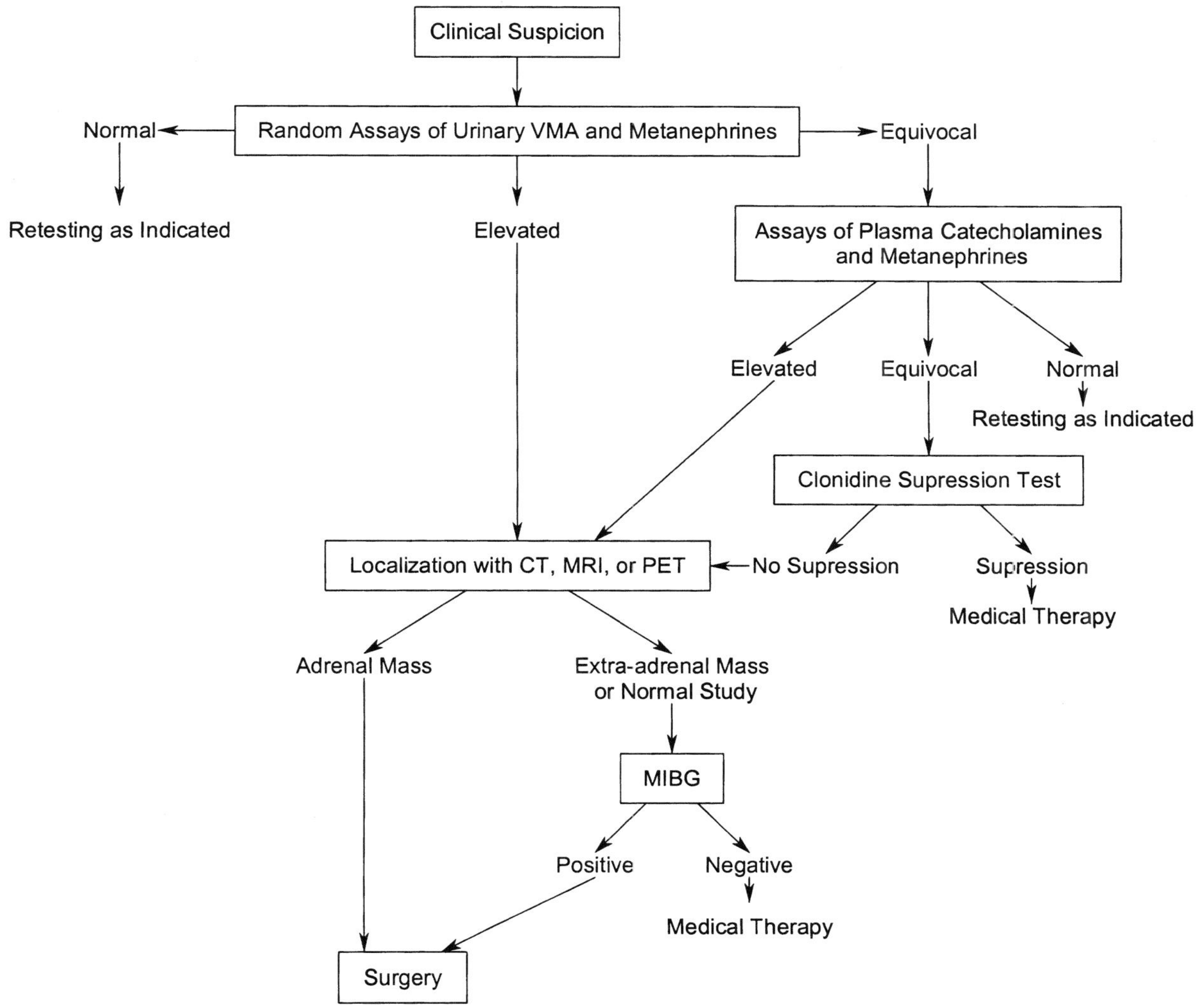

Figure 8 Algorithm for the diagnosis, localization, and treatment of pheochromocytoma.

ing completeness of tumor resection. These two requirements cannot be met with long-acting adrenergic blockers. The concern that high intra-abdominal pressures from pneumoperitoneum would render the control of arterial pressure and heart rate more difficult has been disproven, as the doses of adrenergic receptor blockers needed for laparoscopic adrenalectomies do not differ from those with the conventional open approaches (Table 2).

In bilateral adrenal pheochromocytomas, open transperitoneal resection can be accomplished through an upper midline or bilateral subcostal incision. Extra-adrenal abdominal pheochromocytomas should be preferentially approached through open laparotomy. Laparoscopic experience with bilateral simultaneous adrenalectomy is limited but feasible. Extra-adrenal tumors are often multiple and are potentially malignant and laparoscopic resection should be avoided until the risk of port-site implantation of tumor cells has been disproven by prospective, randomized trials.

In the past 9 years we performed 35 laparoscopic adrenalectomies using the lateral transperitoneal approach with 3 conversions to open. In the same time period 11 pheochromocytomas were resected by the open method because of large tumor size, malignancy, recent stroke, advanced pulmonary disease, and cardiomyopathy. These are relative contra-indications for the laparoscopic method, with recent stroke and myocardial infarction posing special risks because of the increased intracranial pressure and reduction in cardiac output as a result of pneumoperitoneum.

In synchronous bilateral adrenal tumors, frequently seen in patients with familial disease, complete resection of both adrenals is mandatory. Those who advocate orthotopic preservation of adrenal tissue ignore the genesis of tumors from diffuse or nodular medullary hyperplasia. Subtotal resection leads to predictable recurrence within 3 years. Heterotopic autotransplantation of histologically proven pure adrenocortical tissue is an option, even though autografting has achieved limited success.

The debate over removal of the contralateral normal-appearing adrenal in inherited pheochromocytoma will likely continue. The arguments favoring prophylactic resection are predictable high recurrence, morbidity of a second operation, risk of rupture of hemangiomas during hypertensive crises in VHL patients, risk of morbidity or mortality with accidental trauma and lack of compliance with follow-up. Although almost all prophylactically resected adrenals display medullary hyperplasia, we and others advocate close surveillance and metachronous surgery for clinical, biochemical, and imaging evidence of recurrent disease.

All patients with sporadic pheochromocytoma should have lifelong surveillance to detect recurrence and possible association with inherited syndromes Adults who present with sporadic pheochromocytoma should be screened with serum calcitonin, calcium, and parathyroid hormone to exclude MEN 2A and should have ophthalmological examination to rule out the diagnosis of VHL. Children and adolescents should undergo the same screening, with the addition of genetic testing. Patients with sporadic extra-adrenal tumors should be investigated for multiplicity, malignancy, and coexisting paragangliomas. Those with established inherited neoplasia syndromes and their families should undergo screening for the presence of and surveillance for the development of pheochromocytoma using clinical parameters and, if necessary, imaging. Patients diagnosed with pheochromocytoma as part of an inherited syndrome should undergo lifelong testing for recurrence and for development of the other components of the neoplastic syndromes. Pheochromocytoma can be the first manifestation in inherited cancer syndromes, and simultaneous clinical expression of the neoplastic syndromes is the exception rather than the rule.

Malignant pheochromocytoma is rare—about 10% in this and other series. About one half of all malignant tumors arise from extra-adrenal sites in the abdomen, mediastinum, or neck. Unlike adrenocortical tumors, size and angiolymphatic extension are not always predictive of malignant pheochromocytoma. Palliative debulking with optimal antiadrenergic therapy offers long survival.

REFERENCES

1. Hume DM. Pheochromocytoma in the adult and in the child. Am J Surg 1960; 99:458–496.
2. Smithwick RR, Greer WER, Robertson CW, Wilkins RW. Pheochromocytoma: a discussion of symptoms, signs and procedures of diagnostic value. N Engl J Med 1950; 242:252.
3. Lenders JWM, Keiser HR, Goldstein DS, et al. Plasma metanephrines in the diagnosis of pheochromocytoma. Ann Intern Med 1995; 123:101–109.
4. Eisenhofer G, Lenders JWM, Linehan WM, et al. Plasma normetanephrine and metanephrine for detecting pheochromocytoma in von Hippel-Lindau disease and multiple endocrine neoplasia type 2. N Engl J Med 1999; 340:1872–1879.
5. Stackpole RH, Melicow MM, Uson AC. Pheochromocytoma in children: report of 9 cases and review of the first 100 published cases with follow-up studies. J Pediatr 1963; 63:315–330.
6. Gitlow SE, Pertsemlidis D, Dziedzic SW. Pheochromocytoma. In: Krieger DT, Bardin CW, eds. Current Therapy in Endocrinology. Philadelphia: BC Decker, 1983-1984:110–114.
7. Gitlow SE, Pertsemlidis D, Dziedzic SW. Pheochromocytoma. In: Krieger DT, Bardin CW, eds. Current Therapy in Endocrinology and Metabolism. Philadelphia: BC Decker, 1988:148–152.
8. Neumann HPH, Bausch B, McWhinney SR, et al. Germline mutations in nonsyndromic pheochromocytoma. N Engl J Med 2002; 346:1459–1470.
9. Pertsemlidis D. Laparoscopic versus open adrenalectomy in pheochromocytoma. In: Bruch HP Koeckerling F, Bouchard R, Schug-Pass C, eds. Bologna: Monduzzi Editore, 2000:65–74.
10. Curley SA, Lott ST, Luca JW, Frazier ML, Killary AM. Surgical decision-making affected by clinical and genetic screening of a novel kindred with von Hippel-Lindau disease and pancreatic islet cell tumors. Ann Surg 1998; 227:229–235.
11. Libutti SK, Choyke PL, Bartlett DL, et al. Pancreatic neuroendocrine tumors associated with von Hippel-Lindau disease: diagnostic and management recommendations. Surgery 1998; 124(6):1153–1159.
12. Carney JA, Sheps SG, Gordon H. The triad of gastric leiomyosarcoma, functioning extra-adrenal paraganglioma and pulmonary chondroma. N Engl J Med 1977; 296:1517–1518.
13. Manger WM, Gifford RW Jr. Pheochromocytoma New York: Springer Verlag, 1977.

14. Pick L. Das Ganglioma Embryonale Sympathicum (Sympathoma Embryonale), eine typische boesartige Geschwulstform des sympathisches Nervensystem. Berl Klin Wochenschr 1912; 49:16–22.
15. Armstrong MD, Shaw KNF, Wall PR. The phenolic acids in human urine. J Biol Chem 1956; 218:293.
16. Axelrod J. O-Methylation of epinephrine and other catechols. Science 1957; 126:400.
17. Gitlow SE, Mendlowitz M, Khassis S, Cohen G, Sha J. The diagnosis of pheochromocytoma by determination of urinary 3-methoxy-4-hydroxy-mandelic acid. J Clin Invest 1960; 39:221–226.
18. Gitlow SE, Mendlowitz M, Kruk E, Khassis S. Diagnosis of pheochromocytoma by assay of catecholamine metabolites. Circ Res 1961; 9:746–754.
19. Gitlow SE, Mendlowitz M, Wilk EK, Wilk S, Wolf RL, Bertani LM. Excretion of catecholamine metabolites by normal children. J Lab Clin Invest 1968; 72:612–620.
20. Sipple JH. The association of pheochromocytoma with carcinoma of the thyroid gland. Am J Med 1961; 31:163.
21. Eng C. The RET proto-oncogene in multiple endocrine neoplasias type 2 and Hirschsprung's disease. N Engl J Med 1996; 335:943–951.
22. Ricardi VM. Neurofibromatosis: past, present, and future. N Engl J Med 1991; 324:1283–1285.
23. Couch V, Lindor N, Karnes PS, Michels VV. Von Hippel-Lindau disease. Mayo Clin Proc 2000; 75:265–272.
24. Arguiar RCT, Cox G, Pomeroy SL, Dahia RLM. Analysis of the SDHD gene, the susceptibility gene for familial paraganglioma syndrome (PGLI) in pheochromocytoma. J Clin Endocrinol Metab 2001; 86:2890–2894.
25. Lamiell JM, Salazar FG, Hsia YE. Von Hippel-Lindau disease affecting 43 members of a single kindred. Medicine (Balt) 1989; 68:1–29.
26. Maher ER, Yates ER, Harries R. Clinical features and natural history of von Hippel-Lindau disease. Quart J Med 1990; 77:1151–1163.
27. Kalff V, Shapiro B, Lloyd R, et al. The spectrum of pheochromocytoma in hypertensive patients with neurofibromatosis. Arch Intern Med 1982; 142:2092–2098.
28. Griffiths DFR, Williams GT, Williams ED. Duodenal carcinoid tumors, pheochromocytoma and neurofibromatosis; islet cell tumors, pheochromocytoma and von Hippel-Lindau complex: two distinctive neuroendocrine syndromes. Quart J Med 1987; 245:769–782.
29. Howe JR, Norton JA, Wells SA Jr. Prevalence of pheochromocytoma and hyperparathyroidism in multiple endocrine neoplasia type 2A: results of long-term follow-up. Surgery 1993; 114:1070–1077.
30. Cohen MS, Phay JE, DeBenedetti MK, et al. Gastrointestinal manifestations of multiple endocrine neoplasia type 2. 113th Annual Session of the Southern Surgical Association, Hot Springs, VA, Dec 2–5, 2001.
31. Trump DL, Livingston JN, Brylin DB. Watery diarrhea syndrome in an adult with ganglioneuroma-pheochromocytoma: identification of vasoactive intestinal polypeptide, calcitonin and catecholamines and assessment of their biologic activity. Cancer 1977; 40:15–26.
32. Sackel SG, Manson JE, Hazawi SJ, Burakoff R. Watery diarrhea syndrome due to an adrenal pheochromocytoma secreting vasoactive intestinal polypeptide. Dig Dis Sci 1985; 30:1201–1207.
33. Fisher BM, MacPhee GJA, Davies DL, et al. A case of watery diarrhoea syndrome due to an adrenal pheochromocytoma secreting vasoactive intestinal polypeptide with coincidental autoimmune thyroid disease. Acta Endocrinol 1987; 114:340–344.
34. Herrera MF, Stone E, Deitel M, Asa SL. Pheochromocytoma producing multiple vasoactive peptides. Arch Surg 1992; 127:105–108.
35. Wilkenfeld C, Cohen M, Lansman SL, Courtney M, Dische MR, Pertsemlidis D, et al. Heart transplantation for end-stage cardiomyopathy caused by an occult pheochromocytoma. J Heart Lung Transpl 1992; 11:363–366.
36. Inabnet WB, Caragliano P, Pertsemlidis D. Pheochromocytoma: inherited associations, bilaterality and cortex preservation. Surgery 2000; 128(6):1007–1011.
37. Pertsemlidis D, Gitlow SE, Siegel W, Kark AE. Pheochromocytoma: 1) specificity of laboratory diagnostic tests. 2) safeguards during operative removal. Ann Surg 1969; 169:376–385.
38. Lenders JWM, Pacak K, Walther MM, et al. Biochemical diagnosis of pheochromocytoma. JAMA 2002; 287: 1427–1434.
39. Young WF Jr. Pheochromocytoma and primary aldosteronism: diagnostic approaches. Endocrinol Metab Clin North Am 1997; 26(4):801–827.
40. Gitlow SE, Mendlowitz M, Wilk EK, et al. Excretion of catecholamine metabolites by normal children and those with familial dysautonomia. J Clin Invest 1965; 44:1049.
41. Bravo EL, Tarazi RC, Fouad FM, Vidt DG, Gifford RWJ. Clonidine-suppression test: a useful aid in the diagnosis of pheochromocytoma. N Engl J Med 1981; 305:623–626.
42. Yeh HC. Ultrasonography of normal adrenal glands and small adrenal masses. Am J Roentgenol 1980; 1135: 1167–1177.
43. Korobkin M, Brodeur FJ, Francis IR, et al. Delayed enhanced CT for differentiation of benign from malignant adrenal masses. Radiology 1996; 200:737–742.
44. Raisanen J, Shapiro B, Glazer GM, et al. Plasma catecholamines in pheochromocytoma: effect of urographic contrast media. Am J Roentgenol 1984; 143:43–46.
45. Mukherjee JJ, Peppercorn PD, Reznek RH, et al. Pheochromocytoma: effect of nonionic contrast medium in CT on circulating catecholamine levels. Radiology 1997; 202:227–231.
46. Shapiro B, Copp JE, Sisson JC, et al. 131-Iodine-metaiodobenzylguanidine for the locating of suspected

phaeochromocytoma: experience in 400 cases. J Nucl Med 1985:576–585.
47. Hoefnagel CA. Metaiodobenzylguanidine and somatostatin in oncology. Eur J Nucl Med 1994; 21:561–581.
48. Seregni E, Chiti A, Bombardieri E. Radionuclide imaging of neuroendocrine tumours: biological basis and diagnostic results. Eur J Nucl Med 1998; 25:639–658.
49. Proye C, Thevenin D, Cecat P, et al. Exclusive use of calcium channel blockers in preoperative and intraoperative control of pheochromocytomas: hemodynamics and free catecholamine assays in ten consecutive patients. Surgery 1989; 106:1149–1154.
50. Boutros AR, Bravo EL, Zanettin G, Straffon RA. Perioperative management of 63 patients with pheochromocytoma. Cleve Clin J Med 1990; 57:613–617.
51. Johns VJ, Brunjes S. Pheochromocytoma. Am J Cardiol 1962; 9:120–125.
52. Sjoerdsma A, Engelman K, Waldmann TA, Cooperman LH, Hammond WG. Pheochromocytoma: current concepts of diagnosis and treatment; combined clinical staff conference at the National Institutes of Health. Ann Intern Med 1996; 65:1302–1306.
53. Newell KA, Prinz RA, Brooks MH, et al. Plasma catecholamine changes during excision of pheochromocytoma. Surgery 1988; 104:1064–1073.
54. Gabrielson G, Guffin A, Kaplan J, Pertsemlidis D, Iberti T. Continuous intravenous infusions of phentolamine and esmolol for preoperative and intraoperative adrenergic blockade in patients with pheochromocytoma. J Cardiothoracic anesthesia 1987; 6:554.
55. Baxter Healthcare Corporation: Brochure. Sodium Nitroprusside Injection. Greenfield, IL.
56. Rosenthal RJ, Friedman RL, Phillips EH. Intraabdominal pressure, intracranial pressure and hemodynamics. In: Rosenthal RJ, Friedman RL, Phillips EH, eds. Pathophysiology of Pneumoperitoneum. Berlin: Springer Verlag, 1998:85–98.
57. Mitty HA, Yeh HC. Radiology of the Adrenals with Sonography and CT. Philadelphia: Saunders Company, 1982.
58. Pertsemlidis D. Minimal access versus open adrenalectomy. Surg Endosc 1995; 9:384–386.
59. Carney JA, Sizemore GW, Sheps SG. Adrenal medullary disease in multiple endocrine neoplasia type 2: pheochromocytoma and its precursors. Am J Clin Pathol 1976; 66:279.
60. Neumann HPH, Berger DP, Sigmund G, et al. Pheochromocytoma, multiple endocrine neoplasia type 2 and von Hippel-Lindau disease. N Engl J Med 1993; 329:1531–1538.
61. Latif F, Tory K, Gnaza J, et al. Identification of the von Hippel-Lindau disease tumor suppressor gene. Science 1993; 260:1317–1320.
62. Curley SA, Lott ST, Luca JW, et al. Surgical decision making affected by clinical and genetic screening of a novel kindred with von Hippel-Lindau disease and pancreatic islet cell tumors. Ann Surg 1998; 227:229–235.
63. Walther MM, Herring J, Enquist E, et al. von Recklinghausen's disease and pheochromocytoma. J Urol 1999; 162:1582–1586.
64. Barsh GS. Hereditary disorders. In: Leder P, Clayton DA, Rubenstein E, eds. Scientific American. Introduction to Molecular Medicine. New York: Scientific American, 220-224
65. Lack EE. Pathology of Adrenal and Extra-adrenal Paraganglia. Philadelphia: WB Saunders, 1994:1–14.
66. Moulton JS, Moulton JS. CT of adrenal glands. Sem Roentgen 1988; 23:288.
67. Stenstroem G, Svaerdsudd K. Pheochromocytoma in children 1958–1981: an analysis of the National Cancer Registry. Acta Med Scand 1986; 220:225.
68. Melicow MM. One-hundred cases of pheochromocytoma (107 tumors) at the Columbia-Presbyterian Medical Center 1926–1976: a clinicopathological analysis. Cancer 1977; 40:1987–2004.
69. Fries JG, Chamberlin JA. Extra-adrenal pheochromocytoma: literature review and report of a cervical pheochromocytoma. Surgery 1968; 63:268–279.
70. Glenn F, Gray GF. Functional tumors of the organ of Zuckerkandl. Ann Surg 1976; 183:578–586.
71. Khan O, Williams G, Chisholm GD, Welbourn RB. Pheochromocytoma of the urinary bladder. J Roy Soc Med 1982; 75:17.
72. Scott HW Jr, Halter SA. Oncologic aspects of pheochromocytoma: the importance of follow-up. Surgery 1984; 96:1061–1066.
73. van Heerden JA, Sizemore GW, Carney JA, et al. Surgical management of the adrenal glands in the multiple endocrine neoplasia 2 syndrome. World J Surg 1984; 8:612.
74. Modlin IM, Farndon JR, Shepherd A, et al. Pheochromocytoma in 72 patients: clinical and diagnostic features, treatment and long-term results. Br J Surg 1979; 66:465.
75. Mahoney EM, Harrison JH. Malignant pheochromocytoma: clinical course and treatment. J Urol 1977; 118: 225–229.
76. Sclafani LM, Woodruff JM, Brennan MF. Extraadrenal retroperitoneal paragangliomas: natural history and response to treatment. Surgery 1990; 108:1124–1130.
77. Thompson NW, Allo MD, Shapiro B, et al. Extraadrenal and metastatic pheochromocytoma: the role of I-131 meta-iodobenzylguanidine (I-131 MIBG) in localization and management. World J Surg 1984; 8:605–611.
78. Hayes WS, Davidson AJ, Grimley PM, et al. Extraadrenal retroperitoneal paraganglioma: clinical, pathological and CT findings. AJR 1990; 155:1247–1250.

79. van Heerden JA, Sheps BH, Sheedy PF, et al. Pheochromocytoma: current status and changing trends. Surgery 1982; 91:367–373.
80. Averbuch SD, Steakly CS, Young RC, et al. Malignant pheochromocytoma: effective treatment with a combination of cyclophosphamide, vincristine and dacarbazine. Ann Intern Med 1988; 109:267–273.
81. Shapiro B, Copp JE, Sissan JC, et al. Iodine-131 metaiodobenzylguanidine for the locating of suspected pheochromocytoma: experience in 400 cases. J Nucl Med 1985; 26:576–585.
82. Sisson JC. Radiopharmacuetical treatment of pheochromocytoma. Ann NY Acad Sci 2002; 970:54–60.
83. Schenker JG, Chowers I. Pheochromocytoma and pregnancy. Obstet Gynecol Surg 1971; 26:739–746.
84. Schenker JG, Granat M. Pheochromocytoma and pregnancy — an updated appraisal. Aust NZ J Obstet Gynaecol 1982; 22:1–10.
85. Harper MA, Murnaghan GA, Kennedy L, et al. Pheochromocytoma in pregnancy: five cases and a review of the literature. Br J Obstet Gynaecol 1989; 996:594–606.
86. Freier DT, Thompson NW. Pheochromocytoma and pregnancy. Surgery 1993; 114:1148–1152.
87. Brunt LM. Phaeochromocytoma in pregnancy. Br J Surg 2001; 88:481–483.

37

Techniques of Conventional Open Adrenalectomy

Demetrius Pertsemlidis and David S. Pertsemlidis

Mount Sinai School of Medicine, New York University, New York, New York, U.S.A.

1 SURGICAL ANATOMY AND ACCESS TO THE ADRENALS

The adrenal glands are small (4–5 g each, 4–6 cm long, 2–3 cm wide) and are hidden in the uppermost paraspinal recess of the retroperitoneum at the level of the 11th and 12th ribs. The topographic relationship of the adrenals to the kidneys, aorta, and inferior vena cava is shown in Figure 1. The renal arteries are posterior and slightly superior to the renal veins, and one third to one half of the right adrenal gland is retrocaval. The glands are covered anteriorly by Gerota's fascia and are surrounded by fibrofatty tissue. Lipochrome pigment conveys the golden yellow color to the cortex and the less intense pale yellow color to the surrounding fat.

The arterial supply is comprised of 50–60 branches from the inferior phrenic, aorta, and renal arteries, forming a subcapsular plexus (Fig. 2). The main right adrenal vein, about 1 cm long, enters the cava on the posterior or posterolateral side at a distance of 6–7 cm from the junction of the renal vein and cava, occasionally joined by an accessory hepatic vein before entry. The main left adrenal vein, about 2–3 cm long, joins the inferior phrenic before entering the renal vein along its superior wall, at a distance of about 10 cm from the hilus (Fig. 3). Emissary veins connecting the central vein with the pericapsular venous plexus and with renal capsular veins provide alternate pathways for venous outflow at times of stress and protection of the gland from hemorrhage.

The adrenal glands are not easily accessible through either the conventional open or endoscopic approaches. The partially retrocaval and retrohepatic location of the right, the para-aortic, retropancreatic, and juxtasplenic position of the left, their small size, and the surrounding periadrenal and perinephric fat render their exposure difficult.

Three open approaches to the adrenals, the retroperitoneal lumbar, retroperitoneal posterior, and transperitoneal anterior, have dominated our practice. The anterior transperitoneal access remains the optimal approach to malignant and large adrenal tumors. These lesions are highly vascular and are often surrounded by pericapsular desmoplastic reaction, rendering the dissection bloody and difficult. Extra-adrenal pheochromocytomas should be preferentially resected through open laparotomy as their difficult anatomical location along the aorta, often between the aorta and cava, and the high propensity for malignancy demand precise vascular and oncological dissection. Peri-adrenal tumors are at times inseparable from the gland and have to be resected en bloc.

2 RETROPERITONEAL LATERAL APPROACH

2.1 Right Adrenalectomy

The patient arrives in the operating room with established peripheral arterial, central venous, and, in selec-

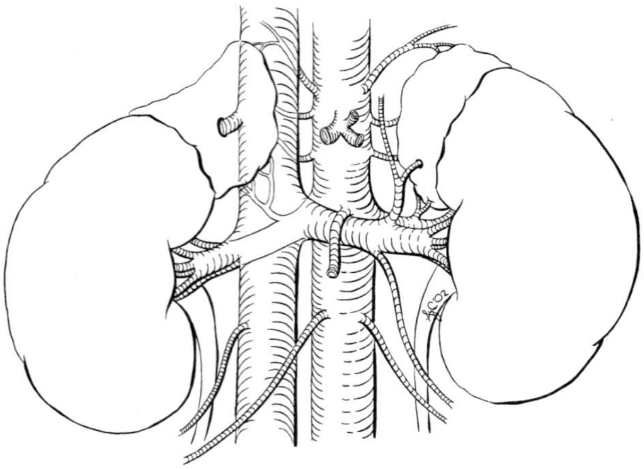

Figure 1 Anatomical relationship of the left and right adrenal glands to the kidneys, aorta, and inferior vena cava. Note the partially retrocaval location of the right gland.

ted cases, pulmonary artery catheters. Anesthetic induction, endotracheal intubation, and insertion of urinary catheter are performed in supine position. The patient is then placed in a left lateral position with the brachial plexus protected by an axillary roll and the right arm suspended on an arm rest. The table is flexed to expose the lumbar region (Fig. 4). Antibiotic prophylaxis against *Staphylococcus aureus* is given within one hour before the incision.

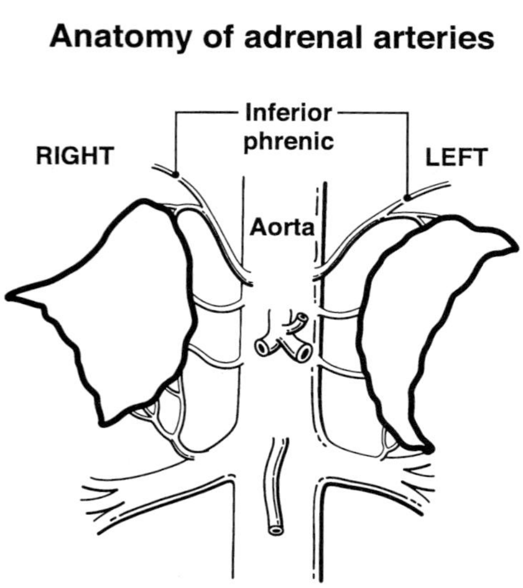

Figure 2 The blood supply to the adrenals is from numerous branches of the aorta inferior phrenic and renal arteries, forming a subcapsular plexus.

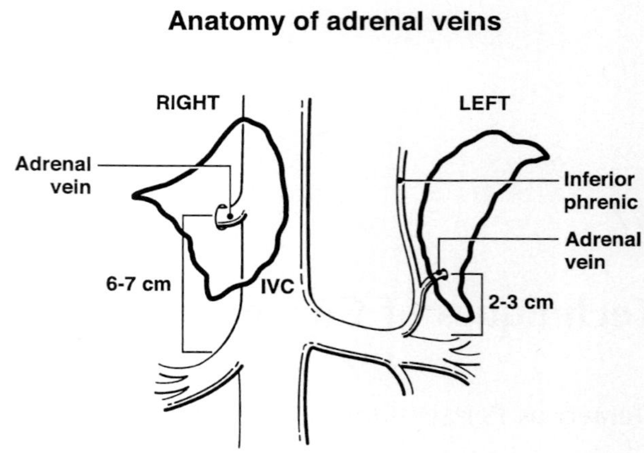

Figure 3 The venous drainage of the adrenals is through a main vein and numerous emissary veins that protect the gland from hemorrhage. Note the significant difference in length between the right and left adrenal veins.

The transverse skin incision is placed along the course of the eleventh rib and extends from the lateral margin of the rectus sheath to the costal angle (Fig. 4). Division of the external oblique and latissimus dorsi is followed by cutting the internal oblique, transversus, and the posterior inferior serratus muscles (Fig. 5). The lumbodorsal fascia enveloping the quadratus lumborum may have to be divided to facilitate the exposure. The lowest intercostal nerves should be preserved whenever possible.

Subperiosteal mobilization and transection of the 11th and, if needed, the 12th ribs should be close to the costal angle (Fig. 6). Inadvertent entry into the pleura is common and inconsequential if recognized and closed with the lung inflated.

The peritoneum covering the liver, duodenum, and right colon is separated from the para-renal fat (Fig. 7), which is excised to expose the kidney (Fig. 8). Division of Gerota's fascia (Fig. 9) is followed by excision of the perinephric adipose tissue to facilitate mobility and retraction of the kidney.

The anatomical landmarks are the inferior vena cava and renal vein. The mobilized kidney is retracted to expose the adrenal gland. Dissection along the lateral avascular margin is followed by separation of the posterior surface of the gland from the upper pole of the kidney. In the apical region, the inferior phrenic vessels are isolated and divided between clips. The freeing of the lateral, posterior, and apical planes is a major advantage as it permits gentle retraction of the adrenal to expose the planes along the renal vessels and cava. These are vascular planes demanding ligation and divi-

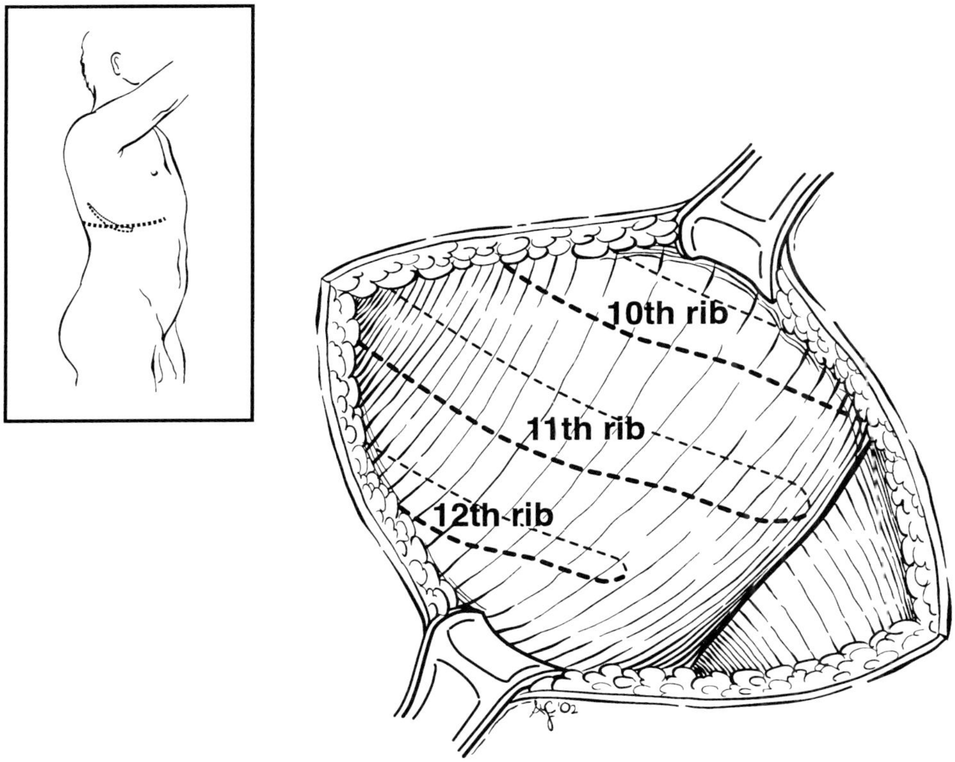

Figure 4 The transverse skin incision for the retroperitoneal lateral approach to the right adrenal is centered over the 11th rib and extends from lateral edge of rectus sheath to costal angle.

sion of small renal and aortic arterial branches and tributaries to the renal vein and cava before the short main renal vein can be exposed (Fig. 10). During dissection along the renal vein, the posterior and slightly superior renal artery and the difficult exposure of the junction of the renal vein and cava may pose problems. Retraction of the mobilized adrenal and cava exposes the para-caval and retro-caval planes to permit easy ligation and division of the main vein (Fig. 11).

In case of accidental tear of the main adrenal vein, usually at its confluence with the cava, a Satinsky vascular clamp can be used for partial occlusion of the cava and suture ligation of the tear. Occasionally, there are small hepatic venous tributaries to the cava, which are not difficult to recognize and treat. The adequacy of exposure of the inferior vena cava and the completeness of hemostasis are shown in Figure 12.

2.2 Left Adrenalectomy

The approach to the left adrenal is a mirror image of that to the right side in the initial steps.

The peritoneum covering the descending colon, splenic flexure, pancreas, and spleen is separated from the para-renal fat and kidney. The anatomical landmarks are the renal vein inferiorly and the aorta medially (Figs. 3, 13).

The sequence of dissection should be similar to that on the right side. The thick wall of the aorta makes the dissection along the para-aortic plane easier than along the inferior vena cava. The relatively long main adrenal vein should be ligated and divided distal to the confluence with the inferior phrenic vein (Figs. 3, 13).

Closure of the incision on either side is done, after restoring the horizontal position, with running sutures separately for the deep and superficial muscle layers.

3 OPEN ANTERIOR TRANSPERITONEAL APPROACH

The anterior transperitoneal approach is familiar to general and endocrine surgeons. The surgical exposure of the adrenals differs from the extraperitoneal ap-

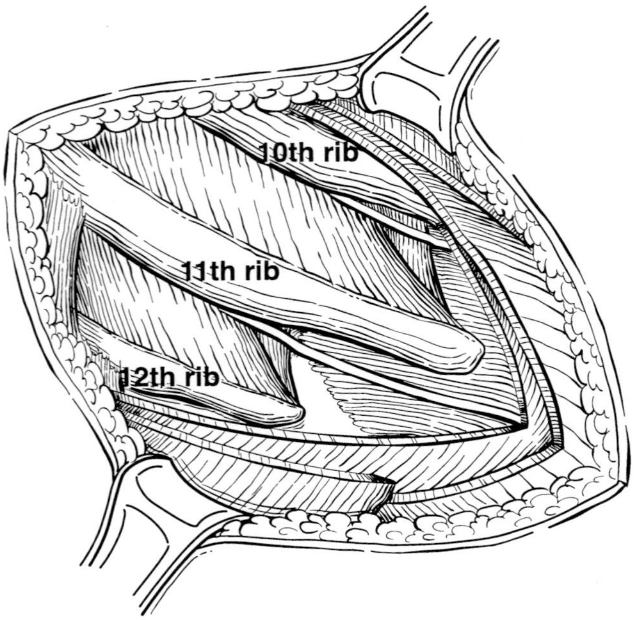

Figure 5 Exposure of the 11th rib requires division of the external oblique and latissimus dorsi, internal oblique, transversus, and posterior inferior serratus muscles.

proaches, but the suprarenal dissection is similar. The retropancreatic position of the left and the partially retrocaval location of the right combined with proximity to major vessels pose a greater challenge, especially with large tumors. Adrenal and extra-adrenal tumors may grow near or around the renal vessels and may be difficult to resect without disrupting renal blood flow.

A midline incision allows access to both adrenals, para-aortic, and pelvic regions, whereas subcostal incisions are better suited for unilateral adrenalectomy.

3.1 Right Adrenalectomy

The exposure of the right adrenal requires mobilization and retraction of the hepatic flexure of the colon and duodenum to expose the inferior vena cava. In large tumors the coronary ligament of the liver is divided to facilitate its retraction. Once the kidney is exposed and stripped of its para-renal and peri-nephric fat, retraction exposes the adrenal gland. The renal vein is exposed and the inferior vena cava is medially retracted to uncover the retrocaval portion of the gland. Sequential freeing of the lateral, posterior, and apical por-

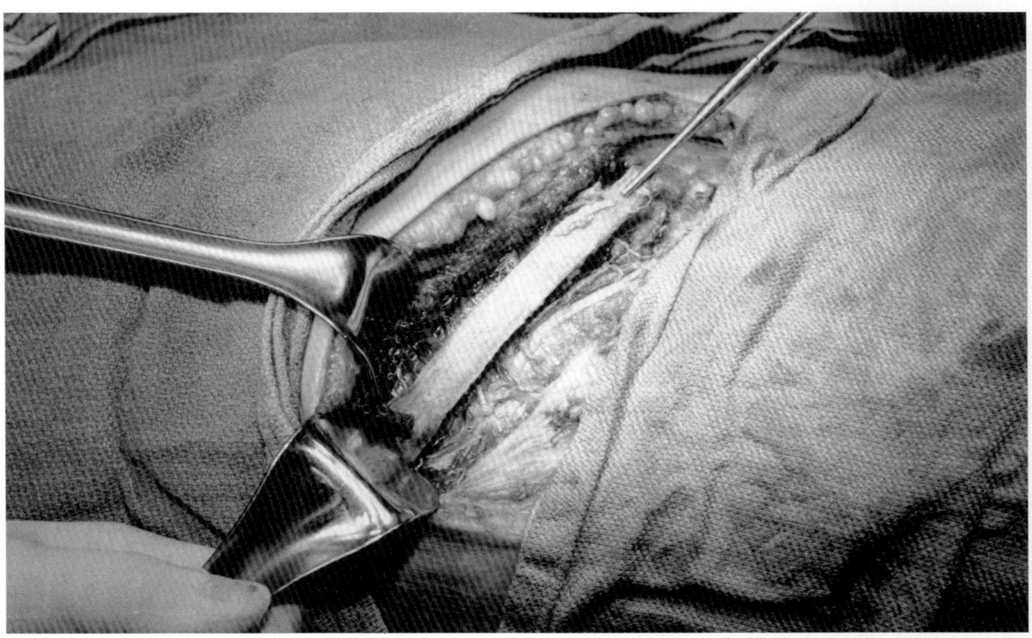

Figure 6 With the periosteum incised, the 11th rib can be elevated and transected close to the costal angle. Entry into the pleura is common and is easily recognized and repaired. Care is taken to avoid injury to the lowest intercostals nerves.

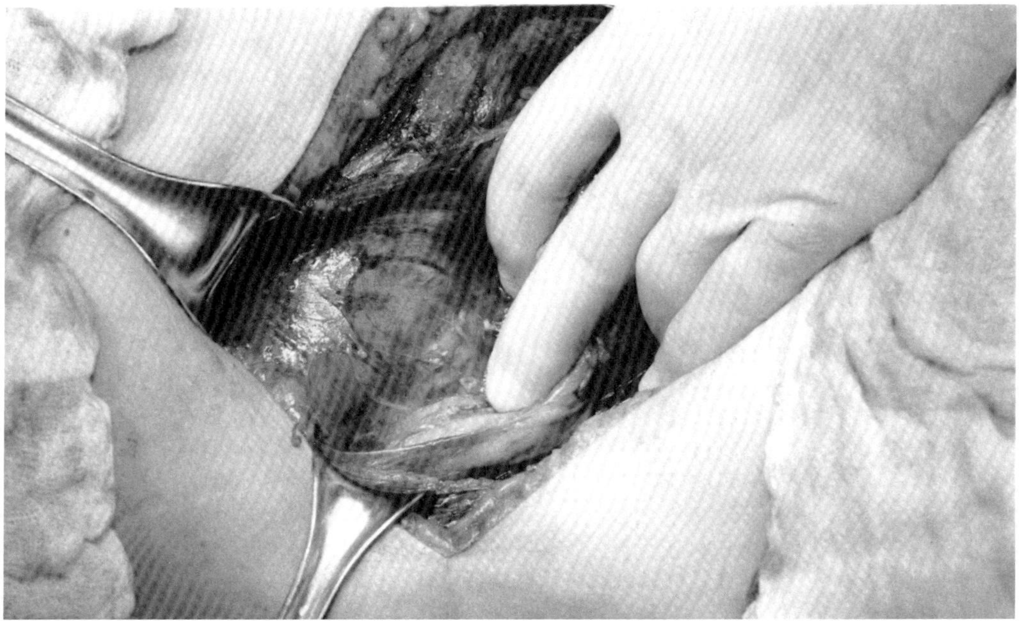

Figure 7 The plane between the pararenal fat and peritoneum is developed using blunt techniques. The liver, being retracted superiorly, can be seen through the thin veil of peritoneum.

tions of the gland is followed by dissection along the renal vein and cava. The main adrenal vein is ligated and cut.

3.2 Left Adrenalectomy

Access to the left supra-renal space is accomplished by entering the lesser sac through the gastrocolic omentum. Separation of the transverse mesocolon from the distal pancreas is followed by division of the lienocolic ligament to free the splenic flexure of the colon.

Retraction of the distal pancreas and spleen exposes the supra-renal space. The two landmarks, the renal vein and aorta, are identified after stripping the perinephric and para-renal adipose tissue.

The dissection around the adrenal is similar to the right side, leading to the main adrenal vein, which is divided between clips.

Draining is not required, and closure of the incision is performed with standard techniques.

3.3 Bilateral Adrenalectomy

Resection of both adrenals can be performed simultaneously. Intravenous cortisol is given before removal of the second adrenal and postoperative substitution with stress doses of cortisol is necessary.

3.4 Heterotopic Autotransplantation of Adrenocortical Tissue After Bilateral Adrenalectomy for Pheochromocytoma

Cortex-sparing techniques, whether orthotopic preservation or heterotopic autotransplantation, are applicable to simultaneous and metachronous adrenalectomy in patients with bilateral disease. The ratio of cortex to medulla is about 10 : 1, allowing easy harvesting of pure cortical tissue for autotransplantation into a peripheral muscle.

Subcapsular segments of cortex are harvested immediately after removal of the gland and preserved in numbered containers filled with iced saline. Slices immediately below the preserved cortical sections are sent for frozen section histology to verify absence of medulla. Following histologically confirmed purity of cortical tissue, the corresponding segments are minced into 1–2 mm fragments and implanted into pockets of the abdominal rectus muscles. Adrenocorticotropic hormone given twice weekly is used to stimulate cellular growth, and the time interval until autografting becomes successful is 6–24 months.

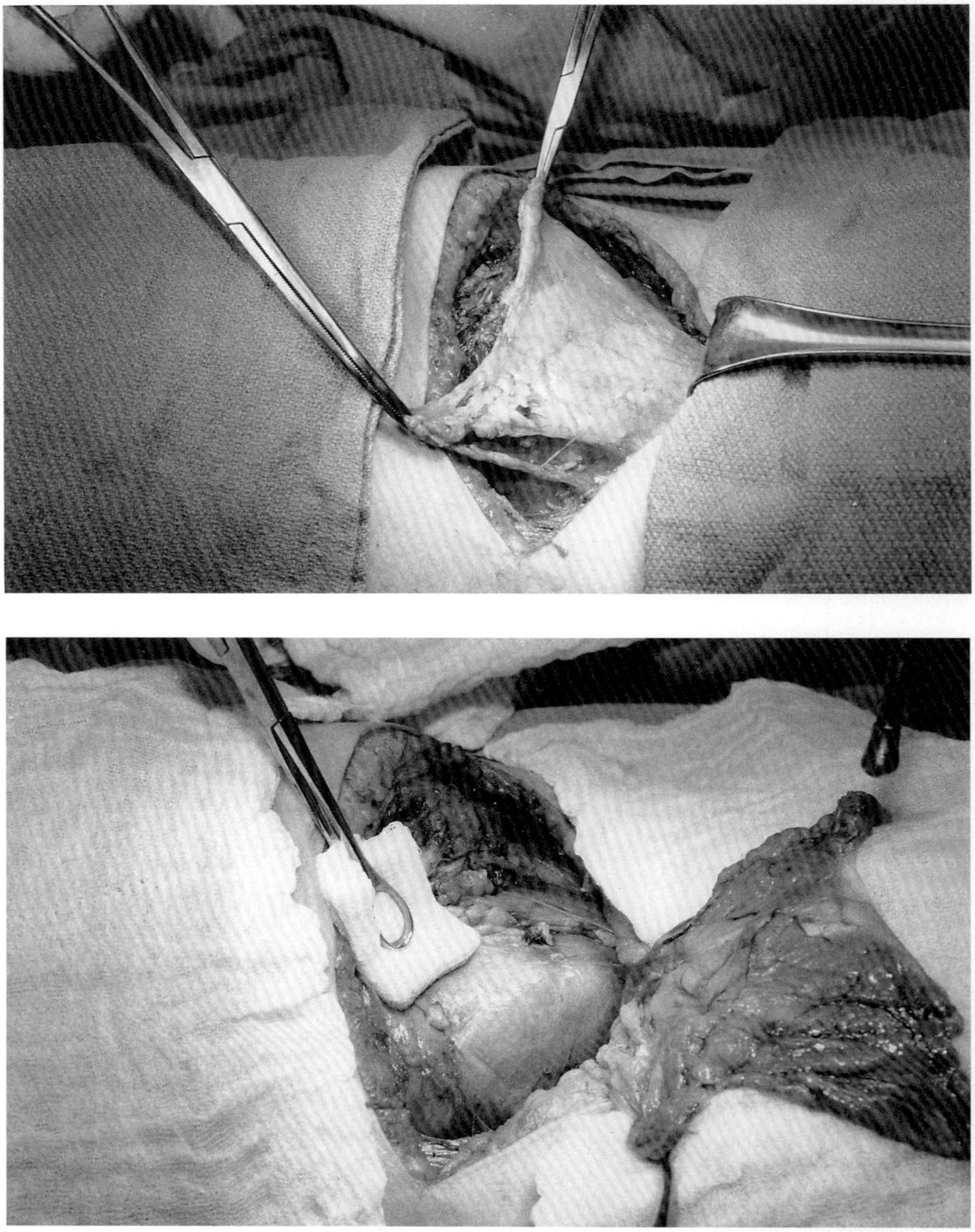

Figure 8 The pararenal fat is fully mobilized and excised, exposing the kidney. The kidney, still covered by Gerota's fascia, is being retracted.

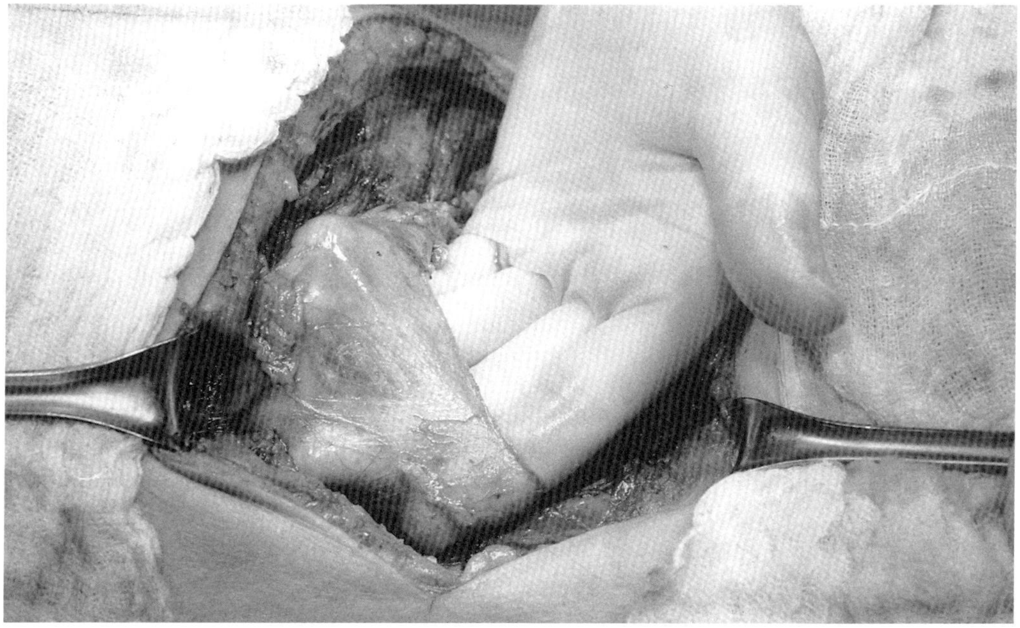

Figure 9 Gerota's fascia is divided and perinephric fat is excised to further allow retraction of the kidney.

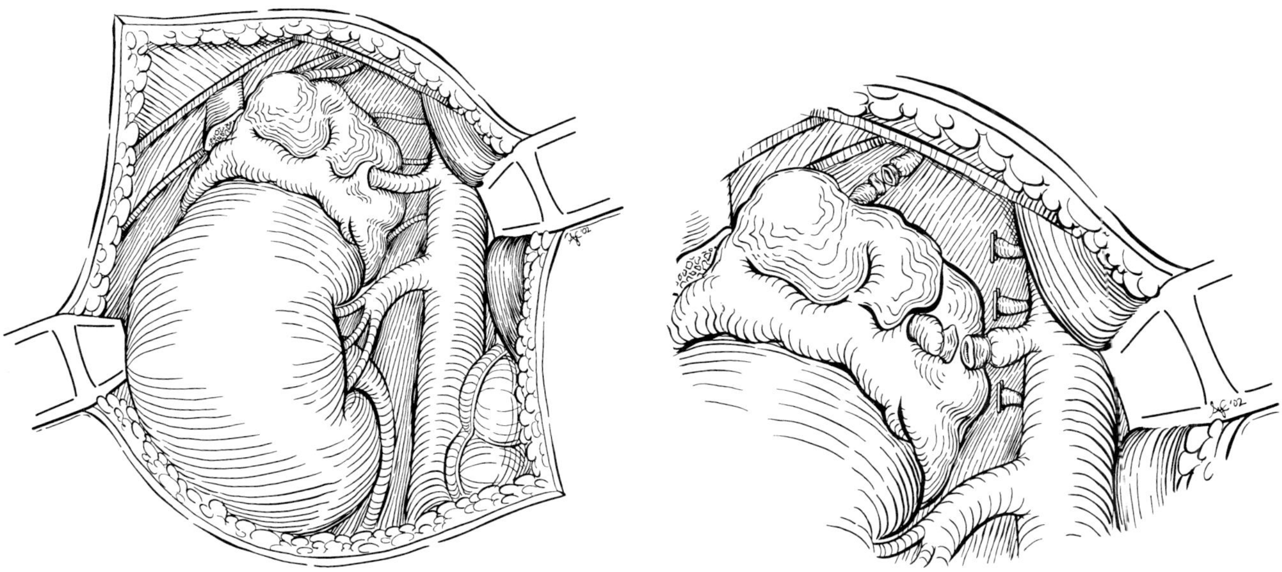

Figure 10 (A,B), Dissection continues in the avascular planes laterally and posteriorly prior to isolation and division of the inferior phrenic vessels. Division of small renal and aortic arterial branches and of small renal and caval venous tributaries is essential to safe dissection of the adrenal vein. The retrocaval location of the medial gland and the posterior or posterolateral junction of the adrenal vein and cava make this the most challenging phase of the operation.

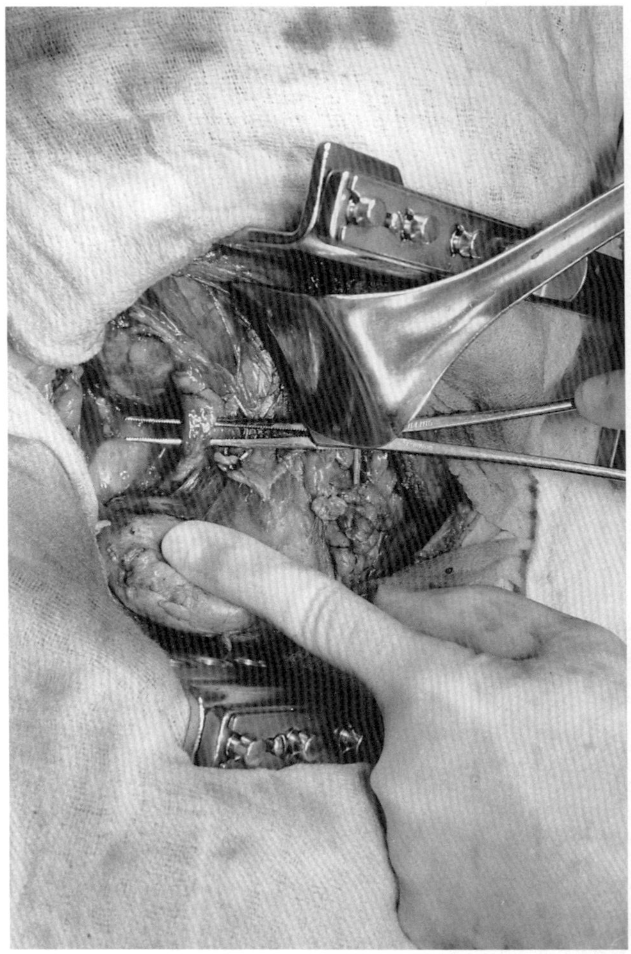

Figure 11 With the gland retracted infero-laterally and the venous confluence identified, the adrenal vein can be ligated and divided.

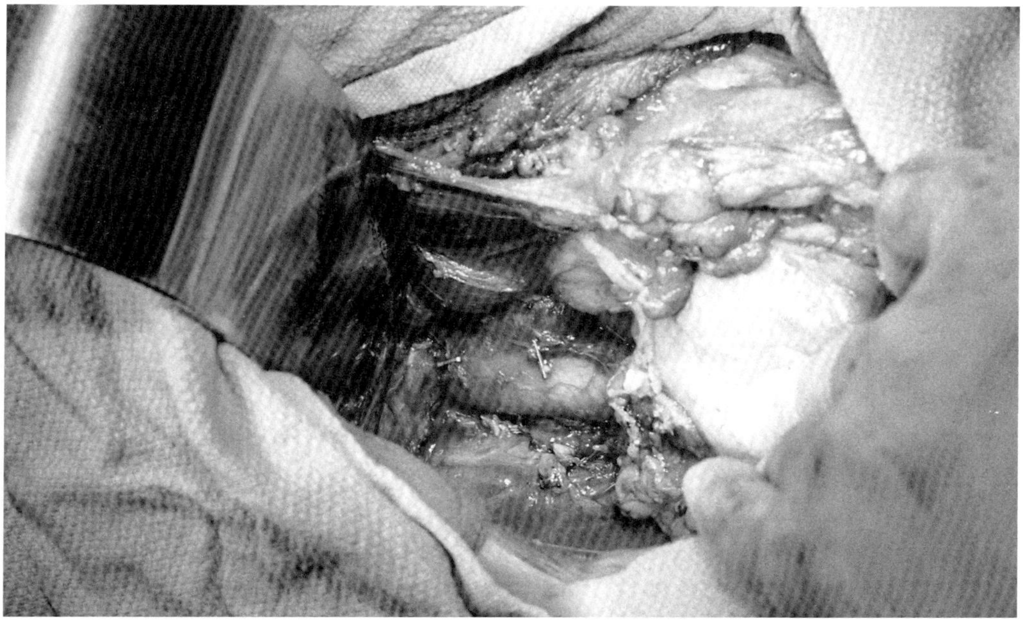

Figure 12 With the tumor removed, the exposure of the vena cava is demonstrated, with clips visible on the inferior phrenic and adrenal veins. Hemostasis is assured, and routine drainage is not indicated.

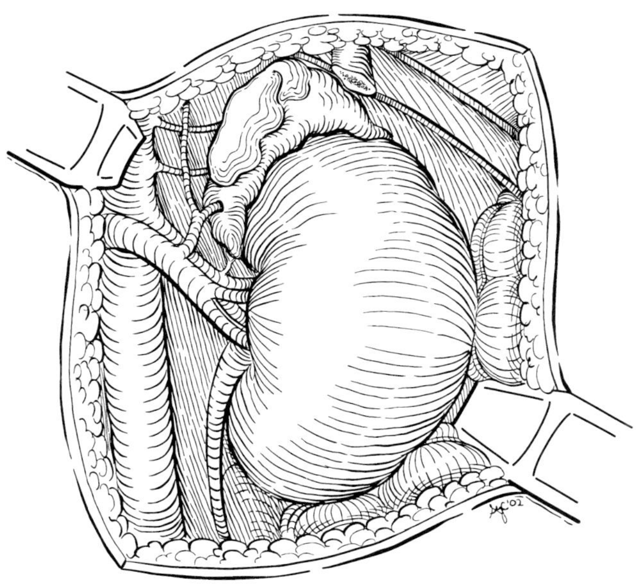

Figure 13 The pertinent landmarks in left adrenalectomy are the renal vein and aorta. Although the thick wall of the aorta and the greater length of the adrenal vein allow for easier dissection on the left, the principles and techniques are unchanged.

38

Laparoscopic Adrenalectomy with the Transabdominal Lateral Approach

Ahmad Assalia and Michel Gagner

Mount Sinai School of Medicine, New York University, New York, New York, U.S.A.

1 INTRODUCTION

Since its first description in 1992 (1), laparoscopic adrenalectomy has proven to be the procedure of choice for the surgical treatment of benign adrenal disease. Multiple reports have consistently demonstrated the benefits of this surgery, including decreased analgesic requirements, less blood loss and shorter hospital stay over the conventional approach (2–8). These results were not surprising considering that the procedure avoids an upper abdominal incision, does not require any reconstruction, benefits from magnification and clarity of view, is commonly performed for benign disease and mostly involves small, easily extractable specimens. Proper application of minimally invasive surgery to the adrenal gland must take into account expertise in both endocrine and laparoscopic surgery. For successful adrenalectomy, one must have knowledge of the anatomy and disease process, maintain meticulous hemostasis and delicately handle tissue.

The alternative open conventional adrenalectomy invariably requires large incisions, and rib resections with the posterior approaches, resulting in significant postoperative morbidity including chronic pain syndromes because of injury to intercostal and other nerves (9). Although those conventional approaches will undoubtedly be still required for certain adrenal pathologies, laparoscopic adrenalectomy, eliminating many of the problems of open surgery, has become the gold standard for treatment of most adrenal diseases.

2 INDICATIONS

The indications for laparoscopic adrenalectomy are basically the same as those for open adrenalectomy (Table 1). Laparoscopic adrenalectomy has been reported in several other conditions (10–12), but is not currently considered standard. These include neuroblastoma and congenital adrenal hyperplasia in children and isolated adrenal metastases.

General contraindications for laparoscopy include uncorrectable/untreated coagulopathy and unacceptable cardiopulmonary risk, previous surgery or trauma in the direct vicinity of the adrenal gland, diaphragmatic hernia, and surgeon's inexperience (3). Obesity and previous major intra-abdominal surgery are no longer a contraindication for laparoscopic adrenalectomy.

Currently, in experienced hands, the only specific absolute contraindication is known large adrenocortical carcinoma with frank tumor invasion to adjacent structures like vena cava, kidney, or diaphragm. In these cases, an open procedure is preferred in order to allow an *en bloc* resection and node dissection to be performed.

Table 1 Indications for Laparoscopic Transabdominal Lateral Decubitus Tehnique

I	Functional adrenal cortical masses
	(1) Cushing syndrome caused by benign cortisol-producing adenoma
	(2) Cushing's disease after failed pituitary surgery, or after failure to control or to find an ectopic-ACTH producing tumor
	(3) Aldosterone producing adenoma (Conn's syndrome)
	(4) Rare virilizing/feminizing tumors
II	Functional medullary adrenal masses
	(1) Benign adrenal pheochromocytoma
III	Nonfunctional adrenal tumors
	(1) Benign looking Incidentalomas (nonfunctioning adenomas) confined to the adrenal glands and meeting accepted criteria for adrenalectomy (size > 4cm at presentation or growth in follow up
	(2) Benign symptomatic lesions
	(3) Rare entities such as cyst and myelolipoma

Although controversy exists over the maximum acceptable tumor size for laparoscopic adrenalectomy, laparoscopy may not be advisable for adrenal tumors larger than 12–14 cm because of the technical difficulties associated with such surgery and the malignant potential of these large tumors.

3 OPERATIVE TECHNIQUE

Detailed knowledge of adrenal anatomy and its common variations is a prerequisite to laparoscopic adrenal surgery. Several laparoscopic approaches to the adrenal glands are demonstrated:

1. Transabdominal lateral (with the patient in the lateral decubitus position)
2. Transabdominal anterior (with the patient in the supine position)
3. Retroperitoneal endoscopic adrenalectomy (lateral or posterior)

Although the retroperitoneal approach is advocated by some, usually practicing urologists (14–17), the technique of choice by most endocrine and general surgeons performing laparoscopic adrenalectomy is the transabdominal lateral approach, originally described by Gagner in 1992 (1,18). In this positioning, the force of gravity helps retract the surrounding organs (including the bowel), and effectively exposes either adrenal gland for laparoscopic intervention. As a result, there is reduced dissection and minimal retraction of the vena cava and other adjacent structure.

The patient is positioned on the table to maximize the distance between the costal margin and the iliac crest. This is achieved by adjusting the laparoscopic operating table in the jackknife position, with the patient placed in the lateral decubitus position with the operated side up. Sufficient padding is placed over pressure points and the patient is strapped and taped in position, avoiding especially a brachial plexus injury or iliac compression. The sterilization of the skin should extend from the nipple to anterior superior iliac spine, and from the midine anteriorly to the spine posteriorly. This allows for conversion to an open procedure should this be necessary.

3.1 Transabdominal Laparoscopic Left Adrenalectomy

Patients are placed in the lateral decubitus position with the left side up (Fig. 1). The surgeon and the assistant stand on the side opposite the diseased gland, facing the abdomen (Fig. 2). A flank cushion is positioned under the patient's right side and the table is flexed so that the left side is hyperextended (Fig. 1). The left arm is extended and suspended. The surgical area is prepared as previously described. An open technique is used to access the abdominal cavity in the left subcostal area at the level of anterior axillary line, and carbon dioxide, up to 15-mm of pressure, is insufflated. One 10-mm trocar is then inserted in this site, and a 30-degree, 10 mm laparoscope is introduced, through which the abdominal cavity is explored, for possible liver metastases, adhesions or contiguous organ involvement/displacement. If the inspection is satisfactory, two more 5 or 10 mm trocars are inserted under direct vision in the flank depending on available instrumentation: one under the 11th rib and one slightly more anterior and medial to the first trocar (Fig. 3).

Often a fourth trocar is needed for retraction and is inserted at the costo-ertebral junction dorsally, since most left adrenalectomies are now performed with three trocars only in more than 80% of the time. All trocars should be at least 5 cm and, and more optimally, 8–10 cm apart. The laparoscope is then inserted in the most anterior trocar and the surgeon will work laterally with a two-hand technique through the other two trocars. Working with the laparoscopic scissors with cautery or the ultrasonic scalpel, in the right hand, and a curved dissector in the left hand, the splenic flexure (or lienocolic ligament) is mobilized medially (Fig. 4) to separate the colon from the inferior pole of the adrenal and expose the lineorenal ligament. Mobilization allows

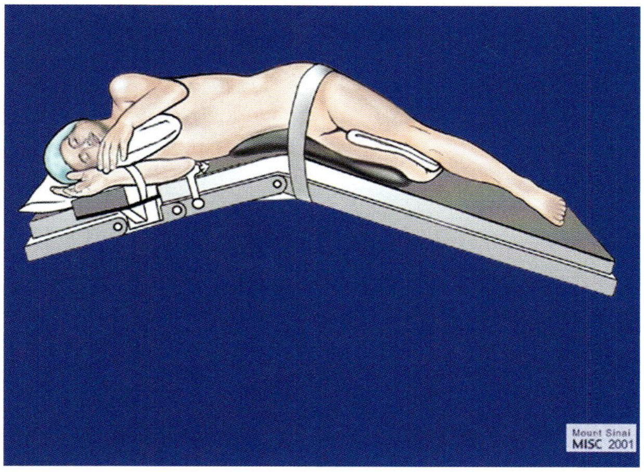

Figure 1 Patient positioning.

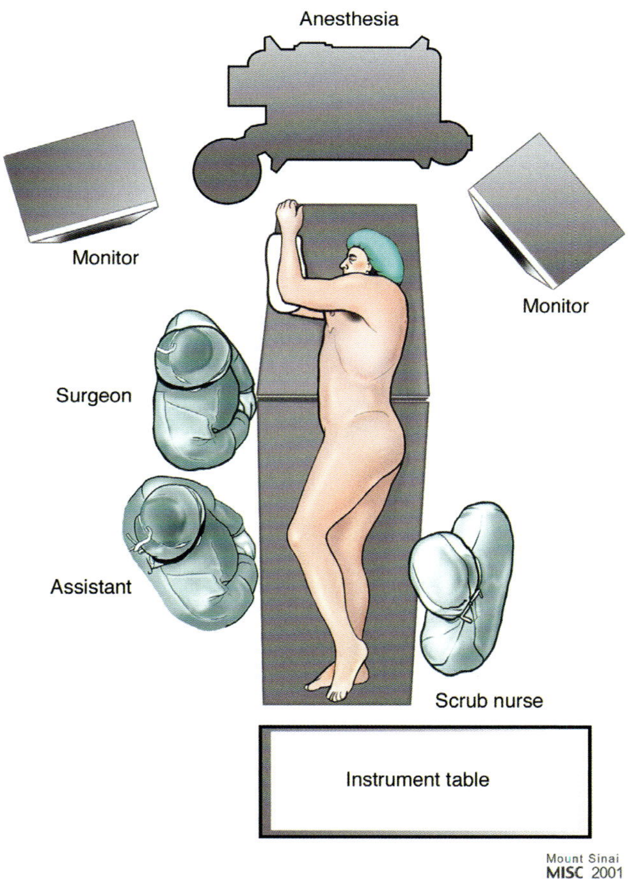

Figure 2 Laparoscopic left adrenalectomy: operating room layout.

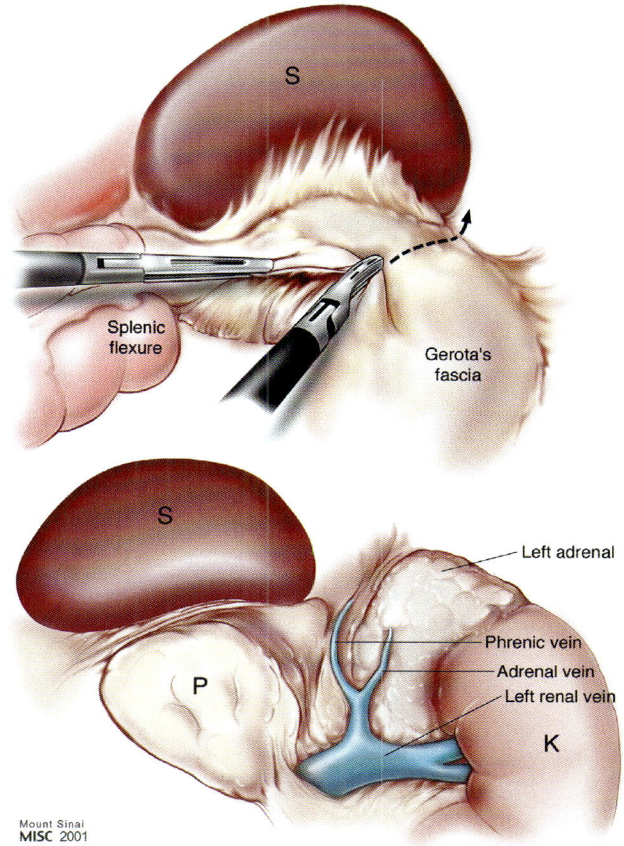

Figure 5 Left adrenal: inferio-superior dissection of the lienorenal ligament and exposure of the adrenal vessels.

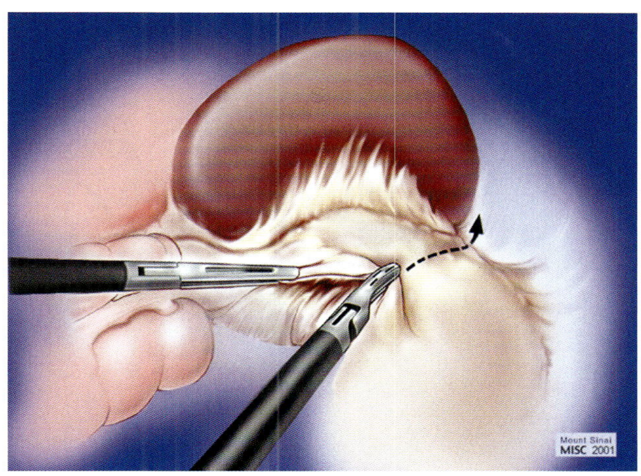

Figure 6 Use of a 5-mm ultrasonic endoscopic shear for division of the lienorenal ligament.

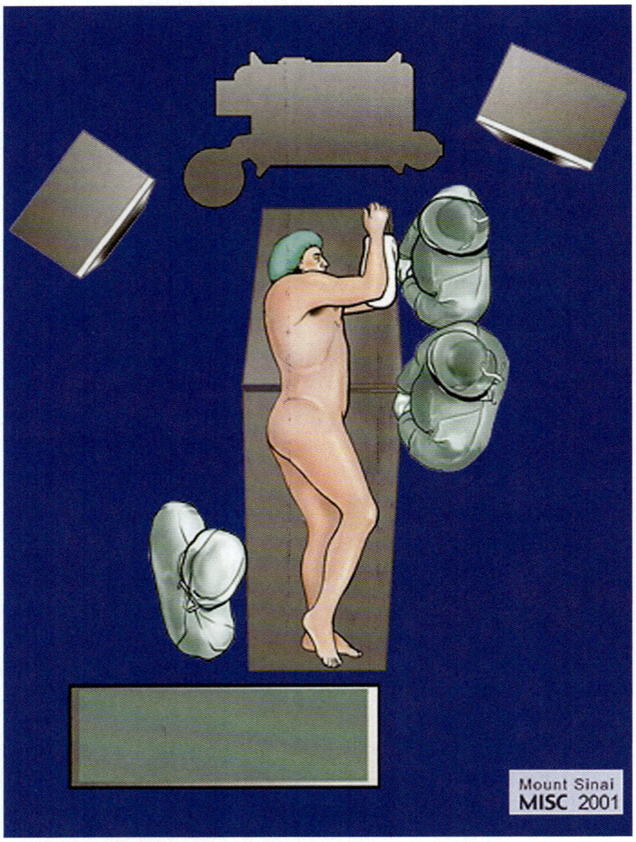

Figure 8 Operating room setup for a laparoscopic right adrenalectomy.

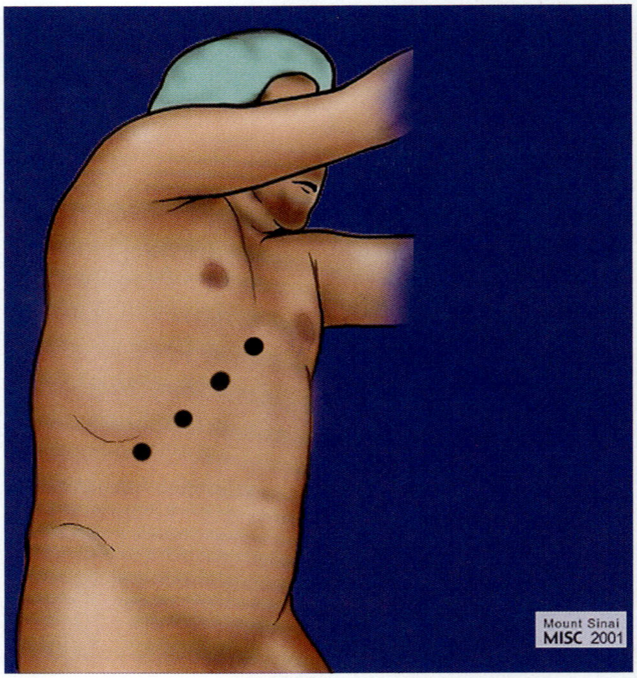

Figure 9 Trocar positions for a laparoscopic right adrenalectomy.

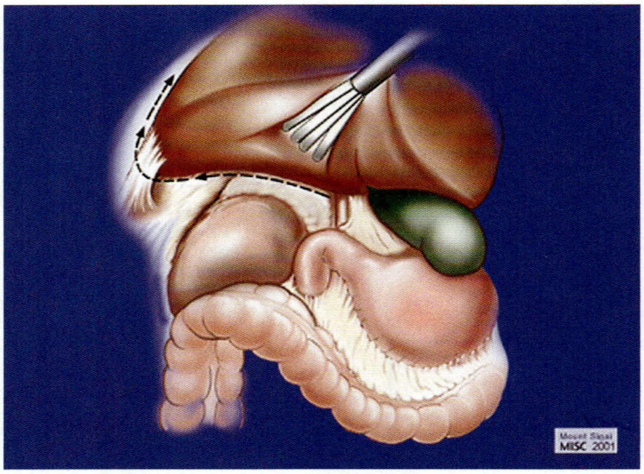

Figure 10 Retraction of the liver: the line of mobilization of the right lobe of the liver is demonstrated including the right triangular ligament.

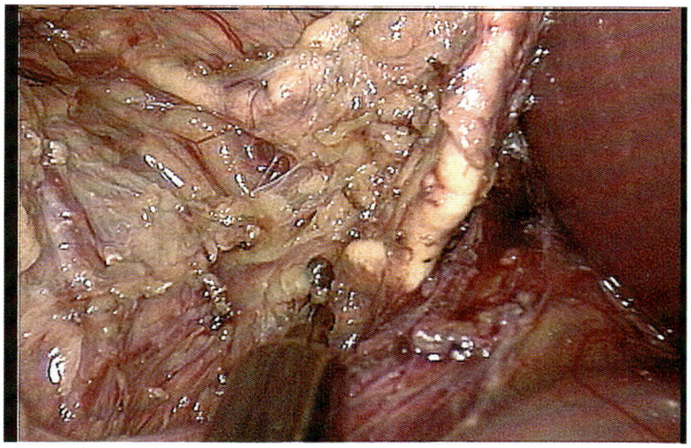

Figure 11 A 5-mm hook instrument (Karl Storz) is used to dissect the small vessels surrounding the inferior pole of the right adrenal gland.

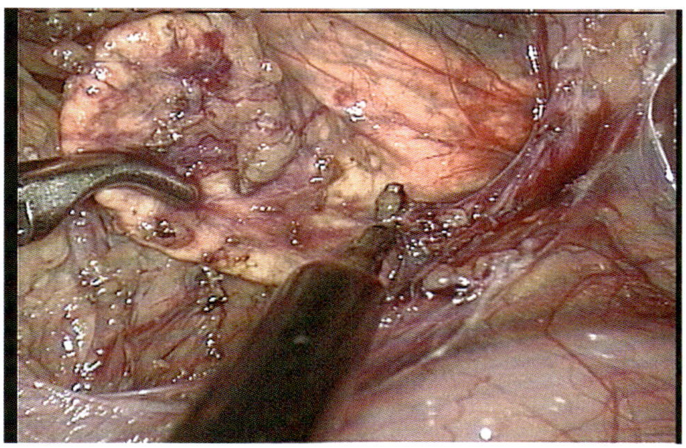

Figure 12 A similar dissection is achieved anteriorly.

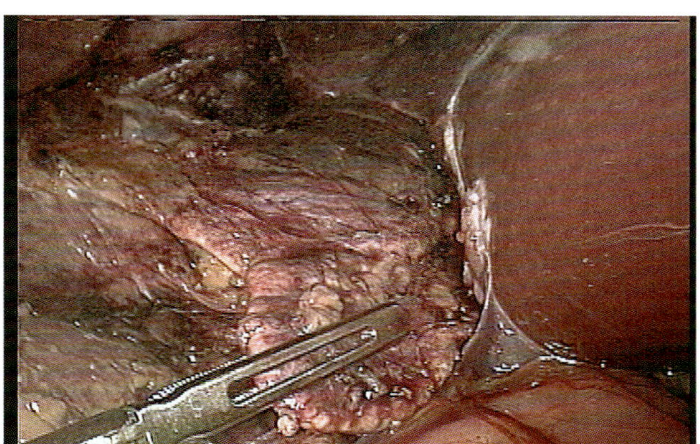

Figure 13 Demonstration of how a Dorsey bowel forcep (Karl Storz) can be used on the right adrenal gland to provide traction, between the gland and the vena cava.

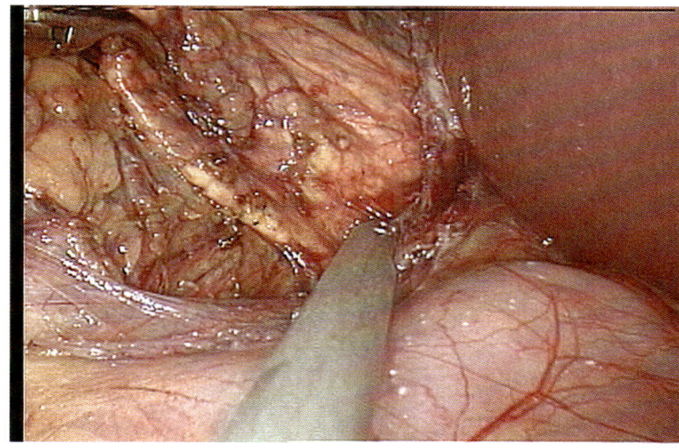

Figure 14 Blunt dissection between the vena cana (next to duodenum) and the right gland, using a 5-mm hydro-dissection cannula.

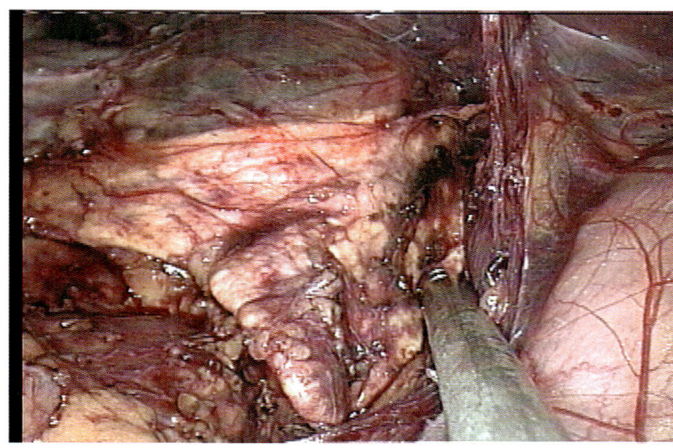

Figure 15 Inferior vena cava exposure.

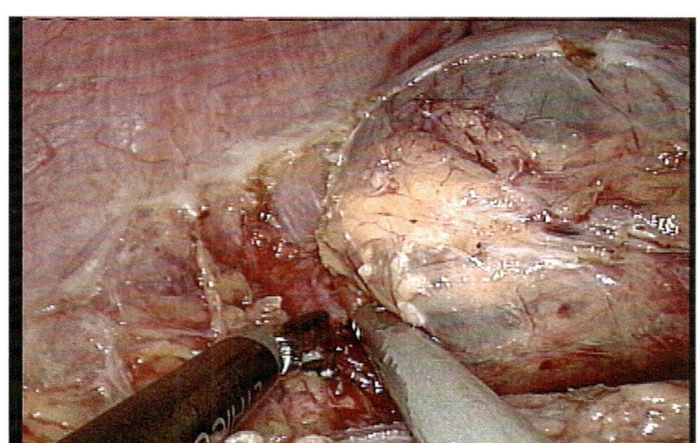

Figure 16 Lateral dissection of a large right pheochromocytoma.

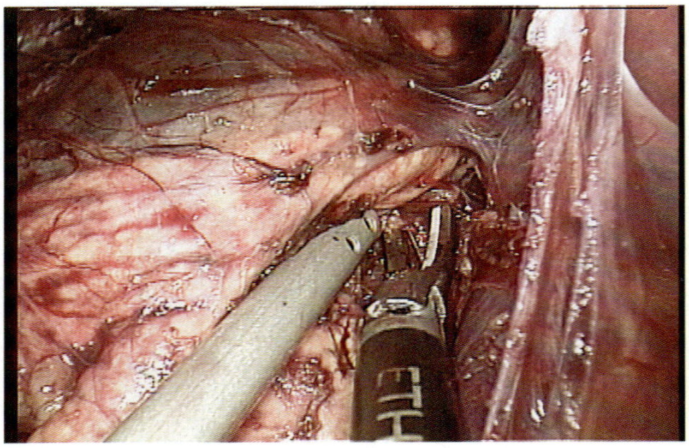

Figure 17 Posterior mobilization behind the right adrenal vein before clipping.

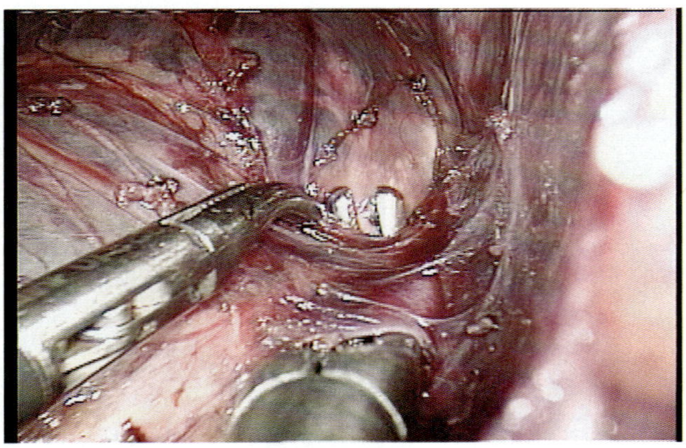

Figure 18 Right adrenal vein dissection using a 10-mm right angle dissector (Karl Storz).

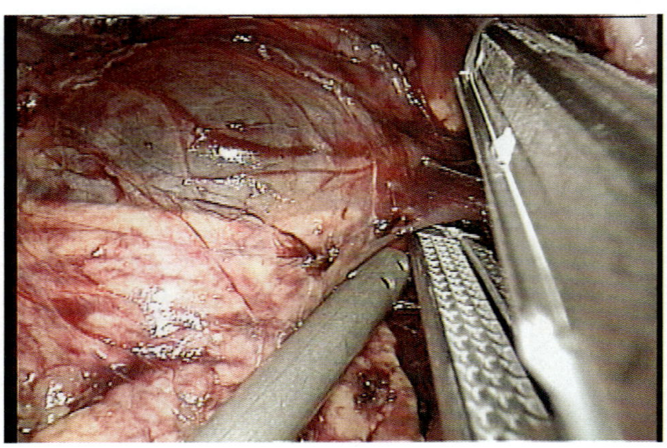

Figure 19 A cautious application of the endoscopic vascular stapler.

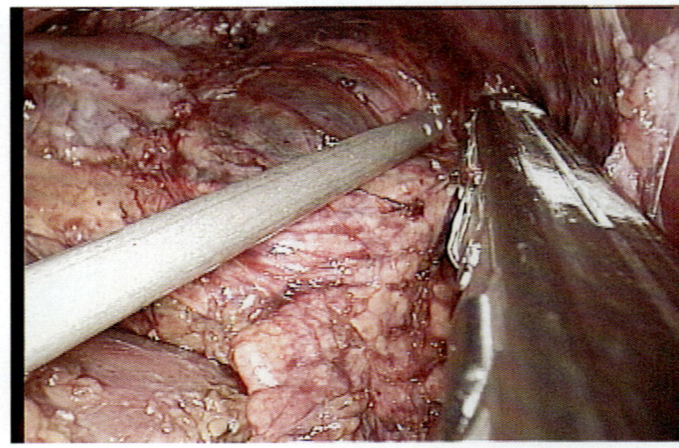

Figure 20 Vascular stapler applied to the right adrenal vein.

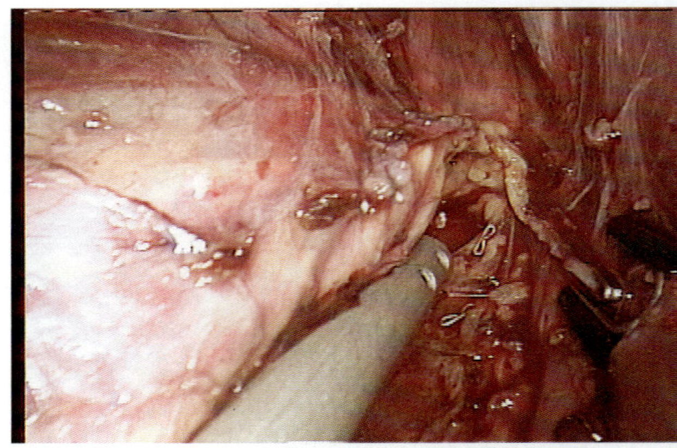

Figure 21 Clips applied to the right adrenal vein stump.

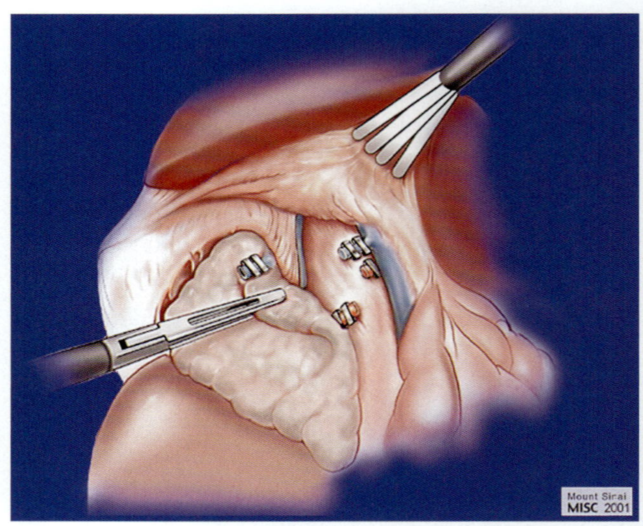

Figure 22 Right adrenal vessel dissection and control.

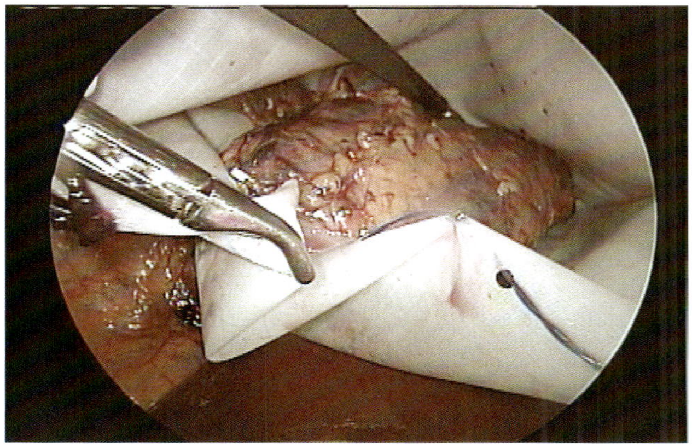

Figure 23 Gland extraction into an impermeable bag.

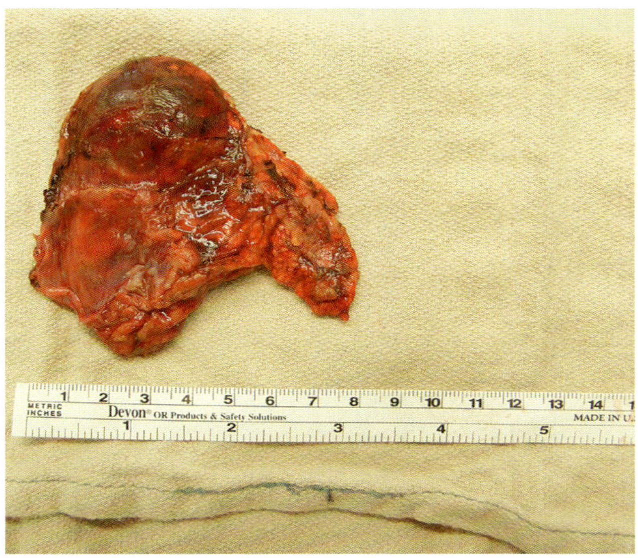

Figure 24 Macroscopic aspects of a resected right adrenal tumor after extraction.

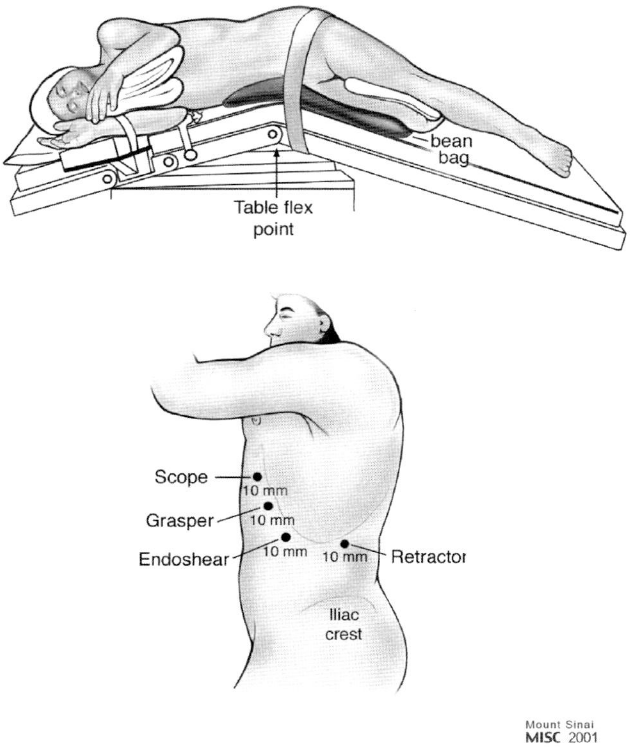

Figure 3 Trocar sites for left laparoscopic adrenalectomy.

instruments to be inserted more easily and helps prevent inadvertent trauma to the colon or spleen during instrument insertion. Next, the lineorenal ligament is incised inferosuperiorly approximately 1 cm from the spleen (Figs. 5, 6). The dissection is carried up to the diaphragm and stopped when the short gastric vessels are encountered posteriorly behind the stomach. This maneuver allows the spleen to fall medially, thus exposing the retroperitoneal space. The lateral edge and anterior portion of the adrenal gland will become visible in the perinephric fat superiorly and medially. If necessary, a fourth 5-mm trocar is inserted dorsally at the costovertebral angle to gently retract large-size spleens, and open the space or to push the left kidney or the surrounding fat downward to expose the inferior pole and lateral edge of the adrenal gland better. This trocar should always be inserted after the previous three because the splenorenal ligament must be divided first, so that the trocar will pass over the lateral and superior border of the kidney. This port, however, is usually not necessary in patients with normal-size spleen. Laparoscopic ultrasound may be used as an adjunct to identify the adrenal gland, the mass within the gland and the adrenal vein (3). The dissection of the adrenal gland can be easy or difficult, depending on the type of perinephric fat. Two types mainly may be encountered: (1) the soft, nonadherent, areolar fat which is easy to dissect, and (2) dense, adherent fat that contains multiple small veins originating from the retroperitoneum. To avoid fracture of the adrenal capsule, it's helpful to leave a little periadrenal fat on the adrenal, so that this tissue, rather than the adrenal itself, can be retracted. Grasping the perinephric fat, dissection of the lateral and anterior part of the adrenal gland is carried out. Hook elecrocautery or ultrasonic scalpel are useful instruments for this phase of dissection. Once the lateral portion of the adrenal gland has been exposed, the patient is moved to the Fowler position to permit further downward migration of the bowel loops and the spleen. Any saline irrigation, bleeding, or oozing will flow downward away from the area of the dissection. The dissection can be continued either inferiorly, so that the left adrenal vein can be clipped early in the dissection, or start superiorly and go down medially to clip the adrenal vein last. The dissection depends on the exposure gained after the spleen has been mobilized, the type of disease, and size of the adrenal mass. In large adrenals (>5 cm), the left adrenal vein may be difficult to visualize. In such cases, dissecting the lateral and superior adrenal poles first will allow better mobilization and make clipping the adrenal vein easier later during the dissection (Fig. 7). In smaller adrenals (<5 cm), it is feasible, and easy, to dissect and clip the adrenal vein. Most left adrenal veins are about 10 mm in diameter and can be clipped with medium to large titanium clips placed with clip applier. With a right-

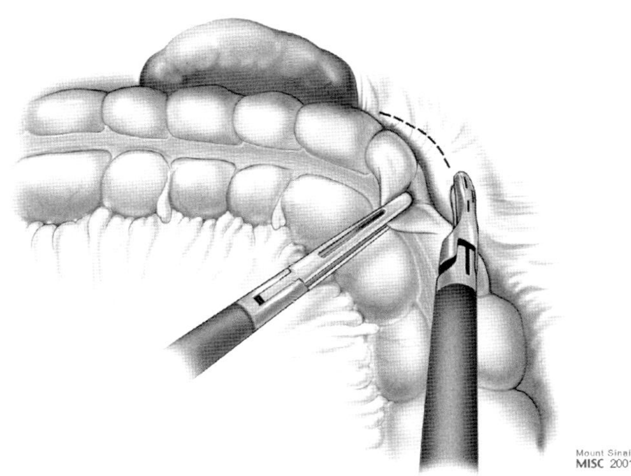

Figure 4 Dissection of splenic flexure.

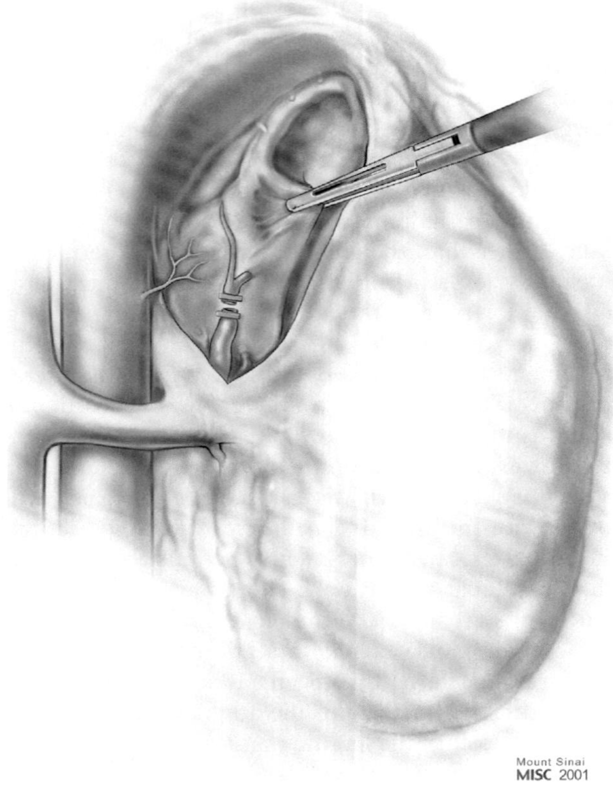

Figure 7 Left adrenal vein clipped and divided.

angle dissector, the adrenal vein is dissected from its insertion into the left adrenal gland. It's not necessary to identify and dissect the origin of the vein from the left renal vein. The adrenal vein is clipped about 1 cm from the renal vein: two clips are placed proximally to the gland and two are positioned distally. The vein is then divided with laparoscopic straight scissors. At this point, adrenal mobilization becomes easy because it is grasped on the perinephric fat with the left-hand grasper; the gland is then pushed upwards and laterally to permit dissection of the medial and superior portions. This dissection is accomplished with hook cautery or ultrasonic scalpel. One should remember that the inferior phrenic arterial branches often require ligation as they approach the superior pole of the left adrenal gland. Once the adrenal gland is free, hemostasis is verified by repeated irrigation and aspiration. The gland is then extracted in total after it has been placed in an appropriately sized impermeable nylon bag. The bag is removed through the most anterior trocar by spreading the abdominal wall musculature using a Kelly clamp. The incision may have to be enlarged to remove large specimens (>4–5 cm) without rupturing the bag. Drainage is seldom necessary unless pancreatic injury is suspected. All fascial incisions are closed with 2–0 absorbable sutures, and skin incisions are closed with 4–0 subcuticular absorbable sutures.

3.2 Transabdominal Laparoscopic Right Adrenalectomy

Patients are positioned in the lateral decubitus position with the right side up (Fig. 8). Pneumoperitoneum is established in the same way as for left adrenalectomy. An open technique is used to access the abdominal cavity approximately 2 cm below and parallel to the costal margin. A 10-mm trocar is inserted at this site for the 30-degree angled laparoscope. Inspection of the abdominal cavity is carried out. Under direct vision three additional 10 mm trocars are inserted 2 cm and parallel to the costal margin (Fig. 9). The second trocar is positioned in the right flank, inferior and posterior to the tip of the 11th rib just above the hepatic flexure of the colon, which seldom needs to be mobilized. The third trocar is then inserted in the most anterior position of the subcostal area between the epigastrium and the anterior axillary line. This most medial trocar should be lateral to the edge of the ipsilateral rectus muscle.

The last trocar is introduced at the either at the tip of the 12th rib or sometimes at the costovertebral subcostal angle after the peritoneal reflection of the lateral edge of the right kidney has been dissected to avoid injury to the right kidney. Four trocars are necessary because the right lobe of the liver must be retracted to expose the most medial aspect of the right adrenal gland. It is, therefore, crucial that the liver retractor be inserted under direct vision, through the most anterior port, so that the right hepatic lobe can be lifted and pushed anteriomedially (Fig. 10) . The laparoscope is removed from the first trocar and inserted in the second trocar, and the surgeon works with the two most lateral trocars. The camera can also be positioned dorsally, and the surgeon works with the two trocars in the middle to obtain another view of the dissection field. This is especially useful for dissecting the superior aspect of the adrenal gland. The liver often must be mobilized to obtain the best exposure of the junction between the adrenal gland and the inferior vena cava. The right lateral hepatic attachments and the triangular ligament are (Fig. 10), therefore, dissected from the diaphragm using laparoscopic scissors or ultrasonic scalpel. This dissection will permit more effective retraction to push the liver medially using a fan or some other atraumatic retractor. This is the key for providing adequate exposure of the right adrenal vein and its entry into the vena cava. We prefer to create a right-angle plane between the anterior aspect of the right kidney and lateral portion of the liver. This plane will provide enough space to work and adequate exposure in case of bleeding. Laparoscopic ultrasound may be of assistance in identifying the anatomy. The right gland is dissected next. If the mass is smaller than 4 cm in diameter, gaining access to the right adrenal vein initially is possible, which permits easier dissection of the rest of the adrenal gland. The inferolateral edge is then mobilized (Fig. 11), and dissection is continued afterwards medially (Fig. 12) and upward (Fig. 13), along the lateral edge of the vena cava (Figs. 14, 15). The adrenal vein should be visualized at this stage. This vein is often short and sometimes broad (Figs. 17, 18). Usually the vein can be clipped with medium to large titanium clips, and at least two should be applied at the vena cava side. If there is not enough space for clips, then a vascular cartridge of 30 or 35 mm laparoscopic stapler is used for secure division of the right adrenal vein (Figs. 19, 20). Smaller veins may be encountered superiorly; these should be clipped or cauterized to prevent bleeding (Figs. 21, 22). The superior pole of the gland is dissected next, and small branches from the inferior phrenic vessels can be clipped or cauterized with hook cautery or ultrasonic scalpel. Again, a fowler position permits all fluids to migrate downward. The lateral border of the gland is then dissected from the perinephric fat using the same instruments (Fig. 16). Meticulous dissection close to the gland will prevent tearing of the lateral branches of the vena cava and other vessels from the retroperitoneum. If a large mass is encountered, we prefer to dissect laterally and superiorly first and then move down along the vena cava to reach the adrenal vein. Once the mass has been dissected free, it is placed in impermeable nylon bag (Figs. 23, 24) and removed through the most anterior trocar site. All wounds are closed as described for the left side. The fascia of the fourth (dorsal) trocar site is not closed because of the depth of this wound.

3.3 Transabdominal Anterior Laparoscopic Adrenalectomy

This approach can be a lengthy procedure due to the difficult dissection of the left colic flexure, spleen and the pancreatic tail on the left side, and the duodenum on the right. In addition, on the right side, the adrenal vein, found posterior to the vena cava, is very difficult to dissect and control. Although in bilateral adrenalectomy it is not necessary to change the position of the patient the average operating time is similar to lateral transabdomonal approach. Nevertheless, because of its drawbacks the majority of the teams have abandoned this approach.

3.4 Bilateral Laparoscopic Adrenalectomy

The indications for bilateral laparoscopic adrenalectomy include the following (19): (1) Cushing's disease refractory to trans-sphenoidal pituitary resection and/or irradiation; (2) cushing's syndrome due to ACTH-independent macronodular or micronodular adrenal hyperplasia; (3) ectopic ACTH syndrome when the primary tumor cannot be resected or medical treatment has failed; (4) Conn's syndrome caused by bilateral adrenal adenomas; and (5) bilateral pheochromocytoma. Other less prevalent relative and possible indications include: (a) unilateral pheochromocytoma in MEN-IIA, due to the fact that in 50% of cases a metachronous lesion will develop in the contralateral side within 10 years of resection of the affected side (20); (b) idiopathic hyperaldosteronism (IHA) caused by bilateral symmetric adrenal hyperplasia refractory to medical treatment; and (c) congenital bilateral adrenal hyperplasia (CAH) which is difficult to manage medically (19).

There are several possible surgical approaches for bilateral laparoscopic adrenalectomy.

3.4.1 Transabdominal Lateral Approach

Is the preferred approach in our opinion. The patient is placed in the lateral decubitus position; usually the left side is performed first because it is easier. After all trocar sites are closed, the patient is repositioned and redraped, to expose the right side. A 15- to 20-minute turnover time is necessary, not significantly adding to the operative length (2). Nevertheless, we prefer this bilateral approach, because gravity aids the dissection when the patient is in the lateral decubitus position, it offers a wide operative field and better control of blood vessels. Furthermore, it may be safer than the retroperitoneal approach for the right adrenal where a better control of a possible major vascular injury (i.e., vena cava) is needed. We have successfully performed bilateral laparoscopic adrenalectomy within a reasonable amount of time using a bilateral lateral technique (3). Utilizing this approach, Chapuis et al. (21), with the largest published series on bilateral laparoscopic adrenalectomy in 24 patients with Cushing's syndrome, reported no major postoperative complications. The operative time have ranged from 243 to 386 minutes for the reported bilateral procedures using this approach.

3.4.2 Retroperitoneal Approach

This can be accomplished using the lateral or the posterior methods described earlier. It's worth to mention, that the few series with data on bilateral laparoscopic lateral and posterior retroperitoneal approaches have not shown greater elevations of carbon dioxide than with the lateral transabdominal approach (22–24).

3.4.3 Anterior Approach

Despite its theoretical advantage in bilateral adrenalectomy, the drawbacks explained above regarding difficulty in exposure and dissection, has led the majority of surgeons to abandon this approach.

No randomized prospective studies have been conducted to compare laparoscopic bilateral adrenalectomy with open bilateral surgery. Even though, the available literature on bilateral laparoscopic adrenalectomy is encouraging with low morbidity and mortality rates (1,3,21,22,25,26). In the setting of Cushing's syndrome, the morbidity and mortality rates of the laparoscopic approach, are noticeably lower than for open surgery (1,3,21,22). The typical operative length for bilateral laparoscopic adrenalectomy, including all approaches) is approximately 300 minutes (19). There have been some reports of operative times longer than 300 minutes, with cases of hypercarbia requiring hyperventilation, but without significant sequelae (22,24). Fernandez-Cruz et al. (27,28) have recommended helium pneumoperitoneum for the bilateral laparoscopic procedure in order to prevent carbon dioxide retention and acidosis. The use of helium may be recommended in patients with pheochromocytoma with previous cardiovascular or respiratory disorders (28).

3.5 Laparoscopic Partial Adrenalectomy

Possible indications for adrenal-sparing surgery include bilateral pheochromocytoma and well-circumscribed bilateral cortisol or aldosterone-producing adenomas. The purpose is to avoid lifelong cortisol replacement therapy (29). The operative technique involves basically the same initial steps as for total adrenalectomy. After exposing the adrenal glands, dissection is first performed at the inferior borders and then carried upwards along the lateral aspect using hook cautery or ultrasonic scalpel and a gentle grasping forceps. One has to preserve as much blood supply as possible. An ultrasound of the gland is then performed using a flexible 7.5 MHz, 10 mm diameter probe, which demonstrates the location of the adrenal vein and arterial supply and confirms the location and borders of the adrenal lesion. It also should be possible to exclude the presence of other nodules or hyperplasia in the adrenal remnant. At this stage, the adrenal lesion can be easily dissected free and elevated. While concomitantly displaying the margins of the tumor with the ultrasound, the harmonic shears are used to bloodlessly transect the adrenal gland away from the lesion. The excised specimen is then placed in a bag, retrieved and sent for immediate histopathologic examination to confirm histology and assess the margins. At least 5-mm rim of normal adrenal tissue is preferred.

3.6 Needlescopic Adrenalectomy

Initially described for dignostic purposes or cholecystectomy, the availability of 2 mm instrumentation and camera technology has triggered the emergence of needlescopic surgery. The rationale behind this technique is to further minimize the abdominal wall trauma, and hence, speeding the convalescence and improving cosmesis. The positioning of the patient and number of trocars are similar to the traditional laparoscopic adrenalectomy. A 10–12 mm trocar is inserted in the superior aspect of the umbilicus to accommodate the 10 mm angled scope under which, most of the procedure is conducted. It also enables the use of bigger instruments should they be required (e.g., vascular endostapler) and the retrieval of the specimen. During these steps, the procedure is monitored through the 2 mm needlescope. On the left side, additional two trocars of 2 mm and 5 mm are used, and on the right side, a fourth 2 mm, trocar is utilized for liver retraction. Placement of the 2-mm ports doesn't require skin incisions. These ports can be readily inserted through needle-like puncture. Thus, at the end of the procedure, these miniature puncture sites require no skin closure, except for Steristrips. The 5 mm port is used by the surgeon's dominant hand in order to accommodate larger instruments such as scissors, electrocautery, suction-irrigation devices and clip-appliers. Dissection is carried out using 2 mm graspers, scissors, and hook electrocautery and vascular control is achieved with elctrocautery (uni-or bipolar) and 5 mm clip-applier.

4 POSTOPERATIVE CARE

Oral fluids are started on the day of surgery and Oral analgesics are provided to help patients tolerate the postoperative pain. However, during the first 12 hours, some patients require parenteral analgesia. The postoperative course is similar to that for laparoscopic cholecystectomy, except that some endocrine disorders will necessitate hormonal support and additional clinical laboratory data. It should be noticed that unexplained hypotension, fever and confusion may be due to acute adrenocortical insufficiency. These patients should have blood drawn for determination of plasma cortisol levels and be immediately treated with 100 mg of hydrocortisone intravenously. Most patients will be ambulatory by the evening of the procedure and the majority will be allowed to leave by the third postoperative day. However, discharge may be delayed in patients who require substantial hormonal support or adjustments of antihypertensive medications.

5 RESULTS

Since 1992, laparoscopic adrenalectomy has gained a worldwide popularity and in a search of the Medline, we were able to retrieve more than 500 articles dealing with laparoscopic adrenalectomy. Table 2 summarizes the reported results of selected large series of laparoscopic adrenalectomies performed with different laparoscopic techniques. Although no prospective randomized series exist, numerous studies have compared laparoscopic with open adrenalectomy (either retrospectively or non-randomised prospectively), documenting the safety, decreased analgesic postoperative requirements, enhanced recovery, shorter hospital stay and cost-effectiveness of the laparoscopic approach (4–8,24,30–39). No differences in patient's population, indications for surgery or mean size of lesions were noticed. Our own experience, presented herein, with 100 procedures in 88 patients (3), further supports the superiority of this procedure.

Table 3 lists the indications and pathology for our procedures. The overall mean age was 46 years (range 17–84 years), and the ratio of female to male was slightly >2:1. Fifty-two of the adrenalectomies were performed in the left and 10 were performed bilaterally. The mean operating time was 132 minutes (range 80–360 minutes). In our initial experience, a right sided procedure required an average of 138 minutes compared to 102 minutes for a left-sided procedure. However, review of the last 30 cases showed the time required for either sides is essentially equal. The time required for bilateral adrenalectomy averaged approximately 45 minutes longer than the combined averages for the unilateral procedure alone. The indications for bilateral adrenalectomy are listed in Table 4. The average length of stay was 2.4 days (range 1–6 days), and the average size of the lesions was 4.95 cm (range 0.7–12 cm). The estimated intraoperative blood loss was approximately 70 ml and the mean number of postoperative narcotic injections was 5.5.

Conversion to open surgery was necessary in three patients (3%). These conversions occurred in our first attempt to laparoscopic adrenalectomy in a patient with 15 cm right adrenal angiomyelolipoma, in a second patient with a locally invasive retroperitoneal sarcoma, and in a third patient with adrenal adenocarcinoma invading the inferior vena cava.

Table 2 Summary of Outcome of Selected Series with Laparoscopic Adrenalectomy

Study	No. of procedures	Operative time (min.)[a]	Blood loss (ml)	Conversion rate (%)	Complication rate (%)	Length of stay (days)	Mortality (%)
Gagner (3), 1997	100	123	70	3	12	2.4	0
Gill (76), 1999	110	188	125	NR[b]	16	1.9	0
Guazzoni (81), 2000	161	160	NR	2.5	5.1	2.8	0
Salomon (80), 2001	115	118	77	0.8	15.5	4	0
Terachi (96), 1997	100	240	77	3	12	NR	0
Manchini (97), 1999	172	132	NR	7	8.7	5.8	1.2
Thompson (6), 1997	50	167	NR	4.5	6	3.1	0
Suzuki (16), 2001	118	166	92	5	12.7	4.6	0
Lezoche (17), 2002	216	100	NR	1.9	2.3	3	0.05
Bonjer (78), 2000	111	114	65	4.5	11	2	0.9
Henry (41), 2000	169	129	NR	5	7.5	5.4	0
Brunt (52), 2001	72	176	107	2.8	19	3	0
Kebebew (98), 2001	176	168	NR	0	5.1	1.7	0
Micoli (99), 2002	137	111	NR	4.3	3.9	3.8	0

[a] Of unilateral procedures.
[b] NR, not recorded.

Table 3 Indications for 100 Laparoscopic Adrenal Procedures

Indication	N
Pheochromocytoma	25
Conn's syndrome	21
Nonfunctional adenoma	20
Cushing's adenoma	13
Cushing's disease	8
Carcinoma	3
Angiomyelolipoma	2
Paraneoplastic hypercortisolism	2
Macronodular hyperplasia	2
Androgen—producing adenoma	2
Others	2

Table 5 Additional Laparoscopic Procedures Performed During Adrenalectomy in 88 Patients

Procedure	Patients (n)
Liver biopsy	8
Cholecystectomy	6
Peri-aortic node dissection	2
Ventral hernia repair	1
CBD exploration	1
Colorectal re-anastomosis	1
Left ovarian cystectomy	1

CBD = common bile duct.

More than half of our patients population (55%) had had previous abdominal surgery. We have not viewed this as a contraindication for laparoscopic approach, and no conversions occurred because of adhesions. We actually have performed one procedure 6 weeks after a laparotomy failed to find the adenoma. In addition, 20 of the 88 patients underwent other associated laparoscopic procedures at the time of their adrenalectomy. These are listed in Table 5.

Of the 100 procedures, 12% had postoperative complications, which are listed in Table 6. Re-operation within 30 days of surgery was required in two occasions (2%) for evacuation of a retroperitoneal hematoma in a patient who had been anticoagulated for mitral vave prosthesis and for postoperative acute cholecystitis in the second case. These procedures were accomplished laparoscopically with uneventful recovery thereafter. There have been no wound complications. There was no mortality.

Injury to structures in the area of dissection are possible (transabdominally or retroperitoneally), adjacent to the adrenals including the kidney, colon, tail of the pancreas, and the stomach on the left side. On the right side, the liver and the duodenum are at risk. Because both adrenals are located in close proximity to major blood vessels (the hilum of kidneys and the vena cava), massive bleeding is a potentially disastrous complication.

Furthermore, dissection high in the abdomen could result in diaphragmatic injury, leading to potential tension pneumothorax. A multi-institutional study by Terachi et al. from Japan, has evaluated 370 patients who underwent laparoscopic adrenalectomy (40). There was no mortality. Overall complications developed in 57 patients (15%), including introperative in 33 patients (9%), and postoperative in 24 patients (6%). Conversion to open surgery was necessary in 13 cases (3.5%). The 33 intraoperative complications involved vascular injury in 22 patients (5.9%), and visceral injury in 11 patients (3%). The 22 vascular injuries involved the vena cava in two patients, renal vein in two patients, adrenal vein in four patients, other adrenal vessels in 11 patients and other vessels in three additional patients. The 11 visceral injuries included the liver in four patients, spleen

Table 4 Indications for Bilateral Laparoscopic Adrenalectomy in 88 Patients Undergoing Adrenalectomy

Indication	Patients (n)
Malignant pheochromocytoma	3
Benign pheochromocytoma	2
Cushing's disease	3
Bilateral adenoma	1
Bilateral macronodular hyperplasia	1

Table 6 Complications Occurring in 100 Laparoscopic Adrenalectomy/Biopsies

Type of complication	N
Postoperative	
Deep venous thrombosis	3
Hematomas	2
Anemia	2
Subdural hematoma	1
Urinary tract infection	1
Colonic pseudo–obstruction	1
Pulmonary edema	1
Acute cholecystitis	1

in three, pancreas in two, gallbladder in one and the adrenal gland in one patient. The 24 postoperative complications involved bleeding in six patients, wound infection in four, atelectasis in three, ileus in two, pneumothorax in one, and other in eight. Most complications were minor and treated laparoscopically. Henry et al. reported the complications of laparoscopic adrenalectomy in 169 consecutive procedures (41). There was no mortality. Twelve patients (7.5%) had significant complications: three peritoneal hematomas requiring (in 2 cases) laparotomy, and (in one case) transfusion; one parietal hematoma; three intraoperative bleeding episodes without need for transfusion; one partial infarction of the spleen; one pneumothorax; one tumor extrraction and two venous throm-boses. Another large multi-institutional study from France (42) reported a similar complication rate of 7.7% occurring in ten patients out of 130 cases of laparoscopic adrenalectomy. Interestingly, neither this study, nor others (40,43–45), have found significant differences between transperitoneal and retroperitoneal approaches, except for the risk of the intraperitoneal visceral injury.

Interestingly, 25% of the pathologies in our series were pheochromocytomas. These tumors were larger than in patients with other diseases: 6.3 cm versus 3.9 cm ($p < 0.05$). In addition, operative time was longer: 2.5 hours versus 1.8 hours ($p < 0.05$). During the removal of these tumors, hypertension occurred in 56% of patients and, hypotension in 52%. Moreover, almost 60% (7/12) of our postoperative complications were observed in this subset. Associated multiple endocrine neoplasia (MEN–IIA) syndrome was identified in six patients, and MEN–IIB in two patients. Several studies have addressed the issue of hemodynamic changes during laparoscopic adrenalectomy for pheochromocytoma compared to open surgery (46–48). The laparoscopic approach has resulted in less (48) or comparable (46,47) hemodynamic changes compared to the traditional open surgery, although patients who underwent laparoscopy had a more rapid postoperative recovery. The retroperitoneal approach seems to offer no advantage over the intraperitoneal approach (49), and carbon dioxide pneumoperitoneum is well tolerated in this subset of patients (47). In a literature review of large series on more than 300 laparoscopic adrenalectomies exclusively for pheochromocytoma, no mortality has been reported to date (28,48,50–61). These cases included familial multiple endocrine hyperplasia syndromes, bilateral pheochromocytoma and extra-adrenal pheochromocytoma. Both transperitoneal and extraperitoneal approaches were used. Although earlier experience was associated with more blood loss, longer operative time and higher complication rate compared to other pathologies (50,51), the more recent large series, demonstrated no significant difference. The occurrence of hypertension postoperatively is rare and in fact, cure of hypertension was achieved in almost all patients.

With regard to the functional outcome in other hormonally active tumors, during our follow-up period (range 1–44 months), patients appear to have responded well to laparoscopic adrenalectomy. Two have been found to have renovascular hypertension and none have had hormonal recurrence. The renal arteriograms showed no stenosis and, in addition, excluded the possibility of superior arteriolar renal occlusions by metal clips. One patient operated upon for Cushing's disease who had a partial response to adrenocorticotropic hormone stimulation, however, was still having serum cortisone levels below the normal range by the end of the follow-up period. Other authors (52,62–65) have uniformly reported excellent results comparable with those of open surgery. The Mayo clinic group reported bilateral laparoscopic adrenalectomy in 19 patients with ACTH–dependent Cushing's syndrome in whom the ACTH-secreting neoplasm couldn't be removed (62). All patients experienced resolution of the signs and symptoms of Cushing's syndrome as well as weight loss, improved glucose tolerance and improved control of blood pressure. No residual cortisol secretion was detected. Similar success rates were reported by others in more than 100 cases with Cushing's disease and syndrome (21,22,25). Rossi et al. (63) reported the effectiveness of laparoscopic adrenalectomy in 30 pateints with primary hyperaldosteronism. Twenty-nine of 30 (95%) patients were rendered normokalemic and persisting hypertension was present in 10 of 30 (33%) patients. In these patients, the hypertension was easily controlled medically. Duration of the hypertension before surgery was a significant risk factor for persistent hypertension. Several other articles specifically focusing on laparoscopic adrenalectomy for aldosteronoma revealed that hypertension was cured or significantly improved in greater than 90% of patients (64,66,67). A recent study by Brunt et al. (52), involving 72 patients with hormonally active adrenal tumors, laparoscopic adrenalectomy resulted in an excellent clinical outcome. Resolution of clinical and biochemical signs was accomplished in 34 of 34 patients with pheochromocytoma, 25 of 26 patients with aldosteronomas, five of five patients with cortisol-producing adenomas and three of three patients with adrenocorticitropic hormone–dependent cushing's syndrome. Two patients with MEN-2 had contralateral pheochromocytomas removed four and five years after the initial surgery. Surprisingly, persistent hypertension necessitating medications was present in 72% of patients with aldosteronomas, although 92% of these patients had significantly improved blood pressure control after surgery. Recurrent hypokalemia developed in one patient (4%) with a cortical nodule in the contralateral adrenal. The authors concluded that the clinical and biochemical cure rates are comparable with those of open adrenalectomy during long term follow-up.

6 MALIGNANCY CONTROVERSY

During aparoscopic adrenalectomy, we have encountered in eight of patients who were treated for malignant diseases, six primaries (three pheochromocytomas and three nonfunctioning tumors that showed microscopic features of carcinoma), and two secondaries, had no evidence of local recurrence during our time period of the follow-up (1–44 months). Laparoscopic adrenalectomy for solitary adrenal metastasis or cancer has also been investigated at few centers, and to date, very few references are available in the literature. The experience from the Cleveland Clinic in 11 patients was reported by Heniford et al. (68). All of the tumors except one were due to metastatic cancer. The metastatic sources included renal cell cancer, lung cancer, colon cancer, and melanoma. The mean size of the tumors was 5.9 cm (range 1.9–12). One patient required conversion to open surgery due to local invasion of the tumor into the vena cava. At a mean follow-up of 8.3 months, there have been no port site or or local recurrences. One patient has developed a new hepatic nodule, 10 of the 11 patients were alive by the time of the report and one has died of extensive brain metastasis from melanoma. Valeri et al. (12), addressing the same issue in a series of eight neoplastic patients with adrenal masses, showed a three-year survival rate of 63% (an adenoma was proved in two cases). Two other reports on laparoscopic adrenalectomy for large (>6 cm) and potentially malignant tumors were recently published and documented favorable outcome (69,70). In the study by Henry et al. (69), out of six patients with adrenocortical carcinoma, only one patient developed liver metastasis six months after surgery and died. The five other patients were disease free with a follow-up ranging from 8 to 83 months. The largest series with the longest follow-up to date, was recently published by Kebebew et al. (71). It included 23 patients who had a laparoscopic approach for suspected and unsuspected malignant adrenal tumors. Six of the patients showed primary adrenal cancers, 13 adrenal metastasis, two lymphomas, and two cases with no evidence of cancer. The tumor resection margin was negative on all adrenalectomies. There were three locoregional recurrences in the six patients with primary adrenal cancer, no port recurrences, and 4 distant recurrences in 13 patients with metastatic adrenal tumors. The disease-free survival was 65% at a mean follow-up time of 3.3 years (range, 1–7 years). Interestingly, these results were comparable with the known results for conventional surgery (72). It is worth mentioning that in all of these studies no major complications occurred, conversions were required only in patients with intraoperative evidence of tumor invasion, the laparoscopic removal achieved free resection margins in all patients and no port site metastasis were reported.

7 ROLE OF LAPAROSCOPIC ULTRASONOGRAPHY

Laparoscopic ultrasonography has been used in 15 selected cases. It showed the location of the adrenal gland after an open surgery failed to find the organ; the presence of a 0.7 cm aldosteronoma, which was disputed before surgery; that no adenoma was present in two cases, necessitating only biopsy and closure rather than adrenalectomy; no vascular, extra-adrenal or lymph node involvement in two large lesions (10 and 12 cm), which then were removed laparoscopically and found to be benign; vascular invasion in one patient with adrenal adenocarcinoma leading to conversion to open successful removal; the invasion of the periadrenal fat by one metastatic cancer that then was removed with negative margins; the right adrenal vein, which facilitated dissection and control in two operations; and bilateral hyperplasia requiring bilateral adrenalectomy. Other groups have reported similar results with the use of laparoscopic ultrasonography in adrenalectomy (73,74). Brunt et al. (74) have utilized this modality during laparoscopic adrenalectomy in 27 patients. They concluded that laparoscopic ultrasound provided useful information to the surgeon in 11 of 28 procedures (39%) by (a) localizing the adrenal gland and tumor and /or guiding the dissection, (b) demonstrating that tumors > 4cm were confined to the gland, and (c) investigating suspected pathology in other organs. Mean time for ultrasound was 10.9 minutes and calculated hospital charges were $602. There were no intraoperative complications. Siperstein et al. (75) found that it was of extreme value in identification of small tumors in obese patients operated on with the posterior technique. Especially in patients with nodular hyperplasia, laparoscopic ultrasound enabled the complete excision of all lesions by demonstrating the absence or presence of residual tumor tissue in the adrenal bed after resection (75). Thus, the information obtained from ultrasonography in many instances can affect the progression of the operation. It involves a simple technique, which can be easily mastered.

8 DISCUSSION

More than a decade after the advent of laparoscopic adrenalectomy, the worldwide accumulated experience indicates that the procedure is safe, successful, and in fact is now considered a well established and the preferred treatment modality for the majority of endocrine and neoplastic disorders affecting the adrenal gland.

The results of laparoscopic adrenalectomy must be compared to those of conventional open surgery. To the best of our knowledge, there are no prospective randomized studies comparing open with laparoscopic adrenalectomy and the excellent results reported in the available retrospective comparative reports, make such a study unnecessary, and possibly non-ethical. In our own retrospective comparative analysis (3), we have found no difference in operating time or adrenal dimensions. The estimated blood loss was 70 ml for the laparoscopic adrenalectomy versus approximately 200 ml for the open procedure. The mean hospital stay for the conventional surgery was nine days versus less than three days in the laparoscopic group. The analgesia requirements and the mean time for ambulation were also significantly lower in the laparoscopic group. Other studies have reported similar outcomes (4–8,24,30–39). The Cleveland Clinic retrospective comparison of 110 laparoscopic adrenalectomies and 100 open cases shows the superior results of the minimally invasive approach (76). Open adrenalectomy was performed by various standard approaches. The laparoscopic group was superior in regard to mean surgical time, mean blood loss, mean narcotic analgesic requirements, mean intensive care unit admissions, mean resumption of oral fluid intake and mean hospital stay. While intraoperative complication rate was similar, there were fewer postoperative complications in the laparoscopic group. Of special interest, is the study by Thompson et al. from the Mayo Clinic (6) who compared laparoscopic transabdominal laparoscopic approach in 50 patients and open posterior approach in 50 well-matched patients. In addition to the known reported advantages of laparoscopy, late incisional neuromuscular complications developed in 54% of the open group, including oblique muscles in 30%, the chronic pain syndrome in 14% and flank numbness in 10%. A recent meta-analysis of the english literature by Brunt (77), has compared the complications of laparoscopic with open adrenalectomy. Complications were tabulated from 50 studies of laparoscopic adrenalectomy involving 1522 patients and 48 studies of open adrenalectomy comprising 2273 patients. Among the reports, 22 compared laparoscopic and open adrenalectomy within a single institution. It was concluded that laparoscopic adrenalectomy has resulted in fewer adrenalectomy-related complications than seen historically with open adrenalectomy. Fewer wound and pulmonary complications and the reduced occurrence of incidental splenectomy are primarily responsible for this improved outcome. Finally, another variable of concern, addressed by several authors, is the cost of the procedure compared to the conventional surgery (5,6,8,31,38). Although Thompson and coworkers (6) have demonstrated higher costs with the laparoscopic procedure, most other reports, in fact, found no significant difference in overall cost between the two approaches. However, it should be noted, that the impact of earlier return to work in patients undergoing the laparoscopic procedure, has not been assessed yet, and future data will, most probably, show lower costs when this is taken into consideration.

As described earlier, the technique of choice by most surgeons performing laparoscopic adrenalectomy is the transabdominal lateral approach. Several authors have successfully documented the feasibility, safety and effectiveness of endoscopic adrenalectomy via the retroperitoneal approach in tumors less than 5–6 cm (14,15, 17,78,79). Since no peritoneum violation or bowel mobilization is required with this approach, it was postulated that this method would be less invasive and, consequently, be associated with better results, especially in small lesions and in obese patients (17,24). Siperstein et al. (15) in a series of 31 patients, concluded that although more demanding, the retroperitoneal approach should be considered in patients with tumors less than 6 cm, bilateral tumors, or extensive previous abdominal surgery. In another large series from the Netherlands, the procedure was described in 111 consecutive cases and showed comparable results with the transabdominal approach (78). These authors recommended the procedure for benign adrenal tumors less than 6 cm. Nevertheless, case history analysis has revealed no apparent difference in patient outcome, morbidity or operative time for the two approaches to the adrenal gland (14,15,44,45,80). Moreover, in our experience and the experience of others (81), no bowel injury or complications developed when using the transperitoneal approach. Comparison between the two techniques, has in fact, indicated no real difference for small masses, although for lesions more than 5–6 cm, the transabdominal route is considered preferable (16). Disadvantages of the retroperitoneal approach include a lack of anatomic landmarks and a restricted working space. This combination of technical difficulties renders the retroperitoneal approach unsuitable for tumors larger than 6 cm. On the other hand, a major advantage of the transperitoneal approach is that the abdominal cavity, and particularly the liver, can be explored. In patients with pheochromocytoma, the liver can be examined by inspection and ultrasound, and suspicious lesions may be biopsied. Moreover, in our personal experience with the retroperitoneal approach, the exposure was inferior to that which an experienced surgeon can readily obtain via the transperitoneal approach to the adrenal gland.

The available data, suggests that there are very few absolute contraindications for laparoscopic adrenalectomy. At the present time, we consider invasive adrenal carcinoma to be the only absolute contraindication for the laparoscopic approach, due to the possible extent and complexity of the operation required. An open technique also may be more desirable for patients with malignant pheochromocytoma when metastatic nodes are present in the peri-aortic chain or close to the bladder. Several authors differentiate between the biologic behavior of adrenal metastasis and primary adrenal cancer as to their suitability for the laparoscopic procedure (51,71). Because solitary adrenal metastasis from an extra-adrenal primary is usually small and confined within the adrenal, the laparoscopic approach has considerable appeal for this specific indication (51). Conversely, adrenal cancer is usually larger and often locally invasive. An important limitation in this regard is that adrenal imaging and even, fine needle aspiration, are often inaccurate enough to diagnose or exclude adrenal malignancy (71). Given that no reliable and accurate preoperative diagnostic test to diagnose adrenal malignancy exists, it is difficult to determine when an open approach should be used. An initial laparoscopic approach can be used to establish the diagnosis with low morbidity and allows curative resection in most instances (71). Laparoscopic ultrasound is a simple and effective intraoperative technical adjunct that may be used to evaluate the nature and invasiveness of the suspected adrenal mass. Obviously, in patients who prove to have local invasion during surgery, the laparoscopic approach should be converted to open procedure in order to allow curative wide radical resection. Interestingly, the limited experience to date, with laparoscopic adrenalectomy in malignant disease is promising, with short term results comparable with those of conventional surgery (69,71). Thus, it appears that a laparoscopic approach is reasonable for metastatic adrenal disease, provided the primary cancer is controlled and there is no evidence of extra-adrenal disease. Similarly, for primary neoplasms, if complete resection is technically feasible, and there is no evidence of local invasion, an initial laparoscopic approach is an acceptable option in experienced hands at selected centers (51, 69,71).

The maximal acceptable size of lesion appropriate for laparoscopic adrenalectomy is another unsettled issue. Although size per se is not definite contraindication, laparoscopy is not advisable in masses larger than 12—14 cm, because of the increased incidence of malignancy and the technical difficulties associated with their removal. The largest lesion that we have resected was 14 cm, but such a mass makes the dissection difficult and is time consuming. The exposure also is problematic because of the limited space available in this area. Frequently, large masses have unusual and numerous retroperitoneal feeding vessels that require tedious and lengthy dissection. Only those surgeons with extensive laparoscopic experience should attempt resection of larger adrenal masses. Generally, the indications and contraindications for laparoscopic adrenalectomy, including the maximal size limit and other issues, are currently dictated largely by the experience of the individual laparoscopic surgeon.

Management recommendations regarding an incidental adrenal mass are still a matter of controversy. Although, generally adrenocortical carcinomas are seen in masses larger than 6 cm, reports are available of incidentally detected cancer in masses 3–5 cm and even smaller (51,82). Another confounding factor is the fact that computed tomography may be associated with 20–40% underestimation of adrenal tumor size compared with actual size on histopathology (82). Definite indications for adrenalectomy include sizes larger than 4 cm, hormonally active lesions, suspicious mass characteristics base on imaging studies, and documented increase in size. In light of the above-mentioned facts and the excellent results of the laparoscopic procedure, we and others (51), propose that laparoscopic adrenalectomy is the preferred management for the young and low operative risk patients, with 3–5 cm adrenal masses. Another argument against the watchful conservative policy in such cases is the observation that most adrenal nodules increase in size with age (51) and the annual need for imaging and biochemical testing throughout their life. Moreover, the patient will be spared the anxiety, expense and time lost from repeated follow-up appointments and the associated studies needed.

At present, we believe it is beyond debate that this minimally invasive technique has become the procedure of choice for hyperaldosteronism (37,63,64), Cushing's syndrome and disease (3,21,22,25,26,62,67), and pheochromocytoma (20,28,48,50,53,54,58).

Bilateral laparoscopic adrenalectomy appears to be safe and effective in patients with pituitary-dependent Cushing's syndrome after failed transsphenoidal surgery and in cases with ectopic ACTH syndrome when the primary tumor cannot be identified or removed (62). It is now obvious that laparoscopic resection of pheochromocytomas can be accomplished safely despite frequent episodes of hemodynamic variability equal to those of historical open control subjects. The expedient recovery, lesser postoperative complications and the lack of endocrinopathy recurrence, makes this approach the procedure of choice for the management of pheochromocytoma (53,57). In addition, a recent publication by Brunt et al. (52) has reported favorable results in cases of unilateral and bilateral familial pheochromocytoma (patients with MEN-2A, MEN-2B, Von Hippel–Lindau and Neurofibromatosis type 1). Another large series from Germany (55), have documented the successful outcome of endoscopic approach in 61 chromaffin neoplasms (52 pheochromocytomas and 9 paragangliomas). The patient population included wide spectrum of this disease: unilateral, hereditary, bilateral, recurrent and multiple tumors. Interestingly, in patients with bilateral disease, partial bilateral adrenalectomy was performed and achieved preservation of the adrenocortical function in 86% of cases, without evidence of recurrence after three years of follow-up. Thus, in patients with hormonally active tumors of the adrenal, the procedure has proved feasible, safe and offered all the advantages of minimally invasive surgery. Additionally, it resulted in an excellent functional outcome and was associated with clinical and biochemical cure rates comparable with those of open surgery during long term follow-up (3,52,53,55,57,62–64).

Recently, newer advances and innovations in the field of laparoscopic adrenalectomy have been introduced. Outpatient laparoscopic adrenalectomy has been performed in selected low risk patients with small adrenal tumors (mainly hyperaldosteronism and excluding pheochromocytoma), with satisfactory results (65,84). To further minimize the morbidity of conventional laparoscopic procedures, Needlescopic technique, utilizing smaller ports, was reported by several groups (84–86). The limited experience to date with small number of patients showed that the procedure was feasible, resulted in improved wound cosmesis, and a trend toward decreased postoperative pain and hospital stay was observed, without prolonging operative time (84). The continued technological advances, offering more effective 2 mm instruments, has the potential to convince more reluctant surgeons to embark on this new technique. Nevertheless, randomized prospective trials comparing needlescopic with conventional laparoscopy are still needed to validate these favorable initial results.

Laparoscopic adrenal-sparing surgery in selected patients with bilateral pheochromocytoma and well-circumscribed bilateral cortisol or aldosterone-producing adenomas (29,59,87–91) was reported. This adrenal sparing approach may be valuable in those who would otherwise require lifelong adrenal replacement therapy after complete adrenal glands extirpation. It was also reported in cases of unilateral aldosterone-producing adenomas (91). Our limited experience (29) and that of others (87–91) confirms the technical feasibility and safety of laparoscopic partial adrenalectomy. It should be noted that recurrence rates in patients with bilateral pheochromocytomas in MEN syndromes, approached 20% (29,90). For this reason it is recommended to avoid adrenal-saving surgery in these instances. Intraoperative ultrasound should be available if adrenal-sparing surgery is planned since it's not possible to rely solely on the direct laparoscopic view. Whenever a clear differentiation between tumor and normal parenchyma is impossible intraoperatively, total adrenalectomy becomes unavoidable. Total adrenalectomy is also undisputed in cases of suspected malignancy. There have been no studies in which failure to preserve adrenal function was clearly associated with main vein ligation, however, every attempt should be made to maintain the main vein during adrenal sparing surgery. In case of severe hypertension during surgery for pheochromocytoma, it has been suggested to temporarily occlude the vein with laparoscopic bulldog clamp (59). Due to the possibility of preserving a better cortical physiologic response to stress stimulation even in cases of unilateral partial resections, adrenal-sparing surgery may represent a valuable alternative to total adrenalectomy for selected indications. However, more data from large prospective series with long-term follow-up is required before drawing definite conclusions.

Another technical advance, further extending the scope of minimally invasive adrenal surgery, is the recent investigation of the thoracoscopic trans-diaphragmatic approach to the adrenal gland (92). Additional novel approaches under investigation are adrenal cryoablation (93) and robotic laparoscopic adrenalectomy (94,95).

Finally, two recent publications have addressed another interesting issue; whether the widespread introduction of laparoscopic adrenalectomy have broadened the indications of the surgical approach to adrenal lesions and changed the pattern of referral (99,100). It has been found that the introduction of laparoscopic adrenalectomy has resulted in an increase in the number of patients referred, and consequently, more adrenalectomies are performed. While one study showed that the criteria for patient selection did not change, but more patients with adrenal metastasis and incidentalomas were operated on laparoscopically (99), the other study, indicated that this was due to increased number of cases with hyperaldosteronism and pheochromocytoma (100). In this study, however, there was no change in the number of operations for incidentalomas and metastasis (100).

9 CONCLUSION

After a decade of worldwide experience, laparoscopic adrenalectomy has successfully achieved maturity. Based on our experience, and that of others, laparoscopic adrenalectomy is a well established technique and is currently the treatment of choice for benign functioning and nonfunctioning neoplasms of the adrenal. Although other laparoscopic approaches are feasible, they have their limitations and offer no clear advantage over the lateral transabdominal approach, the preferred technique practiced by most surgeons performing laparoscopic adrenalectomy. The limited experience with the procedure in malignancy shows some promise. It should be emphasized, however, that its definite role in this regard is yet to be clarified. At the present time, invasive adrenocortical carcinoma and metastatic pheochromocytoma to peri-aortic nodes are the only absolute contraindications. Needless to say, only experienced laparoscopic surgeons should attempt laparoscopic resection of large masses, and generally, the minimally invasive technique is not advisable for lesions greater than 12–14 cm.

REFERENCES

1. Gagner M, Lacroix A, Bolte E. Laparoscopic adrenalectomy in Cushing's syndrome and pheochromocytoma. N Engl J Med 1992; 327:1003.
2. Gagner M, Lacroix A, Prinz RA, et al. Early experience with laparoscopic approach for adrenalectomy. Surgery 1993; 114:1120–1125.
3. Gagner M, Pomp A, Heniford BT, et al. Laparoscopic adrenalectomy. Lessons learned from 100 consecutive procedures. Ann Surg 1997; 226:238–247.
4. Prinz RA. A comparison of laparoscopic and open adrenalectomies. Arch Surg 1995; 130:489–494.
5. Brunt LM, Doherty GM, Norton JA, et al. Laparoscopic adrenalectomy compared to open adrenalectomy for benign adrenal neoplasms. J Am Coll Surg 1996; 183:1–10.
6. Thompson GB, Grant CS, van Heerden JA, et al. Laparoscopic versus open posterior adrenalectomy: a case-control study of 100 patients. Surgery 1997; 122: 1132–1136.
7. Dudley NE, Harrison BJ. Comparison of open posterior versus transperitoneal laparoscopic adrenalectomy. Br J Surg 1999; 86:656–660.
8. Imai T, Kikumori T, Ohiwa M. A case-controlled study of laparoscopic compared with open lateral adrenalectomy. Am J Surg 1999; 178:50–54.
9. Mcleod MK. Complications following adrenal surgery. J Natl Med Assoc 1991; 83:161.
10. Wanaka T, Arai M, Ito M, et al. Surgical treatment for abdominal Neuroblastoma in the laparoscopic era. Surg Endosc 2001; 15:751–754.
11. Castilho LN, Castillo OA, Denes FT, et al. Laparoscopic adrenal surgery in children. J Urol 2002; 168: 221–224.
12. Valeri A, Borrelli A, Presenti L, et al. Adrenal masses in neoplastic patients: the role laparoscopic procedure. Surg Endosc 2001; 15:90–93.
13. Barresi R, Prinz RA. Laparoscopic adrenalectomy. Arch Surg 1999; 134:212–217.
14. Fernandez-Cruz L, Saenz A, Taura P, et al. Retroperitoneal approach in laparoscopic adrenalectomy: is it advantageous? Surg Endosc 1999; 13:86–90.
15. Siperstein AE, Berber E, Engle KL, et al. Laparoscopic posterior adrenalectomy. Technical considerations. Arch Surg 2000; 135:967–971.
16. Suzuki K, Kageyama S, Hirano Y, et al. Comparison of 3 surgical approaches to laparoscopic adrenalectomy: a randomized, background matched analysis. J Urol 2001; 166:437–443.
17. Lezoche E, Guerrieri M, Felicioti F, et al. Anterior, lateral and posterior approaches in endoscopic adrenalectomy. Surg Endosc 2002; 16:96–99.
18. Gagner M, Lacroix A, Bolte E, et al. Laparoscopic adrenalectomy. The importance of a flank approach in the lateral decubitus position. Surg Endosc 1994; 8: 135–138.
19. Marescaux J, Mutter D, Forbes L, et al. Bilateral laparoscopic adrenalectomy. In: Gagner M, Inabnet B, eds. Minimally Invasive Endocrine Surgery. Lippincott Williams & Wilkins, 2002:205–216.
20. Lee JE, Curley SA, Gagel RF, et al. Cortical sparing

adrenalectomy for patients with bilateral pheochromocytoma. Surgery 1996; 120:1064–1071.
21. Chapuis Y, Inabnet B, Abboud B, et al. Bilateral laparoscopic adrenalectomy in Cushing's syndrome. Experience in 24 patients (in French). Ann Chir 1998; 52:35–56.
22. Fernandez-Cruz L, Saenz A, Benarroch G. Laparoscopic unilateral and bilateral adrenalectomy for Cushing's syndrome. Ann Surg 1996; 224:727–736.
23. Walz MK, Pietgen K, Hoermann R, et al. Posterior retroperitoneoscopy as a new minimally invasive approach for adrenalectomy: results of 30 adrenalectomies in 27 patients. World J Surg 1996; 20:769–774.
24. Bonjer HJ, Lange JF, Kazemier G, et al. Comparison of three techniques for adrenalectomy. Br J Surg 1997; 84:679–682.
25. Lanzi R, Montorsi F, Losa M, et al. Laparoscopic bilateral adrenalectomy for persistent Cushing's disease after transsphenoidal surgery. Surgery 1998; 123: 144–150.
26. Ferrer FA, MacGillivray DC, Mlachoff DC, et al. Bilateral laparoscopic adrenalectomy for adrenocorticotropic dependent Cushing's syndrome. J Urol 1997; 157:16–18.
27. Fernandez-Cruz L, Saenz A, Taura P, et al. Pheochromocytoma: laparoscopic approach with CO2 and helium pneumoperitoneum. Endosc Surg Allied Technol 1994; 2:300–304.
28. Fernandez-Cruz L, Saenz A, Pantoja JP. Laparoscopic adrenalectomy for pheochromocytoma. In: Gagner M, Inabnet B, eds. Minimally Invasive Endocrine Surgery. Lippincott Williams & Wilkins, 2002:235–241.
29. Rubino F, Bellantoni R, Gagner M. Laparoscopic adrenal-sparing surgery. In: Gagner M, Inabnet B, eds. Lippincott Williams & Wilkinson, 2002:217–225.
30. Ishikawa Sowa M, Nagayama M, et al. Laparoscopic adrenalectomy : comparison with the conventional approach. Surg Lap Endosc 1997; 7:275–280.
31. Jacobs JK, Goldstein RE, Geer RJ. Laparoscopic adrenalectomy: a new standard of care. Ann Surg 1997; 225:495–502.
32. Linos DA, Stylopoulos N, Boukis M, et al. Anterior, posterior or laparoscopic approach for the management of adrenal disease? Am J Surg 1997; 173:120–125.
33. MacGillivray DC, Shichman SJ, Ferrer FA, et al. A comparison of open vs laparoscopic adrenalectomy. Surg Endosc 1996; 10:987–990.
34. Nash PA, Leibovitch I, Donohue JP. Adrenalectomy via the dorsal approach: a benchmark for laparoscopic adrenalectomy. J Urol 1995; 154:1652–1654.
35. Staren ED, Prinz RA. Adrenalectomy in the era of laparoscopy. Surgery 1996; 120:706–709.
36. Vargas HI, Kavoussi LR, Bartlett DL, et al. Laparoscopic adrenalectomy: a new standard of care. Urology 1997; 49:673–678.
37. Shen WT, Lim RC, Siperstein AE, et al. Laparoscopic vs open adrenalectomy for the treatment of primary hyperaldosteronism. Arch Surg 1999; 134:628–632.
38. Ortega J, Sala C, Garcia S, et al. Cost-effectiveness of laparoscopic vs open adrenalectomy: small savings in an expensive process. J Laparoendosc Adv Surg Tech 2002; 12:1–5.
39. Ichikawa T, Mikami K, Komiya K, et al. Laparoscopic adrenalectomy for functioning adrenal tumors: clinical experience with 38 cases and comparison with open adrenalectomy. Biomed Pharmacother 2000; 54(suppl):178–182.
40. Terachi T, Yoshida O, Matsuda T, et al. Complications of laparoscopic and retroperitoneoscopic adrenalectomies in 370 cases in Japan: a multi-institutional study. Bimed Phamacother 2000; 54(suppl 1):211–214.
41. Henry JF, Defechereux T, Raffaelli M, et al. Complications of laparoscopic adrenalectomy: results of 169 consecutive procedures. World J Surg 2000; 24:1342–1346.
42. Soulie M, Salomon L, Seguin P, et al. Multi-institutional study of complications in 1085 laparoscopic urologic procedures. Urology 2001; 58:899–903.
43. Suzuki K, Ushiyama T, Ihara H, et al. Complications of laparoscopic adrenalectomy in 75 patients treated by the same surgeon. Eur Urol 1999; 36:40–47.
44. Yoneda K, Shiba E, Watanabi T, et al. Laparoscopic adrenalectomy: lateral transabdominal approach vs. posterior retroperitoneal approach. Biomed Pharmacother 2000; 54(suppl 1):215–219.
45. Takeda M. Laparoscopic adrenalectomy: transperitoneal vs. retroperitoneal approaches. Biomed Pharmacother 2000; 54(suppl 1):207–210.
46. Sprung J, O'hara JF, Gill IS, et al. Anesthetic aspects of laparoscopic and open adrenalectomy for pheochromocytoma. Urology 2000; 55:339–343.
47. Inabnet B, Pitre J, Bernard D, et al. Comparison of the hemodynamic parameters of open and laparoscopic adrenalectomy for pheochromocytoma. World J Surg 2000; 24:574–578.
48. Fernandez-Cruz L, Taura P, Saenz A. Laparoscopic approach to pheochromocytoma: hemodynamic changes and catecholamine secretion. World J Surg 1996; 20:762–768.
49. Fernandez-Cruz L, Saenz A, Taura P, et al. Retroperitoneal approach in laparoscopic adrenalectomy. Surg Endosc 1999; 13:86–90.
50. Gagner M, Breton G, Pharand D, et al. Is laparoscopic adrenalectomy indicated for pheochromocytomas? Surgery 1996; 120:1076–1080.
51. Gill IS. The case for laparoscopic adrenalectomy. J Urol 2001; 166:429–435.
52. Brunt LM, Moley JF, Doherty GM, et al. Outcome analysis in patients undergoing laparoscopic adrenalectomy for hormonally active tumors. Surgery 2001; 130:629–634.

53. Kercher KW, Park A, Matthews BD, et al. Laparoscopic adrenalectomy for pheochromocytoma. Surg Endosc 2002; 16:100–102.
54. Brunt LM, Lairmore TC, Doherty GM, et al. Adrenalectomy for familial pheochromocytoma in the laparoscopic era. Ann Surg 2002; 235:713–720.
55. Walz MK, Peitgen K, Neumann H, et al. Endoscopic tretment of solitary, bilateral, multiple and recurrent pheochromocytomas and paragangliomas. World J Surg 2002; 26:1005–1012.
56. Tanaka M, Tokuda N, Koga H, et al. Laparoscopic adrenalectomy for pheochromocytoma: comparison with open adrenalectomy and comparison of laparoscopic surgery for pheohromocytoma versus other adrenal tumors. J Endourol 2000; 14:427–431.
57. Cheah WK, Clark OH, Horn JK, et al. Laparoscopic adrenalectomy for pheochromocytoma. World J Surg 2002; 26:1048–1051.
58. Salomon L, Rabii R, Soulie M, et al. Experience with retroperitoneal laparoscopic adrenalectomy for pheochromocytoma. J Urol 2001; 165:1882–1884.
59. Janetschek G, Finkenstedt G, Gasser R, et al. Laparoscopic surgery for pheochromocytoma: adrenalectomy, partial resection, excision of paragangliomas. J Urol 1998; 160:330–334.
60. Mobius E, Nies C, Ruthmond M. Surgical treatment of pheochromocytomas. Laparoscopic or convetional? Surg Endosc 1999; 13:35–39.
61. Col V, de Canniere L, Collard E, et al. Laparoscopic adrenalectomy for pheochromocytoma: endocrinological and surgical aspects of a new therapeutic approach. Clin Endocrinol 1999; 50:121–125.
62. Vella A, Thompson GB, Grant CS, et al. Laparoscopic adrenalectomy for adrenocorticotropin-dependent Cushing's syndrome. J Clin Endocrinol Metab 2001; 86:1596–1599.
63. Rossi H, Kim A, Prinz RA. Primary hyperaldosteronism in the era of laparoscopic adrenalectomy. Am Surg 2002; 68:253–256.
64. Miyaki, Okuyama A. Surgical management of primary aldosteronism. Biomed Pharmacother 2000; 54(suppl 1):146–149.
65. Edwin B, Reader I, Trondsen E, et al. Outpatient laparoscopic adrenalectomy in patients with Conn's syndrome. Surg Endosc 2001; 15:589–591.
66. Siren J, Haglund C, Huikuri K, et al. Laparoscopic adrenalectomy for primary aldosteronism: clinical experience with 12 patients. Surg Laparosc Endosc 1999; 9: 9–13.
67. Go H, Takeda M, Imai T, et al. Laparoscopic surgery for Cushing's syndrome: comparison with primary aldosteronism. Surgery 1995; 117:11–17.
68. Heniford BT, Arca MJ, Walsh RM, et al. Laparoscopic adrenalectomy for cancer. Semin Surg Oncol 1999; 16:293–306.
69. Henry JF, Sebag F, Iacobone M, et al. Results of laparoscopic adrenalectomy for large and potentially malignant tumors. World J Surg 2002; 26:1043–1047.
70. MacGillivray DC, Whalen GF, Malchoff CD, et al. Laparoscopic resection of large adrenal tumors. Ann Surg Oncol 2002; 9:480–485.
71. Kebebew E, Siperstein AE, Clark OH, et al. Results of laparoscopic adrenalectomy for suspected and unsuspected malignant adrenal neoplasms. Arch Surg 2002; 137:948–953.
72. Vasilopoulou-Sellin R, Schultz PN. Adrenocortical carcinoma: clinical outcome at the end of the 20th century. Cancer 2001; 92:1113–1121.
73. Heniford BT, Iannitti DA, Hale J, et al. The role of intraoperative ultrasonography during laparoscopic adrenalectomy. Surgery 1997; 122:1068–1073.
74. Brunt LM, Bennett HF, Teefey SA, et al. Laparoscopic ultrasound imaging of adrenal tumors during laparoscopic adrenalectomy. Am J Surg 1999; 178: 490–495.
75. Siperstein AE, Berber E. Laparoscopic ultrasonography of the adrenal glands. In: Gagner M, Inabnet B, eds. Lippincot Williams & Wilkinson, 2002:175–183.
76. Gill IS, Schweizer D, Nelson D. Laparoscopic versus open adrenalectomy in 210 patients: Cleveland Clinic experience with 210 cases. J Urol, Suppl 1999; 161:21.
77. Brunt LM. The positive impact of laparoscopic adrenalectomy on complications of adrenal surgery. Endosc Surg 2002; 16:252–257.
78. Bonjer HJ, Sorm V, Berends FJ, et al. Endoscopic retroperitoneal adrenalectomy: lessons learned from 111 consecutive cases. Ann Surg 2000; 232:796–803.
79. Ting AC, Lo CY, Lo CM. Posterior or laparoscopic approach for adrenalectomy. Am J Surg 1998; 175: 488–490.
80. Salomon L, Soulie M, Mouly F, et al. Experience with retroperitoneal laparoscopic adrenalectomy in 115 procedures. J Urol 2001; 166:38–41.
81. Guazzoni G, Cestari A, Montorsi F, et al. Eight experience with transperitoneal laparoscopic adrenal surgery. J Urol 2001; 166:820–824.
82. Linos DA, Stylopoulos N. How accurate is computed tomography in predicting the real size of adrenal tumors? A retrospective study. Arch Surg 1997; 132: 740–743.
83. Gill IS, Hobart M, Schweizer D, et al. Outpatient adrenalectomy. J Urol 2000; 163:717–720.
84. Gill IS, Soble JJ, Sung GT, et al. Needlescopic adrenalectomy: the initial series. Comparison with conventional laparoscopic adrenalectomy. Urology 1998; 52:180–186.
85. Chueh SC, Chen J, Chen SC, et al. Clipless laparoscopic adrenalectomy with needlescopic instruments. J Urol 2002; 167:39–42.
86. Mamazza J, Schlachta CM, Seshadri PA, et al. Needlescopic surgery. A logical evolution from conventional laparoscopic surgery. Surg Endosc 2001; 15:1208–1212.

87. Neumann HPH, Reincke M, Bender BU, et al. Preserved adrenocortical function after laparoscopic bilateral adrenal sparing surgery for hereditary pheochromocytoma. J Clin Endocrinol Metab 1999; 84: 2608–2610.
88. Walz MK, Peitgen K, Saller B, et al. Subtotal adrenalectomy by the posterior retroperitoneoscopic approach. World J Surg 1998; 22:621–627.
89. Imai T, Tanaka Y, Kikumori T, et al. Laparoscopic partial adrenalectomy. Surg Endosc 1999; 13:343–345.
90. Baghai M, Thompson GB, Young WF, et al. Pheochromocytomas and paragangliomas in von Hippel–Lindau disease. Arch Surg 2002; 137:682–689.
91. Al-Sobhi S, Peschel R, Bartsch G, et al. Partial laparoscopic adrenalectomy for aldosterone-producing adenoma: short and long-term results. J Endourol 2000; 14:497–499.
92. Gill IS, Meraney AM, Thomas JC, et al. Thoracoscopic transdiaphragmatic adrenalectomy: the initial experience. J Urol 2001; 165:1875–1881.
93. Schulsinger DA, Sosa RE, Perlmutter AA, et al. Acute and chronic interstitial cryotherapy of the adrenal gland as a treatment modality. J Endourol 1999; 13: 203–299.
94. Gill IS, Sung GT, Hsu TH, et al. Robotic remote laparoscopic nephrectomy and adrenalectomy: the initial experience. J Urol 2000; 164:2082–2085.
95. Young JA, Chapman WHH, Kim VB, et al. Robotic-assisted adrenalectomy for adrenal incidentaloma: case and review of the literature. Surg Laparosc Endosc Percutan Tech 2002; 12:126–130.
96. Terachi T, Matsuda T, Terai A, et al. Transperitoneal laparoscopic adrenalectomy: experience in 100 cases. J Endourol 1997; 11:361–365.
97. Mncini F, Mutter D, Peix JL, et al. Experiences with adrenalectomy in 1997. Apropos of 247 cases. A multicenter prospective study of the French-speaking association of endocrine surgery. Chirurgie 1999; 124:368–374.
98. Kebebew E, Siperstein AE, Duh QY, et al. Laparoscopic adrenalectomy: the optimal surgical approach. J Laparoendosc Adv Surg Tech 2001; 11:409–413.
99. Miccoli P, Raffaelli M, Berti P, et al. Adrenal surgery before and after the introduction of laparoscopic adrenalectomy. Br J Surg 2002; 89:779–782.
100. Sidhu S, Bambach C, Pillinger S, et al. Changing pattern of adrenalectomy at a tertiary referral center 1970–2000. ANZ J Surg 2002; 72:463–466.

39

Retroperitoneoscopic Adrenalectomy

H. Jaap Bonjer and Bruno Sgromo

Erasmus Medical Center, Rotterdam, The Netherlands

1 INTRODUCTION

Adrenal glands are extraperitoneal organs situated almost in the center of the body. Classically, very invasive procedures have been necessary to manage adrenal disease. Endoscopic surgery can play an important role, avoiding large abdominal, lumbar, or thoraco-abdominal incisions. This is of particular importance because the majority of adrenal tumors is small in size and the specimens are readily extractable. Retroperitoneoscopic surgery originates from pneumo-retroperitoneography, a radiological technique, used before the era of computed tomography (CT), based on the injection of air into the para-renal space to enhance the contrast between structures, thereby delineating renal and adrenal tumors. This is possible because the posterior aspect of Gerota's capsule is easily separated from the posterior lumbar fascia as well as from the other fascias. Subsequently, retroperitoneoscopy allows performing diagnostic and operative procedures of kidneys, adrenal glands, renal pelvis, ureters, and great vessels.

The first endoscopic adrenalectomies were performed through transperitoneal access. However, some pioneers such as Mercan (1) developed the extraperitoneal adrenalectomy because the retroperitoneal approach allowed a more direct approach and required less extensive dissection of adjacent organs. In laparoscopic transperitoneal adrenalectomy, retraction of the spleen, the splenic flexure of the colon, and the pancreatic tail is required to expose the left adrenal. Mobilization and retraction of the right lobe of the liver is necessary to reveal the right adrenal in laparoscopic transperitoneal adrenal surgery. The retroperitoneal approach, both in lateral and prone decubitus, obviates opening the peritoneal cavity, reducing manipulation of adjacent organs and, therefore, the possibility of injuries.

Previous abdominal surgery is a relative contraindication for the laparoscopic trans-abdominal approach because of peritoneal adhesions. Intraperitoneal adhesions do not interfere with the retroperitoneal approach. Otherwise, retroperitoneal surgery appears associated with less trauma of the peritoneum and should therefore create fewer adhesions in the peritoneal cavity.

2 ANATOMY

The retroperitoneum is a virtual space, divided in three (four with the renal lodge) parts by connective structures called fascias. The retropubic or Retzius space, the iliac or Bogros space, and the lumbar retroperitoneum can be distinguished. The Retzius space is located posterior to the abdominal rectus muscle and the pubic bone. The lateral boundaries of the Retzius space are the epigastric vessels and the spermatic cord. The urinary bladder is the content of the Retzius space. The iliac or Bogros space is located laterally to the Retzius space. The psoas muscle, the iliac muscle, and the transversus abdominis muscle are its posterior and lateral boundaries. The lumbar space is the cranial extension of Bogros space. The medial boundaries are the caval vein, the aorta, and the vertebral column. The lateral boundaries are the transverse abdominal muscles. The floor of the lumbar space consists of the psoas muscle and the quadratus lumborum muscle. Ventrally Bogros space is covered by the descending colon on the left and ascending colon on the right. The adrenal glands, surrounded by fat, are located in the lumbar retroperitoneum. The lumbar retroperitoneum consists of two virtual spaces: the anterior and the posterior para-renal spaces.

The anterior para-renal space is separated laterally from the posterior para-renal space by the lateroconal fascia, inferiorly from the renal space by Gerota's fascia, and is enclosed by the diaphragm superiorly and posteriorly. Adrenal glands, the tail of the pancreas on the left and the duodenum on the right are located in the anterior para-renal space. The posterior para-renal space is in direct continuity with the iliac retroperitoneal space. The lateroconal fascia is taut between the peritoneal sac and lumbodorsal fascia. To expose the adrenal glands, a wide longitudinal incision of the lateroconal fascia is necessary (2). The origin of the lateroconal fascia is found in the dividing of Gerota's fascia into two parts. The internal layer, which keeps close contact with the renal profile, and the external layer, the lateroconal fascia that goes straight to the diaphragm.

Adrenal glands are small, paired, bilateral, triangular organs situated cranially to the kidneys at the level of the eleventh rib laterally to the first lumbar vertebra.

The left gland is in close relation with the aorta and diaphragmatic crus medially, splenic vessels and the pancreatic tail posteriorly, and with the peritoneum anteriorly. The right gland is placed in a narrow space between vena cava, right kidney, duodenum, right hepatic lobe, and the diaphgragmatic crus.

Adrenal glands receive a very high blood flow from three variable, small arterial branches of the renal artery, aorta, or phrenic artery—respectively, the inferior, middle, and superior adrenal arteries. The right middle adrenal artery has a particular course, arising from the lateral aspect of the aorta and crossing the posterior aspect of the vena cava. The adrenal vein is usually single, emerging from the anterior aspect of the gland, and is a tributary of the caval vein on the right and of the renal vein on the left. The left adrenal vein receives almost constantly, on its posterior aspect, a branch from the inferior phrenic vein. This can be the source of bleeding if not recognized and ligated.

Anatomical variations for both veins and arteries seem to be more frequent on the right side (3,4). The right vein, usually single and tributary of the vena cava, can be doubled or can be a tributary of an inferior hepatic vein.

Lymphatic drainage from the adrenal gland is taken to the para-aortic nodes, first-level nodes, and then to posterior mediastinal lymph nodes by a large number of lymphatics. Nerves are well represented. The posterior aspect of the gland particularly is adjacent to the great splanchnic nerve, and the medial aspect of the adrenal is in contact with the celiac plexus. Those nerves are, together with the adrenal vessels, the only structures maintaining the adrenal glands in a relatively constant position.

3 INDICATIONS

Adrenal pathology encompasses functional and nonfunctional tumors and primary and secondary lesions. Endoscopic techniques have been demonstrated to be safe and effective in all conditions except for adrenal cancer.

Adenomas of the adrenal gland are the most common disease. Of the functionally active adrenal adenomas, Conn's syndrome is the most common, followed by Cushing's syndrome and pheochromocytomas.

Some adrenal neoplasms secrete androgen hormones, which are converted to testosterone by extra-adrenal tissue such as adipose tissue. Androgen secretion is commonly seen in adrenal carcinoma. Another rare condition is congenital adrenal hyperplasia, due to a partial enzymatic defect of 21-hydroxylase.

Incidentalomas represent almost 10% of adrenal pathology, while cancer, metastasis, and adrenal hyperplasia are rare conditions.

Treatment of pheochromocytomas represents a conquest for endoscopic surgery. After initial criticism, it is now recognized that pheochromocytomas can be managed endoscopically as safely as by open surgery. Because 10% of pheochromocytomas are localized outside adrenal glands, preoperative imaging studies are important to assess the exact site of the disease. A combination of (131)I-meta-iodobenzylguanidine (MIBG) scintigraphy with CT or magnetic resonance imaging (MRI) is preferable.

Pheochromocytomas can present in a sporadic form or associated with hereditary syndromes, in particular MEN IIa and IIb, neurofibromatosis, tuberous sclerosis, Sturge-Weber syndrome, and von Hippel-Lindau disease.

In case of paragangliomas, we prefer the open procedure, because in our experience of two paragangliomas, both procedures had to be converted to open surgery. One paraganglioma was located in the renal hilum between the renal artery and vein. Numerous small fragile vessels of the paraganglioma made endoscopic dissection too demanding. The other paraganglioma was located between the caval vein and the aorta. This location could not be readily accessed by retroperitoneoscopy.

Cancer is a relative contraindication to endoscopic procedure. Because of its rarity, no studies have determinated whether laparoscopic and retroperitoneoscopic resection of adrenal cancer is appropriate. However, we believe that radical removal of adrenal cancer offers the only prospect of cure. Therefore, we do not recommend the retroperitoneal approach in patients with adrenal cancer since removal of these usually large tumors cannot be accomplished without manipulation of the tumor (5). For solitary metastasis, usually from lung cancer, the retroperitoneoscopic approach could be considered when the lesion is small.

Another absolute contraindication to retroperitoneoscopy is primary retroperitoneal fibrosis or fibrosis secondary to previous renal or peri-renal surgery.

Obesity is not a contraindication for retroperitoneal adrenalectomy. In our experience, no correlation between obesity, operating time, and blood loss was found. The lumbar retroperitoneum is accessible in obese patients since most fatty tissues are displaced away from the flank in lateral decubitus position (6). However, we consider patients with Cushing's disease the most difficult cases since relatively small adrenal glands are surrounded by abundant fat.

The presence of aptotic kidney, kidney anomalies, and shrunk kidney due to chronic pyelonephritis are not contraindications to retroperitoneal endoscopic surgery, but anatomical landmarks are changed and the surgical field will appear different. The kidney in particular is not only a landmark during dissection but also protects the vena cava on the right side. One should realize that in case of a small right kidney, the caval vein is more liable to injury during dissection.

4 BILATERAL ADRENALECTOMY

Bilateral adrenal hyperplasia due to Cushing's disease is the most frequent indication for bilateral adrenalectomy. Failed pituitary surgery usually precedes adrenal surgery for Cushing's disease. Ectopic unknown adrenocorticotropin hormone (ACTH)–secreting tumors, bilateral pheochromocytomas, and congenital adrenal hyperplasia are other common indications for bilateral adrenalectomy. Hsu and Gil (7) compared two groups of four patients undergoing bilateral laparoscopic adrenalectomy. One group had synchronous bilateral adrenalectomy, while the other had a staged bilateral adrenalectomy. Three of the four patients in both groups underwent retroperitoneal adrenalectomy in lateral decubitus without complications. Between the synchronous and the staged groups, no statistically differences appeared in respect to operative time, blood loss, post-operative narcotic requirement, or hospital stay. However, because of the few series present in literature it is difficult to assess if the staged bilateral adrenalectomy has any advantage with respect to the synchronous bilateral adrenalectomy.

The retroperitoneoscopic posterior approach allows one to perform bilateral adrenalectomies without changing the position, with a reduction in the operative time. However, conversion to open surgery can be demanding when the patient is in the prone position. In our experience with retroperitoneal endoscopic adrenalectomy in lateral decubitus, changing the position of the patient requires less than 15 minutes.

Indications	Contraindications
Adrenal tumor < 6 cm	Adrenal tumor > 6 cm
Conn's syndrome	Prior ipsilateral peri-renal surgery
Cushing's disease and syndrome	Retroperitoneal fibrosis
Pheochromocytoma	Paraganglioma
Incidentaloma	Cancer
Adrenal cyst	
Masculinizing benign tumors	
Myelolipoma	

5 PREOPERATIVE WORK-UP

All adrenal disease requires hormonal investigation. Hypersecretion of adrenocortical hormones or catecholamines should be assessed. Following endocrinologic work-up, imaging of the adrenal mass takes place by thin-collimation computed tomography (8). Intravenous injection of radiopaque dye enhances the resolution of computed tomography. Without intravenous contrast, it can be difficult to distinguish adrenal tissue from aorta and caval vein or surrounding organs. If results of CT are not conclusive, magnetic resonance and nuclear medicine imaging studies should be performed.

MRI can determine the fatty content of adrenal glands, which can be valuable in incidentalomas. In these cases, MRI can identify an incidentaloma as an adenoma.

In a recent study, Honigschnabl et al. (9), analyzed the efficacy of MR imaging in differentiating benign from malignant adrenal masses. MR findings in 229 patients were analyzed and correlated with histopathological findings. The authors concluded that the high accuracy (98%) of MR imaging in characterization of adrenal lesions can offer the advantage of the minimally invasive technique to patients with tumors larger than 5 cm.

Adrenal cancer should be suspected when imaging studies reveal variable density of the tumor, irregular shape of the tumor, or enlarged local lymph nodes.

Invasion of caval or renal vein in adrenal cancer can be imaged by contrast enhanced CT, MRI, or ultrasonography.

Scintigraphic investigations play a major role in the assessment of pheochromocytomas. For pheochromocytomas, CT or MRI combined with MIBG scintigraphy detect pheochromocytomas in 95% (10). For functional adrenocortical tumors, iodo-methylnorcholesterol scintigraphy can assess the presence of bilateral hyperplasia or unilateral hyperactivity.

6 PATIENT PREPARATION

Single shot antibiotic prophylaxis at induction of anesthesia is only employed in patients with hypercortisolism because these patients are more prone to infections. Corticosteroid substitution is started during adrenal surgery in patients with hypercortisolism.

In case of pheochromocytomas, it is mandatory to administrate an á-adrenergic blocking agent for at least 10 days before surgery. If tachycardia occurs, a â-adrenergic blocker is also given. Prophylaxis for deep vein thrombosis is administered preoperatively. A nasogastric tube and a Foley's catheter are placed in the operating room.

7 OPERATIVE TECHNIQUE

Retroperitoneoscopy can be performed using the lateral or flank approach and the posterior approach.

7.1 Lateral Approach

The lateral or flank extraperitoneal approach for adrenal surgery was first described in 1992 by Gaur (11). The advantage of the lateral approach is displacement of the abdominal wall with abdominal organs away from the operative field. After gaining experience with this approach, the anatomical landmarks will be clearer, fascias will be recognized more easily, and the access to the gland will be faster. When conversion is necessary, lumbotomy allows fast access to the operative field.

The patient lies in the lateral decubitus position, and the table is cracked to create the widest space possible between costal margin and iliac crest. This is important to allow free movement of instruments, which can be limited by the prominence of the hip, especially in women. A bean bag or a vacuum mattress is very helpful in maintaining the lateral decubitus position.

The surgeon stands on the abdominal side of the patient for left adrenalectomy and posteriorly to the patient for right adrenalectomy. The assistant stands on the opposite side. The operating room must be ready for a possible conversion to open surgery.

A 2 cm incision is made just caudally to the tip of the 11th rib, the fascia of the external oblique muscle is incised, muscles are split, and after opening of the transversalis fascia, Bogros space is accessed. All the described maneuvers can be done digitally, and the inferior pole of the kidney can be easily palpated (Fig. 1).

In our technique, we employ a transparent dissection balloon, (PDB balloon; Tyco, Norwalk, CT), which is also used for extraperitoneal inguinal hernia repair for creating the retroperitoneal space. After introducing a zero degree endoscope, the insufflation of the retroperitoneal space can be done under endoscopic guidance (Fig. 2). The tip of the dissection balloon is aimed posteriorly to avoid opening the peritoneal sac. The quadratus lumborum muscle is the first anatomical landmark that is discovered during insufflation of the balloon (Figs. 3, 4). Once enough space has been made, the dissection balloon is replaced by a blunt tip inflatable trocar (Origin, Origin Medical System; Tyco, Norwalk, CT). The pneumoretroperitoneum is created at a pressure of 10–12 mmHg, and a second 5 mm trocar is inserted posteriorly. We introduce the second trocar 5–7 cm posteriorly to the first trocar under direct vision to ensure that no injuries occur to the diaphragm.

Using a gentle dissector, the peritoneal sac is mobilized from the antero-lateral abdominal wall in order to make the space to insert the other two trocars. It is very important to maintain the dissection plane as close as possible to the abdominal wall to prevent perforating

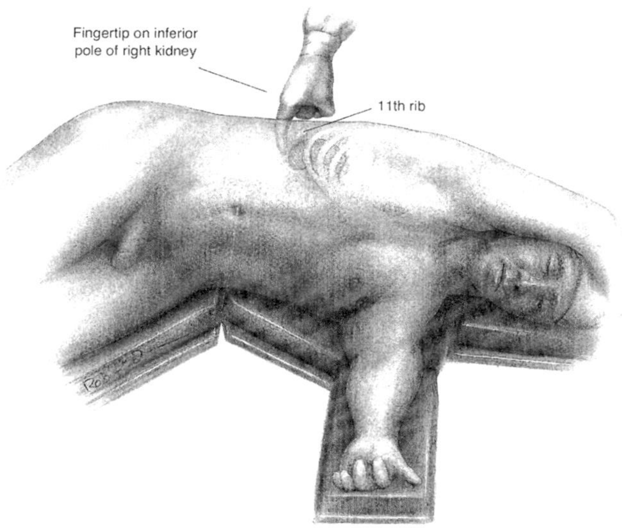

Figure 1 Introducing a finger through the first incision caudally to the tip of the llth rib allows palpation of the lower pole of the kidney.

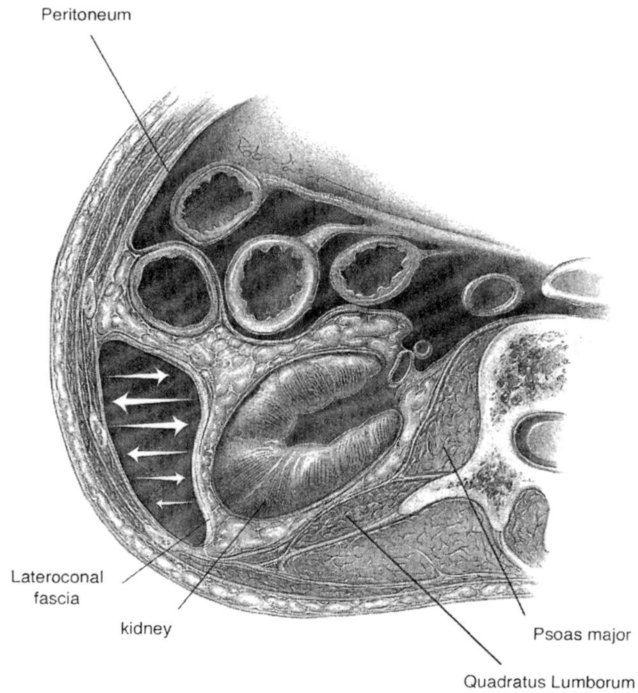

Figure 3 Retroperitoneal space (indicated by arrows) created by balloon dissection.

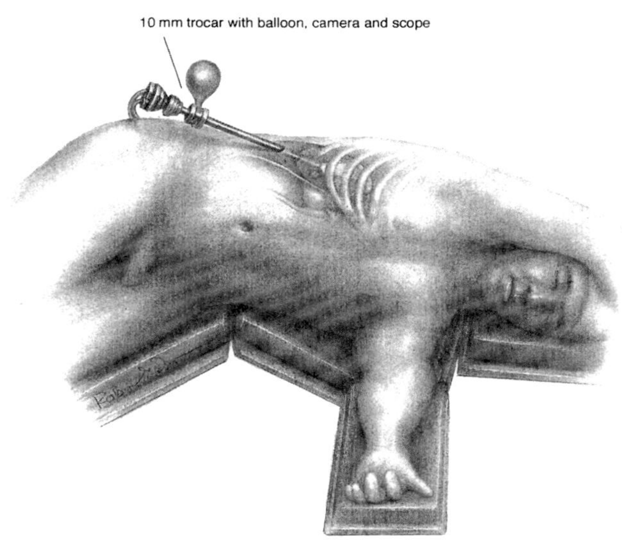

Figure 2 Balloon dissection under endoscopic guidance of the right retroperitoneal space.

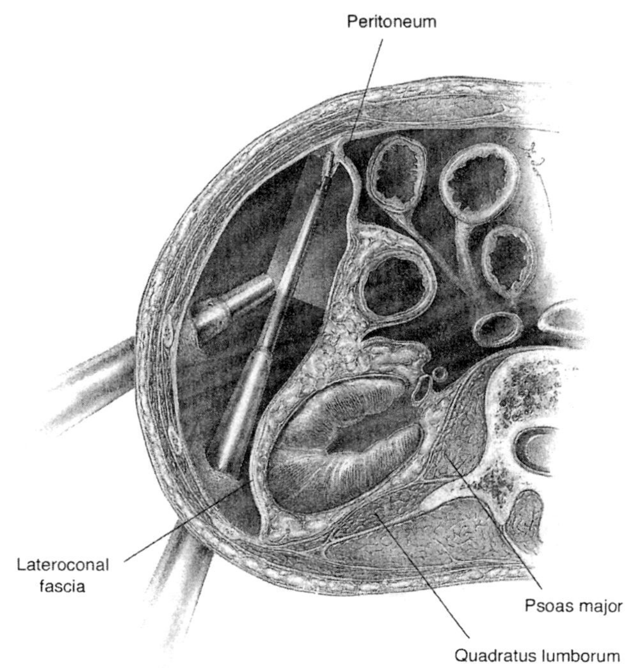

Figure 5 Mobilization of the peritoneal sac to create space for introduction of the third and fourth trocar.

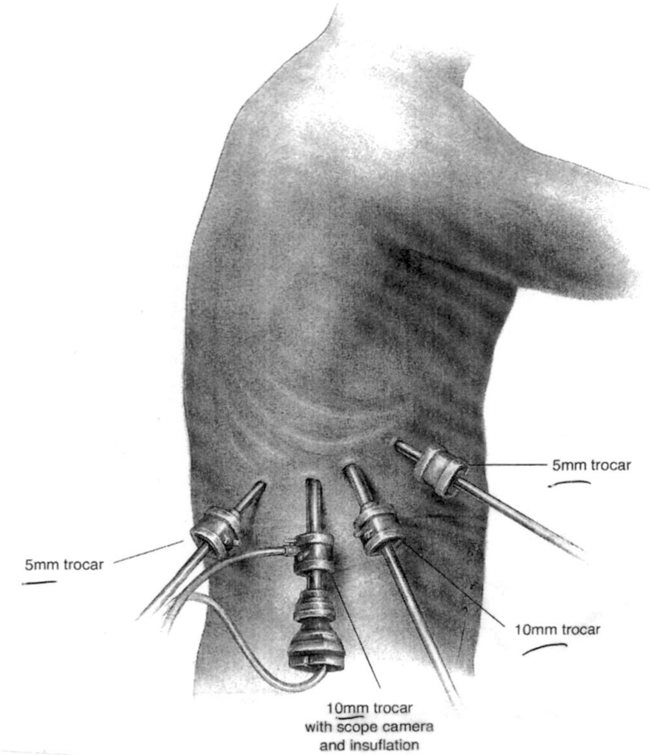

Figure 7 Trocar positioning for right retroperitoneoscopic adrenalectomy.

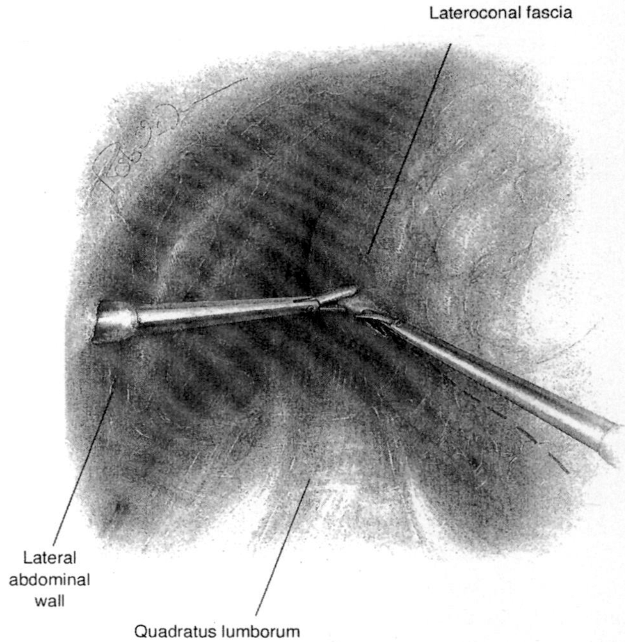

Figure 8 Opening the lateroconal fascia in a longitudinal fashion for right adrenalectomy.

the peritoneal sac (Figs. 5, 6). A 5 mm trocar more medially and a 10 mm trocar between the latter and the first are inserted close to the costal margin (Fig. 7).

Once the Brogos space is opened, the lateroconal fascia is the only structure covering the adrenal glands and the kidney. This white-grey avascular structure has to be incised longitudinally to expose the fatty tissue beneath covering the kidney and the adrenal gland (Figs. 8–11). Subsequently, the upper pole of the kidney should be freed. The created space is defined by the kidney, the peritoneum medially, the quadratus lumborum muscle laterally, the lateral abdominal wall superiorly, and the diaphragm cranially. Teasing all the fat away from the superior renal pole will expose the adrenal gland (Fig. 12). This step and the following dissection can be successfully performed using ultrasonic devices. The gold-yellow adrenal gland will appear in the corner formed on the right by the liver, vena cava and upper renal pole, and on the left by the upper renal pole, aorta, and sometimes by the tail of the pancreas. To avoid pancreatic injury, dissection should be done in a posterior plane during left adrenalectomy.

Particularly if a pheochromocytoma is being removed, delicate handling is required to avoid massive catecolamine delivery into the blood stream. First the anterior and lateral aspects of the adrenal tumor are freed. Subsequently, an attempt is made to elevate the adrenal tumor by gentle indirect retraction (Fig. 13).

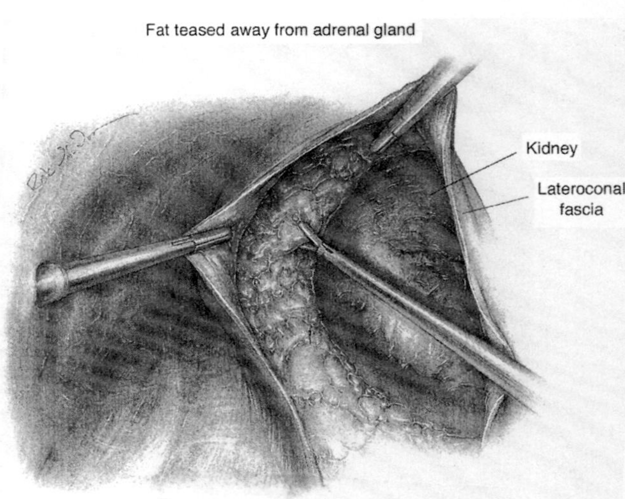

Figure 10 Opening of the lateroconal fascia for right adrenalectomy has been completed.

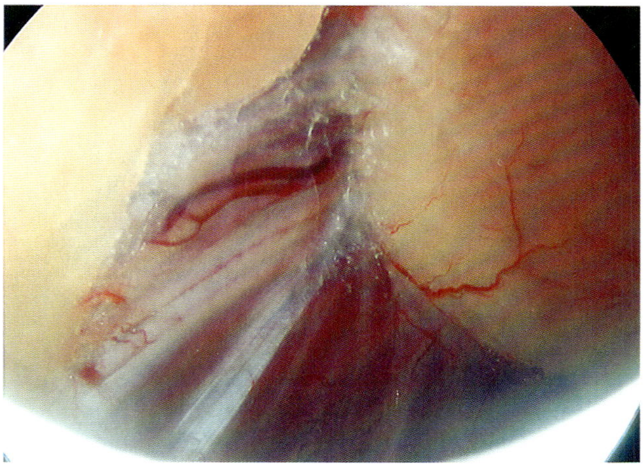

Figure 4 Endoscopic view of quadratus lumborum muscle (bottom picture) during balloon dissection of the retroperitoneal .

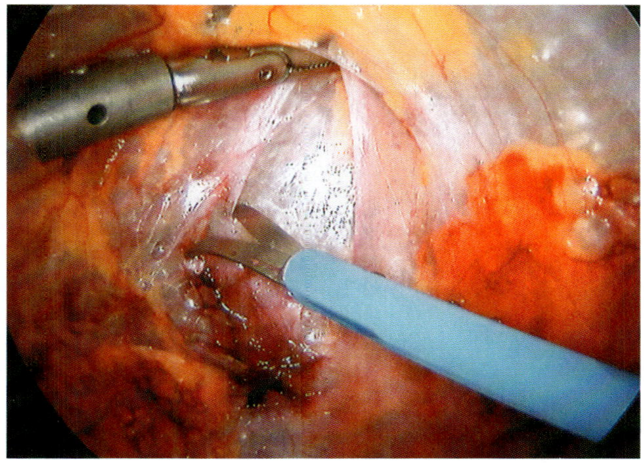

Figure 9 Endoscopic view of opening the lateroconal fascia for left adrenalectomy.

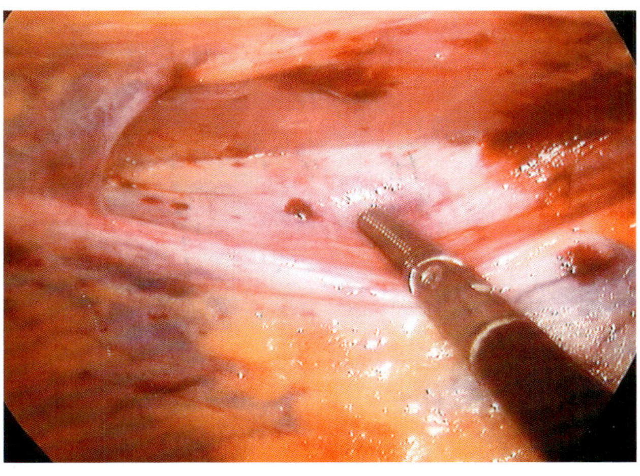

Figure 6 Endoscopic view from lateral to medial during dissection of the peritoneum from the transverse abdominal muscles.

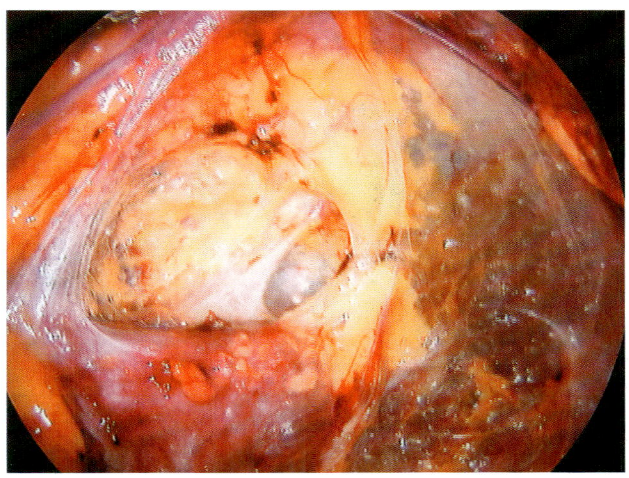

Figure 11 Endoscopic view after completed opening of the lateroconal fascia for left adrenalectomy.

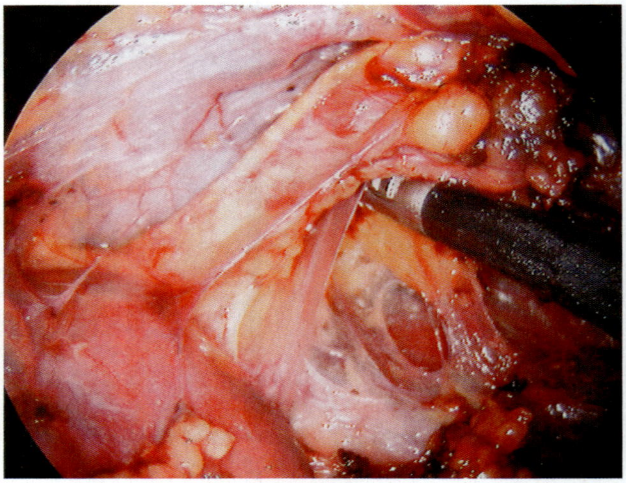

Figure 13 The left adrenal gland is elevated by an endoscopic grasper.

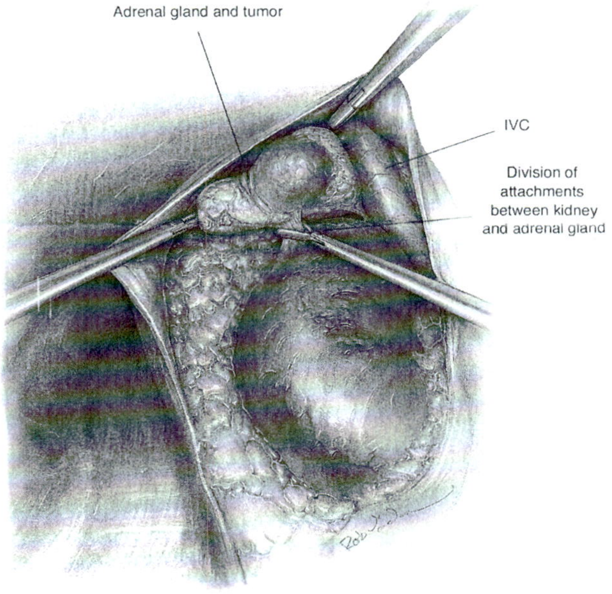

Figure 12 Exposure of the right adrenal gland.

First, the inferior and middle arteries are encountered and then the vein. In our series, we experienced hemodynamic instability in 3 (15%) of 19 patients with a pheochromocytoma, which was well managed by the anesthesiologist. Hemodynamic instability never necessitated conversion of the endoscopic procedure to open surgery. Care should be taken not to ligate the superior branch of the renal artery during dissection of the inferior adrenal artery. Hypertension will follow when a branch of the renal artery is clipped. The adrenal vein on the right side is usually short. Careful dissection is mandatory to gain enough space for a safe ligation of the adrenal vein (Fig. 14). We divide the vein after placing two titanium clips on the vena cava side and one on the adrenal side. On the left side the vein is longer, making its dissection easier than on the right side. Once the vessels have been ligated, the gland can be easily lifted and the dissection can be completed. At the upper aspect of the adrenal gland, small arterial branches, arising from the phrenic artery, can be present. The adrenal tumor is always removed in a plastic bag (Endocatch; USSC, Norwalk, CT) to prevent spillage of adrenal tissue.

7.2 Posterior Approach

The posterior approach to the retroperitoneal space is another surgical option for removing adrenal gland

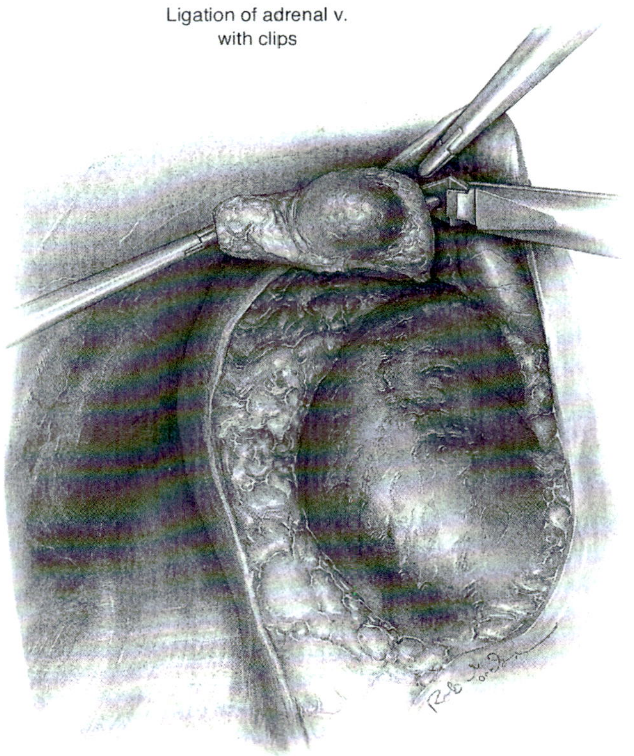

Figure 14 Endoscopic clipping of the right adrenal vein.

disease (Fig. 15). This approach was first described in 1995 by Mercan et al. (1).

After positioning the patient in the prone position, the table is flexed to open the space between the ribs and

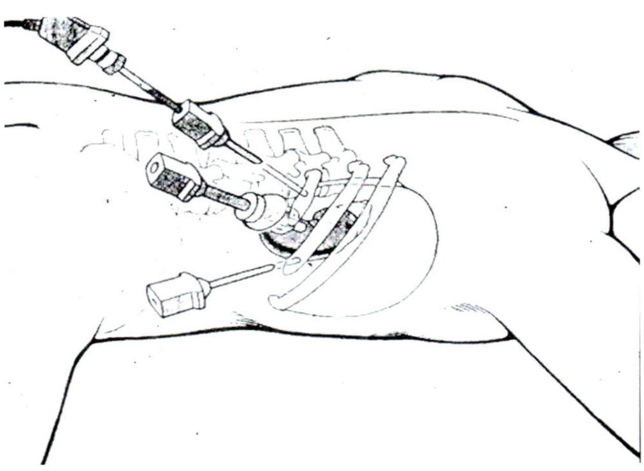

Figure 15 Patient in prone position for right posterior retoperitoneoscopic adrenalectomy.

for adrenal tumors of 5 cm or less.

The postoperative complication rate after endoscopic posterior adrenalectomy was 13%, involving temporary paralysis and hypestesia of the abdominal wall, hematoma, and incisional hernia. Conversion was necessary in 5% of cases because of cardiovascular instability and technical difficulties. Pleural tearing was recognized in four patients but did not require conversion to open surgery.

REFERENCES

1. Mercan S, Seven R, Ozarmagan S, Tezelman S. Endoscopic retroperitoneal adrenalectomy. Surgery 1995; 118: 1071–1075.
2. Himpens J. Endoscopic retroperitoneal surgery. Dig Surg 1998; 15:181–184.
3. Bonjer HJ, Sorm V, Berends FJ, Kazemier G, Steyer-

13. Bonjer HJ, Lange JF, Kazemier G, de Herder WW, Steyerberg EW, Bruining HA. Comparison of three techniques for adrenalectomy. Br J Surg 1997; 84:679–682.
14. Ng CS, Gill IS, Sung GT, Whalley DG, Graham R, Schweizer D. Retroperitoneoscopic surgery is not associated with increased carbon dioxide absorption. J Urol 1999; 162:1268–1272.
15. Bonjer HJ, van der Harst E, Steyerberg EW, de Herder WW, Kazemier G, Mohammedamin RS, Bruining HA. Retroperitoneal adrenalectomy: open or endoscopic? World J Surg 1998; 22:1246–1249.
16. Schell SR, Talamini MA, Udelsman R. Laparoscopic adrenalectomy for nonmalignant disease: improved safety, morbidity, and cost-effectiveness. Surg Endosc 1999; 13:30–34.
17. Darzi A. Retroperitoneoscopy. Oxford Ox 1ST, UK: Pritek S.A.L., Spain, 1996.
18. Gagner M, Inabnet WB. Minimally Invasive Endocrine Surgery. Philadelphia: Lippincott Williams & Wilkins, 2002.

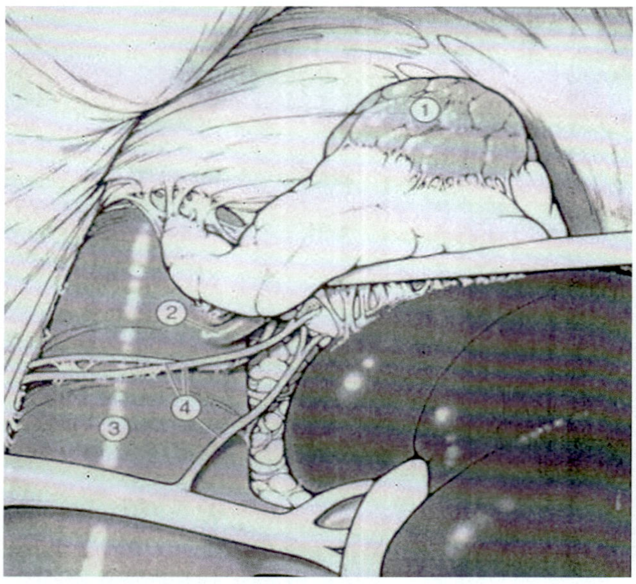

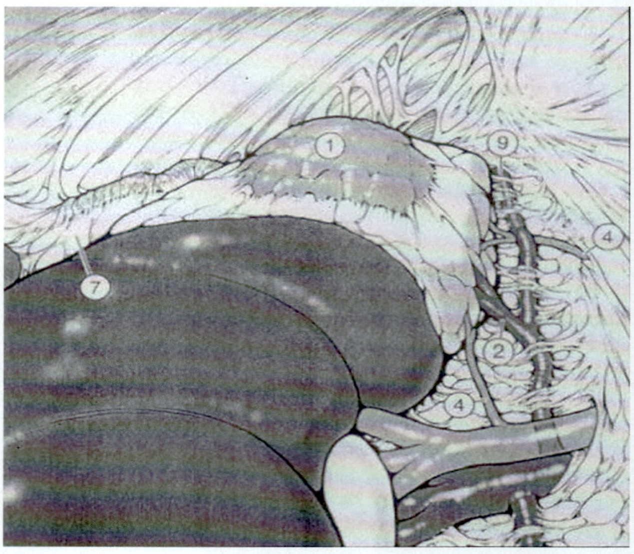

Figure 17 Posterior view of left adrenal anatomy. Left

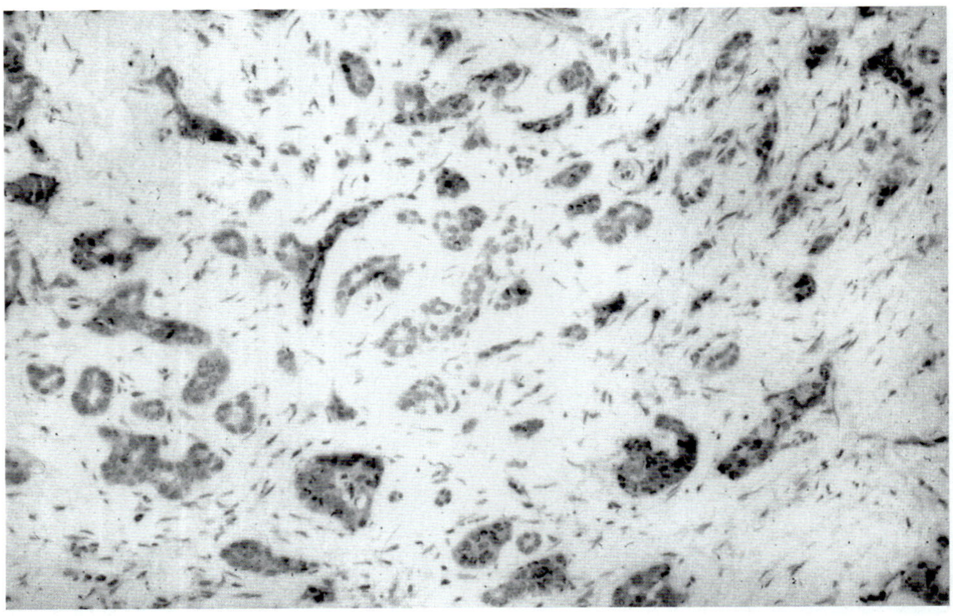

Figure 5 Immunohistochemical stain for gastrin which is positive in this pancreatic neuroendocrine tumor. (Gastrin immunoperoxidase stain ×20.)

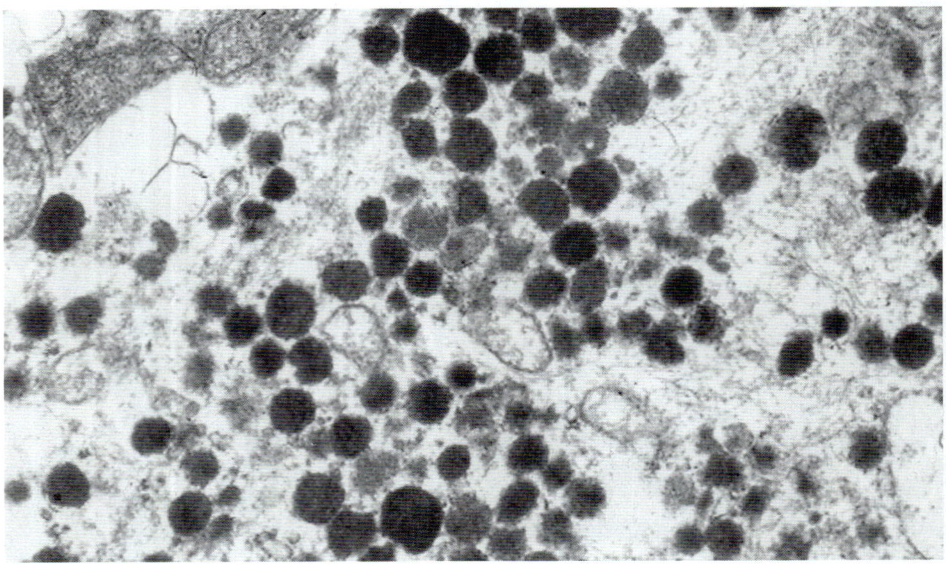

Figure 6 Ultrastructural photomicrograph of a pancreatic gastrinoma. The cytoplasm is filled with dense core neurosecretory granules of varying sizes. (Uranyl acetate/lead citrate ×16000.)

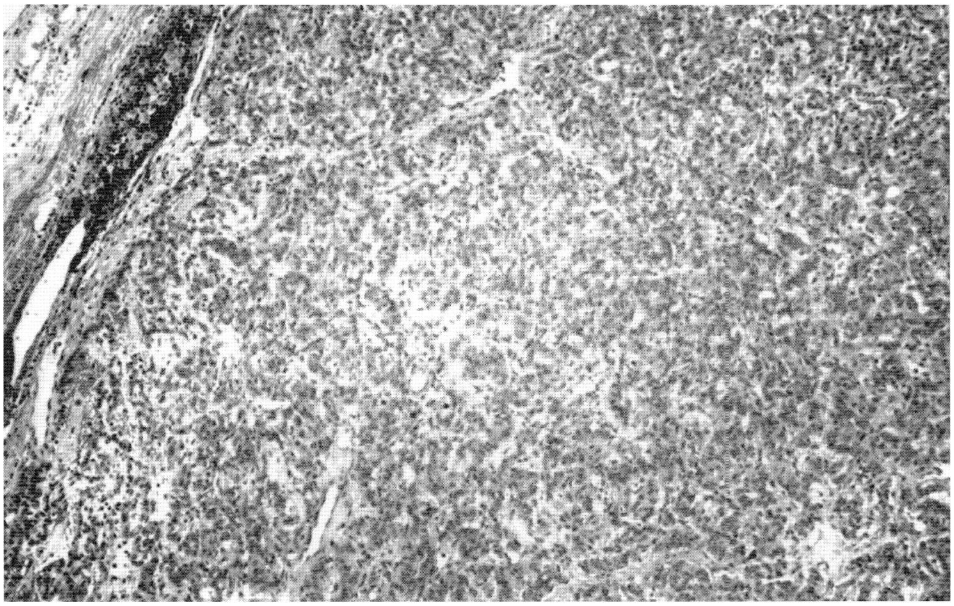

Figure 7 Lymph node with metastatic pancreatic neuroendocrine tumor. (Hemotoxylin/eosin ×10.)

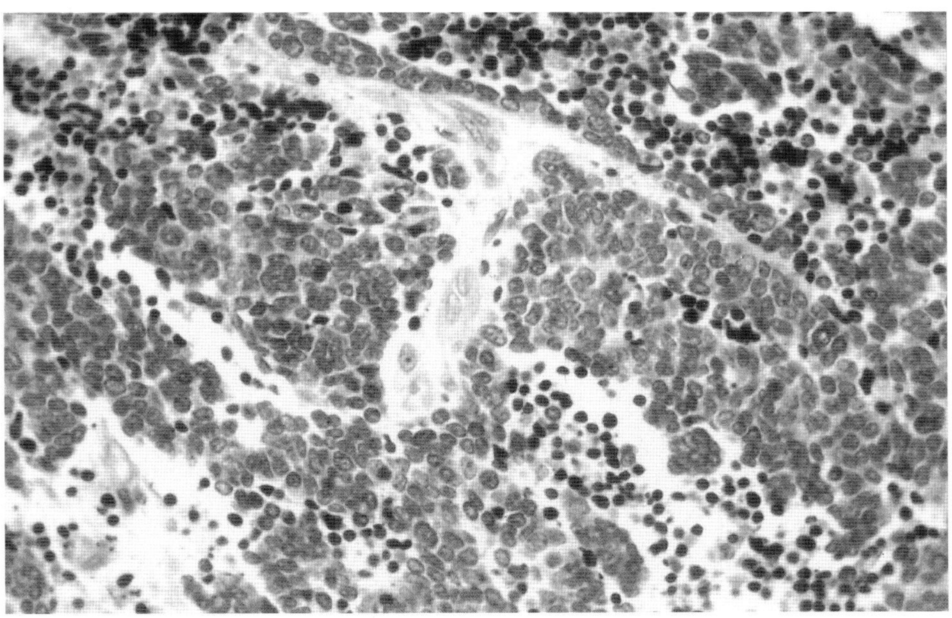

Figure 8 Pancreatic small-cell carcinoma. The tumor is composed of uniform cells with finely clumped chromatin and minimal cytoplasm. (Hemotoxylin/eosin ×40.)

3 GASTRINOMAS

Gastrinomas are the second most common of the functional pancreatic endocrine tumors. In addition to the pancreas, these tumors may arise in extrapancreatic sites and give rise to the Zollinger-Ellison syndrome due to gastrin hypersecretion. These tumors can be found in any pancreatic site but are more common in the gastrinoma triangle, defined by the cystic-hepatic duct confluence, the junction of the second and third portion of the duodenum, and the body of the pancreas. They may be solitary or multiple particularly in MEN I patients. Tumors average in size 2 cm, but lesions smaller than 1 cm can occur. Histologically, there is usually lymphatic/vascular invasion present. Gastrin immunohistochemistry will be positive in the tumor cells, and there may be reaction for other hormones. Ultrstructurally there are electron dense granules of varying size and shape. These are slow-growing tumors, which usually have a malignant course. Metastases may occur many years following detection of the primary tumor.

4 GLUCAGONOMAS

Glucagonomas comprise approximately 5% of the functional pancreatic endocrine tumors and arise from the α cells. These tumors are usually solitary and found in the tail portion of the pancreas. The average size is 7 cm. Immunohistochemical stain for glucagon or a proglucagon peptide will be positive in these tumors and there may be focal positivity for other hormones. The typical α granule on ultrastructural examination will be 180–300 nm with a dense inner core and a surrounding paler rim. Approximately 80% of these cases are malignant, the liver being most often the first site of metastatic spread.

Other functional pancreatic tumors which rarely occur include somatostatinomas and VIPomas (watery diarrhea syndrome) (1–21).

5 SMALL-CELL CARCINOMA OF THE PANCREAS

Small-cell carcinoma is an uncommon primary pancreatic tumor representing approximately 1% of all tumors. It is considered a poorly differentiated endocrine tumor. Elderly men are the usual patient population. Most tumors occur in the head of the pancreas. Grossly, they are large, infiltrative masses with areas of hemmorhage and necrosis and are soft or grey in appearance. Histologically they are similar to the more commonly occurring lung tumors (Fig. 8). The cells are arranged in solid sheets or nests with little appreciable cytoplasm. Nuclei have dense coarse chromatin without prominent nucleoli and may have nuclear molding. Mitotic figures are numerous. Ultrastructurally, there are rare dense core neurosecretory granules. Immunohistochemically, they will react with neuroendocrine markers such as chromogranin and synaptophysin. Hormones are usually not detected. Metastases to either liver lymph nodes or other structures are generally found at the time of presentation (22–24).

REFERENCES

1. Solcia E, Capella C, Kloppel G. Tumors of the pancreas. Atlas of Tumor Pathology, 3rd Series, Fascicle 20. Washington, DC: Armed Forces Institute of Pathology, 1997;145–180.
2. Kloppel G, Heitz PU. Pancreatic endocrine tumors in man. In: Polak JM, ed. Diagnostic Histopathology of Neuroendocrine Tumors. Edinburgh: Churchill Livingstone, 1993:91–121.
3. Howard JN, Moss NH, Rhoads JE. Collective review: hyperinsulinism and islet cell tumors of the pancreas. Int Abstr Surg 1950; 90:417–455.
4. Frantz VK. Tumors of the pancreas. In: Atlas of Tumor Pathology: 1st Series, Fasicle 27–28. Washington, DC: Armed Forces Institute of Pathology, 1959;79–149.
5. Eberle F, Grun R. Multiple endocrine neoplasia, type I (MEN I). Erge Inn Med Kinderheil 1981; 46:76–149.
6. Majewski JT, Wilson SD. The MEN I syndrome: an all or none phenomenon. Surgery 1979; 475–484.
7. Heitz PU, Kasper M, Polak JM, Kloppel G. Pancreatic endocrine tumors. Hum Pathol 1982; 13:263–271.
8. Solcia E, Capella C, Buffa R, Tenti P, Rindi G, Cornaggia M. Antigenic markers of neuroendocrine tumors: their diagnostic and prognostic value. In: Fenoglio CM, Weinstein RS, Kaufman N, eds. New Concepts in Neoplasia as Applied to Diagnostic Pathology. Baltimore: Williams & Wilkins, 1986:242–261.
9. Wilson BS, Lloyd RV. Detection of chromogranin in neuroendocrine cells with a monoclonal antibody. Am J Pathol 1984; 115:458–468.
10. Buffa R, Rindi G, Sessa F, et al. Synaptophysin immunoreactivity and small clear vesicles in neuroendocrine cells and related tumors. Mol Cell Probes 1987; 1:367–381.
11. Cheijfec G, Faulkner S, Grimelius L, et al. Synaptophysin. A new marker for pancreatic neuroendocrine tumors. Am J Surg Pathol 1987; 11:241–247.
12. Bordi C, Bussolati G. Immunoflourescence, histochem-

ical and ultrastructural studies for the detection of multiple endocrine polypeptide tumors of the pancreas. Virchows Arch (Cell Pathol) 1974; 17:13–27.

13. Heitz PU. Pancreatic endocrine tumors. In: Kloppel G, Heitz PU, eds. Pancreatic Pathology. Edinburgh: Churchill-Livingstone, 1984:206–232.
14. Mukai K, Grotting JC, Greider MH, Rosai J. Retrospective study of 77 pancreatic endocrine tumors using the immunoperoxidase method. Am J Surg Pathol 1982; 6:387–399.
15. Broder LE, Carter SK. Pancreatic islet cell carcinoma. I. Clinical features of 52 patients. Am Intern Med 1973; 79:101–107.
16. Cubilla AL, Hajdu SI. Islet cell carcinoma of the pancreas. Arch Pathol 1975; 99:204–207.
17. Kloppel G, Heitz PU. Pancreatic endocrine tumors in man. In: Polak JM, ed. Diagnostic Histopathology of Neuroendocrine Tumors. Edinburgh: Churchill Livingstone, 1993:91–121.
18. Solcia E, Sessa F, Rindi G, Bonato M, Capella C. Pancreatic endocrine tumors: nonfunctioning tumors and tumors with uncommon function. In: Dayal Y, ed. Endocrine Pathology of the Gut and Pancreas. Boca Raton, FL: CRC Press, 1991:105–132.
19. Stefanini P, Carboni M, Patrassi N, Basoli A. Beta islet cell tumors of the pancreas: results of a statistical study on 1,067 cases collected. Surgery 1974; 75:597–609.
20. Greider MH, Rosai J, McGuigan JE. The human pancreatic islet cells and their tumors. II. Ulcerogenic and diarrheogenic tumors. Cancer 1974; 33:1423–1443.
21. Niewenhuijzen Kruseman AC, Knijnenburg G, Brutel de la Rivera G, Bosman FT. Morphology and immunohistochemically defined endocrine function of pancreatic islet cell tumours. Histopathology 1978; 2:389–399.
22. Cubilla AL, Fitzgerald PJ. Tumors of the exocrine pancreas. In: Atlas of Tumor Pathology. Washington, DC: Armed Forces Institute of Pathology, 1984:196–201.
23. O'Connor TP, Held G, Kloppel G. Exocrine pancreatic tumours and their histological classification. A study based on 167 autopsies and 97 surgical cases. Histopathology 1983; 645–661.
24. Reyes CV, Wang T. Undifferentiated small cell carcinoma of the pancreas. Report of a patient with tumor marker studies. Cancer 1992; 70:2500–2502.

41

Ultrasonography of the Pancreas

Hsu-Chong Yeh

Mount Sinai School of Medicine, New York University, New York, New York, U.S.A.

1 ULTRASONOGRAPHIC FEATURES OF THE NORMAL PANCREAS

The pancreas is located in the subdiaphragmatic retroperitoneal space at the level of the first and second lumbar vertebrae. The pancreatic head is located to the right of superior mesenteric vein and medial to the second portion of the duodenum, which can be identified as a fluid- or air-containing structure. The pancreatic body is anterior to the aorta, separated from the latter by retropancreatic and periaortic fat. The superior mesenteric artery and vein pass anterior to the uncinate process and/or posterior to the pancreatic neck and body. The tail of the pancreas extends to near the splenic hilum. The common bile duct runs anterior to the portal vein and enters the inferior aspect of the pancreatic head, then runs inferiorly to join the pancreatic duct close to ampulla.

Normal pancreatic echotexture is hyperechoic relative to that of the liver. The degree of echogenicity is determined mostly by the amount of the fat between the lobules and acinar cells, but to a lesser extent by interlobular fibrous tissue. In the adult, a highly echogenic pancreas is quite common, especially in older age. When echogenicity is similar to peripancreatic fat, the pancreas may not be easily recognized. Visualization of the splenic vein may be greatly helpful in identifying the pancreas in such cases since a large part of pancreas lies immediately anterior to the splenic vein.

The endocrine portion of pancreas is the islets of Langerhans, which are groups of cells scattered throughout the pancreas. They are usually not identifiable on ultrasonography.

2 SCANNING TECHNIQUE

Ideally the patient should fast overnight or for at least 6–8 hours, although in many patients the pancreas is very well visualized without fasting. The purpose of fasting is to prevent gastric contents, especially gas bubbles from obscuring the pancreas. Since the stomach is usually slightly inferior and anterior to the pancreas, scanning from above the pancreas and angling the transducer downward may allow one to visualize the pancreas even if some gas is present in the stomach. Less commonly, the stomach may overlie the pancreas. A firm compression with the transducer during scanning is frequently helpful for visualizing the pancreas in such instances. Sometimes, scanning from below the gas-filled stomach and transverse colon and angling the transducer upward may also be helpful in visualizing the pancreas in such cases. When the volume of gas in the stomach is excessive or difficult to compress because of the large size of the abdomen, drinking a large amount of degassed water or contrast material may sometimes be helpful.

Since the distal part of the tail of the pancreas is located near the splenic hilum, scanning the splenic hilar

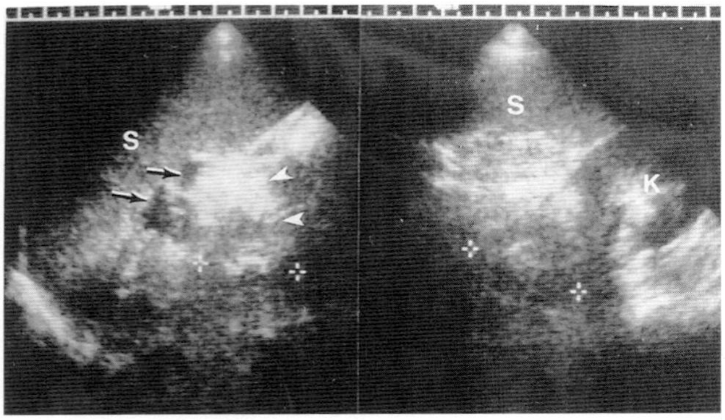

Figure 1 A carcinoid tumor in the tail of pancreas. (Left) Coronal scan from left upper flank region shows a mass (between "+") with central calcifications located in the tail of pancreas (arrowheads), which is inferior to the splenic hilar vessels (arrows). The mass represents a carcinoid tumor. S = spleen. (Right) Transverse scan from left upper flank region shows the mass (between "+") located anterior to the left kidney (K). S = spleen.

area usually clearly visualizes the tail of the pancreas that usually lies immediately inferior to splenic vein. A tumor in the pancreatic tail (Fig. 1) may be seen by this approach.

Intraoperative scanning can be done with a high-frequency (7.5–10 MHz) linear transducer. This will show very good detail of the pancreas and adjacent structures (Fig. 2). The transducer is covered with a sterile sheath, which contains sterile gel. The pancreatic area is filled with sterile saline, and the transducer is placed on or approximately 1 cm above the pancreas (1). The entire pancreas, the pancreatic duct, common bile duct, superior mesenteric artery and vein as well as the inferior vena cava and aorta are usually seen with very good detail.

3 ISLET CELL TUMORS

The islets of Langerhans are the endocrine part of the pancreas. The majority of islet cell tumors are functional, but about one third are non-functioning (2). The most common functional islet cell tumor is insulinoma (60%), followed by gastrinoma (18%), which may cause Zollinger-Ellison syndrome, VIPoma, which produce the WDHA syndrome (watery diarrhea, hypokalemia, and achlorhydria), glucagonomas, somatostatinomas (delta-cell tumors), and carcinoid tumors (Fig. 1), which produce serotonin and an atypical carcinoid syndrome. The functional tumors are frequently small and difficult to detect because hormonal hypersecretion leads to early discovery. About 90% of insulinomas are less than 2 cm in diameter (3) (Fig. 2). Although islet cell tumors have been reported to be most common in the tail of pancreas (54% of 82 tumors) (4), others reported that insulinoma is most commonly found in the pancreatic head (62% of 44 solitary tumors) (1). The detection rate by convetional ultrasonography is only 30–61%. Some small tumors may be difficult to palpate even during surgery.

Intraoperative ultrasonography may be very helpful in such instances. In a series of 28 cases of intraoperative ultrasound scanning, 4 insulinomas, which were not palpable, were visualized by ultrasonography. On the other hand, 2 superficial tumors were obscured in the near field of a 10 MHz transducer, and 2 in the distal pancreatic tail were not scanned because of lack of surgical mobilization of the tail. The sensitivity for detecting insulinomas by intraoperative ultrasonography is 84% compared to 54% for angiography and 30% for computed tomography (CT) (1). The combined sensitivity of intraoperative ultrasonography and surgi-

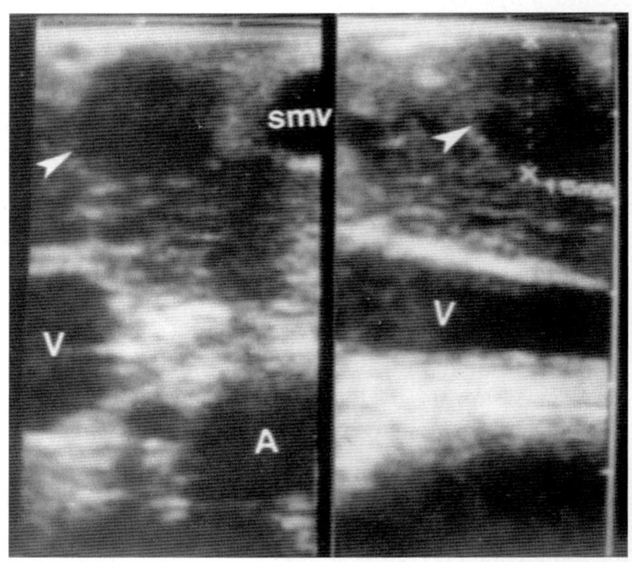

Figure 2 A 1.5 cm insulinoma detected on intraoperative ultrasonography. (Left) Transverse scan shows a small mass (arrowhead) in the head of the pancreas. smv = superior mesenteric vein; V = inferior vena cava; A = aorta. (Right) Longitudinal scan shows the 1.5 cm mass (arrowhead) in the head of pancreas anterior to the inferior vena cava (V).

cal palpation for detecting solitary insulinomas was 100%. Intraoperative ultrasonography may also contribute significantly to the surgical management by precisely demonstrating the relationship of insulinoma to the pancreatic and common bile ducts and pancreatic blood vessels. Intraoperative ultrasonography may differentiate malignant from benign islet cell tumors by demonstrating ill-defined tumor borders, invasion of surrounding pancreatic tissue or the pancreatic duct (5).

Approximately 10% of islet cell tumors are multiple. The sensitivity for detecting multiple islet cell masses is low because many of these tumors may be smaller than 1 cm (1). In a series of 59 insulinomas in 9 patients, the sensitivity for detecting these tumors was as follows: conventional ultrasonography, 15%; intraoperative ultrasonography, 36%; angiography, 29%; CT, 8% (1).

The nonfunctional tumors are easier to detect because they reach a larger size before causing symptoms. They usually range in size from 1 to 20 cm, frequently being more than 10 cm in diameter (5).

The small islet cell tumors are usually hypoechoic homogeneous solid masses, but some larger tumors may be moderately echogenic, heterogeneous, and may contain fluid-filled areas or cystic changes or calcifications (5–9). The homogeneous solid masses are more likely to be functional, and heterogeneous masses with cystic or necrotic areas are more likely to be nonfunctional (2). Solid islet cell tumors were usually indistinguishable from those of adenocarcinoma of the pancreas except that islet cell tumors tend to be hypervascular on color Doppler study, although this is not always true (Fig. 3). Five to 10% of insulomas are malignant. Histologically, these tumors display little evidence of anaplasia and may be impossible to differentiate from benign tumors. The diagnosis is made in the presence of metastases or local invasion (9). The metastases to the liver may appear hypoechoic, near-isoechoic, or hyperechoic and may have cystic changes. Different ultrasono-

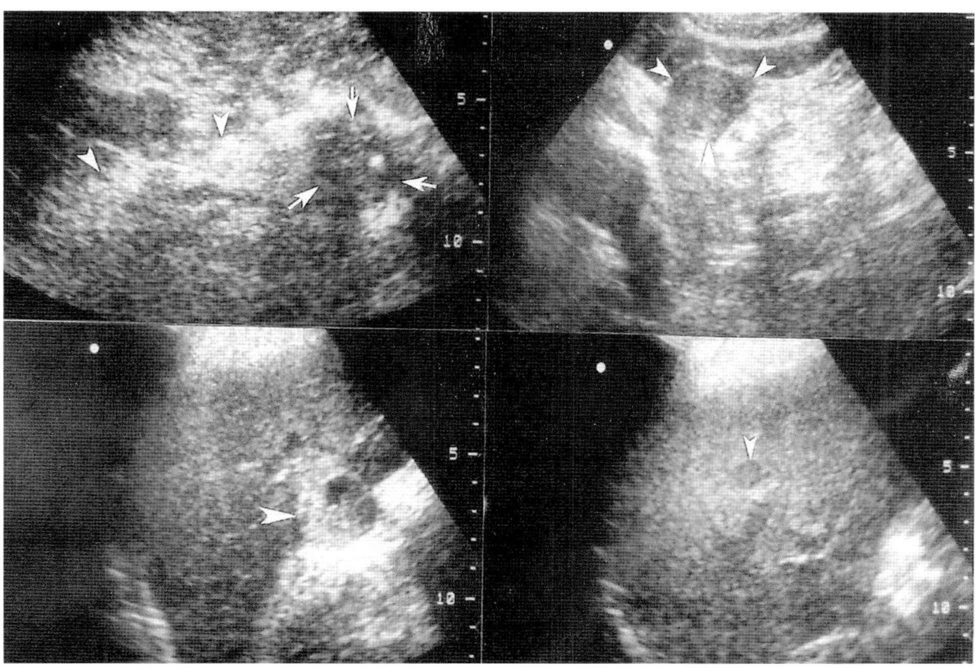

Figure 3 An islet cell carcinoma in the tail of the pancreas with liver metastases. (Top left) Transverse scan shows a mass (arrows) in the tail of the pancreas. The mass contains a small calcification. Arrows = normal head and body of pancreas. Color Doppler study (not shown) did not show hypervascularity in the tumor. (Top right) Sagittal scan shows a near isoechoic mass (arrowheads) in the anterior surface of the left lobe of the liver. (Bottom left) Sagittal scan of right lobe of the liver shows a hyperechoic mass (arrowhead) with a central cavity in the posterior surface of the liver. (Bottom right) Sagittal scan more lateral toward the right shows a small hypoechoic mass (arrowhead) in the liver. The masses in the tail of the pancreas and left lobe of the liver were biopsied under ultrasound guidance, and both proved to be islet cell carcinoma.

graphic features of metastatic lesions may be present in the same liver (Fig. 3).

REFERENCES

1. Galiber AK, Reading CC, Charboneau JW, Sheedy PF, James EM, Gorman B, Grant CS, Heerden JAV, Telander RL. Localization of pancreatic insulinoma: comparison of pre- and intraoperative US with CT and angiography. Radiology 1988; 166:405–408.
2. Gold J, Rosenfield AT, Sostman D, Burrell M, Taylor KJW. Nonfunctioning islet cell tumors of the pancreas: radiographic and ultrasonographic appearances of two cases. Am J Roentgenol 1978; 131:715–717.
3. Fink IJ, Krudy AG, Shawker TH, Norton JA, Gordon P, Doppman JL. Demonstration of an angiographically hypovascular insulinoma with intra-arterial dynamic CT. Am J Roentgenol 1985; 144:555–556.
4. Kruger RL, Dockerty MP. Tumors of the islets of Langerhans. Surg Gyn Obst 1947; 85:495–511.
5. Norton JA, Cromack DR, Shawker TH, Doppman JL, Comi R, Gorden P, Maton PN, Gardna JD. Intraoperative ultrasound localization of islet cell tumors, a prospective comparison to palpation. Ann Surg 1988; 270:160.
6. Raghavendra BN, Glickstein ML. Sonography of islet cell tumor of the pancreas: report of two cases. J Clin Ultrasound 1981; 9:331–333.
7. Fugazzola C, Procacci C, Andreis JCB, Iacono C, Portuese A, Mansueto G, Rasidori E, Zampieri P, Jannucci A, Serio G. The contribution of ultrasonography and computed tomography in the diagnosis of nonfunctioning islet cell tumors of the pancreas. Gastrointest Radiol 1990; 15:139–144.
8. Shawker TH, Doppman JL, Dunnick NR, McCarthy DM. Ultrasonic investigation of pancreatic islet cell tumors. J Ultrasound Med 1982; 1:193–200.
9. Gunther RW, Klose KJ, Ruckert K, Kuhn FP, Beyer J, Klotter HI. Islet-cell tumors: detection of small lesions with computed tomography. Radiology 1983; 148:485–488.
10. Crawford JM, Cotran RS. The pancreas. In: Cotran RS, Kuman SL, Robbins SL, Schoen FJ, eds. Robbins Pathologic Basis of Diseases. 5th ed. Philadelphia: W.B. Saunders, 1994:923.

42

Computed Tomography of the Pancreas

William L. Simpson, Jr. and David S. Mendelson

Mount Sinai School of Medicine, New York University, New York, New York, U.S.A.

1 ANATOMY OF THE PANCREAS

The pancreas is a tongue-shaped retroperitoneal organ (Fig. 1). It is located within the anterior pararenal space along with the ascending and descending colon as well as the duodenum. The pancreas is divided into the uncinate process, head, neck, body, and tail. The long axis of the gland most commonly follows an oblique course with the head at the 8 o'clock position and the tail at 2 o'clock. The normal dimensions of the pancreas depend on many factors, the most important of which is age. The head should measure up to 3.0–3.5 cm, the body up to 2.5 cm, and the tail up to 2.0 cm. Generally the gland tapers in size from head to tail. Fatty infiltration of the gland lobules is common with age. This gives the gland a more lace-like or feathery appearance. The pancreatic duct runs through the entire length of the gland and may measure up to 3.0 mm in the head and gradually tapers to the tail. It is often partially visualized, more commonly in thin section computed tomography (CT). The common bile duct passes through the pancreatic head before it joins the pancreatic duct near the ampulla of Vater. The size of the common bile duct (CBD) in the pancreatic head varies with age as well but should never exceed 10 mm, often attaining the larger diameters on patients post-cholecystectomy.

Anatomically the organ sits posterior to the stomach with the potential space of the lesser sac between them. The left lobe of the liver is anterior as well. The spine, aorta, and inferior vena cava are posterior to the pancreas. The head of the organ sits within the duodenal sweep. The tail extends up into the splenic hilum. The transverse mesocolon attaches to the anterior aspect of the gland.

There are important vascular landmarks related to the pancreas. The splenic vein lies along the dorsal aspect. The splenic vein and superior mesenteric vein join at the portal confluence posterior to the pancreatic head. The uncinate process extends between the superior mesenteric vein and the inferior vena cava (IVC). The splenic artery usu-ally follows a tortuous, serpigenous course behind the organ. It can easily be mistaken for pancreatic cysts or a dilated pancreatic duct on a noncontrast scan by novice observers. Splenic artery calcifications can also be mistaken for pancreatic calcifications. The superior mesenteric artery originates off of the aorta posterior to the body of the pancreas with a fat plane separating the two. The gastroduodenal artery runs along the anterior surface of the pancreatic neck.

2 IMAGING TECHNIQUE

CT imaging of the pancreas has changed with the new developments in CT technology. The goal of scanning a patient with a suspected tumor is not only to establish the diagnosis but also to localize the mass and evaluate for the extent of disease. Noncontrast images of the pancreas are useful for detecting calcifications as eval-

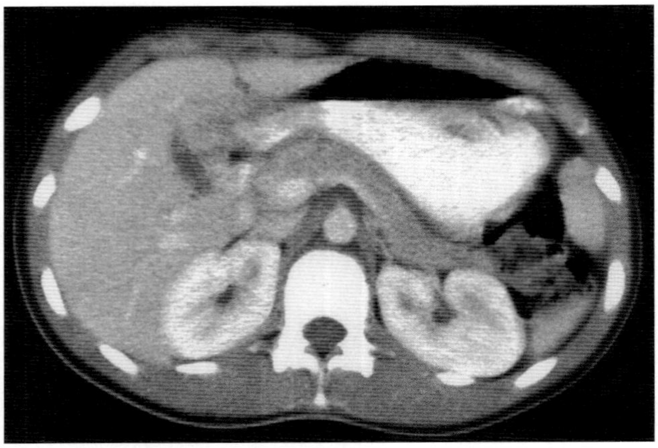

Figure 1 Normal CT appearance of the pancreas.

uating the size and contour of the gland. For most diagnostic studies intravenous contrast enhancement is necessary. The pancreas should be imaged with thin sections—3 mm or less. Helical scanners can cover the pancreas with 3 mm slices in a single breath hold. Multislice scanners can cover the pancreas with as thin as 1 mm slices in one breath hold. The pancreas should be scanned in both the arterial and portal venous phases. An arterial phase scan is obtained by beginning scanning 20–30 seconds after intravenous contrast is injected. The portal venous phase occurs after a 70-second delay. Since the pancreas is a very vascular gland, it enhances readily with contrast. Therefore, most tumors appear as hypo-attenuating lesions in both the arterial and venous phases. However, there are a few tumors that enhance more than the surrounding glandular tissue on the arterial phase—particularly neuroendocrine tumors.

3 NEUROENDOCRINE TUMORS

Most tumors of the pancreas arise from the ductal portion of the gland. These comprise the adenomas and adenocarcinomas. The pancreatic parenchyma gives rise to the neuroendocrine tumors. The majority arises from the islet of Langerhans cells and are also known as islet cell tumors (Fig. 2). They are rare tumors with an incidence of 1.0–1.5 per 100,000 in the general population (1). Approximately half of these tumors are functional, meaning that they produce clinical symptoms from the overproduction of a hormone. The remainder are nonfunctional and come to medical attention due to symptoms from tumor size. The functional tumors include insulinoma, gastrinoma, glucagonoma, vasoactive intestinal peptide-oma (VIPoma), somatostatinoma, growth hormone–releasing factor-oma (GFRoma), adrenocorticotropic hormone-oma (ACTHoma), parathyroid hormone–like-oma (PTHoma), and neurotensinoma. There is only one nonfunctional tumor, namely the pancreatic peptide-oma (PPoma). It produces pancreatic polypeptide and neuron-specific enolase, both of which have no biological activity. Many islet cell tumors are composed of a mixture of more than one cell type.

Insulinomas (Fig. 3) are the most common neuroendocrine tumors of the pancreas. They are predominantly benign (90%) and tend to be solitary and small (<2 cm) (2). Due to their small size they are difficult to localize with CT preoperatively. Sensitivities ranging from 12.5 to 36% have been reported (3–7). However, these studies were performed on conventional dynamic CT scanners using a single phase technique. More recent studies performed on helical scanners with a dual phase technique report sensitivities ranging from 82 to 86% (8,9). Five to 10% of patients with an insulinoma have multiple endocrine neoplasia (MEN)-1 syndrome. MEN-associated insulinomas are more frequently multiple (10).

Gastrimomas are the second most common neuroendocrine tumors (11). The clinical manifestation of the tumor is known as Zollinger-Ellison syndrome. As

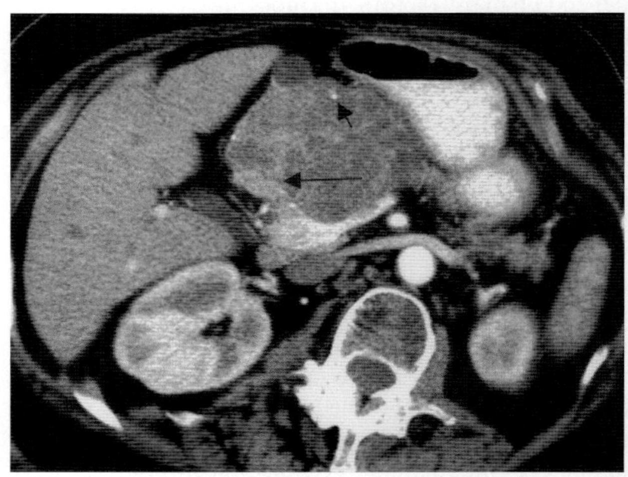

Figure 2 A large nonfunctioning islet cell tumor in the neck/body of the pancreas. The tumor is large as is typical of these tumors since they produce no symptoms except by mass effect. There is both hypervascularity around the periphery of the mass (long arrow) as well as calcification within it (short arrow).

(A)

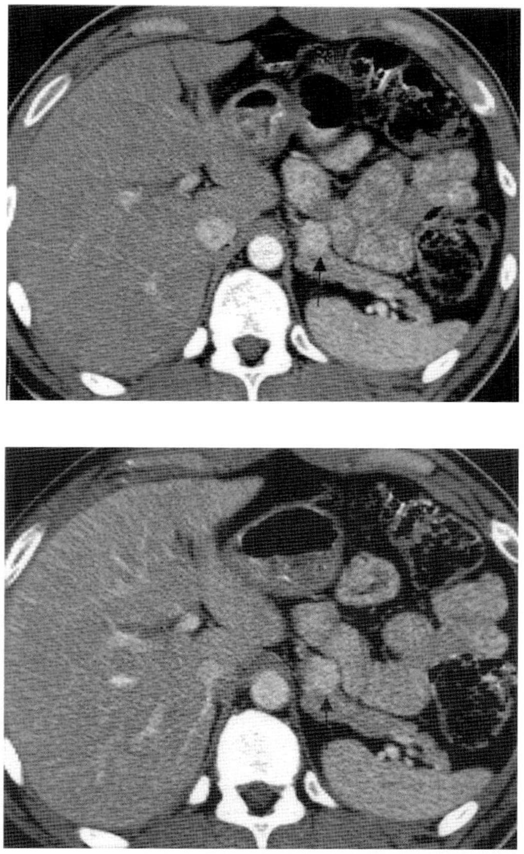

(B)

Figure 3 (A) Insulinoma in the body of the pancreas demonstrates the typical hypervascular enhancement on an arterial phase scan. (B) The mass remains hyperdense compared to the normal pancreatic parenchyma on the portal venous phase scan.

opposed to insulinomas, gastrinomas are predominantly malignant (60–90%) (2). The tumors tend to be small, and preoperative localization is difficult. Roughly 50% of gastrinomas can be localized with CT (12–14), but tumor size is a contributing factor, with the larger ones more easily identified. These commonly appear hypervascular as do the other neuroendocrine tumors. CT can readily detect liver metastasis from malignant tumors (12,15–17). A recent study showed a higher detection rate for gastrinomas when a dual phase helical technique was used (11). Approximately 20% of gastrinomas are associated with MEN-1 (11). In fact, gastrinomas are the most common neuroendocrine tumor of the pancreas associated with MEN-1. As with insulinomas, MEN-associated gastrinomas are frequently multiple and malignant (18). In addition, they are more commonly located in the duodenum (~70%) than in the pancreas (~30%) (19).

Somatostatinomas, glucagonomas, VIPomas, GFRomas, ACTHomas, PTHomas, neurotensinomas, and PPomas are exceedingly rare neuroendocrine tumors. The diagnosis is often delayed due to the nonspecificity of symptoms; therefore, these tumors are often large (>5 cm) at the time of diagnosis and easily detected by CT (20). As is typical for neuroendocrine tumors of the pancreas, they are hypervascular. Calcification is also common in these tumors (21). They have a high incidence of malignancy (22). Each of these tumors can be associated with MEN-1, especially GFRomas (11) and PPomas (23).

REFERENCES

1. Delcore R, Friesen SR. Gastrointestinal neuroendocrine tumors. J Am Coll Surg 1994; 178:187–211.
2. Peplinski GR, Norton JA. Gastrointestinal endocrine cancers and nodal metastases: biological significance and therapeutic implications. Surg Oncol Clin North Am 1996; 5:159–171.
3. Pasieka JL, McLeod MK, Thompson NW, et al. Surgical approach to insulinomas: assessing the need for preoperative localization. Arch Surg 1992; 127:442–447.
4. Dagget PR, Goodburn EA, Kurtz AB, et al. Is preoperative localization of insulinomas necessary? Lancet 1981; 1:483–486
5. Doherty GM, Doppman JL, Shawker JH, et al. Results of a prospective strategy to diagnose, localize and resect insulinomas. Surgery 1991; 110:989–997.
6. Grant CS, van Heerden JA, Charboneau JW, et al. Insulinoma: the value of intraoperative ultrasonography. Arch Surg 1988; 123:843–848.
7. Jensen RT, Norton JA. Endocrine neoplasms of the pancreas. In: Yamada T, Alpers DH, Owyang C, et al., eds. Textbook of Gastroentrology. 3rd ed. Philadelphia: JB Lippincott Co., 1992:2193–2228.
8. Van Hoe L, Gryspeerdt S, Marchal G, et al. Helical CT for the preoperative localization of islet cell tumors of the pancreas. Am J Roentgenol 1995; 165:1437–1439.
9. King AD, Ko GT, Yeung VT, et al. Dual phase spiral CT in the detection of small insulinomas of the pancreas. Br J Radiol 1998; 71:20–23.
10. Demeure MJ, Klonoff DC, Karam JH, et al. Insulinomas associated with multiple endocrine neoplasia type 1: the need for a different surgical approach. Surgery 1991; 110:998–1004.
11. Norton JA. Neuroendocrine tumors of the pancreas and duodenum. Curr Probl Surg 1994; 31:77–164.
12. Jensen RT, Gardner JD, Gastrinoma. In: Go VLW,

DiMango EP, Gardner JD, et al., eds. The Pancreas: Biology, Pathology and Disease. 2d ed. New York: Raven Press, 1993:931–978.
13. Norton JA, Fraker DL, Alexander RA, et al. Surgery to cure the Zollinger-Ellison syndrome. N Engl J Med 1999; 341:635–644.
14. Alexander RA, Fraker DL, Norton JA, et al. Prospective study of somatostatin receptor scintigraphy and its effect on operative outcome in patients with Zollinger-Ellison syndrome. Ann Surg 1998; 228:228–238.
15. Wank SA, Doppman HL, Miller DL, et al. Prospective study of the ability of computerized axial tomography to localize gastrinomas in patients with Zollinger-Ellison syndrome. Gastroenterology 1987;92:905–912.
16. Norton JA, Doherty GD, Fraker DL, et al. Surgical treatment of localized gastrinoma within the liver: a prospective study. Surgery 1998; 124:1145–1152.
17. Gibril F, Reynolds JC, Doppman JL, et al. Somatostatin receptor scintigraphy: its sensitivity compared with that of other imaging methods in detecting primary and metastait gastrinomas: a prospective study. Ann Intern Med 1996; 125:26–34.
18. Mignon M, Ruszniewski P, Podevin P, et al. Current approach to the management of gastrinoma and insulinoma in adults with multiple endocrine neoplasia typeI. World J Surg 1993; 17:489–497.
19. Macfarlane MP, Fraker DL, Alexander HR, et al. A prospective study of surgical resection of duodenal and pancreatic gastrinomsa in MEN-1. Surgery 1995; 118: 973–979.
20. Stanley RJ, Semelka RJ. Pancreas. In: Lee JK, Sagel SS, Stanley RJ, Heiken JP, eds. Computed Body Tomography with MRI Correlation 3d ed.Philadelphia: Lippencott-Raven, 1998:905.
21. Eelkema EA, Stephens DH, Ward EM, et al. CT features of nonfunctioning islet cell carcinoma. Am J Roentgenol 1984; 143:943–948.
22. Wiedenmann B, Jensen RT, Mignon M, et al. General recommendations for the preoperative diagnosis and surgical management of neuroendocrine gastroenteropancreatic tumors. World J Surg 1998; 22:309–318.
23. Strodel WE, Vinik AL, Llyod RV, et al. Pancreatic polypeptide producing tumors. Arch Surg 1984; 119: 508–514.

43

Magnetic Resonance Imaging of Neuroendocrine Pancreatic Tumors

Angela R. Berning and Jeffrey P. Goldman

Mount Sinai School of Medicine, New York University, New York, New York, U.S.A.

1 INTRODUCTION

Neuroendocrine tumors of the pancreas are those arising from the islet cells. They are divided into physiologically functioning or nonfunctioning tumors. The former commonly present with a clinical syndrome resulting from the physiological effects associated with hormone overproduction, and the latter present at a later stage with local complications of a mass or metastatic disease. Less commonly, patients will be evaluated for a known pancreatic mass identified on some other imaging modality.

2 GENERAL MAGNETIC RESONANCE PRINCIPLES

The principle of magnetic resonance imaging (MRI) is based on the inherent motion of hydrogen ion protons within the tissues of the body (1). Each hydrogen ion has a small magnetic field associated with it, which, when placed in the magnetic field of the MRI, spins or precesses at a different rate. The application of an appropriate radio-frequency pulse sequence results in differential motion of the protons and energy exchanges when the protons move to a higher energy state. At the end of the pulse sequence the protons return to their equilibrium state and are said to relax. The term "relaxation time" refers to the rate of this process. This rate is characteristic for a given tissue and is measured in the form of a signal intensity or degree of brightness. The two main relaxation times are T1 and T2.

On T1-weighted images, fluid is generally low in signal intensity, or "dark," and on T2-weighted images fluid has high signal intensity, or is "bright." T1-weighted images are useful for depiction of anatomical detail and is the sequence used after administration of an MR contrast agent (1,2). The most commonly used MR contrast agent is gadopentatate or gadolinium. It is metabolized and excreted in much the same way as iodinated contrast (in computed tomography) but has a much higher safety profile (3,4). T2-weighted images are important in identifying pathology.

The most difficult obstacle for abdominal MRI is overcoming motion artifact from respiration as well as peristalsis (7). Recent technological advances in MRI now allow for breath-hold imaging in almost all sequences, which greatly reduces motion artifact. In abdominal imaging, conventional spin echo (SE) techniques have largely been replaced with gradient-recalled echo (GRE) and fast spin echo (FSE) imaging sequences. On most MR machines these sequences are now standard protocols for T1- and T2-weighted sequences, respectively. Faster imaging also allows for a larger volume to be imaged, or the same volume can be imaged with higher spatial resolution in the same time.

The advantages of MRI over computed tomography (CT) include greater tissue contrast resolution, the ability to obtain multiplanar images, the absence of ionizing radiation, and the lack of nephrotoxity of gadolinium.

A number of studies have compared MR with different modalities in the diagnosis of general pancreatic disease, concluding that while CT is still the modality of choice for pancreatitis, MR has an increasing role in the diagnosis of pancreatic tumors (7,8).

3 MRI OF THE NORMAL PANCREAS

The normal pancreas is intrinsically bright on T1-weighted sequences and similar to or darker than the liver on T2-weighted sequences (9–11) (Figs. 1, 2). This relatively bright signal intensity on T1 is due to aqueous protein contained within the acinar cells (12). With advancing age the pancreas may undergo atro-

(A) (B) (C) (D)

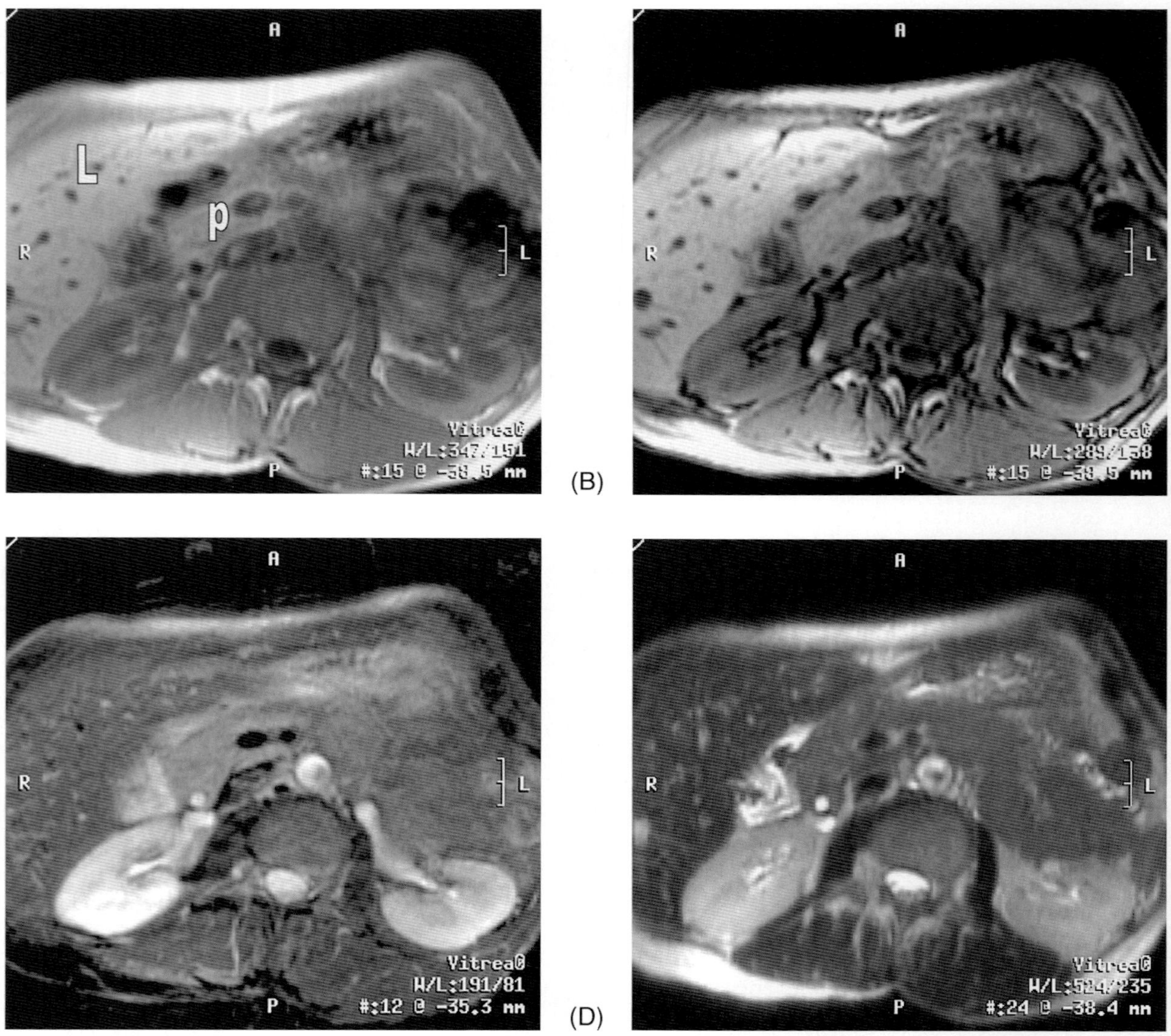

Figure 1 Axial T1 MR images of a normal pancreas (p) both in (A) and out of phase (B) demonstrate the intrinsic brightness of the pancreas, which is similar in intensity to the liver (**L**). On axial T2 fat-suppressed FSE (C) and single-shot (D) sequences, the normal pancreas is dark but still relatively iso-intense with the liver.

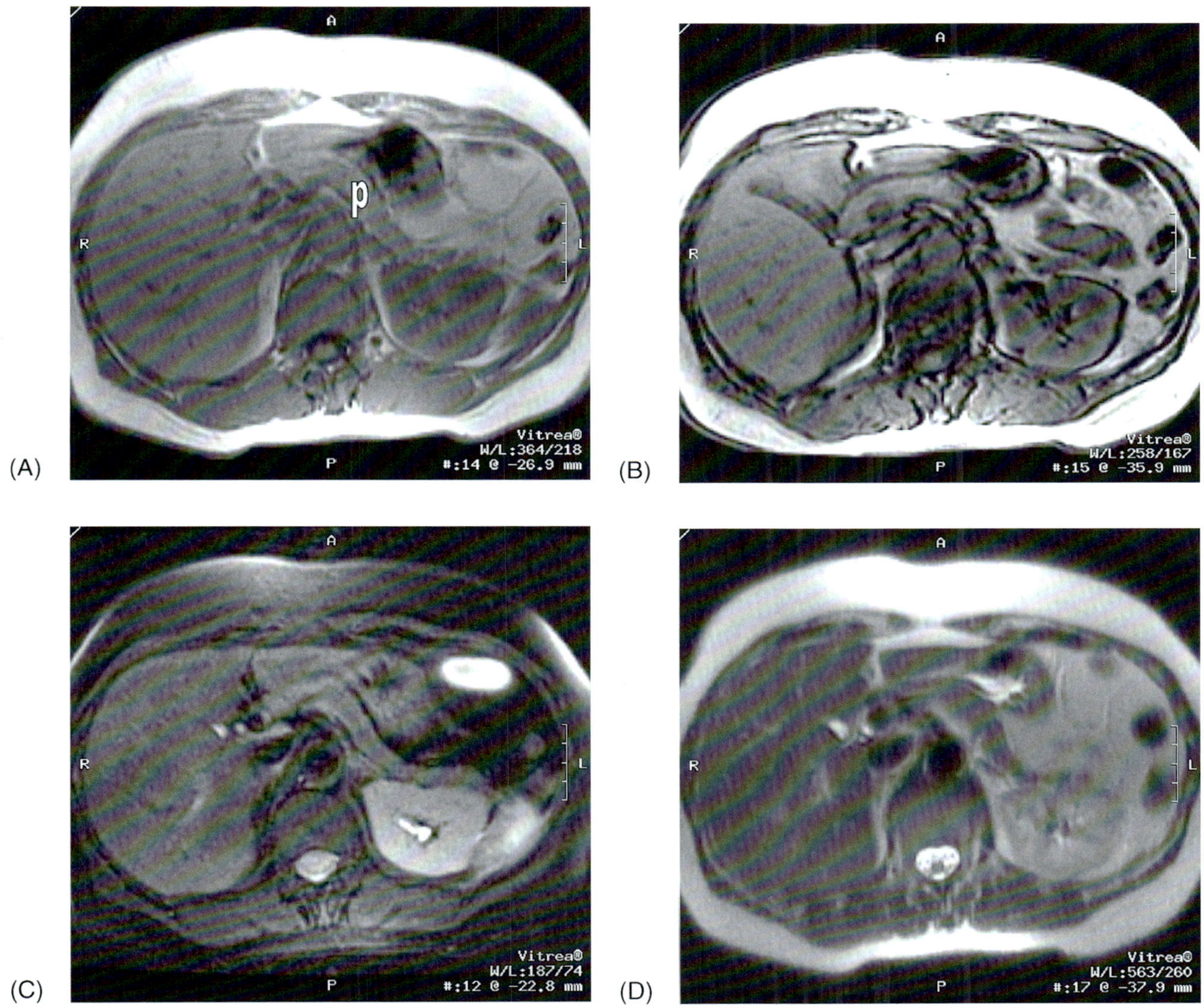

Figure 2 Axial T1 in and out of phase (A and B) and T2 fat-suppressed FSE and single-shot (C and D) sequences in a different patient shows similar characteristics of the normal pancreas (p) as see in Figure 1.

phy, which is due to a combination of fibrosis as well as fatty replacement (13). With advancing age the signal intensity may decrease or increase when compared to that of the liver. Now with improved spatial and contrast resolution, even acinar lobular detail and lesions less than 1 cm in size can usually be delineated on a dedicated pancreas MR study. The pancreatic duct, like the bile duct, follows the signal of fluid and is dark on T1 and bright on T2 (Figs. 3, 4). The pancreas enhances homogeneously with MR contrast agent gadolinium (14) (Figs. 5, 6). As with CT, a bi- or triphasic study has been shown to be the most useful in delineating the pancreas where best pancreatic enhancement occurs almost immediately up to about 15 seconds and of the liver at 25 seconds or later (14) (Fig. 6).

The conspicuity of the pancreas can be increased further by the use of techniques that null the signal from fat such that the surrounding retroperitoneal fat tissue appears dark and the pancreas appears bright (Fig. 7).

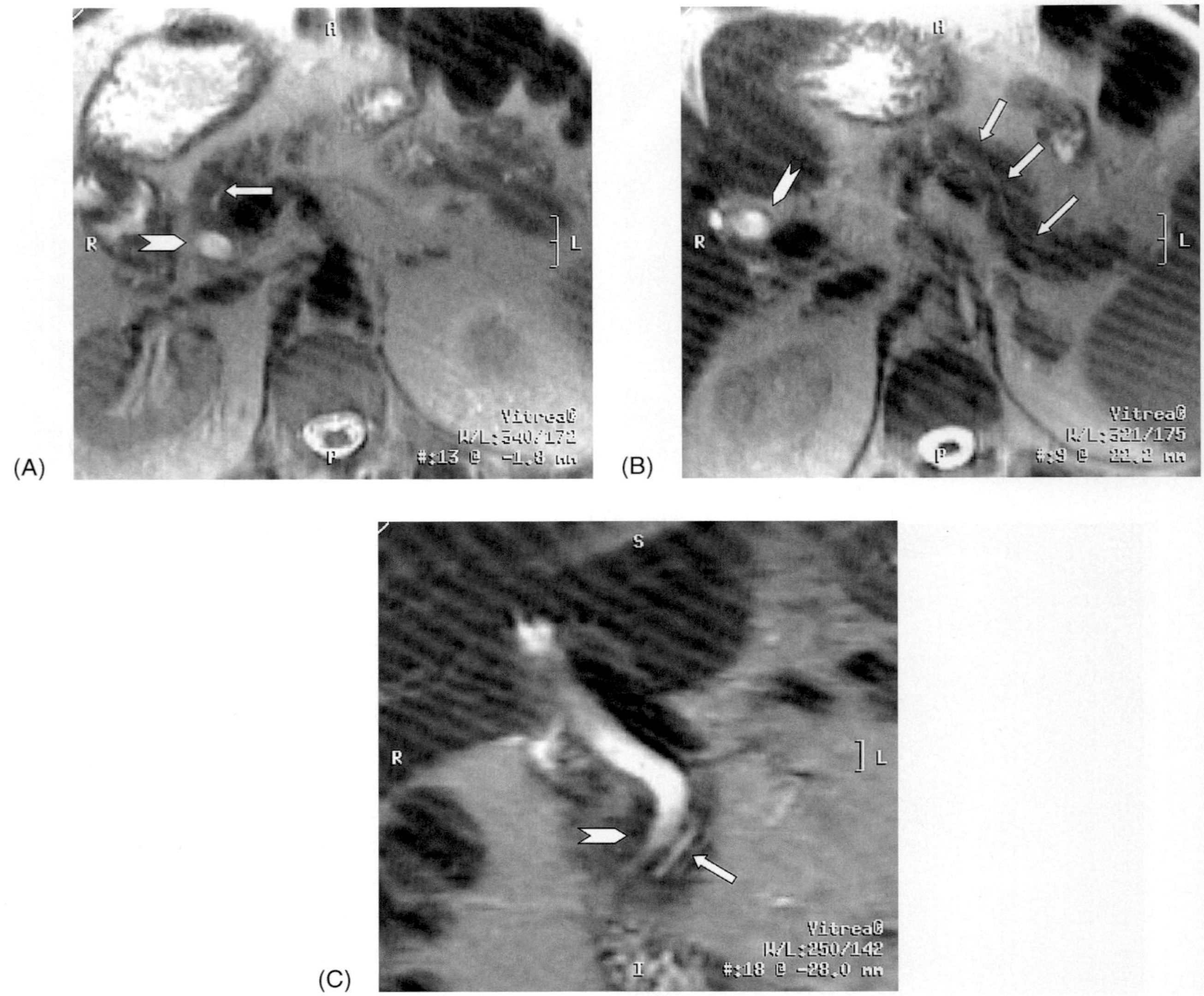

Figure 3 Axial (A and B) and coronal (C) single-shot T2 MR images of a normal pancreatic (small arrows) and common bile duct (arrowhead) which are bright or hyperintense in signal intensity. In A and C the distal common bile duct (CBD) and the pancreatic duct are seen adjacent to one another.

These include fat-suppression (FS) and short tau inversion recovery (STIR) sequences, of which the former has been shown to be the most practicable (15,16).

An examination of the pancreas should, therefore, include high-resolution scans through the pancreas with assessment of the pancreatic duct, associated vasculature, surrounding tissues, and the liver. Slice thickness should be at least 5 mm or less. Imaging is optimal at high field strengths of 1.0 T or greater. It should include the following sequences: T1-weighted, GRE, fat-suppressed sequence both with and without contrast (9,18), a T2-weighted FSE or single-shot (SS) sequence with or without fat suppression, and a thin-slice, single-shot magnetic resonance cholangio-pancreatography (MRCP) sequence in at least one coronal or axial plane to evaluate the pancreatic duct and common bile duct. Postgadolinium images should be in the immediate postcontrast, arterial-capillary blush phase and then at approximately 45 and 90 seconds after contrast (2). Motion from bowel peristalsis can be decreased by using glucagon (19), which should be injected intravenously, and the ingestion of an oral

(A)

(B)

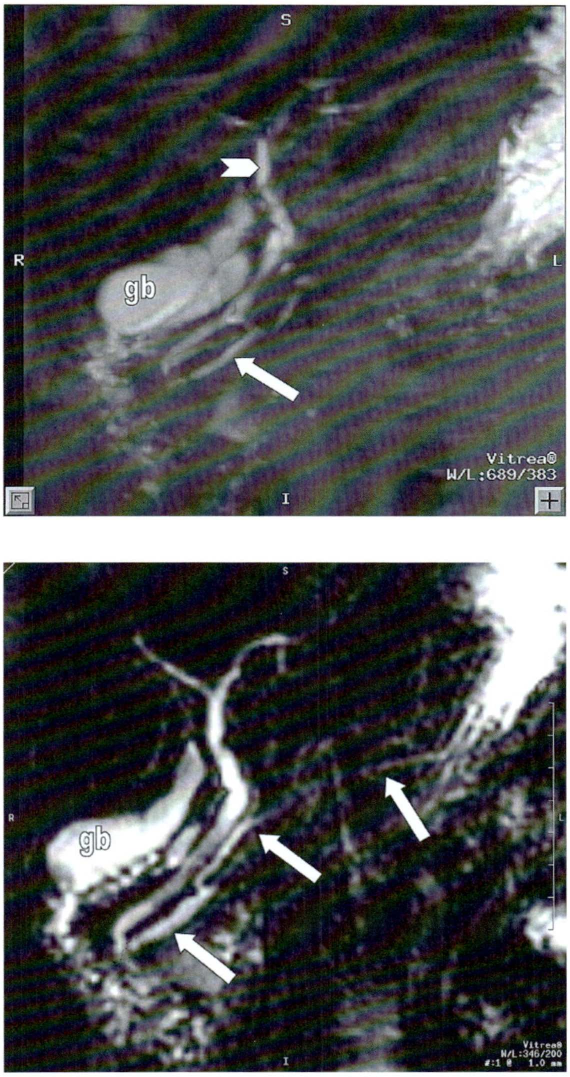

Figure 4 Coronal single shot T2 (A) and thick-slab (B) MR images of the CBD (arrowhead) and pancreatic duct (arrows) in a different patient. Note again that these fluid-containing structures, including the gall bladder (gb), are bright.

contrast agent can further improve differentiation between pancreas and adjacent bowel (20). Plain water is usually sufficient as MR oral agents have not shown to add to the examination (21).

4 MRI OF NEUROENDOCRINE PANCREATIC TUMORS

The use of MRI in the evaluation of neuroendocrine tumors is well documented. The most common appearance is low signal intensity or dark on T1 and intermediate to high signal intensity or bright on T2 sequences (12,19,22,23) (Fig. 8). Tumors usually enhance early, reflecting their vascular nature (Figs. 9, 10). Homogeneous enhancement is most common, although heterogeneous and ring enhancement have also been demonstrated (12,24). This will in part depend on the size of the tumor. The value, however, of differentiating pancreatic masses using enhancement patterns is still debatable, with its main value being in delineating the peri-pancreatic vessels, including the veins, as well as evaluating for metastatic deposits.

These findings have been confirmed by a number of recent comprehensive reviews of the imaging features of neuroendocrine tumors with pathological correlation (24–26). They examined not only the frequency but the spectrum of appearances for various types of pancreatic neuroendocrine tumors. Occasionally some islet cell tumors are high signal on T1 (26), which may be due to complicating hemorrhage. Low signal intensity on T2 has also been demonstrated (27) usually due to an abundance of fibrous tissue, which may also present with lack of enhancement on contrast images (28). In such instances differentiation from ductal-derived (7,29) and, rarely, mixed ductal-acinar cell tumors (30) may be difficult.

Hormone-producing tumors are usually small and benign at presentation. They may be multiple in number and variable in location, following the classic description of being low signal on T1 and high signal on T2. Nonfunctioning tumors tend to be larger on presentation. They are often solitary, and a larger percentage are malignant (31). At least 50% are located within the pancreatic head. They may be complicated and contain areas of calcification and cystic degeneration (32). Cystic change is present in about 42% of tumors greater than 3 cm and will appear as more intense areas of dark and bright signal on T1 and T2 sequences, respectively (25,33) (Fig. 11). More specifically there may be thickening of the cyst wall, irregularity of the inner surface, intense rim enhancement and slight increased signal intensity on T1, usually due to complicating hemorrhage or necrotic tissue (34). In the absence of biochemical evidence of hormonal hypersecretion, differentiation from other pancreatic cystic tumors is impossible and histological, sampling is necessary (35).

Local complications of pancreatic neuroendocrine tumors include invasion of adjacent vessels, most commonly the intrapancreatic portions of the portal and splenic veins, with resultant cavernous transformation of the occluded vessels. Less commonly the renal and superior mesenteric veins may be involved (36). Unlike

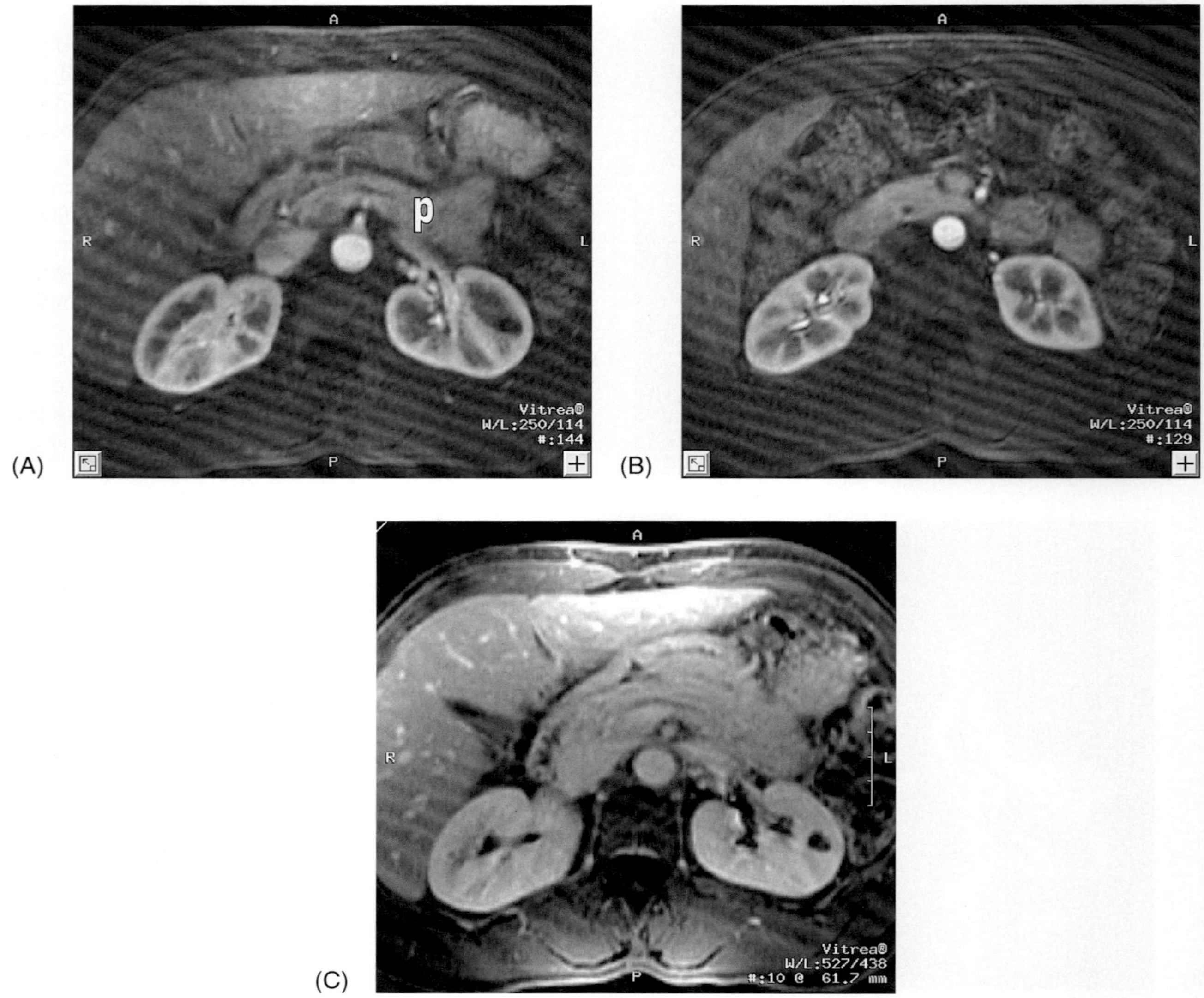

Figure 5 Axial T1 fat-suppressed postgadolinium MR images in the immediate (A and B) and delayed (C) phases. The normal pancreas (p) enhances early and homogeneously.

adenocarcinomas, however, these tumors do not encase the mesenteric vessels and also do not obstruct the pancreatic duct (Fig. 11).

Traditionally CT has been the main form of imaging for pancreatic neuroendocrine tumors. Sonography and contrast-enhanced CT are the most commonly used preoperative imaging methods because of their relatively low cost and widespread availability (37). Historically a number of studies compared the sensitivity and specificity for the detection of islet tumors using different modalities (31,38–41). Results were variable regarding the sensitivity of MR for primary lesion detection. With new advances in MR, however, diagnostic accuracy has markedly improved, and a recent study (27) found that dual-phase CT in the portal venous phase and MR with delayed enhancement are equally effective in detecting islet cell tumors with sensitivities of about 70%. Results do vary slightly, however, depending on sequences used with T1 fat-suppressed gradient echo and T2 FSE sequences demonstrating a sensitivity of 85% for primary lesions (18). Results also vary with the specific type of islet cell tumor being more sensitive for

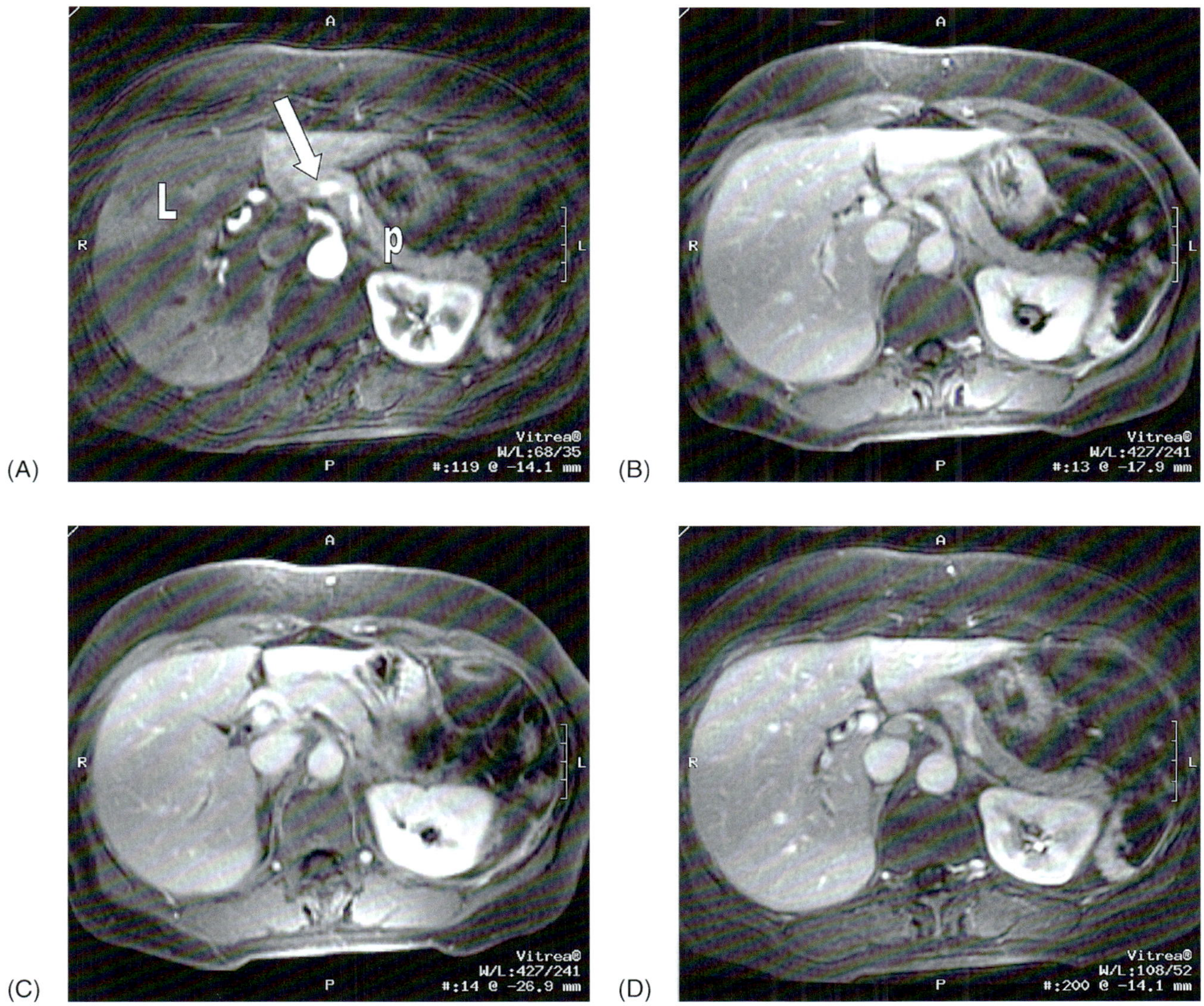

Figure 6 Axial T1 fat-suppressed postgadolinium MR images in a different patient demonstrate optimal enhancement of the pancreas (**P**) and peri-pancreatic vessels (arrow) immediately following contrast injection (A). The liver (**L**) enhances at a slightly later phase (B–D).

insulinomas, which are usually intrapancreatic (42–44), and less sensitive for gastrinomas (19,31,45–47), which are commonly extrapancreatic in location (48).

4.1 Metastases

While the value of MR in the preoperative evaluation of primary tumors is controversial, it has an important role in the evaluation of metastatic disease. Although somatostatin receptor scintigraphy has become the principal modality for detecting metastatic disease (49), MR has been shown to be superior in further localizing and characterizing metastases in the initial staging phase as well as in monitoring response to treatment (40,45).

Metastatic sites include regional lymph nodes, liver, and bone in 50, 30, and 7% of cases, respectively (50). The presence of liver lesions is considered the major criterion for malignancy and a more useful predictor of survival (51,52) as the histology of the primary tumor has been shown to be unreliable (53). Splenic metastases have also been demonstrated in up to 10% of patients, occurring due to the venous communication between

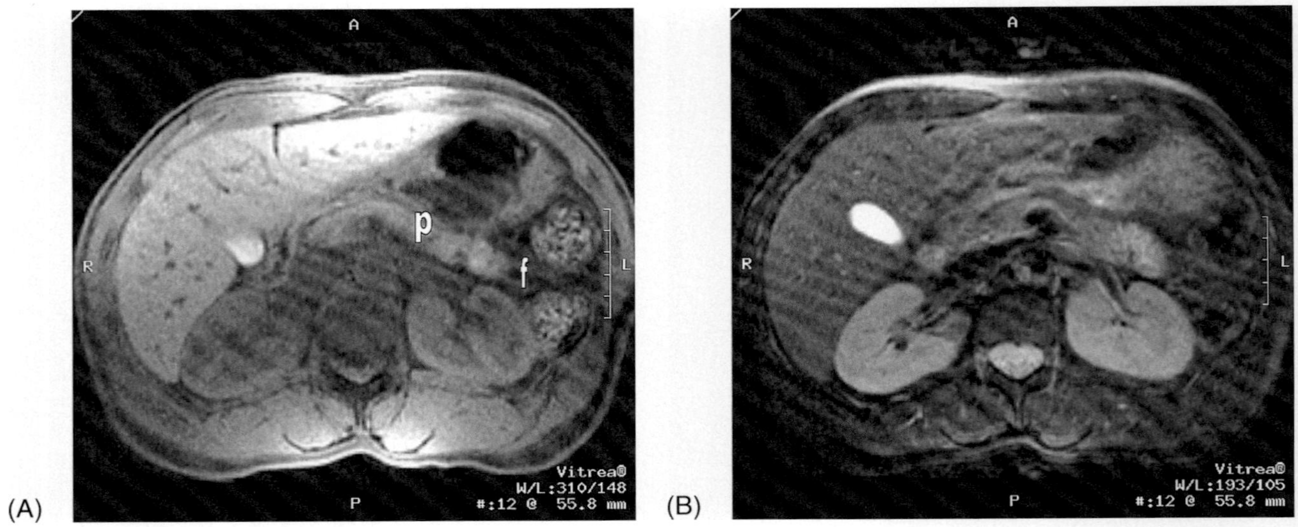

Figure 7 Axial T1 (A) and T2 (B) MR images of a normal pancreas (p), both with fat suppression, which increases the conspicuity of the pancreas by nulling the signal from the surrounding fat (f).

the two organs (24). Bony metastases, which are most commonly located in the axial skeleton (50,54), usually only occur in the presence of liver metastases and also indicate a poor prognosis. Lesions are hypointense on T1 and enhance postcontrast (55). They may also be hyperintense on T2-weighted images (50).

Liver metastases are usually hypointense or isointense on T1 and hyperintense on T2 (Fig. 12). Enhancement with gadolinium is usually early and transient and largely heterogeneous (41,56) and does not show peripheral nodularity (Fig. 13). Most important, in the presence of liver lesions, is the differentiation from hemangiomas and other benign hepatic lesions such as hepatic cysts. This may particularly be difficult in gastrinoma (57) and has also been seen with VIPomas (46), where hepatic metastases are intensely bright on T2 sequences. In most cases the use of a long TE T2-weighted sequence will differentiate metastases as intermediate or low signal intensity, whereas a hemangioma or cyst will remain high in signal intensity (22) (Fig. 11).

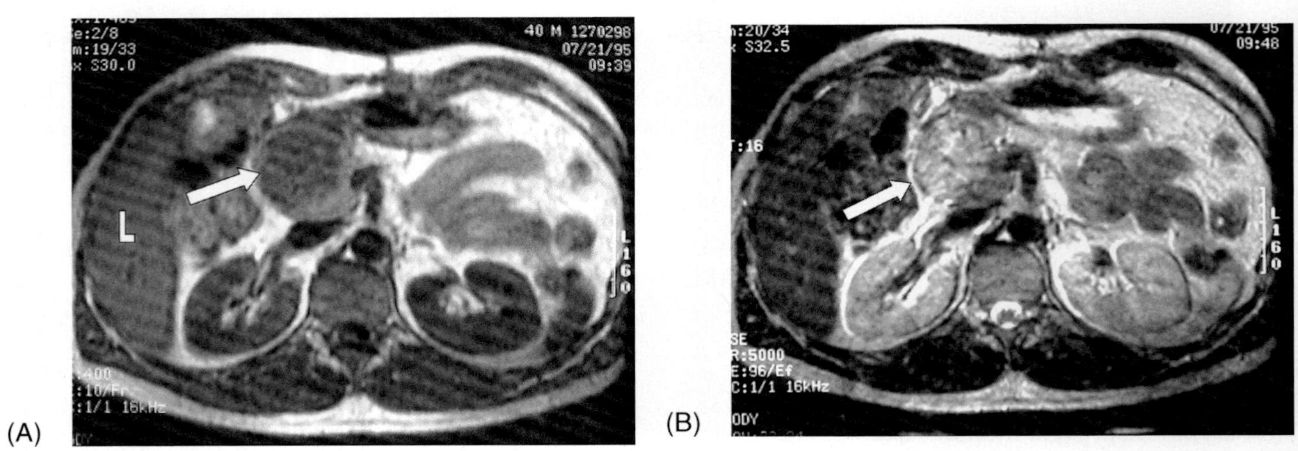

Figure 8 Axial T1 (A) and single-shot T2 (B) MR images of a pancreatic head mass (arrow) which is iso- or hypointense to liver (**L**) on T1 and hyperintense on T2. This was subsequently proven to be an insulinomia. (Courtesy of J. Goldman, Mt. Sinai Medical Center, New York.)

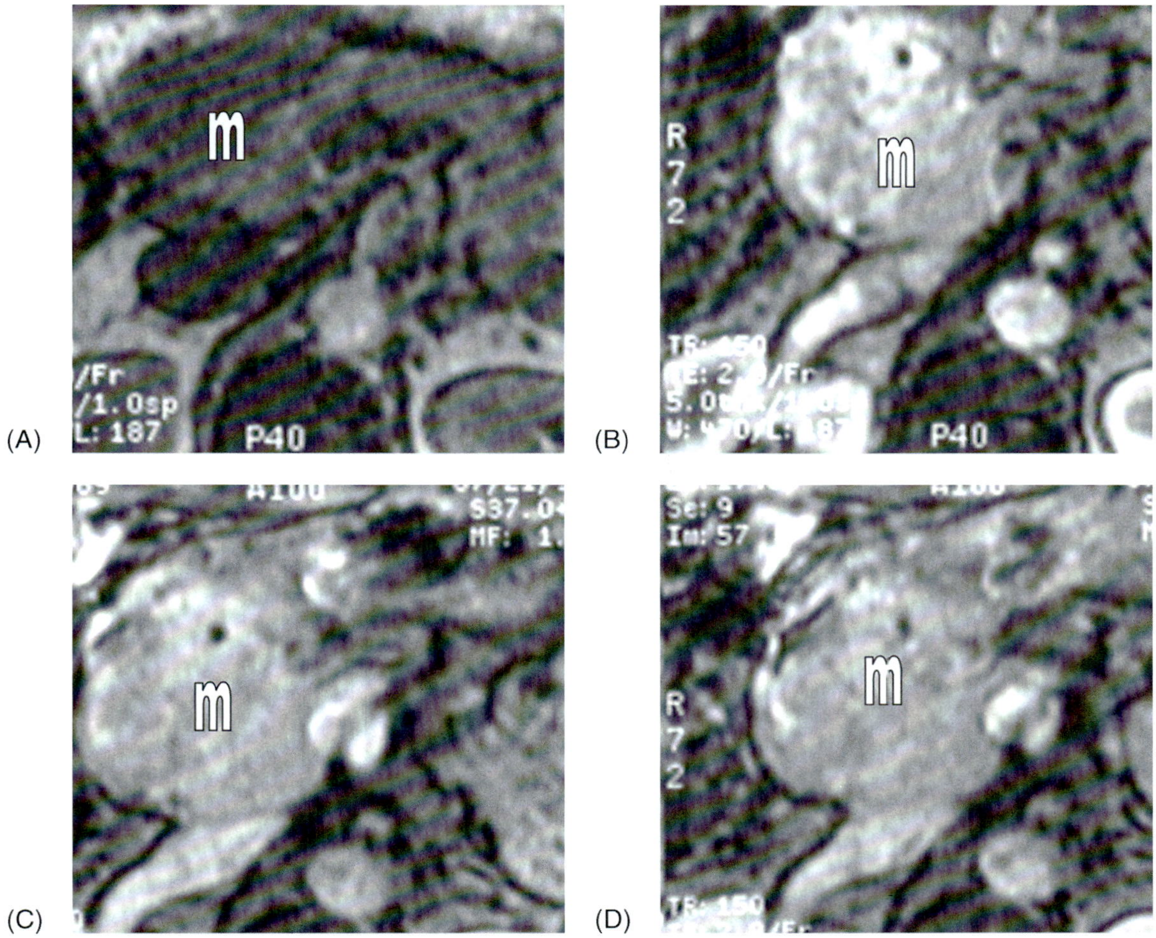

Figure 9 Axial T1 pre (A) and postgadolinium (B–D) MR images of the same patient demonstrating early, but slightly heterogeneous, enhancement of the mass (m). (Courtesy of J. Goldman, Mt. Sinai Medical Center, New York.)

On the nonenhanced sequences, however, their appearances may be identical.

Delayed postcontrast images have been shown to be the most useful in equivocal cases. Metastases are hypointense to normal liver, and hemangiomas show peripheral nodularity and progressive filling-in to produce more intense enhancement over time (57). Some studies have also used MR contrast agents containing superparamagnetic iron oxide particles (58), which has been shown to be useful in the evaluation of hepatic lesions (59). Metastases may also enhance with the intrahepatic contrast agents (60) such as mangafodipir, which, although now used in the liver and biliary tree, were actually initially developed for the pancreas (61–63).

The lungs, mediastinum, peritoneum, and rarely the brain may also be involved in metastatic disease. Apart from the brain, CT is superior in delineating disease extent at these latter sites (64).

4.2 Specific Syndromes

4.2.1 Insulinomas

Insulinomas, the most common (60%) of the islet cell tumors, are single, intrapancreatic, small in size (mean < 2 cm), and benign. About 4% will occur as part of the MEN-1 syndrome (31). They are generally uniformly distributed throughout the pancreas. As with most islet cell tumors, they are usually hypointense or dark on T1 and hyperintense or bright on T2 and homogeneously enhance with gadolinium on immediate postcontrast images (65,66) (Figs. 8, 9). Larger tumors, although uncommon, may show ring enhancement.

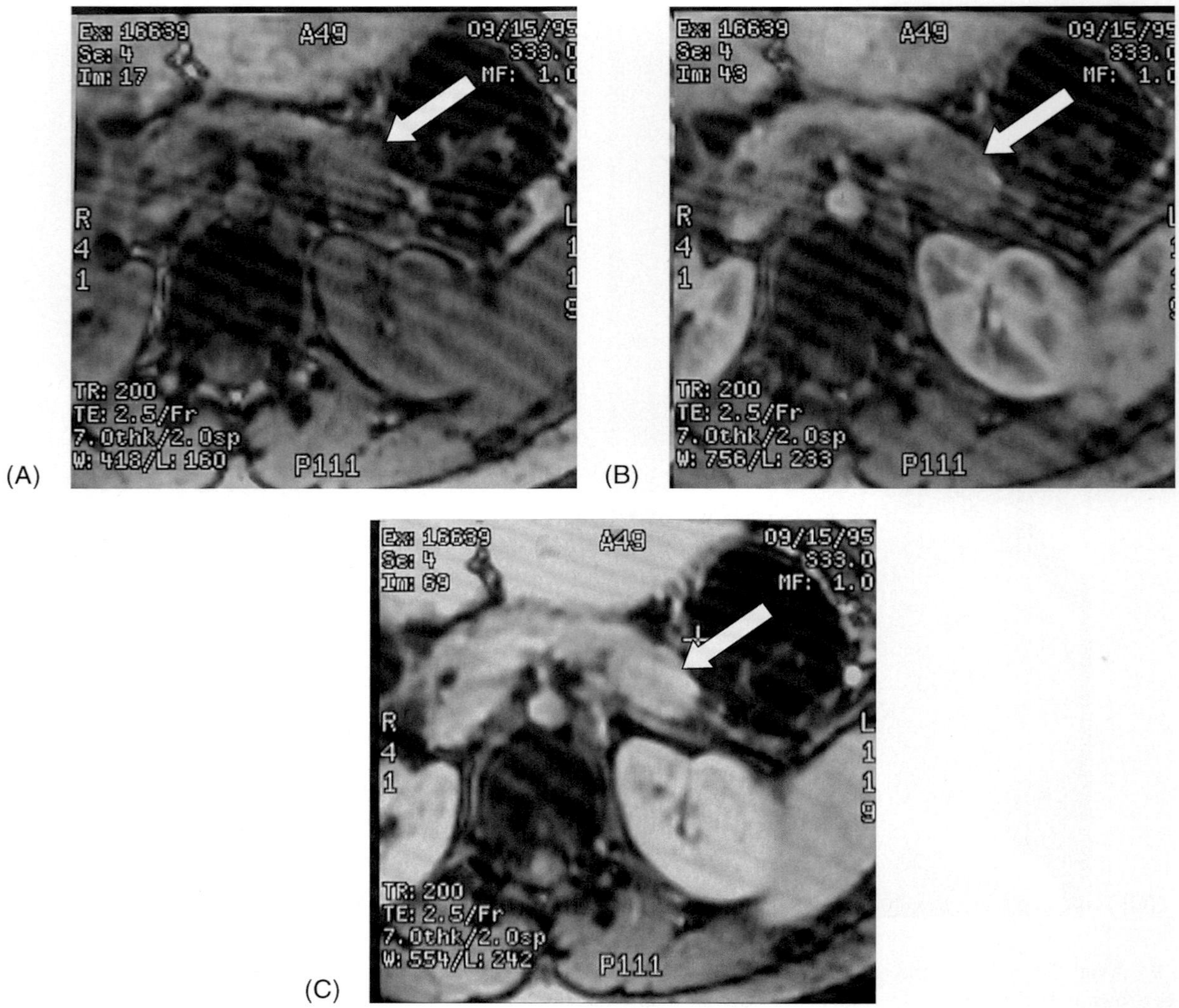

Figure 10 Axial T1 pre- (A) and postgadolinium (B and C) MR images of the primary tumor (arrows) seen in Figures 12 and 13 show homogeneous enhancement with contrast. (Courtesy of J. Goldman, Mt. Sinai Medical Center, New York.)

Displacement rather than invasion of the pancreatic duct (67) has been reported, as has tumor thrombus in the portal vein (68). In rare cases if liver metastases do occur, they may show homogeneous and ring enhancement irrespective of size (12).

4.2.2 Gastrinomas

Gastrinomas account for about 18% of islet cell tumors and are most commonly small in size. Compared to insulinomas, however, they are frequently multiple and extrapancreatic, and at least 60% are malignant. Up to 90% are located within the gastrinoma triangle, and approximately 45% are located within the duodenal wall, thus making preoperative localization much more difficult. Other ectopic sites have been reported (69), including a primary intracardiac location (70). They are usually hypointense or dark on T1, hyperintense or bright on T2, and show ring-like enhancement on immediate postcontrast images. They are generally less vascular than insulinomas. Liver metastases also demonstrate the ring enhancement, which helps to differentiate them from hemangiomas (57).

4.2.3 Glucagonomas, Somatostatinomas, VIPomas, and Other Rare Endocrine Tumors of the Pancreas

These form a small subset of the islet cell tumors and are usually large at presentation. They usually arise in

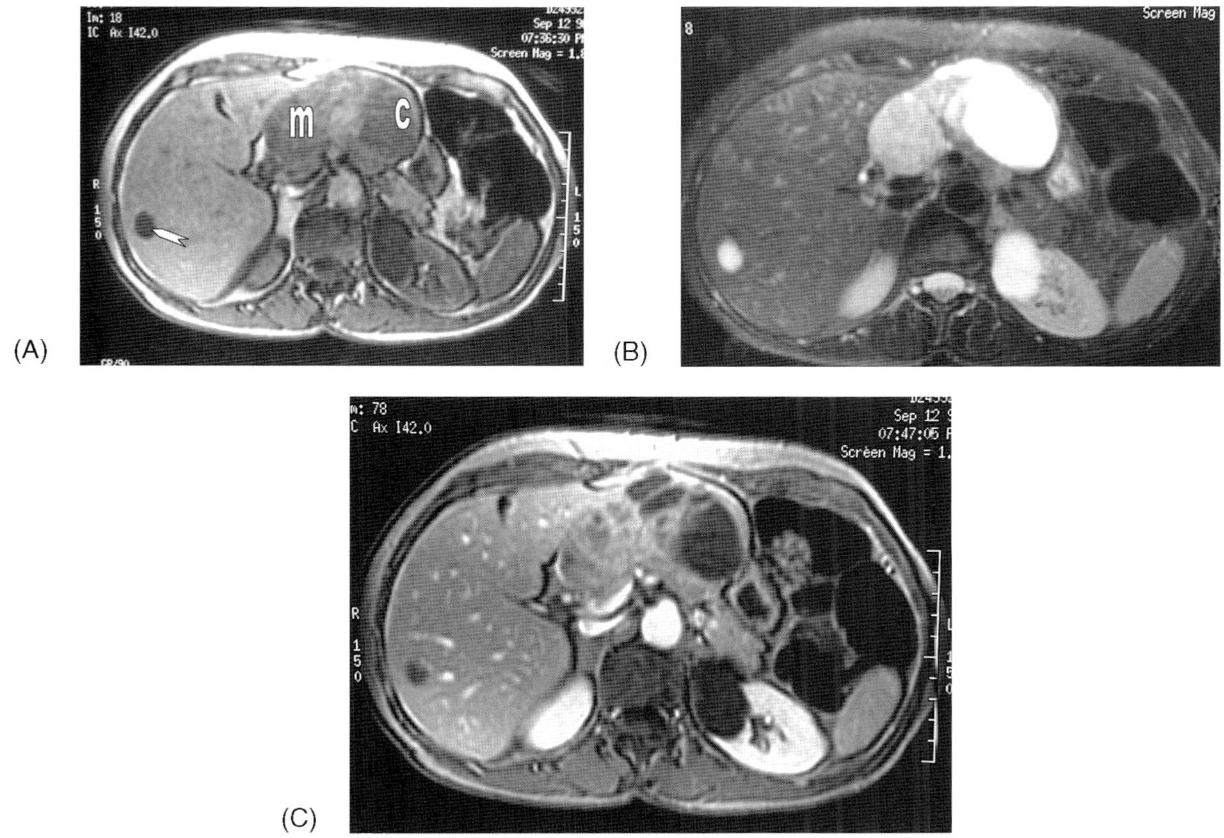

Figure 11 Axial T1 (A), T2 (B), and postgadolinium (C) MR images of a large (>3 cm) mass in the body of the pancreas (m). It contains a large cystic area (c), which follows fluid signal and shows no enhancement with contrast. Note that the mass is draped over, but does not invade, the mesentric vessels, which is typical for islet cell tumors. Incidentally, there is also a lesion in the right lobe of the liver, which also follows the signal of fluid and is in keeping with a hepatic cyst (arrowhead). (Courtesy of J. Goldman, Mt. Sinai Medical Center, New York.)

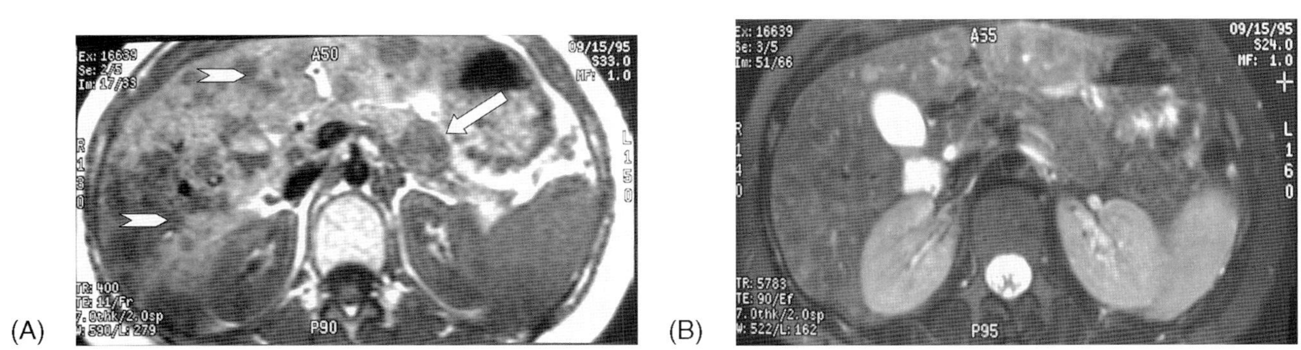

Figure 12 Axial T1 (A) and fat-suppressed T2 (B) MR images demonstrating diffuse hepatic metastases in a patient with a mass in the tail of the pancreas (arrow), which is dark or hypointense on both sequences. Hepatic metastases (arrowheads) are characteristically dark on T1 and bright on T2, but this patient has such diffuse disease that the lesions are no longer focal. (Courtesy of J. Goldman, Mt. Sinai Medical Center, New York.)

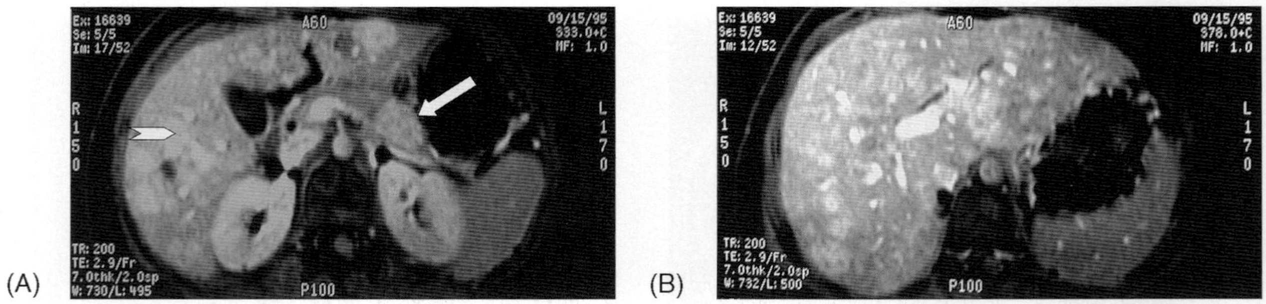

Figure 13 Axial T1 fat-suppressed postgadolinium (A and B) MR images demonstrating marked enhancement of the primary lesion (arrow) (M) and the hepatic metastasis (arrowheads). (Courtesy of J. Goldman, Mt. Sinai Medical Center, New York.)

the body and tail of the pancreas, although ectopic sites have been demonstrated (71,72), and are frequently malignant with metastatic lesions (73–76). Signal intensity characteristics are variable depending on the size of the tumor and the absence or presence of complications.

4.2.4 Association with Non-MEN Inherited Neoplastic Syndromes

Von Hippel-Lindau (VHL) disease is a hereditary syndrome characterized by a predisposition for bilateral and multicentric retinal angiomas, hemangioblastomas in the central nervous system (CNS), renal cell carcinomas, pheochromocytomas, islet cell tumors of the pancreas, endolymphatic sac tumors, as well as cysts in the kidney, pancreas, and epididymis (77,78). The signal intensity of the pancreatic tumor is usually similar to that of primary neuroendocrine tumors.

4.2.5 Differential Diagnoses

Pancreatic Carcinoma. Pancreatic tumors arising from ductal cells are far more common than islet cell tumors but, at times, may be difficult to differentiate from the latter. They are usually dark or hypointense on both T1 and T2 and show variable enhancement. They are also more likely to show areas of hemorrhage, necrosis, and cystic change (7,29) (Fig. 14).

Pancreatic Cysts/Pseudo-Cysts Pancreatic cysts are most commonly associated with a history of

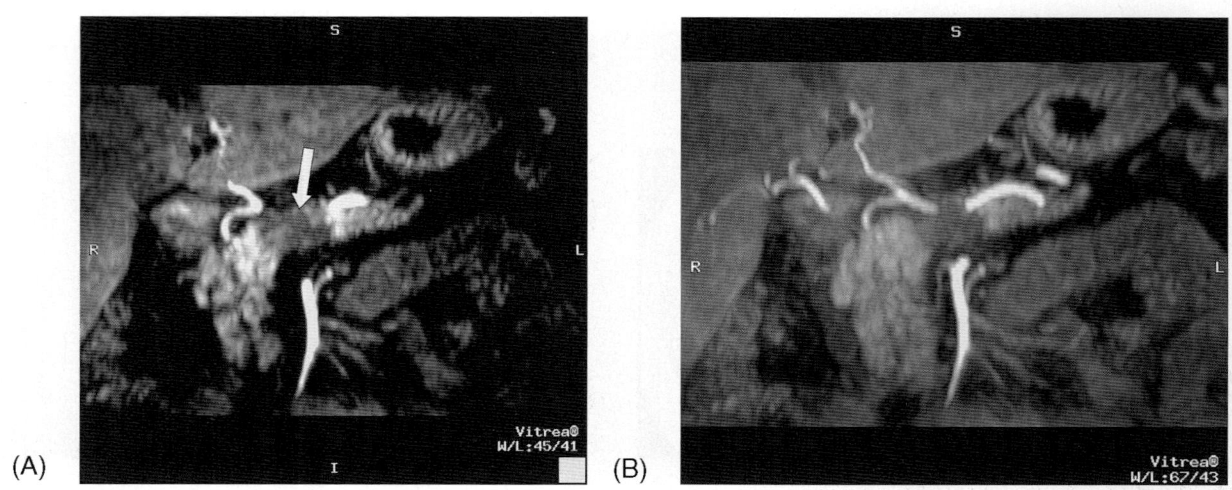

Figure 14 Axial T1 fat-suppressed immediate postgadolinium MR images (A and B) of a hypo-intense mass (arrow) in the body of the pancreas, which was proven to be a ductal-derived tumor. There is almost no enhancement with contrast.

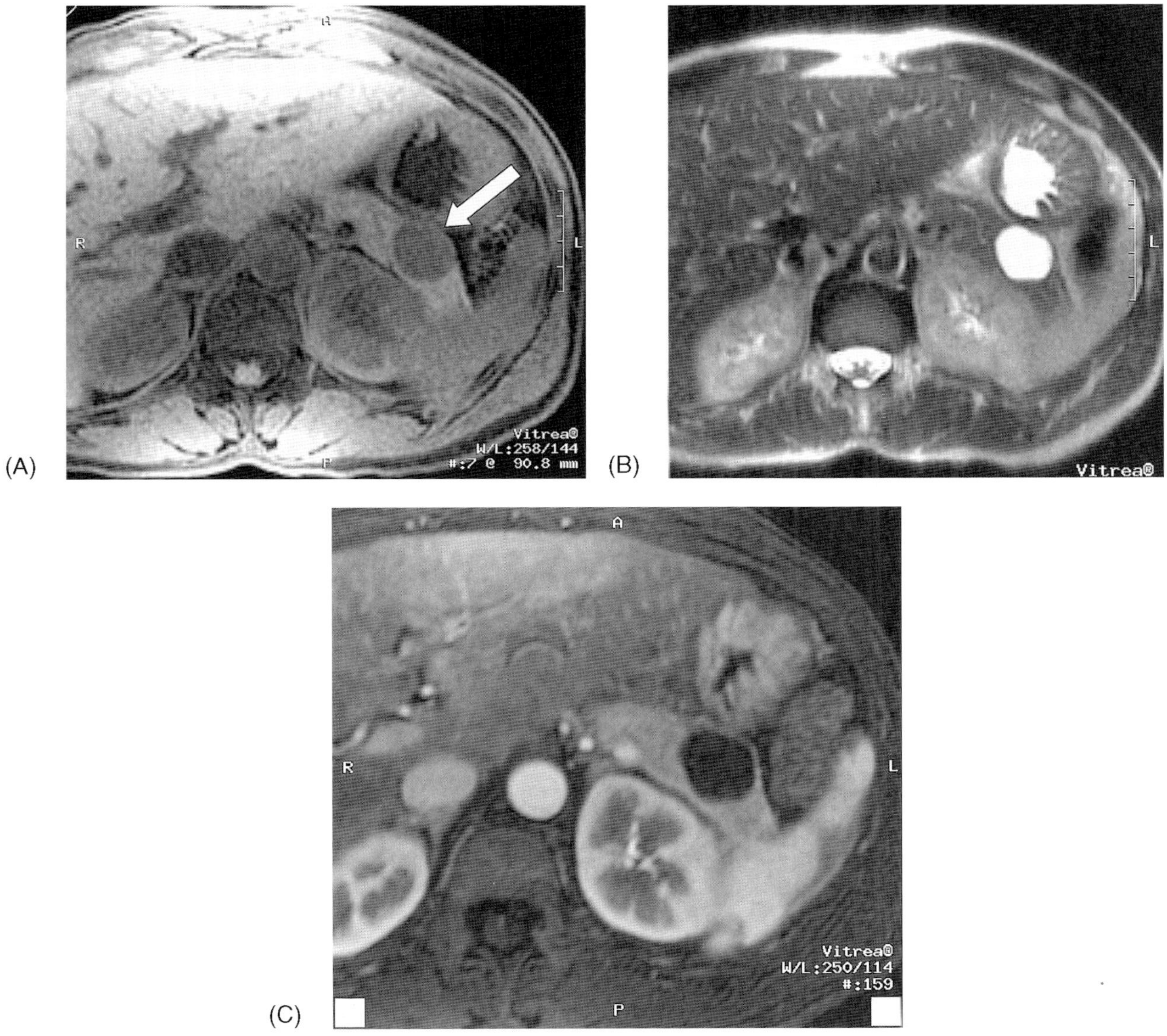

Figure 15 Axial fat-suppressed T1 (A), and single-shot T2 (B), and T1 fat-suppressed postgadolinium (C) MR images of a pseudo-cyst in the tail of the pancreas (arrow).

pancreatitis. Although, like islet cell tumors, they are dark on T1 and bright on T2, they are usually easy to identify as fluid-containing structures and show no enhancement with contrast (12,22,24) (Fig. 15).

5 FUTURE DIRECTIONS

MR is being increasingly utilized in the pre- and post-operative evaluation of pancreatic transplants. The combined use of MR and MR angiography has been found to be as accurate as conventional angiography (79), but the major advantage is the lack of nephrotoxicity of gadolinium and the ability to also evaluate the soft tissue structures.

6 CONCLUSION

Despite all the recent advances in MR technology, the choice of preoperative imaging for pancreatic neuroendocrine tumors remains controversial and will continue to depend on the specific clinical problem, local expertise, and availability of imaging techniques. It should, however, be the examination of choice in patients with compromised renal function or renal disease and probably in pregnant mothers.

ACKNOWLEDGMENT

The authors would like to thank Dr. Emil Cohen for his assistance with presenting the images.

REFERENCES

1. Megibow AJ, Lavelle MT, Rofsky NM. MR imaging of the pancreas. Surg Clin North Am 2001; 81(2):307–320, ix–x.
2. Martin DR, Semelka RC. MR imaging of pancreatic masses. Magnet Reson Imaging Clin North Am 2000; 8(4):787–812.
3. Murphy KJ, Brunberg JA, Cohan RH. Adverse reactions to gadolinium contrast media: a review of 36 cases. AJR Am J Roentgenol 1996; 167(4):847–849.
4. Prince MR, Arnoldus C, Frisoli JK. Nephrotoxicity of high-dose gadolinium compared with iodinated contrast. J Magnet Reson Imaging 1996; 6(1):162–166.
5. Diehl SJ, et al. MR imaging of pancreatic lesions. Comparison of manganese-DPDP and gadolinium chelate. Invest Radiol 1999; 34(9):589–595.
6. Wang C. Mangafodipir trisodium (MnDPDP)-enhanced magnetic resonance imaging of the liver and pancreas. Acta Radiol Suppl 1998; 415:1–31.
7. Semelka RC. Pancreatic disease: prospective comparison of CT,ERCP,and 1.5T MR imaging with dynamic gadolinium enhancement and fat suppression. Radiology 1991; 181:785–791.
8. Sood GK, Gupta RK, Broor SL. Magnetic resonance imaging in pancreatic diseases: comparison with other imaging techniques. Indian J Gastroenterol 1992; 11(2): 59–61.
9. Outwater EK, Siegelman ES. MR imaging of pancreatic disorders. Top Magnet Reson Imaging 1996; 8(5):265–289.
10. Mitchell DG, Winston CB, Outwater EK, et al. Delineation of pancreas with MR imaging: multiobserver comparison of five pulse sequences. J Magnet Reson Imaging 1995; 5:193–199.
11. Semelka RC, Ascher SM. MRI of the pancreas: state of the art. Radiology 1993; 188:593–602.
12. Semelka RC, et al. Islet cell tumors: comparison of dynamic contrast-enhanced CT and MR imaging with dynamic gadolinium enhancement and fat suppression. Radiology 1993; 186(3):799–802.
13. Winston CB, Mitchell DB, Outwater EK, et al. Pancreatic signal intensity on T1-weighted fat saturation MR images. J Comput Assist Tomogr 1995; 5:267–271.
14. Kanematsu M, et al. Pancreas and peripancreatic vessels: effect of imaging delay on gadolinium enhancement at dynamic gradient-recalled-echo MR imaging. Radiology 2000; 215(1):95–102.
15. Kraus BB, Ros PR. Insulinoma: diagnosis with fat-suppressed MR imaging. AJR Am J Roentgenol 1994; 162(1):69–70.
16. Mitchell DG. Liver and pancreas:improved spin-echo T1 contrast. Radiology 1991; 178:67.
17. Mori M, et al. Insulinoma: correlation of short-TI inversion-recovery (STIR) imaging and histopathologic findings. Abdom Imaging 1996; 21(4):337–341.
18. Thoeni RF, et al. Detection of small, functional islet cell tumors in the pancreas: selection of MR imaging sequences for optimal sensitivity. Radiology 2000; 214(2): 483–490.
19. Mitchell DG, et al. MRI of pancreatic gastrinomas. J Comput Assist Tomogr 1992; 16(4):583–585.
20. Pavone P, et al. Pancreatic beta-cell tumors: MRI. J Comput Assist Tomogr 1993; 17(3):403–407.
21. Fink C, et al. [Prospective study to compare high-resolution computed tomography and magnetic resonance imaging in the detection of pancreatic neoplasms: use of intravenous and oral MR contrast media]. Rofo Fortschr Geb Rontgenstr Neuen Bildgeb Verfahr 2001; 173(8):724–730.
22. Carlson B, et al. MRI of pancreatic islet cell carcinoma. J Comput Assist Tomogr 1993; 17(5):735–740.
23. Kelekis NL, Semelka RC. Carcinoma of the pancreatic head area. Diagnostic imaging: magnetic resonance imaging. Rays 1995; 20(3):289–303.
24. Semelka RC, et al. Neuroendocrine tumors of the pancreas: spectrum of appearances on MRI. J Magnet Reson Imaging 2000; 11(2):141–148.
25. Buetow PC, Parrino TV, Buck JL, et al. Islet cell tumors of the pancreas: pathologic-imaging correlation among size, necrosis and cysts, calcification, malignant behaviour and functional status. AJR Am J Roentgenol 1995; 165:1175–1179.
26. Owen NJ, et al. MRI of pancreatic neuroendocrine tumours. Br J Radiol 2001; 74(886):968–973.
27. Ichikawa T, et al. Islet cell tumor of the pancreas: biphasic CT versus MR imaging in tumor detection. Radiology 2000; 216(1):163–171.
28. Iglesias A, et al. Unusual presentation of a pancreatic insulinoma in helical CT and dynamic contrast-enhanced MR imaging: case report. Eur Radiol 2001; 11(6):926–930.
29. Vellet AD, et al. Adenocarcinoma of the pancreatic ducts: comparative evaluation with CT and MR imaging at 1.5 T. Radiology 1992; 183(1):87–95.
30. Okada Y, Mori H, Tsutsumi A. Duct-acinar-islet cell tumor of the pancreas. Pathol Int 1995; 45(9):669–676.

31. King CM, et al. Imaging islet cell tumours. Clin Radiol 1994; 49(5):295–303.
32. Buetow PC, Miller DL, Parrino TV, Buck JL. Islet cell tumors of the pancreas: clinical, radiologic, and pathologic correlation and localisation. Radiographics 1997; 17:453–472.
33. Sohaib SA, et al. Cystic islet cell tumors of the pancreas. AJR Am J Roentgenol 1998; 170(1):217.
34. Takeshita K, et al. Cystic islet cell tumors: radiologic findings in three cases. Abdom Imaging 1994; 19(3): 225–228.
35. Kehagias D, et al. Cystic pancreatic neoplasms: computed tomography and magnetic resonance imaging findings. Int J Pancreatol 2000; 28(3):223–230.
36. Smith TM, et al. Islet cell tumor of the pancreas associated with tumor thrombus in the portal vein. Magnet Reson Imaging 1999; 17(7):1093–1096.
37. Gorman B, Reading CC. Imaging of gastrointestinal neuroendocrine tumors. Semin Ultrasound CT MR 1995; 16(4):331–341.
38. Chirletti P, et al. Topographic diagnosis and surgical treatment of insulinoma. Chir Ital 2000; 52(1):11–16.
39. Moore NR, Rogers CE, Britton BJ. Magnetic resonance imaging of endocrine tumours of the pancreas. Br J Radiol 1995; 68(808):341–347.
40. Aspestrand F, Kolmannskog F, Jacobsen M. CT, MR imaging and angiography in pancreatic apudomas. Acta Radiol 1993; 34(5):468–473.
41. Carriere F, et al. [Role of MRI in the diagnosis of endocrine tumors of the pancreas]. J Radiol 1992; 73(4): 235–242.
42. Liessi G, et al. MRI in insulinomas: preliminary findings. Eur J Radiol 1992; 14(1):46–51.
43. Doherty GM, et al. Results of a prospective strategy to diagnose, localize, and resect insulinomas. Surgery 1991; 110(6):989–997.
44. Angeli E, et al. Value of abdominal sonography and MR imaging at 0.5 T in preoperative detection of pancreatic insulinoma: a comparison with dynamic CT and angiography. Abdom Imaging 1997; 22(3):295–303.
45. Pisegna JR, et al. Prospective comparative study of ability of MR imaging and other imaging modalities to localize tumors in patients with Zollinger-Ellison syndrome. Dig Dis Sci 1993; 38(7):1318–1328.
46. Tjon ATRT, et al. CT and MR imaging of advanced Zollinger-Ellison syndrome. J Comput Assist Tomogr 1989; 13(5):821–828.
47. Frucht H, et al. Gastrinomas: comparison of MR imaging with CT, angiography, and US. Radiology 1989; 171 (3):713–717.
48. Prinz RA. Localization of gastrinomas. Int J Pancreatol 1996; 19(2):79–91.
49. Krenning EP, et al. Somatostatin receptor scintigraphy with [111In-DTPA-D-Phe1]- and [123I- Tyr3]-octreotide: the Rotterdam experience with more than 1000 patients. Eur J Nucl Med 1993; 20(8):716–731.
50. Debray MP, et al. Imaging appearances of metastases from neuroendocrine tumours of the pancreas. Br J Radiol 2001; 74(887):1065–1070.
51. Sutliff VE, et al. Growth of newly diagnosed, untreated metastatic gastrinomas and predictors of growth patterns. J Clin Oncol 1997; 15(6):2420–2431.
52. Masson B, et al. [Somatostatinoma. Apropos of a case]. J Chir (Paris) 1997; 134(1):22–26.
53. Sata N, et al. Malignant insulinoma causing liver metastasis 8 years after the initial surgery: report of a case. Surg Today 1995; 25(7):640–642.
54. Patel N, et al. Skeletal metastasis of malignant glucagonoma mimicking avascular necrosis of the hip scintigraphic and MRI correlation. Clin Nucl Med 1993; 18(1):70–72.
55. Gibril F, et al. Bone metastases in patients with gastrinomas: a prospective study of bone scanning, somatostatin receptor scanning, and magnetic resonance image in their detection, frequency, location, and effect of their detection on management. J Clin Oncol 1998; 16(3):1040–1053.
56. Soyer P, et al. Dynamic Gd-DOTA-enhanced MR imaging of hepatic metastases from pancreatic neuroendocrine tumors. Eur J Radiol 1994; 18(3):180–184.
57. Berger JF, et al. Differentiation between multiple liver hemangiomas and liver metastases of gastrinomas: value of enhanced MRI. J Comput Assist Tomogr 1996; 20(3): 349–355.
58. Vandevenne JE, et al. Insulinoma associated with liver lesions: value of MR imaging. Am J Gastroenterol 1998; 93(9):1559–1562.
59. Vogl TJ, Hammerstingl R, Schwartz W, et al. Superparamagnetic iron oxide-enhanced MR imaging for differential diagnosis of focal liver lesions. Radiology 1996; 198:881–887.
60. Mathieu D, et al. Unexpected MR-T1 enhancement of endocrine liver metastases with mangafodipir. J Magn Reson Imaging 1999; 10(2):193–195.
61. Ahlstrom H, Gehl HB. Overview of MnDPDP as a pancreas-specific contrast agent for MR imaging. Acta Radiol 1997; 38(4 Pt 2):660–664.
62. Gehl HB, et al. Mn-DPDP in MR imaging of pancreatic adenocarcinoma: initial clinical experience. Radiology 1993; 186(3):795–798.
63. Gehl HB, et al. Pancreatic enhancement after low-dose infusion of Mn-DPDP. Radiology 1991; 180(2):337–339.
64. Vasseur B, et al. Peritoneal carcinomatosis in patients with digestive endocrine tumors. Cancer 1996; 78(8): 1686–1692.
65. Chatziioannou A, et al. Imaging and localization of pancreatic insulinomas. Clin Imaging 2001; 25(4):275–283.
66. Beccaria L, et al. Multiple insulinomas of the pancreas: a patient report. J Pediatr Endocrinol Metab 1997; 10 (3):309–314.

67. Kuramitsu T, et al. Poorly vascularized malignant insulinoma displaced the pancreatic ducts around the mass on endoscopic retrograde cholangiopancreatography. Intern Med 2001; 40(1):28–31.
68. Obuz F, Bora S, Sarioglu S. Malignant islet cell tumor of the pancreas associated with portal venous thrombus. Eur Radiol 2001; 11(9):1642–1644.
69. Eshkar NS, et al. Case report: MRI of extrapancreatic gastrinoma. Comput Med Imaging Graph 1995; 19(5): 447–449.
70. Gibril F, et al. Somatostatin receptor scintigraphy: its sensitivity compared with that of other imaging methods in detecting primary and metastatic gastrinomas. A prospective study. Ann Intern Med 1996; 125(1):26–34.
71. De Giorgio R, et al. Asymptomatic glucagonoma presenting with an isolated hepatic nodule. Hepatogastroenterology 1998; 45(22):1093–1096.
72. Tjon ATRT, et al. Imaging features of somatostatinoma: MR, CT, US, and angiography. J Comput Assist Tomogr 1994; 18(3):427–431.
73. Sofka CM, et al. MR imaging of metastatic pancreatic VIPoma. Magn Reson Imaging 1997; 15(10):1205–1208.
74. Tjon ATRT, et al. MR, CT, and ultrasound findings of metastatic vipoma in pancreas. J Comput Assist Tomogr 1989; 13(1):142–144.
75. Kelekis NL, et al. ACTH-secreting islet cell tumor: appearances on dynamic gadolinium-enhanced MRI. Magn Reson Imaging 1995; 13(4):641–644.
76. Amikura K, et al. Role of surgery in management of adrenocorticotropic hormone-producing islet cell tumors of the pancreas. Surgery 1995; 118(6):1125–1130.
77. Hes FJ, Feldberg MA. Von Hippel-Lindau disease: strategies in early detection (renal-, adrenal-, pancreatic masses). Eur Radiol 1999; 9(4):598–610.
78. Mallek R, et al. Contrast MRI in multiple endocrine neoplasia type 1 (MEN) associated with renal cell carcinoma. Eur J Radiol 1990; 10(2):105–108.
79. Boeve WJ, et al. Comparison of contrast enhanced MR-angiography-MRI and digital subtraction angiography in the evaluation of pancreas and/or kidney transplantation patients: initial experience. Magn Reson Imaging 2001; 19(5):595–607.

44

Radionuclide Imaging of the Pancreatic Endocrine Tumors

Chun Ki Kim, Borys R. Krynyckyi, and Josef Machac

Mount Sinai School of Medicine, New York University, New York, New York, U.S.A.

1 INTRODUCTION

Somatostatin receptors (SSR) are expressed by the majority of neuroendocrine tumors, including pancreatic endocrine tumors. Several subtypes of SSR exist. SSR subtype 2 predominance has been found in 80% of pancreatic endocrine tumors (1). Octreotide, a somatostatin analogue used to treat selected symptomatic patients with neuroendocrine tumors, binds to SSR subtype 2 and subtype 5. Indium-111 (In-111)–labeled octreotide is the most commonly used radiotracer for imaging of pancreatic endocrine tumors. Readers interested in details of the imaging protocol are referred to guidelines published by the Society of Nuclear Medicine (2).

Other radiotracers used in selected cases of neuroendorine tumors include iodine-131 (or iodine-123) meta-iodobenzylguanidine (MIBG), a norepinephrine analogue, and fluorine-18 fluorodeoxyglucose (F-18 FDG), a positron-emitting radiotracer. More detailed information regarding these radiotracers is presented in Chapter 31.

This chapter discusses the role of radionuclide imaging in the diagnostic evaluation of pancreatic endocrine tumors. Therapeutic applications of radiolabeled compounds will not be discussed.

2 SOMATOSTAIN RECEPTOR SCINTIGRAPHY

On a normal In-111 octreotide scan, the spleen and kidneys are typically most intense, followed by the liver (Fig. 1). The scan also shows varying levels of radioactivity in the bowel and bladder. The thyroid and pituitary glands are occasionally visualized. The gallbladder is also often visualized, which may be misinterpreted as a hepatic lesion. A fatty meal or cholecystokinin may be given to contract the gallbladder. Activated lymphocytes express somatostatin receptors, so any inflammatory site or recent postsurgical wounds should be carefully evaluated.

Investigators have reported that false-positive findings with somatostain receptor scintigraphy (SRS) is rare (3–5). Although false-positive findings were found to be as high as in 12% in a series (6), these findings would probably not confuse experienced readers. Extra-abdominal false-positive localizations were more common than intra-abdominal. Thyroid disease, breast disease, and granulomatous lung disease were reported to be the most frequent causes of extra-abdominal false-positive uptake. Causes of intra-abdominal false-positive uptake included accessory spleens and uptake in

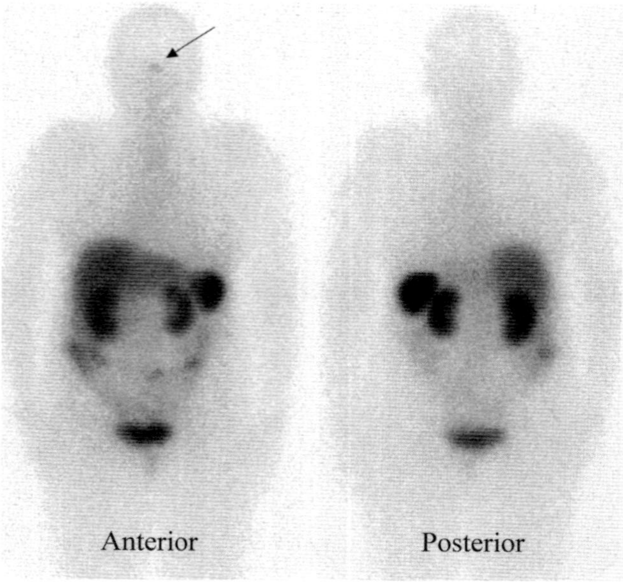

Figure 1 A normal In-111 octreotide scan showing physiological activity in the spleen, kidneys, liver, bowel, and urinary bladder. Minimal activity is seen in the pituitary (arrow), with a trace of activity also noted in the thyroid bed region.

previous surgical sites. Urine activity in dilated renal calyces can also mimic a tumor.

Accurate staging is essential for the optimal management of patients with neuroendocrine tumors (Fig. 2). SRS using In-111 octreotide has been extensively evaluated in patients with pancreatic endocrine tumors for approximately 15 years. In a large European multicenter trial (7), the sensitivity of SRS was 100% for the detection of glucagonomas, 88% for VIPomas, 73% for gastrinomas, 82% for "nonfunctioning" islet cell tumors, but only 46% for insulinomas. Obviously, false-negative studies occur due in part to diminished or absent tumor somatostatin receptors, an inherent limitation (8). Insulinoma cells are reported to express relatively low SSR subtype 2.

Single photon emission computed tomography (SPECT) of the liver and abdomen (Fig. 3) must be performed in all cases as physiological liver and bowel activity may obscure lesions in the liver and abdomen on the planar images. SPECT imaging detected 25% more liver metastases compared with planar imaging (9). SPECT imaging has been reported to improve the sensitivity (87.5% vs. 44% of planar imaging) even for

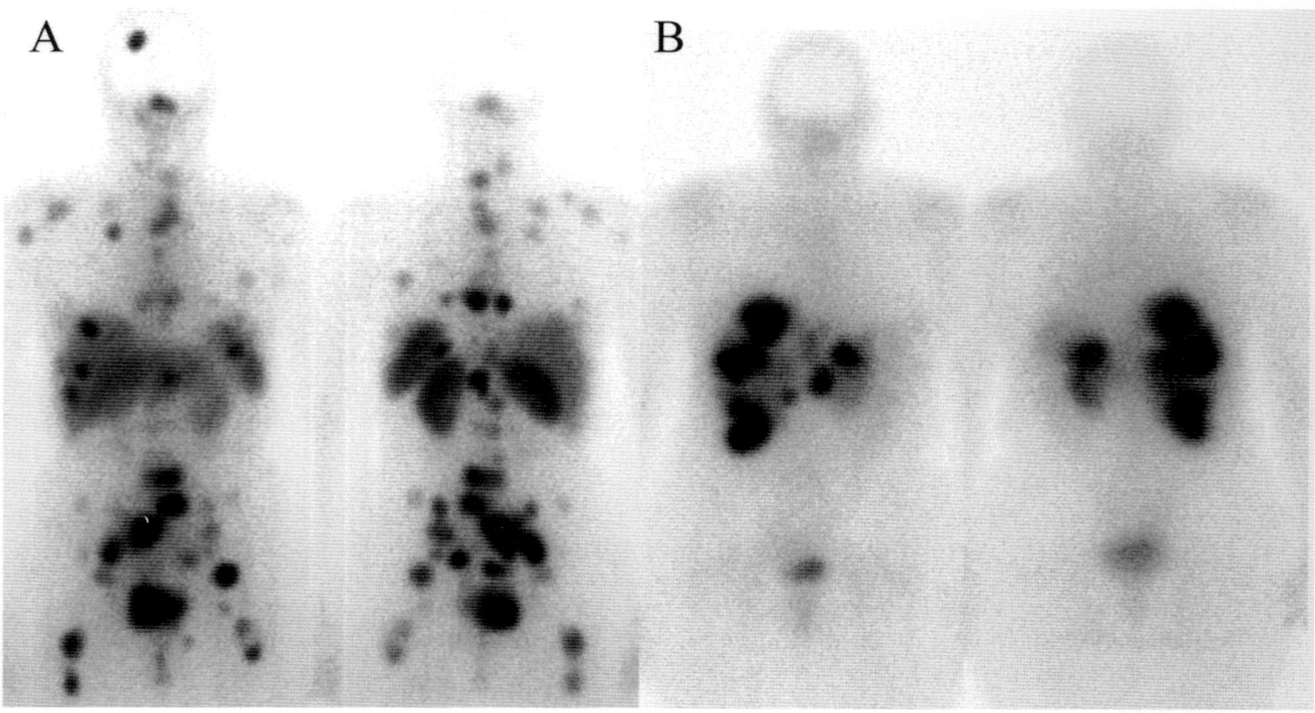

Figure 2 In-111 octreotide scans performed in two patients with gastroenteropancreatic endocrine tumors. Patient A has extensive skeletal metastatic disease, whereas Patient B has multiple large and small metastatic lesions confined to the liver only.

the detection of insulinoma, for which SRS is generally known to be quite insensitive (10).

3 SRS VERSUS CONVENTIONAL IMAGING TECHNIQUES AND CLINICAL ROLES

Several prospective studies have shown that SRS has both higher sensitivity and higher specificity for detecting gastroenteropancreatic (GEP) endocrine tumors. SRS has also been reported to alter the management in a significant proportion of patients.

In a prospective study of 122 patients with Zollinger-Ellison syndrome, SRS altered management in 47% of patients. Primary tumor localization and clarification of equivocal localization results from conventional imaging studies [ultrasonography, computerized tomography (CT), magnetic resonance imaging (MRI), angiography, and bone scan] were the principal reasons for altering management (Fig. 3) (11). In another prospective study including 160 patients with biologically and/or histologically proven GEP tumors, the results of SRS modified patient classification in 38 cases (24%) and changed surgical therapeutic strategy in 40 patients (25%) (12). SRS seems particularly valuable in detecting extrahepatic tumor sites and lymph node metastases not detected by anatomical imaging techniques in patients with gastrinoma as well as other neuroendocrine tumors (13–16). SRS also outperforms CT or ultrasonography in detection of the unknown primary tumor (16).

Most investigators feel that SRS should be the initial imaging modality for patients with pancreatic endocrine tumors because of the ability of SRS to alter clinical management combined with its superior sensitivity, high specificity, simplicity, and cost-effectiveness. Insulinoma would be an exception to this. Endoscopic ultrasonography has been proposed as the first choice of localization method for insulinoma by one group (17). In a preliminary investigation, 8 of 10 insulinomas were detected on iodine-123–labeled vasoactive intestinal peptide (VIP) scintigraphy (18).

4 OTHER CLINICAL ROLES OF SRS

4.1 Prediction of Response to Somatostatin Therapy

It has been suggested that a positive scan predicts a good suppressive effect of octreotide on hormonal hypersecretion by pancreatic endocrine tumors (19).

4.2. Radioguided Intraoperative Probe Localization

It has been reported that intraoperative gamma probe examination is able to reveal small gastroenteropancreatic tumor sites accumulating In-111 octreotide more efficiently than scintigraphy alone. Lesions as small as 5 mm can be detected using the gamma probe (20,21), whereas SPECT imaging failed to visualize any lesion small than 9 mm (21). The feasibility of detecting occult endocrine tumors using radioguided intraoperative probe has also been demonstrated (22).

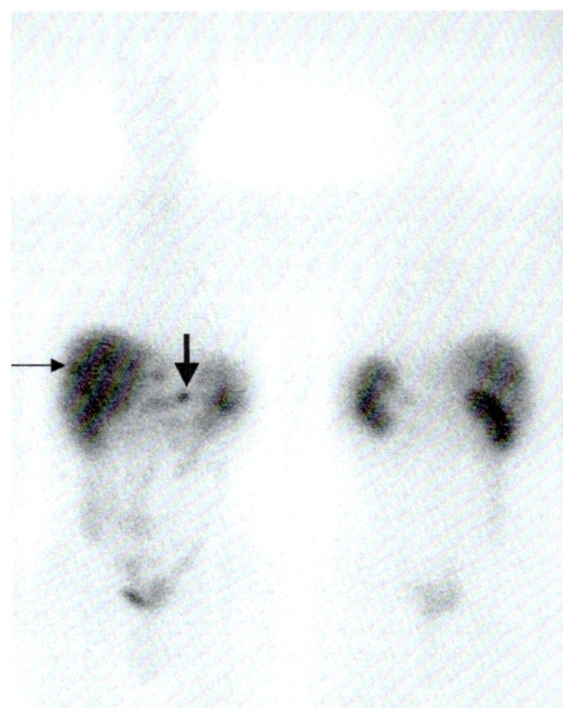

(A)

Figure 3 A patient with Zollinger-Ellison syndrome in whom conventional imaging showed several hepatic lesions but no primary tumor could be found. An In-111 octreotide study was ordered. (A) The whole body planar octreotide images show vague focal activity in the liver (thin arrow) and a focus in the epigastric region (thick arrow), which may represent a part of bowel activity or a tumor. (B) Transverse (2 top panels) and coronal (2 bottom panels) SPECT images clearly demonstrate multiple hepatic lesions as well as a tumor in the pancreatic bed. At surgery, a gastrinoma in the body of pancreas was found.

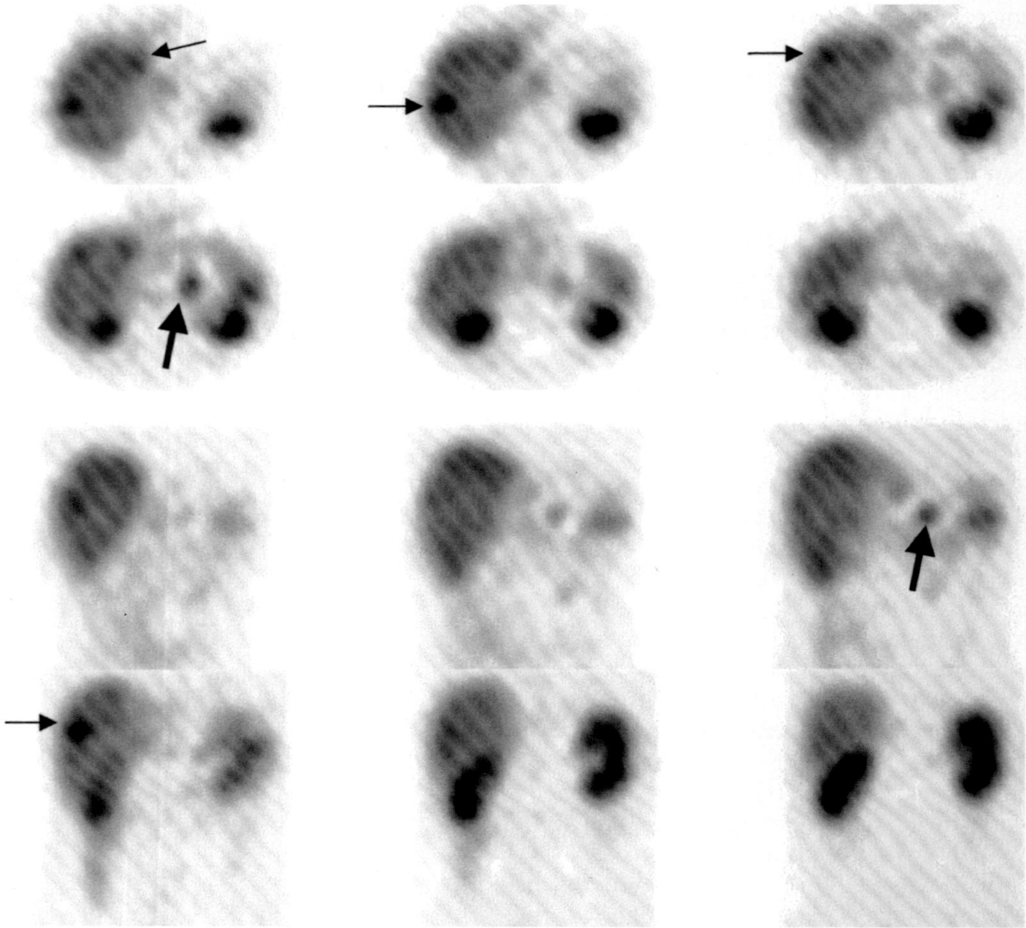

(B)

Figure 3 Continued.

4.3 Differential Diagnosis Between Nonfunctioning Islet Cell Tumors and Pancreatic Duct Cancers

It has been suggested that SRS has a place in the preoperative differential diagnosis of islet cell tumors and pancreatic duct cancers as well as in the follow-up, especially in patients in whom no tumor histological analysis was initially obtained or when the pathological examination of the tumor tissue had not included special staining procedures for neuroendocrine characteristics (23). In this series, SRS visualized the primary pancreatic islet cell tumor as well as previously unrecognized metastases in 31 (65%) of 48 patients, but none of the 26 pancreatic adenocarcinomas or their metastases. Interestingly, SRS revealed metastatic lesions in 5 of the 12 patients who were alive more than 3 years after pancreaticoduodenectomy for pancreatic duct adenocarcinomas. It was subsequently realized that these 5 patients were not operated on for adenocarcinomas but for "nonfunctioning" islet cell tumors.

4.4 Influence of Somatostatin Analogue Therapy on SRS

It has been recommended that somatostatin therapy be withdrawn before scintigraphy because of potential saturation of the receptors by unlabeled somatostatin, which could result in false-negative studies (24). However, more recent studies suggest that tumor-to-background ratio actually increases during treatment with somatostatin analogue compared to the studies performed before the treatment (25,26).

5 OTHER RADIONUCLIDE TECHNIQUES

5.1 SRS Versus Bone Scintigraphy

In a prospective study comparing bone scintigraphy, MRI, and SRS for identifying bone metastases in 115 patients with gastrinomas, SRS and MRI had a higher sensitivity and specificity than bone scintigraphy (27). Between SRS and MRI, SRS was the recommended procedure for screening for bone metastases because bone metastases can occur initially outside the axial skeleton. Another group reported that in patients with GEP tumors, all 19 patients with proven bone metastases had positive SRS and 17 of the 19 had positive bone scintigraphy, although there was no statistically significant difference (28).

5.2 Radiolabeled MIBG Imaging

There is wide variation in the reported sensitivity of MIBG studies in pancreatic endocrine tumors. The reported combined sensitivity (from three reports in the 1980s) is 60% (24). MIBG imaging detected only one of 12 (9%) islet cell carcinomas compared to 11 of 12 patients (92%) with positive octeotide scintigraphy in a recent series (29). Regardless of this variation, SRS is clearly superior in this patient population. MIBG imaging may be helpful in SRS-negative cases.

5.3 Positron Emission Tomography

Fluorine-18 fluorodeoxyglucose is a glucose analogue. Aggressive and proliferative growth of tumors is typically associated with increased uptake of this tracer. As in other tumors, neuroendorine tumors with increased FDG uptake also seem to be characterized by rapid growth or aggressive behavior (30). Other investigators have also shown that well-differentiated neuroendocrine tumors with low proliferative activity tend to concentrate octreotide but not FDG, while less differentiated tumors with high proliferative activity tend to concentrate FDG but not octreotide (31).

6 CONCLUSIONS

Somatostatin receptor scintigraphy using In-111 octreotide is an accurate, cost-effective technique in the diagnostic evaluation of most pancreatic endocrine tumors except for insulinomas. SRS is valuable in the localization of the primary tumor in symptomatic patients, in the localization of occult primary tumors in patients with metastases, in staging for optimal treatment, and in assessing receptor status of the tumor and predicting the outcome of treatment with somatostatin analogue.

REFERENCES

1. de Herder WW, Lamberts SW. Somatostatin and somatostatin analogues: diagnostic and therapeutic uses. Curr Opin Oncol 2002; 14:53–57.
2. Balon HR, Goldsmith SJ, Siegel BA, Silberstein EB, Krenning EP, Lang O, Donohoe KJ. Society of Nuclear Medicine. Procedure guideline for somatostatin receptor scintigraphy with (111)In-pentetreotide. J Nucl Med 2001; 42:1134–1138.
3. Krenning EP, Kwekkeboom DJ, Bakker WH, Breeman WA, Kooij PP, Oei HY, van Hagen M, Postema PT, de Jong M, Reubi JC, et al. Somatostatin receptor scintigraphy with [111In-DTPA-D-Phe1]- and [123I-Tyr3]-octreotide: the Rotterdam experience with more than 1000 patients. Eur J Nucl Med 1993; 20:716–731.
4. Schirmer WJ, Melvin WS, Rush RM, O'Dorisio TM, Pozderac RV, Olsen JO, Ellison EC. Indium-111-pentetreotide scanning versus conventional imaging techniques for the localization of gastrinoma. Surgery 1995; 118: 1105–1113.
5. King CM, Reznek RH, Bomanji J, Ur E, Britton KE, Grossman AB, Besser GM. Imaging neuroendocrine tumours with radiolabeled somatostatin analogues and X-ray computed tomography: a comparative study. Clin Radiol 1993; 48:386–391.
6. Gibril F, Reynolds JC, Chen CC, Yu F, Goebel SU, Serrano J, Doppman JL, Jensen RT. Specificity of somatostatin receptor scintigraphy: a prospective study and effects of false-positive localizations on management in patients with gastrinomas. J Nucl Med 1999; 40:539–553.
7. Krenning EP, Kwekkeboom DJ, Pauwels EK, Kvols LK, Reubi JC. Somatostatin receptor scintigraphy. In: Nuclear Medicine Annual. New York: Raven Press, 1995:1–50.
8. Kvols LK, Brown ML, O'Connor MK, Hung JC, Hayostek RJ, Reubi JC, Lamberts SW. Evaluation of a radiolabeled somatostatin analog (1-123 octreotide) in the detection and localization of carcinoid and islet cell tumors. Radiology 1993; 187:129–133.
9. Le Guludec D, Cadiot G, Lebtahi R, Mignon M. Detection of endocrine tumors of the digestive tract. Value and limitations of scintigraphy of somatostatin receptors. Presse Med 1996; 25:677–682.
10. Schillaci O, Massa R, Scopinaro F. 111In-Pentetreo-

tide scintigraphy in the detection of insulinomas: importance of SPECT imaging. J Nucl Med 2000; 41:459–462.

11. Termanini B, Gibril F, Reynolds JC, Doppman JL, Chen CC, Stewart CA, Sutliff VE, Jensen RT. Value of somatostatin receptor scintigraphy: a prospective study in gastrinoma of its effect on clinical management. Gastroenterology 1997; 112:335–347.
12. Lebtahi R, Cadiot G, Sarda L, Daou D, Faraggi M, Petegnief Y, Mignon M, Le Guludec D. Clinical impact of somatostatin receptor scintigraphy in the management of patients with neuroendocrine gastroenteropancreatic tumors. J Nucl Med 1997; 38:853–858.
13. Alexander HR, Fraker DL, Norton JA, Bartlett DL, Tio L, Benjamin SB, Doppman JL, Goebel SU, Serrano J, Gibril F, Jensen RT. Prospective study of somatostatin receptor scintigraphy and its effect on operative outcome in patients with Zollinger-Ellison syndrome. Ann Surg 1998; 228:228–238.
14. Frilling A, Malago M, tin H, Broelsch CE. Use of somatostatin receptor scintigraphy to image extrahepatic metastases of neuroendocrine tumors. Surgery 1998; 124:1000–1004.
15. Chiti A, Fanti S, Savelli G, Romeo A, Bellanova B, Rodari M, van Graafeiland BJ, Monetti N, Bombardieri E. Comparison of somatostatin receptor imaging, computed tomography and ultrasound in the clinical management of neuroendocrine gastro-entero-pancreatic tumours. Eur J Nucl Med 1998; 25:1396–1403.
16. Shi W, Johnston CF, Buchanan KD, Ferguson WR, Laird JD, Crothers JG, McIlrath EM. Localization of neuroendocrine tumours with [111In] DTPA-octreotide scintigraphy (reoscan): a comparative study with CT and MR imaging. QJM 1998; 91:295–301.
17. Gibril F, Jensen RT. Comparative analysis of diagnostic techniques for localization of gastrointestinal neuroendocrine tumors. Yale J Biol Med 1997; 70:509–522.
18. Virgolini I, Raderer M, Kurtaran A, Angelberger P, Yang Q, Radosavljevic M, Leimer M, Kaserer K, Li SR, Kornek G, Hubsch P, Niederle B, Pidlich J, Scheithauer W, Valent P. 123I-vasoactive intestinal peptide (VIP) receptor scanning: update of imaging results in patients with adenocarcinomas and endocrine tumors of the gastrointestinal tract. Nucl Med Biol 1996; 23:685–692.
19. Lamberts SW, Hofland LJ, van Koetsveld PM, Reubi JC, Bruining HA, Bakker WH, Krenning EP. Parallel in vivo and in vitro detection of functional somatostatin receptors in human endocrine pancreatic tumors: consequences with regard to diagnosis, localization, and therapy. J Clin Endocrinol Metab 1990; 71:566–574.
20. Adams S, Baum RP. Intraoperative use of gamma-detecting probes to localize neuroendocrine tumors. Q J Nucl Med 2000; 44:59–67.
21. Ohrvall U, Westlin JE, Nilsson S, Juhlin C, Rastad J, Lundqvist H, Akerstrom G. Intraoperative gamma detection reveals abdominal endocrine tumors more efficiently than somatostatin receptor scintigraphy. Cancer 1997; 15; 80(suppl 12):2490–2494.
22. Adams S, Baum RP, Hertel A, Wenisch HJ, Staib-Sebler E, Herrmann G, Encke A, Hor G. Intraoperative gamma probe detection of neuroendocrine tumors. J Nucl Med 1998; 39:1155–1160.
23. van Eijck CH, Lamberts SW, Lemaire LC, Jeekel H, Bosman FT, Reubi JC, Bruining HA, Krenning EP. The use of somatostatin receptor scintigraphy in the differential diagnosis of pancreatic duct cancers and islet cell tumors. Ann Surg 1996; 224:119–124.
24. Hoefnagel CA. Metaiodobenzylguanidine and somatostatin in oncology: role in the management of neural crest tumours. Eur J Nucl Med 1994; 21:561–581.
25. Dorr U, Rath U, Sautter-Bihl ML, Guzman G, Bach D, Adrian HJ, Bihl H. Improved visualization of carcinoid liver metastases by indium-111 pentetreotide scintigraphy following treatment with cold somatostatin analogue. Eur J Nucl Med 1993; 20:431–433.
26. Janson ET, Kalkner KM, Eriksson B, Westlin JE, Oberg K. Somatostatin receptor scintigraphy during treatment with lanreotide in patients with neuroendocrine tumors. Nucl Med Biol 1999; 26:877–882.
27. Gibril F, Doppman JL, Reynolds JC, Chen CC, Sutliff VE, Yu F, Serrano J, Venzon DJ, Jensen RT. Bone metastases in patients with gastrinomas: a prospective study of bone scanning, somatostatin receptor scanning, and magnetic resonance image in their detection, frequency, location, and effect of their detection on management. J Clin Oncol 1998; 16:1040–1053.
28. Lebtahi R, Cadiot G, Delahaye N, Genin R, Daou D, Peker MC, Chosidow D, Faraggi M, Mignon M, Le Guludec D. Detection of bone metastases in patients with endocrine gastroenteropancreatic tumors: bone scintigraphy compared with somatostatin receptor scintigraphy. J Nucl Med 1999; 40:1602–1608.
29. Kaltsas G, Korbonits M, Heintz E, Mukherjee JJ, Jenkins PJ, Chew SL, Reznek R, Monson JP, Besser GM, Foley R, Britton KE, Grossman AB. Comparison of somatostatin analog and meta-iodobenzylguanidine radionuclides in the diagnosis and localization of advanced neuroendocrine tumors. J Clin Endocrinol Metab 2001; 86:895–902.
30. Pasquali C, Rubello D, Sperti C, Gasparoni P, Liessi G, Chierichetti F, Ferlin G, Pedrazzoli S. Neuroendocrine tumor imaging: can 18F-fluorodeoxyglucose positron emission tomography detect tumors with poor prognosis and aggressive behavior? World J Surg 1998; 22: 588–592.
31. Adams S, Baum R, Rink T, Schumm-Drager PM, Usadel KH, Hor G. Limited value of fluorine-18 fluorodeoxyglucose positron emission tomography for the imaging of neuroendocrine tumours. Eur J Nucl Med 1998; 25:79–83.

45

Insulinoma

Per Hellman

University Hospital, Uppsala, Sweden

1 INTRODUCTION

Insulinomas are fascinating tumors in terms of their great diversity in symptoms, the difficulties in establishing the diagnosis, and the operative challenge. Although many patients present with obvious symptoms and a clear biochemical diagnosis and the operation is straightforward, other cases may offer the surgeon great difficulties. The main problems are the sometimes nonspecific symptoms not recognized as hypoglycemia, with potential devastating consequences, including permanent hypoglycemic brain damage, the sometimes difficult localization procedures as well as need for correct intraoperative decisions, and the potential of malignancy or multiple tumors as in multiple endocrine neoplasia type 1 (MEN-1). Insulinoma is the most common of several causes for organic hyperinsulinism. A review of this small, often benign, but still dangerous tumor is presented in this chapter.

2 HISTORY

The accumulation of knowledge about insulin and insulin-producing tumors began in the 1920s, when Banting and Best discovered insulin (1), and the first attempt to surgically cure a patient with an unresectable insulin-producing tumor was performed by William J. Mayo (2), followed by the first successful resection of an insulinoma (3). The development of precise diagnostic methods, the introduction of sensitive localization tools, and minimally invasive surgical techniques have all improved our management of these patients.

3 DEMOGRAPHICS

Insulinoma is one of several causes for organic hyperinsulinism. The annual incidence is low—about 4 in 1 million population (4). Epidemiological data of classical insulinoma patients describe a median age of approximately 48 years, but with a considerable range. In the literature, patients from 8 to 88 years of age are reported. Slightly more than half are females (~58%), 7% are ultimately found to suffer from MEN-1, and approximately 8–10% are found to be malignant (4–6).

4 CLINICAL FEATURES

The classical symptoms related to insulinoma described by Whipple and Frautz (7) are (1) symptoms from hypoglycemia like feeling of hunger, tremor, dizziness, etc., (2) plasma glucose levels less than 50 mg/dL, and (3) relief of symptoms after glucose administration. In a recent survey of 65 patients operated on for organic hyperinsulinism, the majority of the patients suffered from these symptoms. However, a majority of the patients also had other symptoms that proved misleading (6). The symptoms are classically divided into neuroglycopenic and sympathethic. The neurological symptoms are the most common, but also most diverse, and range from blurring of vision, diplopia, and headache to paresthesia or even paralysis, most often in the legs (8). The patients often undergo thorough neurological investigations before the diagnosis of hypoglycemia is clear. Some patients also suffer from multiple seizures and may be diagnosed as having epilepsy. In various reports, a fourth to a third of the patients had received different neurological diagnoses before the hypoglycemia was appreciated (6,9). Psychological symptoms may be most apparent to the relatives of hypoglycemic patients. They often described personality changes, various degrees of confusion, and aggressiveness or dementia-like behavior, which often occur fleetingly and are sometimes difficult to recognize, except by the closest relatives. Hypoglycemia may lead to coma in about a third of the patients. Hypoglycemia, whether associated with coma or not, has the risk of causing permanent brain damage and persistent personality changes even after a surgically successful operation (5). Although Whipple's symptomatic triad often is present, it is often not recognized immediately. The neuroglycopenic symptoms, which may be vague and difficult to appreciate, are often the only signs of the underlying insulinoma and should always suggest a diagnosis of hypoglycemia due to organic hyperinsulinism (8).

The neuroglycopenic symptoms may be accompanied by a sympathethic neural response with sweating, weakness, hunger, tremor, nausea, and palpitations. Another common symptom is weight gain, a result of the increased intake of carbohydrates over a long time period. The symptoms may vary among the hypoglycemic individuals, although each patient seems to respond similarly during each attack. The symptoms may lead to various incidents among the patients, including the relatively high frequency of patients involved in traffic accidents (6). The onset of symptoms may precede the diagnosis by a considerably long interval—in one European study an average of 3.1 years and in the Mayo Clinic series 46 months—and individual patients may have suffered several decades before diagnosis, as was the case of one patient in the Mayo series who had a 52-year-long history (6,10).

5 PHYSIOLOGY AND PATHOPHYSIOLOGY

Proinsulin is produced in the pancreatic β cell and before secretion cleaved into insulin and the remaining C-peptide (11). The secretory granules consist of equal molar amounts of insulin and C-peptide, which is important in the diagnostic assay (see below). In addition, exogenously administered insulin contains no C-peptide, which together with the longer half-life of C-peptide makes serum levels of this cleavage product an important marker to discover the occasional patients with facticious hypoglycemia due to self-administration of insulin or oral sulfonylurea preparations. Such individuals do occur (12) and are reported among patients who have undergone diagnostic and even operative procedures for supposed organic hyperinsulinism and hypoglycemia (6,13).

The unregulated autonomous secretion of insulin is characteristic of an insulin-producing tumor. Thus, even though serum glucose levels decline, and may worsen during fasting or physical exercise, the insulin level remains at the same level, although not necessary pathologically high. Although the most frequent tumor is the small (< 2 cm) and benign one, other patients present with larger and obviously malignant and metastatic tumors. Patients with such insulin-producing malignant tumors have poor survival prospects, often less than 1 year, and unless a life-saving procedure is needed, surgery is rarely performed. Some patients suffer from large pancreatic tumors classified as nonfunctioning, and many patients with malignant tumors may secrete a high proportion of proinsulin, proposed as a marker of a more malignant feature.

Occasional ovarian carcinomas may rarely produce insulin. In addition, insulin growth factor-II may, if secreted in sufficient amounts, also cause hypoglycemia by binding to the insulin receptors. Such a mechanism may rarely be seen in hepatocellular carcinoma and breast carcinoma (14,15).

The cause for insulinoma is obscure. In a minority of patients, hereditary genomic derangements are present, such as mutation in the menin gene in MEN-1. In one series this gene was not found to be involved in sporadic cases (16). Other reports demonstrate a gain at chromosome locus 9q34 in insulinomas and a potential tumor suppressor gene on chromosome 3p in the development of malignant tumors (17,18).

6 BIOCHEMICAL ASSAYS

6.1 Basal Measurements

The traditional diagnostic approach in suspected insulin-producing tumors includes measurements of s-glucose (and s-insulin) during a crisis, after a prolonged fast, and during physical exercise. Basal levels during a symptomatic event are in many cases diagnostic (6), and the diagnosis of insulinoma should be suspected if glucose levels are less than 40 mg/dL (2 mmol/L). In addition, a normal serum glucose level during a crisis excludes insulinoma as a diagnosis. Serum insulin is nowadays measured by highly sensitive immunoradiometric or enzyme-linked immunological methods. The s-insulin level may, however, not be raised when measured during a hypoglycemic attack; in one series only 10 out of 29 patients had elevated s-insulin (6). However, lack of feedback regulation of insulin secretion in patients with hypoglycemia implies that a detectable s-insulin in patients with s-glucose < 40 mg/dL (2 mmol/L) supports a diagnosis of insulinoma (19). Some authors have advocated measurements of the insulin/glucose ratio as a more sensitive diagnostic tool (10,20). The limitations for the successful use of this method are supported by the finding that only 2 out 15 patients reported by Hellman et al. (6) reached the proposed pathological ratio of 0.4 (s-glucose measured in mg/dL and s-insulin in μU/mL), and in a Mayo series only 19% had a ratio of < 0.3 (19). Proinsulin may be selectively measured by specific assays, and also reported to be pathologically high in insulinoma patients (21). The normal ratio of proinsulin/insulin of 20% is thus exceeded in insulinoma patients, and ratios above 50% have been proposed to indicate malignancy, consistent with excess secretion of the more immature proinsulin peptide. However, there are few reports in the literature that clarify this approach.

In patients who have cross-reacting circulating insulin autoantibodies, diagnostic testing is difficult, and the results may mimic insulinoma (22). On the other hand, C-peptide levels may still be indicative of the diagnosis in these patients.

6.2 Provocative Testing

6.2.1 Fasting Test

The most frequently used diagnostic test is a prolonged fast aimed at lasting 48–72 hours (5,20). The fast must be supervised since the patient may develop symptoms, but also to hinder patients from taking food to reduce the developing symptoms. The latter is not unusual and must be clearly explained to the patients. It is unusual that patients with insulinomas reach 72 hours of fasting. In one series only 2 out of 56 patients managed to suffer through the 48 hours the test was planned for (6). Diagnostic assays of the fasting test are s-glucose and s-insulin levels, as well as the insulin/glucose ratio. Supportive are developing neuroglycopenic symptoms. The diagnosis of organic hyperinsulinism has been reported to be precise in 70–80% after a 24-hour, in 90–95% after a 48-hour, and in 98–100% after a 72-hour fast (23,24). The test is discontinued when the patient develops severe symptoms. Blood samples for s-glucose and s-insulin measurements are drawn initially and regularly during the fasting period. In addition, samples for C-peptide levels, β-hydroxybutyrate, and sulfonylurea are drawn to detect signs of exogenously administered drugs. In case of an insulinoma, insulin/glucose ratios during a fast should slowly rise as the s-glucose levels falls, since the autonomous s-insulin level remains. Thus, a pathological insulin/glucose ratio profile is indicative of an insulinoma (25). In one series the insulin/glucose ratios were above 0.4 in 86% of the patients at the end of the fast (6). The fasting test has a high positive predictive value, while a negative result is difficult to interpret and does occur in patients who had successful resection of insulinoma. Also, unusually low levels of s-insulin in association with hypoglycemia have been documented in insulinoma patients (26).

If the diagnosis is still uncertain after the fasting test, the test should be repeated. In addition, there are a number of different provocative tests that can be used.

6.2.2 Tolbutamide Test

Tolbutamide stimulates insulin secretion and causes a hypoglycemic response and seems to cause an exaggerated release of insulin from insulinoma cells compared to normal β cells. If tolbutamide is infused during a 2-minute period, s-glucose should decrease by 50% after 30 minutes followed by a return to normal levels. Sustained hypoglycemia and associated hyperinsulinemia 3 hours after tolbutamide infusion is indicative of insulinoma. The test is positive in 80% of the cases (10), but is rarely used nowadays.

6.2.3 C-Peptide Suppression Test

Exogenous insulin—not containing C-peptide—is infused to produce hypoglycemia less than 40 mg/dL. Normal individuals suppress their endogenous insulin/C-peptide secretion during the infusion, while insulinoma patients present with persistently elevated C-peptide levels, due to the autonomous secretion from the tumor (27). However, the test is not specific for insulinoma (28), and is rarely used.

7 LOCALIZATION

7.1 Noninvasive Methods

7.1.1 Background

The majority of the literature has concluded that the best method for localizing an insulinoma is intraoperative palpation and intraoperative ultrasound.

Therefore, some authors have questioned the use of preoperative localization procedures (29). However, preoperative radiological examinations should always be performed, not for localization of the insulinoma, but to rule out hepatic and lymph node metastases. Indeed, there are authors who conclude that preoperative localization procedures are helpful in selected cases (20). An obvious fact is that none of the noninvasive localization procedures used—transabdominal ultrasound (US), computed tomography (CT), magnetic resonance imaging (MRI), octreoscan (OCT), or positron-emission tomography (PET)—have been a success. Sensitivity figures ranging from 11 to 64% have been reported in different series (9,13,20,30–32). All authors agree that indications for surgery is a clear biochemical diagnosis and that preoperative localization is unnecessary. However, in certain situations, especially in cases of reoperation, localization, including invasive methods, may be very helpful. Reoperation may be needed in the minority of patients who have undergone a negative open laparotomy or laparoscopy (insulinoma "not found"?, nesidioblastosis?), who develop recurrent insulinomas and possibly suffer from malignant insulinomas or unrecognized MEN-1.

7.1.2 Transabdominal Ultrasound

Transabdominal ultrasound is extremely operator-dependent and based on the patient's habitus, which are the main limitations with this method. However, it is cheap, and some authors describe an almost acceptable sensitivity (64%) (9), even though range is wide (8–64%), and many reports call attention to a comparably high false-positive rate (9,13,20,30–33).

7.1.3 Computed Tomography

CT is a readily available method, and is useful in determining extrapancreatic spread of disease, although the sensitivity for localization of the insulinoma is poor. However, the technique is constantly improving, with new scanners, software, dynamic scanning techniques with intravenous contrast, etc.

7.1.4 Magnetic Resonance Imaging

A few authors report up to 100% sensitivity with gadolinium-enhanced and fat-suppressed MRI, but the technique is not widely used (34,35).

7.1.5 Somatostatin Receptor Scintigraphy and PET

Somatostatin receptor scintigraphy is useful for detection of most abdominal endocrine tumors due to the comparably high expression levels of somatostatin receptors. However, while most endocrine tumors are 80–100% sensitive, the level of detection for insulinomas remains at about 60% (36,37). This is most likely explained by the somewhat lower expression of somatostatin receptors in these tumors compared to other abdominal as well as pancreatic endocrine tumors. Injection of isotope-labeled somatostatin analogs (octreotide) and intraoperative detection of the primary as well as secondary tumors using a hand-held gamma counter may be useful in the future. A few reports reveal that development of this technique is currently taking place (38,39).

PET may be used with different tracers, where 5-hydroxy-tryptophane (HTP) and possibly 18F-fluorodeoxyglucose (FDG) are useful for neuroendocrine pancreatic tumors (40). However, the success for insulinomas is low, and few series are hitherto reported.

7.2 Invasive Methods

Invasive methods are arterial angiography, transhepatic portal venous sampling, selective arterial calcium stimulation, the promising endoscopic ultrasonography, and finally the widely used intraoperative sonography and palpation.

7.2.1 Endoscopic Ultrasound (EUS)

Endoscopic ultrasound (EUS) is an improvement of the transabdominal ultrasound. This method is perhaps even more operator-dependent than the regular ultrasound, but nevertheless has a high accuracy in the right hands (Fig. 1). Thus, both disappointing and impressive sensitivity rates are reported (41–44). The technique will most likely be increasingly used in the future. Two main instruments are available—one with a rotating radial scanner allowing constant visualization of 360° and one with a sector scanner.

7.2.2 Intraoperative Palpation and Ultrasound

The main and most important localization methods that always should be used are the intraoperative thorough palpation of the entire pancreas and intraoperative ultrasound (IOUS) (Figs. 2–7). The sensitivity of palpation varies between 75 and 95% but is dependent on the experience of the surgeon (9). The most difficult insulinomas to palpate are the smaller tumors in the pancreatic head, which emphasize the importance of a complete mobilization of the entire pancreas. IOUS has been proven successful with sensitivity rates around 75–90% without palpation (45,46). However, the combined technique of palpation and

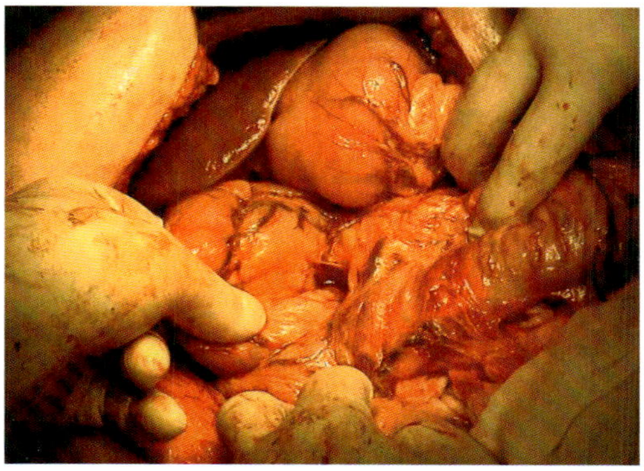

Figure 2 Intraoperative palpation of the pancreatic head after a thorough Kocher's mobilization.

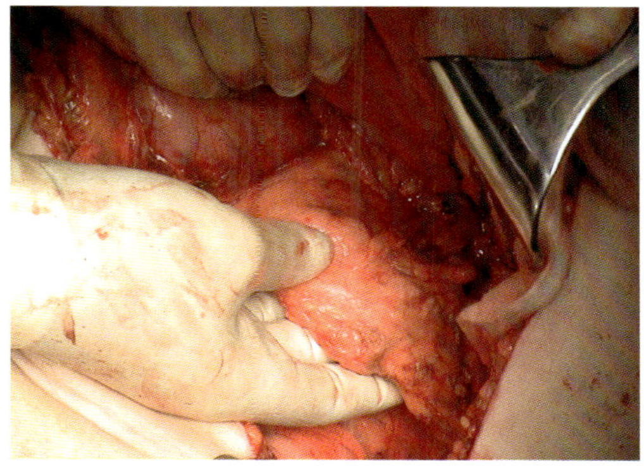

Figure 3 Intraoperative palpation of the pancreatic body and tail after opening of the lesser sac and mobilization of the left pancreas.

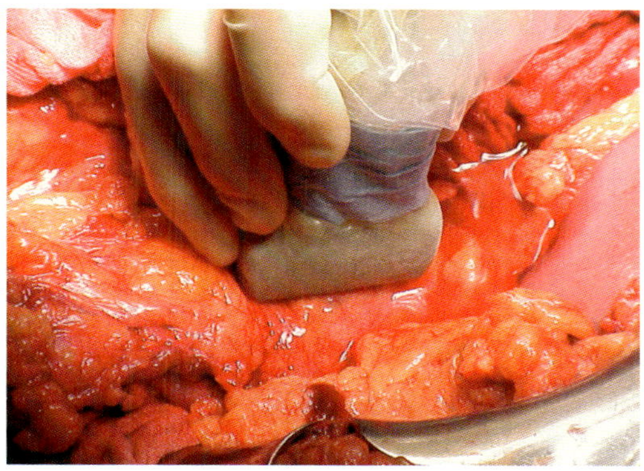

Figure 4 Intraoperative ultrasound of the pancreas. The ultrasonic probe may be applied in direct contact with the pancreatic surface. Resolution may be enhanced by introduction of saline into the operative field.

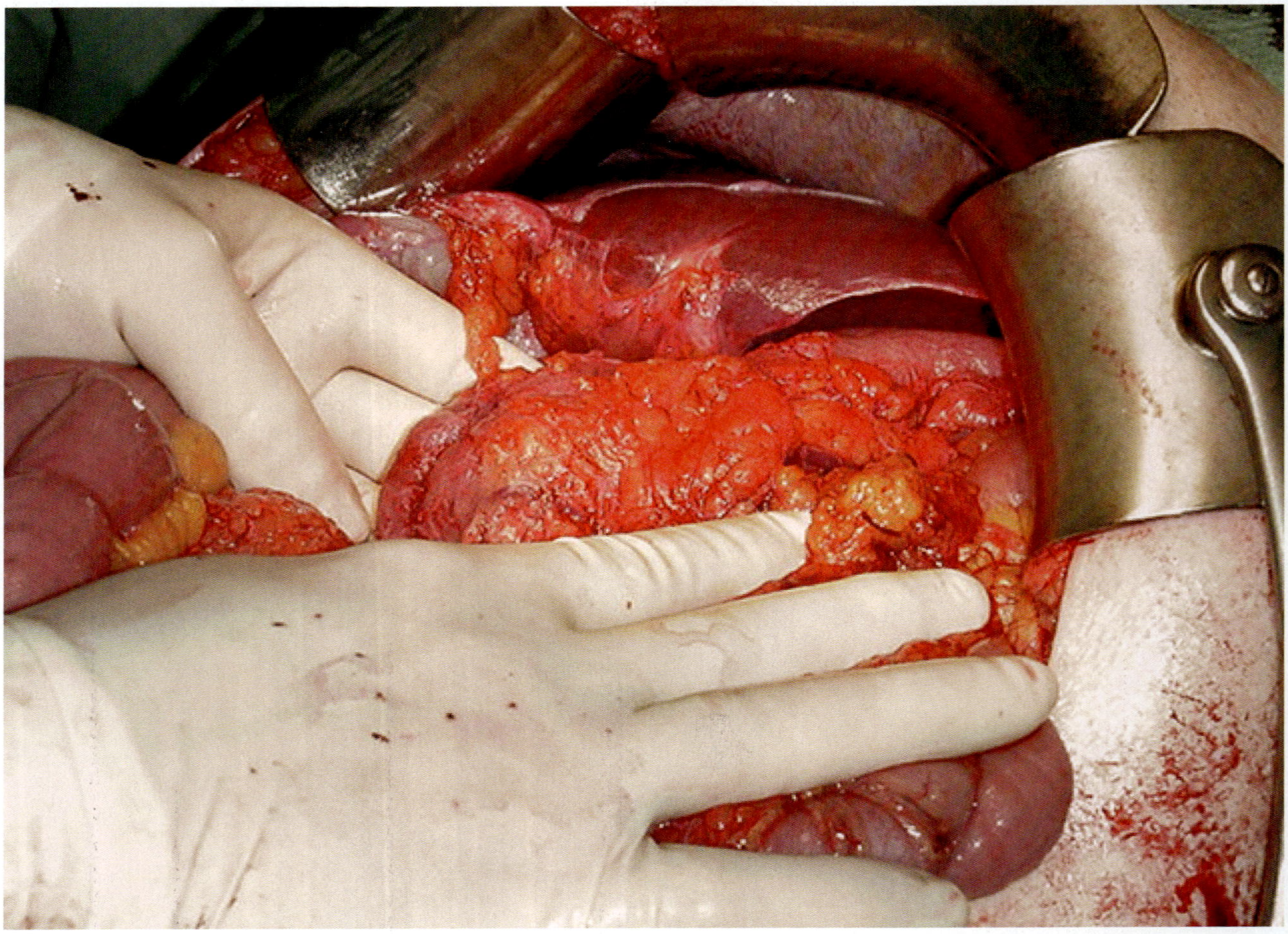

Figure 7 Bimanual palpation of the pancreas, allowing sensitive examination of the tissue.

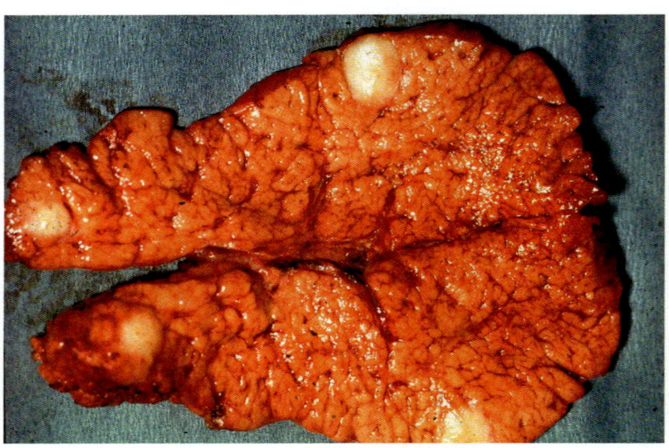

Figure 9 Multiple tumors in a specimen from a patient with MEN-1.

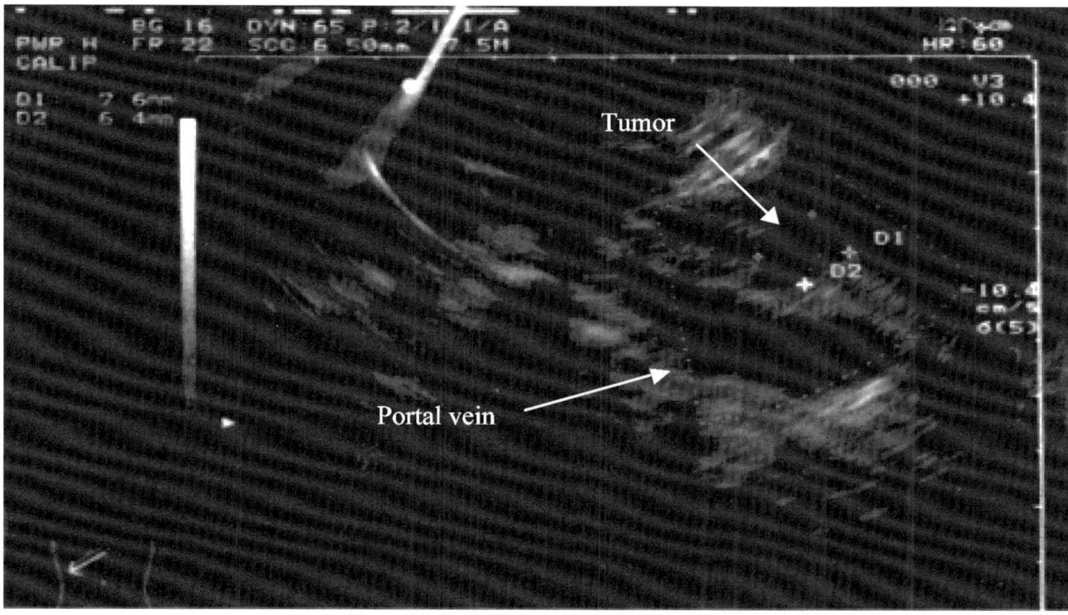

Figure 1 Endoscopic ultrasound picture of a 7.6 × 6.4 mm insulinoma not recognized by transabdominal ultrasound or CT. The endoscopic ultrasound was performed with a radial scanner on the Pentax FG-32 endoscope, at 7.5 MHz, with the probe in the prepyloric area of the stomach.

ultrasound enhance the sensitivity to nearly 100%. Many authors describe the introduction of IOUS as a breakthrough in the surgical handling of these tumors (47). At the Mayo Clinic, IOUS is being used as the main localization procedure, although a preoperative transabdominal US is also performed (19). The success of IOUS is also supported by several series, including one from Düsseldorf with only one failure in 65 cases (6). IOUS also defines the relationship of the pancreatic and bile ducts, and the portal vein to the tumor, which is important in the decision making regarding the type of resection.

7.2.3 Arterial Angiography

Before the era of IOUS, the most sensitive method and the gold standard for localization of insulinoma was arteriography. Indeed, as late as 1998 it was recommended by the American College of Surgeons as the best diagnostic method in these patients. The background for success is the high vascularity of insulinomas, which may be readily seen on the radiographic images as a distinctive blush (48). In different series the sensitivity is not as high as initially stated, with rates between 29 and 75%, possibly relating to different expertise with the method (6,13,20,31,49). The use of this method has declined in recent years, and it is being utilized in selected cases only.

7.2.4 Selective Arterial Calcium Stimulation with Hepatic Venous Sampling

Calcium stimulates insulin secretion and may be used to increase the insulin release from insulinomas (50). This is a feature of the Imamura test, initially used for regionalization of gastrinomas. In this method, a catheter

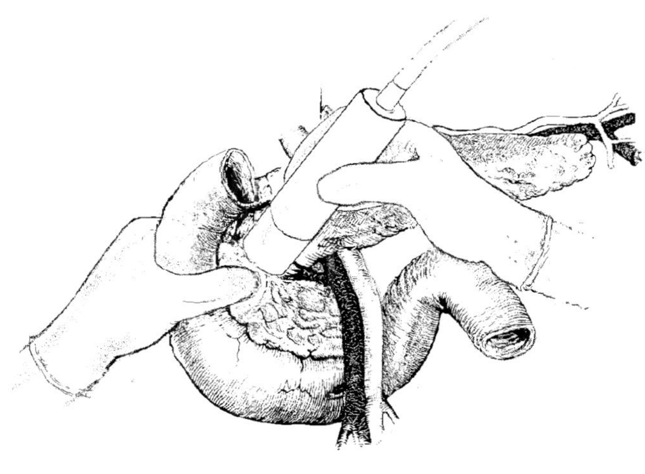

Figure 5 Schematic picture of intraoperative palpation of the pancreatic head in conjunction with ultrasound. A thorough search using these techniques simultaneously is preferred.

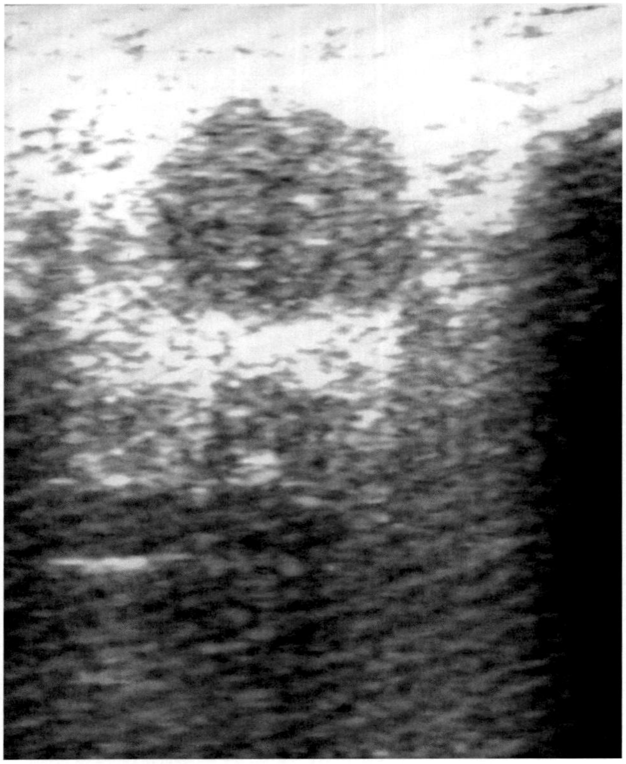

Figure 6 Ultrasonic picture of insulinoma found during intraoperative ultrasound and verified with palpation.

is placed in the gastroduodenal, splenic, common hepatic, and superior meseneteric arteries, through which calcium gluconate is infused, leading to selective stimulation of different parts of the pancreas. A venous catheter is placed in a hepatic vein through which blood samples are drawn before injection as well as after 30, 60, and 120 seconds (Fig. 8). Regionalization of the insulinoma is possible after evaluation of the insulin concentrations in the samples collected after stimulation of different parts of the pancreas (51). Some authors, including investigators at the National Institutes of Health (NIH), report a high success rate of precise regionalization, while the Mayo Clinic seems more hesitant to adopt this method (19,52,53). An advantage of the method is the technical similarity to regular arteriography, which is performed at the same session.

7.2.5 Transhepatic Portal Venous Sampling

Previously, portal venous sampling was used as a regionalizing method taking advantage of the fact that insulin is secreted into the portal venous system. Nowadays this method is rarely used, except in complicated reoperative cases. The method has a high sensitivity for regionalization to the head, body, or tail. The transhepatic catheter is introduced into the portal, splenic, and superior mesenteric veins, and multiple samples are drawn for assays of insulin. In the right hands, sensitivity rates up to 80–100% have been reported (9,20,33). The main disadvantage is the morbidity from the transhepatic instrumentation, as well as the time span of the learning curve (24).

7.3 Recommendations

Local traditions influence the preoperative localization procedures, which should not be initiated unless the diagnosis is clear. In a previously unoperated patient, a CT scan is useful to screen for extrapancreatic spread, although one should not anticipate localization of the primary tumor. Transcutaneous abdominal ultrasound may also be performed for the same reason. If EUS is available, it may be added to the preoperative work-up, because of the greater sensitivity of this modality. Whether these procedures are negative or positive, the next localization procedures are the intraoperative palpation and IOUS. A vast majority of the patients (up to 98%) is cured when using this algorithm. In patients where neither the pre- nor the intraoperative localization procedure is successful, and in those who present with recurrent hypoglycemia, other approaches are indicated. Intraoperative failure to find an insulinoma should not lead to blind resections of the pancreas, but rather to closing the abdominal wound. These patients should undergo repeated diagnostic and localization efforts as before the initial operation (CT, transabdominal US, EUS). In such situations localization efforts should be thorough, including use of selective arterial calcium stimulation in conjunction with conventional arterial angiography. In a personal series, we found the evasive tumor in the pancreatic head by repeated EUS, allowing cure after pancreaticoduodenectomy. PET scan and somatostatin receptor scintigraphy has been proven useful in occasional cases. In addition, a thorough search for hereditary disease (MEN-1), including evaluation of the parathyroid and pituitary function, should be performed. These patients may express several small tumors throughout the entire pancreas, which may be missed during the intraoperative imaging. However, the microadenomas in the MEN-1 pancreas rarely cause hypoglycemia (54). Nevertheless, one may consider sequencing of the MEN-1 gene, which is now available. If regionalization of the insulin production is clear, one may proceed with a reoperation, either a left-sided pancreatic resection or

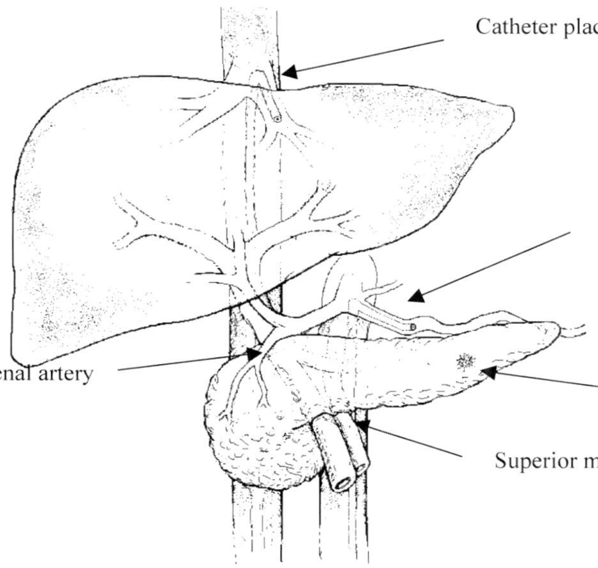

Figure 8 Schematic drawing of selective arterial calcium stimulation with hepatic venous sampling. Through the catheter, which may be placed into the gastroduodenal, splenic (as in the drawing), superior mesenteric arteries, or even to evaluate liver metastases into the common hepatic artery, calcium is infused. Blood samples are drawn in a catheter placed in the hepatic veins. This method is preferentially used in selected patients only, for instance before a reoperation, and may be performed in conjunction with a regular arterial angiography.

a pancreaticoduodenectomy. In the extremely rare but doubtful cases, other procedures like transhepatic portal venous sampling may be performed.

8 PATHOLOGY

While most cases of organic hyperinsulinism are due to the classical solitary benign insulinoma, multiple or malignant tumors may also appear. In addition, a minority of patients may suffer from adult nesidioblastosis associated with considerable difficulties in localization and surgical decision making. A number of published series have documented that up to a fourth or even a third of patients operated on for organic hyperinsulinism may harbor findings other than a benign solitary insulinoma (6,55).

8.1 Benign Solitary Insulinoma

The tumor size may range from 0.1 to 10 cm, the overwhelming majority averaging 1.5 cm in size, and 90% less than 2 cm. They are usually yellow-brownish and have a pseudo-capsule, which allows extirpation without seriously affecting the surrounding normal pancreas. They may reside anywhere in the pancreas, and ectopic location is extremely rare. The detection of insulin is generally obvious in postoperative immunohistochemistry, but may be surprisingly low in selected cases, perhaps due to the rapid flux and high turnover of the peptides. In other cases greater detection of proinsulin is seen. This marker has been coupled to higher risk of malignancy, although clearly benign cases also express more proinsulin than insulin.

8.2 Multiple Insulinomas and MEN-1

Multiple tumors are present in 7–17% of different series of patients. In such cases, MEN-1 must be suspected, especially in younger patients. Among all patients with organic hyperinsulinism about 4–10% has MEN-1 (56). To avoid intraoperative surprises, all patients with organic hyperinsulinism should be evaluated for possible MEN-1, including a thorough family history, and search for hyperparathyroidism, which is the most common associated manifestation. However, in a recent report 6 out of 8 patients with multiple insulinomas could not be proven to have MEN-1, in 2 cases also after genetic sequencing (6). Thus, it appears that there are other sporadic or hereditary causes for multiple insulinomas than MEN-1. It should also be noted that the MEN-1 patients usually demonstrate a number of pancreatic tumors, ranging in size from microscopically small over the whole pancreas to largely invasive and malignant tumors (Fig. 9). These tumors may produce a variety of hormones. Subsets of these tumors may produce insulin, sometimes due to the size of the tumor, in large enough amounts to cause organic hyperinsulinism with the classical symptoms thereof (54).

8.3 Malignant Insulinomas

Malignant insulinomas may be discovered pre- or intraoperatively by the finding of metastases or tumor infiltration, or postoperatively by the pathologist who detects microscopic infiltration. The rate of malignancy is about 8–10% in different series (6,57,58). Unless the tumor is widely spread, tumor resection is indicated to reduce troublesome hypoglycemia. Since a number of tumors are found to be malignant only in the histopathological examination of the specimen, one may argue against enucleation as the procedure of choice in order to comply with oncological principles. However, these findings are extremely rare and do not justify pancreatic resections in all cases. Instead one may consider enucleation including a rim of normal pancreatic tissue in cases where the pseudocapsular margin is unclear or the size is >2 cm. In case of noncurative extended enucleation a reoperative resection may have to be performed. In case of liver metastases these should be treated with any of the available methods (surgical resection, radiofrequency ablation, liver embolization, chemotherapy). Some patients with malignant insulinomas, however, have a rapidly progressing disease and short survival prospects and do not benefit from surgery (59).

8.4 Adult Nesidioblastosis

This disease is widely debated, with some authors questioning its presence and others finding impressive rates among their patients with organic hyperinsulinism (19,26). However, histopathological examinations have classified a pattern seen in such adult patients with hypertrophy of islet cells and hormonally active cells budding off the ductular epithelium (60). In addition, surgical resection of the pancreas have clearly benefited such patients (6). In a Japanese survey of 1085 cases with hypoglycemia due to hyperinsulinism, 44 cases with signs of nesidioblastosis were found (4.1%). Interesting, in 28 of these cases (2.8%) a concomitant insulinoma was also found (55). A similar case was observed in the Düsseldorf series (6), in which the author participated. To be noted are findings in autopsy material of normoglycemic patients bearing histopathological similarities to nesidioblastosis, indicating that this diagnosis may be an extreme variant of normal histology. However, it should be suspected that patients with MEN-1 were included in these reports.

Patients with nesidioblastosis may be among those with negative preoperative localization attempts, negative IOUS, and intraoperative palpation. It has been widely debated how to manage such patients, but most authors seem to agree that the abdomen should be closed and repeated, extensive testing should be performed (see above).

9 MEDICAL TREATMENT

The ultimate goal for the medical treatment is to avoid hypoglycemic episodes. Therefore, the patient should be told to have frequent meals and snacks and to avoid prolonged intervals without intake of carbohydrates. This means that the patient has to wake up at night for a meal. Diazoxide is an antihypertensive and hyperglycemic drug, which suppresses insulin secretion and enhances glycogenolysis (61). In a patient with a benign insulinoma it is usually possible to avoid this drug. It is also important to await introduction of diazoxide until after the diagnosis of organic hyperinsulinism is clear to avoid difficult work-up. However, in malignant disease one often has to introduce the drug early, which has a number of negative effects: edema, hypotension, weight gain, nausea, and hirsutism. Diazoxide may be necessary in patients with malignant insulinoma, which is not resectable. There are few alternatives; although somatostatin analogues may inhibit insulin secretion, success is limited since these tumors express a lower number of somatostatin receptors. Glucagon may be used as a hyperglycemic drug, and verapamil, which interferes with the calcium channels in the insulin-producing cells, has been used in cases of malignant insulinomas as well as adult nesidioblastosis (62,63).

10 SURGICAL APPROACH

10.1 Exploration

A bilateral subcostal incision is made. A thorough examination of the peritoneal cavity is performed to rule out metastatic disease. The first aim is to perform a thorough visualization and exploration of the entire pancreas. A Kocher's maneuver is performed, after retraction of the hepatic colonic flexure, if necessary. The mobilization of the pancreatic head should be complete until the aorta can be palpated with the fingers. The mobilization of duodenum continues downward to include the third horizontal part. The mesentery of the transverse colon should be dissected away, and the superior mesenteric vein and its tributaries should be exposed. The lesser sac is now entered, either by lifting the major omentum from the transverse colon and retracting it upwards together with the stomach, or by dividing the gastrocolic ligament, distal to the gastro-epiploic vessels, but well away from the colonic mesentery. The lower border of the pancreatic body and tail is now visualized. The adhesions between the posterior surface of the stomach and the anterior surface of the pancreas are divided. The peritoneum along the inferior border of the pancreas is incised, the transverse mesocolon separated, and the distal pancreas mobilized by using blunt technique. The splenic artery should be identified along its entire course. The far end of the tail may be mobilized together with the spleen after dividing the lieno-colic ligament. The tail can now be lifted up together with the spleen. After this thorough mobilization of the pancreas, bimanual palpation and IOUS is performed (Figs. 2–7). Thus, even if an insulinoma is found early in the course, the whole pancreas should be examined to avoid missing multiple tumors. The tumors are usually visible on the surface but are occasionally embedded within the parenchyma. IOUS is performed not only to scan the whole pancreas for tumors, but also to examine the course of the pancreatic and bile ducts, as well as the relation of the tumor to the vessels, mainly the portal and splenic veins.

10.2 Selecting the Resection Procedure

Pancreatic surgery has been associated with a high complication rate, mostly from leakage of pancreatic fluid and development of fistulas and pseudocysts. These complications as well as the history of high morbidity after pancreaticoduodenectomies have had a hampering effect on the performance of pancreatric surgery, sometimes creating a conservative attitude. However, modern techniques, novel suture materials, and refinement of indications have reduced the rate of complications after pancreatic surgery.

Different authors reported an increased risk of leakage when handling insulinomas in the pancreatic head, whether by enucleation or resection (6,58). It is concluded that for pancreatic head tumors it is important to define the relationship of the pancreatic and bile ducts and the vessels to the tumor. If the tumor is well away from these structures, enucleation is the method of choice. Even though it is rarely needed for insulinomas, a pancreaticoduodenectomy can be performed, even for benign disease. Recent improvement in surgical techniques, postoperative care, and surgical expertise have made this operation possible with minimal morbidity and mortality (64,65).

Some authors have noticed higher risk of fistula formation after enucleation in the pancreatic neck (66). This was attributed to the oblique course of the pancreatic duct and the confluence with the accessory duct of Santorini in this part of the pancreas. Again, IOUS is helpful in clarifying the anatomical landmarks. The majority of the tumors in the uncinate process of the head, the neck, as well as the body of the pancreas may be enucleated. If the selection of the type of procedure is difficult, a resection should be performed. Alternatives that may be rarely used are duodenum-preserving resection of the pancreatic head and neck (Beger's procedure) or central pancreatectomy (67,68).

Tumors in the pancreatic tail may also be enucleated, especially the ones close to the body or protruding from the margin of the pancreas, but a liberal attitude towards a spleen-preserving left-sided pancreatic resection is suggested.

In case of multiple tumors or findings of malignancy, resection is proposed. While many authors advocate a left-sided resection up to the portal vein and enucleations from the pancreatic head, others have suggested a more radical extended subtotal pancreatic resection, especially in families where malignant pancreatic tumors are known to occur (54). However, if MEN-1 is suspected intraoperatively, a left-sided resection combined with enucleations from the head is sufficient, followed by a thorough postoperative work-up to confirm the diagnosis and proceed with extended pancreatic reresection later.

10.3 Enucleation

The insulinomas usually have a pseudocapsule making it possible to enter a plane between the tumor and the surrounding normal pancreatic tissue. If the tumor is found to have unclear margins during the dissection and suspicions of malignancy appear, conversion to a resective procedure is proposed. By using a meticulous technique, fine instruments, and multiple ligations with polypropylene 5-0 or 6-0, a safe enucleation can be performed (Fig. 10). If there is suspicion of injury to the pancreatic duct, intravenous secretin will visualise extravasation of pancreatic fluid from the resected area. An injured duct may be closed using fine sutures (N. Thompson, personal communication), or, alternatively, the operation is converted to a resection. Helpful in the dissection is to lift the pancreas with one hand and, if possible, pull the tumor upwards with a stitch placed through it. The defect should not be closed, since injury

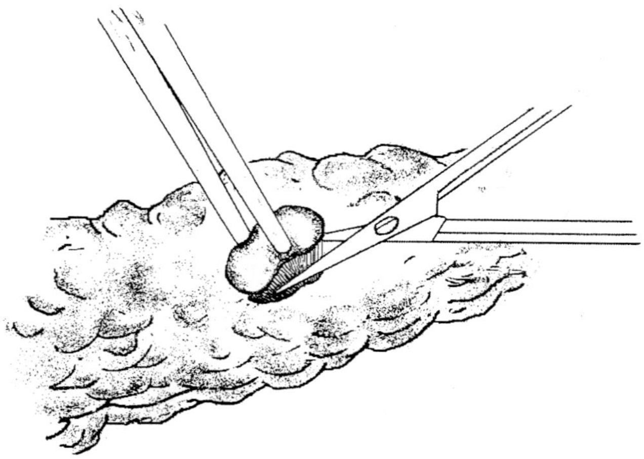

Figure 10 Schematic drawing of an enucleation of an insulinoma. Meticulous technique and fine instruments and sutures should be used.

to the pancreatic tissue is likely to result in development of a pancreatic pseudocyst. It is wise to put some fibrin glue and possibly an omental flap to cover the defect. The area of enucleation should be carefully drained.

10.4 Left-Sided Pancreatic Resection

A spleen-preserving left-sided pancreatic resection is a safe procedure (69). The pancreatic tail is mobilized from the splenic vessels, often by dividing several smaller branches. A thorough search for the main pancreatic duct in the remaining pancreas is suggested, since ligation of this presumably reduces the risk of postoperative leakage. The pancreas may be cut with a scalpel according to the "fish-mouth" technique. Smaller bleeders should be suture ligated with polypropylene 5-0 or 6-0. The cut edge is then carefully closed with sutures, avoiding large bites of pancreatic tissue in order to reduce the risk of devascularization. Fibrin glue is applied to the cut edge, and the area is carefully drained.

10.5 Pylorus-Preserving Pancreaticoduodenectomy

The pylorus-preserving pancreaticoduodenectomy is a modification of the classical Whipple's procedure. In selected large and invasive cases an extended operation including resection of the mesenteric and portal veins may be needed (70). In brief, after thorough examination of the entire pancreas, attention is drawn to the pancreatic head, and the common bile duct, common hepatic artery and portal vein are exposed and isolated. The portal vein is freed and followed underneath the pancreatic neck. A similar dissection is performed from below to isolate the mesenteric vein until the two veins are separated from the pancreatic neck using blunt dissection. The next step is ligation and division of the gastroduodenal artery, and the common hepatic artery is dissected away from the suprapancreatic area. To allow isolation of the uncinate process, the arterial branches and venous tributaries of the mesenteric vessels should be divided. Three structures now have to be divided: (1) jejunum, approximately 20 cm inferior to Treitz's ligament; (2) duodenum; (3) common bile duct. The latter is usually divided immediately above the entrance of the cystic duct, making a cholecystectomy necessary. Jejunum is divided with a stapler while the proximal duodenum is divided with a scalpel after clamping the antrum. Duodenum and the proximal jejunum are transposed to the right. Pancreas is now divided over the portal vein, and the pancreatic duct identified in the preserved part. The specimen is now free, and the reconstruction phase begins. An end-to-side pancreaticojejunostomy is performed using polydioxanone 4-0 and the classical invaginating technique with an inner row of sutures between the jejunal mucosa and the pancreatic rim, including the edges of the pancreatic duct, and an outer layer between jejunal serosa approximately 1 cm from the cut opening in the side of the gut and the pancreatic capsule. One may insert a small 3 cm piece of a pediatric feeding tube into the duct before closing the anastomosis. An end-to-side hepaticojejunostomy is constructed with polydioxanone 4-0 in a single layer. If the hepatic duct is narrow one may consider using a stent to avoid stricture of the anastomosis. The catheter is passed down in the jejunal loop for about 10 cm before exiting through the intestinal and abdominal walls. The duodenojejunostomy is also constructed end-to-side with a single layer of running sutures of polydioxanone 4-0. A drain is used and positioned near the pancreatic and biliary anastomoses.

10.6 Minimally Invasive Techniques

The development of laparoscopic surgery has also made it possible to enucleate insulinomas and perform distal pancreatic resections (71–75). The key to a technically successful laparoscopic operation of an insulinoma is a thorough exploration of the entire pancreas. As in open surgery, even though one tumor may be immediately seen, one has to examine the whole pancreas for the possibility of multiple tumors. Since bimanual palpation is impossible, one has to rely on laparoscopic ultrasound imaging (73). The mobilization of the head of the pancreas, including the Kocher maneuver, entry into the lesser sac and mobilization of the pancreatic tail demand high expertise in laparoscopic techniques. There are only a few reports with small numbers of patients describing success using the laparoscopic approach for insulinomas. The success rate of IOUS without palpation during open surgery is 75–90%, but it reaches 100% with bimanual palpation. The usual demands when introducing a laparoscopic procedure is that it should not only be possible to perform, but also be at least as successful as the corresponding open one. A pure laparoscopic approach to insulinomas may therefore presumably be less successful since bimanual palpation is impossible. However, recent development of hand-port devices which allows introduction of one of the surgeon's hands into the abdomen and still keeping the intraabdominal gas pressure up during a laparoscopic procedure may lead to new operative approaches for insulinoma. Thus, the introduced hand may unimanually palpate the pancreas, and the success rate for this approach in conjunction with laparoscopic ultrasound has to be evaluated in the future.

10.7 Complications

Pancreatic surgery has been associated with a number of complications, mainly intraperitoneal leakage of pancreatic fluid or development of pancreatic fistula (76,77). Less frequently, a pseudocyst may develop. These complications have had a hampering effect on pancreatic surgery, sometimes creating a conservative attitude toward surgical treatment. However, serious attempts have been made to modify the surgical technique to reduce the number and severity of these complications. Different postoperative medical and surgical interventions for management of fistulas and pseudocysts have also been discussed (77,78). Nowadays pancreatic surgery is performed more safely, and excellent series have been reported with minimal morbidity and mortality (6,77). Most authors have reported that postoperative drainage containing high amylase concentrations in most cases resolve spontaneously. In some cases one may leave the drain in place while the patient is fed. There seems to be no indication for somatostatin (or analogue) treatment in these cases; This statement is supported by a prospective randomized trial using octreotide to prevent pancreatic fistulas after pancreaticoduodenectomy (78). If the drainage does not resolve, various reoperative methods may be used to correct the leak.

10.8 Postoperative Management

Once the insulinoma is resected, the blood glucose levels rise while on glucose-free intravenous solutions, which may be used as an intraoperative parameter to verify success. In fact, in some cases insulin may have to be given, with frequent assays of serum glucose postoperatively. Drains may be removed if the output is less than 20 mL/day, or higher if the fluid contains low amylase concentrations.

11 ADDITIONAL THERAPY

Malignant insulinomas are rare and may be very difficult to manage. In some patients the resection may be complete, but the patient has to be under surveillance. Median disease-free survival after a curative resection in one study was 5 years, but after recurrence, median survival was 19 months (4). Several studies have advocated an aggressive approach towards these tumors, with repeated resections and use of debulking or cytoreductive surgery. However, some authors propose that at least 90% of the tumor has to be resected in order to achieve true palliation. The aggressive surgical approach should be accompanied by chemotherapy using adriamycin and streptozocin, which have had excellent results in several studies (79,80). For massive liver metastases, embolization may be considered. Some patients suffer from a highly malignant variant with a high proliferative index (measured with, for example, immunohistochemistry using antibodies directed against Ki-67) and short survival, which has to be taken into account when planning the treatment.

ACKNOWLEDGMENTS

I am thankful to Prof. Göran Åkerström for careful reading and commenting on the manuscript, as well as Drs. Ola Hessman and Björn Hellman for help with the illustrations.

REFERENCES

1. Banting F, Best C. Internal secretion of the pancreas. J Lab Med 1922; 7:251–252.
2. Wilder R, Allan F, Power M. Carcinoma of the islets of the pancreas: hyperinsulinism and hypoglycemia. JAMA 1927; 89:348–349.
3. Howland G, Campbell W, Maltby E. Dysinsulinism:

convulsions and coma due to islet cell tumor of the pancreas with operation and cure. JAMA 1929; 93:674–675.
4. Service F, McMahon M, O'Brien P, Ballard DJ. Functioning insulinoma—incidence, recurrence, and long-term survival of patients: a 60-year study. Mayo Clin Proc 1991; 66:711–719.
5. Stefanini P, Carboni M, Patrassi N. Beta-islet tumors of the pancreas: results of a study on 1,067 cases. Surgery 1974; 75:597–609.
6. Hellman P, Goretzki P, Simon D, Dotzenrath C, Röher H. Therapeutic experience of 65 cases with organic hyperinsulinism. Langenbeck's Arch Surg 2000; 385:329–336.
7. Whipple A, Frautz V. Adenomas of islet cells with hyperinsulinism: a review. Ann Surg 1935; 101:1299–1335.
8. Dizon AM, Kowalyk S, Hoogwerf BJ. Neuroglycopenic and other symptoms in patients with insulinomas. Am J Med 1999; 106:307–310.
9. Doherty GM, Doppman JL, Shawker TH, Miller DL, Eastman RC, Gorden P, Norton JA. Results of a prospective strategy to diagnose, localize, and resect insulinomas. Surgery 1991; 110:987–989.
10. Service FJ, Dale AJ, Elveback LR, Jiang NS. Insulinoma: clinical and diagnostic features of 60 consecutive cases. Mayo Clin Proc 1976; 51:417–429.
11. Gorden PJ. Plasma insulin: fluctuations in the "big" insulin component in man after glucose and other stimuli. J Clin Invest 1969; 48:2225–2234.
12. Waickus CM, de Bustros A, Shakil A. Recognizing factitious hypoglycemia in the family practice setting. J Am Board Fam Pract 1999; 12:133–136.
13. Grama D, Eriksson B, Mårtensson H, Cedermark B, Ahrén B, Kristoffersson A, Rastad J, Öberg K, Åkerström G. Clinical characteristics, treatment and survival in patients with pancreatic tumors causing hormonal syndromes. World J Surg 1992; 16:632–639.
14. Bessell EM, Selby C, Ellis IO. Severe hypoglycaemia caused by raised insulin-like growth factor II in disseminated breast cancer. J Clin Pathol 1999; 52:780–781.
15. Hizuka N, Fukuda I, Takano K, Okubo Y, Asakawa-Yasumoto K, Demura H. Serum insulin-like growth factor II in 44 patients with non-islet cell tumor hypoglycemia. Endocr J 1998; 45(suppl):S61–S65.
16. Cupisti K, Hoppner W, Dotzenrath C, Simon D, Berndt I, Roher HD, Goretzki PE. Lack of MEN1 gene mutations in 27 sporadic insulinomas. Eur J Clin Invest 2000; 30:325–329.
17. Hessman O, Lindberg D, Einarsson A, Lillhager P, Carling T, Grimelius L, Eriksson B, Akerstrom G, Westin G, Skogseid B. Genetic alterations on 3p, 11q13, and 18q in nonfamilial and MEN 1-associated pancreatic endocrine tumors. Genes Chromosomes Cancer 1999; 26: 258–264.
18. Speel EJ, Scheidweiler AF, Zhao J, Matter C, Saremaslani P, Roth J, Heitz PU, Komminoth P. Genetic evidence for early divergence of small functioning and nonfunctioning endocrine pancreatic tumors: gain of 9Q34 is an early event in insulinomas. Cancer Res 2001; 61:5186–5192.
19. Grant C. Insulinoma. In: Doherty G, Skogseid B, eds. Surgical Endocrinology. Philadelphia: Lippincott, Williams & Wilkins, 2001:345–360.
20. Pasieka JL, McLeod MK, Thompson NW, Burney RE. Surgical approach to insulinomas. Assessing the need for preoperative localization. Arch Surg 1992; 127:442–447.
21. Gutman RA, Lazarus NR, Penhos JC, Fajans S, Recant L. Circulating proinsulin-like material in patients with functioning insulinomas. N Engl J Med 1971; 284: 1003–1008.
22. Lohmann T, Kratzsch J, Kellner K, Witzigmann H, Hauss J, Paschke R. Severe hypoglycemia due to insulin autoimmune syndrome with insulin autoantibodies crossreactive to proinsulin. Exp Clin Endocrinol Diabetes 2001; 109:245–248.
23. van Heerden J, Edis A, Service F. The surgical aspects of insulinomas. Ann Surg 1979; 189:677–682.
24. Wayne J, Tanaka R, Kaplan E. Insulinomas. In: Clark O, Duh Q, eds. Textbook of Endocrine Surgery. Philadelphia: W.B. Saunders Company, 1997:557–591.
25. Merimee T, Tyson J. Hypoglycemia in man: pathological and physiological variants. Diabetes 1977; 26:161.
26. Fajans SAI. Insulin-producing islet cell tumors. Endocinol Metab Clin North Am 1989; 18:45–74.
27. Service FJ, O'Brien PC, Kao PC, Young WF Jr. C-peptide suppression test: effects of gender, age, and body mass index: implications for the diagnosis of insulinoma. J Clin Endocrinol Metab 1992; 74:204–210.
28. Wasada T, Katsumori K, Saeki A, Kuroki H, Arii H, Saito S, Omori Y. Lack of C-peptide suppression by exogenous hyperinsulinemia in subjects with symptoms suggesting reactive hypoglycemia. Endocr J 1996; 43:639–644.
29. Daggett PR, Goodburn EA, Kurtz AB, Le Quesne LP, Morris DV, Nabarro JD, Raphael MJ. Is preoperative localisation of insulinomas necessary? Lancet 1981; 1: 483–486.
30. Angelini L, Bezzi M, Tucci G, Lirici MM, Candiani F, Rubaltelli L, Tremolada C, Tamburrano G, Fegiz G. The ultrasonic detection of insulinomas during surgical exploration of the pancreas. World J Surg 1987; 11:642–647.
31. Grant CS, Charboneau JW, Reading CC, James EM, Galiber A. Insulinoma: the value of intraoperative ultrasonography. Wien Klin Wochenschr 1988; 100:376–380.
32. Menegaux F, Schmitt G, Mercadier M, Chigot JP. Pancreatic insulinomas. Am J Surg 1993; 165:243–248.
33. Bottger TC, Junginger T. Is preoperative radiographic localization of islet cell tumors in patients with insulinoma necessary? World J Surg 1993; 17:427–432.
34. Semelka R, Cumming M, Shoenut J. Comparison of dynamic contrast-enhanced CT and MR imaging with dynamic gadolinium enhancement and fat suppression. Radiology 1993; 186:799–802.
35. Pavone P, Mitchell DG, Leonetti F, Di Girolamo M,

Cardone G, Catalano C, Tamburrano G, Passariello R. Pancreatic beta-cell tumors: MRI. J Comput Assist Tomogr 1993; 17:403–407.

36. Krenning EP, Kwekkeboom DJ, Bakker WH, Breeman WA, Kooij PP, Oei HY, van Hagen M, Postema PT, de Jong M, Reubi JC. Somatostatin receptor scintigraphy with [111In-DTPA-D-Phe1]- and [123I-Tyr3]-octreotide: the Rotterdam experience with more than 1000 patients. Eur J Nucl Med 1993; 20:716–731.
37. Ur E, Bomanji J, Mather SJ, Britton KE, Wass JA, Grossman AB, Besser GM. Localization of neuroendocrine tumours and insulinomas using radiolabelled somatostatin analogues, 123I-Tyr3-octreotide and 111In-pentatreotide. Clin Endocrinol (Oxf) 1993; 38: 501–506.
38. Woltering EA, Barrie R, O'Dorisio TM, O'Dorisio MS, Nance R, Cook DM. Detection of occult gastrinomas with iodine 125-labeled lanreotide and intraoperative gamma detection. Surgery 1994; 116:1139–1147.
39. Ohrvall U, Westlin JE, Nilsson S, Juhlin C, Rastad J, Lundqvist H, Akerstrom G. Intraoperative gamma detection reveals abdominal endocrine tumors more efficiently than somatostatin receptor scintigraphy. Cancer 1997; 80: 2490–2494.
40. Eriksson B, Bergstrom M, Orlefors H, Sundin A, Oberg K, Langstrom B. Use of PET in neuroendocrine tumors. In vivo applications and in vitro studies. Q J Nucl Med 2000; 44:68–76.
41. Anderson MA, Carpenter S, Thompson NW, Nostrant TT, Elta GH, Scheiman JM. Endoscopic ultrasound is highly accurate and directs management in patients with neuroendocrine tumors of the pancreas. Am J Gastroenterol 2000; 95:2271–2277.
42. Ardengh JC, Rosenbaum P, Ganc AJ, Goldenberg A, Lobo EJ, Malheiros CA, Rahal F, Ferrari AP. Role of EUS in the preoperative localization of insulinomas compared with spiral CT. Gastrointest Endosc 2000; 51: 552–555.
43. Zimmer T, Scherubl H, Faiss S, Stolzel U, Riecken EO, Wiedenmann B. Endoscopic ultrasonography of neuroendocrine tumours. Digestion 2000; 62:45–50.
44. Thompson NW, Czako PF, Fritts LL, Bude R, Bansal R, Nostrant TT, Scheiman JM. Role of endoscopic ultrasonography in the localization of insulinomas and gastrinomas. Surgery 1994; 116:1131–1138.
45. Böttger T, Weber W, Beyer J, Junginger T. Value of tumor localization in patients with insulinoma. World J Surg 1990; 14:107–114.
46. Zeiger MA, Shawker TH, Norton JA. Use of intraoperative ultrasonography to localize islet cell tumors. World J Surg 1993; 17:448–454.
47. Norton J, Shawker T, Doppman J, Miller D, Fraker D, Cromack D. Localization and surgical treatment of occult insulinomas. Ann Surg 1990; 212:615–620.
48. Kaplan EL, Lee CH. Recent advances in the diagnosis and treatment of insulinomas. Surg Clin North Am 1979; 59: 119–129.
49. Demeure M, Klonoff D, Karam J, Duh Q, Clark O. Insulinomas asociated with multiple endocrine neoplasia type I: the need for a different surgical approach. Surgery 1991; 110:998–1002.
50. Kaplan E. Calcium infusion. A new provocative test for insulinomas. Ann Surg 1979; 190:501–507.
51. Doppman J, Miller D, Chang R, et al. Insulinomas: localization with selective intra-arterial injection of calcium. Radiology 1991; 178:237–241.
52. Defreyne L, Moser C, Scheidt T, Kubale R, Meessen S, Koch B, Kramann B. Intra-arterial calcium provocation for the preoperative diagnosis of the location of an occult insulinoma. Dtsch Med Wochenschr 1992; 117:1829–1837.
53. Doppman J, Chang R, Fraker D. Localization of insulinomas to regions of the pancreas by intra-arterial stimulation with calcium. Ann Intern Med 1995; 123: 269–273.
54. Skogseid B, Rastad J, Åkerström G. Pancreatic endocrine tumors in multiple endocrine neoplasia type 1. In: Skogseid B, Doherty G, eds. Surgical Endocrinology. Philadelphia: Lipincott, Williams & Wilkins, 2001:511–524.
55. Soga J, Yakuwa Y, Osaka M. Insulinoma/hypoglycemic syndrome: a statistical evaluation of 1085 reported cases of a Japanese series. J Exp Clin Cancer Res 1998; 17:379–388.
56. Sheppard BC, Norton JA, Doppman JL, Maton PN, Gardner JD, Jensen RT. Management of islet cell tumors in patients with multiple endocrine neoplasia: a prospective study. Surgery 1989; 106:1108–1117.
57. Lo CY, Lam KY, Kung AW, Lam KS, Tung PH, Fan ST. Pancreatic insulinomas. A 15-year experience. Arch Surg 1997; 132:926–930.
58. Boukhman MP, Karam JH, Shaver J, Siperstein AE, Duh QY, Clark OH. Insulinoma—experience from 1950 to 1995. West J Med 1998; 169:98–104.
59. Jensen RT. Natural history of digestive endocrine tumors. In: Mignon M, Colombel J, eds. Recent Advances in the Pathophysiology and Management of Inflammatory Bowel Diseases and Digestive Endocrine Tumors. Paris: John Libbey Eurotext, 1999:192–219.
60. Service F, Natt N, Thompson G, Grant C, van Heerden J, Andrews J, Lorenz E, Terzic A, Lloyd R. Noninsulinoma pancreatogenous hypoglycemia: a novel syndrome of hyperinsulinemic hypoglycemia in adults independent of mutations in Kir6.2 and SUR1 genes. J Clin Endocrinol Metab 1999; 84:1582–1589.
61. Fajans S, Floyd J Jr, Thiffault C. Further studies on diazoxide suppression of insulin release from abnormal and normal islet tissue in man. Ann NY Acad Sci 1968; 150:261–280.
62. Stehouwer CD, Lems WF, Fischer HR, Hackeng WH. Malignant insulinoma: is combined treatment with verapamil and the long-acting somatostatin analogue octreotide (SMS 201-995) more effective than single therapy with either drug? Neth J Med 1989; 35:86–94.

63. Witteles RM, Straus IF, Sugg SL, Koka MR, Costa EA, Kaplan EL. Adult-onset nesidioblastosis causing hypoglycemia: an important clinical entity and continuing treatment dilemma. Arch Surg 2001; 136:656–663.
64. Cameron J, Pitt H, Yeo C, Lillemore K, Kaufman H, Coleman J. One hundred forty-five consecutive pancreaticoduodenectomies without mortality. Surgery 1993; 217:430–438.
65. Barnes S, Lillemoe K, Kaufman H, Sauter P, Yeo C, Talamini M, Pitt H, Cameron J. Pancreaticoduodenectomy for benign disease. Am J Surg 1996; 171:131–135.
66. Huai JC, Zhang W, Niu HO, Su ZX, McNamara JJ, Machi J. Localization and surgical treatment of pancreatic insulinomas guided by intraoperative ultrasound. Am J Surg 1998; 175:18–21.
67. Beger HG, Schlosser W, Siech M, Poch B. The surgical management of chronic pancreatitis: duodenum-preserving pancreatectomy. Adv Surg 1999; 32:87–104.
68. Warshaw A, Rattner D, Fernandez-del Castillo C, Z'graggen K. Middle segment pancreatectomy. A novel technique for conserving pancreatic tissue. Arch Surg 1998; 133:327–331.
69. Lillemoe K, Kaushal S, Cameron J, Sohn T, Pitt H, Yeo C. Distal pancreatectomy: indications and outcomes in 235 patients. Ann Surg 1999; 229:693–700.
70. Hellman P, Andersson M, Rastad J, Juhlin C, Karacagil S, Eriksson B, Skogseid B, Akerstrom G. Surgical strategy for large or malignant endocrine pancreatic tumors. World J Surg 2000; 24:1353–1360.
71. Vezakis A, Davides D, Larvin M, McMahon MJ. Laparoscopic surgery combined with preservation of the spleen for distal pancreatic tumors. Surg Endosc 1999; 13:26–29.
72. Gagner M, Pomp A, Herrera MF. Early experience with laparoscopic resections of islet cell tumors. Surgery 1996; 120:1051–1054.
73. Iihara M, Kanbe M, Okamoto T, Ito Y, Obara T. Laparoscopic ultrasonography for resection of insulinomas. Surgery 2001; 130:1086–1091.
74. Fernandez-Cruz L, Herrera M, Saenz A, Pantoja JP, Astudillo E, Sierra M. Laparoscopic pancreatic surgery in patients with neuroendocrine tumours: indications and limits. Best Pract Res Clin Endocrinol Metab 2001; 15:161–175.
75. Berends FJ, Cuesta MA, Kazemier G, van Eijck CH, de Herder WW, van Muiswinkel JM, Bruining HA, Bonjer HJ. Laparoscopic detection and resection of insulinomas. Surgery 2000; 128:386–391.
76. Fraker DL, Alexander HR. The surgical approach to endocrine tumors of the pancreas. Semin Gastrointest Dis 1995; 6:102–113.
77. Yeo C. Management of complications following pancreaticoduodenectomy. Surg Clin North Am 1995; 75: 913–924.
78. Lowy A, Lee J, Pisters P, Davidson B, Fenoglio C, Stanford P, Jinnah R, Evans D. Prospective, randomized trial of octreotide to prevent pancreatic fistula after pancreaticoduodenectomy for malignant disease. Ann Surg 1997; 226:632–641.
79. Eriksson B. Systemic therapy for neuroendocrine tumors of the pancreas. In: Doherty G, Skogseid B, eds. Surgical Endocrinology. Philadelphia, PA: Lippincott, Williams & Wilkins, 2001:393–404.
80. Moertel C, Lefkopoplou M, Lipsitz S. Streptozocin-doxorubicin, streptozocin-fluorouracil, or chlorozotocin in the treatment of advanced islet-cell carcinoma. N Engl J Med 1992; 326:519–523.

46

Hyperinsulinism

Stephen E. Dolgin

Mount Sinai School of Medicine, New York University, New York, New York, U.S.A.

Hypoglycemia is especially dangerous to the developing brain of the newborn. Frequently, cases of neonatal hypoglycemia result from easily managed self-limited causes. Less often, hypoglycemia persists and can be extremely difficult to control. Severe persistent hypoglycemia of the newborn is usually due to excessive production of insulin from the pancreas. An insulinoma is almost never present. The underlying condition causing persistent hypoglycemic hyperinsulinism had, until fairly recently, been widely attributed to diffuse hyperplasia of islet cells and was designated nesidioblastosis. That term is no longer acceptable, since the pathogenesis has been revisited. Some alternate expressions used to name this rare but morbid condition are strikingly unwieldy. Some authors, for instance, choose persistent pancreatogenous hypoglycemic hyperinsulinism of infancy without insulinoma. This bulky expression denotes that the condition excludes transient cases, exogenous sources of insulin, and the unexpected insulinoma. Some have proposed a much simpler expression intended to mean exactly the same thing: hyperinsulinism.

1 CLINICAL PRESENTATION

Symptoms of hypoglycemia include those described as adrenergic, such as sweating and tachycardia, and those described as neuroglycopenic, such as seizures and coma. In older patients neuroglycopenic symptoms include headaches, fatigue, and behavioral and cognitive dysfunction. One definition of hypoglycemia in the neonate is a serum glucose concentration of $\leq$40 mg/dL.

Often hypoglycemia in the newborn is short-lived. Infants of diabetic mothers commonly demonstrate transient hypoglycemia because the fetal pancreas may have been exposed to high glucose concentrations and was therefore conditioned to produce high amounts of insulin. When severe hypoglycemia persists in the newborn, the cause is most often hyperinsulinism. This is a rare problem affecting about one in 50,000 people. When the onset of persistent hypoglycemia is quite soon after birth, the cases are typically the most severe and refractory to medical management.

Newborns with hyperinsulinism are often large for gestational age. Certain features help distinguish hyperinsulinism from other causes of hypoglycemia. The critical blood sample, the one drawn when the patient is hypoglycemic, may show an inappropriately elevated insulin concentration of greater than 5 μU/mL. These patients have a marked glycemic response after intravenous glucagon administration. A rise in the serum glucose concentration of 30 mg/dL or more after intravenous glucagon is supportive of hyperinsulinism as opposed to other causes of hypoglycemia. In the patient with hyperinsulinism, free fatty acids and ketone levels are low.

2 PATHOLOGICAL BASIS OF HYPERINSULINISM

The underlying pathological condition in a newborn whose hyperinsulinism persists is almost never a true insulinoma. Controversy has surrounded the actual underlying histopathology. The term nesidioblastosis, applied broadly to the congenitally abnormal pancreas producing excessive insulin, was conceived in 1939, curiously, in a paper actually about focal pancreatic lesions (1). The author, Laidlaw, called the lesions nesidioblastomas. Laidlaw speculated that if such lesions were multiple in a pancreas, the condition could be called nesidioblastosis. Laidlaw recognized islet cells budding from pancreatic ductal cells. The term nesidioblastosis is suffering a slow death because the histological finding described by Laidlaw has not consistently been associated with hyperinsulinism. The finding of β cells budding from epithelium (ductulo-insular complexes) is characteristic of the fetal developmental process. It persists as a developmental stage postnatally (2). It is reproduced in many states of injury, including pancreatic duct obstruction, and in recovery from these conditions. This histological condition has been recognized in the normal pancreas of newborns and infants. In the view of many pathologists, the finding of nesidioblastosis does not correlate with hypoglycemia (3–5).

Not only does this diffuse condition exist without hyperinsulinism, but centers with extensive experience have found that about one third of young children with hyperinsulinism have unifocal lesions. (6; N. S. Adzick, personal communication). Since nesidioblastosis implies diffuse hyperplasia of β cells throughout the pancreas, it has become an inappropriate term when applied broadly to patients with hyperinsulinism.

The focal lesions being discovered are not adenomas. Unlike true adenomas, these focal lesions do not represent the proliferation of a single cell type. Rather, they have been described histopathologically as focal adenomatous hyperplasia. They are described as conglomerations of otherwise normal islets with centralized β cells and non-β cells in the periphery. These focal lesions are, grossly, much smaller than insulinomas, measuring only a few millimeters. They are not discernible by modern imaging studies, and they are most often not visible to gross examination. The β cell nuclei appear normal. These small lesions crowd the exocrine pancreas. The remainder of the pancreas is histologically normal.

The centers most actively studying patients with hyperinsulinism still find a diffuse lesion in the majority of children. Bizarre and large β cell nuclei are noted throughout the gland, which is therefore described as being in an "activated state."

3 MEDICAL MANAGEMENT

When a newborn suffers hyperinsulinism, maximal steps are taken to correct the hypoglycemia in order to protect the developing brain. These steps include provision of glucose at rates greatly exceeding the normal demands. The normal newborn typically requires about 6 mg of glucose per kg of body weight per minute. The patient with hyperinsulinism frequently requires a central venous catheter to provide two to four times that amount of glucose. This supplements provision of enteral glucose often by nasogastric tube or gastrostomy.

Numerous agents have been used to control the hyperinsulinism. Diazoxide has been the standard first choice and has had some success in select patients. It is probably least useful in children with the onset of severe hypoglycemia in the neonatal period. Diazoxide interferes with the SUR-K_{ir} receptors (a receptor complex called sulfonylurea receptor–potassium internal rectifier) on the insulin-producing β cell membrane. That complex of receptors helps control insulin secretion. Reviewing their results in a large number of children with hyperinsulinism, the group from Paris and Brussels showed that their success was largely limited to patients with onset of hypoglycemia at a somewhat later age (7). They could effectively control the hypoglycemia with diazoxide in only one of 31 patients whose hypoglycemia began in the neonatal period. They were able to control the hypoglycemia in 12 of 39 children with early infantile onset and all 7 of the uncommon "late-infantile" cases. These authors concluded that diazoxide is useful when hyperinsulinism occurs in infants and children, but not in newborns. Some patients with hyperinsulinism have defects in the SUR–K_{ir} receptor system, and these may be the ones who do not respond to diazoxide. At present, testing for this defect has had very little role in the clinical management of these patients. When the team from Paris and Brussels reported 52 neonates treated surgically for hyperinsulinism, they noted that during the 13 years of their study, 11 patients with hyperinsulinism were treated successfully with diazoxide (8). Perhaps patients with abnormalities in the sulfonylurea receptor complex are those presenting with hyperinsulinism at the earliest ages explaining the resistance to diazoxide.

Assorted other medications have been utilized, including steroids, calcium channel blockers, and octreotide. A group in Israel has championed octreotide (9).

However, octreotide use demands either continuous subcutaneous infusion or four daily injections. Of 15 patients receiving octreotide in that study, 7 ultimately underwent resection.

4 OPERATIVE APPROACH IN RECENT DECADES

Medical steps usually fail to successfully and permanently control hypoglycemia from early-onset hyperinsulinism. Operative interventions have been required in most such cases. Imaging techniques have totally failed in identifying lesions. Although efforts to refine modern imaging techniques continue, so far the lesions causing hyperinsulinism in the youngest patients have not been detectable by available technology. For those patients with diffuse lesions, it is understandable that imaging would be fruitless. Unfortunately, the focal lesions also provide a marked obstacle to effective imaging because they are so extremely small and preserve normal pancreatic architecture.

For a few decades surgeons debated the extent of pancreatic resection that would best serve these patients. Historically, surgeons have performed extensive pancreatic resections believing the condition to be a diffuse hyperplasia of β cells and generally considering lesser resections to yield unacceptable persistent hypoglycemia. While inadequate resection allows persistent hypoglycemia with the threat of cumulative ongoing neurological damage, excessive resection carries the increased risk of diabetes mellitus and pancreatic exocrine insufficiency. Long-term follow-up of these patients is necessary to clarify the extent of the morbidity from extensive resections. Several groups have found relatively late onset of diabetes mellitus in young patients long after pancreatic resection (10,11).

The terminology surgeons have used to describe the extent of resection has been quite murky. Sometimes authors quantify the resection as between 70 and 98% pancreatectomy and often define these quantities poorly. Qualitative terms, also often poorly defined, include left-sided pancreatectomy, subtotal pancreatectomy, and near-total pancreatectomy. Attempts have been made to define these assorted terms anatomically, although the inherent variability in gross morphology of the child's pancreas imposes inevitable inaccuracy. An autopsy study specifically designed to determine the variability of the infant's pancreas showed that anatomical landmarks often used to quantify a resection are quite variable (12). For instance, when all pancreatic tissue to the left of the superior mesenteric vessels was weighed and compared to the weight of the gland, this amount ranged from about 32 to about 67%. When all pancreatic tissue to the left of the pancreatico-duodenal vessels was assessed, that amount varied from 43 to 96%.

The group at the Children's Hospital of Philadelphia did provide clear anatomical definitions for resections named by different numbered percentages. They reviewed 35 years of surgical care for hyperinsulinism in 1999 (13). Since 1980, 95% pancreatectomy was the operation they usually performed in this series. This they defined as resection of the entire pancreas except for the tissue to the right of the common bile duct and a "thin rim along the second portion of the duodenum and pancreatico-duodenal arteries." When persistent hypoglycemia demanded a second operation ("re-resection"), they favored a 98% pancreatectomy, which "leaves only small islands of the pancreas along the pancreatico-duodenal arteries."

Often, the more extensive operations have seemed to be the only way to control the hypoglycemia from hyperinsulinism (13–15). In many series, recurrence was relatively common with less aggressive operations. By carefully ligating branches from the splenic vessels and preserving the vessels to the spleen, splenectomy generally has not been preformed during extensive pancreatic resections by pediatric surgeons for hyperinsulinism.

In multiple series from multiple centers, some children suffered irreversible neurological injury before resections. Others had persistent hypoglycemia postoperatively, although in some it was easier to control than before the resections. Diabetes mellitus occurred in some after extensive pancreatic resections. Some patients were cured with little morbidity.

5 PRESENT OPERATIVE APPROACH

A sea change in the surgical approach to hyperinsulinism is unfolding. A few centers focused on this condition, sporting teams of endocrinologists, radiologists, pathologists, and surgeons, are rewriting the approach to hyperinsulinism. The histopathology underlying hyperinsulinism is no longer called nesidioblastosis. It is in fact a diffuse abnormality in only two thirds of these patients. One third of the patients have small (2.5–7 mg) focal lesions called focal adenomatous hyperplasia (6; N. S. Adzick, personal communication).

Although imaging has not yet been successful in identifying these lesions, arteriography and venography have been utilized preoperatively. These techniques, requiring considerable sophistication when applied to the neonate, do not image the lesions with the type of blush sometimes seen in insulinomas. Rather, they aid in localization through chemical sampling. This includes selective pancreatic venous sampling. A transhepatic catheter is inserted into the hepatic veins and threaded sequentially into the venous drainage of different sites in the pancreas. Blood is drawn for concomitant insulin and glucose determination. In addition, differential sequential arterial stimulation is performed with a catheter manipulated into the different arterial branches subserving different sites in the pancreas. Concomitant samples from a venous catheter in the inferior vena cava near the hepatic veins help determine if there are focal or diffuse sites of excessive insulin production. Agents utilized to stimulate insulin secretion include calcium and tolbutamide. By measuring venous concentrations of insulin and glucose at different sites of the pancreas and by stimulating specific sites in the pancreas through arterial catheters and measuring the insulin response, it is sometimes possible to differentiate focal from diffuse lesions and localize the focal lesions to the specific areas of the pancreas. These preoperative studies are neither perfect nor available for newborns at most medical centers.

At exploration, the surgeon, in a rather laborious procedure, exposes the entire pancreas and either palpates and sees a small irregular lesion, aided by magnifying glasses, or excises a 1 cm block of tissue in the region proposed by the preoperative angiographic studies. Many intraoperative biopsies are done to guide the operative choices.

The pathologists distinguish by frozen section the focal lesions. These small focal lesions are described as conglomerations of otherwise normal islets crowding the exocrine pancreas. The remainder of the gland is normal, in a "resting state." If the focal lesion resides in the head of the pancreas, a distal duct to jejunum anastomosis has been utilized in some cases. A choledochoduodenostomy has restored bile flow in others. In about two thirds of the cases the lesion is diffuse. The histopathological findings include numerous diffusely represented abnormal β cells with large bizarre nuclei, suggesting hyperfunction (the activated state). Extensive resection remains the standard choice for those patients. The extent of this resection remains a balancing act between too little, leaving persistent hypoglycemia, and too much, resulting in diabetes mellitus and possibly pancreatic exocrine insufficiency.

Operations for hyperinsulism have been done when medical management for hyperinsulism has failed. Despite the risks of operative management, the ongoing threat to the brain demands a more effective approach when nonoperative steps are failing.

The first major published series with this sophisticated approach came from the productive group in Paris and Brussels. They reported 45 patients treated with partial resections for the focal form of hyperinsulinism (6). This group contends that patients with the focal form of hyperinsulinism always have an abnormality on the chromosomes "with the loss of maternal alleles from chromosome 11p15." This results in an "unbalanced expression of imprinted genes involved in the control of cell growth" and "somatic reduction to hemi or homozygosity of a paternally inherited mutation of the gene for the sulfonylurea, which leads to hyperinsulinism." This association may imply that these children will not respond effectively to diazoxide, which works through the SUR receptor. In fact, diazoxide was ineffective in 91% of these 45 patients. It is this subset of patients with the focal form that consistently can do very well after appropriately guided limited resection without risk of subsequent diabetes mellitus. Even this remarkably experienced team could not effectively localize the lesion preoperatively in 11 of the 45 newborns with focal adenomatous hyperplasia.

6 REVISITING EARLIER SERIES

With this modern approach in mind, earlier series can be reassessed. For instance, extensive resections of the pancreas done for presumed diffuse lesions may have worked successfully in some cases when a focal lesion was included in the resection. In retrospect, some of the successes might have been managed by less morbid resections limited to the site of the focal lesion. Ninety-eight percent reresection may have been effective in diffuse cases refractory to lesser resection because, as presumed, the diffuse malfunction persisted in the residual pancreatic remnant. However, cases of persistent hypoglycemia could just as well have represented unifocal lesions located in the head of the pancreas near the duodenum, left in place at the initial resection, but included in the more extensive reresection.

At present, an infant with hyperinsulinism should be managed at a center capable of distinguishing focal from diffuse forms and performing the appropriate resection. As the molecular biological information accrues, the future promises better preoperative differentiation between patients who will respond to medical treatment and those who will benefit from resection. The best approach for the patient with refractory hyperinsulinism from a diffuse lesion remains, at present, an extensive pancreatic resection. The outlook for these patients remains guarded, while for those with focal lesions results have been excellent.

7 HYPERINSULINISM IN ADULTS: AGONAL RESPIRATIONS OF NESIDIOBLASTOSIS

Reports have appeared identifying small but increasing numbers of adults with pancreatogenous hypoglycemic hyperinsulinism without insulinoma (adult-onset hyperinsulinism) (16,17). These unusual patients defy preoperative imaging since no focal lesion is identifiable. The patients behave a bit differently than patients with insulinomas. The positive response to a 72-hour fast, characteristic of patients with insulinomas, is often not present in these patients. During the period when 10 adults with hyperinsulinism were treated at the Mayo Clinic, 200 with insulinomas were managed there (16). Only one of these 200 patients with insulinomas had a negative 72-hour fast. On the other hand, this test was negative in 8 of the 10 without insulinoma (and not done in one). Although imaging was unrevealing, insulin measurement in the hepatic vein showed an at least twofold increase when any site in the pancreas was stimulated by arterial injection of calcium. The histopathology showed diffuse islet enlargement and islets budding from ducts. All were managed by left-sided resections of variable extent. All but one of these patients were relieved of their neuroglycopenic symptoms after the operation.

Use of the term nesidioblastosis to describe adults with hyperinsulinism should be discouraged since this histopathological term does not correlate with hyperinsulinism. It will be interesting to learn if any adults with hyperinsulinism have focal adenomatous hyperplasia and can be cured with limited resections.

REFERENCES

1. Laidlaw GF. Nesidioblastoma, the islet tumor of the pancreas. Am J Pathol 1938; 14:125–134.
2. Jaffe R, Hashida Y, Yunis EJ. The endocrine pancreas of the neonate and infant. In: Rosenberg HS, Bernstein J, eds. Perspectives in Pediatric Pathology. Vol. 7. New York: Masson Publishing, 1982:137–165.
3. Jaffe R, Hashida Y, Yunis EJ. Pancreatic pathology in hyperinsulinemic hypoglycemia of infancy. Lab Invest 1980; 42:356–365.
4. Witte DP, Greider MH, DeSchryver-Kecskemeti K, Kissane JM, White NH. The juvenile human endocrine pancreas: normal v idiopathic hyperinsulinemic hypoglyce-mia. Semin Diagn Pathol 1984; 1:30–42.
5. Rahier J, Guiot Y, Sempoux C. Persistent hyperinsulinaemic hypoglycaemia of infancy: a heterogeneous syndrome unrelated to nesidioblastosis. Arch Dis Child Fetal Neonatal Ed 2000; 82:F108–F112.
6. Crétolle C, Nihoul-Fékété C, Jan D, Nassogne MC, Saudubray JM, Brunelle F, Rahier J. Partial elective pancreatectomy is curative in focal form of permanent hyperinsulinemic hypoglycaemia in infancy: a report of 45 cases from 1983 to 2000. J Pediatr Surg 2002; 37:155–158.
7. Touati G, Poggi-Travert F, Ogier De Baulny H, Rahier J, Brunelle F, Nihoul-Fekete C, Czernichow P, Saudubray JM. Long-term treatment of persistent hyperinsulinaemic hypoglycaemia of infancy with diazoxide: a retrospective review of 77 cases and analysis of efficacy-predicting criteria. Eur J Pediatr 1998; 157:628–633.
8. De Lonlay-Debeney P, Poggi-Travert F, Fournet J-C, Sempoux G, Vici CD, Brunelle F, Touati G, Rahier J, Junien C, Nihoul-Fékété C, Robert J-J, Saudubray J-M. Clinical features of 52 neonates with hyperinsulinism. N Engl J Med 1999; 340:1169–1175.
9. Glaser B, Hirsch HJ, Landau H. Persistent hyperinsulinemic hypoglycemia of infancy: long-term octreotide treatment without pancreatectomy. J Pediatr 1993; 123:644–650.
10. Shilyansky J, Fisher S, Cutz E, Perlman K, Filler RM. Is 95% pancreatectomy the procedure of choice for treatment of persistent hyperinsulinemic hypoglycemia of the neonate? J Pediatr Surg 1997; 32:342–346.
11. Leibowitz G, Glaser B, Higazi AA, Salameh M, Cerasi E, Landau H. Hyperinsulinemic hypoglycemia of infancy (nesidioblastosis) in clinical remission: high incidence of diabetes mellitus and persistent β-cell dysfunction at long-term follow-up. J Clin Endocrinol Metab 1995; 80:386–392.
12. Reyes GA, Fowler CL, Pokorny WJ. Pancreatic anatomy in children: emphasis on its importance to pancreatectomy. J Pediatr Surg 1993; 28:712–715.
13. Lovvorn HN III, Nance ML, Ferry RJ Jr, Stolte L, Baker L, O'Neill JA Jr, Shnaufer L, Stanley CA, Adzick NS. Congenital hyperinsulinism and the surgeon: Lessons learned over 35 years. J Pediatr Surg 1999; 34:786–793.
14. Spitz L, Bhargava RK, Grant DB, Leonard JV. Surgical treatment of hyperinsulinaemic hypoglycaemia in infancy and childhood. Arch Dis Child 1992; 67:201–205.
15. Kramer JL, Bell MJ, DeSchryner K, Bower RJ, Ternberg JL, White NH. Clinical and histologic indications for extensive pancreatic resection in nesidioblastosis. Am J Surg 1982; 143:116–119.
16. Thompson GB, Service FJ, Andrews JC, Lloyd RV, Natt N, Van Heerden JA, Grant CS. Noninsulinoma pancreatogenous hypoglycemia syndrome: an update in 10 surgically treated patients. Surgery 2000; 128:937–945.
17. Witteles RM, Straus FH II, Sugg SL, Koka MR, Costa EA, Kaplan EL. Adult–onset nesidioblastosis causing hypoglycemia. Arch Surg 2001; 136:656–663.

47

Gastrinomas and Other Rare Pancreatic Endocrine Tumors

Sydney S. Guo and Mark P. Sawicki

West Los Angeles Veterans Administration Hospital and David Geffen School of Medicine at UCLA, Los Angeles, California, U.S.A.

1 THE MAGNITUDE OF THE PROBLEM

There are few other tumors that have held the interest and fascination of surgeons and internists like gastrinomas. Since first reported in 1955, gastrinomas have challenged the traditional thinking in oncology. The relatively high frequency of multiple primary tumors and the potential for tumors to arise from many different locations are both unique attributes of gastrinoma. In addition, gastrinomas continue to defy established oncological principles and classifications even in the current molecular era. For example, it has been shown that sporadic gastrinomas at different sites are monoclonal (1), and thus probably represent systemic disease. However, clinical experience from several centers suggests that multiple gastrinomas even with lymph node involvement are "curable" by surgery (2–4). Although gastrinomas are rare, they have stimulated clinicians and led to significant clinical advances in biochemical assays, imaging, and tumor biology (5). In time, gastrinomas will lead to new advances in our understanding of tumor genetics, cell biology, stem cells, and new avenues for cancer treatment.

2 RISK FACTORS

The only risk factor for the development of gastrinoma is a family history of multiple endocrine neoplasia type 1 (MEN1). Approximately 25% of patients with gastrinoma have concurrent MEN1. Since the cloning of the *MEN1* gene in 1997, genetic testing is now feasible. However, because there has not been a consensus developed as to the recommended treatment for gastrinomas in the setting of MEN1, routine genetic testing is not useful.

3 DEMOGRAPHICS

Sporadic gastrinomas occur with a slight male preponderance (6). Age of onset is approximately 50 years (7). This is contrasted with the age of onset for MEN1 syndrome, which is approximately 30 years (8).

4 CLINICAL FEATURES

Gastrinomas are neuroendocrine tumors that secrete the hormone gastrin in excess and result in the classic Zollinger–Ellison syndrome (ZES). First described in 1955, ZES includes the triad of diffuse gastroduodenal ulcerations, gastric hypersecretion, and pancreatic islet tumors (9). Other prominent symptoms include diarrhea, reflux esophagitis, and severe abdominal pain (Table 1). Patients with ZES have more severe acid secretion compared to patients with uncomplicated peptic ulcer disease. This results in increased severity of symp-

Table 1 Zollinger–Ellison Syndrome Signs and Symptoms

Abdominal pain
Diarrhea
Peptic ulcers
Reflux esophagitis
Complications of hyperacidity
Bleeding
Perforation
Obstruction
Radiological findings
Hypertrophic gastric rugal folds
Multiple ulcers
Unusual ulcer locations
Pancreatic mass

toms such as increased number of ulcers, ulcers occasionally at atypical locations (e.g., jejunal ulcers), and increased pain. Failure to respond to conventional medical ulcer treatment and/or recurrence after adequate therapy should also raise suspicion of ZES. Unlike typical peptic ulcer disease, diarrhea is a prominent symptom in ZES and will respond to antacid therapy. Diarrhea occurs in ZES when large quantities of acid enter the duodenum and small bowel, damaging the small bowel mucosa as well as destroying pancreatic enzymes. Both events lead to malabsorption and subsequent diarrhea.

Gastrinomas may occur sporadically (75%) or as part of the multiple endocrine MEN1 syndrome (25%) (10). MEN1 is an autosomal-dominant syndrome characterized by parathyroid hyperplasia, pituitary adenomas, pancreatic endocrine tumors, and other neuroendocrine tumors (10). Differentiation between sporadic and familial gastrinomas depends on the presence of family history as well as a high clinical suspicion, as pancreatic endocrine tumors may infrequently be the first manifestation of the MEN1 syndrome. It is important to make this distinction because the clinical management of sporadic and MEN1-associated ZES differs. Although multiple tumors are frequently found even in sporadic gastrinomas, these can often be resected for cure, and surgery should be aggressively pursued unless there is extensive hepatic involvement. However, patients with ZES in the context of MEN1 have multiple small tumors that are difficult to completely excise, and surgical exploration in these patients should be based on case-by-case considerations.

The majority of gastrinomas (85%) occur in the gastrinoma triangle (11) (Fig. 1), which is an anatomical area bordered by imaginary lines connecting (1) the junction of cystic and common bile ducts, (2) the junction between the second and third portion of the duodenum, and (3) the junction between the neck and body of the pancreas. Within this area, gastrinomas are known to originate from the pancreas, duodenum, and surrounding soft tissue including lymph nodes. Although the majority of gastrinomas occur in the gastrinoma triangle, they can also occur to the left of the superior mesenteric vessels; these gastrinomas tend to metastasize to the liver more frequently than those found within the triangle (12). Duodenal gastrinomas are submucosal and are found most commonly in the first and second portions but can reside in all four portions of the duodenum. Primary nodal gastrinomas have also been described (13). Furthermore, ectopic primary gastrinomas have been resected from liver, common bile duct, jejunum, pylorus, antral mucosa, omentum, ovary, and even heart (14–18).

Gastrinomas may be benign or malignant (4). When malignant, they may metastasize to adjacent lymph nodes or to the liver and less commonly to bone. Experience from several centers suggests that lymph node metastasis, a traditional indicator of systemic disease and an important prognostic indicator in most other tumors, does not seem to have significant impact on patient survival in ZES (Fig. 2) (2–4,19). Resection of the primary tumor(s) and lymph node(s) is the only curative treatment for gastrinomas. When this is not possible, aggressive surgical exploration and resection has been shown to limit the potential for metastatic spread. However, gastrinomas, even when metastatic to the liver, can have an indolent course characterized by slow growth (4). In a recent study of 19 ZES patients with hepatic involvement, only 42% showed rapid growth, while 32% demonstrated slow growth, and 26% had no growth (20). With the availability of powerful proton pump inhibitors (PPI) to control acid hypersecretion, the main determinant of patient survival is now tumor burden and not acid-related complications (7).

Insulinomas and gastrinomas occur with approximately the same frequency among pancreatic endocrine tumors (21). Nonfunctional islet tumors occur in approximately 36–53% of all islet tumors (22,23). Other types of functional pancreatic endocrine tumors are exceedingly rare. These include glucagonomas, VIPomas, and somatostatinomas. Most of these tumors are large and metastatic at presentation, and surgical cure is often not possible. However, debulking procedures may be indicated to lessen the pain and hormonal overproduction and to palliate local mass effects causing obstruction (gastrointestinal or biliary tracts).

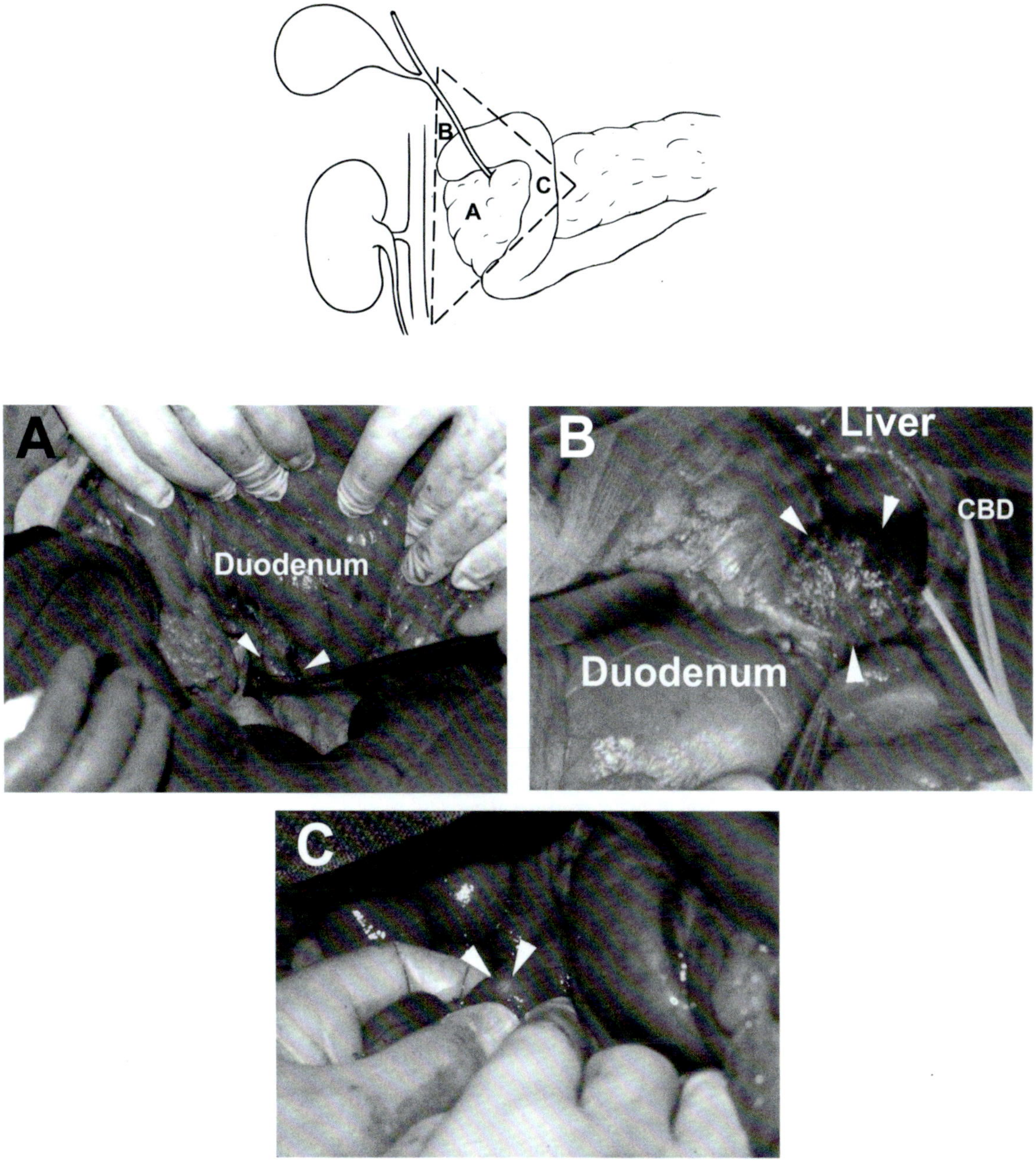

Figure 1 Gastrinoma triangle. The majority of gastrinomas (85%) occur in the gastrinoma triangle, which is an anatomical area bordered by imaginary lines connecting (1) the junction of cystic and common bile ducts, (2) the junction between the second and third portion of the duodenum, and (3) the junction between the neck and body of the pancreas. (A) Retropancreatic gastrinoma. The duodenum is reflected by the Kocher maneuver to expose the gastrinoma. Approximate tumor size: 1.5 × 1 cm. (B) Hepatoduodenal ligament gastrinoma. The common bile duct is encircled with vessel loops. Approximate tumor size: 3 × 3.5 cm. (C) Duodenal gastrinoma. Approximate tumor size: 0.5 × 0.5 cm. CBD, common bile duct; SB, small bowel. Arrowheads point to tumors.

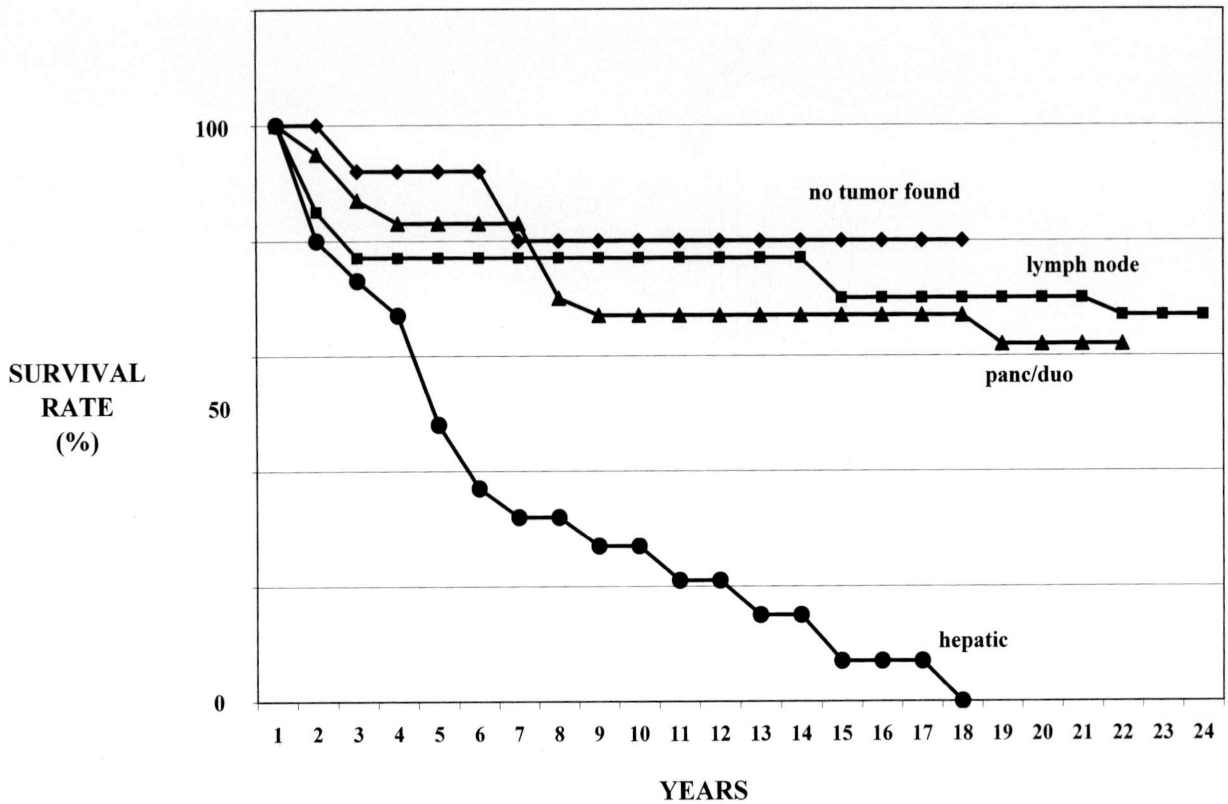

Figure 2 Survival of patients with ZES—influences of intraoperative findings. Patients with either (1) no tumor found, (2) tumor found in lymph node(s) only, (3) tumor found in the peri-pancreatic/duodenal area only, or (4) hepatic involvement were followed and studied. (Data from Ref. 19.)

5 PHYSIOLOGY

Gastrin is a hormone produced by G-cells that reside in the antrum of stomach. Gastrin is found in pancreatic islets in fetal life, but it is unknown whether gastrin is present in the normal adult pancreas (24,25). Gastrin may also be demonstrated in a variety of neuroendocrine tumors by sensitive pathological staining. However, only gastrinomas secrete sufficient amount of gastrin to cause symptoms of ZES.

In the context of the MEN1 syndrome, there can be both hypercalcemia and hypergastrinemia. Calcium is a known stimulant of gastrin release, and calcium has been used as a provocative test in the diagnosis of gastrinomas. In MEN1, the hypercalcemia tends to exacerbate the elevated gastrin and acid production. However, the exact mechanism of this stimulation remains unclear. There is evidence that gastrinomas express calcium-sensing receptors (26), and release gastrin in response to extracellular calcium level. Calcium has also been shown to increase acid secretion by parietal cells independently of gastrin, histamine, or acetylcholine (27). Therefore, in MEN1 patients, parathyroidectomy alone may partially relieve their ulcer diathesis by decreasing both gastrin and acid production, even if the gastrinoma is unresectable (28).

Gastrin also has trophic effects on susceptible cells, and gastric carcinoids may arise from the transformation of enterochromaffin-like (ECL) cells in the context of chronic hypergastrinemia in the setting of ZES. Frequent and regular endoscopy is required to monitor the growth of these carcinoid tumors, and resection is indicated when there is significant growth. Similarly, it has been proposed that hypergastrinemia may be involved in the tumorigenesis of colon adenocarcinoma, but this association has not been definitively demonstrated (29–31).

Several investigators have studied the genetic and molecular alterations of gastrinomas and other pancreatic endocrine tumors (Table 2). The *MEN1* gene is frequently mutated (loss-of-function mutations) in pancreatic endocrine tumors, especially gastrinomas (10,32).

Table 2 Molecular Defects in Gastrinomas and Other Pancreatic Endocrine Tumors

Chromosome deletions	Tumor suppressors	Oncogenes
Chromosome 1	*MEN1*—mutated in 25%	Cyclin D1 – overexpressed
Chromosome 3	*Smad4/DPC* – mutated in 50%	*HER-2/neu* – amplified
	P16 – promoter hypermethylated	
	P27 – overexpressed	
	P53 – rare mutations	

Chromosome 1 and chromosome 3 are also frequently deleted in these tumors and predict malignant behavior of sporadic pancreatic endocrine tumors (33,34). Key oncogenes such as cyclin D1 (35) and HER-2-neu (36), as well as tumor suppressors p16/INK4 (37,38), p27/KIP1 (39,40), Smad4/DPC (41), and p53 (42) are also altered in gastrinomas as well as other types of pancreatic endocrine tumors.

6 BIOCHEMICAL ASSAYS

Because the physical examination is usually not specific for gastrinoma, the diagnosis of ZES rests mainly on biochemical assays and imaging (Fig. 3). A fasting serum gastrin level (radioimmunoassay) is usually the first diagnostic test obtained, and in most instances a confirmatory secretin stimulation test should be performed (Table 3). Whereas a normal fasting serum gastrin is < 150 pg/mL, patients with ZES may have levels greater than 1000 pg/mL. In patients with fasting serum gastrin levels between these extremes, it is essential to rule out other causes of hypergastrinemia. Concurrent gastric outlet obstruction, *Helicobacter pylori* infection, renal insufficiency, and hyperlipidemia all may lead to elevated levels of gastrin. Patients with atrophic gastritis/pernicious anemia may also have hypergastrinemia without ZES as G-cells increase the secretion of gastrin to compensate for the decreased acid production. It is for the same reason that patients on proton-pump inhibitor (PPI) therapy and patients status postvagotomy may have elevated serum gastrin. Primary diffuse G-cell hyperplasia, or pseudo-Zollinger-Ellison syndrome, may also lead to elevated fasting serum gastrin level and increased basal acid secretion. A recent study of 239 patients showed that in ZES patients, but not in MEN1 patients, the initial fasting serum gastrin correlates with the size of the primary tumor, the frequency of lymph node and liver metastasis, and survival (43).

In patients with normal or intermediate levels of fasting serum gastrin, a secretin stimulation test is obtained (Fig. 4) (44). Administration of secretin (2 units/kg intravenously) followed by a rise in serum gastrin level of greater than 200 pg/mL or a greater than twofold increase within 15 minutes is diagnostic of ZES in 90% of patients. This test is sensitive and specific, as other causes of hypergastrinemia mentioned above do not respond to secretin with the paradoxical rise in gastrin level. The calcium stimulation test can also differentiate ZES from other causes of hypergastrinemia (45,46). However, this test is less sensitive and less specific than the secretin test (47), and is associated with many systemic side effects (primarily cardiac) from hypercalcemia.

Measurement of basal acid output (BAO) and maximal acid output (MAO) may also be useful in the management of patients with ZES (48,49). Because ZES patients are chronically exposed to high levels of gastrin, their BAO is expected to be high and not very responsive to further exposure to pentagastrin used in the provocative test. Their BAO/MAO ratio is therefore close to 1.0. However, even after curative resection, some ZES patients have persistently elevated BAO and MAO. This is due to the trophic effects of chronic high gastrinemia on the parietal cell mass. Therefore, the fasting serum gastrin and secretin stimulation test, and not BAO and MAO, are used to assess the adequacy of tumor resection. Postoperative fasting serum gastrin and secretin stimulation tests are both independent and significant predictors of 5-year cure (50). BAO and MAO remain useful indices in following ZES patients maintained on antisecretory therapy.

In patients with ZES in the context of suspected MEN1 syndrome, it is important to obtain serum calcium and parathormone (PTH) levels, as well as a prolactin level, to rule out synchronous parathyroid and pituitary disease. Surgical correction of hypercalcemia should precede exploration for gastrinomas to lessen general anesthetic risks. Furthermore, because hypercalcemia exacerbates gastrin and acid production (see above), parathyroidectomy should precede gastrinoma resection, and parathyroidectomy should be performed even if the gastrinoma is deemed unresectable (i.e., diffuse metastatic disease) (28).

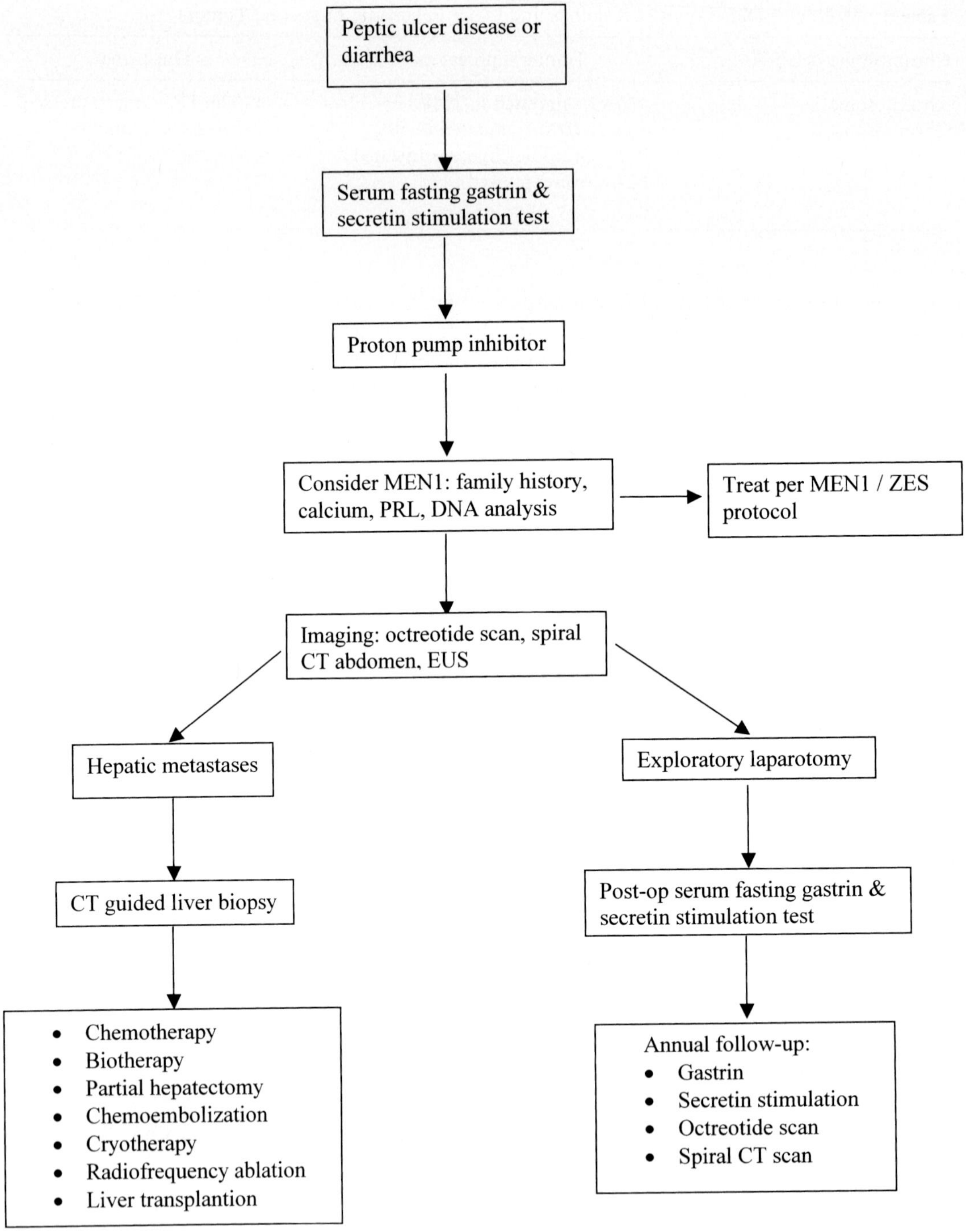

Figure 3 Suggested clinical management pathway. MEN1, multiple endocrine neoplasia, type-1; PRL, prolactin; ZES, Zollinger–Ellison syndrome; EUS, endoscopic ultrasound.

Table 3 Indications for Obtaining Serum Gastrin Measurement

Ulcer disease refractory to medical management
Recurrent ulcer disease after successful treatment
Family history of MEN1
Concurrent hypercalcemia
Concurrent nephrolithiasis
Ulcer disease in children
Pancreatic mass
Unexplained chronic diarrhea
Atypical ulcers

7 SERUM MOLECULAR MARKERS

Serum gastrin and chromogranin A (CgA) levels have been used to assess the response to and completeness of surgical therapy in ZES patients. Both are very sensitive and correlate with the presence of disease (51). The serum gastrin level, however, better correlates to tumor burden and therefore is more useful (51). Stabile and colleagues have suggested that whereas gastrin is a product of the tumor itself, CgA elevation is caused by the trophic effect of gastrin on gastric enterochromaffinlike cells (52). The use of serum gastrin in the diagnosis of ZES is discussed above. Chromogranin A has a specificity for gastrinoma of approximately 65% (51) and is therefore best used to follow the response to treatment in patients with known ZES.

8 LOCALIZATION BY IMAGING

Preoperative localization of pancreatic endocrine tumors (Fig. 5) is an important step in the management of these patients. As discussed earlier, surgical approach should be aggressive because it represents the only chance of cure for these patients. However, when there is extensive hepatic involvement, the decision for surgical exploration should be made on a case-by-case

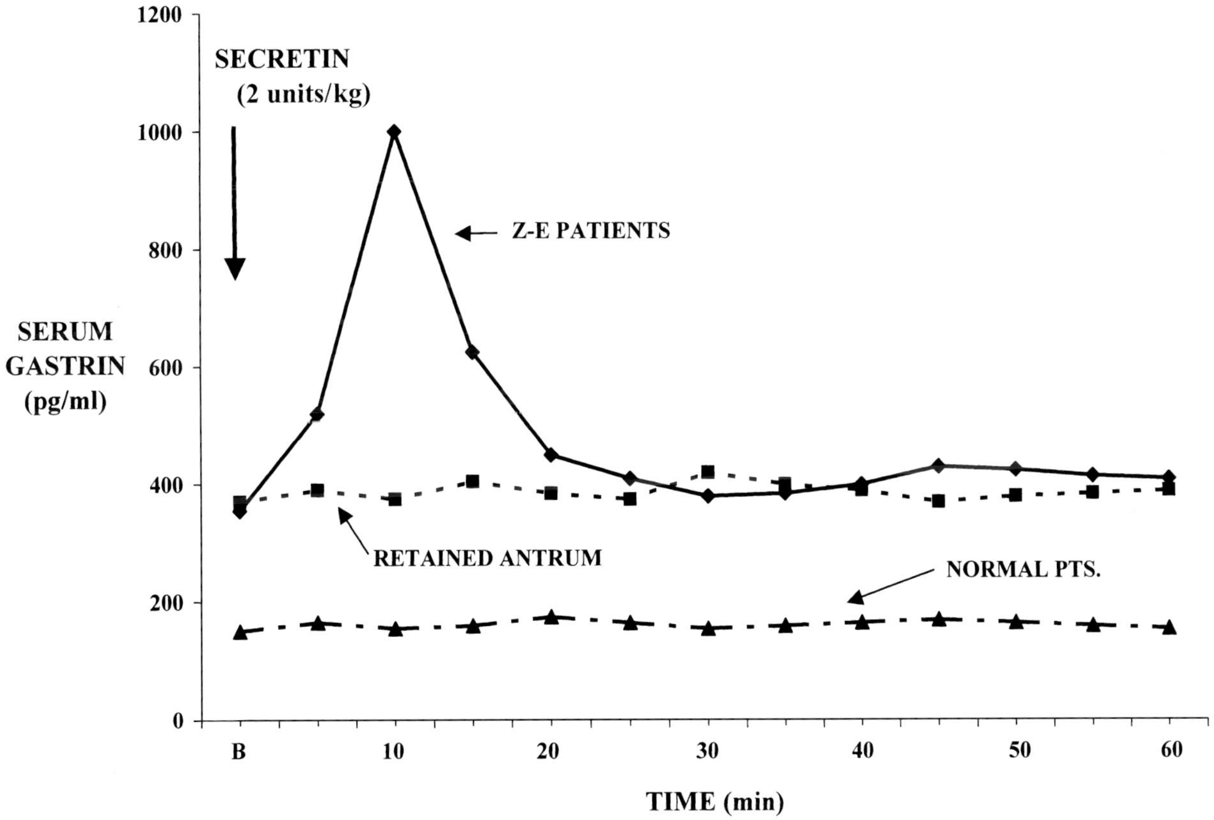

Figure 4 Secretin provocative test. Secretin is given at 2 units/kg intravenously, and the level of serum gastrin is measured over time. A rise in serum gastrin level of greater than 200 pg/mL or a greater than twofold increase within 15 minutes is diagnostic of ZES in 90% of patients. This test is sensitive and specific, as other causes of hypergastrinemia do not respond to secretin with the paradoxical rise in gastrin level. B, baseline. (From Ref. 44.)

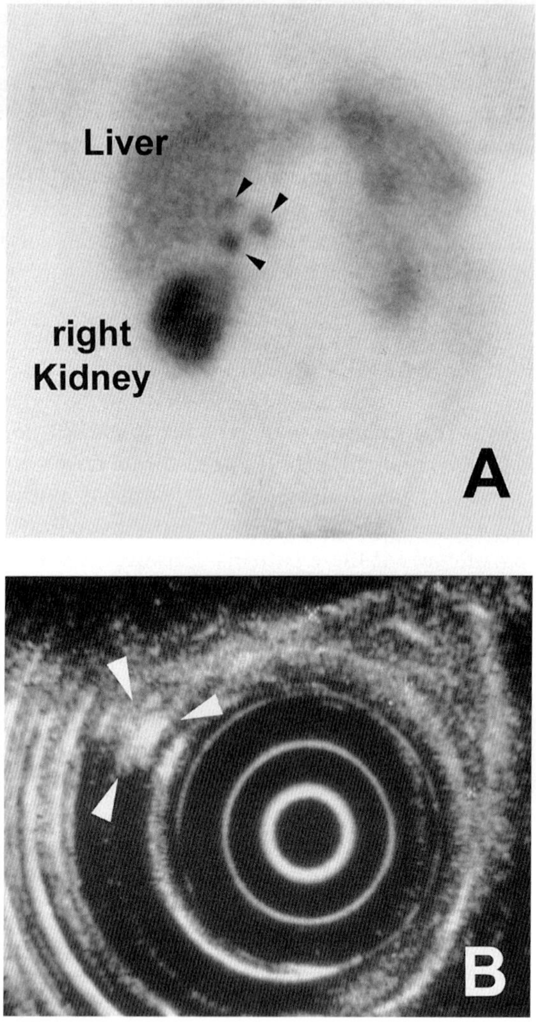

Figure 5 Preoperative localization studies. (A) Somatostatin receptor scintigraphy (SRS) demonstrating three somatostain receptor-positive tumors in the gastrinoma triangle area. (B) Endoscopic ultrasound (EUS) demonstrating a tumor in the wall of duodenum. Arrowheads point to tumors.

basis. Generally, octreoscan, endoscopic ultrasound, and a computed tomography (CT) scan or magnetic resonance imaging (MRI) should be performed in all patients. Other, more invasive studies may be considered, but in our experience the risks outweigh the benefits.

Often, the first imaging modality obtained is a CT scan because it is noninvasive and widely available. CT scan (spiral CT with pancreatic phase protocol) will usually demonstrate the tumor if it is greater than 3 cm in diameter, and it is helpful in visualizing hepatic metastases (53,54). Certainly, current CT imaging is more sensitive than these early reports may suggest. MRI, especially short-time inversion recovery (STIR)-MRI may be more sensitive in demonstrating both primary tumors and hepatic metastases than CT scan (55). All patients should have either an MRI or a CT scan. The decision should be determined by the institution's experience and available technology.

The most useful imaging modality is the somatostatin receptor scintigraphy (SRS, also known as OctreoScan). Using ^{111}In-pentetreotide, a recent large study of 146 ZES patients demonstrated that SRS has a false-positive rate of 12%, a sensitivity of 71% and a specificity of 86%, a positive predictive value of 85%, and a negative predictive value of 52% (56). Because it is a whole body scan, it has the advantage of localizing ectopic pancreatic endocrine tumors. Bony metastases are also detected by SRS, which obviates the use of bone scans. Many authors have thus recommended SRS as the first-line imaging modality for pancreatic endocrine tumors. However, because an experienced surgeon can detect approximately 30% more gastrinomas at surgery, SRS does not have an impact on the disease-free rate (57).

A new localization test that is gaining wide use is endoscopic ultrasound (EUS). A recent study of 82 patients with pancreatic endocrine tumors who underwent EUS showed that EUS has a sensitivity of 94%, an accuracy of 97%, and a specificity of 95% for pancreatic endocrine tumors (58). EUS was able to detect insulinomas, gastrinomas, as well as one glucagonoma and one somatostatinoma in this series, encompassing both pancreatic endocrine tumors that occur mostly in the head of pancreas and tumors that occur uniformly throughout the entire pancreas. The disadvantage of EUS as compared to SRS is that it is not as reliable in localizing extrapancreatic tumors, which is frequently the circumstance with sporadic gastrinomas.

Other localization studies include the invasive modalities of selective arteriography with or without intra-arterial injection of secretin/calcium and selective venous sampling. These studies are limited to large academic centers and are invasive in nature. They are thus used only in difficult cases of pancreatic endocrine tumors.

The positron emission tomography (PET) scan has emerged on the horizon as an exciting and promising diagnostic study for pancreatic endocrine tumors. The PET scan utilizes the uptake of labeled tracers that are metabolic substrates for tumors and the subsequent metabolic breakdown of the tracers to generate signals. Two such tracers, ^{11}C-L-DOPA and ^{11}C-5-HTP, have shown early promising results and performed better than ^{18}F-FDG in diagnosing pancreatic endocrine tumors (59–62). Furthermore, because the generation of signals is based on regional tumor metabolism, PET scans can also be used to monitor the efficacy of therapy. A combined PET/CT scan merges metabolic and anatomical information, and has been preliminarily applied to other areas of oncology (63,64). This seems to be a promising modality in preoperative localization and may be useful to image pancreatic endocrine tumors.

9 STAGING

Standardized tumor, node, metastasis (TNM) staging for gastrinomas and other pancreatic neuroendocrine tumors has been proposed but is still in evolution and not universally utilized (65). To a large extent, this is due to the rarity of these tumors and the difficulty in predicting a given tumor's biological behavior based upon traditional pathological criteria. Biological behavior of these tumors is dependent on the particular type of tumor and a variety of other factors. Gastrinomas are the most difficult to clearly define. From a practical standpoint, the most important criteria for determining gastrinoma resectability for cure is the presence of distant metastases involving liver or bone. For gastrinomas, lymph node involvement is controversial with regard to impact on respectability for cure and is thought to represent "primary nodal tumors" in some cases (4,19). In addition, primary liver gastrinomas have been reported, thus defying traditional assessment of these tumors (4,66,67). Moreover, it has been suggested that like other endocrine tumors there are both benign and malignant forms of the disease (4,68). Finally, there may be multiple primary tumors. Nongastrinomas appear to be more straightforward with regard to lymph node involvement and distant metastases.

For the moment, it is best to fully characterize each ZES patient with regard to size and exact location of primary tumor; the size, accurate location, and number of tumors within lymph nodes; and the full extent of distant metastases, particularly the exact location and number of hepatic metastases. Moreover, it is equally important to carefully follow-up (lifetime) patients to identify both persistent and recurrent disease.

10 SURGICAL APPROACH

10.1 Gastrinoma

The optimal treatment for sporadic gastrinomas, as for other neuroendocrine tumors, is complete surgical excision. Sporadic gastrinomas are now diagnosed early because of both increased awareness and better diagnostic tests (69). Consequently, surgical resection for cure is more likely. Patient selection for surgery is based upon the presence of MEN1 syndrome and preoperative imaging studies (19,70). Patients with MEN1 syndrome and gastrinoma without hepatic metastases may be considered for surgical exploration in selected cases. Patients with extensive liver involvement by preoperative imaging are not candidates for curative excision unless they have (rarely) evidence that the liver contains the primary tumor.

Preoperative imaging in sporadic gastrinoma patients is principally important to identify liver metastases. As for other types of tumors, if the preoperative studies localize the tumor, this information should be used in directing the abdominal exploration. Imaging (conventional and octreotide scan) is positive in approximately 70% of patients. Patients without liver metastases or MEN1 should be explored regardless of whether preoperative imaging demonstrates the primary tumor (s).

Exploration is usually performed through a midline incision, although a bilateral subcostal incision may be appropriate for selected patients depending upon their body habitus. Laparoscopy to look for liver metastases as well as exploration may be considered if the surgeon has sufficient experience with this approach. Since the vast majority of gastrinomas (85%) are found within the gastrinoma triangle, initial exploration should be directed there (Fig. 1) and any tumor identified by preoperative imaging studies (11). Perform a Kocher maneuver to expose the duodenum and pancreatic head. The colon hepatic flexure may need to be mobilized inferiorly to effectively expose this region. The head of the pancreas should be bimanually palpated. Fat and attachments to the colon or stomach should be cleared to allow careful inspection. Small suspicious nodules can be safely enucleated and sent for frozen section histology. These nodules can vary in size from 5 mm to several centimeters, and there may be more than one tumor present. Although we have enucleated gastrinomas as large 4 cm, larger masses may require pancreaticoduodenectomy to avoid pancreatic duct leak and excessive bleeding. If more than one tumor is identified, these should be individually excised rather than attempting a "radical oncological resection." In sharp contrast to its sensitivity for identifying pancreatic insulinomas, we have not found intraoperative ultrasonography helpful in localizing gastrinomas.

Next, the duodenum should be carefully palpated. Many small occult gastrinomas are often found within the wall of the duodenum. Most often they are in the second portion, but can be identified within any portion of the duodenum. Gastrinomas are rarely in the stomach or proximal jejunum, although these areas should not be overlooked. A useful technique to identify these tumors is to transilluminate the bowel with an upper endoscope (71). They will appear as a dark spot against the lighter red background of the bowel. Brunner's gland adenomas and heterotopic pancreas have a similar appearance, but they can be distinguished by frozen section biopsy. Performing duodenotomy, which should be performed even if duodenal transillumination fails to reveal tumor, can also identify small duodenal gastrinomas. The duodenotomy (longitudinal 3 cm) is made at the junction of the second and first portions of the duodenum, and the entire duodenum should be palpated. It is important to remember these tumors are submucosal and do not have the typical mucosal appearance of a gastrointestinal adenocarcinoma.

Next, all lymph nodes around the pancreatic head, in particular, the retropancreatic lymph nodes, should be excised. This includes lymph nodes along the inferior vena cava and medial border of the aorta. The hepatoduodenal ligament should be thoroughly explored. All lymphatic tissue should be sent for frozen section. Dissection should proceed towards the hilum of the liver, excising all suspicious masses and lymph nodes.

The liver should be carefully palpated. Suspicious nodules should be removed by wedge resection. Formal hepatic lobectomy may be necessary in selected cases where a single large metastasis is present. Generally, patients who have liver involvement have extensive disease at presentation and curative resection is not feasible. Rarely, a liver primary gastrinoma is present and curative resection can be accomplished. The remainder of the pancreas should be carefully palpated. Tumors within the body and tail are more often malignant. The lesser sack should be entered through the avascular fusion within gastrocolic ligament on the left side of the abdomen. The pancreas body and tail should be mobilized and palpated. The splenic hilum should be carefully inspected.

The remainder of the exploration should include the stomach, proximal jejunum, greater omentum, kidneys, and ovaries. It is important to remember that gastrinomas may be multiple, extrapancreatic, and extraintestinal in location. Thorough search is mandatory.

In approximately 10% of patients, exploration fails to lead to localization of the primary tumor or, if a tumor is found, the patient may still be hypergastrinemic postoperatively. These experiences have led us to emphasize the following general guidelines for exploration. Perform a thorough evaluation of the abdomen, but focus on the gastrinoma triangle. Some gastrinomas may be within the liver and may never be identified unless imaging studies are positive and can direct surgical exploration. The most likely location of a missed gastrinoma is within the duodenum, and careful and exhaustive inspection should always be performed there. Most gastrinomas are extrapancreatic in sharp contrast to their classification as "pancreatic neuroendocrine or islet tumors," and every nodule and lymph node, without exception, should be sent for frozen section biopsy.

Since a patient may have multiple tumors, either as multiple primaries or micrometastases, there clearly is a need to determine completeness of resection at the time of operation. A rapid gastrin radioimmunoassay that yields results in 60 minutes can be used to assess completeness of resection (72,73), but has not gained wide acceptance. Prior to initiation of exploration, a baseline study is performed with injection of secretin (2 u/kg) and measurement of serum gastrin at 2, 4, and 6 minutes. The study is then repeated after the surgeon is convinced he has excised all gastrinoma tissue. The utility of such a test is to direct the surgeon to further explore the patient with the intent of identifying and resecting additional tumor. Long-term studies need to validate this approach.

Radioguided surgery ideally would improve gastrinoma cure rates (74). Unfortunately, some gastrinomas are not identified by octreotide scan. Furthermore, a given patient may have multiple tumors, only some of which may label effectively with octreotide. Nonetheless, with further refinements in the hand-held gamma probe technology as well as better tumor markers, this technique may prove valuable.

Life-long follow-up is essential for patients with sporadic gastrinoma. Repeat serum fasting gastrin levels should be obtained immediately after surgery and at 6 months. Thereafter, these biochemical tests should be repeated annually with imaging studies. For patients with recurrent disease, usually the secretin stimulation test will be positive before elevation of the baseline fasting gastrin. Proton pump inhibitor therapy should be continued through the initial postoperative period to avoid rebound hyperacidity in the face of possible persistent hypergastrinemia. As much as 50% of patients may have persistent hypergastrinemia after excision for cure (75). We reserve reoperation for patients who have persistent hypergastrinemia and have tumor identifiable by imaging studies.

10.2 Nongastrinoma

Like gastrinomas, the optimal treatment for nongastrinoma pancreatic neuroendocrine tumors is complete surgical excision. In contrast to gastrinomas, these tumors are symptomatic due to their size and readily identified by imaging studies. These tumors are usually malignant and rarely extrapancreatic. In contrast to gastrinomas, surgical exploration and formal pancreatic resection should be performed rather than tumor enucleation. (Insulinomas discussed in Ch. 45.)

11 MEDICAL THERAPY

Patients with gastrinoma should be immediately treated with antacid therapy with either proton pump inhibitors or H2-receptor antagonists. Octreotide may also be added to the regimen. Once stabilized, they should be evaluated for surgical therapy. Patients who cannot be cured surgically must continue with medical therapy. The proton pump inhibitors [omeprazole (76,77), lansoprazole (78–80), pantoprazole oral (81) and intravenous (82), rabeprazole (83)] are the most effective medications for controlling acid secretion and are preferred to H2-receptor antagonists [cimetidine (84), ranitidine (85), famotidine (86), nizatidine (87)]. Proton pump inhibitors are vastly superior because they require less frequent dosing, have less tachyphylaxis, and breakthrough hyperacidity is uncommon (77,88–92). Measurement of gastric acid production is generally recommended to initially monitor efficacy of the antacid therapy (93). Gastric acid secretion should be less than 10 mEq/h for the hour prior to the next dose. If not, the dose should be increased until acid secretion is sufficiently suppressed. Patients with previous acid-reducing surgical procedures should have lower acid production (< 5 mEq/h). It is important to use sufficient drug to control acid production to avoid acute complications related to peptic ulcer disease such as bleeding and perforation. Compared to nongastrinoma patients, higher doses of these medications may be required to achieve ulcer and esophagitis healing and control diarrhea and pain. *Helicobactor pylori* is not a risk factor for peptic ulceration in ZE patients, and, based upon current studies, patients do not need routine antimicrobial therapy (94). The potential complications of prolonged use of potent antacid therapy include malabsorption of vitamin B_{12}. Patients should be monitored periodically for the development of B_{12} deficiency and anemia (95). In rats treated for 2 years with omeprazole, gastric ECLomas developed, which raises a concern for ZE patients who may require life-long therapy (96). Gastric carcinoids arising as a consequence of antacid therapy, however, have not been convincingly demonstrated in humans (97).

12 CHEMOTHERAPY, BIOTHERAPY, AND RADIATION THERAPY

Standard chemotherapy is at best modestly effective, and, as for most solid tumors, better therapies need to be developed. Tumors may respond for 2–3 years but eventually become resistant. Because of the rarity of these tumors, few prospective randomized controlled trials have been published. The response to chemotherapy is particularly difficult to evaluate because often no distinction is made between the various types of neuroendocrine tumors and carcinoids included in the trial. In addition, often patients with gastrinoma in lymph node are considered to have malignant disease and are grouped with patients with liver metastases. Clearly, surgical survival data demonstrates that these two patient groups have vastly different survival expectations (Fig. 2).

Of the standard chemotherapy agents tested, streptozocin (STZ)-based therapies have been the most effective, and combination therapy is generally better than STZ alone (98–101). One of the larger randomized cooperative group trial comparing STZ/doxorubicin, STZ/fluorouracil (5FU), and chlorozotocin (CTZ) demonstrated a 69% response rate and improved median survival with the STZ/doxorubicin combination (102). This study is often quoted as the best available therapy trial, but results (retrospective analysis) using a similar regimen at another institution have challenged this recommendation (103). Other regimens have been less effective or ineffective. DTIC (5-dimethyltriazeno-imidazole-4-carboxamide)-based therapies have a modest response (104–106). Single-agent therapy with either carboplatin, mitoxantrone, or etoposide is not effective (107–109).

Biotherapy with interferon-α, which has been used extensively to treat carcinoids, is thought to have some efficacy in a few small phase II trials with pancreatic neuroendocrine tumors (110). Interferon-α combined with octreotide is the most effective regimen reported (111,112). Interferon-α either alone (113) or combined with 5-FU (114) has minimal activity. These trials frequently suffer from the same limitations hindering chemotherapy trials: nonrandomized, small sample size, heterogeneous tumor types included, and inadequate distinction between liver and lymph node involvement. Similar to the streptozotocin based chemotherapy clinical trials described above, randomized control trials need to be performed to determine what role, if any, interferon-α has in treatment of sporadic gastrinomas and other neuroendocrine tumors.

Octreotide, a long-acting synthetic analogue of somatostatin, potently inhibits both the secretion and the peripheral actions of hormones and biological amines produced by neuroendocrine tumors. Octreotide, however, does not have a clearly defined role in the treatment of gastrinoma as it does for other endocrine tumors such as carcinoid. This is primarily because antacid therapy with proton pump inhibitors is very effective in controlling symptoms of Zollinger-Ellison syndrome. Octreotide is administered parenterally three times daily and the injections can be painful, which reduces patient compliance. In addition, there is tachyphylaxis with long-term therapy. Similar to other proton pump inhibitors and the H2-receptor antagonists, the omeprazole dose must be titrated to effect. Therapy can be monitored by improvement in symptoms and reduction in serum gastrin levels, which is more convenient than monitoring gastric acid production. Once the patient has demonstrated a response to octreotide, he should be converted to one of the longer-acting preparations (either octreotide LAR or lanreotide) (115, 116). The efficacy is the same for both octreotide and the longer-acting preparations, and patient compliance should be higher with monthly (octreotide LAR) or twice-monthly injections [lanreotide (117)].

There have been anecdotal reports of octreotide inhibiting tumor progression, but there has not been a randomized control trial showing a survival advantage (118–121). A recent prospective study of octreotide therapy in 15 patients with gastrinoma hepatic metastases demonstrated either tumor stabilization or a decrease in tumor size in approximately 50% of patients studied (115). If octreotide were proven effective biotherapy, it might be a reasonable alternative to standard chemotherapy or be used as an adjunct to other therapies such as chemoembolization of liver metastases. In addition, it could have a role in prevention or treatment of gastric ECLomas that might arise with long-term antacid therapy.

Because of the high affinity of octreotide for gastrinomas, there is great promise of radionuclide therapy with radiolabeled somatostatin analogues. This radioligand is internalized into the tumor cell and can induce cell cytotoxicity. Preclinical and phase I trials suggest that radiolabeled somatostatin analogs [DOTA, Tyr(3)] octreotide and [DOTA, Tyr(3)]octreotate may be effective in a subset of patients with gastrinoma (122). Further work in this area is essential to determine whether this strategy will be effective.

13 PALLIATIVE THERAPY

Patients with hepatic or other distant metastatic disease can have an indolent course, and every effort should be made to surgically resect all identifiable tumors. Medical therapy with proton pump inhibitors and octreotide will generally control the ravages of peptic ulcer disease in ZES. Rarely, total gastrectomy may be required. Lesser procedures such as vagotomy and antrectomy are not recommended. Likewise, blind resection of the pancreas is usually ineffective. Isolated hepatic or lung metastases should be resected with curative intent (123). Chemotherapy or biotherapy, although not curative, should be offered, as some patients will respond to therapy.

Patients with extensive liver involvement pose a great challenge. One surgical option is liver transplantation. Although it is encouraging that some patients have achieved prolonged survival, unfortunately, this is a risky procedure, and in the immune-compromised state many of these patients may later succumb to recurrent disease (124,125). Transplantation should be reserved for patients who are not candidates for other cytoreductive therapies. Radiofrequency ablation or cryosurgery alone or in combination with partial hepatectomy or chemoembolization may also be considered (126,127).

Transcatheter arterial chemoembolization (TACE) is an alternative procedure. Because the liver has a dual vascular supply and hepatic metastases derive the majority of blood from the hepatic artery, the regional delivery of chemotherapy can achieve higher tumor doses than systemic therapy. The hepatic artery embolization of tumor vessels can induce selective metastasis ischemia and necrosis. The combination of these two strategies, or chemoembolization, may be synergistic (128–134). Such an approach may palliate the symptoms of many patients with liver-dominant metastases.

14 PROGNOSIS

14.1 Gastrinoma

Functional endocrine tumors pose two different problems with regard to treatment and prognosis: control of hormone-related symptoms and control of tumor progression. ZES cure is defined as surgical resection of all gross tumor with resolution of symptoms, normal postoperative fasting serum gastrin levels, and a negative postoperative secretin stimulation test (19). ZES cure rates vary from center to center (34–85%) (19,67), but using current treatment strategies with earlier diagnosis and aggressive surgical management survival is much better than historically thought (135). Some patients, however, who are not surgically "cured" never have progression of their disease, and their survival can be similar to patients who have been surgically "cured." In one large prospective series, the overall survival during a 15-year follow-up period was excellent with 16% of patients having ZES-related cause of death (7). The hormonal effects of their gastrinoma may be controlled with antacid therapy and octreotide. Consequently, patients rarely die as a consequence of the hormonal effects of their tumors. As long as the tumor does not distantly metastasize, they may survive with their tumor controlled with medical therapy.

The prognosis for patients with sporadic gastrinoma is primarily determined by the presence of distant (liver and bone) metastases at the time of operation (4). In fact, it is unusual for a patient who does not have liver metastases at the time of initial exploration to later develop liver metastases (< 10%) (4,7,19). We have found that patients with primary tumor located to the left of the mesenteric vessels more often (20% vs. 40%) have liver metastases (12). Generally, patients can be placed into one of four broad groups. The first group consists of patients with a clear diagnosis of gastrinoma, who are found to have a pancreatic, duodenal, or peripancreatic primary tumor that is resected at operation. The second group has tumor within lymph node(s). Gastrinoma in a lymph node may represent either a so-called nodal primary tumor or metastatic disease (19). In either circumstance, these patients have similar survival rates to patients within the first group. The third group (~ 10%) consists of patients in which no tumor is identifiable at exploration. These patients, like those in the first two groups, have a favorable prognosis. The fourth group (~ 20%) has liver metastases at the time of operation. These patients have a less favorable prognosis, but these tumors can be slow growing and should be treated aggressively (20,123).

14.2 Nongastrinoma

Most other pancreatic endocrine tumors, with the notable exception of insulinomas, have a poor prognosis. Surgical resection is the only means to a cure. Chemotherapy, biotherapy, and hepatic cytoreduction should be attempted in advanced cases. These tumors can be quite aggressive, however, and the patient will often eventually succumb to inanition from hepatic metastases.

REFERENCES

1. Goebel SU, Vortmeyer AO, Zhuang Z, Serrano J, Jensen RT, Lubensky IA. Identical clonality of sporadic gastrinomas at multiple sites. Cancer Res 2000; 60(1): 60–63.
2. Kisker O, Bastian D, Bartsch D, Nies C, Rothmund M. Localization, malignant potential, and surgical management of gastrinomas. World J Surg 1998; 22(7):651–657.
3. Norton JA, Alexander HR, Fraker DL, Venzon DJ, Gibril F, Jensen RT. Comparison of surgical results in patients with advanced and limited disease with multiple endocrine neoplasia type 1 and Zollinger-Ellison syndrome. Ann Surg 2001; 234(4):495–505.
4. Stabile BE, Passaro E Jr. Benign and malignant gastrinoma. Am J Surg 1985; 149(1):144–150.
5. Passaro E Jr, Stabile BE, Howard TJ. Contributions of the Zollinger-Ellison syndrome. Am J Surg 1991; 161(2):203–206.
6. Mignon M, Ruszniewski P, Haffar S, Rigaud D, Rene E, Bonfils S. Current approach to the management of tumoral process in patients with gastrinoma. World J Surg 1986; 10(4):703–710.
7. Yu F, Venzon DJ, Serrano J, Goebel SU, Doppman JL, Gibril F, Jensen RT. Prospective study of the clinical course, prognostic factors, causes of death, and survival in patients with long-standing Zollinger-Ellison syndrome. J Clin Oncol 1999; 17(2):615–630.
8. Brandi ML, Gagel RF, Angeli A, Bilezikian JP, Beck-Peccoz P, Bordi C, Conte-Devolx B, Falchetti A, Gheri RG, Libroia A, Lips CJ, Lombardi G, Mannelli M, Pacini F, Ponder BA, Raue F, Skogseid B, Tamburrano G, Thakker RV, Thompson NW, Tomassetti P, Tonelli F, Wells SA Jr, Marx SJ. Guidelines for diagnosis and therapy of MEN type 1 and type 2. J Clin Endocrinol Metab 2001; 86(12):5658–5671.
9. Zollinger RM, Ellison EH. Primary peptic ulcerations of the jejunum associated with islet cell tumors of the pancreas. Ann Surg 1955; 142:709.
10. Guo SS, Sawicki MP. Molecular and genetic mechanisms of tumorigenesis in multiple endocrine neoplasia type-1. Mol Endocrinol 2001; 15(10):1653–1664.
11. Stabile BE, Morrow DJ, Passaro E Jr. The gastrinoma triangle: operative implications. Am J Surg 1984; 147(1):25–31.
12. Howard TJ, Sawicki MP, Stabile BE, Watt PC, Passaro E Jr. Biologic behavior of sporadic gastrinoma located to the right and left of the superior mesenteric artery. Am J Surg 1993; 165(1):101–105.
13. Herrmann ME, Ciesla MC, Chejfec G, DeJong SA, Yong SL. Primary nodal gastrinomas. Arch Pathol Lab Med 2000; 124(6):832–835.
14. Bordi C, Corleto VD, Azzoni C, Pizzi S, Ferraro G, Gibril F, Delle Fave G, Jensen RT. The antral mucosa as a new site for endocrine tumors in multiple endocrine neoplasia type 1 and Zollinger-Ellison syndromes. J Clin Endocrinol Metab 2001; 86(5):2236–2242.
15. Gibril F, Curtis LT, Termanini B, Fritsch MK, Lubensky IA, Doppman JL, Jensen RT. Primary

cardiac gastrinoma causing Zollinger-Ellison syndrome. Gastroenterology 1997; 112(2):567–574.
16. Hirasawa K, Yamada M, Kitagawa M, Takehira Y, Tamakoshi K, Nakamura T, Kawamura K, Takagi M, Murohisa B, Ozawa T, Hanai H, Kaneko E. Ovarian mucinous cystadenocarcinoma as a cause of Zollinger-Ellison syndrome: report of a case and review of the literature. Am J Gastroenterol 2000; 95(5):1348–1351.
17. Wu PC, Alexander HR, Bartlett DL, Doppman JL, Fraker DL, Norton JA, Gibril F, Fogt F, Jensen RT. A prospective analysis of the frequency, location, and curability of ectopic (nonpancreaticoduodenal, nonnodal) gastrinoma. Surgery 1997; 122(6):1176–1182.
18. Bhagavan BS, Slavin RE, Goldberg J, Rao RN. Ectopic gastrinoma and Zollinger-Ellison syndrome. Hum Pathol 1986; 17(6):584–592.
19. Howard TJ, Zinner MJ, Stabile BE, Passaro E Jr. Gastrinoma excision for cure. A prospective analysis. Ann Surg 1990; 211(1):9–14.
20. Sutliff VE, Doppman JL, Gibril F, Venzon DJ, Yu F, Serrano J, Jensen RT. Growth of newly diagnosed, untreated metastatic gastrinomas and predictors of growth patterns. J Clin Oncol 1997; 15(6):2420–2431.
21. Eriksson B, Oberg K, Skogseid B. Neuroendocrine pancreatic tumors. Clinical findings in a prospective study of 84 patients. Acta Oncol 1989; 28(3):373–377.
22. Kloppel G, Heitz PU. Pancreatic endocrine tumors. Pathol Res Pract 1988; 183(2):155–168.
23. Lo CY, van Heerden JA, Thompson GB, Grant CS, Soreide JA, Harmsen WS. Islet cell carcinoma of the pancreas. World J Surg 1996; 20(7):878–883.
24. Dubois PM, Paulin C, Chayvialle JA. Identification of gastrin-secreting cells and cholecystokinin-secreting cells in the gastrointestinal tract of the human fetus and adult man. Cell Tissue Res 1976; 175(3):351–356.
25. Track NS, Creutzfeldt C, Litzenberger J, Neuhoff C, Arnold R, Creutzfeldt W. Appearance of gastrin and somatostatin in the human fetal stomach, duodenum and pancreas. Digestion 1979; 19(5):292–306.
26. Goebel SU, Peghini PL, Goldsmith PK, Spiegel AM, Gibril F, Raffeld M, Jensen RT, Serrano J. Expression of the calcium-sensing receptor in gastrinomas. J Clin Endocrinol Metab 2000; 85(11):4131–4137.
27. Geibel JP, Wagner CA, Caroppo R, Qureshi I, Gloeckner J, Manuelidis L, Kirchhoff P, Radebold K. The stomach divalent ion-sensing receptor scar is a modulator of gas-tric acid secretion. J Biol Chem 2001; 276(43):39549–39552.
28. Norton JA, Cornelius MJ, Doppman JL, Maton PN, Gardner JD, Jensen RT. Effect of parathyroidectomy in patients with hyperparathyroidism, Zollinger-Ellison syndrome, and multiple endocrine neoplasia type I: a prospective study. Surgery 1987; 102(6):958–966.
29. Carroll RE, Matkowskyj KA, Chakrabarti S, McDonald TJ, Benya RV. Aberrant expression of gastrin-releasing peptide and its receptor by well-differentiated colon cancers in humans. Am J Physiol 1999; 276(3 pt 1): G655–G665.
30. Saurin JC, Nemoz-Gaillard E, Sordat B, Cuber JC, Coy DH, Abello J, Chayvialle JA. Bombesin stimulates adhesion, spreading, lamellipodia formation, and proliferation in the human colon carcinoma Isreco1 cell line. Cancer Res 1999; 59(4):962–967.
31. Watson SA, Smith AM. Hypergastrinemia promotes adenoma progression in the APC(Min−/+) mouse model of familial adenomatous polyposis. Cancer Res 2001; 61(2):625–631.
32. Wang EH, Ebrahimi SA, Wu AY, Kashefi C, Passaro E Jr, Sawicki MP. Mutation of the MENIN gene in sporadic pancreatic endocrine tumors. Cancer Res 1998; 58(19):4417–4420.
33. Guo SS, Arora C, Shimoide AT, Sawicki MP. Frequent deletion of chromosome 3 in malignant sporadic pancreatic endocrine tumors. Mol Cell Endocrinol 2002; 190(1–2):109–114.
34. Guo SS, Wu AY, Sawicki MP. Deletion of chromosome 1, but not mutation of MEN-1, predicts prognosis in sporadic pancreatic endocrine tumors. World J Surg 2002; 26(7).
35. Chung DC, Brown SB, Graeme-Cook F, Seto M, Warshaw AL, Jensen RT, Arnold A. Overexpression of cyclin D1 occurs frequently in human pancreatic endocrine tumors. J Clin Endocrinol Metab 2000; 85(11):4373–4378.
36. Evers BM, Rady PL, Sandoval K, Arany I, Tyring SK, Sanchez RL, Nealon WH, Townsend CM Jr, Thompson JC. Gastrinomas demonstrate amplification of the HER-2/neu proto-oncogene. Ann Surg 1994; 219(6): 596–601.
37. Muscarella P, Melvin WS, Fisher WE, Foor J, Ellison EC, Herman JG, Schirmer WJ, Hitchcock CL, DeYoung BR, Weghorst CM. Genetic alterations in gastrinomas and nonfunctioning pancreatic neuroendocrine tumors: an analysis of p16/MTS1 tumor suppressor gene inactivation. Cancer Res 1998; 58(2): 237–240.
38. Serrano J, Goebel SU, Peghini PL, Lubensky IA, Gibril F, Jensen RT. Alterations in the p16INK4a/CDKN2A tumor suppressor gene in gastrinomas. J Clin Endocrinol Metab 2000; 85(11):4146–4156.
39. Canavese G, Azzoni C, Pizzi S, Corleto VD, Pasquali C, Davoli C, Crafa P, DelleFave G, Bordi C. p27: a potential main inhibitor of cell proliferation in digestive endocrine tumors but not a marker of benign behavior. Hum Pathol 2001; 32(10):1094–1101.
40. Guo SS, Wu X, Shimoide AT, Wong J, Sawicki MP. Anomalous overexpression of p27(Kip1) in sporadic pancreatic endocrine tumors. J Surg Res 2001; 96(2):284–288.
41. Bartsch D, Hahn SA, Danichevski KD, Ramaswamy A, Bastian D, Galehdari H, Barth P, Schmiegel W, Simon B, Rothmund M. Mutations of the DPC4/

Smad4 gene in neuroendocrine pancreatic tumors. Oncogene 1999; 18(14):2367–2371.
42. Lin HJ, French SW, Reichenbach D, Wan YJ, Passaro E Jr, Sawicki MP. Novel p53 mutation in a malignant tumor secreting vasoactive intestinal peptide. Arch Pathol Lab Med 1997; 121(2):125–128.
43. Berger AC, Gibril F, Venzon DJ, Doppman JL, Norton JA, Libutti SK, Bartlett DL, Jensen RT, Alexander HR. Prognostic value of initial fasting serum gastrin levels in patients with Zollinger-Ellison syndrome. J Clin Oncol 2001; 19(12):3051–3057.
44. Isenberg JI, Walsh JH, Passaro E Jr, Moore EW, Grossman MI. Unusual effect of secretin on serum gastrin, serum calcium, and gastric acid secretion in a patient with suspected Zollinger-Ellison syndrome. Gastroenterology 1972; 62(4):626–631.
45. Basso N, Passaro E Jr. Calcium-stimulated gastric secretion in the Zollinger-Ellison syndrome. Arch Surg 1970; 101(3):399–402.
46. Passaro E Jr, Basso N, Walsh JH. Calcium challenge in the Zollinger-Ellison syndrome. Surgery 1972; 72(1):60–67.
47. Frucht H, Howard JM, Slaff JI, Wank SA, McCarthy DM, Maton PN, Vinayek R, Gardner JD, Jensen RT. Secretin and calcium provocative tests in the Zollinger-Ellison syndrome. A prospective study. Ann Intern Med 1989; 111(9):713–722.
48. Fraker DL, Norton JA, Saeed ZA, Maton PN, Gardner JD, Jensen RT. A prospective study of perioperative and postoperative control of acid hypersecretion in patients with Zollinger-Ellison syndrome undergoing gastrinoma resection. Surgery 1988; 104(6):1054–1063.
49. Pisegna JR, Norton JA, Slimak GG, Metz DC, Maton PN, Gardner JD, Jensen RT. Effects of curative gastrinoma resection on gastric secretory function and antisecretory drug requirement in the Zollinger-Ellison syndrome. Gastroenterology 1992; 102(3):767–778.
50. Alexander HR, Bartlett DL, Venzon DJ, Libutti SK, Doppman JL, Fraker DL, Norton JA, Gibril F, Jensen RT. Analysis of factors associated with long-term (five or more years) cure in patients undergoing operation for Zollinger-Ellison syndrome. Surgery 1998; 124(6):1160–1166.
51. Goebel SU, Serrano J, Yu F, Gibril F, Venzon DJ, Jensen RT. Prospective study of the value of serum chromogranin A or serum gastrin levels in the assessment of the presence, extent, or growth of gastrinomas. Cancer 1999; 85(7):1470–1483.
52. Stabile BE, Howard TJ, Passaro E Jr, O'Connor DT. Source of plasma chromogranin A elevation in gastrinoma patients. Arch Surg 1990; 125(4):451–453.
53. Pisegna JR, Doppman JL, Norton JA, Metz DC, Jensen RT. Prospective comparative study of ability of MR imaging and other imaging modalities to localize tumors in patients with Zollinger-Ellison syndrome. Dig Dis Sci 1993; 38(7):1318–1328.
54. Wank SA, Doppman JL, Miller DL, Collen MJ, Maton PN, Vinayek R, Slaff JI, Norton JA, Gardner JD, Jensen RT. Prospective study of the ability of computed axial tomography to localize gastrinomas in patients with Zollinger-Ellison syndrome. Gastroenterology 1987; 92(4):905–912.
55. Modlin IM, Tang LH. Approaches to the diagnosis of gut neuroendocrine tumors: the last word (today). Gastroenterology 1997; 112(2):583–590.
56. Gibril F, Reynolds JC, Chen CC, Yu F, Goebel SU, Serrano J, Doppman JL, Jensen RT. Specificity of somatostatin receptor scintigraphy: a prospective study and effects of false-positive localizations on management in patients with gastrinomas. J Nucl Med 1999; 40(4):539–553.
57. Alexander HR, Fraker DL, Norton JA, Bartlett DL, Tio L, Benjamin SB, Doppman JL, Goebel SU, Serrano J, Gibril F, Jensen RT. Prospective study of somatostatin receptor scintigraphy and its effect on operative outcome in patients with Zollinger-Ellison syndrome. Ann Surg 1998; 228(2):228–238.
58. Anderson MA, Carpenter S, Thompson NW, Nostrant TT, Elta GH, Scheiman JM. Endoscopic ultrasound is highly accurate and directs management in patients with neuroendocrine tumors of the pancreas. Am J Gastroenterol 2000; 95(9):2271–2277.
59. Ahlstrom H, Eriksson B, Bergstrom M, Bjurling P, Langstrom B, Oberg K. Pancreatic neuroendocrine tumors: diagnosis with PET. Radiology 1995; 195(2): 333–337.
60. Bombardieri E, Maccauro M, De Deckere E, Savelli G, Chiti A. Nuclear medicine imaging of neuroendocrine tumours. Ann Oncol 2001; 12(suppl 2):S51–S61.
61. Eriksson B, Bergstrom M, Orlefors H, Sundin A, Oberg K, Langstrom B. Use of PET in neuroendocrine tumors. In vivo applications and in vitro studies. Q J Nucl Med 2000; 44(1):68–76.
62. Orlefors H, Sundin A, Ahlstrom H, Bjurling P, Bergstrom M, Lilja A, Langstrom B, Oberg K, Eriksson B. Positron emission tomography with 5-hydroxytryprophan in neuroendocrine tumors. J Clin Oncol 1998; 16(7):2534–2541.
63. Charron M, Beyer T, Bohnen NN, Kinahan PE, Dachille M, Jerin J, Nutt R, Meltzer CC, Villemagne V, Townsend DW. Image analysis in patients with cancer studied with a combined PET and CT scanner. Clin Nucl Med 2000; 25(11):905–910.
64. Makhija S, Howden N, Edwards R, Kelley J, Townsend DW, Meltzer CC. Positron emission tomography/computed tomography imaging for the detection of recurrent ovarian and fallopian tube carcinoma: a retrospective review. Gynecol Oncol 2002; 85(1):53–58.
65. Ellison EC. Zollinger-Ellison syndrome. In: Cameron JL, ed. Current Surgical Therapy. St. Louis: Mosby, Inc., 1998:83–90.

66. Tiomny E, Brill S, Baratz M, Messer G, Greif F, Moshkowitz M, Gilat T. Primary liver gastrinoma. J Clin Gastroenterol 1997; 24(3):188–191.
67. Norton JA, Fraker DL, Alexander HR, Venzon DJ, Doppman JL, Serrano J, Goebel SU, Peghini PL, Roy PK, Gibril F, Jensen RT. Surgery to cure the Zollinger-Ellison syndrome. N Engl J Med 1999; 341(9):635–644.
68. Passaro E Jr, Howard TJ, Sawicki MP, Watt PC, Stabile BE. The origin of sporadic gastrinomas within the gastrinoma triangle: a theory. Arch Surg 1998; 133(1):13–16.
69. Howard TJ, Passaro E Jr. Gastrinoma. New medical and surgical approaches. Surg Clin North Am 1989; 69(3):667–681.
70. Norton JA, Fraker DL, Alexander HR, Venzon DJ, Doppman JL, Serrano J, Goebel SU, Peghini PL, Roy PK, Gibril F, Jensen RT. Surgery to cure the Zollinger-Ellison syndrome. N Engl J Med 1999; 341(9):635–644.
71. Norton JA. Intraoperative methods to stage and localize pancreatic and duodenal tumors. Ann Oncol 1999; 10(suppl 4):182–184.
72. Kato M, Imamura M, Hosotani R, Shimada Y, Doi R, Itami A, Komoto I, Kosaka TT, Konishi J. Curative resection of microgastrinomas based on the intraoperative secretin test. World J Surg 2000; 24(11): 1425–1430.
73. Proye C, Pattou F, Carnaille B, Paris JC, D'Herbomez M, Marchandise X. Intraoperative gastrin measurements during surgical management of patients with gastrinomas: experience with 20 cases. World J Surg 1998; 22(7):643–649.
74. Schirmer WJ, O'Dorisio TM, Schirmer TP, Mojzisik CM, Hinkle GH, Martin EW. Intraoperative localization of neuroendocrine tumors with 125I-TYR[3]-octreotide and a hand-held gamma-detecting probe. Surgery 1993; 114(4):745–751.
75. Fishbeyn VA, Norton JA, Benya RV, Pisegna JR, Venzon DJ, Metz DC, Jensen RT. Assessment and prediction of long-term cure in patients with the Zollinger-Ellison syndrome: the best approach. Ann Intern Med 1993; 119(3):199–206.
76. Termanini B, Gibril F, Stewart CA, Weber HC, Jensen RT. A prospective study of the effectiveness of low dose omeprazole as initial therapy in Zollinger-Ellison syndrome. Aliment Pharmacol Ther 1996; 10(1):61–71.
77. Metz DC, Strader DB, Orbuch M, Koviack PD, Feigenbaum KM, Jensen RT. Use of omeprazole in Zollinger-Ellison syndrome: a prospective nine- year study of efficacy and safety. Aliment Pharmacol Ther 1993; 7(6):597–610.
78. Hirschowitz BI, Simmons J, Mohnen J. Long-term lansoprazole control of gastric acid and pepsin secretion in ZE and non-ZE hypersecretors: a prospective 10-year study. Aliment Pharmacol Ther 2001; 15(11):1795–1806.
79. Jensen RT, Metz DC, Koviack PD, Feigenbaum KM. Prospective study of the long-term efficacy and safety of lansoprazole in patients with the Zollinger-Ellison syndrome. Aliment Pharmacol Ther 1993; 7(suppl 1):41–50.
80. Metz DC, Pisegna JR, Ringham GL, Feigenbaum K, Koviack PD, Maton PN, Gardner JD, Jensen RT. Prospective study of efficacy and safety of lansoprazole in Zollinger-Ellison syndrome. Dig Dis Sci 1993; 38(2): 245–256.
81. Desir B, Poitras P. Oral pantoprazole for acid suppression in the treatment of patients with Zollinger-Ellison syndrome. Can J Gastroenterol 2001; 15(12): 795–798.
82. Lew EA, Pisegna JR, Starr JA, Soffer EF, Forsmark C, Modlin IM, Walsh JH, Beg M, Bochenek W, Metz DC. Intravenous pantoprazole rapidly controls gastric acid hypersecretion in patients with Zollinger-Ellison syndrome. Gastroenterology 2000; 118(4):696–704.
83. Carswell CI, Goa KL. Rabeprazole: an update of its use in acid-related disorders. Drugs 2001; 61(15):2327–2356.
84. Bonfils S, Mignon M, Gratton J. Cimetidine treatment of acute and chronic Zollinger-Ellison syndrome. World J Surg 1979; 3(5):597–604.
85. Jensen RT, Collen MJ, McArthur KE, Howard JM, Maton PN, Cherner JA, Gardner JD. Comparison of the effectiveness of ranitidine and cimetidine in inhibiting acid secretion in patients with gastric hypersecretory states. Am J Med 1984; 77(5B):90–105.
86. Howard JM, Vinayek R, Maton PN, Wank SA, Gardner JD, Jensen RT. Famotidine: effective treatment of Zollinger-Ellison syndrome. J Clin Gastroenterol 1987; 9(suppl 2): 23–25.
87. Levendoglu H, Mehta B, Wait C, Reddy G, Hatcher C. Nizatidine: a new histamine receptor blocker in the treatment of active duodenal ulcers. Am J Gastroenterol 1986; 81(12):1167–1170.
88. Stabile BE, Ippoliti AF, Walsh JH, Passaro E Jr. Failure of histamine H2-receptor antagonist therapy in Zollinger-Ellison syndrome. Am J Surg 1983; 145(1): 17–23.
89. McArthur KE, Collen MJ, Maton PN, Cherner JA, Howard JM, Ciarleglio CA, Cornelius MJ, Jensen RT, Gardner JD. Omeprazole: effective, convenient therapy for Zollinger-Ellison syndrome. Gastroenterology 1985; 88(4):939–944.
90. Lamers CB. Present experiences with omeprazole in the Zollinger-Ellison syndrome. Scand J Gastroenterol Suppl 1986; 118:123–128.
91. Delchier JC, Soule JC, Mignon M, Goldfain D, Cortot A, Travers B, Isal JP, Bader JP. Effectiveness of omeprazole in seven patients with Zollinger-Ellison syndrome resistant to histamine H2-receptor antagonists. Dig Dis Sci 1986; 31(7):693–699.
92. Meijer JL, Jansen JB, Lamers CB. Omeprazole in the treatment of Zollinger-Ellison syndrome and histamine

H2-antagonist refractory ulcers. Digestion 1989; 44 (suppl 1):31–39.
93. Metz DC, Pisegna JR, Fishbeyn VA, Benya RV, Jensen RT. Control of gastric acid hypersecretion in the management of patients with Zollinger-Ellison syndrome. World J Surg 1993; 17(4):468–480.
94. Weber HC, Venzon DJ, Jensen RT, Metz DC. Studies on the interrelation between Zollinger-Ellison syndrome, Helicobacter pylori, and proton pump inhibitor therapy. Gastroenterology 1997; 112(1):84–91.
95. Termanini B, Gibril F, Sutliff VE, Yu F, Venzon DJ, Jensen RT. Effect of long-term gastric acid suppressive therapy on serum vitamin B12 levels in patients with Zollinger-Ellison syndrome. Am J Med 1998; 104(5): 422–430.
96. Havu N. Enterochromaffin-like cell carcinoids of gastric mucosa in rats after life-long inhibition of gastric secretion. Digestion 1986; 35(suppl 1):42–55.
97. Solvell L. The clinical safety of omeprazole. Digestion 1990; 47(suppl 1):59–63.
98. Rivera E, Ajani JA. Doxorubicin, streptozocin, and 5-fluorouracil chemotherapy for patients with metastatic islet-cell carcinoma. Am J Clin Oncol 1998; 21(1):36–38.
99. Frame J, Kelsen D, Kemeny N, Cheng E, Niedzwiecki D, Heelan R, Lippermann R. A phase II trial of streptozotocin and adriamycin in advanced APUD tumors. Am J Clin Oncol 1988; 11(4):490–495.
100. von Schrenck T, Howard JM, Doppman JL, Norton JA, Maton PN, Smith FP, Vinayek R, Frucht H, Wank SA, Gardner JD. Prospective study of chemotherapy in patients with metastatic gastrinoma. Gastroenterology 1988; 94(6):1326–1334.
101. Moertel CG, Hanley JA, Johnson LA. Streptozocin alone compared with streptozocin plus fluorouracil in the treatment of advanced islet-cell carcinoma. N Engl J Med 1980; 303(21):1189–1194.
102. Moertel CG, Lefkopoulo M, Lipsitz S, Hahn RG, Klaassen D. Streptozocin-doxorubicin, streptozocin-fluorouracil or chlorozotocin in the treatment of advanced islet-cell carcinoma. N Engl J Med 1992; 326(8):519–523.
103. Cheng PN, Saltz LB. Failure to confirm major objective antitumor activity for streptozocin and doxorubicin in the treatment of patients with advanced islet cell carcinoma. Cancer 1999; 86(6):944–948.
104. Ramanathan RK, Cnaan A, Hahn RG, Carbone PP, Haller DG. Phase II trial of dacarbazine (DTIC) in advanced pancreatic islet cell carcinoma. Study of the Eastern Cooperative Oncology Group-E6282. Ann Oncol 2001; 12(8):1139–1143.
105. Altimari AF, Badrinath K, Reisel HJ, Prinz RA. DTIC therapy in patients with malignant intra-abdominal neuroendocrine tumors. Surgery 1987; 102(6):1009–1017.
106. Kessinger A, Foley JF, Lemon HM. Therapy of malignant APUD cell tumors. Effectiveness of DTIC. Cancer 1983; 51(5):790–794.
107. Neijt JP, Lacave AJ, Splinter TA, Taal BG, Veenhof CH, Sahmoud T, Lips CJ. Mitoxantrone in metastatic apudomas: a phase II study of the EORTC Gastro-intestinal Cancer Cooperative Group. Br J Cancer 1995; 71(1):106–108.
108. Saltz L, Lauwers G, Wiseberg J, Kelsen D. A phase II trial of carboplatin in patients with advanced APUD tumors. Cancer 1993; 72(2):619–622.
109. Kelsen D, Fiore J, Heelan R, Cheng E, Magill G. Phase II trial of etoposide in APUD tumors. Cancer Treat Rep 1987; 71(3):305–307.
110. Oberg K. Interferon in the management of neuro-endocrine GEP-tumors: a review. Digestion 2000; 62(suppl 1):92–97.
111. Frank M, Klose KJ, Wied M, Ishaque N, Schade-Brittinger C, Arnold R. Combination therapy with octreotide and alpha-interferon: effect on tumor growth in metastatic endocrine gastroenteropancreatic tumors. Am J Gastroenterol 1999; 94(5):1381–1387.
112. Fjallskog ML, Sundin A, Westlin JE, Oberg K, Janson ET, Eriksson B. Treatment of malignant endocrine pancreatic tumors with a combination of alpha-interferon and somatostatin analogs. Med Oncol 2002; 19(1):35–42.
113. Pisegna JR, Slimak GG, Doppman JL, Strader DB, Metz DC, Benya RV, Orbuch M, Fishbeyn VA, Fraker DL, Norton JA. An evaluation of human recombinant alpha interferon in patients with metastatic gastrinoma. Gastroenterology 1993; 105(4):1179–1183.
114. Saltz L, Kemeny N, Schwartz G, Kelsen D. A phase II trial of alpha-interferon and 5-fluorouracil in patients with advanced carcinoid and islet cell tumors. Cancer 1994; 74(3):958–961.
115. Shojamanesh H, Gibril F, Louie A, Ojeaburu JV, Bashir S, Abou-Saif A, Jensen RT. Prospective study of the antitumor efficacy of long-term octreotide treatment in patients with progressive metastatic gastrinoma. Cancer 2002; 94(2):331–343.
116. Ricci S, Antonuzzo A, Galli L, Orlandini C, Ferdeghini M, Boni G, Roncella M, Mosca F, Conte PF. Long-acting depot lanreotide in the treatment of patients with advanced neuroendocrine tumors. Am J Clin Oncol 2000; 23(4):412–415.
117. Wymenga AN, Eriksson B, Salmela PI, Jacobsen MB, Van Cutsem EJ, Fiasse RH, Valimaki MJ, Renstrup J, de Vries EG, Oberg KE. Efficacy and safety of prolonged-release lanreotide in patients with gastro-intestinal neuroendocrine tumors and hormone-related symptoms. J Clin Oncol 1999; 17(4):1111.
118. Aparicio-Pages MN, Verspaget HW, Pena AS, Jansen JB, Lamers CB. Natural killer cell activity in patients with neuroendocrine tumours of the gastrointestinal tract; relation with circulating gastrointestinal hormones. Neuropeptides 1991; 20(1):1–7.

119. Arnold R, Trautmann ME, Creutzfeldt W, Benning R, Benning M, Neuhaus C, Jurgensen R, Stein K, Schafer H, Bruns C, Dennler HJ. Somatostatin analogue octreotide and inhibition of tumour growth in metastatic endocrine gastroenteropancreatic tumours. Gut 1996; 38(3):430–438.
120. Saltz L, Trochanowski B, Buckley M, Heffernan B, Niedzwiecki D, Tao Y, Kelsen D. Octreotide as an antineoplastic agent in the treatment of functional and nonfunctional neuroendocrine tumors. Cancer 1993; 72(1):244–248.
121. Eriksson B, Renstrup J, Imam H, Oberg K. High-dose treatment with lanreotide of patients with advanced neuroendocrine gastrointestinal tumors: clinical and biological effects. Ann Oncol 1997; 8(10):1041–1044.
122. De Jong M, Valkema R, Jamar F, Kvols LK, Kwekkeboom DJ, Breeman WA, Bakker WH, Smith C, Pauwels S, Krenning EP. Somatostatin receptor-targeted radionuclide therapy of tumors: preclinical and clinical findings. Semin Nucl Med 2002; 32(2):133–140.
123. Norton JA, Doherty GM, Fraker DL, Alexander HR, Doppman JL, Venzon DJ, Gibril F, Jensen RT. Surgical treatment of localized gastrinoma within the liver: a prospective study. Surgery 1998; 124(6):1145–1152.
124. Makowka L, Tzakis AG, Mazzaferro V, Teperman L, Demetris AJ, Iwatsuki S, Starzl TE. Transplantation of the liver for metastatic endocrine tumors of the intestine and pancreas. Surg Gynecol Obstet 1989; 168(2):107–111.
125. Dousset B, Saint-Marc O, Pitre J, Soubrane O, Houssin D, Chapuis Y. Metastatic endocrine tumors: medical treatment, surgical resection, or liver transplantation. World J Surg 1996; 20(7):908–914.
126. Chung MH, Pisegna J, Spirt M, Giuliano AE, Ye W, Ramming KP, Bilchik AJ. Hepatic cytoreduction followed by a novel long-acting somatostatin analog: a paradigm for intractable neuroendocrine tumors metastatic to the liver. Surgery 2001; 130(6):954–962.
127. McEntee GP, Nagorney DM, Kvols LK, Moertel CG, Grant CS. Cytoreductive hepatic surgery for neuroendocrine tumors. Surgery 1990; 108(6):1091–1096.
128. Yao KA, Talamonti MS, Nemcek A, Angelos P, Chrisman H, Skarda J, Benson AB, Rao S, Joehl RJ. Indications and results of liver resection and hepatic chemoembolization for metastatic gastrointestinal neuroendocrine tumors. Surgery 2001; 130(4):677–682.
129. Dominguez S, Denys A, Madeira I, Hammel P, Vilgrain V, Menu Y, Bernades P, Ruszniewski P. Hepatic arterial chemoembolization with streptozotocin in patients with metastatic digestive endocrine tumours. Eur J Gastroenterol Hepatol 2000; 12(2):151–157.
130. Kim YH, Ajani JA, Carrasco CH, Dumas P, Richli W, Lawrence D, Chuang V, Wallace S. Selective hepatic arterial chemoembolization for liver metastases in patients with carcinoid tumor or islet cell carcinoma. Cancer Invest 1999; 17(7):474–478.
131. Falconi M, Bassi C, Bonora A, Sartori N, Procacci C, Talamini G, Mansueto GC, Pederzoli P. Role of chemoembolization in synchronous liver metastases from pancreatic endocrine tumours. Dig Surg 1999; 16(1):32–38.
132. Perry LJ, Stuart K, Stokes KR, Clouse ME. Hepatic arterial chemoembolization for metastatic neuroendocrine tumors. Surgery 1994; 116(6):1111–1116.
133. Tomassetti P, Del Vecchio E, Faccioli P, Ricci S, Gambari PI, Roversi R, Barbara L. Treatment of liver metastases of an endocrine pancreatic tumor by hepatic artery chemoembolization with streptozotocin. J Clin Gastroenterol 1994; 18(2):170–172.
134. Clouse ME, Perry L, Stuart K, Stokes KR. Hepatic arterial chemoembolization for metastatic neuroendocrine tumors. Digestion 1994; 55(suppl 3):92–97.
135. Zollinger RM. Gastrinoma: factors influencing prognosis. Surgery 1985; 97(1):49–54.

48

Techniques of Conventional Open Pancreatic Surgery

Demetrius Pertsemlidis and David S. Pertsemlidis

Mount Sinai School of Medicine, New York University, New York, New York, U.S.A.

Pancreatic surgical procedures range from enucleation of solitary small peripheral subcapsular tumors to segmental or total pancreatectomy. Accurate localization and protection of the pancreatic and biliary ducts in enucleations and segmental resections are the keys to successful outcome. Patients undergoing distal pancreatectomies should have vaccinations against pneumococcal and meningococcal infections, antibiotic prophylaxis, and cleansing of the colon prior to surgery. Open pancreatic surgery is performed through midline or subcostal incisions.

1 SURGICAL ANATOMY

The pancreas extends from the duodenal sweep to the splenic hilus and has a triangular configuration (Fig. 1). It is surrounded by the gastric antrum, duodenum, jejunum, transverse mesocolon, and spleen (Fig. 2). The posterior surface is adjacent to the right kidney and hilus, the inferior vena cava, and aorta, and the superior mesenteric vessels lie between the neck of the pancreas and the uncinate process. The distal bile duct traverses the pancreatic head. The blood supply is derived from the celiac trunk and the superior mesenteric artery and the venous flow parallels the arteries, draining into the splenic, superior mesenteric, and portal veins.

2 MOBILIZATION OF THE PANCREAS

Entry into the lesser sac exposes most of the pancreas (Fig. 3). The anterior surface of the pancreatic head is exposed after ligation and division of the epiploic (omental) vessels and blunt separation of the transverse mesocolon, which is draped over the anterior pancreas (Fig. 4). The entire duodenum is mobilized down to the third portion until the middle colic and superior mesenteric veins are exposed. The posterior pancreatic surface is separated from the inferior vena cava and aorta, and the superior mesenteric vessels are freed from the body of the pancreas along avascular planes (Figs. 5,6). The distal pancreas is separated from the transverse mesocolon, and the lienocolic ligament is divided.

Unless the entire anterior and posterior surfaces are freed, inspection, palpation, and ultrasonographic examination of the pancreas is inadequate. More than 90% of pancreatic endocrine tumors can be localized by preoperative imaging and intraoperative manual and ultrasonographic examination of the thoroughly mobilized pancreas.

3 ENUCLEATION OF TUMORS

Small peripheral subcapsular tumors can be enucleated after intraoperative sonographic determination of prox-

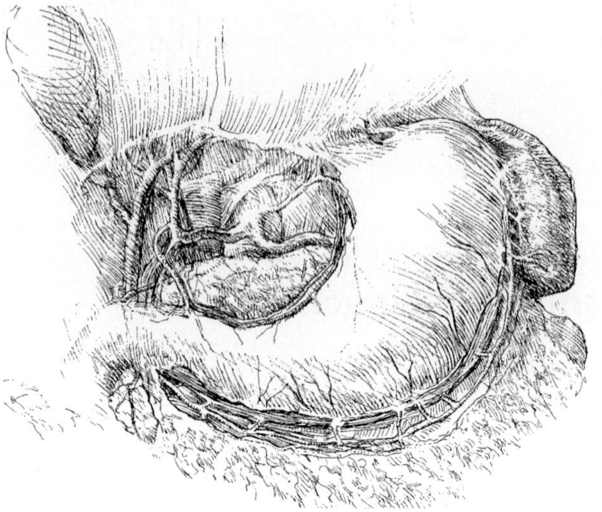

Figure 1 The pancreas, stomach, spleen, and biliary structures shown in situ. The locations of the gastroduodenal artery, gastroepiploic arcade, and common bile duct must be appreciated prior to entry into the lesser sac, mobilization of the duodenum, and portal dissection.

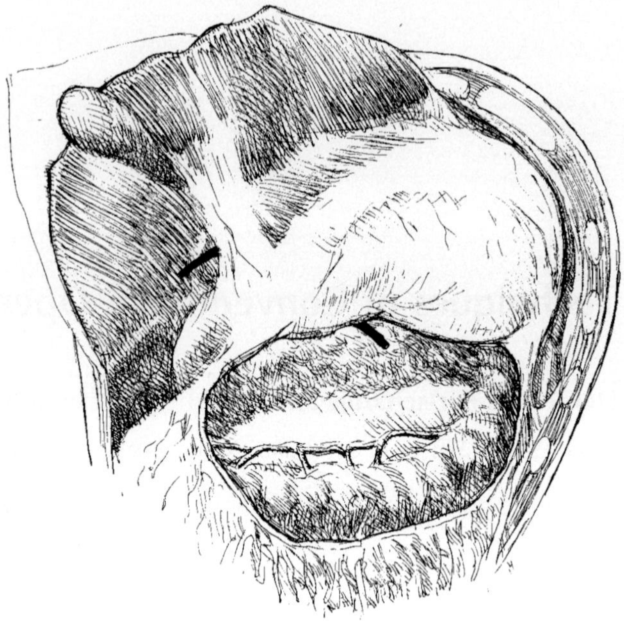

Figure 3 With the stomach elevated, the broad attachment of the transverse mesocolon to the pancreas is appreciated. A probe is depicted in the epiploic foramen.

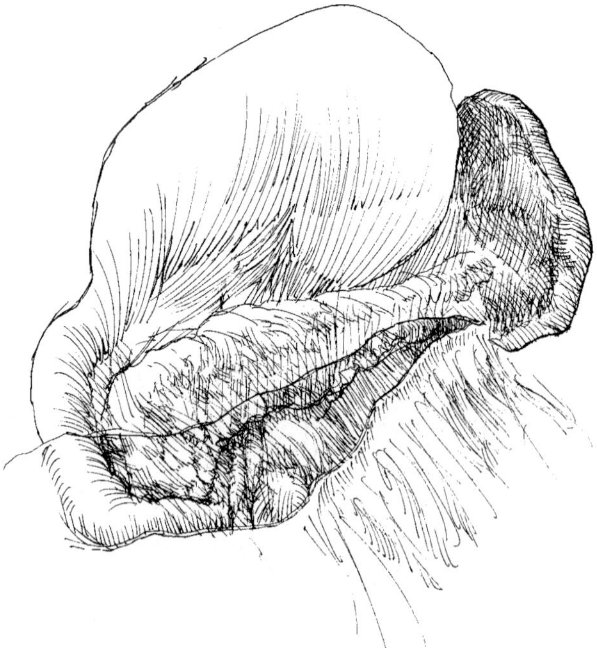

Figure 2 The gastrocolic omentum has been incised and the lesser sac entered.

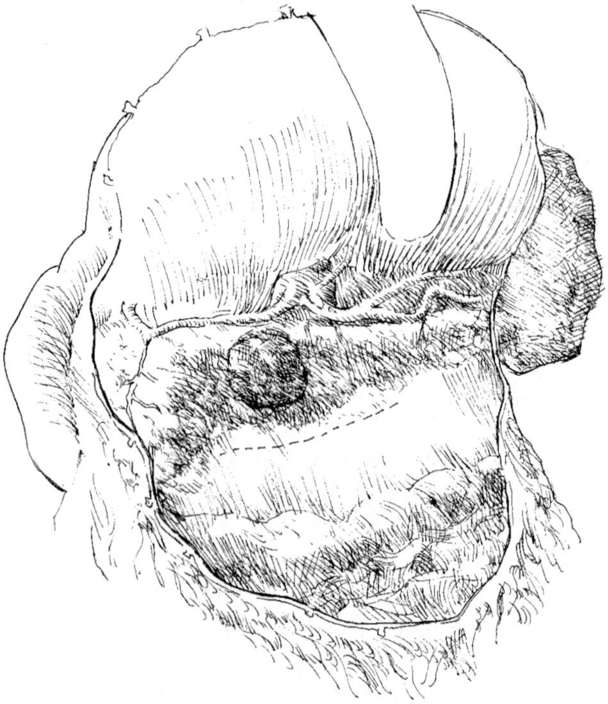

Figure 4 Exposure of the anterior surface of the pancreas has been performed. The transverse mesocolon is to be incised, exposing the inferior border of the pancreas.

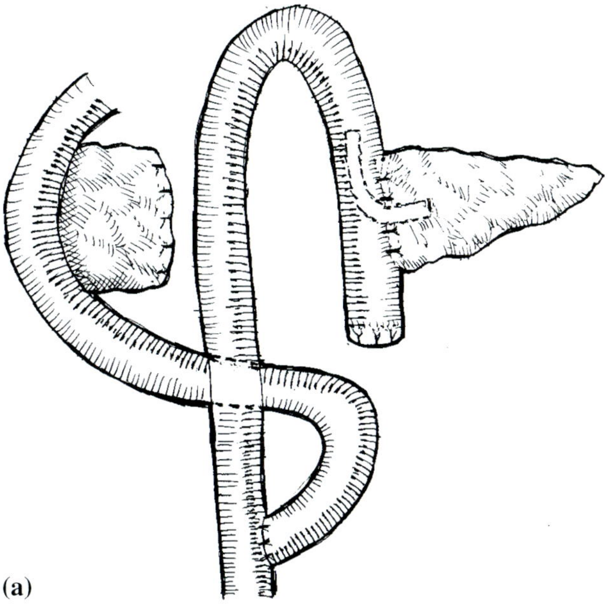

(a)

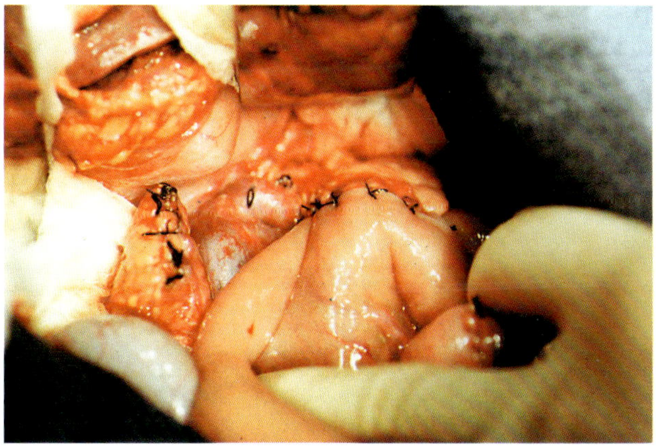

(b)

Figure 9 (a) Central pancreatectomy has been performed with closure of the cephalic stump and construction of a Roux-Y end-to-side pancreaticojejunostomy 40–50 cm from the jejunojejunostomy. Stenting of the duct, usually with a pediatric feeding tube, is depicted. (b) Central pancreatectomy has been performed with closure of the cephalic stump and construction of a Roux-Y end-to-side pancreaticojejunostomy 40–50 cm from the jejunojejunostomy. The anterior surface of the SMV is seen between the pancreatic stump and efferent jejunal limb.

stump in a seromuscular pocket of the jejunum. The seromuscular plane is created with injection of saline and blunt separation of the muscular layer down to submucosa. The intramural pocket should conform to the size of the pancreatic stump, and the mucosal opening should be equal to the size of the duct. The posterior suture line should be done first and the anterior closure after the duct to mucosa anastomosis using interrupted 2-0 silk (Figure 9).

6 PANCREATICO-DUODENECTOMY

The steps in the exposure and mobilization of the pancreas have been described at the beginning of this chapter. Resectability is determined after ascertaining absence of distant metastases and during separation of the pancreas from the major vessels.

6.1 Resectional Phase

With an extended Kocher maneuver completed and the SMV exposed, the dissection in the hepatoduodenal ligament is begun. The gastroduodenal artery is ligated and divided. Cholecystectomy is performed and the common hepatic duct is transected above the junction with the cystic duct. The portal vein is exposed and bluntly separated from the duodenum, hepatic artery, and bile duct. During dissection within the hepatoduodenal ligament, attention should be paid to possible vascular aberrations, particularly if preoperative imaging raised questions of anomalous anatomy.

Pancreatico-duodenectomy can be performed with or without preservation of the pylorus, depending on the extent of the tumor, adequate blood supply to the proximal duodenum, and preference of the surgeon. The distal stomach or proximal duodenum is divided with a stapler and the proximal jejunum is freed after dividing the ligament of Treitz. The jejunal mesentery and vessels are ligated and cut, and the jejunum and distal duodenum are transposed to the right side. The mesenteric defect is closed to prevent internal herniation.

Dissection along the uncinate process is the Achilles' heel of this procedure. Major bleeding during or after operation can occur from branches of the superior mesenteric artery or from the venous tributaries of the mesenteric and portal veins. In extended pancreatico-duodenectomy, segments of the superior mesenteric or portal veins may have to be resected and interposition of internal iliac vein graft may be necessary. After placement of traction sutures, the pancreas is transected with scalpel or electrocautery (Fig. 10).

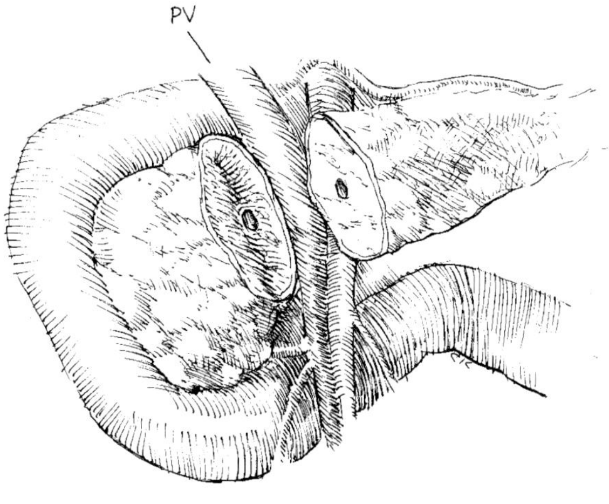

Figure 10 The resectional stage of the pancreaticoduodenectomy is complete with the duodenum mobilized, common hepatic duct, stomach, and jejunum divided, and the pancreas transected. Division of the venous tributaries to the portal vein (PV) and superior mesenteric vein and separation of the specimen from the lateral border of the superior mesenteric artery are crucial as arterial injury is a major and avoidable cause of postoperative hemorrhage.

6.2 Restorative Phase

The proximal jejunum is transposed into the supra-colic space through the transverse mesocolon. An enterotomy is made about 10 cm from the blind end, large enough to accommodate the pancreatic stump. An end-to-side pancreatico-jejunostomy is constructed with interrupted 2-0 silk sutures approximating pancreatic capsule to full thickness jejunum. A dilated pancreatic duct can be used for duct-to-mucosa anastomosis with the described technique (Fig. 11) while stenting of the anastomosis is used routinely in small pancreatic ducts. The two types of pancreatico-jejunal anastomoses are equally effective.

An end-to-side hepatico-jejunostomy is constructed using a single layer of absorbable suture. Stents or t-tubes are not routinely used. Gastrointestinal continuity is restored with an end-to-side antecolic anastomosis of either the distal stomach or proximal duodenum to the jejunum at a distance of 30–40 cm from the bilio-enteric anastomosis. The gastroenteric anastomosis can be of the Polya or Hofmeister type using stapling or hand-sewn techniques.

The opening in the transverse mesocolon should be closed around the transposed jejunum to prevent internal herniation, and drainage of the hepatico- and pancreatico-jejunostomies is required.

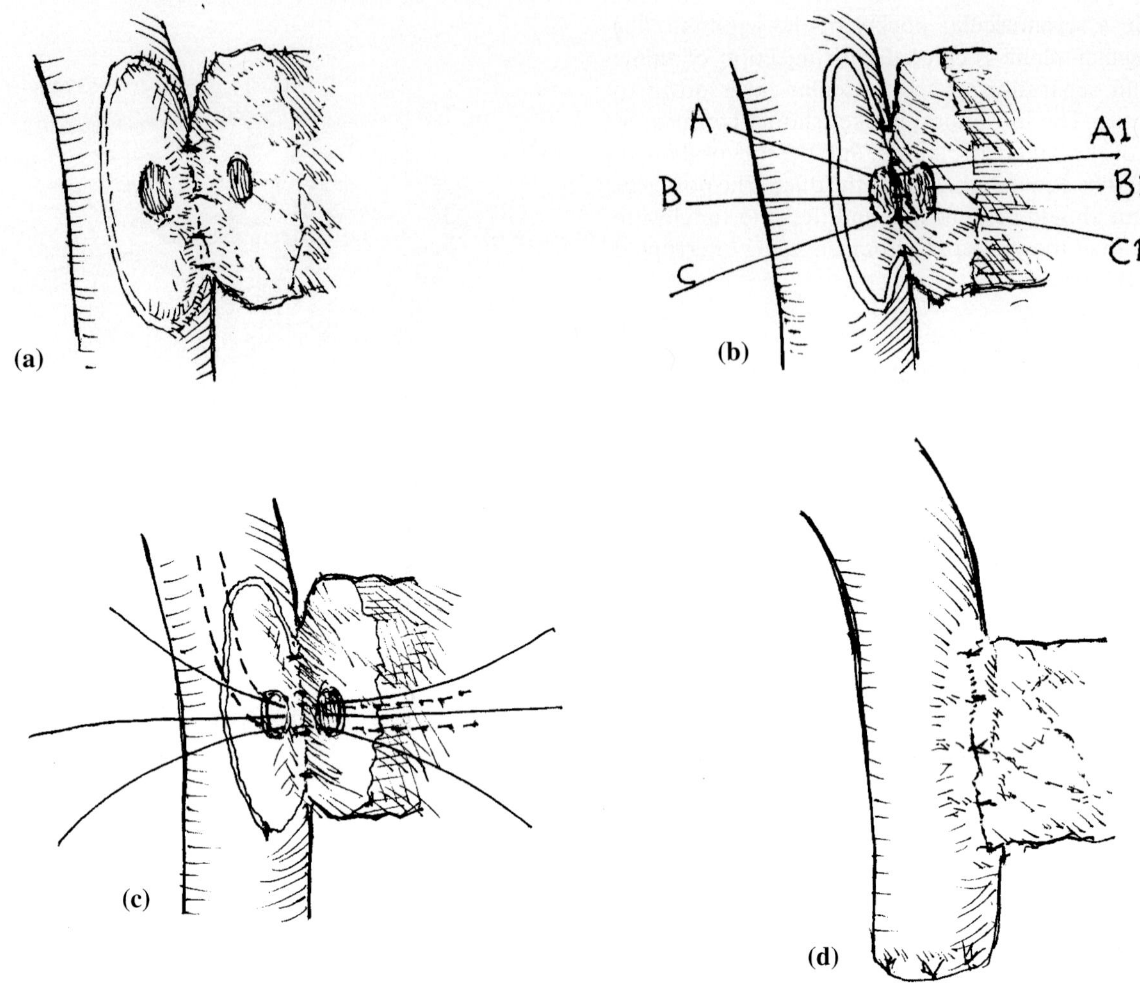

Figure 11 (a–d) End-to-side pancreaticojejunostomy is constructed on a dilated duct using duct-to-mucosa anastomosis. Dotted lines indicate stent location, but stenting is routinely performed only in ducts of normal caliber.

49

Laparoscopic Management of Pancreatic Islet Cell Tumors

Michel Gagner and William B. Inabnet

Mount Sinai School of Medicine, New York University, New York, New York, U.S.A.

Christine A. Chu

Bay Area Surgical Associates, Inc., and John Muir/Mount Diablo Health System, Walnut Creek, California, U.S.A.

1 INTRODUCTION

Laparoscopy was first used for visual examination of the pancreas in 1911; this was revisited in 1972 where again examination of the pancreas using laparoscopy was suggested (1,2). The advent of laparoscopic ultrasonography (3–5), along with improvement of surgeons' technical capabilities, have established a new chapter in the diagnosis, staging, and management of unresectable pancreatic carcinoma (6–8). This approach was, however, slow to gain acceptance for resection of malignant pancreatic lesions due to the high morbidity and mortality in operating on this retroperitoneal structure. A new milestone in pancreatic surgery was set by Gagner and Pomp in 1993 (9) when they challenged the surgical field and explored unbroken territories. They performed a laparoscopic pylorus-preserving pancreatoduodenectomy for a patient with chronic pancreatitis localized in the head of the pancreas with pancreas divisum. Although technically feasible, the laparoscopic Whipple procedure did not improve the postoperative outcome or shorten the postoperative recovery period. Attention was then drawn to more benign lesions, including laparoscopic distal pancreatectomy with splenectomy for chronic pancreatitis (10) and laparoscopic resections of islet cell tumors by enucleation or distal pancreatectomy (11). Laparoscopic pancreatic surgery began to gain acceptance and popularity (12) in the mid-1990s. Laparoscopic distal pancreatectomy or enucleation was felt to be technically feasible, safe, and seemed to benefit patients by shortening their hospital stay with no recurrence of disease (11,13–15). Hand-assisted techniques were also attempted with success (16,17). There is a growing worldwide interest in performing laparoscopic enucleation or distal pancreatectomy for islet cell tumors (18–34).

2 INDICATIONS FOR ISLET CELL TUMOR REMOVAL

In 1869, Paul Langerhans described islands of richly innervated characteristic cells distributed throughout the pancreas. Each islet is a well-organized, micro-organ consisting of several different cell types that are arranged in a typical format. In the core are insulin-producing beta-cells (β-cells). The peripheral zone contains various peptides, including alpha-cells (α-cells) that produce glucagon and delta-cells (δ-cells) that produce somatostatin. Other polypeptides that are secreted include pancreatic polypeptide, vasoactive intestinal peptide (VIP), and growth hormone–releasing factor, just to name a few.

Insulinoma is by far the most common islet cell tumor. More than 90% of these are benign, often solitary, and distributed about a third each in the head, body, and tail of the pancreas. It measures < 1 cm in about 40% and < 2 cm in 90% of cases. In situ, the lesion usually appears darker in color than the surrounding pancreas and is frequently found to have a network of small vessels around it. Patients can present with a spectrum of neurological, cardiovascular, and gastrointestinal symptoms due to hypoglycemia and catecholamine release. The classic finding is the Whipple's triad, whereby the patient experiences (a) hypoglycemia during fasting or exertion, (b) blood sugar < 45 mg/dL at the time of symptoms, and (c) symptoms ameliorated by oral or intravenous glucose. Diagnostic studies include elevated serum insulin level (normal < 30 μU/mL), insulin-to-glucose ratio of ≥1.0, and C-peptide suppression test. Provocative tests may be necessary in equivocal studies with high clinical suspicion. These include intravenous tolbutamide test (80% sensitivity), intramuscular glucagon test (70% sensitive), oral glucose tolerance test (60% sensitive), and intravenous calcium infusion test. Preoperative localization studies remain controversial as intraoperative ultrasound has 75–90% sensitivity. Depending on localization, surgical management should be enucleation or distal pancreatectomy with or without splenectomy (35).

Glucagonoma derives from alpha-cells and is usually found in patients over 50 years of age. Patients may present with the classic necrolytic migratory erythema whereby there is migratory, scaling rash with intense puritus, usually in the groin and lower extremities. The plasma glucagon level can exceed 1000 pg/mL The lesion tends to be large (> 4 cm), malignant, and found within the body and tail of the pancreas. About 70% of patients are found to have liver metastasis at the time of diagnosis (36).

Other pancreatic endocrine lesions are rare, tend to be large, and have a higher malignant potential, i.e., gastrinomas. These lesions may be better approached via a standard laparotomy.

3 PREOPERATIVE CONSIDERATIONS

Patients undergo standard preoperative work-up, including conventional blood tests, chest radiograph, electrocardiogram, and computed tomography (CT) scan. Preoperative endoscopic ultrasound (EUS) is performed in most cases. In anticipation of possible splenectomy, triple vaccination against *S pneumoniae, H influenzae,* and *N meningitidis* is routinely administered. A modern state-of-the art operating room is equally important and must be equipped with high flow insufflators, Xenon light sources, a digital mixer that permits switching from laparoscopic view to laparoscopic ultrasonography, or have them on the same screen in a split mode (Fig. 1).

4 SURGICAL TECHNIQUE

The patient is under general anesthesia and should have large intravenous access for aggressive resuscitation; an arterial line may also facilitate hormone monitoring during the procedure. The patient is positioned in a supine, split-leg fashion with anchoring supports at both feet. Foam wedges should be placed under the left flank to elevate the retroperitoneal structures. In some cases, a steeper right-sided decubitus with the left side up about 45 degrees is necessary. In fact, the degree of patient rotation is variable and primarily determined by surgeon preference, similar to the variation of patient position for laparoscopic splenectomy. However, patients are generally positioned with more rotation of the left side upwards for a distal pancreatectomy compared with an enucleation procedure. Foley catheter, venodyne boots, and an orogastric tube should be in place prior to final positioning. The surgeon stands between the patient's legs, with the scrub nurse to the patient's left side and the first assistant to the patient's right. Two video monitors, placed above each of the patient's shoulders, are usually used (Fig. 1).

The initial 10 mm port should be placed at supra-umbilicus and pneumoperitoneum established to 15 mm Hg. A state-of-the art 3-chip or digital camera coupled with a 30-degree angle scope is used (Figs. 2, 3); a general inspection of the abdomen should be performed to eliminate metastasis, especially on the liver surface. A total of five trocars are generally required, though the precise number and size of trocars may vary depending on the patient's body habitus, the surgeon's comfort, and the size of the available instruments. In order to use an endoscopic linear stapler and perform laparoscopic ultrasonography, a 12 mm port is necessary. This port should be placed on the left side at mid-clavicular line just below the level of umbilicus to facilitate smooth insertion of the stapler across the pancreas and thorough scanning with the ultrasonographic probe. The remaining cannulae are usually 5 mm ports for Maryland dissector (Fig. 4), curved scissors (Fig. 5), and retracting instruments.

4.1 Exposure and Mobilization of the Pancreas

With the patient in slight reverse Trendelenburg, the stomach is grasped and the gastrocolic ligament and distal inferior short gastric vessels lateral to the gastroepiploic artery are divided (Fig. 6). The splenic flexure of the colon is also mobilized. These can be performed using the ultrasonic dissector, bipolar cauthery (Ligasure, Valleylab, Boulder, CO) or simple diathermy and/or clips. Once access to the lesser sac is achieved, the posterior peritoneum is then incised along the inferior and superior borders of the body and tail of the pancreas using both sharp and blunt techniques.

A high-definition linear array laparoscopic ultrasound probe is then inserted via the 12 mm port (Fig. 7). A systematic approach in localizing the lesion is essential. Most surgeons prefer a 6.5–7.5 MHz frequency to scan the ventral and dorsal surfaces of the head, body, and tail of the pancreas searching for the lesion, which should appear hypoechoic (Fig. 8). Its spatial relationship to surrounding structures such as pancreatic duct, splenic vessels, portal vein, superior mesenteric vessels, and spleen should be noted.

4.2 Laparoscopic Distal Pancreatectomy with Splenectomy

The splenic vessels are divided at the planned line of pancreatic transection, using either clips or endoscopic staplers (2.0 or 2.5 mm in height and 45 mm in length; TycoHealthcare, Norwalk, CT). The pancreas and splenic vein are usually divided as a single unit with an endoscopic stapler, and the vein stump doubly secured

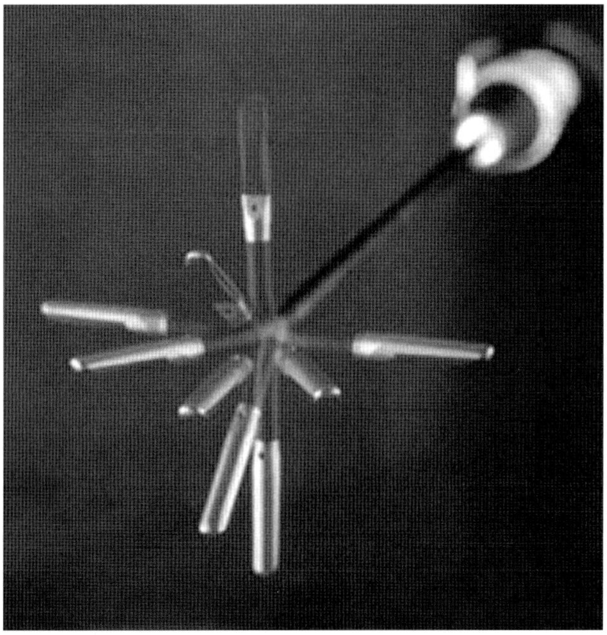

Figure 7 Laparoscopic probe.

with clips if possible. The pancreas is then mobilized from body to tail, in retrograde fashion (Fig. 9).

For resection of lesions in the tail of the pancreas an alternative approach is sometimes taken, in which the spleen and pancreas are mobilized prior to division of the splenic vessels and the pancreas. Ligamentous

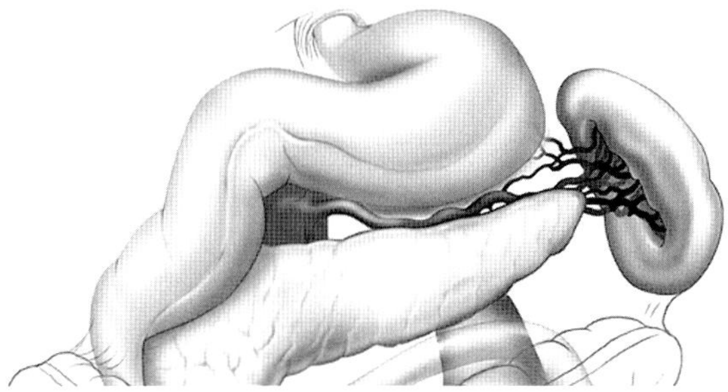

Figure 6 Exposure of the lesser sac content by opening the gastrocolic ligament.

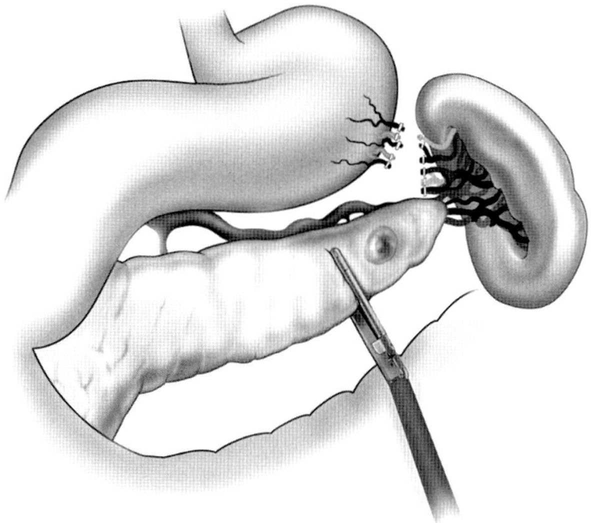

Figure 9 Laparoscopic distal pancreatectomy; the linear stapler divides and closes the pancreatic parenchyma.

attachments of the spleen are divided, and the posterior spleen and tail of the pancreas are mobilized from the retroperitoneum, dissecting from lateral to medial, in an antegrade direction along the pancreas (Fig. 10).

After transecting the pancreas, the proximal stump is inspected for hemostasis and to ensure closure of the main pancreatic duct. If a patent duct is visualized, it is suture ligated intracorporeally, using a fine nonabsorbable, monofilament suture . Oversewing the proximal stump with a fine, nonabsorbable, monofilament, running suture may improve hemostasis and decrease leakage. The technique of buttressing an endoscopic mechanical stapler with strips of bovine pericardium has been shown to have preliminary success in resection of pulmonary bullous areas (37,38). Applying a similar technique to pancreatic transection may decrease postoperative leak. Specimens are removed from the abdomen using sturdy, nonporous laparoscopic retrieval bags to prevent tissue spillage. When the opening of the retrieval bag is pulled out above the abdominal wall, ring forceps are used to morcellate the spleen while preventing intra-abdominal spillage. The umbilical trocar site is enlarged to 2.0–2.5 cm for removal of the pancreatic specimen. The abdomen is reinsufflated to check for hemostasis and a closed suction drain placed near the pancreas. Trocar sites greater than 5 mm diameter are closed. Splenectomy may be indicated when the lesion is at the very tip of the pancreas or when preservation of splenic vessels is not feasible. At times when the vein is densely adhered to the dorsal surface of the pancreas, it may be more feasible to divide it as a single unit with an endoscopic vascular stapler.

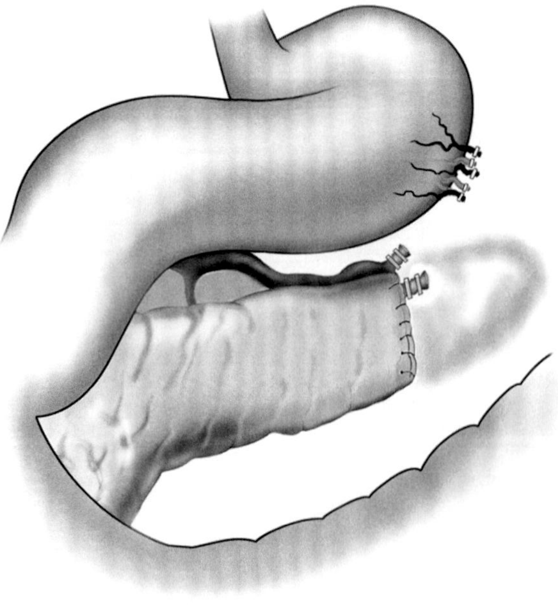

Figure 10 Laparoscopic distal pancreatectomy with en bloc splenectomy.

4.3 Laparoscopic Distal Pancreatectomy with Splenic Preservation

Following the laparoscopic exposure of the pancreas described above, the inferior border of the pancreas is dissected from the retroperitoneal fat until the splenic vein is reached posteriorly and superiorly. The tail of the pancreas is then gently grasped with 5 mm atraumatic forceps and retracted anteriorly and inferiorly to expose the transverse branches of the splenic artery and vein. These vessels are divided with the ultrasonic shears or 5 mm titanium clips until the desired length of pancreas is achieved. The entire pancreatic tail and body are mobilized, up to the portal vein if necessary. The pancreas is transected with an endoscopic linear stapler (Fig. 11). Occasionally, it is transected with an ultrasonic shear (Ethicon EndoSurgery, Cincinnati, OH) or bipolar device (Ligasure, Valleylab, Boulder, CO) to decrease blood loss. The specimen is extracted in a rigid plastic bag through a minimally enlarged umbilical incision. Laparoscopic distal pancreatectomy with or without splenectomy should be performed when enucleation is not feasible or indicated.

4.4 Laparoscopic Distal Pancreatectomy with Splenic Vessels and Spleen Preservation

The spleen-preserving techniques are particularly indicated for patients with benign diseases, since lymphadenectomy is expected to be insufficient for curative intent in malignancies (39).

Dissecting and clipping the superior edge of the pancreas from the vessels emerging from the splenic vein and artery is the most commonly performed splenic preservation technique (Figs. 12–15). This technique requires a longer operative time and laparoscopic surgical expertise, and, unfortunately, vascular damage when performing this procedure might occur due to the delicate maneuvers necessary in the upper margin of the pancreas.

4.5 Laparoscopic Enucleation of Islet Cell Tumors

Laparoscopic enucleation should be performed on lesions felt to be benign, technically achievable due to its surface location or its physical distance away from vital structures. LIOUS is routinely used to confirm the

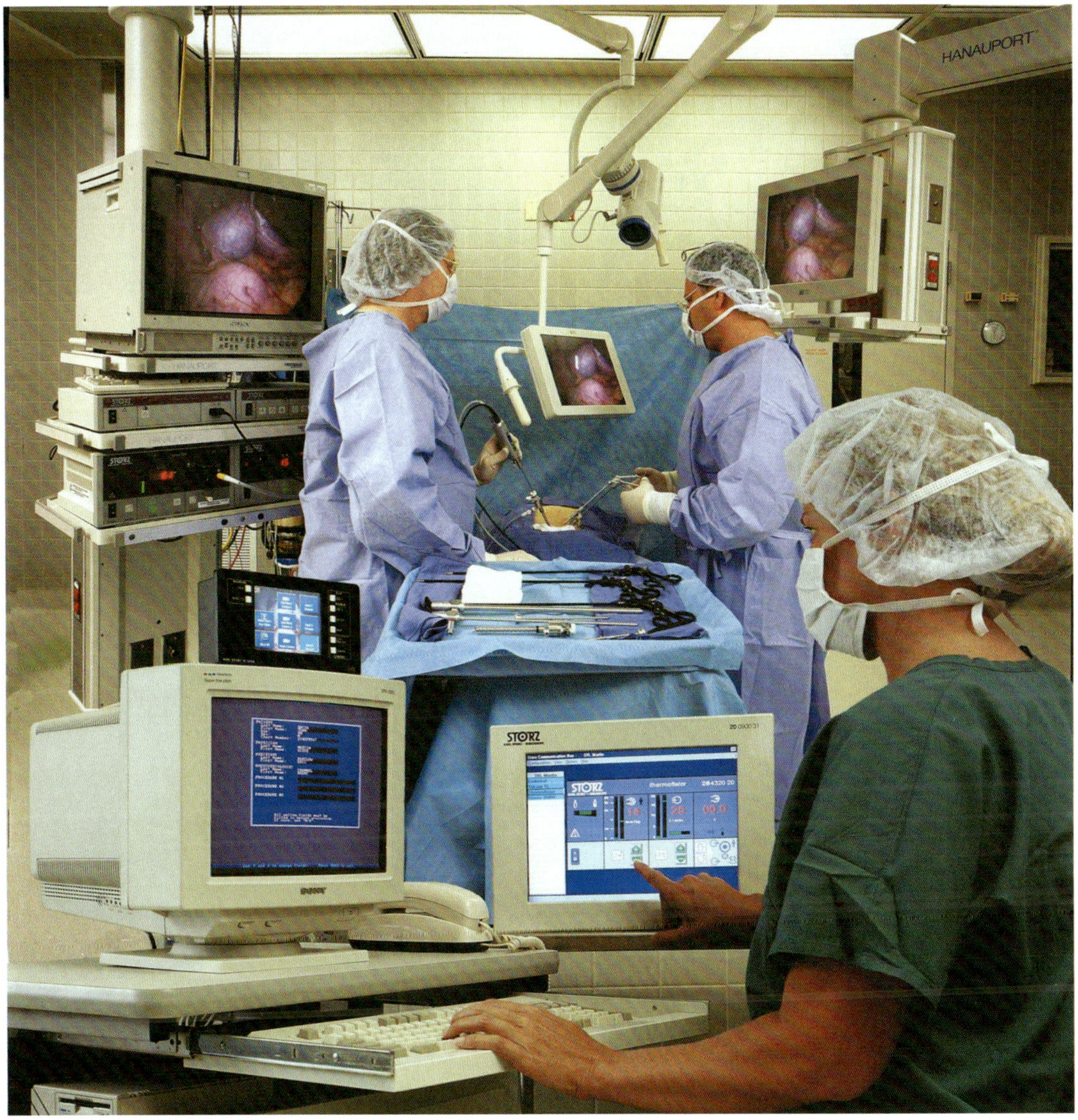

Figure 1 Minimally invasive surgery operating room. Suspended flat screens and booms for insufflators, light sources, and digital video systems are part of the new ergonomic environment. (Courtesy of Karl Storz Endoscopy.)

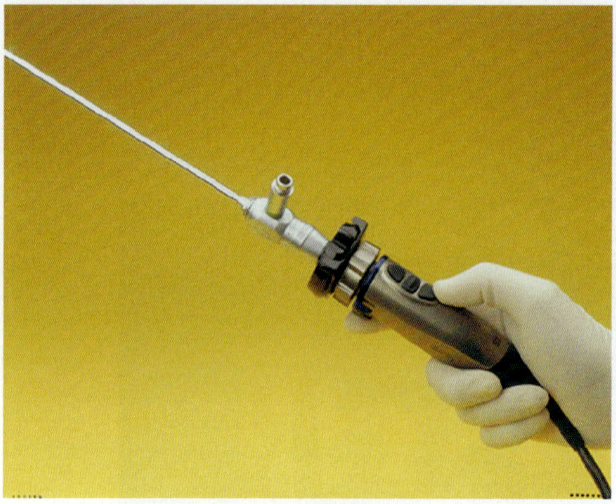

Figure 2 Digital camera mounted with a 5 mm laparoscope. (Courtesy of Karl Storz Endoscopy.)

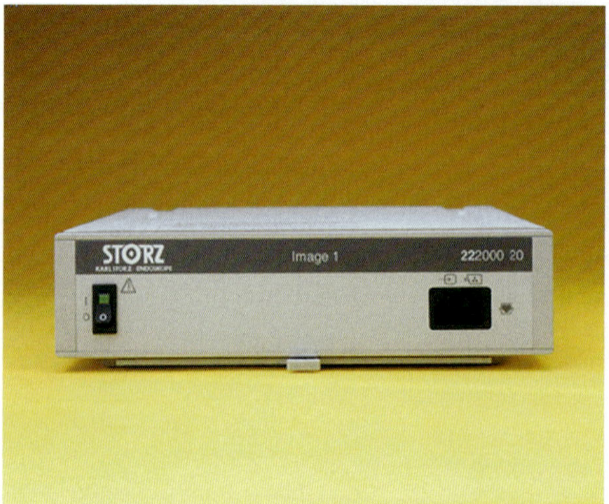

Figure 3 Digital camera ampificator. (Courtesy of Karl Storz Endoscopy.)

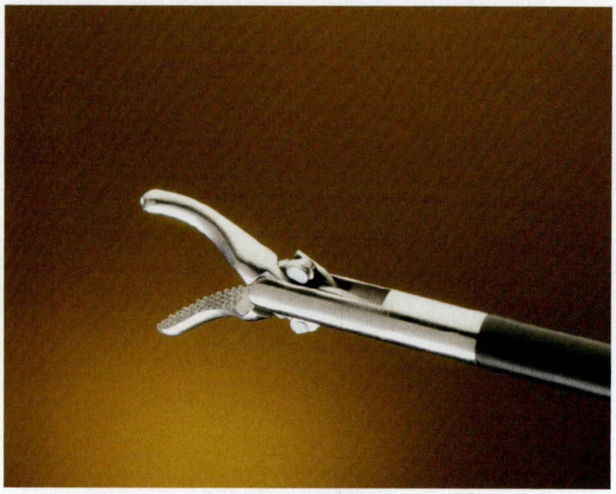

Figure 4 A laparoscopic curve dissector. (Courtesy of Karl Storz Endoscopy.)

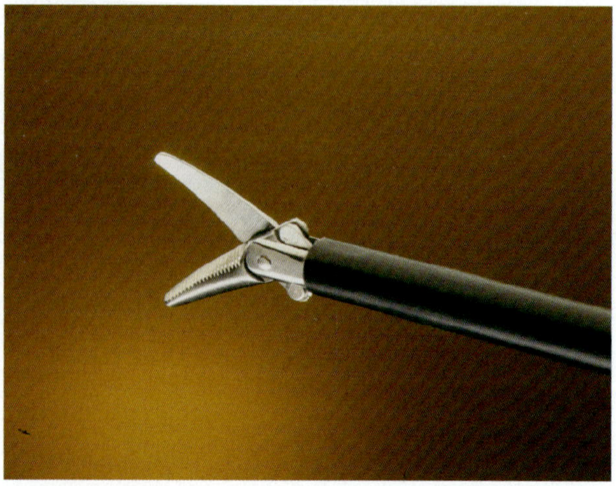

Figure 5 A laparoscopic curved scissor. (Courtesy of Karl Storz Endoscopy.)

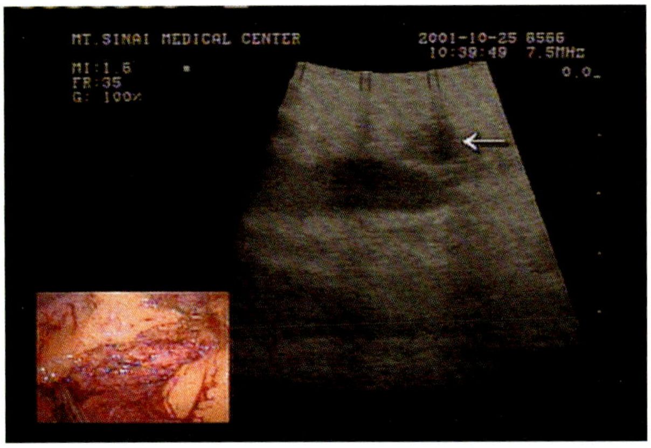

Figure 8 Laparoscopic ultrasonography on the anterior body of the pancreas, looking for an islet cell tumor. Note the split image of the laparoscope and of the laparoscopic ultrasonography.

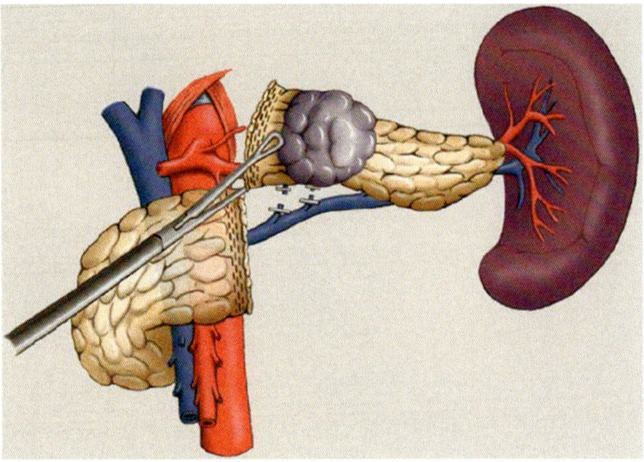

Figure 12 Laparoscopic distal pancreatectomy with spleen and splenic vessels preservation.

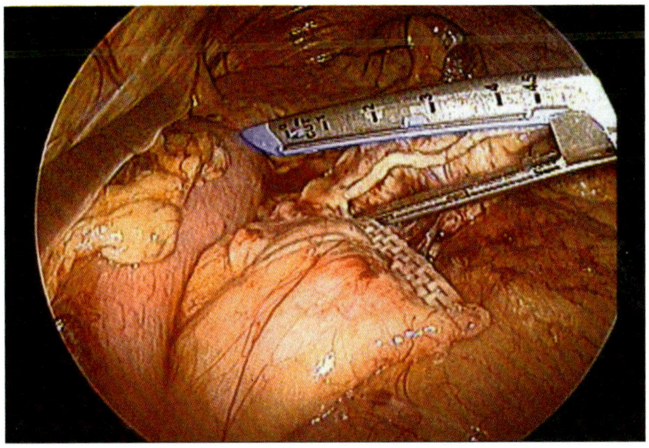

Figure 11 Laparoscopic distal pancreatectomy with splenic preservation; stapler across the pancreas.

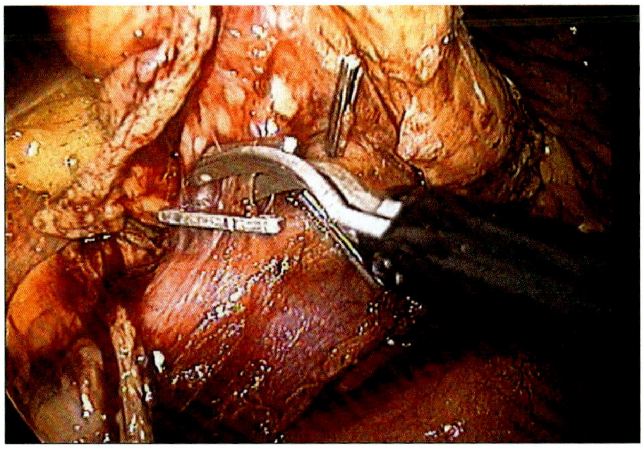

Figure 13 Endoshears dividing small pancreatic vessel branches.

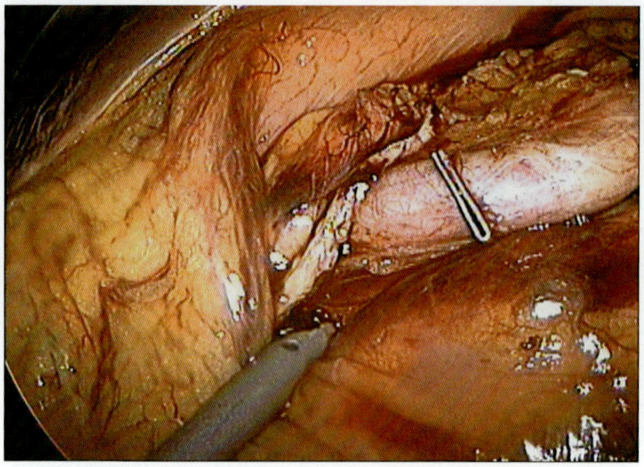

Figure 14 Titanium clips on arterial branch.

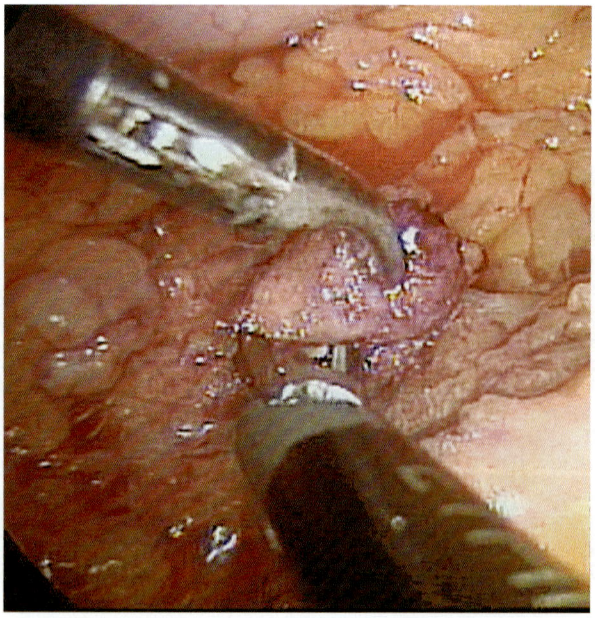

Figure 17 Enucleation using ultrasonic shears.

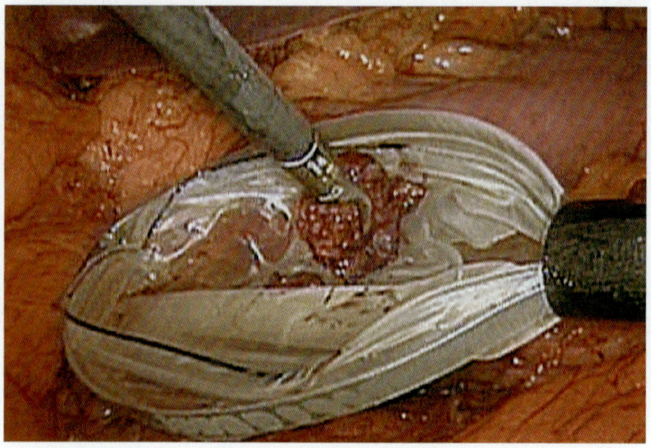

Figure 18 Extraction using an impermeable bag.

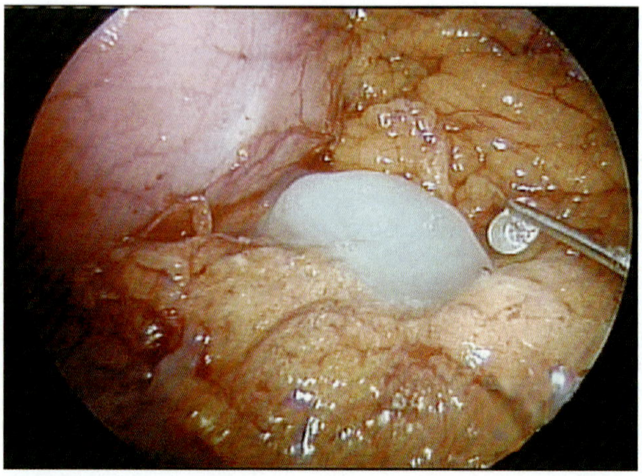

Figure 19 Application of fibrin glue to the enucleation site—a preventive method to avoid a pancreatic fistula.

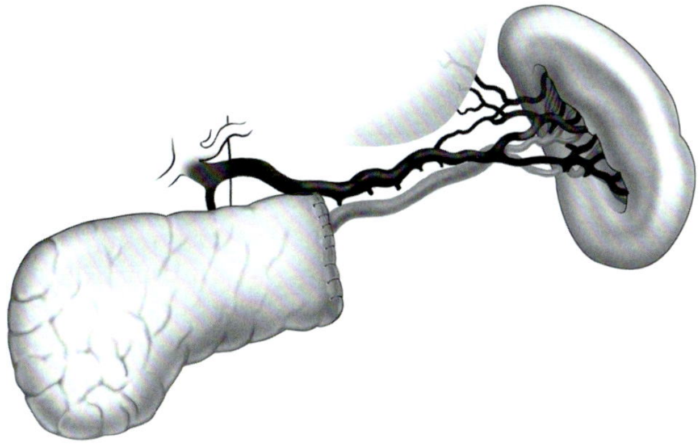

Figure 15 Splenic vessel branch dissection.

location and relationship to the pancreatic duct and peripancreatic vessels. Once the islet cell tumor is localized, the dissection is carried out between the tumor and the normal parenchyma using an electrocautery hook or ultrasonic coagulating shears (Figs. 16, 17). Since insulinomas tend to have a vascular network, it is useful to dissect with electrocautery hook or ultrasonic device in one hand, while retracting and exposing with a suction tip in the other. A margin of normal parenchymal tissue should be included. The pancreatic vessels feeding the tumor are ligated with medium to large titanium clips. Once the tumor is completely enucleated, it is extracted in a small sterile bag through the 12 mm port (Fig. 18). A closed suction drain is placed in the lesser sac at the enucleation site. Depending on the depth of the defect and general appearance of the surrounding tissue, the enucleated crater may be filled with fibrin glue, though its efficacy in decreasing postoperative leak has not been determined (Fig. 19) (40,41).

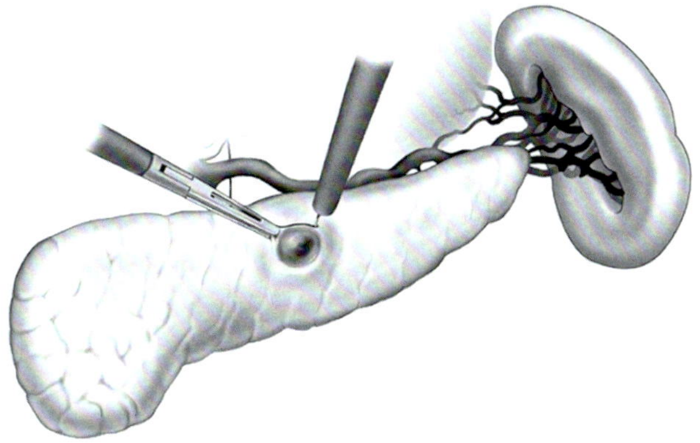

Figure 16 Demonstration on the use of a laparoscopic hook with cauthery for enucleation of an islet cell neoplasm.

4.6 Hand-Assisted Laparoscopic Pancreatectomy

Conventional laparoscopy has been proven to be difficult in cases involving large tumors, massive intraoperative bleeding, dense adhesions, malignant diseases (43), and obesity (42). Hand-assisted laparoscopic surgery may have an advantage in these groups of patients (43). This technique basically involves the assistance of the surgeon's nondominant hand while still performing a laparoscopic procedure. It can be used either as the initial or as an intermediary step in cases in which the surgeon faces technical difficulties (34).

Although only a few such cases have been reported, the advantages described include the possibility of using the assistance of the hand for dissection (palpate and identify tissues) (42,44), to mobilize large organs (44), for access to the utilization of instruments (42), for protection of the wound during the extraction of malignant specimens (42), to shorten the operative time required, and to utilize of the fingers to rapidly stop unexpected bleeding.

4.7 Postoperative Care

Nasogastric tubes are removed intraoperatively in all patients. Clear fluids are routinely begun on the evening of surgery. Patients are advanced to a regular diet after they pass flatus. Fluid from the closed suction drain is routinely sent for amylase level determination on postoperative day 3. The drain is removed when it contain only serous fluid and the amylase level is approximately equal to serum level.

4.8 Complications

The incidence of bleeding in pancreatic open resections reported by Halloran et al. in 2002 was found to be 4.8% (45). Factors like dense adhesions between the pancreas and the vessels (e.g., chronic pancreatitis) (46,11), increase the incidence of intraoperative hemorrhage. To prevent bleeding, ligature of the splenic artery as close as possible to its origin might reduce the risk of major bleeding and could also be used as an attempt to reduce the size of the spleen (47), facilitating the subsequent steps of the operation. Hemorrhage is a threatening complication that can also occur postoperatively and manifest itself as a sero-sanguineous fluid coming out from the drain or, if severe, with hemodynamic instability. Reoperation is the rule for the latter group of patients, while a conservative management can be achieved for the former one.

Pancreatic fistula is a notorious complication of distal pancreatectomies and enucleations, showing a higher incidence among the latter group of patients. Fistulization is the most common complication reported in laparoscopic series (17.9%) and seems to be higher than those reported in open series [10.4% (45), 5% (48)]. The symptoms of this complication will primarily depend on the fistula output, varying from small peripancreatic collections up to high output fistulas, requiring total parenteral nutrition, somatostatin analogs, or even reoperation.

Distal pancreatectomies for chronic pancreatitis usually carry a lower incidence of pancreatic fistula or leak due to the firm consistency of the gland (34) as opposed to a normal, soft pancreas.

There is consensus about leaving a drain near the pancreatic stump, which helps manage a pancreatic fistula and prevents pancreatic ascites. The utilization of somatostatin analogs (Sandostatin. Novartis AG, Switzerland) has been proposed to prevent fistulas or accelerate their closure. This proposed attempt to reduce the complication has not been confirmed to be effective; multiple trials had different outcome (45). If a fistula happens to occur, its management does not differ from the standard treatments. In general, external pancreatic fistulas are managed conservatively with continuous aspiration from the drain, clinical surveillance, octreotide and enteral or even total parenteral nutrition, as most (>80%) fistulas have a successful outcome and close nonoperatively (49). Reoperation might be required in those cases that do not respond to conservative medical management (49). Fortunately, based on the literature, these kinds of fistulas rarely occur after a laparoscopic resection.

Occasionally a fistula will manifest itself as a fluid collection near the pancreatic stump or enucleated area. These collections are best treated percutaneously due to lowered morbidity and mortality rates (50) instead of reoperation. The success rate for percutaneous drainage in postoperative pancreatic infected collections was reported by Cinat et al. to be 75% (51). Abdominal pain, fever, and leukocytosis are the most common presenting symptoms. In these cases, surgery must be strongly considered when a second percutaneous attempt has failed (51). Splenic abcesses often follow splenic-preserving procedures for spleen salvage. In his original description, Warshaw had 1 splenic abscess out of 22 patients, which occurred after 8 weeks. Splenomegaly might be a contraindication for this procedure, since these kinds of spleens require a greater vascular supply and short gastric vessels alone might be insufficient.

Splenic abscesses will present with abdominal pain and fever, Tc99 sulfur colloid spleen scan will show abnormal uptakes and CT scan reveal sufficient or insufficient blood flow (52). Depending on each particular case, either drainage (53) or splenectomy (54) might be performed to treat these patients.

Infarction of the spleen can follow a pancreatic resection and happens only after splenic-preserving procedures, but could also appear after conventional spleen-sparing distal pancreatectomy. We recommend looking at the spleen before finishing the procedure and evaluating the need for splenectomy if major ischemia exists, since it can lead to abscess formation or severe postoperative pain. In Gagner's series, one patient presented with ischemic spleen after a spleen-sparing distal pancreatectomy, which necessitated removal (34).

4.9 Mount Sinai Series

Indications for laparoscopic pancreatic resection included cystic lesions (10 patients) neuroendocrine tumors (7), chronic pancreatitis (1), and schwannoma (1). Pathological diagnoses of the cystic lesions are cystadenocarcinoma (1), serous cystadenoma (2), mucinous cystadenoma (5), ductal papillary hyperplasia (1), lymphoid cyst (1), and congenital cyst (1). An unsuspected small pancreatic adenocarcinoma was discovered in the distal pancreatectomy specimen for chronic pancreatitis. Of the neuroendocrine tumors, four were insulinomas and three were nonfunctioning islet cell tumors (34) (Table 1).

The median operating time was 4.4 hours (range 1.6–6.6). Median blood loss was 200 mL (range 20–4000). Four patients (21%) received blood transfusions during

Table 1 Types of Tumor Removed by Laparoscopic Distal Pancreatectomy, Mount Sinai Series

Tumor type	No.
Chronic pancreatitis	8
Pancreatic adenocarcinoma	3 (1)
Neuroendocrine tumors:	59
Insulinoma	49 (6)
Nonfunctioning tumor	6 (3)
Gastrinoma	2
VIPoma	1
Functioning tumor in MEN-1	1
Cystic pancreatic lesion:	58
Mucinous cystadenoma	34 (5)
Serous cystadenoma	18 (2)
Cystadenocarcinoma	2 (1)
Ductal papillary hyperplasia	2 (1)
Lymphoid cyst	1 (1)
Congenital cyst	1 (1)
Schwannoma	1
Nesidioblastoma	1

Table 2 Intraoperative Data and Types of Technique

Variables	Literature	Mount Sinai experience
Mean operative time[a]	3.7 h	4.1 h
Range	1.7–6.6 h	1.6–6.6 h
Median blood loss	300 mL	200 mL
Range[b]	100–733 mL	20–4000 mL
Type of resection[c]		
Distal pancreatectomy with splenectomy	57 (43.8%)	13 (59%)
Distal pancreatectomy with spleen preservation	46 (35.4%)	4 (18%)
Enucleation	27 (20.8%)	5 (18%)
Technique[d]		
Completed laparoscopically	123 (86.6%)	20 (90.9%)[e]
Converted to laparotomy	19 (13.3%)	2 (9%)

[a] Literature total 137 patients.
[b] Literature range is the mean range of series.
[c] Literature total 125 patients.
[d] Literature total 128 patients.
[e] One patient converted to hand-assisted.

the hospital stay. Distal pancreatectomy with splenectomy was performed in 12 patients (63%). Spleen-preserving procedures were planned preoperatively in 4 of 15 patients (27%) undergoing distal pancreatectomy. Three of four spleens (75%) were successfully preserved, and one was removed because it appeared ischemic following completion of the pancreatic resection. Five patients (18%) underwent laparoscopic enucleation of islet cell tumors (Table 2).

Sixteen of 19 (84%) pancreatic resections were completed laparoscopically. One distal pancreatectomy adhered to the splenic vein and artery. Two patients (11%) were converted from laparoscopic (5%) to a hand-assisted technique because the cystic mass was densely to open procedures: one due to bleeding, and the second for a suspicion of malignancy in a patient with a 6 cm solid tumor on CT scan in which splenic hilar invasion was discovered at laparoscopy. Cystadenocarcinoma of the pancreatic tail was confirmed pathologically.

The major morbidity rate was 16%, and the minor morbidity rate was 10%, for a total morbidity of 26%. There were two minor postoperative complications: superficial phlebitis and prolonged ileus. Pancreatic fistulas developed postoperatively in three patients (16%): one patient who had an enucleation (25%), one patient who underwent distal pancreatectomy with splenectomy (8%), and one patient after spleen-preserving distal pancreatectomy (33%). Two of the patients with fistulas had the longest hospital stays of 18 and 26 days, respectively. The third patient had an initial hospital stay of 5 days and was readmitted to hospital several days later. All three patients were treated with CT-guided percutaneous drainage of a peripancreatic collection and total parenteral nutrition (TPN). They were discharged home on TPN until the fistula closed.

There were no late postoperative complications and no deaths within 30 days of surgery. The median length

Table 3 Laparoscopic Pancreatic Series: Postoperative Results

First author, year	No.	Morbidity (%)	Minor complication (%)	Major complication (%)	Leak (%)	Mortality after 30 days (%)	Hospital stay (days)	Ref.
Gagner, 2002	22	31.5	13.5	18	18	0	7	34
Fernandez-Cruz, 2002	18	27.7	0	27.7	27.7	0	5	61
Melotti, 2002	25	32.4	13.6	18.8	18.1	0	9	62
Fabre, 2002	13	38	23	15	15	0	7	63
Ferraina, 2002	5	20	0	20	20	0	5.3	64
Shinchi, 2001	2	0	0	0	0	0	7	43
Lo, 2000	3	33	0	33	33	0	NR	27
Mahon, 2001	3	0	0	0	0	0	4.7	65
Berends, 2000	10	50	20	30	20	0	7	26
Salky, 2000	7	28	28	0	0	0	4	13
Vezakis, 1999	6	33	0	33	33	0	34.5	25
Park, 1999	5	20	0	20	20	NR	5	22
Chapuis, 1998	5	20	8	31	8	0	4.7	15
Cuschieri, 1996	5	40	20	20	20	0	12	
Total	142	31.6	10.8	20	17.9	0 (n = 137)	7.4 (n = 139)	

Table 4 Laparoscopic Distal Pancreatectomy and Enucleation Series: Peri-Operative Data

First author, year	No.	Operation time (h)	Enucleation	Distal pancreatectomy	Pancreatectomy "spleen preserving"	Conversion (%)	Ref.
Gagner, 2002	22	4.1	5	17	4	13.5	34
Fernandez-Cruz, 2002	18	4.5	4	14	10	11.1	61
Melotti, 2002	25	2.8	3	22	17	0	62
Fabre, 2002	13	4.7	0	11	10	15.4	63
Ferraina, 2002	5	3.2	2	3	3	0	64
Shinchi, 2001	2	6.6	0	2	0	NR	43
Lo, 2000	3	NR	1	1	1	33	27
Mahon, 2001	3	1.7	0	3	2	0	65
Berends, 2000	10	3	5	1	NR	40	26
Salky, 2000	7	3.7	—	—	—	—	13
Vezakis, 1999	6	5.0	0	6	5	33	25
Park, 1999	5	5,0	0	5	NR	NR	22
Chapuis, 1998	5	2.4	3	2	—	20	66
Gagner, 1997	13	4	4	9	—	30.7	15
Cuschieri, 1996	5	4.5	0	5	5	0	12
Total	142	1.7–6.6 (range)	27	103	57	14.8[a] (n = 128)	

[a] The conversion rate of 142 patients is 13.3.

of postoperative hospital stay (LOS) was 6 days (range 1–26 days). In patients who had an uncomplicated course, the mean LOS was 5 days, whereas patients with complications had a mean LOS of 12 days, although this difference was not statistically significant.

4.10 Discussion and Review of the Literature

Since distal pancreatectomy is similar to adrenalectomy in that a relatively large incision is required to remove a small lesion, the potential benefits of the minimal access approach are therefore substantial. The operative and postoperative results of laparoscopic pancreatic resection appear to be acceptable. Operative times of just over 4 hours are identical to open pancreatectomy series (48).

Patients generally have minimal postoperative pain, a very short-lasting ileus, and a quick return to normal activity. An average of 7 days postoperative hospital stay compares favorably with the 10–15 days reported in open series (48,55). Total morbidity of 26% may appear high, but it is actually at the low end of the range of morbidities reported in other open and laparoscopic series (20–60%) (Tables 3, 4) (15,48,55,56).

The 16–18% pancreatic fistula rate in Mount Sinai series may also seem high, but the denominator is small. Broughan et al. reported a low fistula rate (6%) in a

Table 5 Open Distal Pancreatectomy Series: Postoperative Results

First author, year	No.	Operation time (h)	Morbidity (%)	Minor complication (%)	Major complication (%)	Leak (%)	Mortality after 30 days (%)	Hospital stay (days)	Ref.
Lillemoe, 1999	235	4.3	31	NR	31	5	0,9	10	48
Benoist, 1999	40	NR	63	5	58	23	0	15	55
Broughan, 1986	84	—	24	—	24	6	3.6	—	57
Total	359	4.3 (n = 235)	32.9 (n = 359)	5 (n = 40)	32.3 (n = 359)	7.2 (n = 359)	1.4 (n = 359)	10.7 (n = 275)	

relatively large series of 84 patients with an open resection (Table 5) (57).

The laparoscopic procedures may have a complication rate of 31%, similar to recent series of open pancreatic procedures (33%) (48,55,57) Only 29 patients (20%) had a major complication following the laparoscopic procedures, and these complications were mostly due to a pancreatic leak (86%) (Table 6). The leak rate (mean 17.9%; range 0–33%) seems higher when compared with the same open series (mean 7.2%; range 5–23%). An appropriate control of fistulas and peripancreatic collections was always possible with CT-guided percutaneous drainage. Only in two cases did the pancreatic leak lead to reoperation. In addition, the

Table 6 Reported Complications Following a Laparoscopic Distal Pancreatectomy

First author (Ref.)	No. cases	Surgery	Complication	Treatment
Cuschieri (10)	5	5 DP+S	1 Pancreatic fistula	Resolved spontaneously
Gagner (11)	7	3 E	1 Major bleeding (splenic vein)[a]	Multiple titanium clips
		4 DP	Small infected collection[a]	Percutaneous drainage
Vezakis (25)	4	4 DP	2 Pancreatic fistula	Percutaneous drainage and PN
Ueno (67)	1	1 DP	Small splenic infarct (1 month)	Resolved spontaneously
Cuschieri (42)	4	2 HADP+S	1 Intraop. bleeding	Conversion
		1 HACG	—	—
		1 HACJ	—	—
Patterson (34)	17	10 DP+S	1 Intra-op bleeding	Conversion
			1 Pancreatic fistula	CT-guided percutaneous drainage and PN
		3 DP	1 Pancreatic fistula	
		4 E	1 Pancreatic fistula	
Fabre (63)	13	13 DP	2 Intraop bleeding from splenic vein	Conversion (1 splenectomy)
			1 Pancreatic fistula	Conservative
			2 Liquid cysts	
			1 Bleeding from trocar	Reoperation
Fernandez-Cruz (54)	11	5 DP	Perforated duodenal ulcer	Reoperation
		2 LIGD	—	—
		4 TCG	—	—
Park (22)	28	9 CGLSA	1 Myocardial infarction	Death
			1 Necrotizing pancreatitis	Multiple (open) debridement
		5 MLIGCG	—	—
		11 TCG	2 Postop bleeding	Transfusion
		3 LCJ	—	—
	23	21 DP	2 Intraop bleeding	Transfusion
			1 Pancreatic fistula	Percutaneous drainage
		2 HADP	1 Wound infection	NR
Gramatica (68)	9	4 E	1 Pancreatic fistula	Resolved spontaneously
		4 DP	1 Pleural effusion	
		1 DP+S	1 Fluid collection	
Mahon (65)	3	2 DP	Urinary retention	Catheterization
		1 DP+S		
Fernandez-Cruz (61)	16	4 E	2 Pancreatic fistula	Drainage
		12 DP	3 Pancreatic fistula	Drainage
			1 Splenic abscess	Splenectomy
			1 Intraop bleeding	Controlled w/stapler

DP: Distal pancreatectomy; S: splenectomy; CGLSA: cyst gastrostomy by the lesser sac approach; MLIGCG: mini-laparoscopic intragastric cyst gastrostomy; TCG: transgastric cyst gastrostomy; LCJ: laparoscopic cyst jejunostomy; HADP: hand-assisted distal pancreatectomy; HACG: hand-assisted cyst gastrostomy; HACJ: hand-assisted cyst jejunostomy; E: enucleation; NR: nonreferred; PN: parenteral nutrition; LIGD: lsaparoscopic intragastric drainage.

[a] Surgery not specified.

pancreatic leak rate was higher in the enucleation patients than the distal pancreatectomy patients. In addition there were 9 patients (11%) with intra-abdominal infections in that series, which are usually associated with pancreatic leaks, therefore the true pancreatic leak rate is probably underestimated. Thus, the rate of postoperative pancreatic fistula formation in the Mount Sinai series is comparable to open series. It is interesting that all three of the pancreatic leaks presented as peripancreatic collections, despite the presence of a functioning closed-suction drain in each patient. One could speculate that this phenomenon is due to decreased adhesion formation after laparoscopic versus open surgery and therefore an increased risk of fluid collection formation if a pancreatic leak occurs.

The consistency of the pancreatic parenchyma has previously been shown to correlate with the pancreatic fistula rate after distal pancreatectomy (58,59). The firm pancreas as seen in chronic pancreatitis is associated with a lower fistula or leak rate than the normal, soft pancreas. The large open series reported by Lillemoe et al. had only a 5% incidence of fistula formation, but 24% of their patients were the low-risk group with chronic pancreatitis. In the Mount Sinai series, only 1 of 19 patients (5%) had chronic pancreatitis, and thus our fistula rate is expected to be higher than the 5% incidence in Lillemoe et al. study (48).

Pancreatic lesions requiring resection should be carefully evaluated and selected for a laparoscopic approach. Laparoscopic distal pancreatectomy for adenocarcinoma of the pancreatic tail is controversial. Unfortunately, patients with these lesions rarely present with curable disease. Laparoscopic resection for islet cell neoplasms and cystic lesions is feasible, but they are not widely performed. Insulinomas are ideal lesions for laparoscopic resection as they are usually single and benign. Proven principles of open pancreatic surgery must be adhered to in laparoscopic resection, and insulinomas close to the pancreatic duct should be resected rather than enucleated. In retrospect, this was probably the case in our patient who developed a pancreatic fistula after enucleation of a 1.5 cm insulinoma from the neck of the pancreas.

Laparoscopic pancreaticoduodenal resection (palliative) was successfully attempted for a malignant islet cell tumor invading the duodenal lumen and causing bleeding by Gagner in 1997, while he was at the Cleveland Clinic, during a live surgery for the AHPBA (American Hepato-Pancreato-Biliary Association). First performed in 1993 (9), laparoscopic pancreaticoduodenectomy remains in question because of the technical difficulty and the prolonged operating time, which may outweigh the potential benefits of the minimal access approach (60). In the series of 10 patients, the operative time required to perform a laparoscopic Whipple procedure averaged 8.5 hours, the rate of conversion to laparotomy was 40%, and the mean hospital stay was 22.3 days (15). Huscher from San Giovanni Hospital in Rome has recently revisited this procedure and may have better results due to improved instrumentations than were available 10 years ago. This will need to be confirmed by multiple teams and compared with open surgery.

5 CONCLUSION

One decade after the first laparoscopic pancreatic resection, the literature continues to show encouraging outcomes for laparoscopic distal pancreatectomies and enucleations. These procedures are technically feasible and result in acceptable complication and mortality rates. As with other laparoscopic procedures, the benefits include reduced postoperative pain, better cosmetic results, shorter hospitalization, and lower rate of major complications. Laparoscopic enucleation or distal pancreatectomy with or without splenectomy is technically feasible, safe, and benefits patients. The ability to avoid a large incision and perform resection of an islet cell tumor that is predominantly small and benign is a meaningful advantage of laparoscopic surgery. Localization of these lesions by intraoperative inspection of the pancreas and contact ultrasonography has added significant merit to this approach.

At the current time, given the small number of patients included in the series, the relatively short follow-up, and the possible increased risk of pancreatic leak, the laparoscopic approach needs further study.

REFERENCES

1. Bernheim B. Organoscopy. Cystoscopy of the abdominal cavity. Ann Surg 1911; 53:764–767.
2. Meyer-Burg J. [Laparoscopic examination of the pancreas]. Rev Esp Enferm Apar Dig 1972; 38:697–704.
3. Hirata K, Mima S, Fukuda M. [High-resolution ultrasonography in cancer diagnosis—advances and indication of intraluminal sonography]. Gan To Kagaku Ryoho 1986; 13:1661–1667.
4. Cuesta MA, Meijer S, Borgstein PJ, Sibinga Mulder L, Sikkenk AC. Laparoscopic ultrasonography for hepatobiliary and pancreatic malignancy. Br J Surg 1993; 80: 1571–1574.
5. Murugiah M, Paterson-Brown S, Windsor JA, Miles WF, Garden OJ. Early experience of laparoscopic ultra-

sonography in the management of pancreatic carcinoma. Surg Endosc 1993; 7:177–181.

6. Cuschieri A. Laparoscopic surgery of the pancreas. J R Coll Surg Edinb 1994; 39:178–184.
7. Gouma DJ, de Wit LT, Nieveen van Dijkum E, Van Delden O, Bemelman WA, Rauws EA, Van Lanschot JJ, Obertop H. Laparoscopic ultrasonography for staging of gastrointestinal malignancy. Scand J Gastroenterol Suppl 1996; 218:43–49.
8. Pietrabissa A, Di Candio G, Giulianotti PC, Mosca F. Laparoscopic exposure of the pancreas and staging of pancreatic cancer. Semin Laparosc Surg 1996; 3:3–9.
9. Gagner M, Pomp A. Laparoscopic pylorus-preserving pancreatoduodenectomy. Surg Endosc 1994; 8:408–410.
10. Cuschieri A, Jakimowicz JJ, van Spreeuwel J. Laparoscopic distal 70% pancreatectomy and splenectomy for chronic pancreatitis. Ann Surg 1996; 223:280–285.
11. Gagner M, Pomp A, Herrera MF. Early experience with laparoscopic resections of islet cell tumors. Surgery 1996; 120:1051–1054.
12. Cuschieri A. Laparoscopic pancreatic resections. Semin Laparosc Surg 1996; 3:15–20.
13. Salky BA, Edye M. Laparoscopic pancreatectomy. Surg Clin North Am 1996; 76:539–545.
14. Sussman LA, Christie R, Whittle DE. Laparoscopic excision of distal pancreas including insulinoma. Aust NZ J Surg 1996; 66:414–416.
15. Gagner M, Pomp A. Laparoscopic pancreatic resection: Is it worthwhile?. J Gastrointest Surg 1997; 1:20–26.
16. Klingler PJ, Hinder RA, Menke DM, Smith SL. Hand-assisted laparoscopic distal pancreatectomy for pancreatic cystadenoma. Surg Laparosc Endosc 1998; 8:180–184.
17. Gagner M, Gentileschi P. Hand-assisted laparoscopic pancreatic resection. Semin Laparosc Surg 2001; 8:114–125.
18. Yoshida T, Bandoh T, Ninomiya K, Matsumoto T, Baatar D, Kitano S. Laparoscopic enucleation of a pancreatic insulinoma: report of a case. Surg Today 1998; 28:1188–1191.
19. Collins R, Schlinkert RT, Roust L. Laparoscopic resection of an insulinoma. J Laparoendosc Adv Surg Tech A 1999; 9:429–431.
20. Dexter SP, Martin IG, Leindler L, Fowler R, McMahon MJ. Laparoscopic enucleation of a solitary pancreatic insulinoma. Surg Endosc 1999; 13:406–408.
21. Marescaux J, Mutter D, Vix M, Leroy J. Endoscopic surgery: ideal for endocrine surgery? World J Surg 1999; 23:825–834.
22. Park A, Schwartz R, Tandan V, Anvari M. Laparoscopic pancreatic surgery. Am J Surg 1999; 177:158–163.
23. Underwood RA, Soper NJ. Current status of laparoscopic surgery of the pancreas. J Hepatobiliary Pancreat Surg 1999; 6:154–164.
24. Van Nieuwenhove Y, Delvaux G. Laparoscopic management of neuroendocrine tumours of the pancreas. Acta Chir Belg. 1999; 99:249–252.
25. Vezakis A, Davides D, Larvin M, McMahon MJ. Laparoscopic surgery combined with preservation of the spleen for distal pancreatic tumors. Surg Endosc 1999; 13:26–29.
26. Berends FJ, Cuesta MA, Kazemier G, van Eijck CH, de Herder WW, van Muiswinkel JM, Bruining HA, Bonjer HJ. Laparoscopic detection and resection of insulinomas. Surgery 2000; 128:386–391.
27. Lo CY, Lo CM, Fan ST. Role of laparoscopic ultrasonography in intraoperative localization of pancreatic insulinoma. Surg Endosc 2000; 14:1131–1135.
28. Raeburn CD, McIntyre RC Jr. Laparoscopic approach to adrenal and endocrine pancreatic tumors. Surg Clin North Am 2000; 80:1427–1441.
29. Spitz JD, Lilly MC, Tetik C, Arregui ME. Ultrasound-guided laparoscopic resection of pancreatic islet cell tumors. Surg Laparosc Endosc Percutan Tech 2000; 10:168–173.
30. Cogliandolo A, Pidoto RR, Causse X, Kerdraon R, Saint Marc O. Minimally invasive management of insulinomas. A case report. Surg Endosc 2001; 15:1042.
31. Furihata M, Tagaya N, Kubota K. Laparoscopic enucleation of insulinoma in the pancreas: case report and review of the literature. Surg Laparosc Endosc Percutan Tech 2001; 11:279–283.
32. Gentileschi P, Gagner M. Laparoscopic pancreatic resection. Chir Ital 2001; 53:279–289.
33. Iihara M, Kanbe M, Okamoto T, Ito Y, Obara T. Laparoscopic ultrasonography for resection of insulinomas. Surgery 2001; 130:1086–1091.
34. Patterson EJ, Gagner M, Salky B, Inabnet WB, Brower S, Edye M, Gurland B, Reiner M, Pertsemlides D. Laparoscopic pancreatic resection: single-institution experience of 19 patients. J Am Coll Surg 2001; 193: 281–287.
35. Falconi M, Molinari E, Carbognin G, Zamboni G, Bassi C, Pederzoli P. What preoperative assessment is necessary for insulinomas? Calculating the degree of waste: an analysis of 29 cases. Chir Ital 2002; 54(5):597–604.
36. Chu QD, Al-Kasspooles MF, Smith JL, Nava HR, Douglass HO Jr, Driscoll D, Gibbs JF. Is glucagonoma of the pancreas a curable disease? Int J Pancreatol 2001; 29(3):155–162.
37. Santambrogio L, Nosotti M, Baisi A, Bellaviti N, Pavoni G, Rosso L. Buttressing staple lines with bovine pericardium in lung resection for bullous emphysema. Scand Cardiovasc J 1998; 32:297–299.
38. Olmos-Zuniga JR, Jasso-Victoria R, Sotres-Vega A, Gaxiola-Gaxiola M, Cedillo-Ley I, Argote-Greene LM, Santillan-Doherty P. Suture-line reinforcement with glutaraldehyde-preserved bovine pericardium for non-anatomic resection of lung tissue. J Invest Surg 2001; 14:161–168.
39. Warshaw A. Conservation of the spleen with distal pancreatectomy. Arch Surg 1988; 123:550–553.

40. Tashiro S, Murata E, Hiraoka T, Nakakuma K, Watanabe E, Miyauchi Y. New technique for pancreaticojejunostomy using a biological adhesive. Br J Surg 1987; 74:392–394.
41. Hiraoka T, Kanemitsu K, Tsuji T, Saitoh N, Takamori H, Akamine T, Miyauchi Y. A method for safe pancreaticojejunostomy. Am J Surg 1993; 165:270–272.
42. Cuschieri A. Laparoscopic hand-assisted surgery for hepatic and pancreatic disease. Surg Endosc 2000; 14:991–996.
43. Shinchi H, Takao S, Noma H, et al. Hand-assisted laparoscopic distal pancreatectomy with mini-laparotomy for distal pancreatic cystadenoma. Sugr Laparosc Endosc Percut Tech 2000; 11(2):139–143.
44. Klinger P, Hinder R, Menke DM, et al. Hand-assisted laparoscopic distal pancreatectomy for pancreatic cystadenoma. Surg Laparosc Endosc 1998; 3:180–184.
45. Halloran CM, Ghanch P, Bosennet L, Hartley MN, Sutton R, Neoptolemos JP. Complications of pancreatic cancer resection. Dig Surg 2002; 19(2):138–146.
46. Aldridge M, Williamson R. Distal pancreatectomy with and without splenectomy. Br J Surg 1991; 78:976–979.
47. Cuschieri A, Jackimowicz J, van Spreeuwel J. Laparoscopic distal 70% pancreatectomy and splenectomy for chronic pancreatitis. Ann Surg 1996; 3:280–285.
48. Lillemoe KD, Kaushal S, Cameron, et al. Distal pancreatectomy: indications and outcomes in 235 patients. Ann Surg 229:693-700.
49. Ridgeway MG, Stabile BE. Surgical management and treatment of pancreatic fistulas. Surg Clin North Am 1996; 76(5):1159–1173.
50. McLean TR, Simmons K, Svensson LG. Management of postoperative intra-abdominal abscesses by routine percutaneous drainage. Surg Gynecol Obstet 1993; 176(2): 167–171.
51. Cinat M, Wilson S, Din A. Determinants for successful percutaneous image-guided drainage of intra-abdominal abscess. Arch Surg 2002; 137(7).
52. Watanabe Y, Motomichi S, Kikkawa H, et al. Spleen-preserving laparoscopic distal pancreatectomy for cystic adenoma. Hepato Gastroenterol 2002; 49, 148–152.
53. Warshaw A. Conservation of the spleen with distal pancreatectomy. Arch Surg 1988; 123:550–553.
54. Fernandez-Cruz L, Saenz A, Astudillo E, et al. Laparoscopic pancreatic surgery in patients with chronic pancreatitis. Surg Endosc 2002; 16:996–1003.
55. Benoist S, Dugue L, Sauvanet A, Valverde A, Mauvais F, Paye F, Farges O, Belghiti J. Is there a role of preservation of the spleen in distal pancreatectomy? J Am Coll. Surg. 1999; 188:255–260.
56. Cuschieri A. Laparoscopic pancreatic resections. Semin Laparosc Surg 1996; 3(1):15–20.
57. Broughan TA, Leslie JD, Soto JM, Hermann RE. Pancreatic islet cell tumors. Surgery 1986; 99(6):671–678.
58. Buchler M, Friess H, Klempa I, Hermanek P, Sulkowski U, Becker H, Schafmayer A, Baca I, Lorenz D, Meister R. Role of octreotide in the prevention of postoperative complications following pancreatic resection. Am J Surg. 1992; 163(1):125–130.
59. Montorsi M, Zago M, Mosca F, Capussotti L, Zotti E, Ribotta G, Fegiz G, Fissi S, Roviaro G, Peracchia A. Efficacy of octreotide in the prevention of pancreatic fistula after elective pancreatic resections: a prospective, controlled, randomized clinical trial. Surgery 1995; 117(1):26–31.
60. Cuschieri A. Whither minimal access surgery: tribulations and expectations. Am J Surg 1995; 169:9–19.
61. Fernandez-Cruz L, Saenz A , Astrdillo E, Martinez I, Hoyos S, Pantoja JP, Navarro. Outcome of laparoscopic pancreatic surgery: endocrine and nonendocrine tumors. World J Surg, 2002 (DOI:10.1007/s00268-002-6673-).
62. Melotti G, Piccoli M, Bassi C, Falconi M, Bonilauri S, Lazzaretti MG, Fettucciari V. L'approccio laparoscopico ai tumori cistici del corpo-coda del pancreas: indicazioni e tecnica. Osp Ital Chir 2000; 6:411–415.
63. Fabre JM, Dulucq JL, Vacher C, Lemoine MC, Wintringer P, Nocca D, Burgel JS, Domergue J. Is laparoscopic left pancreatic resection justified? Surg Endosc, 2002 (DOI: 10.1007/s00464-001-9206-3).
64. Ferraina P, Ferraro A, Merello Lardies J, Cuenca Abente F. Academia Argentina de Cirugia 2002.
65. Mahon D, Allen E, Rhodes M. Laparoscopic distal pancreatectomy. Three cases of insulinomas. Surg Endosc 2002; 16:700–702.
66. Chapuis Y, Bigourdan JM, Massault PP, Pitre J, Palazzo L. Exérèse d'un insulinome pancreatique sous coelioscopie. Chirugie 1998; 123(5):461–467.
67. Ueno T, Oka M, Nishihara K, et al. Laparoscopic distal pancreatectomy with preservation of the spleen. Surg Laparosc Endosc Percut Tech 1999; 4:290–293.
68. Gramatica L, Herrera M, Mercado-Luna A, et al. Videolaparoscopic resection of insulinomas: experience in two institutions. World J Surg 2002; 26:1297–1300.

50

Multiple Endocrine Neoplasia and Other Familial Endocrine Tumor Syndromes

Charles A. G. Proye

University of Lille II and Hôpital Claude Huriez, Lille, France

Stephen G. Farrell

University of Melbourne and St. Vincent's Hospital, Melbourne, Australia

1 INTRODUCTION

The multiple endocrine neoplasia (MEN) syndromes are rare and fascinating autosomal dominant inherited conditions, each characterized by a cluster of endocrine neoplasms. The first recognizable description of MEN1, by Erdheim (1) in 1903, was of a patient with acromegaly and four enlarged parathyroid glands. In 1954, Wermer (2) described the syndrome of familial pituitary, parathyroid, and pancreatic islet cell neoplasia and coined the term "adenomatosis" of the endocrine glands. Wermer's syndrome is synonymous with MEN1.

MEN2 is dominated by the development of medullary thyroid cancer and pheochromocytoma. Hyperparathyroidism is less common and relatively insignificant in MEN2A and does not occur in MEN2B. Individuals with MEN2B have a marfanoid habitus and pathognomonic facies. Familial medullary thyroid cancer (FMTC) is a variant of MEN2 without associated features.

Sipple (3) first described the association of thyroid carcinoma and phaeochromocytoma in 1961, and the MEN2A syndrome is sometimes referred to as Sipple's syndrome. In 1968 Gorlin et al. (4) and Steiner et al. (5) described the MEN2B syndrome.

Although largely unrecognized until recently, increased awareness of these syndromes led to concerted efforts to determine the cause, natural history, and optimal management. Determination of the genes responsible for MEN1 and MEN2 has dramatically altered the management of these syndromes, especially MEN2. In the case of MEN1, genetic testing determines which kindred members are carriers of the mutant gene and therefore require screening and early management of endocrine tumors. MEN2 is possibly the finest model yet of a condition in which genetic testing allows specific surgical prophylaxis against tumor development.

1.1 Background

MEN1 results from a germline mutation of the *MEN1* gene. Subsequent somatic mutation of the wild-type allele causes loss of function of this growth-suppressor gene. In MEN2, germline mutation confers a gain of function in the *RET* proto-oncogene. In both MEN1 and MEN2 penetrance is almost complete in carriers of the mutant gene, while the disease expression is varied. Interestingly, in MEN2 a strong genotype-phenotype correlation is found, while in MEN1 no such correlation is found. Both MEN1 and MEN2 may also arise as de novo mutations, which are then heritable. The variation in expression of MEN1 is remarkable. While hyperparathyroidism (HPT) is the most common initial manifestation, the other associated lesions may present in any order, or not at all.

Before the genetic revolution, the diagnosis of MEN1 required confirmation of the presence of two of the three major associated endocrinopathies in an index case and one lesion in a relative. There were frequent cases of uncertainty. The lack of a ubiquitous, early biological marker of disease meant that all kindred members required repeated, intensive screening with biochemical tests and imaging.

In MEN2A, diagnosis in an index case was also unlikely prior to development of a second tumor. However, screening in kindreds was simpler than in MEN1, if not perfect. Basal and pentagastrin-stimulated calcitonin levels usually became positive well before clinical evidence of medullary thyroid cancer (MTC). But pentagastrin-stimulated calcitonin testing is unpleasant, and positive results did not universally occur at an early stage of disease. Conversely, false-positive results sometimes occurred.

Historically, complications due to hormone secretion were the major causes of morbidity and mortality in MEN1: in particular, peptic ulcer due to gastrinoma and hypoglycemia due to insulinoma. In MEN2, hypertensive stroke and cardiac disease due to pheochromocytoma were frequent causes of death, but medullary carcinoma was the main cause of death. Modern medical and surgical treatment has altered the natural history of both syndromes, and now malignant transformation is the most significant clinical problem: pancreatico-duodenal malignancy in MEN1 and MTC in MEN2.

The minimally invasive revolution in surgery has had the most impact on MEN2A. Laparoscopic adrenalectomy has become the preferred approach to benign adrenal tumors, including bilateral pheochromocytoma. However, the approach to MTC, which demands lymph node dissection, is necessarily via an adequate open exploration. Similarly, there is little enthusiasm for parathyroidectomy and thymectomy by either video-assisted or endoscopic means in MEN1. Pancreatico-duodenal disease is multifocal, and while only one of the tumors may be responsible for a clinical syndrome such as hyperinsulinemia, difficulty in identifying the secreting lesion precludes laparoscopic pancreatic tumor enucleation. Furthermore, most surgeons would, by preference, perform more extensive surgery such as left pancreatectomy plus enucleation of any cephalic tumors for insulinoma in MEN1. Such surgery might be performed laparoscopically in some patients, by some surgeons, perhaps with robot assistance, but the day has not yet arrived when this is a routine option.

While hyperparathyroidism is the common feature of MEN1 and MEN2A, it is of major clinical importance usually only in MEN1. It is the most common first expression of MEN1 and usually requires surgery, the appropriate extent of which is debated. Radical excision risks troublesome hypocalcemia in young patients, while less radical excision risks persistence or recurrence. In contrast, in MEN2A the main concern with respect to the parathyroid glands is usually the preservation of adequate function after thyroidectomy for treatment or prophylaxis of medullary thyroid cancer.

Despite greatly increased knowledge of the genetics and natural history of the MEN syndromes and a significant body of experience in management of these rare syndromes in specialist centers, there remain controversies. The major contentious issues are:

1. The timing and extent of surgery for the Zollinger-Ellison syndrome (ZES) in MEN1
2. The extent of lymph node surgery for clinical MTC in MEN2
3. The age at which prophylactic thyroidectomy should be performed in gene carriers in MEN2
4. The role of lymph node clearance associated with prophylactic thyroidectomy for MEN2

2 MULTIPLE ENDOCRINE NEOPLASIA TYPE 1 (WERMER'S SYNDROME)

Multiple endocrine neoplasia is characterized by the development of endocrine neoplasms of the parathyroid, pancreas, and pituitary. The true prevalence of this condition is unknown. Shepherd (6) has emphasized the existence of unrecognized MEN1. The sporadic occurrence of each of the component disorders is indeed much more common than in association with MEN1. Peptic ulcer, for example, is a very common disease, usually treated adequately by modern medications, and unless it presents in an unusual fashion may not evoke MEN1. Many cases of endocrine tumor are either asymptomatic or minimally symptomatic and may go entirely unrecognized during the life of the patient. Variable expression of the syndrome is such that the associated endocrinopathies often present metachronously and may be separated by many years: 39 years in one reported case (7).

In 1982 only 3 patients with MEN1 were known in Tasmania, an Australian island with a population of about 450,000. Thorough investigation of relatives led to the discovery of about 250 cases within 10 years—a prevalence of about 1 in 1800. There may be yet more undiagnosed cases in different families. Reported estimated rates in other countries vary from 1 in 5000 to1 in 500,000 (8,9).

2.1 Genetics

The *MEN1* gene was first cloned in 1997 by Chandrasekharappa et al. (10). It is situated on the long arm of chromosome 11 at 11q13. It contains 10 exons and encodes a 610-amino-acid protein, menin. The means by which menin acts as a tumor suppressor are not understood. Agarwal et al. (11) have shown that menin interacts with the activating protein 1 (AP1) transcription factor JunD and represses JunD-activated transcription. *MEN1* mutations are enormously diverse, occurring in and around the open reading frame of *MEN1* with a different mutation found for most families. More than 250 mutations have been identified. When subsequent somatic mutation or loss of the second *MEN1* allele occurs in a cell, neoplastic clonal expansion may occur. Loss of function of both alleles is evident in about a quarter of sporadic varieties of MEN1 tumors (12).

Genetic mutations at the *MEN1* locus have been identified in 80–90% of families with clinical MEN1 (13). The difficulty in testing for MEN1 in the proband is that there are no hot spots. Failure to find a genetic mutation in a proband does not exclude MEN1. More extensive testing of the gene may be required. Unlike in MEN2, no general correlation between genotype and phenotype has yet been found, but some mutations may be harbingers of a more aggressive disease (14).

2.2 Clinical Features

In MEN1, more than 90% of individuals develop hyperparathyroidism by the age of 35, 30–75% develop clinically significant pancreatico-duodenal tumors (while more than 80% have demonstrable lesions at necropsy), and 15–30% develop clinically significant pituitary tumors. Approximately 80% of individuals express some clinical form of the syndrome by the age of 50, although occasionally no clinical expression occurs despite being a gene carrier (15).

The first manifestation of the syndrome is hyperparathyroidism in 43% of patients, pancreatico-duodenal tumor in 33%, and pituitary tumor in 23%. About 40% of gastrinomas and 5% of insulinomas occur in the setting of MEN1.

A number of other lesions are associated with the syndrome. These include adrenal cortical tumors, cutaneous or visceral (angio)lipomas, facial angiofibromas, collagenomas, foregut-derived carcinoids, rarely pheochromocytoma, fibrosarcoma, meningioma, and ependymoma (Table 1).

2.3 Hyperparathyroidism in MEN1

While hyperparathyroidism is the feature that most often leads to diagnosis of MEN1 and occurs in virtually 100% of gene carriers by the age of 50 (12), only 2–4% of patients with primary hyperparathyroidism have MEN1 (12,16). In general only patients with a suggestive family history, patients younger than 40 years of age, and those with multigland disease should be considered for further clinical or genetic investigation. The age of onset and clinical severity of HPT is markedly varied, but HPT usually occurs around 20–25 years of age and is present in 90% by 35 years of age (12). Burgess et al. (17) have shown significant osteoporosis even in young women with MEN1 HPT. Significant and symptomatic hypercalcemia is common and may even lead to hypercalcemic crisis.

The pathological nature of HPT in MEN1 is not entirely clear. The distinction between adenoma and hyperplasia is not straightforward, and no universal or reliable tools for the pathologist exist. Some authors have reported the possibility of single gland disease in MEN1 (18–20). Friedman et al. (21) showed the monoclonality of most parathyroid lesions in MEN1. On this basis it might be argued that independent tumors arise, possibly on the background of hyperplasia. However, because of the invariable development of four-gland

Table 1 Clinical Characteristics of MEN1 Syndrome

Key features
Primary hyperparathyroidism: >95%
Pancreatic/duodenal endocrine tumour: 30–75%
Pituitary tumor: 20–40%
Other features
Adrenocortical tumors
Bronchial, thymic, and gastric carcinoids
(Angio)Lipomas
Cutaneous angiofibromas and collagenomas
Ependymomas
Clinical diagnosis
Two key features in index case
One key feature in relative

disease over time and histological features consistent with hyperplasia including the absence of a rim of normal tissue, we and other authors continue to view this disease as nodular hyperplasia (22,23). Marked asymmetry of the glands is noted; some appear normal early in the disease (24). However, all glands are eventually involved, and recurrence of HPT in those patients treated by resection of only enlarged glands is very high (20,25). Some authors have proposed the existence of a circulating mitogenic factor for parathyroid tissue in MEN1 (26).

There is a possibility that a new class of drugs, calcimimetics, may alter or delay the indications for surgery by lowering serum calcium through stimulation of calcium receptors (27).

2.3.1 Surgery for Hyperparathyroidism in MEN1

The indication for surgery is the presence of demonstrable hyperparathyroidism whether or not it is symptomatic. Two different surgical strategies are practiced by experts in this field. The first is subtotal parathyroidectomy (24,28), which is our preferred strategy (see below); the second is total parathyroidectomy with autograft (30). It is clear that performance of anything less than subtotal parathyroidectomy results in a high rate of recurrence and cannot be supported (28).

Preoperative localization prior to initial parathyroid surgery has little place in MEN syndromes because of the need for complete exploration and thymectomy. Localizing studies including sestamibi scintigraphy are less accurate in multigland disease than in the typical uniglandular disease of sporadic HPT. Nevertheless, sestamibi scan may be useful if it identifies a mediastinal lesion inaccessible to cervical thymectomy or a submandibular lesion, best seen on oblique views, which allow separation of the image of the undescended parathyroid from the salivary gland.

Whatever the surgical strategy, the thymus should be resected as completely as possible using the transcervical route for two reasons. First, in MEN1 supernumerary parathyroids are found in the mediastinal thymus in about 30% of cases (28). Second, especially in men, thymic carcinoid tumours develop in 5% of cases and may be lethal. Normally 6–10 cm of mediastinal thymus can be extracted via the neck.

If exploration fails to find one of the glands, it is preferable to have available intraoperative PTH assay to confirm biological cure in perhaps 2% of cases with only 3 glands. In our experience a drop in PTH by 50% at 10 minutes is not an adequate marker of cure in patients with multigland disease including MEN1. A fall of PTH to subnormal levels is required to be confident of long term-cure.

2.3.2 Subtotal Parathyroidectomy

The surgical strategy should be to identify all four parathyroid glands and any supernumerary glands. The thymus and all of the parathyroids should be resected, leaving a well-vascularized remnant of the most normal gland (Fig. 1). The remnant should be the size of one or two normal glands (30–60 mg), marked by a metal clip and/or permanent suture. Preferably the remnant should be an inferior parathyroid because of its more superficial location in the neck and greater distance from the recurrent laryngeal nerve, which reduces difficulty and risk in case of reoperation or alcohol ablation. It is not necessary to leave a remnant in proportion to the overall volume of parathyroid tissue. Larger remnants lead to recurrent disease. Cryopreservation of parathyroid tissue should be available because of the risk of hypoparathyroidism after initial or reoperative surgery. In the absence of significant bone disease, calcium replacement is not usually required in the early postoperative period.

2.3.3 Total Parathyroidectomy and Autograft

All four glands should be identified and excised. Supernumerary glands should also be removed and a cervical thymectomy carried out. The autograft is prepared from fresh parathyroid by dicing about 60 mg of the most normal parathyroid tissue into multiple morsels about 1 × 2 mm in size. These are individually implanted into pockets in the brachioradialis muscle of the non-dominant forearm. Each pocket is marked with a metal clip or permanent suture. The autograft should not be into the sternomastoid muscle because of the difficulty in distinguishing the source of recurrent HPT by either sestamibi scan or venous sampling in this situation.

2.3.4 Comparison of Subtotal Parathyroidectomy with Total Parathyroidectomy and Autograft

The advantage of subtotal parathyroidectomy is the low overall rate of permanent hypocalcemia [12.7% Arnalsteen (28)] for the entire group of patients, including those who have had reoperation for recurrent HPT. In most cases, therefore, there is no need for autotransplantation of cryopreserved tissue. The disadvantage is the frequent recurrence of hypercalcemia in the long term [43% at 15 years (28); 50% (12)]. However, we view this outcome as achieving prolonged normocalcemia

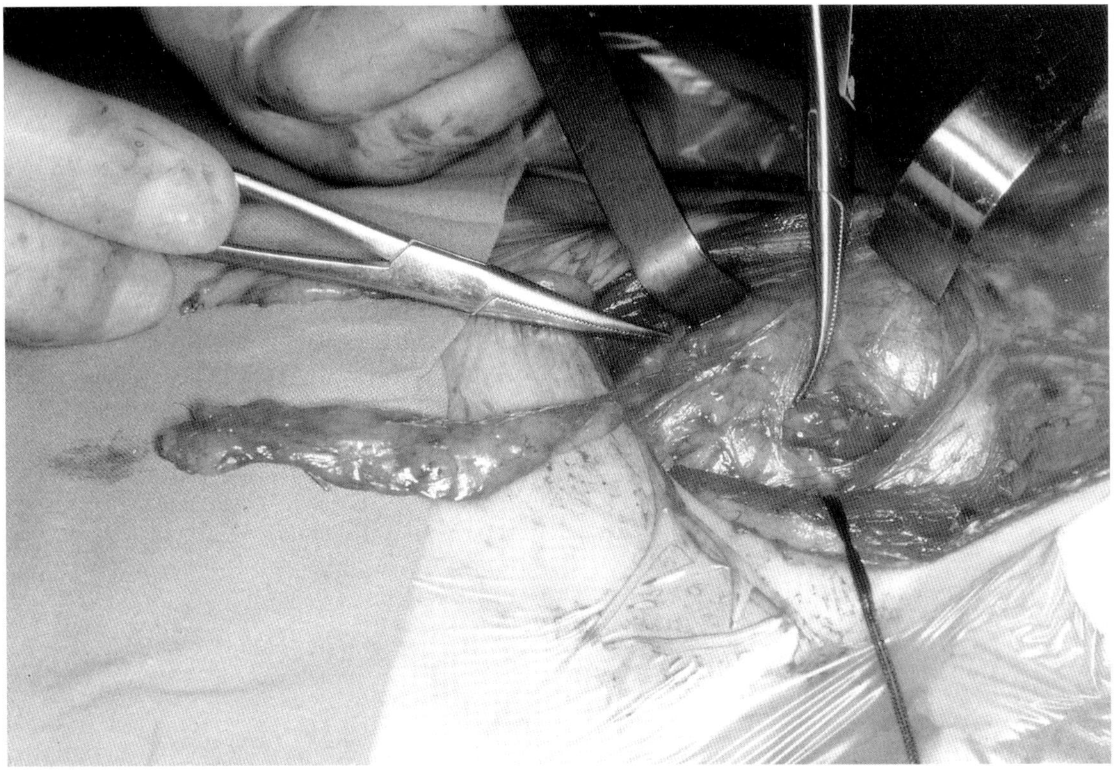

Figure 1 Dissection for subtotal parathyroidectomy in MEN1 showing the thymic horns, the inferior thyroid artery (black silk), and superior and inferior parathyroid glands (forceps). The recurrent nerve, not seen here, lies behind the superior parathyroid. Note the lateral approach (strap muscles lie medially).

(> 6 yr) in most patients. Reoperation may be required in some patients with recurrent hypercalcemia.

Disease recurrence may be due to unidentified supernumerary glands anywhere in the neck, mediastinal disease or hyperplasia of the remnant, under the stimulus of the genetic mutation. It is important to note that many descriptions of subtotal parathyroidectomy in the literature are not the equivalent of our modern definition of the operation (above). Some authors have not excised the thymus, and others have included in their category of subtotal parathyroidectomy, resections of one or two glands (29). In our reported experience (28) of 79 patients with HPT and MEN1, 9 have had reoperation for recurrent hypercalcemia, 3 of these twice. None of these patients remained hypercalcemic after adequate surgery. Of note, 4 of 13 patients who had only resection of enlarged glands performed at initial surgery elsewhere had recurrence requiring reoperation. This compares with 5 of 66 patients who had a subtotal parathyroidectomy.

The proposed advantage of total parathyroidectomy with forearm autograft is a higher rate of long-term cure of hypercalcemia (30). However, with respect to the control of hypercalcemia, total parathyroidectomy cannot be expected to improve upon the results of subtotal parathyroidectomy because most failures are due to unrecognized supernumerary disease, not hyperplasia of the remnant (20).

If recurrence occurs, possible hyperfunction of the autograft can be assessed by the Casanova test (31). A pneumatic tourniquet is applied to the upper, grafted arm, cutting the graft off from the circulation. Venous samples for PTH are taken from the opposite arm. A significant fall in PTH levels in these samples demonstrates that it is the graft that is hyperfunctioning. There is the additional advantage that the neck does not necessarily need to be re-explored in case of recurrence.

The disadvantage is reliance upon autograft function and cryopreserved tissue if the autograft fails. Saxe et al. (32) reported a 10% failure rate of fresh parathyroid autografts in a review of the subject. The initial success of cryopreserved autografts ranges from 50 to 80% in the literature (30,33–35). In a literature review of the results of subtotal versus total parathyroidectomy for secondary hyperparathyroidism, Al-Sobhi and Clark (36) found the rate of permanent hypocalcemia to be 15% of 257 patients and 24% of 211 patients, respectively.

Our experience with autografting has not been as favorable as that of Wells and others. We have had significant failure rates of both primary (<20%) and cryopreserved autografts (>50%). A further disadvantage of the technique is that resection of hyperfunctioning graft is in fact not straightforward but can be an awkward procedure. There is great variation in the size of the grafted tissue, which can be difficult to identify and selectively resect, without risking further reimplantation. Even with the aid of intraoperative isotope detection to try to ensure completeness of excision, we have generally found that a small "fillet" of muscle needs to be removed for adequate local control.

2.3.5 Reoperation for Persistent or Recurrent Disease

The first step is to review the original operation notes and pathology reports (which it should be remembered can be very misleading!), along with all previous localisation studies. The surgeon must keep in mind the possibility of multiple sites of recurrence. New localization studies are essential, regardless of the deductions made from original notes. We routinely commence with sestamibi scan and ultrasonography ± fine needle aspiration (FNA) of suspected neck lesions for PTH assay. For mediastinal lesions we use magnetic resonance imaging (MRI) and computed tomography (CT). When localization by these methods fails or weakly suggests mediastinal disease, we use selective venous sampling to regionalize the lesion(s) or corroborate other results. We consider a step-up, or highest value to background ratio of 2 in the neck and of 1.4 in the mediastinum, to be significant provided there is a gradient observed (and not an isolated, possibly spurious result).

In the case of reoperation in the neck, our aim is to remove *all* parathyroid tissue and cryopreserve it for possible delayed autograft in the event of hypocalcemia which does not recover after 6–8 weeks. We do not perform immediate autograft because of the high risk of persistent functioning tissue even after reoperation. Saxe et al. (37) reported that 69% of patients remained normocalcemic or hypercalcemic after total parathyroidectomy without autograft at reoperation for primary HPT due to hyperplasia. If no significant neck disease is found and the PTH does not fall, we explore the mediastinum by sternotomy. In principle, this entails excision of all anterior mediastinal fatty and lymphatic tissue. If preoperative imaging demonstrates a posterior lesion, the posterior mediastinum and the aortopulmonary window should be examined for rare ectopic lesions (38).

If the patient has had a total parathyroidectomy and forearm autograft, we perform a Casanova test along with sestamibi scan and ultrasound of the neck and forearm as the initial investigations. This helps to determine whether there is hyperfunctioning tissue in the forearm and/or neck. If there is hyperfunctioning tissue in the forearm, this should be totally excised and cryopreserved. In our experience of this situation, there is usually an impressive initial response, but this is often followed by evidence of persistent disease either in the forearm or in the neck (unmasked by the removal of the forearm, grafted tissue). Subsequent, painstaking reoperation on the forearm and or the neck is often required.

2.4 Pancreas and Duodenum

Endocrine pancreatic and duodenal lesions affect 30–75% of individuals in clinical series (12,39). In autopsy series these tumors are found in more than 80% of patients. They are nearly always multiple, and most of the lesions in a given patient remain asymptomatic (Fig. 2). Typically, clinical syndromes are found from the age of 40, but Shepherd (6) has stressed that clinical syndromes due to neuroendocrine pancreatic and duodenal tumours may present in teenagers. Biochemical evidence of pancreatico-duodenal endocrine tumors precedes the clinical occurrence of disease by, on average, about 20 years (39). Malignant disease occurs in appproximately 40% of patients and is the leading cause of death in MEN1, often in middle age (40,41). At the time of onset of symptoms related to functioning pancreatic neuroendocrine tumor, approximately 50% of patients will have malignant disease (42). Malignant disease typically runs an indolent clinical course over many years.

Pancreatic and duodenal lesions in MEN1 are true tumors. The specter of islet cell hyperplasia as a virtually untreatable cause of endocrine pancreatic syndromes in MEN1 has disappeared. Hyperplasia is itself a response to the hypersecreting tumor and is not responsible for clinical syndromes (43,44). Thompson et al. (45) have shown that there is, early in the course of the disease and spread throughout the gland, a range of lesions from nesidioblastosis and hyperplasia through micro- and macroadenomas to carcinoma. In their experience there

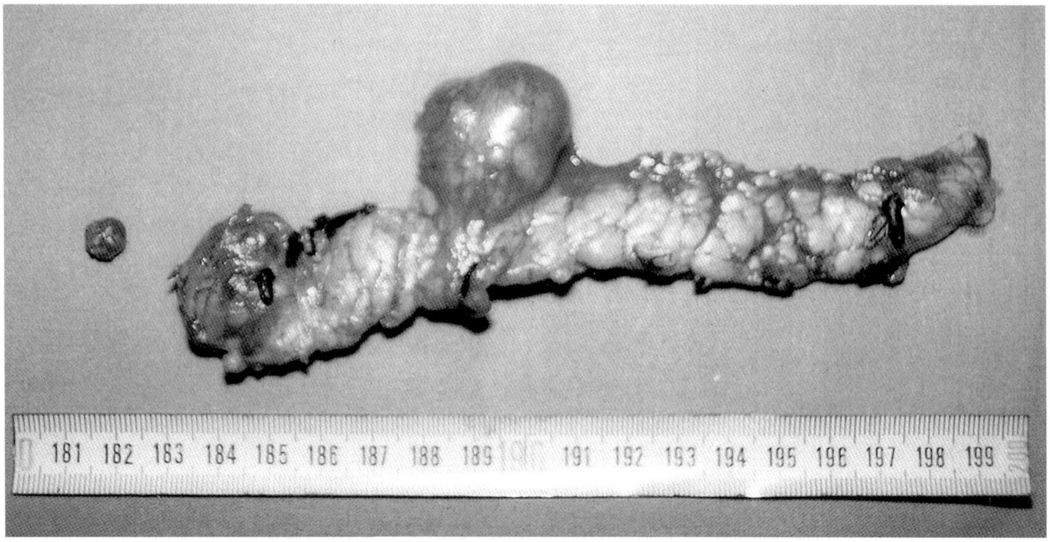

Figure 2 Spleen preserving subtotal pancreatectomy and enucleation of tumor of the head of pancreas. The large lesion was a functioning insulinoma. Multiple microadenomas were seen on histopathology.

are always discrete tumors which stain for the symptomatic hormone, and, in contrast, the hyperplastic tissue does not stain for this hormone.

In MEN1, much more than in sporadic disease, a single tumor may secrete a multitude of hormones. Clinical evidence of this is usually a sign of malignancy.

Approximately one third of endocrine pancreatic tumours are cystic or predominantly cystic. Therefore, diagnosis of cystadenoma of the pancreas in MEN1 on the basis of imaging studies should be regarded with scepticism.

The clinical syndromes, diagnosis, and differential diagnosis of apparently sporadic gastrinomas and insulinomas and other islet cell tumors are covered in detail elsewhere in this book. In cases where MEN1 can be confirmed, the management of these patients is quite different from the management of sporadic disease. When a genetic diagnosis of MEN1 precedes clinical disease, management is aimed at screening.

2.4.1 Gastrinomas

Of the functioning lesions, gastrinoma is the most common, occurring in up to 60% of patients with MEN1 (15). Some 25–50% of gastrinomas occur in the setting of MEN1. The majority are malignant, and approximately half have metastasized at the time of clinical presentation (46). The vast majority are situated in the gastrinoma triangle described by Stabile et al. (47). In MEN1 90% of gastrinomas are in the duodenum. Early reports of sporadic and MEN1 gastrinomas significantly underestimate the frequency of duodenal lesions because they were not systematically sought by duodenotomy. In MEN1, there are in fact multiple duodenal, submucosal tumors, usually less than 5 mm in size, predominantly in the first and second part of the duodenum but ranging from the gastric antrum through to the first part of the jejunum. They are frequently impossible to feel, except with a finger on the mucosal surface of the duodenum. These duodenal microadenomas have a high propensity to malignancy (>50%), which is characterized by early spread to the paraduodenal, peripancreatic, and gastrohepatic lymph nodes (48). Local invasion of the duodenum occurs in less than 50% of cases and is typically limited, with 16% extending into the muscularis mucosae and 27% into the muscularis propria (49). Metastasis to lymph nodes confers a poorer prognosis but is still consistent with long-term survival. Distant metastasis to the liver occurs late in the course of disease in about 10% of cases and is a marker of poorer prognosis than lymph node metastasis.

True pancreatic gastrinomas are uncommon and are, in a sense, ectopic since the normal adult pancreas does not produce gastrin (gastrin may be found in foetal islet cells). They have a tendency to grow larger than the duodenal lesions and, at sizes greater than 1 cm, they are increasingly likely to metastasise to the liver (50).

The features of gastrinoma conferring a poorer prognosis are pancreatic (rather than duodenal) tumor, metastases, ectopic Cushing's syndrome, and high gastrin level.

2.4.2 Insulinomas

Insulinoma is the second most common functioning tumor of the pancreas in the setting of MEN1, occuring in 10–20% of patients (51). The hypoglycemic effects of proinsulin and insulin in these patients can be life threatening. Diazoxide and careful dietary manipulation are only partially successful in controlling symptoms. The syndrome is often due to one functioning lesion, as determined by intense insulin immunostaining, but many other nonfunctioning or minimally secreting lesions may be present (45). Insulinomas occur throughout the pancreas with equal distribution. Lesions typically begin to be symptomatic at small size, often less than 1 cm. About one third are associated with another functioning islet cell tumor, usually gastrinoma. They are malignant in less than 20% of cases in MEN1 (51). Metastatic spread is to both the regional lymph nodes and more commonly, the liver.

Four to 8% of insulinomas are found in association with MEN1. When insulinoma arises in a young patient, and especially if multiple neuroendocrine tumors are found, the diagnosis of MEN1 should be considered. Shepherd has shown that insulinoma may precede hyperparathyroidism in MEN1 (6).

2.4.3 Glucagonoma and Vasoactive Intestinal Peptideoma

Glucagonoma and vasoactive intestinal peptideoma (VIPoma) are rare, perhaps 10% occurring in the setting of MEN1. The tumors are frequently larger than 2 cm. About 60% are malignant, and they occur most often in the body and tail of the pancreas.

2.4.4 Nonfunctioning Tumors

Nonfunctioning tumors are the most common of all islet cell tumors in MEN1, and typically the pancreas harbors numerous micro- and macroadenomas. Larger tumors (>3 cm) are likely to be malignant and may sometimes be aggressive. In index cases, these tumors are likely to be large at presentation because it is not until they cause symptoms from mass effect that they are discovered. However, in a screened population, either elevation of chromogranin A and hPP or a small mass lesion should be identified early in the course of the tumor.

2.4.5 Surgery for MEN1 Pancreatico-Duodenal Tumors

It is vital to keep in mind that pancreatic and duodenal disease in MEN1 is multifocal by definition and that nothing short of total pancreaticoduodenectomy could be hoped to be curative. The potential morbidity and mortality of this strategy prohibit it as a prophylactic measure. Neither persistence nor recurrence of disease necessarily implies a poor prognosis, as frequently even malignant disease has a protracted course (52). On the other hand, pancreatic endocrine cancer is the leading cause of death in MEN1 today. Doherty et al. (41) reported that 46% of patients in 34 kindreds died as a result of malignant endocrine tumors at a mean age of 47 years and that islet cell tumors were the main cause of death. Resection of tumors prior to the occurrence of distant metastasis could possibly alter long-term survival. There is general consensus with respect to the surgical management of insulinomas, VIPomas, and glucagonomas in MEN1. Management of gastrinomas is controversial.

Surgery for Insulinomas, Glucagonomas, and VIPomas. Insulinomas, glucagonomas, and VIPomas, in particular, share common features. They are located in the pancreas and produce a florid and life-threatening clinical syndrome. Medical treatment becomes increasingly unsatisfactory if the tumor is allowed to grow unchecked. Glucagonomas and VIPomas are highly likely to be malignant, while insulinoma may be malignant in up to 20% of cases.

They should therefore always be resected unless there is significant untreatable liver metastasis. It may be possible to cure the syndrome by enucleation of small tumors, but this is not considered wise practice. In the setting of multiple pancreatic lesions, it is difficult to determine accurately the source of the excess hormone, and the wrong lesion may be excised. Enucleation is unacceptable treatment for potentially malignant lesions and, futhermore, the remaining pancreatic pathology is ignored by such management.

There is near consensus (51,53,54) that for most of these lesions, the best option is a spleen-preserving subtotal pancreatectomy, transecting the pancreas to the right of the portal vein. Tumors in the head of the pancreas should be enucleated using intraoperative ultrasound to aid identification of lesions and the pancreatic ductal system. Some authors also recommend a lymph node dissection (55) routinely or if any pancreatic lesion greater than 3 cm is identified. The apparent advantage of this approach is that the bulk of the tumor-producing pancreas and tumors of the head are removed and the syndrome is cured. Complication rates are acceptable, with rare deaths and a morbidity of 20–30%, mostly due to pancreatic fistula. Diabetes should occur in less than 10%. Recurrent lesions can be managed on their merits, when the need arises.

For large and malignant lesions of the head of the pancreas, various forms of resection of the head of the pancreas are indicated whenever possible. In the absence of metastatic disease, life expectancy is good (56). Resection and reconstruction of involved vascular structures (e.g., superior mesenteric vein) is sometimes indicated (57).

In the case of insulinoma, intraoperative glucose monitoring is essential to avoid hypoglycemia. Intraoperative portal venous insulin testing can be used as a predictor of successful resection (58). A further modification is the use of intraoperative secretin stimulation to confirm the completeness of resection. Contrary to the results observed in gastrinomas, secretin does not stimulate the insulin-secreting tumor but normal islet cells, free from the negative feedback of the tumor. Thus, after resection, if the injection of secretin produces a rise in insulin secretion, the absence of residual tumor is confirmed (59,60).

Surgery for Gastrinomas. The indications for surgery and extent of surgery for gastrinoma are a most contentious subject of debate at present. Whatever the operative strategy, the syndrome must be well controlled with proton pump inhibitors before surgery. There are two points of general agreement.

1. Operate on the parathyroid glands first. Reduction in serum calcium has the effect of reducing the stimulatory effect of calcium on the gastrinoma.
2. Do not operate if metastatic disease in the liver is extensive and not amenable to excision or ablative therapy.

All other points are debatable. There are four main management strategies:

1. Observe these patients, treat them with proton pump inhibitors and do not operate unless there is an associated insulinoma (or VIPoma or glucagonoma) that is not responsive to medical treatment (61).
2. Operate only when imaging demonstrates a lesion greater than 3 cm (52,62).
3. Operate in all cases with a clinical syndrome regardless of preoperative imaging studies, provided there is no evidence of distant metastasis. Operate also for asymptomatic tumors identified by imaging (63–65).
4. Operate in young patients as soon as screening tests identify elevated tumoral hormones (chromogranin A, human pancreatic polypeptide, gastrin, etc.) or a mass lesion seen on echoendoscopy. It is hoped by this strategy to prevent the occurrence of metastasis from malignant tumors that may arise (42).

The first approach, somewhat nihilistic, is founded on the fact that the genetic trait is ubiquitous, that the pathology is diffuse, and the prospect of long-lasting cure by surgery is remote, while surgery may produce significant complications. This is the approach of many physicians and perhaps half of the surgeons with expertise in this field (53).

The second protocol is also founded on the belief that the prospect for long-term cure of Zollinger-Ellison (ZES) by surgery is remote because of multiple lesions and recurrent if not persistent disease. Thus, surgery is proposed for mass lesions to excise potential cancers, not necessarily to cure the hormone secretion. This is the view of Norton et al., who have reported that virtually no patients with MEN1 are cured of ZES by surgery (52). But this approach has its disadvantages, and they are major ones. By the time operation is eventually undertaken, metastases are frequently present. Imaging is often positive due to pancreatic primary or metastatic disease but rarely due to the duodenal tumors which are the usual cause of the syndrome. It seems rather odd to wait for a tumor to become in all probability incurable before operating on it. On the other hand, Norton et al. (52) report that the survival after surgery and resection of patients with advanced disease is the same as in patients with limited disease. The mean follow-up, however, was only 7 years.

The third strategy, proposed by Thompson, is that adopted by many surgeons, and may produce long-term remissions, giving the appearance of cure. In his series of 43 patients with neuroendocrine pancreaticoduodenal tumors, 37 of whom had gastrinomas, only one patient (with ZES) developed metastasis to the liver after operation (66). The 5-, 10-, and 15-year survival in his series is 97, 94, and 94%, respectively. There are a number of arguments in favor of this approach:

1. Most neuroendocrine pancreatic tumors can be identified before they reach 3 cm in size. Most tumors can therefore be resected before they metastasize.
2. Most, if not all patients with ZES, have duodenal microadenomas that are the cause of hypergas-

trinemia. Half of the patients with duodenal microadenomas will have lymph node metastases. Thorough exploration of the duodenum and resection of potentially involved lymph nodes will result in clinical cure of hypergastrinaemia in a majority of patients, and only 10% or fewer of these patients will develop liver metastases.

3. Nearly all tumors of the head and uncinate process of the pancreas can be identified by intraoperative ultrasound (IOUS) and are amenable to enucleation. The body and tail of the pancreas can be resected readily. Thus, all tumors greater than several millimeters in size can be simultaneously treated.

The last approach, recommended by the Uppsala group (42), is the most radical and is not yet supported by adequate evidence for us to consider prophylactic pancreatectomy in MEN1. Can early resection prevent the occurrence of cancer? And is the apparent benefit seen in the early studies more than just a lead-time bias? We do not know. If reresection is performed for recurrent ZES or tumors found by imaging, perhaps one can keep a step ahead of the development of cancer. There is no doubt that part of the apparent benefit arises from lead-time bias from operating on screen detected patients at an average age of 20 years younger than those operated on for clinically significant or mass lesions. The concern many others have is that this type of surgery is accompanied but a significant morbidity and occasional mortality. Exposure of patients to these risks 20 years before otherwise necessary is a bold step. Only long-term comparative studies will answer the questions.

The "Thompson" Operation for ZES. Our approach is based on that of Thompson (Figs. 3,4) (63). The steps of the operation are:

1. Subtotal pancreatectomy, with the line of section to the right of the portal vein, in order to remove all contained tumors, whether gastrin secreting or not, and some of which are or may become malignant.
2. Enucleation of all tumors of the head of the pancreas, whether palpable, detected by intraoperative ultrasound, or by intraoperative isotope detection.

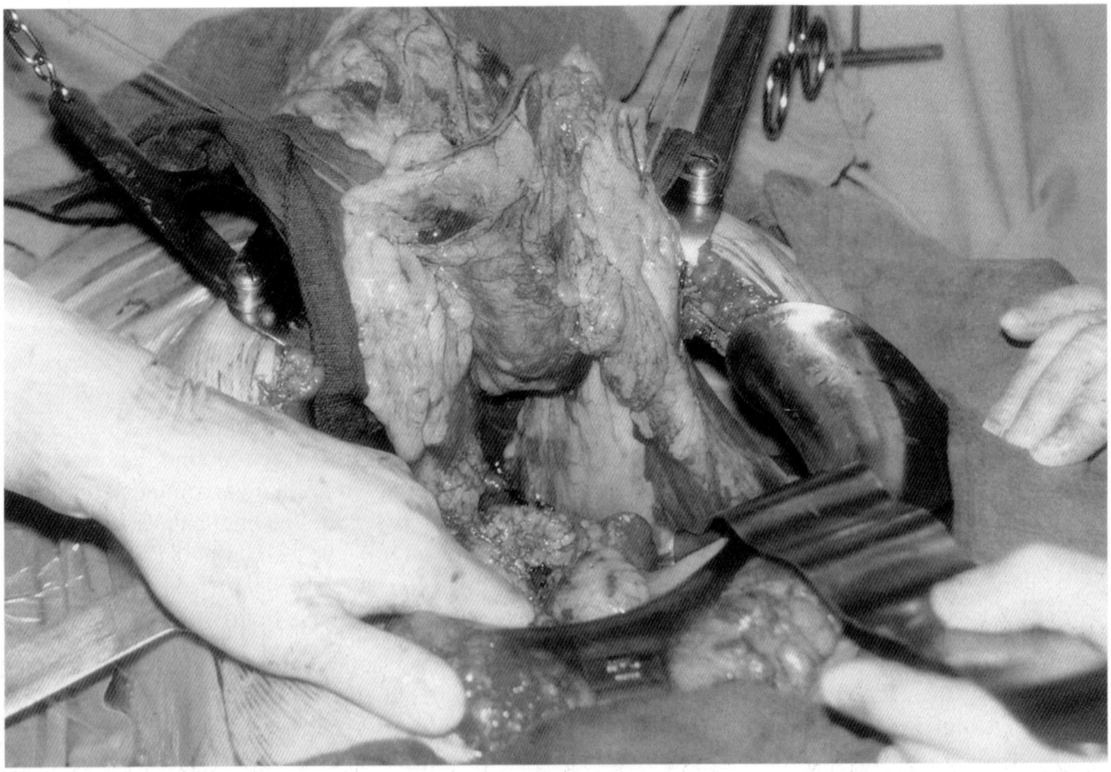

Figure 3 Surgical exposure for the Thompson operation. Bilateral subcostal incision. Stomach and omentum elevated. A large tumor of the body of the pancreas is visible.

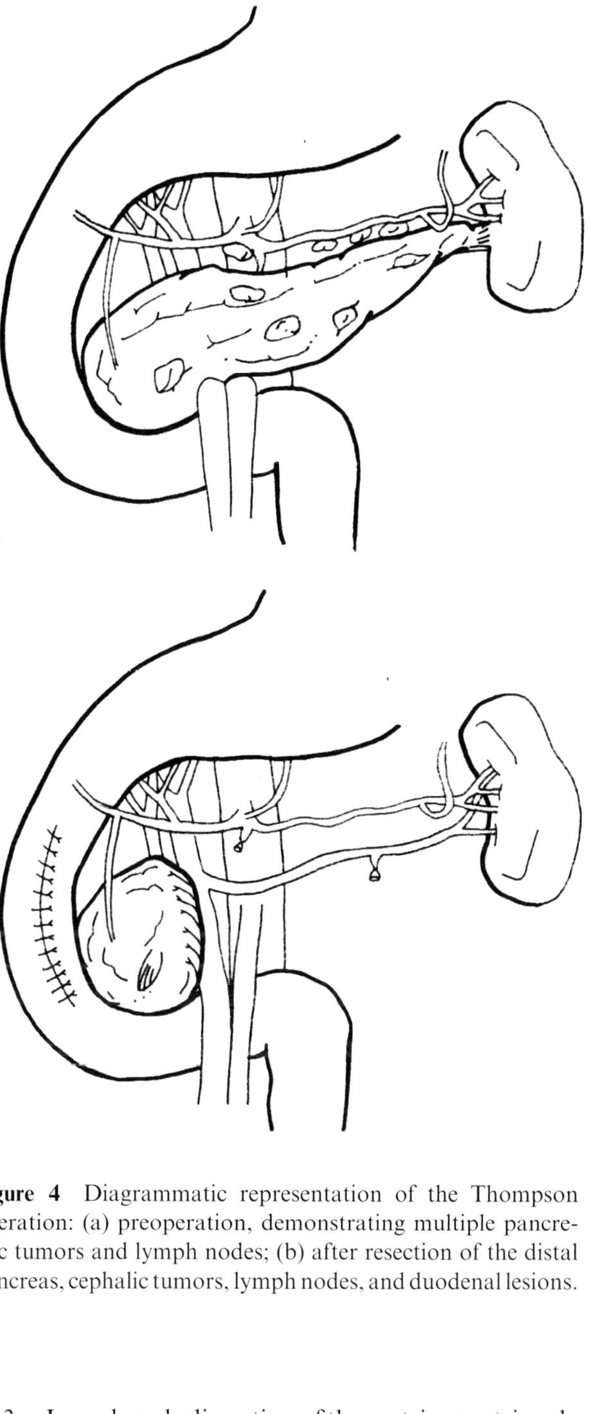

Figure 4 Diagrammatic representation of the Thompson operation: (a) preoperation, demonstrating multiple pancreatic tumors and lymph nodes; (b) after resection of the distal pancreas, cephalic tumors, lymph nodes, and duodenal lesions.

3. Lymph node dissection of the gastrinoma triangle and frozen section examination. If there are involved nodes, there is certainly at least one malignant duodenal gastrinoma, and the hope for cure is reduced. If not, there is still very likely one or more duodenal gastrinomas, and the chance of cure is greater.
4. Routine duodenotomy and excision of all microgastrinomas which are found by endoscopic transillumination and palpation. Transillumination of the duodenum allows recognition of about 60% of lesions but is no substitute for routine duodenotomy whatever the pancreatic and lymph node findings. Submucosal resection is usually adequate but full thickness local excision may be required. Extended resection is not usually indicated. If duodenotomy is negative, the first jejunal loop should be opened.
5. Cholecystectomy because of possible future, unresectable, malignant disease. There is a risk of somatostatin-induced gallstone disease due to stasis, and the possible need for chemoembolization of liver metastases, which may cause gallbladder necrosis.
6. Secretin testing (67) to verify the completeness of resection. We measure basal and stimulated gastrin levels in peripheral venous blood (it is not necessary to take portal venous samples because gastrin is metabolized in the kidney, not the liver). We use 2 U/kg of secretin, injected into a peripheral vein, and make serial measurements. Four minutes after injection, a rise in gastrin to less than 80 pg/mL or a rise of $<20\%$ from the level prior to excision confirms cure (68).
7. Adrenal tumors should be excised—certainly those greater than 4 cm.

This therapeutic strategy results in normal basal gastrin levels in two thirds of patients and normal stimulated levels in 33% of cases with a follow-up of up to 10 years (69). These results are much the same as those achieved by the National Institutes of Health (NIH) group for sporadic ZES and for which they strongly advocate surgery because of a survival benefit (46). There are few indications for proximal pancreaticoduodenectomy, but they include periampullary tumors, large, invasive tumors, massive nodal involvement and possibly multiple duodenal tumors, and a positive intraoperative secretin test (70).

In our practice we perform parathyroidectomy and pancreatic surgery in the same operative session. We begin with parathyroidectomy, and if the operation proves to be particularly laborious or intraoperative PTH assessment is suggestive of mediastinal or other unresected disease, the pancreatic surgery can be deferred to another day.

2.4.6 Preoperative Localization

Given the multiplicity and frequent small size of lesions and that our surgical strategy for all pancreatico-duodenal disease in MEN1 involves full exploration of the pancreas (and duodenum in ZES) with the aid of ultrasound, there is little useful information that can be gained preoperatively. Identification of liver metastases is the single most important reason for imaging as it may preclude surgery. CT, endoscopic ultrasound (EUS), and octreotide scan may be used to provide advanced warning of atypical findings, such as a large tumor of the head of the pancreas, which may lead to a different operative strategy.

2.4.7 Management of Metastatic Pancreatico-Duodenal Disease in MEN1

Surgery for metastases may be considered if they are favorably located for resection. Five-year survival after hepatic resection of metastases from sporadic pancreatic neuroendocrine tumors may be extended from 28% to 79% (71). It is rare to find suitable cases in MEN1.

Medical therapy may be required for symptomatic control of hypersecretion. The most common medical therapies are diazoxide for insulinoma, proton pump inhibitors for gastrinoma, and somatostatin for VIPoma. Long-acting somatostin analogues have become a major component of palliation of neuroendocrine tumors. Other therapeutic options include chemotherapy, interferon-α, chemoembolization and radioisotope-labeled somatostatin analogues. These are described elsewhere in this book.

Hepatic transplantation has been performed for metastatic endocrine pancreatic tumors, sometimes in association with islet cell transplants. Except for the series of Pichlmayr et al. (72), who achieved a survival of 82% at 5 years, the results have been disappointing. There were no cases with MEN1 in the series, and the indication for transplantation and immunosuppression in a condition with a genetic predisposition to cancer must be questioned.

Ablative therapy has been available in many forms for a long time. Recently radiofrequency ablation of hepatic lesions has shown promising results. It is suitable for multiple lesions, but not more than about 10. It is more focused and more successful in appropriate patients and safer than chemoembolization.

2.5 Pituitary Lesions

Anterior pituitary lesions are one of the three main features of the MEN1 syndrome. The prevalence in MEN1 is about 30% in screened patients and 70% at autopsy. About two thirds are microadenomas. Prolactinoma is by far the most common lesion followed by growth hormone–secreting tumor. Nearly all anterior pituitary tumor types have been reported in MEN1. Treatment is similar to that of sporadic tumors. Many of the prolactinomas respond well to medical therapy.

2.6 Foregut-Derived Carcinoids

Thymic carcinoid occurs in less than 5% of MEN1 patients, usually in males and often with familial clustering (73). It may be aggressively malignant, apparently moreso in MEN1 than sporadic tumors.

Bronchial carcinoid occurs in about 5% of patients, and is seen mostly in females. CT or MRI is useful in the diagnosis or screening for these lesions.

Type II gastric enterochromaffin-like cell (ECL) carcinoids are mainly found in patients with ZES and MEN1 during endoscopy. They are common (30–50%), multiple (90%), small (usually <1.5 cm), and are associated with a proliferation of extratumoral ECL cells from which the tumor is thought to originate (74,75). In 90% invasion is limited to the submucosa, but metastases to lymph nodes occur in 30% and to the liver in 10%. It is proposed that they arise as a result of gastrin and acid stimulation of increased histamine production in MEN1 ZES. These lesions rarely secrete hormones. They are apparently in part genetically determined by mutation of *MEN1*, because they are rarely seen in sporadic ZES (75). Gauger and Thompson reported two cases, which spontaneously regressed after resection of the gastrinoma (66). They have occasionally been reported to be aggressive malignancies. It is not clear whether proton-pump inhibitors have any direct effect on the natural history of these tumors.

2.7 Adrenal Cortical Lesions

These occur in about 40% of patients and are often bilateral, hyperplastic, and nonsecreting. Adenomas with an indolent clinical course (10–20%) and aggressive carcinomas (5%) may also occur (76,77). Adrenal lesions are usually seen only in patients who also have pancreatic lesions. Previously most groups have had a conservative approach to these adrenal lesions. As a result of some unexpected cases of rapid growth and death from malignant adrenal disease, a more active policy of resection during pancreatic surgery, otherwise regular screening, and resection at 4 cm is now warranted.

2.8 Other Lesions

Perhaps one third of patients have cutaneous or visceral (angio)lipomas. These are encapsulated and typically do not recur after surgery. Large visceral lipomas are uncommon.

Cutaneous angiofibromas and collagenomas appear to be very common (78). They occur in at least 80% of patients and are often found on the face. Ependymoma, meningioma, fibrosarcoma, pheochromocytoma, and other lesions have been reported more commonly in MEN1 than in control populations but remain uncommon in MEN1.

2.9 Screening for MEN1

The aims and elements of different screening protocols reflect the resources and management philosophies of the groups involved. For example, the Uppsala group, which has a policy of early surgical intervention for pancreatic disease, has an aggressive and extensive screening protocol to identify this disease (42). The most effective initial step is to determine gene carriers by genetic testing. The hormone assays and imaging studies can be rationalized according to the clinical impact of the disease being screened and the cost-effectiveness of the tests (Table 2). Parathyroid disease is easily screened with annual ionized calcium or corrected calcium and PTH. Screening should certainly begin by 10 years of age and should be life-long as gene carriers may manifest the disorders at any age.

Screening for pituitary disease is also relatively straightforward; a typical program might be annual prolactin and insulin-like growth factor 1, with annual MRI studies for 2 or 3 years. Screening should begin at around 5 years of age, as the earliest reported morbid and potentially treatable lesion was an aggressive pituitary macroadenoma at the age of 5 years (79).

Table 2 Screening Protocol for MEN1

Biochemical screening: annual, essential
Serum calcium (prefer ionized) and PTH
Glucose with simultaneous insulin, proinsulin, and glucagon
Gastrin (+secretin stimulation test)
Prolactin and IGF-1
Biochemical screening: comprehensive
Pancreatic polypeptide
Chromogranin A
VIP
Urinary 5-HIAA (Hydroxyindole acetic acid)
$\alpha+\beta$ HCG (Human chorionic gonadotropin)
Calcitonin
Meal test[a]
Imaging: 2–3 yearly, essential
High-quality contrast enhanced spiral CT of chest and abdomen
MRI of pituitary
Endoscopic ultrasound of the pancreas
Imaging: optional
Upper gastrointestinal endoscopy
Octreotide scan

[a] See text for explanation.

With respect to pancreatico-duodenal disease, insulinoma, gastrinoma, and any pancreatic lesions greater than 1 cm have the most impact on patients, and thus screening should at least aim to detect subclinical insulinoma and gastrinoma and tumors of this size. A minimal program would thus include annual fasting glucose with simultaneous insulin and proinsulin, gastrin with secretin stimulation test, and high-quality CT scan every 2–3 years.

Glucose, proinsulin, and insulin testing during a 72-hour supervised fast may be indicated to confirm the diagnosis of insulinoma. Endoscopic ultrasound is the most sensitive imaging study for pancreatic tumors, being able to detect lesions of around 3 mm in size in favorable patients and should be considered along with CT. Some groups use 111 IN-DTPA octreotide scan. It is perhaps most useful in identifying metastases, but will detect also around 80% of tumors greater than 1 cm in size (80). Most duodenal microadenomas will not be detected by CT or octreotide scan, and EUS has only been able to detect perhaps one half to two thirds of lesions. However, when combined, octreotide scan and EUS may have a sensitivity as high as 94% (81). Screening for pancreatic disease should begin in teenagers.

More rigorous biochemical screening may include glucagon, chromogranin A, hPP, hCG, and VIP. The standardized carbohydrate-rich meal test may be used to elicit a stimulated rise in hPP and gastrin in the presence of a pancreatic tumor, regardless of which peptide hormone is dominantly secreted (82).

2.10 Burin Syndrome and Other Variants of MEN1

This variant of MEN1 produces pituitary tumors, HPT, and carcinoid tumors but not pancreatic tumors. Familial acromegaly can coexist with prolactinoma in this syndrome.

3 MULTIPLE ENDOCRINE NEOPLASIA TYPE 2

MEN2 is an autosomal dominant syndrome characterized by the development of medullary thyroid carcinoma (MTC) but also notable for pheochromocytoma and to a lesser extent hyperparathyroidism. There are three major and distinct variants: MEN2A, MEN2B,

Table 3 Clinical Characteristics of MEN2 Syndromes

Syndrome	Characteristics
MEN2A	MTC: >90% by age 60 Pheochromocytoma: 50% (25% bilateral) Hyperparathyroidism: 20% (codon 634)
MEN2B	MTC: Age <5 years Phaeochromocytoma Intestinal and submucosal ganglioneuromas Characteristic facies and marfanoid habitus
FMTC	MTC: least aggressive MEN2 variant
MEN2A and cutaneous lichen amyloidosis	MEN2A Pruritic lesions of the upper back
MEN2A or FMTC and Hirschsprung's disease	MEN2A or FMTC Hirschsprung's disease

and familial medullary thyroid cancer (FMTC) (Table 3). MEN2A represents over 75% of MEN2. There are perhaps fewer than 1000 kindreds identified worldwide (83). Rare variants have been described. These include MEN2A with cutaneous lichen amyloidosis and MEN2A or FMTC with Hirschsprung's disease.

MEN2 syndromes result in disease related death in perhaps 50% of index cases because of delayed treatment of MTC until after clinical recognition and sudden death from pheochromocytoma. Because of the great advances in genetics it is now possible to perform prophylactic thyroidectomy to prevent MTC and to screen for and excise pheochromocytoma before morbidity arises. It is not yet certain that prophylactic thyroidectomy can remove the risk of MTC for life because follow-up has not yet been lifelong in an adequate number of cases. But evidence is already present that the risk of death and morbidity is greatly reduced, even when "prophylactic" surgery is undertaken after malignancy has occurred (84).

3.1 Genetics

The first identification in MEN2 of mutations of the *RET* proto-oncogene was made by Mulligan et al. (85) and Donis–Keller et al. (86) in 1993. The following year Mulligan et al. (87) reported evidence of a correlation between specific mutations and phenotypes (Table 4). The *RET* gene is located near the centromere of chromosome 10 and encodes ret, a membrane-bound tyrosine kinase enzyme. MEN2 results from germline mutations, which change one amino acid. Mutations may occur in both the extracellular and intracellular domain sites of the gene. The result is activation of ret by either homodimerization of the extracellular component (which normally occurs as a result of ligand binding) or by activating the enzyme's intracellular catalytic site.

Genetic testing in MEN2 is far simpler than for MEN1 and is extremely reliable. The false-positive and false-negative rates are very low. A positive genetic test on two separate occasions, to minimize the risk of sample mix-up (especially between family members with the same name) and contamination of DNA, has a positive predictive value close to 100%.

A mutation can be identified in the *RET* gene in 98% of index cases. A limited number of mutations has been identified, involving exons 10,11,13,14,15, and 16. These are the only exons requiring routine testing. The recent development of a specific microarray kit, which was

Table 4 Genotype-Phenotype Correlation in MEN2

	Mutation					
Syndrome	Exon 10	Exon 11	Exon 13	Exon 14	Exon 15	Exon 16
MEN2A	609,611 618,620	630,634 635,637	790		891	
MEN2A and CLA		634				
MEN2A and Hirschsprung's	609,618 620					
MEN2B				804	883	918,922
FMTC	609,611 618,620	630	768,790 791	804		

CLA, cutaneous lichen amyloidosis.

successful in identifying the mutations in all Korean families with MEN2, may facilitate the genetic testing in MEN2 (88).

3.2 Multiple Endocrine Neoplasia Type 2A (Sipple's Syndrome)

MEN2A is a clinical syndrome of MTC in 90% of cases, pheochromocytoma in 50%, and multigland parathyroid disease in 20–30% (89–91). Prior to recognition of the syndrome and screening of family members, death from MTC occurred in about 20% of cases. Sudden death from pheochromocytoma was equally frequent. New index cases arising from sporadic mutations and unrecognized kindreds still result in late presentations and death from MTC and from pheochromocytoma (92,93).

3.2.1 Pheochromocytoma

Pheochromocytoma in MEN2 once carried a significant morbidity and a mortality rate of about 20%. Never should medullary carcinoma of the thyroid be tackled before exclusion of, or excision of pheochromocytoma.

Pheochromocytomas occur in 42% of patients with MEN2, with a wide family variation, between 6 and 100% (89,92,94). In 60% of patients with pheochromocytoma there is a synchronous or metachronous contralateral pheochromocytoma (Fig. 5). In 10–27% of cases they are the presenting lesion, occurring 10 years prior to MTC in 8.5% of cases (93). They are ectopic in 4% and malignant in 3% of cases. They preferentially secrete adrenaline rather than noradrenaline (92), which may explain the frequent absence of hypertension.

Apparently sporadic pheochromocytoma may have a germline genetic cause in 5–15% of cases. Pheochromocytoma has been found in kindreds with all *RET* mutations except codons 609, 768, 804, and 891. Codon 634 mutation carriers have a 60% likelihood of developing pheochromocytoma, which has been found as early as 5–10 years of age. Screening for pheochromocytoma can be stratified by risk according to mutation, just as for MTC (53).

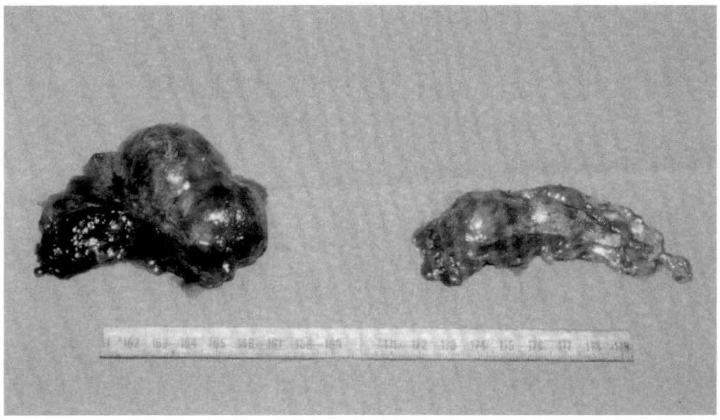

Figure 5 Surgical specimen. Bilateral adrenalectomy for phaeochromocytoma in MEN2A.

Screening for early evidence of pheochromocytoma in MEN2 should begin in teenagers. 24-hour urine collection for catecholamines and metanephrines or assay of venous blood for plasma methoxy-derivatives are the best diagnostic tests. Combined urinary and plasma tests are the most sensitive. MIBG scanning in combination with CT or MRI is useful for localization and to look for multiple lesions, metastases, and nonfunctioning tumours.

Preoperative preparation is a vital issue in surgical management of pheochromocytoma. There is little consensus as to the optimal preparation as apparently a number of regimens are effective. We prefer to prepare patients with a calcium channel blocker, and, intraoperatively, intravenous calcium channel blocker is used as required. We have found this to be a better preparation, associated with less perioperative instability and postoperative hypotension (95).

Adrenal medullary hyperplasia is nearly a constant feature of MEN2. Tumors may be multiple: unilateral, bilateral, and in approximately 50% of cases of unilateral pheochromocytoma, a lesion develops in the contralateral gland after an average interval of 7 years (96). Some groups have therefore advocated systematic bilateral adrenalectomy in MEN2 (97). The main objections to this strategy are that the patient risks addisonian crisis in up to 25% of cases (96,98). Steroid-dependent patients still occasionally die today because of addisonian crisis (98,99). Perhaps 50% of patients will have no clinical need for bilateral surgery. Screening for development of another pheochromocytoma has shown no increase in morbidity due to delayed diagnosis.

Surgical Approach. The traditional approach to pheochromocytoma in the setting of MEN2 was a large midline or bi-subcostal incision allowing bilateral adrenal examination and exploration of all sites of possible paragangliomas and nodal and liver metastasis prior to resection of the tumor. Now that laparoscopic surgery is the optimal approach and preoperative localization is undertaken, routine exploration of the entire abdomen is no longer necessary. Modern imaging with CT, MRI, and MIBG has virtually eliminated the finding of unexpected multifocal, malignant, or metastatic disease (100).

Adrenal resection for pheochromocytoma requires minimal handling to avoid hypertensive crises and, generally, early control of venous drainage. Where possible the periadrenal fat should be resected with the tumor to minimize the risk of capsular rupture and spread of the tumor. There is no evidence that patients are more unstable during laparoscopy than at open surgery and perhaps the contrary is true (101). Rare, malignant lesions may require open, en bloc resection of adjacent organs and lymph nodes.

Most authors would now perform bilateral adrenalectomy, when indicated, laparoscopically. An alternative surgical option is total removal of one adrenal and subtotal resection of the gland on the other side to preserve function. In the series of Lee et al. (99), metachronous tumors in the remnant occurred in 21% of patients, with a follow-up of 11 years, but this may result in no survival disadvantage to the patient, and the risk of addisonian crisis is reduced. Subtotal adrenalectomy can also be performed laparoscopically.

3.2.2 Medullary Thyroid Cancer

Medullary cancer of the thyroid is genetically linked in 29% of cases. Of these, 60% arise in MEN2A, 5% in MEN2B, and 35% occur without any other association and therefore are putatively familial medullary thyroid cancer (FMTC). MTC is a nearly constant finding in MEN2A (89,94).

What is the value of genetic evaluation in cases of apparently sporadic MTC? In practice, if the patient is >40 years of age and there is a unifocal tumor, the likelihood of apparently sporadic MTC being due to MEN2 is around 2% and MEN2 accounts for only 7% of all apparently sporadic MTC (102). Nevertheless, the importance of a positive genetic test for MEN2 means that most patients with MTC should be tested.

By the age of 60 years about 90% of individuals with MEN2A will have clinical MTC. Often, however, it presents much earlier and may be found in children. MTC is the usual first stigma of MEN2A and the most common syndrome-related cause of death today.

A palpable tumor is unusual before 10 years of age, but when the tumour is greater than 2 cm in size it is usually incurable because of unresectable metastases to mediastinal nodes or distant organs. Nevertheless, surgery is the mainstay of treatment for clinically evident disease because MTC does not take up radioactive iodine and is not responsive to chemotherapy, radiotherapy, or hormonal treatment.

Histopathology and Biochemistry. MTC in MEN2 variants is characteristically multifocal and arises in a background of clear-cell hyperplasia (CCH). Conversely, in sporadic MTC, 20% of tumors are bilateral but without CCH. The progression from CCH to MTC is very variable and may be precocious as in MEN2B or never clinically evident. The aggressiveness of the disease depends upon the genetic mutation. The tumor secretes calcitonin but also a number of other peptide hormones. The basal or pentagastrin-stimulated calcitonin level is nearly always elevated in the presence of MTC. According to Wells et al., tumors greater than 5 mm in size can always be biochemically detected (103). Elevated calcitonin is a marker of persistent disease after surgery for MTC.

Clinical MTC, even tumors less than 1 cm in size, is associated with high rates (>70%) of nodal invasion: to the central compartment (level VI), upper mediastinal (level VII), and ipslateral and contralateral neck lymph nodes (levels II–V). Distant metastasis is primarily to the liver, central mediastinal lymph nodes, and lungs in order of frequency. Node involvement is more extensive in MEN2 than in sporadic disease (104).

Surgery for Clinical MTC in MEN2. Total thyroidectomy plus central lymph node dissection and thymectomy en bloc is required in all cases. Management of the parathyroid glands is discussed below. The indications for ipsilateral, contralateral, and mediastinal lymph node dissections have been debated in the absence of clinically involved nodes, but we, and other surgeons (105), would routinely perform such extended lymph node clearance for clinical MTC.

Some surgeons determine the extent of nodal clearance by the results of basal and stimulated calcitonin tests, the size of the primary tumor, and the presence of central lymphadenopathy (104).

When serum calcitonin is very high (>5000 pg/mL) the likelihood of distant metastatic disease is great. In these cases, staging of the disease by CT scan of the chest and abdomen is indicated. If CT staging is negative, laparoscopy to identify liver metastasis is indicated prior to thyroidectomy. The finding of metastatic disease changes the goal of surgery from possible cure to local control of disease. It is important to remember that distant metastasis is not incompatible with long-term survival, as many cases of MTC are relatively indolent despite their tendency to metastasize early. Death from tumor growth in the neck by invasion of the trachea, vocal cord palsies, and carotid blowout can often be prevented by total thyroidectomy and central node clearance.

Detailed description of total thyroidectomy with extensive lymph node dissection for MTC can be found elsewhere in this book.

Prophylactic Thyroid Surgery for Gene Carriers. Prior to the genetic revolution, the indication for prophylactic surgery was limited by the lack of sensitivity and specificity of the pentagastrin stimulation test. In the experience of the Groupe d'Etude des Tumeurs a Calcitonine (GETC) (106), this test has not been sufficiently reliable because of false positives and inability to differentiate CCH from MTC. Causes of false-positive results include C-cell hyperplasia in thyroiditis, normal physiological elevation in men over 50, smoking, and renal insufficiency. Kindred members without MEN2 have undergone surgery on the basis of falsely elevated calcitonin testing (106). Conversely, by the time stimulated calcitonin testing becomes positive, some patients will have nodal metastasis (107).

Confirmation of the MEN2 mutation should be sought and is a strong indication for prophylactic thyroid surgery (108). Carriers have a very high risk of developing a potentially lethal tumor. Prophylactic surgery in teenagers, on the basis of calcitonin testing, has shown evidence of cure, in most cases, at long-term follow-up (90,109).

Wells and colleagues (84) in 1994 (Table 5) were the first to report prophylactic thyroidectomy on the basis of positive genetic testing in "at-risk" children. The absence of nodal involvement in the 13 patients in this series has given hope for cure in these patients. However, in 10 of the patients, macroscopic or microscopic MTC was found, and thus the operation was effectively therapeutic, not prophylactic. These patients had an average age of 13 years. In 3 of 6 of these patients, who also had negative pentagastrin tests, microscopic MTC was already present. In a separate report at 3-years follow-up of 18 patients having precocious prophylactic thyroidectomy (average age 10 years) for a genetic diagnosis of MEN2A, no patient had biochemical evidence of disease (110).

The extent of nodal dissection in children undergoing prophylactic surgery is the subject of debate. Can nodal surgery be omitted in some cases? Only a small proportion of children (3 of 55) had nodal involvement in the Saint-Louis group (84), and the children were older than the currently recommended age for prophylactic surgery. The risk of nodal disease as determined by genotype and the age of the child at the time of surgery may be used to decide the need for node dissection in individual cases (111).

Some surgeons routinely clear the central neck compartment lymph nodes because they wish to avoid the possibility of reoperating in the central compartment. If prophylactic total thyroidectomy and central node clearance with thymectomy is to be performed in children, it is important that the complications of surgery do not outweigh the benefit of prophylaxis.

Recently, pooled experience with MEN2 patients (53,112) has led to provisional categorization of very high, high, and intermediate risk groups for carriers of MEN2 according to the mutation identified (Table 6). The risk group determines the optimum age for prophylactic surgery. The very high risk group is that of children with MEN2B and/or *RET* mutations of codon 883, 918, and 922. Surgery for these children should be in infancy (see below). In the high risk group with *RET* mutations of codon 611, 618, 620, and 634, surgery is recommended before 5 years of age. In some patients with codon 634 mutations, positive lymph nodes have been found at the age of 5 (113), while in others microscopic MTC has been found at the age of 2 (114). For this high risk group, there is possibly a trade between age at surgery and extent of surgery—either earlier surgery without nodal clearance or later surgery with clearance. Some groups rely on the results of provocative tests to determine which patients should undergo node dissection. No case of a negative pentagastrin stimulation test with positive nodes has been reported by GETC.

Children with *RET* mutations in codon 609,768, 790,791,804, and 891 have intermediate risk. The natural history of MTC in carriers of these mutations is variable, but generally MTC develops at a later age and grows more slowly. Lymph node metastasis and death has been seen in patients with each of these mutations

Table 5 Early Results of Prophylactic Thyroidectomy in MEN2A

Number of carriers/subjects/families	Basal calcitonin elevated	Positive penta-gastrin test	Number of total thyroidectomies (+ node dissection)	Histopathology				
					Macro MTC	Micro MTC	CCH	Node Pos.
21/132/7	0	9	13(+)	Pg+ = 7	3	4		0
				Pg− = 6	1	2	3	0

Source: Ref. 84.

Table 6 Correlation of MEN2 Mutation and Risk of MTC

Risk group	Mutations	Recommended age for surgery
Very high	883,918,922	1 month to 1 year
High	611,618,620,634	2–5 years
Intermediate	609,768,790,791, 804,891	5–10 years

except codons 790 and 791 (115). They should all undergo total thyroidectomy; however, this can be delayed beyond 5 years of age. Some groups recommend 10 years of age, and others wait for provocation testing to become positive. The age at which provocation tests become positive is usually between 3 and 35 years, with fewer than 5% converting after this age, according to Raue and Frank-Raue (116).

In patients with a positive provocation test but normal baseline calcitonin, there is rarely nodal involvement [e.g., only 1 of 34 patients in the series of Gimm et al. (107)]. Similarly, Murat et al. (106) found that when the stimulation test was positive but the level was less than 130 pg/mL, none of 20 patients had nodal involvement. There seems to be little advantage in delaying surgery beyond late adolescence regardless of the test results as continued life-long testing will be required and there is the possibility of missing the opportunity to cure the disease.

Consequently, is it necessary to perform central node clearance for prophylactic surgery in MEN2A? For the moment, the answer is yes in the patient over 10 years of age or if there is a positive pentagastrin test or if there is a codon 634 mutation. Up to the age of 5 years, systematic node clearance may not be necessary, particularly for non-634 mutations.

Reoperation for MTC. MTC is unfortunately not responsive to standard chemotherapeutic regimens, radiotherapy, or hormone therapy. Control of diarrhea can be partially achieved with octreotide.

Reoperation is indicated in a number of situations. Even in the absence of macroscopic disease in the neck and mediastinum, if calcitonin levels remain elevated postoperatively, and initial surgery did not consist of extensive lymph node dissection, reoperation is indicated unless macroscopic distant metastases are present (104). In this circumstance completion total thyroidectomy, if not already performed, central node, lateral node, and selective mediastinal node clearance is required. The technique of microdissection as originally described by Tisell et al. (117) and practiced by others (105), including ourselves, is recommended.

When macroscopic disease is present in the neck, surgery may be indicated to avoid local complications.

Mediastinal node dissection via sternotomy is controversial because of a slight increase in morbidity and lack of evidence that it alters the natural history of the disease. Mediastinal nodes are just as likely to be involved as lateral neck nodes and may be involved when lateral nodes are uninvolved (i.e., "skip nodes") (105). At least the central compartment should be cleared down to the level of the brachiocephalic veins. This strategy results in normalization of the pentagastrin stimulation test in 38% of cases at 1 year (104).

3.2.3 Hyperparathyroidism

HPT is reported in 17–40% (mean 22%) of cases of MEN2A (89,118). It often has a late presentation, around 40 years of age, and reveals the syndrome in only 8% of cases. Frequently patients are normocalcemic and the HPT is not clinically significant. HPT in MEN2 is genetically determined, is not a response to calcitonin, and is highly associated with a mutation of codon 634. It manifests in 73% of patients with this mutation (119). Mutations in codons 609, 611, 618, 620, 790, and 791 are less frequently associated with HPT. Those with codon 768, 804, and 891 mutations rarely develop HPT.

Apparently single gland disease was observed at initial operation in 37% of cases (20). The secretory function of these glands is variable. During cervicotomy for MTC, in about two thirds of cases one finds one or more enlarged parathyroid glands which are hyperplastic on histology without any evidence of hypercalcemia. In 15% of cases PTH is inappropriately elevated in the presence of normocalcemia.

With respect to the parathyroid glands, the primary surgical concern in MEN2A is to avoid hypocalcemia after thyroid surgery for MTC or its prophylaxis. Adequate thyroid surgery requires thymectomy with central node clearance. In normocalcemic patients it is our practice to try to leave the (normal) superior glands in situ and transplant to the sternomastoid muscle the (normal) inferior glands, which are resected en bloc with the thyroid, lymph nodes, and thymus. Any enlarged parathyroid glands should also be excised, leaving an adequate amount of vascularized parathyroid tissue. In hypercalcemic patients, subtotal parathyroidectomy or total parathyroidectomy with autograft to the nondominant forearm may be indicated. Other surgeons practice routine total parathyroidectomy and autografting to the sternomastoid or forearm to facilitate radical neck clearance without concern for the vascularity of the parathyroids (104).

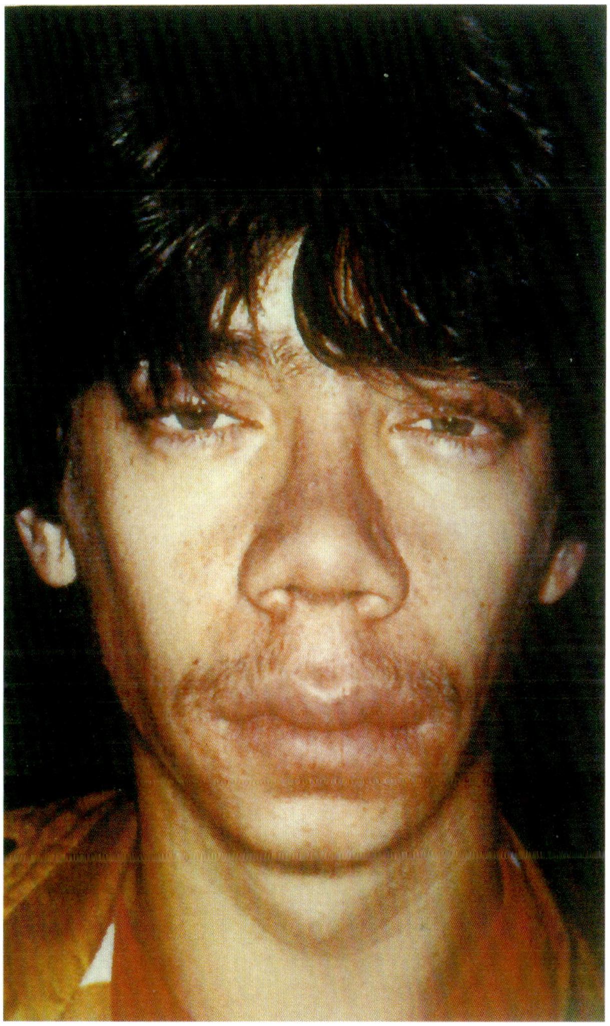

Figure 6 MEN2B. Thickened lips and characteristic facies.

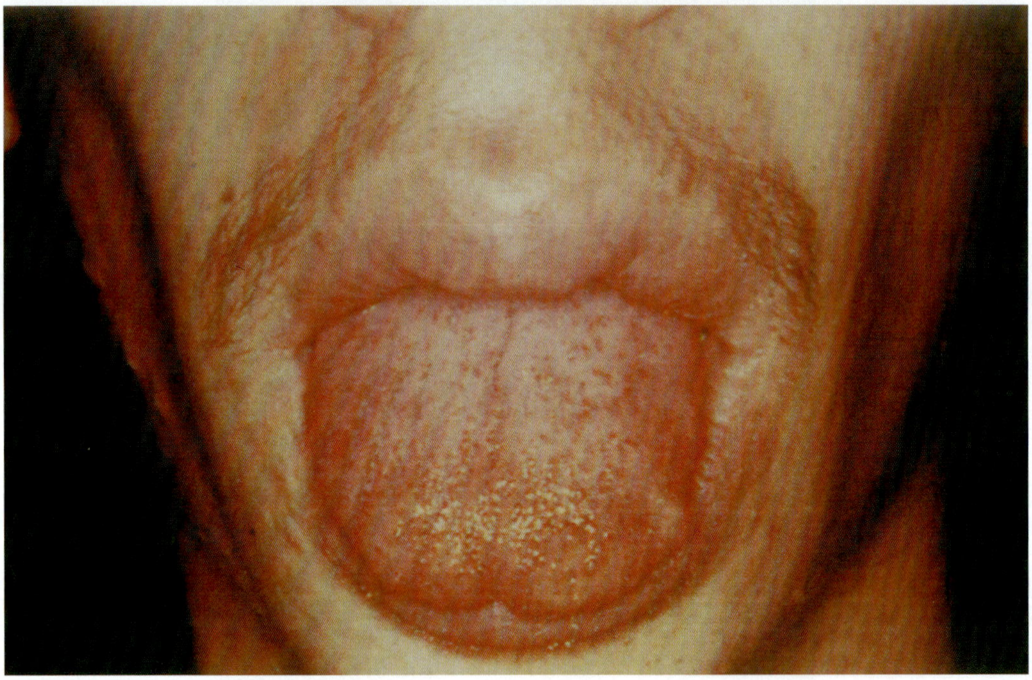

Figure 7 MEN2B. Submucosal neuromas of the tongue.

3.3 MEN2A with Hirschsprung's Disease

Mutations of the *RET* proto-oncogene, which are inactivating by nature, are known to cause Hirschsprung's disease. Activating mutations of codons 609, 618, and 620 have been found in patients with MEN2A and Hirschsprung's disease. There have been rare cases of Hirschsprung's disease with activating mutations of these codons yet no features of MEN2A disease.

3.4 MEN2A with Cutaneous Lichen Amyloidosis

This is a rare variant of MEN2A with the addition of pruritic, macular, cutaneous lesions of the interscapular region of the upper back. It is associated with mutation of codon 634.

3.5 Multiple Endocrine Neoplasia Type 2B (Gorlin or Steiner's Syndrome)

MEN2B is much less common than MEN2A. The clinical course of the syndrome is dominated by that of the associated MTC, which is more aggressive in this disease than in any other clinical settings. Diarrhea from hormone secretion by metastatic MTC can be troublesome despite octreotide therapy. The other major morbid component of the syndrome is intestinal ganglioneuromatosis. Pheochromocytoma is observed in about one half of patients, at a later age of onset than the MTC. It may not have time to manifest in many cases. Hyperparathyroidism is not a feature of MEN2B. There appears to be an equal sex distribution. Sporadic germline mutation is the cause of the syndrome in about 50% of cases. Kindreds may be short-lived due to the lethality of the mutation. The distinctive features of this syndrome are the characteristic facies and marfanoid habitus, which are usually present from infancy and allow instant diagnosis if recognized (Figs. 6,7). The full syndrome was described by a number of groups (4,5), but it is perhaps the name of Gorlin that is most associated with MEN2B.

The condition is sufficiently rare that frequently the diagnosis is delayed. The most striking feature is thickened lips and eyelids as a result of submucosal neural tumors. The tongue is nodular and dentition usually deranged. Adults are characteristically marfanoid. Neural hypertrophy is most evident in the retina as seen by slit lamp examination. Orthopedic problems including pes cavus and talipes may be the initial presentation. During infancy and childhood, megacolon development due to intestinal ganglioneuromatosis may necessitate surgery in 50% or more of patients (121). Commonly, the appearance of a lump in the neck, which gives rise to the diagnosis of MTC, is the trigger to the diagnosis of MEN2B. Pheochromocytoma may occasionally be diagnosed before any other feature of the syndrome is recognized. MTC in MEN2B typically presents in childhood with apparently aggressive disease, having nodal and distant metastases. It is well recognized that infants with MEN2B may have MTC, suggesting the possibility of malignant change in utero. Despite metastatic disease, patients may live for many years with minimal morbidity due to indolent behavior of their tumor.

MEN2B is associated almost exclusively with a mutation of the codon 918 in the intracellular domain of the *RET* proto-oncogene located on chromosome 10. Other rarer mutations occur in codons 883 and 922.

The surgical strategy for MTC in MEN2B is similar to that of MEN2A. In sporadic or index cases, surgery is carried out at diagnosis. The presence of a functioning pheochromocytoma must be sought and treated before thyroid surgery! In sporadic cases, surgery consists of total thyroidectomy with central compartment and upper mediastinal node clearance, thymectomy, and bilateral neck dissection.

Prophylactic surgery should be performed probably before the age of 1 year and perhaps in the first few months. Microscopic MTC is commonly found within the first year of life, and lymph node metastasis in infants has also been described (109). Total thyroidectomy with central node dissection is performed in this setting. Lymph node involvement indicates the need for more extensive lymph node clearance.

Occasional children present with true "short segment" Hirschsprung's disease. Others with intestinal ganglioneuromatosis may present a pseudo-Hirschsprung's disease. Gene analysis in these patients allows prophylactic thyroidectomy for cure at an early age (120).

3.6 Familial Medullary Thyroid Cancer

In this variant of MEN2, no other features are expressed. The MTC is similar to that of other MEN2 syndromes, i.e., multifocal, arising in a background of CCH, and metastasizing readily. There is some variation of clinical course within this group, due in part to the existence of a number of different genetic mutations, but in general onset is at a later age and the clinical course is more indolent than in MEN2A. Mutations of many codons in both the extracellular and intracellular domains of the *RET* proto-oncogene have been associated with FMTC (Table 4). There is overlap of the genetic mutations in MEN2A and FMTC, and thus the two conditions cannot be differentiated by the genotype in all cases. There is a danger that MEN2A may be misdiagnosed as FMTC due to lack of expression of other features during the lifetime of kindred members. To avoid the possibility of missing the opportunity to screen for pheochromocytoma, there are strict inclusion criteria which can be applied before confirming FMTC (53). There should be more than 10 carriers in the kindred and multiple carriers or affected members over the age of 50 who have been thoroughly investigated.

Prophylactic thyroid surgery should be undertaken in FMTC at the appropriate age determined by mutation analysis just as in MEN2A.

3.7 Mixed MEN1 and MEN2

Rare observations of apparent mixed syndromes such as ZES and pheochromocytoma (122) are difficult to explain now that the genetic basis of each condition has been clearly determined.They are probably variants of MEN1.

4 OTHER ENDOCRINE TUMOUR SYNDROMES

4.1 Familial Hyperparathyroidism and Hyperparathyroid–Jaw Tumor Syndrome

Huang et al. (123) reported 51 cases of familial hyperparathyroidism without MEN. Hypercalcemia in these patients is often severe and associated with complications. Multiple gland disease was found in 45% of cases and supernumerary glands in 29%. Persistent or recurrent HPT was observed in 20% of cases after surgery.

There is no doubt that there is genetic heterogeneity in this group of patients (123). Wassif et al. (124) reported a large family with HPT characterized by metachronous adenoma development and in one case carcinomatous change. Five affected family members were genetically tested, none of whom had mutations in the *MEN1* gene or the *RET* gene. Tsukada et al. (125) recently reviewed mutations of the MEN1 gene. It appears that some missense mutations are specifically associated with familial hyperparathyroidism.

Jackson et al. (126) described the HPT–jaw tumor syndrome. This consists of primary HPT and mandibular fibrous tumors inherited in an autosomal dominant fashion: the gene is located at 1q21-32 (127). These are not the brown tumors of HPT and do not disappear after parathyroid surgery. The clinical expression of this condition is often delayed beyond the age of 40 years. The parathyroid disease may take the form of adenoma(s), carcinoma $\pm$ adenoma(s), and hyperplasia. The glands are frequently cystic. One variant is described with familial cancer of the parathyroid.

The principles of surgery in this group are the same as for MEN1. These syndromes should generally be regarded as multiglandular for the purpose of surgical strategy. Subtotal parathyroidectomy, thymectomy, and a search for supernumerary glands including opening the carotid sheaths is recommended. Where a family history of parathyroid cancer exists, surgery should be undertaken at the first sign of hyperparathyroidism. Jaw tumors require resection.

4.2 Familial Hypocalciuric Hypercalcemia and Neonatal Hypercalcemia

While these disorders are not due to endocrine tumors, they are included here because familial hypocalciuric hypercalcemia (FHH) is the major differential diagnosis of primary hyperparathyroidism. The syndrome of familial benign hypercalcemia was described in 1972 by Foley et al. (128). The principal characteristic is modest hypercalcemia, which is generally asymptomatic and typically begins in childhood. There is associated mild hypermagnesemia and hypophosphatemia. The urinary calcium is inappropriately low in relation to the serum level. Serum PTH is usually normal but inappropriate to the serum calcium level (129,130). The glands are apparently normal macroscopically and histologically (129). The condition is hereditary, transmitted as an autosomal dominant pattern. The prevalence is not well known. In 1980 Marx et al. (131) reported 9% of patients operated without success for primary HPT had in fact FHH. According to Toss et al. (132), in a region of Sweden, 1 in 10,000 of the population had this condition, while 3 in 10,000 had primary HPT.

Hypercalcemia is relatively stable throughout life except in infancy, where the serum calcium level may be a little higher (133). Daily calcium excretion is usually less than 100 mg per 24 hours with a lowered ratio of calcium clearance to creatinine clearance. A calcium clearance/creatinine clearance ratio of <0.01 suggests FHH, while a ratio of >0.02 suggests HPT (129–131).

Severe neonatal hypercalcemia, on the other hand, is rare and classically presents with extreme, symptomatic, and sometimes fatal hypercalcemia. Recently genetic studies have shown that these syndromes represent the heterozygous and homozygous form of the same disorder of calcium receptor function for which the gene lies at chromosome 3q. The parathyroid cells and renal tubular cells are less than normally sensitive to ambient calcium, resulting in higher urinary conservation of calcium and an elevated serum level. From a surgical point of view the difference between the two forms is major. In the case of severe neonatal hypercalcemia, the intervention must be as early as possible and requires total parathyroidectomy and thymectomy with parathyroid cryopreservation if one wishes to avoid persistent hypercalcemia and high associated mortality (134). Some authors, however, counsel a conservative approach if possible (133), as it appears there may be variants in which the neonatal hypercalcemia may ameliorate with time. In the case of FHH, the hypercalcemia is usually modest, with few clinical features. Surgery should be avoided because less than total parathyroidectomy results in persistent hypercalcemia (129), while total parathyroidectomy results in hypoparathyroidism (129,131) and no clinical benefit.

4.3 Familial Nonmedullary Thyroid Cancer

Familial papillary thyroid cancer is becoming more widely recognized (135). While sporadic papillary cancers are frequently associated with RET-ptc mutations, genetic studies have not yet located the gene(s) responsible for familial disease. About 6% of all patients with papillary cancers have a family history. At least 90% of FNMTC is papillary cancer. The majority of reports suggest that the familial forms are more aggressive than sporadic disease (136).

Familial Hürthle cell carcinoma is rare. It has been associated in some cases with mutations at 19p13.2 (137).

4.4 Inherited Pheochromocytoma and Paraganglioma Syndromes Other Than MEN 2

4.4.1 Neurofibromatosis Type 1 (Von Recklinghausen's Disease)

Neurofibromatosis (NF) type 1 is an autosomal dominant disorder arising from mutations of the NF tumor suppressor gene at chromosome 17q11. This is a large gene with many mutations identified over its entire length. No genotype-phenotype correlation has yet been found.

The disease occurs in about 1 in 3500 people. The predominant features of the disease are benign cutaneous neurofibromas and café-au-lait spots. Less than 4% of NF patients develop pheochromocytoma, which is bilateral in about 10% of cases and malignant in 10% of cases (138). They are usually intra-adrenal (96%) and may be of mixed pathology such as neuroblastoma and ganglioneuroma.

In the syndrome of von Recklinghausen's neurofibromatosis, periampullary duodenal somatostatinomas with psammomatous calcification sometimes occur and are virtually pathognomonic, occasionally being the presenting lesion (139). Unusual groupings of endocrine tumors are occasionally seen. Examples are association of NF with MTC and HPT (Fig. 8), which have been observed by the senior author.

4.4.2 Von Hippel–Lindau Syndrome

Von Hippel–Lindau Syndrome (VHL) is a relatively rare, autosomal dominant cancer syndrome with an incidence of about 1 in 35,000. The VHL tumor suppressor gene is located at chromosome 3p25–26. A great number of mutations have been identified. The gene mutation leads to an upregulation of vascular endothelial growth factor (VEGF). The syndrome is characterized by retinal angiomas (55%), medullary angioblastomas (55–85%), and renal cell carcinoma (30%) (140). Families with a missense mutation generally also have pheochromocytomas and are classed as VHL type 2. Families with other mutations and without pheochromocytoma are classed as VHL type 1 (140).

Pheochromocytomas are observed in 42% of cases of VHL. They are bilateral in about 50% and are frequently ectopic, in particular intrathoracic (141). Pancreatic tumors are also common (20–55%) and are usually cystic and nonfunctioning but may be solid and functioning. The majority of the endocrine pancreatic tumors are benign, and 8% of the pheochromocytomas are malignant. As many as 20% of all pheochromocytomas may in fact be due to VHL (140). About a quarter of patients with VHL do not have a family history but are de novo cases.

4.4.3 The Familial Paragangliomas, Pheochromocytomas, and Succinate Dehydrogenase Deficiencies

Recent studies have shown that a significant proportion of familial pheochromocytoma is due to mutation of the succinate dehydrogenase gene. Succinate dehydrogenase has four subunit components: SDHA, SDHB, SDHC, and SDHD. Mutations in SDHC and SDHD are associated with familial paraganglioma (142), and SDHB has recently been associated with both familial paraganglioma and phaeochromocytoma (143).

Extra-adrenal pheochromocytomas or paragangliomas arise from the same neural crest–derived cells as adrenal medullary pheochromocytoma. They occur in a young population, between 10 and 30 years of age,

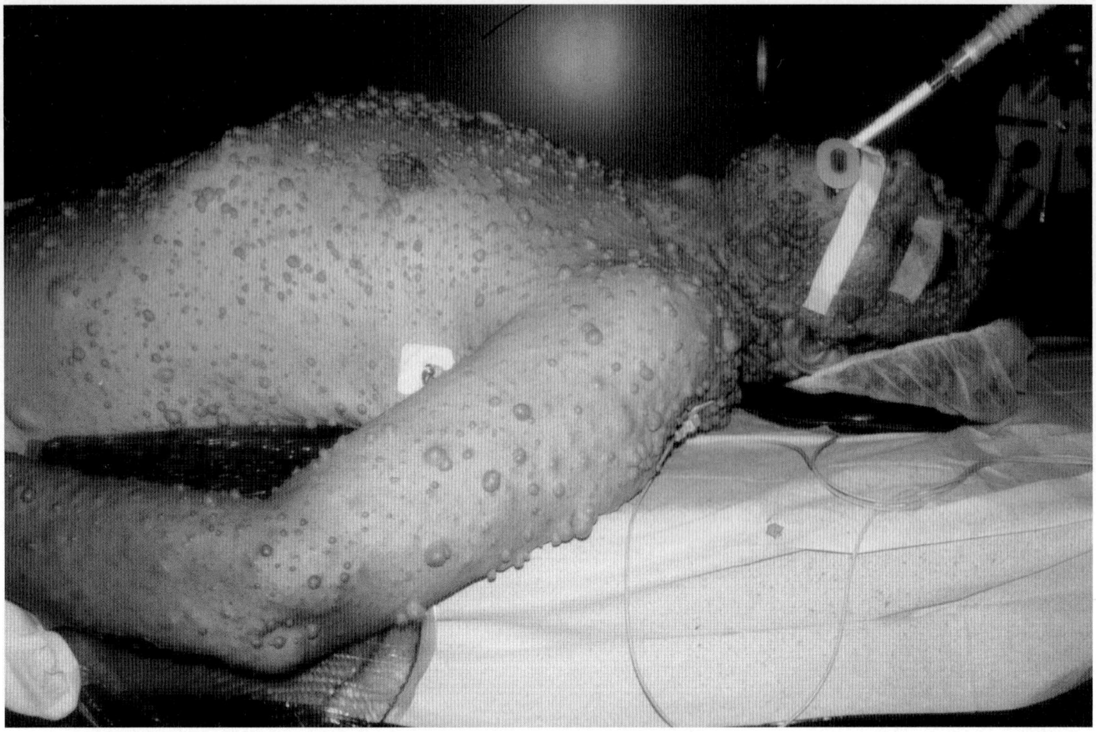

Figure 8 Neurofibromatosis type 1. This patient had an operation for medullary thyroid cancer.

and they are multiple in 15–24% of cases. Only 1% of paraganglionomas of the head and neck secrete catecholamines, while intrathoracic, intra-abdominal, retroperitoneal, and pelvic lesions are usually secretory. They are more often malignant than adrenal phaeochromocytomas: about 40% versus 10% in the literature (144) and 59% versus 18% in our experience. These tumors arise from the vagus and glossopharyngeal parasympathetic ganglia, the sympathetic paravertebral chain including the organ of Zuckerkandl, the carotid and aortic bodies, the wall of the jugular vein, tympanic plexus and visceral autonomic ganglia such as in the bladder. Paragangliomas are rarely amenable to laparoscopic surgery because of their unusual locations, hypervascularity, and frequent multiplicity of lesions.

A comparison of the characteristics of phaeochromocytoma in MEN2A, VHL, NF type 1, and succinate dehydrogenase deficiency is shown in Table 7.

4.5 Cowden Syndrome

This syndrome, named after Rachel Cowden, who was the first described patient, is due to mutation of the *PTEN* gene and is characterized by multiple hamartomas, breast cancer, characteristic facies, and sometimes an intellectual deficit. The cutaneous lesions are facial papules, oral mucosal papillomatosis, and acral keratosis. In both men and women there is an association with differentiated carcinoma of the thyroid and with HPT (145).

4.6 Tuberous Sclerosis

In the syndrome of tuberous sclerosis, an autosomal dominant phakomatosis, angiomyelolipomas, occa-

Table 7 Characteristics of Familial Pheochromocytomas

	Mean age	Bilaterality %	Ectopic %	Malignant %
MEN2A	40(14–68) index 26 screened	60	4	3
VHL	28(5–58)	50	15	<10
NF1	42(1.5–74)	10	4	10
SDD	20(10–30)	20	>80	50

SDD, succinate dehydrogenase deficiency.

sional adrenal pheochromocytomas, and occasional cases of insulinoma have been described. Two different genes have been associated with the syndrome.

4.7 Familial Adenomatous Polyposis

Familial adenomatous polyposis is an autosomal dominant syndrome of multiple colonic polyps with a high rate of malignant transformation. The gene responsible is the *FAP* gene at chromosome 5q21. Small intestinal adenocarcinoma, in particular at the ampulla of Vater, is the next most significant tumor, occurring in 10% of cases. In Gardner's syndrome, which is a variant, there are also osteomas and desmoid tumors and epidermoid cysts. There is an association with papillary carcinoma of the thyroid. The Leeds Castle polyposis group (146) (an international workshop group) had collected 69 such cases by 1991. Of these, the majority were papillary but were not uncommonly the follicular variant of papillary or "mixed papillary and follicular." Occasional apparently purely follicular carcinomas were noted. The papillary lesions were typically multicentric and cribriform. There is no doubt that they occur more commonly than in matched populations, with approximately 100-fold relative risk. There is a further association with adrenal cortical adenomas.

4.8 Carney Triad or Complex

In 1985 Carney et al. (147) published a report of 40 cases in which there was an association of cardiac (72%), cutaneous (45%), and breast (30%) myxomas with muco-cutaneous lentigines (65%), melanotic schwannomas, Cushing's sydrome due to pigmented macronodular adrenocortical hyperplasia (45%), acromegaly (10%), and Sertoli cell testicular tumors (56%). The prognosis is largely determined by the presence of the cardiac myxomas, which are late presenting and often multiple and tend to recur after excision. Cushing's syndrome in these patients may be cured by bilateral adenalectomy. Testicular tumors are frequently bilateral and multicentric and often occur in children. Screening for lesions should begin at about the age of 5 because of early and severe manifestations of the syndrome.

4.9 Carney Syndrome

This syndrome is an association of pulmonary chondroma, gastric leiomyosarcoma (Fig. 9), and functioning extra-adrenal paraganglioma (148). It does not appear to be inherited.

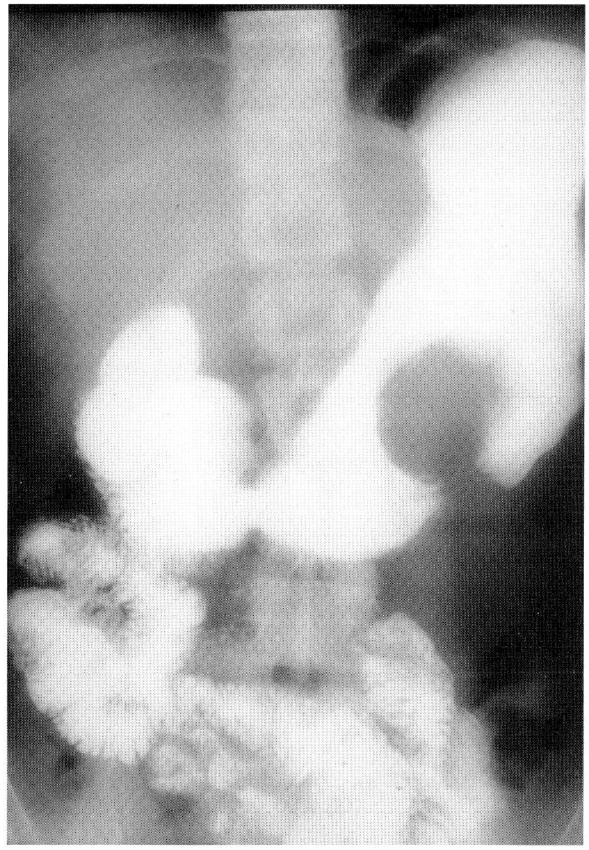

Figure 9 Gastric leiomyosarcoma in Carney syndrome.

4.10 Ataxia–Telangiectasia Syndrome

Ataxia–telangiectasia (AT) is a rare autosomal recessive disorder characterized by progressive neuronal degeneration, immunological deficiency, radio-sensitivity, and an increased risk of cancer. Several studies have confirmed that AT heterozygosis increases the risk of breast cancer and there is also an association with papillary thyroid cancer.

4.11 Li–Fraumeni Syndrome

The Li–Fraumeni syndrome is caused by a mutation in the *p53* gene located on chromosome 17p13. This gene acts as a tumor suppressor gene and is vital to the process of apoptosis of abnormal cells formed by mitosis. A wide range of tumors, including sarcoma, breast cancer, and lung cancer may arise as a result. There is a frequent association with carcinoma of the adrenal cortex.

4.12 Familial Glucocorticoid Remediable Hyperaldosteronism

Approximately 50 families with a precocious and severe hypertension, hypokalemia, and hyperaldosteronism have been reported. This may give rise to an asymmetrical nodular hyperplasia of the adrenal glands. Surgery is not indicated, and therapy with steroids is appropriate (149). Therapy with dexamethasone relieves the hypertension and hyperaldosteronism.

4.13 Familial Carcinoid Syndrome

Oberg reported four families in which midgut carcinoids developed over two generations. These were not associated with known genetic defects including *MEN1* (150).

4.14 Noonan Syndrome

This is an autosomal dominant or sporadic syndrome due to mutation at chromosome 12, which may affect both sexes and has a phenotype similar to Turner's syndrome. There is an association with neurofibromatosis and pheochromocytoma (151).

4.15 Beckwith–Wiedeman Syndrome

This is a congenital syndrome of hemihypertrophy, macroglossia, gigantism, and omphalocele with visceromegaly. Postnatal hypoglycemia due to islet cell hyperplasia/nesidioblastosis, pancreatoblastoma, adrenal cortical carcinoma, Cushing's syndrome, and Wilms' tumor are some of the many associations of this syndrome. The syndrome is generally sporadic but may be inherited in a minority of cases.

REFERENCES

1. Erdheim J. Zur normalen und pathologischen Histologie der Glandula thyroidea, Parathyroidea und Hypophyse. Beitr Pathol Anat 1930; 33:158–236.
2. Wermer P. Genetic aspects of adenomatosis of endocrine glands. Am J Med 1954; 16:363–371.
3. Sipple JH. The association of phaeochromocytoma with carcinoma of the thyroid gland. Am J Med 1961; 31:163–166.
4. Gorlin RJ, Sedano HO, Vickers RA, Cervenka J. Multiple mucosal neuroma, phaeochromocytoma, and medullary carcinoma of the thyroid: a syndrome. Cancer 1968; 22:293–299.
5. Steiner AL, Goodman AD, Powers SR. Study of a kindred with phaeochromocytoma, medullary thyroid carcinoma, hyperparathyroidism and Cushing's disease: multiple endocrine neoplasia, type 2. Medicine 1968; 47:371–409.
6. Shepherd JJ. The natural history of multiple endocrine neoplasia type 1. Highly uncommon or highly unrecognised? Arch Surg 1991; 126:935–952.
7. Zollinger RM, Ellison EC, O'Dorisio TM, Sparks J. Thirty years' experience with gastrinoma. World J Surg 1984; 8:427–435.
8. Kraimps JL, Duh QY, Demeure M, Clark OH. Hyperparathyroidism in multiple endocrine neoplasia syndrome. Surgery 1992; 112:1080–1086.
9. Lips CJM, Vasen HFA, Lamers CBHW. Multiple endocrine neoplasia syndromes. Critical reviews in oncology and haematology 1984; 2:117–184.
10. Chandrasekharappa SC, Guru SC, Manickam P, Olufemi SE, Collins FS, Emmert-Buck MR, Debelenko LV, Zhuang Z, Lubensky IA, Liotta LA, Crabtree JS, Wang Y, Roe BA, Weisemann J, Boguski MS, Agarwal SK, Kester MB, Kim YS, Heppner C, Dong Q, Spiegel AM, Burns AL, Marx SJ. Positional cloning of the gene for multiple endocrine neoplasia-type 1. Science 1997; 276:404–407.
11. Agarwal SK, Guru SC, Heppner C, Erdos MR, Collins RM, Park SY, Saggar S, Chandrasekharappa SC, Collins FS, Spiegel AM, Marx SJ, Burns AL. Menin interacts with the AP1 transcription factor JunD and represses JunD-activated transcription. Cell 1999; 96: 143–152.
12. Marx SJ. Multiple endocrine neoplasia type 1. In: Scriver CR, Beaudet AL, Sly WS, Valle D, eds. The Metabolic and Molecular Basis of Inherited Disease. 8th ed. New York: McGraw-Hill, 2001:943–966.
13. Calendar A, Zhang CX, Porchet N, Gaudray P. Genetic abnormalities in multiple endocrine neoplasia type 1. In: Doherty GM, Skogseid B, eds. Surgical Endocrinology. Philadelphia: Lippincottt, Williams and Wilkins, 2001:479.
14. Bartsch DK, Langer P, Wild A, Schilling T, Celik I, Rothmund M, Nies C. Pancreaticoduodenal endocrine tumours in multiple endocrine neoplasia type 1: surgery or surveillance? Surgery 2000; 128:958–966.
15. Burgess JR, Greenway TM, Shepherd JJ. Expression of the MEN1 gene in a large kindred with multiple endocrine neoplasia type 1. J Int Med 1998; 243:465–470.
16. Uchino S, Noguchi S, Sato M, Yamashita H, Yamashita H, Watanabe S, Murakami T, Toda M, Ohshima A, Futata T, Mizukoshi T, Koike E, Takatsu K, Terao K, Wakiya S, Nagatomo M, Adachi M. Screening of the MEN1 gene and discovery of germ-line and so-

matic mutations in apparently sporadic parathyroid tumors. Cancer Res 2000; 60:5553–5557.
17. Burgess JR, David R, Greenway TM, Parameswaran V, Shepherd JJ. Osteoporosis in multiple endocrine neoplasia type 1. Arch Surg 1999; 134:1119–1123.
18. Allo M, Thompson NW. Familial hyperparathyroidism caused by solitary adenomas. Surgery 1982; 92: 486–490.
19. van Heerden JA, Kent RB III, Sizemore GW, Grant CS, ReMine WH. Primary hyperparathyroidism in patients with multiple endocrine neoplasia syndromes. Surgical experience 1983; 118:533–536.
20. Kraimps JL, Duh QY, Demeure M, Clark OH. Hyperparathyroidism in multiple endocrine neoplasia syndrome. Surgery 1992; 112:1080–1088.
21. Friedman E, Sakaguchi K, Bale AE, Falchetti A, Streeten E, Zimering MB, Weinstein LS, McBride WO, Nakamura Y, Brandi ML. Clonality of parathyroid tumors in familial multiple endocrine neoplasia type 1. N Engl J Med 1989; 321:213–218.
22. Kraimps JL, Barbier J. Familial hyperparathyroidism in multiple endocrine neoplasia syndromes. In: Clark OH, Duh QY, eds. Textbook of Endocrine Surgery. Philadelphia: WB Saunders, 1997:381.
23. Duh QY. Surgical approach to primary hyperparathyroidism (bilateral approach). In: Clark OH, Duh QY, eds. Textbook of Endocrine Surgery. Philadelphia: WB Saunders, 1997:357.
24. O'Riordain DS, O'Brien T, Grant CS, Weaver A, Gharib H, van Heerden JA. Surgical management of primary hyperparathyroidism in multiple endocrine neoplasia types 1 and 2. Surgery 1993; 114:1031–1037.
25. van Heerden JA, Grant CS. Surgical treatment of primary hyperparathyroidism: an institutional perspective. World J Surg 1991; 15:688–692.
26. Brandi ML, Aurbach GD, Fitzpatrick LA, Quarto R, Spiegel AM, Bliziotes MM, Norton JA, Doppman JL, Marx SJ. Parathyroid mitogenic activity in plasma from patients with familial multiple endocrine neoplasia type 1. N Engl J Med 1986; 314:1287–1293.
27. Silverberg SJ, Bone HG III, Marriott TB, Locker FG, Thys-Jacobs S, Dziem G, Kaatz S, Sanguinetti EL, Bilezikian JP. Short-term inhibition of parathyroid hormone secretion by a calcium-receptor agonist in patients with primary hyperparathyroidism. N Engl J Med 1997; 337:1506–1510.
28. Arnalsteen LC, Alesina PF, Quievreux JL, Farrell SG, Pattou FN, Carnaille BM, Cardot-Bauters CM, Wemeau JL, Proye CAG. Long term results of less than total parathyroidectomy for hyperparathyroidism in multiple endocrine neoplasia type 1 (MEN1). Surgery 2002; 132:1119–1125.
29. Hellman P, Skogseid B, Juhlin C, Akerstrom G, Rastad J. Findings and long term results of parathyroid surgery in multiple endocrine neoplasia type 1. World J Surg 1992; 16:718–723.
30. Wells SA Jr, Farndon JR, Dale JK, Leight GS, Dilley WG. Long-term evaluation of patients with primary parathyroid hyperplasia managed by total parathyroidectomy and heterotopic autotransplantation. Ann Surg 1980; 192:451–458.
31. Casanova D, Sarfati E, De Francisco A, Amado JA, Arias M, Dubost C. Secondary hyperparathyroidism: diagnosis of site of recurrence. World J Surg 1991; 15:546–549.
32. Saxe AW, Gibson GW, Kay S. Characterisation of a simplified method of cryopreserving human parathyroid tissue. Surgery 1990; 108:1033–1039.
33. Carty SE, Norton JA. Management of patients with persistent or recurrent primary hyperparathyroidism. World J Surg 1991; 15:716–723.
34. Saxe AW, Brennan MF. Reoperative parathyroid surgery for primary hyperparathyroidism caused by multiple-gland disease: total parathyroidectomy and autotransplantation with cryopreserved tissue. Surgery 1982; 91:616–621.
35. Wagner PK, Seesko HG, Rothmund M. Replantation of cryopreserved human parathyroid tissue. World J Surg 1991; 15:751–755.
36. Al-Sobhi S, Clark OH. Parathyroid hyperplasia: parathyroidectomy. In: Clark OH, Duh QY, eds. Textbook of Endocrine Surgery. Philadelphia: WB Saunders, 1997:372.
37. Saxe AW, Spiegel AM, Marx SJ, Brennan MF. Deferred parathyroid autografts with cryopreserved tissue after reoperative parathyroid surgery. World J Surg 1982; 117:538–543.
38. Proye C, Lefebvre J, Bourdelle-Hego M-F, Francois M, Carnaille B, Foucher C, Durieu JP, Quievreux JL, Gough I. Adenome parathyroidien mediastinal moyen de la fenetre aorto-pulmonaire. Chirurgie 1988; 114: 166–173.
39. Skogseid B, Eriksson B, Lundqvist G, Lorelius LE, Rastad J, Wide L, Akerstrom G, Oberg K. Multiple endocrine neoplasia type 1: a 10-year prospective screening study in four kindreds. J Clin Endocrinol Metab 1991; 73:281–287.
40. Dean PG, van Heerden JA, Farley DR, Thompson GB, Grant CS, Marasen WS, Ilstrup DM. Are patients with multiple endocrine neoplasia type 1 prone to premature death? World J Surg 2000; 24:1437–1441.
41. Doherty GM, Olson JA, Frisella MM, Lairmore TC, Wells SA Jr, Norton JA. Lethality of multiple endocrine neoplasia type I. World J Surg 1998; 22:581–586.
42. Skogseid B, Oberg K, Eriksson B, Juhlin C, Granberg D, Akerstrom G, Rastad J. Surgery for asymptomatic pancreatic lesion in multiple endocrine neoplasia type I. World J Surg 1996; 20:872–877.
43. Le Bodic MF, Heymann MF, Lecomte M, Berger N, Berger F, Louvel A, De Micco C, Patey M, De Mascarel A, Burtin F, Saint-Andre JP. Immunohistochemical study of 100 pancreatic tumors in 28 patients with

multiple endocrine neoplasia, type I. Am J Surg Pathol 1996; 20:1378–1384.
44. Goudsward WB, Houthoff HJ, Koudstaal J, Zwierstra RP. Nesidioblastosis and endocrine hyperplasia of the pancreas. A secondary phenomenon. Human Pathol 1986; 17:46–54.
45. Thompson NW, Lloyd RV, Nishiyama RH, Vinik AI, Strodel WE, Allo MD, Eckhauser FE, Talpos G, Mervak T. MEN I pancreas: a histological and immunohistochemical study. World J Surg 1984; 8:561–574.
46. Norton JA, Fraker DL, Alexander HR, Venzon DJ, Doppman JL, Serrano J, Goebel SU, Peghini PL, Roy PK, Gibril F, Jensen RT. Surgery to cure the Zollinger-Ellison syndrome. N Engl J Med 1999; 341:635–644.
47. Stabile BE, Morrow DJ, Passaro E. The gastrinoma triangle, operative implications. Am J Surg 1984; 147: 25–31.
48. Friesen SR. Are "aberrant nodal gastrinomas" pathologically similar to "lateral aberrant thyroid" nodules? Surgery 1990; 107:236–238.
49. Thom AK, Norton JA, Axiotis CA, Jensen RT. Location, incidence, and malignant potential of duodenal gastrinomas. Surgery 1991; 110:1086–1091.
50. Cadiot G, Vuagnat A, Doukhan I, Murat A, Bonnaud G, Delemer B, Thiefin G, Beckers A, Veyrac M, Proye C, Ruszniewski P, Mignon M. Prognostic factors in patients with Zollinger-Ellison syndrome and multiple endocrine neoplasia type 1. Groupe d'Etude des Neoplasies Endocriniennes Multiples (GENEM and groupe de Recherche et d'Etude du Syndrome de Zollinger-Ellison (GRESZE). Gastroenterology 1999; 116:286–293.
51. Cougard P, Goudet P, Peix JL, Henry JF, Sarfati E, Proye C, Calender A. et le GENEM Les insulinomes dans les neoplasies endocriniennes multiples de type 1 (NEM1). A propos D'une serie de 44 cas du groupe D'etude des neoplasies endocriniennes multiples (GENEM). Ann Chir 2000; 125:118–123.
52. Norton JA, Alexander HR, Fraker DI, Venzon DJ, Gibril F, Jensen RT. Comparison of surgical results in patients with advanced and limited disease with multiple endocrine neoplasia type 1 and Zollinger-Ellison syndrome. Ann Surg 2001; 234:495–505.
53. Brandi ML, Gagel RF, Angeli A, Bilezekian JP, Beck-Peccoz P, Bordi C, Conte-Devolx B, Falchetti A, Gheri RG, Libroia A, Lips CJM, Lombardi G, Manelli M, Pacini F, Ponder BAJ, Raue F, Skogseid B, Tamburrano G, Thakker RV, Thompson NW, Tomassetti P, Tonelli F, Wells SA, Marx SJ. Guidelines for diagnosis and therapy of MEN type 1 and type 2. J Clin Endocrinol Metab 2001; 86:5658–5671.
54. Proye C. Endocrine tumours of the pancreas: an update. Aust NZ J Surg 1998; 68:90–100.
55. Bartsch DK, Langer P, Wild A, Schilling T, Celik I, Rothmund M, Nies C. Pancreaticoduodenal endocrine tumours in multiple endocrine neoplasia type 1: surgery or surveillance? Surgery 2000; 128:958–966.
56. Hellman P, Anderson M, Rastad J, Juhlin C, Karacagil S, Eriksson B, Skogseid B, Akerstrom G. Surgical strategy for large or malignant endocrine pancreatic tumours. World J Surg 2000; 24:1353–1360.
57. Lairmore TC, Chen VY, De Benedetti MK, Gillanders WE, Norton JA, Doherty GM. Duodenopancreatic resections in patients with multiple endocrine neoplasia type 1. Ann Surg 2000; 231:909–918.
58. Proye C, Pattou F, Carnaille B, Lefebvre J, Decoulx M, d'Herbomez M. Intraoperative insulin measurement during surgical management of insulinomas. World J Surg 1998; 22:1218–1224.
59. Imamura M, Hattori Y, Nishida O, Honda T, Shimada Y, Miyahara T, Wagata T, Baba N, Tobe T. Unresponsiveness of insulinoma cells to secretin: significance of the secretin test in patients with insulinoma. Pancreas 1990; 5:467–473.
60. Kato M, Immamura M, Hasotani R, Shimada Y, Doi R, Itami A, Komoto I, Kosaka T, Konisimi I. Curative resection of microgastrinomas based on the intraoperative secretin test. World J Surg 2000; 24: 1425–1430.
61. Mignon M, Ruszniewski P, Podevin P, Sabbagh L, Cadiot G, Rigsud D, Bonfils S. Current approach to the management of gastrinoma and insulinoma in adults with multiple endocrine neoplasia type 1. World J Surg 1993; 17:489–497.
62. McFarlane MP, Fraker DI, Alexander HR, Norton JA, Lubensky I, Jensen RT. Prospective study of surgical resection of duodenal and pancreatic gastrinomas in multiple endocrine neoplasia type 1. Surgery 1995; 118:973–980.
63. Thompson NW, Pasieka J, Fukunchi A. Duodenal microgastrinomas, duodenotomy and duodenal exploration in the surgical management of Zollinger-Ellison syndrome. World J Surg 1993; 17:455–462.
64. Wiedenmann B, Jensen RT, Mignon M, Modlin CI, Skogseid B, Doherty G, Oberg K. Preoperative diagnosis and surgical management of neuroendocrine gastroenteropancreatic tumours: general recommendations by a consensus workshop. World J Surg 1998; 22:309–318.
65. Lowney JK, Frisella MM, Lairmore TC, Doherty GM. Pancreatic islet cell tumour metastasis in multiple endocrine neoplasia type 1: correlation with primary tumour size. Surgery 1998; 124:1043–1048.
66. Gauger PG, Thompson NW. Early surgical intervention and strategy in patients with multiple endocrine neoplasia type1. Best Prac Res Clin Endocrinol Metab 2001; 15:213–223.
67. Imamura M, Takahashi K. Use of selective arterial secretin injection test to guide surgery in patients with Zollinger-Ellison syndrome. World J Surg 1993; 17: 433–438.

68. Proye C, Pattou F, Carnaille B, Paris J-C, d'Herbomez M, Marchandise X. Intraoperative gastrin measurements during surgical management of gastrinomas: experience with 20 cases. World J Surg 1998; 22:643–650.
69. Thompson NW. Current concepts in the surgical management of multiple endocrine neoplasia type 1 pancreatico-duodenal disease. Results in the treatment of 40 patients with Zollinger-Ellison syndrome, hypoglycaemia or both. J Intern Med 1998; 243:495–500.
70. Delcore R, Friesen SR. Role of pancreaticoduodenectomy in the management of primary duodenal wall gastrinomas in patients with the Zollinger-Ellison syndrome. Surgery 1992; 112:1016–1023.
71. McEntee GP, Nagorney DM, Kvole LK, Moertel CG, Grant CS. Cytoreductive hepatic surgery for neuroendocrine tumours. Surgery 1990; 108:1091–1096.
72. Pichlmayr R, Weimann A, Oldhafer KJ, Schlitt HJ, Klempnauer J, Bornscheuer A, Chavan A, Schmoll E, Lang H, Tusch G, Ringe B. Role of liver transplantation in the treatment of unresectable liver cancer. World J Surg 1995; 19:807–813.
73. Teh BT, McArdle J, Chan SP, Menon J, Hartley L, Pullan P, Ho J, Khir A, Wilkinson S, Larsson C, Cameron D, Shepherd J. Clinicopathologic studies of thymic carcinoids in multiple endocrine neoplasia type 1. Medicine 1997; 76:21–29.
74. Rindi G, Bordi C, Rappel S, La Rosa S, Stolte M, Solcia E. Gastric carcinoids and neuroendocrine carcinomas: pathogenesis, pathology, and behavior. World J Surg 1996; 20:168–172.
75. Jensen RT. Management of the Zollinger-Ellison syndrome in patients with multiple endocrine neoplasia type 1. J Intern Med 1998; 243:477–488.
76. Skogseid B, Rastad J, Gobl A, Larsson C, Backlin K, Juhlin C, Akerstrom G, Oberg K. Adrenal lesion in multiple endocrine neoplasia type 1. Surgery 1995; 118: 1077–1082.
77. Burgess JR, Harle RA, Tucker P, Parameswaran V, Davies P, Greenaway TM, Shepherd JJ. Adrenal lesions in a large kindred with multiple endocrine neoplasia type 1. Arch Surg 1996; 131:699–702.
78. Darling TN, Skarulis MC, Steinberg SM, Marx SJ, Spiegel AM, Turner M. Multiple facial angiofibromas and collagenomas in patients with multiple endocrine neoplasia type 1. Arch Dermatol 1997; 133:853–857.
79. Stratakis CA, Schussheim DH, Freedman SM, Keil MF, Pack SD, Agarwal SK, Skarulis MC, Weil RJ, Lubensky IA, Zhuang Z, Oldfield EH, Marx SJ. Pituitary macroadenoma in a 5 year old: an early expression of MEN1. J Clin Endocrinol Metab 2000; 85: 4776–4780.
80. Cadiot G, Lebtahi R, Sarda L, Bonnaud G, Marmuse JP, Vissuzaine C, Ruszniewski P, Le Guludec D, Mignon M. Preoperative detection of duodenal gastrinomas and peripancreatic lymph nodes by somatostatin receptor scintigraphy. Groupe D'etude Du Syndrome De Zollinger-Ellison. Gastroenterology 1996; 111:845–854.
81. Proye C, Malvaux P, Pattou F, Filoche B, Godchaux JM, Maunoury V, Palazzo L, Huglo D, Lefebvre J, Paris JC. Noninvasive imaging of insulinomas and gastrinomas with endoscopic ultrasonography and somatostatin receptor scintigraphy. Surgery 1998; 124: 1134–1143.
82. Skogseid B, Oberg K, Benson L, Lindgren PG, Lorelius LE, Lundquist G, Wide L, Wilander E. A standardized meal stimulation test of the endocrine pancreas for early detection of pancreatic endocrine tumors in multiple endocrine neoplasia type 1 syndrome: five years experience. J Clin Endocrinol Metab 1987; 64:1233–1240.
83. Eng C, Clayton D, Schuffenecker I, Lenoir G, Cote G, Gagel RF, van Amstel HK, Lips CJ, Nishisho I, Takai SI, Marsh DJ, Robinson BG, Frank-Raue K, Raue F, Xue F, Noll WW, Romei C, Pacini F, Fink M, Niederle B, Zedenius J, Nordenskjold M, Komminoth P, Hendy GN, Mulligan LM, et al. The relationship between specific RET proto-oncogene mutations and disease phenotype in multiple endocrine neoplasia type 2. International RET mutation consortium analysis. JAMA 1996; 276:1575–1579.
84. Wells SA Jr, Chi DD, Toshima K, Dehner LP, Coffin CM, Dowton SB, Ivanovich JL, De Benedetti MK, Dilley WG, Moley JF, Norton JA, Donis-keller H. Predictive DNA testing and prophylactic thyroidectomy in patients at risk for multiple endocrine neoplasia type 2A. Ann Surg 1994; 220:237–247.
85. Mulligan LM, Kwok JB, Healey CS, Elsdon MJ, Eng C, Gardner E, Love DR, Mole SE, Moore JK, Papi L, Ponder MA, Telenius H, Tunnacliffe A, Ponder BAJ. Germ-line mutations of the RET proto-oncogene in multiple endocrine neoplasia type 2A. Nature 1993; 363:458–460.
86 Donis-Keller H, Dou S, Chi D, Carlson KM, Toshima K, Lairmore TC, Howe JR, Moley JF, Goodfellow P, Wells SA Jr. Mutations in the RET proto-oncogene are associated with MEN 2A and FMTC. Hum Mol Genet 1993; 2:851–856.
87. Mulligan LM, Eng C, Healey CS, Clayton D, Kwok JB, Gardner E, Ponder MA, Frilling A, Jackson CE, Lehnert H. Specific mutations of the RET proto-oncogene are related to disease phenotype in MEN 2A and FMTC. Nat Genet 1994; 6:70–74.
88. Kim IJ, Kang HC, Park JH, Ku JL, Lee JS, Kwon HJ, Yoon KA, Heo SC, Yang HY, Cho BY, Kim SY, Oh SK, Youn YK, Park DJ, Lee MS, Lee KW, Park JG. RET oligonucleotide microarray for the detection of RET mutations in multiple endocrine neoplasia type 2 syndromes. Clin Cancer Res 2002; 8:457–463.
89. Howe JR, Norton JA, Wells SA Jr. Prevalence of pheochromocytoma and hyperparathyroidism in multiple endocrine neoplasia type 2A: results of long-term follow-up. Surgery 1993; 114:1070–1077.

90. Gagel RF, Tashjian AH Jr, Cummings T, Papathanasopoulos N, Kaplan MM, DeLellis RA, Wolfe HJ, Reichlin S. The clinical outcome of prospective screening for multiple endocrine neoplasia type 2A. An 18-year experience. N Engl J Med 1988; 318:478–484.
91. Schuffeneker I, Virally-Monod M, Brohet R, le Groupe D'Etude des Tumeurs a Calcitonine. Risk and penetrance of primary hyperparathyroidism in multiple endocrine neoplasia type 2A families with mutations at codon 634 of the RET proto-oncogene. J Clin Endocrinol Metab 1998; 83:487–491.
92. Casanova S, Rosenberg-Bourgin M, Farkas D, Calmettes C, Feingold N, Heshmati HM, Cohen R, Conte-Devolx B, Guillausseau PJ, Houdent C, et al. Phaeochromocytoma in multiple endocrine neoplasia type 2 A: survey of 100 cases. Clin Endocrinol (Oxf) 1993; 38:531–537.
93. Modigliani E, Vasen HM, Raue K, Dralle H, Frilling A, Gheri RG, Brandi ML, Limbert E, Niederle B, Forgas L. Pheochromocytoma in multiple endocrine neoplasia type 2: European study. The Euromen Study Group. J Intern Med 1995; 238:363–367.
94. Raue F, Frank-Raue K, Grauer A. Multiple endocrine neoplasia type 2. Clinical features and screening. Endocrinol Metab Clin North Am 1994; 23:137–156.
95. Proye C, Thevenin D, Cecat P, Petillot P, Carnaille B, Verin P, Sautier M, Racadot N. Exclusive use of calcium channel blockers in the preoperative and intraoperative control of phaeochromocytomas: haemodynamics and free catecholamine assays in ten consecutive patients. Surgey 1989; 106:1149–1154.
96. Lairmore TC, Ball DW, Baylin SB, Wells SA. Management of Phaeochromocytomas in patients with multiple endocrine neoplasia type 2 syndromes. Ann Surg 1993; 217:595–601.
97. van Heerden JA, Sizemore GW, Carney JA, Grant CS, ReMine WH, Sheps SG. Surgical management of the adrenal glands in the multiple endocrine neoplasia type II syndrome. World J Surg 1984; 8:612–621.
98. De Graaf JS, Dullaart RP, Zwierstra RP. Complications after bilateral adrenalectomy for phaeochromocytoma in multiple endocrine neoplasia type 2: a plea to conserve adrenal function. Eur J Surg 1999; 165: 843–846.
99. Lee JE, Curley SA, Gagel RF, Evans DB, Hickey RC. Cortical sparing adrenalectomy for patients with bilateral phaeochromocytomas. Surgery 1996; 120:1064–1071.
100. Pattou FN, Combermale FP, Poirette JF, Carnaille B, Wemeau JL, Huglo D, Ernst O, Proye C. Questionability of the benefits of routine laparotomy as the surgical approach for phaeochromocytomas and abdominal paraganglionomas. Surgery 1996; 120:1006–1012.
101. Fernandez-Cruz L, Taura P, Saenz A, Benarroch G, Sabater L. Laparoscopic approach to pheochromocytoma: hemodynamic changes and catecholamine secretion. World J Surg 1996; 20:762–768.
102. Eng C, Mulligan LM, Smith DP, Healey CS, Frilling A, Raue F, Neumann HP, Ponder MA, Ponder BA. Low frequency of germline mutations in the RET proto-oncogene in patients with apparently sporadic medullary thyroid carcinoma. Clin Endocrinol (Oxf) 1995; 43:123–127.
103. Wells SA Jr, Dilley WG, Farndon JA, Leight GS, Baylin SB. Early diagnosis and treatment of medullary thyroid carcinoma. Arch Int Med 1985; 145:1248–1252.
104. Moley JF, Albinson C. Medullary thyroid carcinoma and the multiple endocrine neoplasia type 2 syndromes. In: Clark OH, Duh QY, eds. Textbook of Endocrine Surgery. Philadelphia: WB Saunders, 1997:541.
105. Dralle H. Medullary thyroid cancer. P Heinman lecture. IAES conference, Brussels, 2001.
106. Murat A, Modigliani E, Conte-Devolx B, Rohmer V, Leclerc L, Guilhem I, Bigorgne JC, Boneu A, Maes B, Chabre O, Niccoli P, Schuffenecker I, Giraud S. Early therapeutic management of patients genetically predisposed to medullary thyroid cancer. Ann Chir 1998; 52:455–460.
107. Gimm O, Ukkat J, Dralle H. Determinative factors of biochemical cure after primary and reoperative surgery for sporadic medullary thyroid carcinoma. World J Surg 1998; 22:562–568.
108. Ukkat J, Lorenz K, Hinze R, Thomusch O, Dralle H. Importance of early screening and prophylactic thyroidectomy in asymptomatic non index RET germline carriers. World J Surg 2001; 25:713–717.
109. Skinner MA, DeBenedetti MK, Moley JF, Norton JA, Wells SA. Medullary thyroid cancer in children with multiple endocrine neoplasia types 2A and 2B. J Pediatr Surg 1996; 31:177–181.
110. Wells SA, Skinner MA. Prophylactic thyroidectomy, based on direct genetic testing, in patients at risk for multiple endocrine neoplasia type 2 syndromes. Exp Clin Endocrinol Diabetes 1998; 106:29–34.
111. Dralle H, Gimm O, Simon D, Frank-Raue K, Gortz G, Niederle B, Wahl RA, Koch B, Walgenbach S, Hampel R, Ritter MM, Spelsberg F, Heiss A, Hinze R, Hoppner W. Prophylactic thyroidectomy in 75 children and adolescents with hereditary medullary thyroid carcinoma: German and Austrian experience. World J Surg 1998; 22:744–749.
112. Kikumori T, Evans D, Lee J, Cote G, Gagel R. Genetic abnormalities in multiple endocrine neoplasia type 2. In: Doherty G, Skogseid B, eds. Surgical Endocrinology. Philadelphia: Lippincott, Williams and Wilkins, 2001:531.
113. Gill JR, Reyes-Mugica M, Iyengar S, Kidd KK, Touloukian RJ, Smith C, Keller MS, Genel M. Early presentation of metastatic medullary carcinoma in

multiple endocrine neoplasia, type IIA: implications for therapy. J Pediatr 1996; 129:459–464.
114. Modigliani E, Cohen R, Campos JM, Conte-Devolx B, Maes B, Boneu A, Schlumberger M, Bigorgne JC, Dumontier P, Leclerc L, Corcuff B, Guilhem I. Prognostic factors for survival and for biochemical cure in medullary thyroid carcinoma: results in 899 patients. The GETC Study Group. Groupe d'Etude des Tumeurs a Calcitonine. Clin Endocrinol (Oxf) 1998; 48:265–273.
115. O Gimm, J Ukkat, BE Niederle, M Bockhorn, A Frilling, B Niederle, H Dralle, Ret proto-oncogene mutations affecting codon 790/791: a mild form of MEN2A? Surgery 2002; 132:952–959.
116. Raue F, Frank-Raue K. Biochemical parameters in diagnosis and follow up of patients with multiple endocrine neoplasia type 2. Acta Chir Austr 1997; 29:9–11.
117. Tisell LE, Hansson G, Jansson S, Salander H. Reoperation in the treatment of asymptomatic metastasizing medullary thyroid carcinoma. Surgery 1986; 99: 60–66.
118. Kraimps JL, Denizot A, Carnaille B, Henry JF, Proye C, Bacourt F, Sarfati E, Dupond JL, Maes B, Travagli JP, Boneu A, Roger P, Houdent C, Barbier J, Modigliani E. Primary hyperparathyroidism in multiple endocrine neoplasia type IIa: retrospective French multicentric study. Groupe d'Etude des Tumeurs a Calcitonine (GETC, French Calcitonin Tumors Study Group), French Association of Endocrine Surgeons. World J Surg 1996; 20:808–812.
119. Schuffeneker I, Virally-Monod M, Brohet R. le Groupe D'Etude des Tumeurs a Calcitonine. Risk and penetrance of primary hyperparathyroidism in multiple endocrine neoplasia type 2A families with mutations at codon 634 of the RET proto-oncogene. J Clin Endocrinol Metab 1998; 83:487–491.
120. Romeo G, Ceccherini I, Celli J, Priolo M, Betsos N, Bonardi G, Seri M, Yin L, Lerone M, Jasonni V, Martucciello G. Association of multiple endocrine neoplasia type 2 and Hirschsprung disease. J Intern Med 1998; 242:515–520.
121. O'Riordain DS, O'Brien T, Crotty TB, Gharib H, Grant CS, van Heerden JA. Multiple endocrine neoplasia type 2B: more than an endocrine disorder. Surgery 1995; 118:936–942.
122. Tamasawa N, Terada A, Kodama T, Ishigame M, Ishimaru K, Hishida R, Satoh T, Takebe K, Sasaki M, Imamura K. Pheochromocytoma with multiple islet cell carcinoma. Presse Med 1994; 23:32–34.
123. Huang SM, Duh QY, Shaver J, Siperstein AE, Kraimps JL, Clark OH. Familial hyperparathyroidism without multiple endocrine neoplasia. World J Surg 1997; 21:22–29.
124. Wassif WS, Moniz CF, Friedman E, Wong S, Weber G, Nordenskjold M, Peters T, Larsson C. Familial isolated hyperparathyroidism: a distinct genetic entity with an increased risk of parathyroid cancer. J Clin Endocrinol Metab 1993; 77:1485–1489.
125. Tsukada T, Yamaguchi K, Kameya T. The MEN1 gene and associated disease: an update. Endocr Pathol 2001; 12:259–273.
126. Jackson CE, Norum RA, Boyd SB, Talpos GB, Wilson SD, Taggart RT, Mallette LE. Hereditary hyperparathyroidism and multiple ossifying jaw fibromas: a clinically and genetically distinct syndrome. Surgery 1990; 108:1006–1012.
127. Teh BT, Farnebo F, Twigg S, Hoog A, Kytola S, Korpi-Hyovalti E, Wong FK, Nordenstrom J, Grimelius L, Sandelin K, Robinson B, Farnebo LO, Larsson C. Familial isolated hyperparathyroidism maps to the hyperparathyroidism-jaw tumor locus in 1q21-q32 in a subset of families. J Clin Endocrinol Metab 1998; 83:2114–2120.
128. Foley TP, Harrison HC, Arnaud CD, Harrison HE. Familial benign hypercalcaeimia. J Pediatr 1972; 81: 1060–1067.
129. Law WM Jr, Heath H III. Familial benign hypercalcemia (hypocalciuric hypercalcemia). Clinical and pathogenetic studies in 21 families 1985; 102:511–519.
130. Lyons TJ, Crookest PF, Postlethwaite PW, Sheridan B, Brown RC, Atkinson AB. Familial hypocalciuric hypercalcaemia as a differential diagnosis of hyperparathyroidism: studies of a large kindred and review of the surgical experience in the condition. Br J Surg 1986; 73:183–192.
131. Marx SJ, Stock JL, Attie MF, Downs RW, Gardner DG, Brown EM, Spiegel AM, Doppman JL, Brennan MF. Familial hypocalciuric hypercalcaemia: recognition among patients referred after unsuccessful parathyroid exploration. Ann Int Med 1980; 92:351–356.
132. Toss G, Arnqvist H, Larsson L, Nilsson O. Familial hypocalciuric hypercalcaemia: a study of four kindreds. J Intern Med 1989; 225:201–206.
133. Page LA, Haddow JE. Self-limited neonatal hyperparathyroidism in familial hypocalciuric hypercalcaemia. J Pediatr 1987; 111:261–264.
134. Blair JW, Carachi R. Neonatal primary hyperparathyroidism: a case report and review of the literature. Eur J Pediatr Surg 1991; 1:110–114.
135. Musholt TJ, Musholt PB, Petrich T, Oetting G, Knapp WH, Klempnauer J. Papillary thyroid carcinoma: genetics, criteria for diagnosis, clinical features and surgical treatment. World J Surg 2000; 24:1409–1417.
136. Takami H, Ozaki O, Ito K. Familial nonmedullary thyroid cancer: an emerging entity that warrants aggressive treatment. Arch Surg 1996; 131:676.
137. Alsanea O, Clark OH. Familial thyroid cancer. Curr Opin Oncol 2001; 13:44–51.
138. Walther MM, Herring J, Enquist E, Keiser HR, Lineham WM. Von Recklinghausen's disease and phaeochromocytomas. J Urol 1999; 162:1582–1586.
139. Wheeler MH, Curley IR, Williams ED. The association

of neurofibromatosis, phaeochromocytoma and somatostainoma-rich duodenal carcinoid. Surgery 1986; 100:1163–1169.

140. Neumann HP, Wiestler OD. Clustering of features of Von Hippel-Lindau syndrome: evidence for a complex genetic lesion. Lancet 1991; 337:1052–1054.
141. Walther MM, Reiter R, Keiser HR, Choyke PL, Venzon D, Hurley K, Gnarra JR, Reynolds JC, Glenn GM, Zbar B, Lineham WM. Clinical and genetic characterisation of phaeochromocytoma in von Hippel Lindau families:comparison with sporadic phaeochromocytoma gives insight into natural history of phaeochromocytoma. J Urol 1999; 162:659–664.
142. Gimm O, Armanios M, Dziema H, Neumann HPH, Eng C. Somatic and occult germline mutations in SDHD, a mitochondrial compex II gene, in non-familial phaeochromocytoma. Cancer Res 2000; 60:6822–6825.
143. Astuti D, Latif F, Dallol A, Dahia PL, Douglas F, George E, Skkoldberg F, Husebye ES, Eng C, Maher ER. Gene mutations in the sucinate dehydrogenase subunit SDHB cause susceptibility to familial phaeochromocytoma and to familial paraganglioma. Am J Hum Genet 2001; 69:49–54.
144. O'Riordain DS, Young WF, Grant CS, Carney JA, van Heerden JA. Clinical spectrum and outcome of extra-adrenal phaeochromocytoma. World J Surg 1996; 20: 916–922.
145. Mallory SB. Cowden syndrome (multiple hamartoma syndrome). Dermatol Clin 1995; 13:27–31.
146. Leeds Castle Polyposis GroupAbstracts from the fourth biannual meeting of the Leeds Castle Polyposis Group. May 9-11, 1991, Fort Lauderdale, Florida. Int J Colorectal Dis 1991; 6:224–236.
147. Carney JA, Gordon H, Carpenter PC, Shenoy BV, Go VL. The complex of myxomas, spotty pigmentation, and endocrine overactivity. Medicine (Baltimore) 1985; 64:270–283.
148. Carney JA. The triad of gastric epitheliod leiomyosarcoma, pulmonary chondroma and functional extra-adrenal paraganglionoma. A five year review. Medicine 1983; 62:159–164.
149. Ganguly A. Glucocorticoid-suppressible hyperaldosteronism: an update. Am J Med 1990; 88:321–324.
150. Oberg K. Carcinoid and flushing syndromes. In: Doherty G, Skogseid B, eds. Surgical Endocrinology. Philadelphia: Lippincott, Williams and Wilkins, 2001:405.
151. Noonan JA. Noonan syndrome. An update and review for the primary pediatrician. Clin Pediatr (Phila) 1994; 33:548–555.

51

Carcinoid Tumors

Irvin M. Modlin, Kevin Lye, and Mark Kidd

Yale University School of Medicine, New Haven, Connecticut, U.S.A.

1 OVERVIEW

Carcinoid tumors are slow-growing malignancies with distinct biological and clinical characteristics. Because these tumors derive from neuroendocrine cell compartments, their frequency of occurrence correlates with the site-density of neuroendocrine cells. As such, over 60% of carcinoid tumors arise along the largest human endocrine organ, the intestine. Another common location is the bronchopulmonary system (25%), reflecting the high density of Kulchitsky cells in the respiratory epithelium. Other carcinoid tumors, however, occur infrequently and in obscure sites; their biological and clinical characteristics may not be as apparent.

The clinical manifestations of carcinoid tumors are often either vague or absent. Nevertheless, in approximately 10% of patients these tumors secrete bioactive mediators, which may engender various elements characteristic of the carcinoid syndrome. Symptoms generally manifest following metastasis to the liver but may commonly occur in primary ovarian or retroperitoneal carcinoid tumors. After localization and biochemical characterization, the bioactivity of these tumors should be blocked by the somatostatin analogue octreotide, sometimes in combination with other pharmacological antagonists, with a goal of symptom control and increased safety of primary tumor resection. If curative resection is not feasible, then a cytoreductive management scheme should be employed, which includes surgical debulking and, when necessary, hepatic arterial embolization, followed by palliation with octreotide. Newer therapeutic modalities, such as receptor-based isotope therapy, are under investigation.

Since carcinoid tumors differ substantially from conventional gastrointestinal adenocarcinomas in their pathophysiology and outcome, it is imperative that the surgeon consider the biology of these lesions in defining appropriate therapy. This chapter will briefly focus on these aspects of carcinoid tumors and will outline primary management options. An algorithm for choice among these options will be presented, and the effect of this algorithm on patient outcome will be summarized. In addition, the management of specific or unusual presentations of enterological carcinoid tumors will be described.

2 HISTORICAL PERSPECTIVES

Although Langhans (1) described a gut carcinoid tumor in 1867, it was not until 1888 that Lubarsch (2) became the first to describe such a lesion in detail (Fig. 1). At that time, Lubarsch described the microscopic features of multiple tumors of the ileum, but regarded them as carcinomas. Two years later, Ransom (3) provided the first detailed descriptions of the classical symptoms of carcinoid syndrome in a patient with an ileal carcinoid tumor and hepatic metastases. Oberndorfer (4) first used the word *Karzinoide* in 1907 to distinguish these neoplasms, which he believed to be benign, from malig-

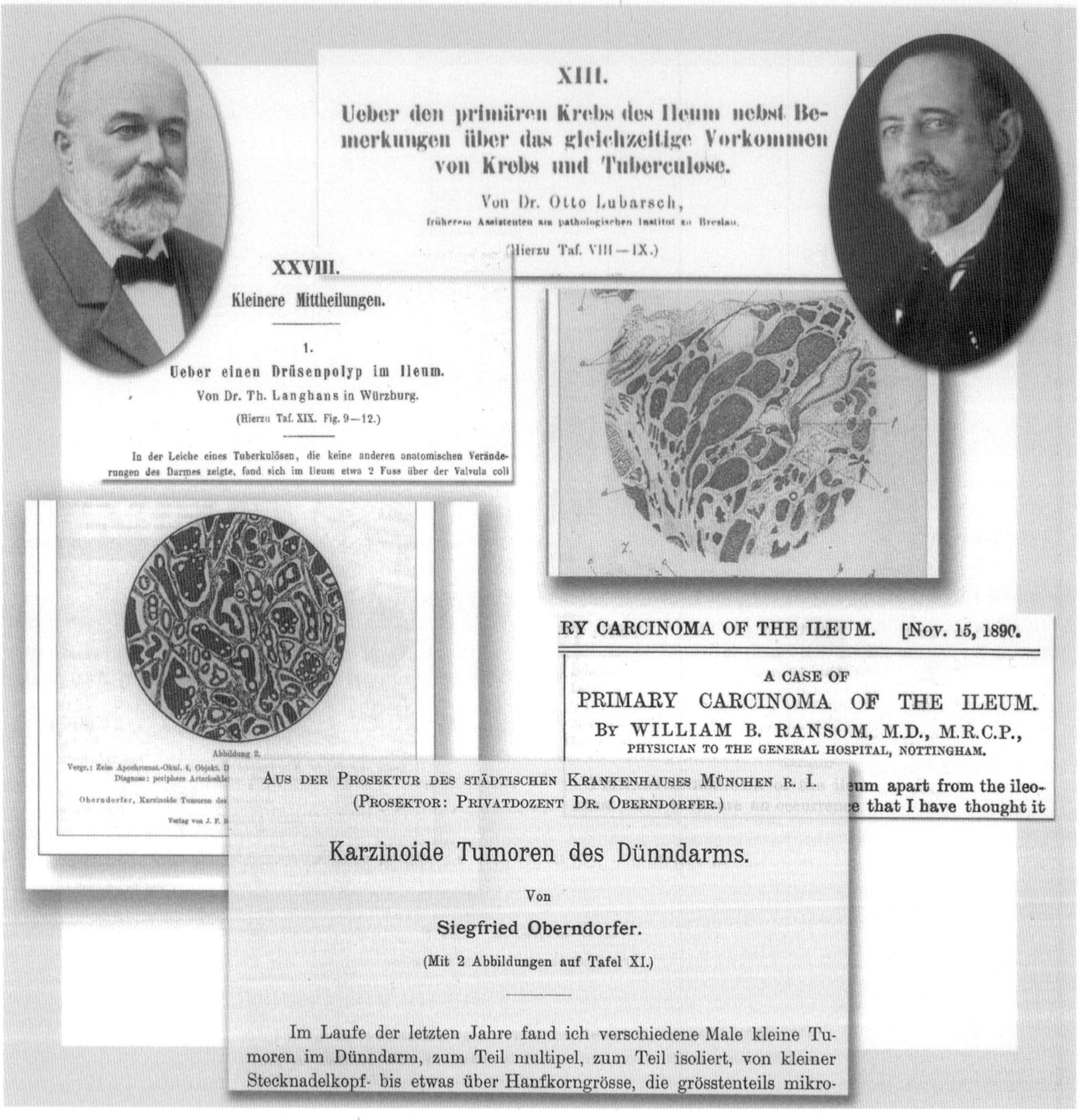
XIII.
Ueber den primären Krebs des Ileum nebst Bemerkungen über das gleichzeitige Vorkommen von Krebs und Tuberculose.
Von Dr. Otto Lubarsch,
früherem Assistenten am pathologischen Institut zu Breslau.
(Hierzu Taf. VIII—IX.)
XXVIII.
Kleinere Mittheilungen.
1.
Ueber einen Drüsenpolyp im Ileum.
Von Dr. Th. Langhans in Würzburg.
(Hierzu Taf. XIX. Fig. 9—12.)
In der Leiche eines Tuberkulösen, die keine anderen anatomischen Veränderungen des Darmes zeigte, fand sich im Ileum etwa 2 Fuss über der Valvula coli
RY CARCINOMA OF THE ILEUM. [Nov. 15, 1890.
A CASE OF
PRIMARY CARCINOMA OF THE ILEUM.
By WILLIAM B. RANSOM, M.D., M.R.C.P.,
PHYSICIAN TO THE GENERAL HOSPITAL, NOTTINGHAM.
eum apart from the ileo-
e that I have thought it
Abbildung 2.
Aus der Prosektur des städtischen Krankenhauses München r. I.
(Prosektor: Privatdozent Dr. Oberndorfer.)
Karzinoide Tumoren des Dünndarms.
Von
Siegfried Oberndorfer.
(Mit 2 Abbildungen auf Tafel XI.)
Im Laufe der letzten Jahre fand ich verschiedene Male kleine Tumoren im Dünndarm, zum Teil multipel, zum Teil isoliert, von kleiner Stecknadelkopf- bis etwas über Hanfkorngrösse, die grösstenteils mikro-

Figure 1 Prominent figures in the early recognition of carcinoid disease. The report of Theodor Langhans (1839–1915) (top left) in 1867 of an intriguing ileal tumor was referred to by Otto Lubarsch (1860–1933) (top right) in 1888. Two years later, William Ransom (1860–1909) described a patient with what is now recognized as the classical carcinoid syndrome. Siegfried Oberndorfer (1876–1944) coined the term *Karzinoide* in 1907 to describe these characterstic lesions; the histological diagrams in his work closely resemble those of Lubarsch from some 20 years prior.

nant adenocarcinoma, with its distinctly different biological behavior and prognostic implications. The recognition of carcinoids as endocrine-related tumors was outlined by Gosset and Masson in 1914 (5). However, it was only in 1963 that Williams and Sandler (6) classified carcinoids according to their anatomical site of origin: (a) foregut carcinoids (respiratory tract, stomach, duodenum, biliary system, and pancreas), (b) midgut carcinoids (small bowel, appendix, cecum, and proximal colon), and (c) hindgut carcinoids (distal colon and rectum). However, with the subsequent introduction of immunohistochemistry and the refinement of diagnostic imaging methods (computed tomography, magnetic resonance imaging, and SPECT-based somatostatin receptor scintigraphy) over the past two decades (7), the management of neuroendocrine tumors has advanced significantly.

In recent years it has become apparent that the term "carcinoid" represents a wide spectrum of neoplasms originating from a variety of neuroendocrine cell types. It has become apparent that this archaic descriptor fails to convey the pathological spectrum of such neoplasms with their wide array of secretory products.

Although the precise identification of the specific cell type of each neuroendocrine tumor of the gastrointestinal tract is far from complete, the widespread use of endoscopy, ultrasonography, and other advanced imaging modalities has significantly enhanced the identification of previously undetectable lesions and allowed a more accurate delineation of metastases. As a consequence, there has been an apparent statistical increase in enterological carcinoid tumor incidence over the last 20 years (16).

Almost half a century after Gosset and Masson initially detailed the derivation of these tumors from cells with argentaffin-staining properties, Erspamer and Asero (8) in 1952 identified the primary secretory product of the gut enterochromaffin (EC) cell as 5-hydroxytryptamine (serotonin). Lembeck (9) later isolated serotonin from a human ileal carcinoid tumor and proposed that this bioactive amine caused the hormonal symptoms of the carcinoid syndrome.

Elucidation of the embryological origin of the EC cell, which in turn gives rise to the midgut carcinoid tumor, has not been without controversy. In the first half of the twentieth century, Masson (10) proposed that argentaffin cells originated from gut endoderm, while Danisch (11) argued on the basis of morphology that these cells must derive and migrate from the visceral abdominal neural plexus. In 1966, Pearse (12) proposed that enterochromaffin cells, like all cells that exhibit amine precursor uptake and decarboxylation (APUD), derived embryologically from the neural crest and then migrated into the gut during cellular maturation. Although the unifying concept of APUD cells served to emphasize the production of bioactive amines by tumors derived from these cells, this theory of common origin has since proven to be flawed (13).

3 NEUROENDOCRINE GUT BIOLOGY

The gastrointestinal tract is the largest neuroendocrine system in the body. Unlike other endocrine organs, the endocrine cells of the gut are dispersed singly throughout the tract from the gastro-esophageal junction to the rectum. In some instances these cells have a brush border accessing the gut lumen, while in other cases access is limited to surrounding cells, blood vessels, and nerves. One particular point of interest in the pathobiology of gastrointestinal endocrine cells is their relation to carcinoid tumors. A number of observations have supported the hypothesis that these neoplasms and naïve endocrine cells arise from the same progenitor cell: (a) characteristic similarities between normal endocrine cells and carcinoid tumor cells are demonstrable by specific staining; (b) electron microscopy studies have revealed almost identical neuroendocrine granules in naïve and neoplastic cells; and (c) immunocytochemistry of the peptide products supports the histogenesis of gastrointestinal carcinoid tumors.

Each type of endocrine cell may produce one or more bioactive products (peptides), although in many instances the exact products and their precise functions remain without full delineation. These peptides are transmitted to their sites of action by any of three main pathways: endocrine, paracrine, or neurocrine. Peptides for which an endocrine function has been proven include gastrin, secretin, cholecystokinin, peptide YY, and somatostatin. Those for which a hormonal role is very likely, but not unequivocally proven, include gastric inhibitory polypeptide (GIP), motilin, and glucagon-like peptide-1 (GLP-1). Peptides secreted from typical endocrine cells but for which an endocrine function has yet not been identified with certainty include neurotensin, enteroglucagon, and GLP-2.

Gastrin has a pivotal role in that it directly regulates gastric enterochromaffin-like (ECL) cell proliferation and histamine release. Histamine stimulates the acid secretion of parietal cells and exerts a substantial trophic effect on the ECL cells of the stomach. Recently, peptide YY has been implicated in the inhibition of peripheral gastric acid secretion. Of considerable clinical relevance is somatostatin, which is secreted by D cells in the stomach and small intestine. In broad terms, somatostatin appears to function as a general inhibitor of many gastrointestinal functions, either directly or indirectly influencing motility, secretion, and absorption.

4 DEMOGRAPHICS

Carcinoid tumors are enigmatic, slow growing malignancies which occur most frequently (67%) in the gastrointestinal tract (Fig. 2). Gastrointestinal carcinoids are not rare, arising in 1.68 of every 100,000 people (14). Carcinoid is, in fact, the most common endocrine gut tumor (15). Carcinoid lesions are usually identified histologically by their affinity for silver salts, by general neuroendocrine markers, or, more specifically, by immunocytochemistry using antibodies against their specific cellular products. Within the gut, the most frequent sites of origin are the small bowel (25–28%), rectum (9–15%), appendix (4–12%), and stomach (4–5%). Sites of less frequent occurrence include the esophagus (0.04% of all carcinoid tumors), gallbladder (0.18%), biliary tract (0.23%), liver (0.3–0.4%), and pancreas (0.7%) (14,16,17).

In many instances these neoplasms are detected incidentally at the time of noninvasive imaging or at surgery for other gastrointestinal disorders. The tendency for metastatic spread does correlate with tumor size and is substantially higher in lesions larger than 2.0 cm. An association with synchronous noncarcinoid neoplasms is noted in 8–22% of lesions (14,18); adenocarcinoma of the colon is the most common second primary tumor (19). At initial clinical presentation, an incomplete evaluation could miss a second primary

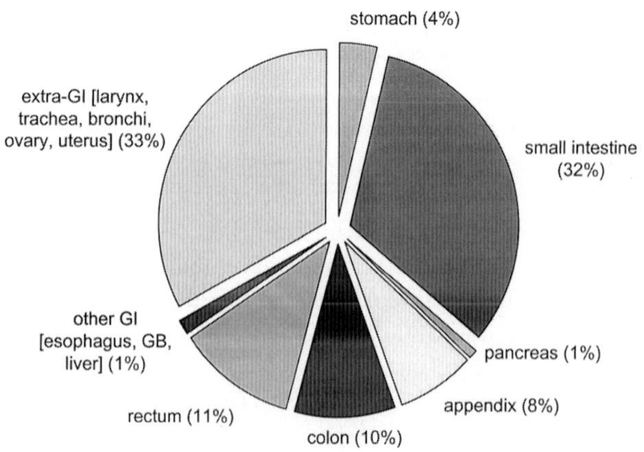

Figure 2 Distribution of 10,878 carcinoid tumors by site. (From Ref. 44.)

lesion that may necessitate a radically different therapy. Similarly, such patients should be followed aggressively for the development of new metachronous primary gut tumors, whereas the appearance of a carcinoid recurrence or metastasis should prompt attempts at tissue or biochemical diagnosis to be sure that the supposed carcinoid is not, in fact, a distinct adenocarcinoma.

5 CLINICAL FEATURES

5.1 Clinical Manifestations

Carcinoid lesions are the most common enterological endocrine tumors, comprising approximately 50% of all neuroendocrine tumors of the gastrointestinal tract. The presence of these lesions may be undetectable for years without obvious signs or symptoms. Evidence for this observation is supported by their relatively high incidence in large autopsy series (16). The occurrence of symptoms can be attributed either to local tumor effects or to the bioactive products of the neoplasm. Symptoms caused by local tumor effects include vague and nonspecific abdominal pain, which is often undiagnosed or leads to erroneous diagnoses. A relatively large percentage of carcinoid tumors are found as multiple lesions, suggesting that a common growth factor stimulus may influence similar stem cells in different locations throughout the body. A widely variable clinical picture may be evident, depending on the combination of bioactive substances secreted by the tumor.

The humoral secretion of tryptamines from primary midgut carcinoids and mesenteric lymph node metastases is generally countered by monoamine oxidase activity during initial hepatic passage; secreted products of retroperitoneal or ovarian carcinoids may bypass the liver and therefore cause systemic symptoms without metastases (20). Midgut carcinoid tumors are generally advanced at diagnosis unless they are discovered incidentally. Mucosal lesions may ulcerate and present with bleeding. Direct obstruction of the small bowel is uncommon except by very large tumors. However, small bowel obstruction is not rare in patients with bioactive carcinoid tumors. Intra-abdominal and retroperitoneal fibrosis are often clinically impressive and have been attributed to secretory products of these tumors such as serotonin. The humorally stimulated overproduction of extracellular matrix within the bowel wall, the mesentery, and the retroperitoneum may cause marked cicatrization, which may kink and obstruct the bowel. Such fibrosis may also result in intestinal ischemia or infarction, while ureteral obstruction may also occur (21).

5.2 Carcinoid Syndrome

The classical carcinoid syndrome occurs in fewer than 10% of patients (22); its most typical clinical manifestations include cutaneous flushing and gut hypermotility with secretory diarrhea, which occurs in up 75% of individuals (23). Less frequent findings include bronchoconstrictive wheezing, myopathy, increased skin pigmentation, and cardiac valvular abnormalities (24–27). These symptoms may be paroxysmal and wax or wane with time or, alternatively, may respond intermittently to a particular trigger agent, such as alcohol, aged cheese, coffee, or exercise. A common feature of all carcinoid tumors is a significant association with other noncarcinoid tumors of various histological types. It has been proposed that some of the bioactive agents secreted by such neoplasms function as growth factors which may promote phenotypic changes in susceptible cells and hence induce neoplastic transformation. This may be consistent not only with the role of neuroendocrine cells in the regulation of secretion and motility, but also in cell proliferation and differentiation.

The observed frequency of carcinoid syndrome symptoms varies with the intensity with which physicians seek them and the nature of the documented series. Investigation of such symptoms should suggest the possibility of a carcinoid tumor. Although diarrhea and flushing are the most common systemic symptoms, a third of patients with elevated serotonin levels may lack either symptom (28). The characteristic carcinoid facial flush is frequently accompanied by lacrimation and may be induced by small amounts of alcohol or coffee. Clinical evaluation of these patients must also explore the possibility of synchronous or metachronous gastrointestinal tumors.

6 BIOCHEMICAL CHARACTERIZATION AND DIAGNOSTIC FEATURES

6.1 Histology

Carcinoid tumors share unifying biological characteristics at clinical, histological, and epidemiological levels. Clinically, these tumors commonly present with a protean variety of classical symptoms. When such symptoms are not identifiable, the agents secreted may be biologically inactive, secreted in small amounts, inactivated by the liver, or may be of a subtle metabolic nature not currently detectable. Histologically, these tumors are composed of small epithelioid cells with basophilic nuclei and slow growth potential, characterized by a low mitotic index. Carcinoid tumor cells may be distinguished by their characteristic neuroendocrine secretory granules; they stain immunocytochemically with a variety of neuroendocrine markers, such as synaptophysin, neuron-specific enolase, and chromogranin A (29). The classic argyrophilic staining is found in a majority of neuroendocrine tumors, whereas argentaffin staining is relatively specific for midgut carcinoid tumors containing serotonin (24). Epidemiologically, carcinoid tumors are compatible with a substantially longer life expectancy than adenocarcinomas of a similar stage. The presence of severe hormonal symptoms in patients who may live for years with such tumors has prompted palliative cytoreduction in patients for whom complete extirpation is not feasible. Therapeutic methods allowing this cytoreduction without open surgical procedures are under investigation.

6.2 Composite Tumors

Increasing pathological sophistication has led to the identification of a genus of adenocarcinoid gastrointestinal tumors, most common in the appendix, but also found elsewhere in the gastrointestinal tract. These rare tumors, which contain elements resembling both adenocarcinoma and carcinoid tumor, are often termed composite or collision tumors depending on whether the disparate tumor elements are intermixed or simply in close contact (30). Although such tumors may display biochemical evidence of bioactive secretion, they are not typically accompanied by clinical evidence of the carcinoid syndrome. Although the rarity of composite tumors precludes definitive life table analysis, their natural history appears to resemble that of gastrointestinal adenocarcinomas, and they should therefore be treated accordingly.

6.3 Biochemistry

Since carcinoid tumors frequently present with obscure clinical manifestations, an extensive series of investigatory procedures are often undertaken before the correct diagnosis is finally established. The diagnostic strategies employed usually depend on the individual clinical presentation. If a classical symptom complex can be identified, the relevant specific peptides and amines should be measured. Thus, in gastric carcinoids, elevated plasma histamine levels may be seen, while small bowel lesions may exhibit increased levels of plasma substance P, serotonin, or increased urinary 5-hydroxy-indoleacetic acid (5-HIAA). If results are equivocal, these tests should be repeated and the *nonspecific* plasma markers of neuroendocrine tumors, such as pancreatic polypeptide and chromogranin, should be measured.

Classical biochemical identification of carcinoid tumors has involved quantitation of 24-hour urinary excretion of 5-HIAA. With a normal range of 2–8 mg per 24 hours, this test has been reported to have 73% sensitivity and a specificity of 100% (31). In our clinical laboratory, this test is considered strongly positive only if urinary 5-HIAA is greater than 30 mg/d. Feldman has detailed the techniques and precautions involved in this test. Measurement of plasma or urinary serotonin, substance P, neurotensin, chromogranins, or β-human chorionic gonadotropin may also prove useful in the diagnosis of selected patients. Biochemical testing has primarily been used to diagnose carcinoid tumors and is now providing information for the development of target-specific pharmacological antagonism.

6.4 Pentagastrin Provocation

For patients in whom biochemical evaluation is negative or equivocal, yet strong clinical suspicion for carcinoid persists, provocation testing may substantiate the diagnosis. Provocatory tests originated with observations that small doses of epinephrine or norepinephrine could recreate carcinoid flushing (32). Although the epinephrine challenge reveals both biochemical and clinical evidence of carcinoid syndrome in some patients, the test is neither sensitive nor specific. Pentagastrin stimulation tests have now evolved into a more accurate means of biochemically demonstrating an occult carcinoid tumor. It is likely that pentagastrin acts as an endogenous catecholamine test by liberating epinephrine, norepinephrine, and dopamine from the adrenal glands. Pentagastrin does not appear to have a direct effect on serotonin release from carcinoid tumor cells. Such provocation testing may also demonstrate the completeness of octreotide blockade in patients with established carcinoid syndrome before undergoing tumor manipulation or general anesthesia (33).

6.5 Provocative Testing and Scintigraphy

If the nonspecific plasma markers of neuroendocrine tumors (pancreatic polypeptide or chromogranin) are elevated and urinary 5-HIAA and plasma amines (substance P and serotonin) levels are unremarkable, the use of a provocative study such as the pentagastrin test may be of value (34). If the provocative study is positive or one of the above amines is initially elevated, the precise localization of the primary tumor and its metastases should be undertaken, utilizing somatostatin receptor (SST_R) scintigraphy. Intravenous ^{111}In-labeled octreotide can identify neuroendocrine tumors expressing somatostatin receptors, particularly of the subtypes 2 and 5, for which octreotide has a particularly high affinity (35). The sensitivity of somatostatin receptor scintigraphy (SRS) can be further enhanced by the simultaneous use of single positron emission computed tomography (SPECT) imaging. Although intraoperative gamma detection has been utilized and was initially considered to be potentially superior to SST_R scintigraphy in the detection of small endocrine lesions, the lack thus far of appropriate collimators has resulted in a disappointing early experience.

7 SITE-SPECIFIC DISEASE

7.1 Overview

Consistent with their endodermal origin, carcinoid tumors are historically classified according to foregut, midgut, or hindgut derivation. Foregut endocrine cells give rise to carcinoid tumors in the respiratory tract, the stomach, the first part of the duodenum, and the pancreas (Fig. 3). Midgut carcinoid tumors appear in the bowel from the second part of the duodenum through the ascending colon and appendix, whereas hindgut carcinoids appear in the transverse and descending colon and rectum. Carcinoid tumors from different segments of the embryological gut typically differ in the character of their bioactive products. These differences in secreted agents result in differences in symptoms and immunohistochemical staining patterns, and variations in anatomical location and venous drainage may further alter clinical presentations. Most notably, foregut carcinoids characteristically present early with local symptoms in the bronchial tract (cough, wheezing, hemoptysis, or infection distal to the tumor). Bronchial carcinoids frequently produce unusual systemic symptoms such as atypical and severe flushing (36) or no systemic symptoms at all, because of a low serotonin content and a variety of unusual bioactive agents. Kallikrein secretion, which induces bradykinin-like peptides and hypersecretion of histamine, has been linked to the atypical bronchial carcinoid flush. Midgut tumors most commonly produce serotonin and tachykinins but often cause systemic symptoms (diarrhea,

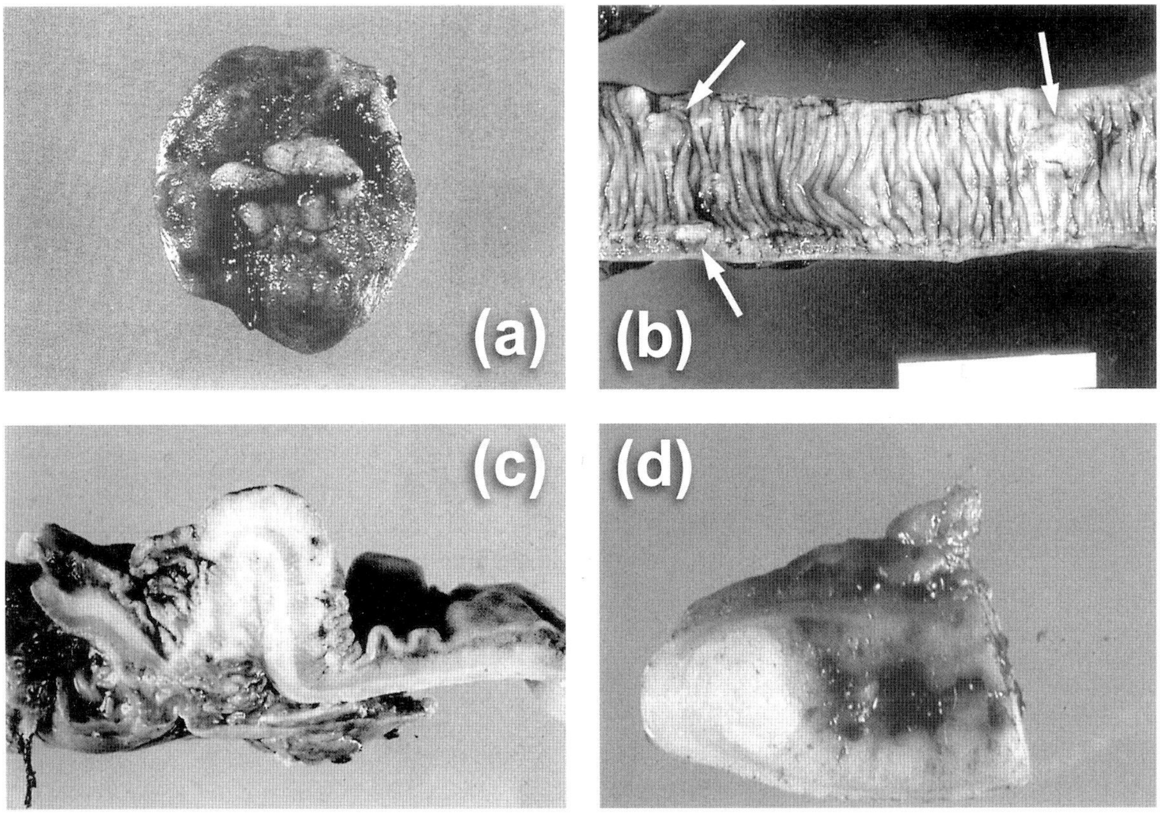

Figure 3 Gross pathological appearance of some carcinoid tumors. (a) Gastric fundus demonstrating typical carcinoid lesion with intact mucosa and focal gastritis. (b) Ileal carcinoid lesions (arrows) with overt ulceration of the largest lesion (right). (c) Knuckle of bowel formed by characteristic ileal carcinoid lesion, with muscular hypertrophy and direct serosal involvement. (d) Appendiceal tip exhibiting classic focal carcinoid nodule.

flushing, wheezing, right-sided valvular disease, and cutaneous telangiectasias) only after metastasis to the liver. An exception to this is the appendiceal carcinoid, which is a relatively benign lesion that rarely produces serotonin. These tumors present with local symptoms such as acute appendicular obstruction. Hindgut tumors characteristically synthesize and store several hormones or proforms of hormones not clearly proven to be secreted into the circulation. The substances immunolocalized to these tumor cells may include somatostatin, tachykinins, glicentin, and peptide YY (37).

Most carcinoids derive from the embryological midgut. Indeed, one meta-analysis of 3718 collective cases (38) found 45% of the tumors to be in the appendix and 28% within the jejunum or ileum. Conversely, 34% of small intestinal neoplasms and 77% of neoplasms of the appendix are carcinoids. Although Meckel's diverticulum is relatively uncommon, among Meckel's diverticular tumors, carcinoid is the most common and may occur in up to 13% of all diverticula.

7.2 Esophagus

The first description of an esophageal carcinoid was noted in 1969 by Brenner et al. (39), and to date only 17 patients have been reported; the average age at diagnosis is 58 years (range 30–82) (40,41). Esophageal carcinoid lesions exhibit a marked male predominance with a male:female ratio of 6:1.

Most esophageal carcinoids occur in the lower third of the esophagus or at the gastroesophageal junction; this parallels the distribution of endocrine cells. Such lesions arise in the submucosa but have generally invaded the esophageal wall at the time of presentation. Local lymph node metastases are a common feature and are present in approximately 50% of patients.

Patients usually present with nonspecific symptoms, which may be indicative of a carcinoid neoplasm, including dysphagia (64%), weight loss (43%), pain (14%), reflux esophagitis (14%), fatigue (7%), and melenic stools (7%) (40). However, the occurrence of the carcinoid syndrome is rare for patients with esophageal carcinoid.

Immunohistochemical studies may reveal immunoreactivity for neuron-specific enolase (NSE), vasoactive intestinal peptide (VIP), and serotonin (40). Interestingly, many tumors are not positive for argentaffin and argyrophilic staining. An association with Barrett's esophagitis has been described (42); an increased number of endocrine cells has been found in the setting of Barrett's metaplasia and may therefore lead to an increased incidence of esophageal carcinoids.

The diagnostic algorithm is similar to that of all esophageal masses and includes endoscopy with biopsy and computed tomography to exclude distant metastases. Barium studies may also be useful to assess the extent of the lesion. Evaluation of 5-HIAA in a 24-hour urine collection is not recommended, as only 25% of such patients exhibit elevated levels (40).

Esophageal carcinoids exhibit a malignant nature with a high degree of local spread and a relatively poor outcome compared to that of colonic carcinoids (15). Survival correlates well with the stage of the disease; whereas most stage I and II patients are tumor-free after an interventional procedure, most stage III and IV patients ultimately die of the disease process.

Most of the 17 patients described above underwent subtotal esophagectomy with gastroesophageal anastomosis; local excision was performed for one small esophageal lesion, with survival of this patient 8 years after the initial procedure.

7.3 Stomach

Gastric carcinoid tumors were previously thought to be extremely rare lesions. In literature from the preendoscopic era, they comprised only 0.3% of all gastric tumors and 1.9% of all gastrointestinal carcinoids. More recent studies have reported that as many as 10–30% of all carcinoids may occur in the stomach. In addition, it has been noted that gastric carcinoids exhibit an increased incidence in individuals with atrophic gastritis and pernicious anemia or in those with a combined Zollinger-Ellison syndrome and MEN1 (ZES-MEN1) (43). This apparent increase may represent either an improvement in diagnostic techniques, increased awareness of carcinoid disease, or a true increase in incidence. Indeed, a 40-year analysis of 265 gastric carcinoid tumors from the National Cancer Institute (NCI) database revealed an increase in gastric carcinoids among all gastric malignancies from 0.3 to 0.54% (17). In the same study, the percentage of gastric carcinoids among all gastrointestinal carcinoids increased from 2.4 to 5.6% over a 20-year period (1969–1979). The average age at diagnosis remained relatively unchanged (62.4 vs. 63.8 y).

Although earlier reports have suggested that approximately one half of gastric carcinoid tumors are not localized to the stomach at diagnosis (17), recent analysis of the National Cancer Institute's Surveillance, Epidemiology, and End Results (SEER) database, with case data on 501 gastric carcinoid tumors, indicates that among such tumors diagnosed during the 1992–1999 period, 67.5% were solitary, 3.1% were regionalized, and 6.5% were associated with distant metastases (44). In addition, an association with other noncarcinoid neoplasms was evident in 20.5% of these cases.

Hypergastrinemia-associated gastric carcinoid tumors (those of type A chronic atrophic gastritis and ZES-MEN1 patients) typically have a good prognosis (45), are generally noninvasive, and metastasize in only a small percentage (7.6–12%) of individuals. Sporadic gastric carcinoid tumors often display markedly aggressive local biological behavior and tend to demonstrate distant metastases. The 5-year survival rate is significantly higher for localized disease (64.3%) and for lesions with regional metastases (29.9%) than for lesions with distant metastases (10%) (17). Although the tendency to metastasize correlates with tumor size, minute primary tumors have been reported with spread. Factors predicting aggressive behavior in sporadic tumors include moderate cellular atypia, 2 or more mitoses per 10 high-powered fields, angioinvasion, and transmural invasion of the gastric wall (46).

Patients with gastric carcinoid tumors generally present with a variety of nonspecific symptoms and signs, including pain, vomiting, upper gastrointestinal bleeding, dyspepsia, anemia, heme-positive stools, and gastric polyps at endoscopy. It is very unusual for gastric carcinoids to exhibit symptoms of the carcinoid syndrome (47). The appearance of such symptoms is usually associated with sporadic gastric carcinoid tumors, which behave as neuroendocrine carcinomas.

As such, three distinct gastric carcinoid tumor types have been proposed in light of the distinct pathobiological behaviors of these tumors: (a) gastric carcinoids associated with type A chronic atrophic gastritis (CAG/A), (b) gastric carcinoids associated with a ZES-MEN1, and (c) sporadic gastric carcinoids. Gastric carcinoids arising in CAG/A patients (type I tumors) and ZES-

MEN1 patients (type II tumors) are usually associated with hypergastrinemia (48); histologically, these tumors consist mainly of ECL cells. Type I lesions are the most frequent and comprise approximately 65% of all gastric carcinoids. These tumors are localized in the oxyntic mucosa (gastric body and fundus) in individuals with CAG/A with or without pernicious anemia.

One characteristic feature of gastric carcinoid tumors is a multiplicity of small lesions of low malignant potential. In patients with type II tumors (ZES-MEN1), numerous small lesions, together with argyrophil cell hyperplasia or dysplasia, are evident throughout the entire nonatrophic oxyntic mucosa, in contrast to the flattened mucosa of CAG/A patients (49). Sporadic carcinoid lesions (type III tumors) are encountered less frequently (21%) and display a moderately aggressive behavior with invasive growth and a high incidence of metastasis. They are almost invariably solitary large lesions that evolve within normal gastric mucosa and in association with normal plasma gastrin levels.

Histopathologically, gastric carcinoid tumors comprise a variety of cell types including enterochromaffin, enterochromaffin-like, and X cells. They display growth patterns similar to those observed in carcinoid tumors from other locations and include trabecular or gyriform, medullary or solid, glandular or rosette-like growth, or a mixture of these types. Over 80% of gastric carcinoids are argyrophilic, but only a minority (14%) stain positively for argentaffin (50). Immunohistochemically, chromogranin, synaptophysin, and Leu-7 are present in over 90% of cases, whereas neuron-specific enolase and serotonin are detectable in only 60% and 34%, respectively.

Neuroendocrine carcinomas, previously known as atypical carcinoids, represent an aggressive neuroendocrine neoplasm that bears greater resemblance to sporadic carcinoids than to hypergastrinemia-associated tumors. These lesions display invasive growth, metastasize with great frequency, and progress rapidly.

Upper gastrointestinal endoscopy with biopsy is the most useful diagnostic tool. Gastric carcinoids are typically small, rounded, submucosal masses, which are often yellow in color (51). In patients with multiple tumors, numerous small, erythematous nodules may be seen. Solitary lesions are often found as large and ulcerated erythematous nodules. Barium contrast studies are useful in diagnosing polypoid tumors, and endoscopic ultrasound may be of value in identifying submucosal lesions and determining the degree of transmural spread.

The overall 5-year survival rate in gastric carcinoid tumors of types I, II, and III is 68.1% when the lesion is localized, 34.9% with regional spread, and 10.0% with distant metastases (44). There is, however, a far higher survival rate for the type I subgroup.

Hypergastrinemia-associated lesions less than 1.0 cm in size and fewer than three to five in number should initially be managed by endoscopic excision if possible (52). If a lesion is larger than 1.0 cm, more than five lesions are present, or recurrence at a site of endoscopic polypectomy is present, local excision of the lesions and antrectomy to eliminate the trophic stimulus (gastrin) that promotes tumor growth should be performed. Regression of gastric carcinoids has been reported after antrectomy alone. Nevertheless, such regression is not always the case, and the criteria for predicting whether this will occur remain ill-defined. Either endoscopic polypectomy or surgical excision and antrectomy should be followed by surveillance endoscopy with biopsy at 6-month intervals. Sporadic lesions and neuroendocrine carcinomas require aggressive surgical management upon diagnosis; complete or partial gastrectomy with regional lymph node dissection is mandatory in such cases (53).

7.4 Duodenum

The small intestine is the most frequent location for carcinoid tumors, and lesions of this organ comprise between 26.8 and 28.7% of all carcinoids in large series (16). However, it is likely that the real incidence of small intestinal carcinoids is even higher, given the relatively large number of asymptomatic and thus undetected lesions. In addition, small bowel carcinoids are the second most frequent neoplasm encountered in the small intestine, after adenocarcinomas.

In an autopsy series by Berge and Linell, carcinoids comprised 95% of all small intestinal primary tumors; 88% were incidental (54). Such lesions occur 6.5–8.4 times more frequently in the ileum than in the duodenum and jejunum (55), and their relative frequency increases in the aboral direction. This is distinct from adenocarcinomas, most of which occur in the duodenum and decrease in the aboral direction. The male:female incidence ratio shows a slight predominance for women (between 1.1 and 1.6), and the average age at diagnosis of small intestinal carcinoid is 64.2 years (16).

The majority of patients present with dyspepsia suggestive of duodenal ulceration. In some circumstances anemia from covert bleeding can occur; rarely, a major gastrointestinal bleed precedes carcinoid diagnosis.

Five major types of neuroendocrine tumors are identifiable in the duodenum. Gastrin-producing tumors with a trabecular pattern (type I) are most frequent, and occur preferentially in the proximal duodenum. In one third of patients, an association with Zollinger-Ellison syndrome and multiple endocrine neoplasia type 1 (ZES-MEN1) is evident. Somatostatin-producing tumors (type II) are second in frequency, have a predilection for the ampulla of Vater, and are often a component of neurofibromatosis. Histologically, type II lesions demonstrate a glandular structure and exhibit psammoma bodies. Gangliocytic paragangliomas (type III) are characterized by their nonfunctioning behavior and frequently occur in the ampullary or periampullary regions. Such lesions are predominantly immunocytochemically somatostatin- and pancreatic polypeptide–positive, and usually are benign (56). Tumors producing serotonin and other hormones such as calcitonin and pancreatic polypeptide (type IV) are rare. These are usually small lesions residing outside of the ampulla and lack signs and symptoms of infiltrative growth. Poorly differentiated neuroendocrine carcinomas (type V) are quite rare and highly malignant neoplasms, usually occurring in the ampulla of Vater. A notable feature of duodenal carcinoids is their association with von Recklinghausen's disease, Zollinger-Ellison syndrome, and multiple endocrine neoplasia (57).

Burke et al. (58) have characterized the histological and immunohistochemical features of 65 duodenal carcinoids. The majority of such tumors showed a mixture of cribiform, insular, glandular, solid, and trabecular growth patterns. Eighty-five percent of the examined neoplasms were argyrophilic, while the remainder stained positive for argentaffin positivity. Over 80% showed a positive staining for chromogranin, Leu-7, and neuron-specific enolase. In addition, 47% of these duodenal carcinoids were positive for somatostatin, 56% for gastrin, 39% for serotonin, 19% for calcitonin, while fewer than 5% were positive for either insulin, pancreatic polypeptide, adrenocorticotropic hormone, or glucagon. That the immunocytochemical profile of duodenal carcinoids is similar to that of normal duodenal mucosa lends credence to the previously noted position that mucosal endocrine cells are the site of origin for transformed carcinoid precursors.

Negative prognostic features associated with metastases in duodenal carcinoids include tumor size of >2 cm, involvement of the muscularis propria, and the presence of mitotic figures (59). Small duodenal carcinoids may be resected endoscopically with good outcome, although bleeding is a common hazard.

Small lesions of <2 cm should ideally be aggressively treated, although the ability of an individual patient to withstand a pancreatico-duodenal resection requires careful consideration. In the case of larger lesions a similar policy may be adopted, although the likelihood of metastases usually precludes curative resection. Occasionally the endoscopic biopsy of a small (<0.5 cm) "suspicious" nodule in the duodenum may yield the diagnosis of carcinoid tumor. Endoscopic excision may be considered in such circumstances, although there is little formal data to support such an option. In elderly or unfit persons, however, this consideration may be reasonable.

7.5 Jejunum and Ileum

The prognosis of small bowel carcinoids reflects the malignant nature of the tumor with early dissemination to both lymph nodes and the liver. Jejuno-ileal carcinoids, in particular, have a relatively poor 5-year survival rate (55%) compared with other gastrointestinal carcinoids. One explanation may derive from the fact that carcinoids of the rectum, the duodenum, and the stomach are now detectable earlier by endoscopy, whereas jejuno-ileal carcinoids are only evident when they become symptomatic. These mid-bowel lesions often exhibit transmural invasion and metastases at the time of diagnosis. The overall male:female ratio for carcinoid of the small intestine is 1.10 (44). Incidence among white males is 0.67 per 100,000 population per year (1.28 among African American males). Incidence among white females is somewhat lower, with an analogous increased incidence among African American females as well: 0.48 and 0.76 per 100,000 population per year, respectively (14,16).

The clinical presentation of jejuno-ileal carcinoids differs from those occurring in other sites of the gut. Such tumors are usually at an advanced stage at the time of presentation; in many instances they are detected at surgery for unexplained bowel obstruction or during exploration of the small bowel in search of a primary tumor once distant metastases have been detected. However, in the majority of individuals the diagnosis of carcinoid is not made prior to surgery. The carcinoid syndrome is reported to occur in up to 18% of patients with jejuno-ileal carcinoids (60); this is rarely evident in carcinoids of the duodenum.

Extensive liver metastases without a carcinoid syndrome may also occur. This suggests the nonsecretory nature of certain tumors. An association with other noncarcinoid neoplasms is evident in 16.6% of distal small bowel carcinoids and constitutes the largest percentage of such incidence among all gastrointestinal carcinoids.

Jejunal and ileal carcinoids typically display an insular growth pattern (type I), which consists of solid nests or cords of cells with clearly defined boundaries (55). The trabecular pattern (type II) consists of narrow cell bands forming ribbons and regularly anastomosing along a highly differentiated vascular network. The third type demonstrates a glandular pattern, consisting of cells arranged in alveolar, acinar, or rosette patterns with glandular cavities or pseudocavities. Type IV and V carcinoids consist of undifferentiated and mixed cells, respectively. The frequency of multicentricity lies between 26 and 30% (55,61).

Lundqvist and Wilander (62) describe endocrine cell hyperplasia and small proliferating endocrine cell aggregates within the mucosal crypts in association with the small intestinal carcinoids, suggesting that such lesions originate from an intraepithelially located endocrine cell and subsequently infiltrate through the basement membrane into the lamina propria. Transmural invasion is a common feature contributing to the aggressive clinical behavior of the neoplasm. The tumor cells characteristically display arggrophilic and argentaffin positivity, and the vast majority of all small bowel carcinoids are "classical" ileal carcinoids, with production of serotonin and substance P. Enteroglucagon-, pancreatic polypeptide–, and peptide YY–producing tumors are exceptionally rare. In addition, over 85% of distal small bowel tumors exhibit positive reactions for chromogranin, Leu-7, neuron-specific enolase, and serotonin (55). Carcinoembryonic antigen is present in about two thirds of ileal and jejunal carcinoids, prostatic acid phosphatase in about 20%, and S-100 protein in 7%.

In jejuno-ileal carcinoids, several factors have been postulated as predictors of their relatively malignant nature, including distant metastases at the time of surgery, rate of mitosis, lesion multiplicity, female gender, depth of invasion, and the presence of carcinoid syndrome (55). Tumor size is the most predictive correlate for the frequency of nonlocalized disease.

In general, the carcinoid syndrome is clinically apparent once hepatic metastases are present; this initiates clinical investigation. The 5-year survival rate of patients with hepatic tumor spread is 20–30%. An increased median survival (4.4 years) is evident in patients with jejuno-ileal carcinoids exhibiting a mixed insular and glandular histological pattern (63). In contrast, patients with an undifferentiated cellular atypia have a median survival of only 6 months. In lesions with pure insular and trabecular patterns, an intermediate prognosis is evident, with a median survival time of 2.9 and 2.5 years, respectively.

Metastatic spread to the regional lymph nodes is often noted at the time of diagnosis of the small bowel carcinoid. Thus, wide resection of the primary tumor, including regional lymph nodes, is advisable. Since multicentric lesions, liver metastases, and other noncarcinoid malignancies may occur, a careful search should be undertaken at surgery even in the presence of a small primary tumor. Even if liver metastases are present at diagnosis during surgery, the primary tumor should be resected to avoid complications such as bowel obstruction, bleeding, and perforation.

7.6 Appendix

Although appendiceal carcinoids were previously recognized as the most frequently occurring carcinoid tumors, their relative frequency appears to have decreased over time (4.7–18.9% of all carcinoid tumors and 7.4–25.7% of all gastrointestinal carcinoids) (16). This may be secondary to a decreased surgical commitment to appendectomy over the past two decades In addition, the relative frequency of appendiceal carcinoids compared with all tumors of the appendix has decreased over the past 30 years, from 40% to 15.2% during the most recent decade (44). Identification of an appendiceal carcinoid occurs in 5–6 per 1000 appendectomies (6), but the exact incidence is not known because many such lesions remain asymptomatic.

Berge and Linell identified appendiceal carcinoids in 0.04% of individuals in an autopsy series of 16,294 cases between 1958 and 1969 (54). The true number is assumed to be much higher, as the use of immunocytochemistry to detect neuroendocrine lesions is a relatively recent development. Although a marked female predominance (over 80%) has been reported, one series of 820 patients revealed an age-adjusted male:female ratio of only 0.47 (22). Appendiceal carcinoids present in a younger patient population than other gastrointestinal carcinoid tumors, with a median age of 42.2 years, reflecting the role of appendectomy in the identification of such lesions (16,64).

A minority of these tumors present with signs and symptoms of acute appendicitis; the carcinoid syndrome is very rarely observed. In such circumstances, these symptoms are usually associated with widespread metastases of the primary tumor, predominantly to the liver or retroperitoneum.

Appendiceal carcinoids may be divided into two types: EC-cell argentaffin carcinoids and nonargentaffin L-cell tumors, with the majority of lesions identified as EC-cell tumors producing serotonin and substance P and exhibiting a typical insular pattern. The nonargentaffin L-cell tumors are much less common, producing glicentin-related peptides (enteroglucagons), pancreatic polypeptide, and peptide YY, and usually have a trabecular growth pattern. Occasional instances of positive immunostaining for vasoactive intestinal polypeptide (VIP) and adrenocorticotropic hormone (ACTH) have been reported. A variant of the true appendiceal carcinoid is the so-called mucinous carcinoid or adenocarcinoid. These mixed lesions exhibit macroscopic similarities to true carcinoids, but possess morphological features suggestive of both carcinoid and glandular differentiation. The growth of appendiceal carcinoids is exclusively in the lamina propria, beneath the epithelial crypt of the submucosa, and in the lamina muscularis mucosa; these lesions appear to have a relatively benign clinical and biological nature. In 1928, Masson identified the subepithelial Kulchitsky cells as the origin of appendiceal carcinoid tumors and demonstrated that these cells exhibit both endocrine and neural characteristics (65). With modern immunocytochemical techniques it has been demonstrated that these subepithelial neurosecretory cells are an integral part of the subepithelial nerve plexus. Shaw et al. (66) provided further evidence of the neuroectodermal origin of appendiceal carcinoids, reporting that subepithelial neuroendocrine cells of the appendix were more numerous towards the tip, while epithelial neuroendocrine cells were evenly distributed throughout the organ. This is consistent with the observation that 70–80% of appendiceal carcinoids occur at the tip, 5–20% in the body, and only 7–8% at the base of the organ. The complete absence of subepithelial neuroendocrine cells in the appendiceal specimens surgically removed from patients with total aganglionosis further supports this concept of neural origin.

Appendiceal carcinoid patients are generally young, and it is noteworthy that in the Mayo Clinic series the patients with larger tumors and metastases were younger (29 years) than those with smaller and clinically benign lesions (42 years) (67). Associated noncarcinoid tumors are evident in 17.9% of lesions, the third highest percentage in the gastrointestinal tract after small intestinal and gastric carcinoids.

Carcinoid tumors of the appendix are usually discovered as an incidental finding during surgery performed for other reasons. The diagnosis is often made at laparotomy or laparoscopy, undertaken to evaluate nonspecific symptoms or for those of appendicitis.

Patients with appendiceal carcinoids have the best prognosis among all types of carcinoids, and the relatively benign course of these tumors may reflect either the anatomical site of the lesion, its early detection and removal, or the biology of the tumor itself. The most predictive determinants of survival are the factors that influence metastatic development; in this respect, the size of the primary tumor is the most reliable determinant of the risk of metastases. Appendiceal carcinoids smaller than 2.0 cm rarely metastasize (< 3%), while the risk of metastatic spread is considerably higher in lesions of >2.0 cm (30–60%) (67). Furthermore, the metastatic potential depends greatly upon the depth of penetration and the site of origin. Mesoappendiceal invasion is reported to occur more frequently in patients with distant and lymph node metastases. However, some reports have suggested that the invasion of the mesoappendix is not a reliable predictor of metastatic potential (68,69).

Surgery is the treatment of choice in carcinoids of the appendix. Lesions of <1.0 cm have an exceedingly small risk of metastatic spread, and simple appendectomy without further follow-up is generally accepted as the most appropriate treatment (67,70). In tumors >2.0 cm, a more aggressive resection, consisting of a right hemicolectomy or ileocolectomy and lymph node dissection, is ideal. The same procedures should be performed in tumors with vascular invasion, involvement of the mesoappendix, or nodal spread (71). Right hemicolectomy has also been advocated in cases of appendiceal carcinoids involving the base of the organ. However, instances of patients with incomplete excision of tumors of the base of the appendix remaining disease-free for 17–30 years after the operation have been reported (72,73). In elderly patients or those at high operative risk, a simple appendectomy may be justified, even when the lesion is larger than 2.0 cm. For appendiceal carcinoids 1.0–2.0 cm in size, the appropriate treatment depends on several factors. A more radical approach is recommended in the following circumstances: younger patients, tumor extension into the mesoappendix, lymphatic metastases, or tumor location near the base of the appendix. The 5-year survival rates for localized lesions, regional spread, and distant metastases are 90.7, 81.5, and 28.2%, respectively (44).

7.7 Meckel's Diverticulum

The most common developmental abnormality of the gastrointestinal tract, Meckel's diverticulum is a vestigial remnant of the omphalomesenteric duct. Johann Friedrich Meckel (74) reported this anomaly in 1809, although the German surgeon Wilhelm Fabry of Hilden is noted to have reported this unusual diverticulum of the small intestine in 1598 (75). In 1962 Thorek (76) described his theory of Meckel's diverticula (now seen only as a first-order approximation) as follows: 2% of the population, 2 feet from the ileocecal valve, 2 inches in length, 2 times as common in males compared to females, 2 types of ectopic tissue (gastric and pancreatic), and 2 types of complication (hemorrhage and inflammation). After sarcoma, carcinoids are the second most common tumor arising from Meckel's diverticula (77). Three fourths of patients with Meckel's diverticulum carcinoid are male (78). Roughly 50% of patients with known liver metastases develop symptoms of the carcinoid syndrome. Common symptoms among such patients include abdominal pain (33%), diarrhea (19%), gastrointestinal bleeding (19%), weight loss (11%), and nausea or emesis (8%) (78). Meckel's diverticula are unusual sites for both benign and malignant neoplasms (79); the incidence of carcinoid in a Meckel's diverticulum is between 0.3 and 1.7%. Seventy percent of patients with carcinoid of Meckel's diverticula are diagnosed at laparotomy. Overall 5-year survival is 50% but decreases to 21% with liver metastases (80). Multiple synchronous diverticular lesions have also been noted (81). Metastases to lymph nodes and the liver are noted in approximately 25% of diverticular carcinoid cases. Since most of these lesions are found by chance and are often small, surgical management of noncomplicated diverticular carcinoid includes simple excision of the diverticulum and a wedge of adjoining mesentery. Larger lesions should be treated using the principles applied to the management of ileal carcinoid tumors.

7.8 Colon

Carcinoid tumors of the colon comprise 4.4–13% of all carcinoid cases and occur most frequently (39–47%) in the cecum (82,83). It is probable that some cecal lesions are initially of appendiceal origin and have extended into the cecum. A female predominance is noted, with a male:female ratio of 0.66. The average age at the time of diagnosis is 70 years (16).

Around 6% of patients with colonic carcinoids are asymptomatic (84). The remainder of patients typically complain of abdominal pain, ranging from vague and generalized to severe. Over half of patients complain of nonspecific symptoms such as weight loss and weakness, but occasionally diarrhea or rectal bleeding may occur, suggesting a tumor location distal to the hepatic flexure. Diarrhea as a part of the carcinoid syndrome itself is very rare (3%) in these patients.

In general, carcinoids of the colon resemble those of the rectum. However, colonic lesions exhibit a more undifferentiated pattern with clinically more aggressive features, whereas well-differentiated histological patterns, such as insular, trabecular, and glandular types, are less common.

Size criteria are of little use in the assessment of the prognosis of colonic carcinoid tumors, since the majority of these lesions exceed a size of 2.0 cm and involve the muscularis propria at presentation (84). As such, colonic carcinoids exhibit the poorest prognosis among all gastrointestinal carcinoid tumors, with an overall 5-year survival of only 33–42%. Nuclear mitotic rate, overall tumor grade, and the histological pattern of the neoplasm also influence survival. Associated noncarcinoid tumors occur in 18.9% of patients (16).

Diagnosis of colonic carcinoid is usually made by colonoscopy and biopsy, though occasionally a double-contrast barium enema may be of use.

A local excision can only be recommended in the minority of patients who present with a tumor size of <2.0 cm. Analysis of Connecticut tumor registry data noted that only one out of six tumors with a size of >2 cm was nonlocalized, whereas metastases were evident in more than two thirds of patients with a tumor of >2 cm in diameter (82). With this, a wide resection, including lymph node dissection, is advocated for most patients. Excision should follow the principles of colonic adenocarcinoma resection.

7.9 Rectum

Rectal carcinoids comprise 21.2% of all carcinoid tumors and represent the second largest group of gut carcinoids. No specific gender predominance is noted; the average age at diagnosis is markedly lower than for colonic carcinoids (56.7 vs. 70 years) (14,16). The age-adjusted incidence rates of rectal carcinoids is three to four times higher in African Americans compared to American white populations.

Approximately 50% of patients with rectal carcinoids are asymptomatic. When complaints are present, they usually manifest as a discomfort in the anorectal area, with some degree of constipation, bleeding, or a change in bowel habits. Rarely, rectal pain and pruritus ani may occur. In general, rectal carcinoids identified as small, mobile, submucosal nodules or focal areas of submucosal thickening and are typically first observed after a bleeding episode and subsequent endoscopy.

Although metastatic spread is a common feature in colonic carcinoids (yielding the second highest percentage of nonlocalized lesions at the time of diagnosis of all carcinoid tumors), rectal carcinoids present with metastasis in only 7–20% of cases (44). Tumors larger than 1.0 cm are more likely to have metastasized at the time of diagnosis (Table 1). Rectal carcinoids are associated with noncarcinoid tumors in 15.6% of cases.

Macroscopically, rectal carcinoid lesions are usually nodular, though occasionally they may be polypoid or sessile (85). The most common histological pattern is that of the ribbon type, followed by mixed and acinar patterns. On light microscopy, rectal carcinoid cells are small to intermediate in size, arranged in clusters, and typically demonstrate extensive necrosis. At the ultrastructural level, neurosecretory granules 80–200 nm in diameter are occasionally observed. Rarely, mucus-secreting cells may be found, and may even obfuscate diagnosis of a pure carcinoid tumor in some instances. Occasionally, rarer forms of carcinoids, such as goblet cell carcinoids and adenocarcinoids, are identified.

Although most carcinoids of the rectum immunohistochemically exhibit numerous amines and peptides in parallel to the normal mucosa of the rectum, presentation with clinical symptoms or the carcinoid syndrome is very rare (86). The majority of such tumors are argyrophil-positive by the Grimelius stain; only a few are argentaffin-positive. Immunohistochemical identification in rectal carcinoids of somatostatin, glicentin, pancreatic polypeptide, peptide YY, enkephalin, endorphin, and serotonin has been described. Prostate-specific acid phosphatase is expressed by rectal carcinoids, and occasionally these tumors may also exhibit high levels of serotonin or glucagon (87,88). They display moderate neurofilament staining, and more than 70% stain positive for chromogranins. More than 50% of rectal carcinoids stain positively for neuron-specific enolase, although the pattern of staining may be quite variable. There is a marked variability in staining with S-100 and Leu-7, in contrast to the positive reaction exhibited by carcinoid tumors of the foregut and midgut. Classic tumor markers, such as CA 19-9, CA 50, carcinoembryonic antigen, and α-fetoprotein (AFP), are consistently absent (89).

Several parameters have been suggested as predictive criteria in the assessment of the malignant nature of rectal carcinoid neoplasms, including tumor size, histological growth pattern (90), histological microinvasiveness, presenting symptoms, and DNA ploidy (91). Of these, tumor size and microinvasiveness are the two most important prognostic factors (18).

On physical examination, findings are usually nonspecific; digital rectal examination is mandatory, as this may occasionally detect a tumor mass. Since most rectal vault tumors lie in the anterior and lateral portions of the lower one third of the rectum, the majority of such tumors are amenable to palpation. Nonetheless, most tumors are identified during proctoscopy and sigmoidoscopy.

Due to their low propensity to metastasize, rectal carcinoids have a relatively favorable prognosis, with a 5-year survival rate of 82% (Table 2). Approximately 80% of rectal carcinoid lesions are < 1.0 cm in size, submucosal, and show no metastatic spread; for such lesions a minor procedure (proctoscopic or transanal resection) can be advocated (92). For tumors 1.0–2.0 cm in size (approximately 10% of cases) without evidence of lymph node metastasis, a wide excision with a meticulous evaluation to exclude muscular invasion is recommended.

If the neoplasm is ≥2.0 cm (10% of cases) or muscular invasion or lymph node metastases are present, radical surgery (low anterior resection with total mesorectal excision, or abdomino-perineal resection) should be performed. The management of patients with rectal carcinoids >2.0 cm with hepatic and lymph node me-

Table 1 Relationship Between Carcinoid Tumor Size and Percentage Cases with Metastatic Spread by Site

	Metastatic spread (%)					
	Tumor < 1 cm		Tumor 1–2 cm		Tumor > 2 cm	
	LN	Liver	LN	Liver	LN	Liver
Stomach	0	0	0	0	100	100
Small intestine	17	9	64	16	82	58
Appendix	0	0	3	0	21	24
Colon	—	—	13	25	79	39
Rectum	3	0	7	7	64	45

LN = lymph node metastases; Liver = liver metastases.
Source: Ref. 18.

Table 2 Five-Year Survival Rates of Carcinoid Tumors of the Foregut, Midgut, and Hindgut

	5-year survival (%)				
Carcinoid site	Localized	Regional	Distant	Unstaged	All stages
Foregut (stomach, liver, GB, pancreas, trachea/bronchi/lung)	80.0 ± 0.9	68.7 ± 2.0	18.2 ± 2.3	56.4 ± 3.0	70.0 ± 0.8
Foregut (GI sites only)	65.6 ± 2.9	27.9 ± 6.8	17.4 ± 3.7	59.6 ± 4.8	51.3 ± 2.2
Midgut (small intestine, appendix, colon)	67.1 ± 1.3	65.8 ± 1.3	35.6 ± 1.5	49.8 ± 3.4	57.0 ± 0.8
Midgut (small intestine, appendix)	65.8 ± 1.5	68.8 ± 1.4	39.7 ± 1.8	43.0 ± 4.1	59.1 ± 29.6
Hindgut (rectum)	87.4 ± 1.2	40.9 ± 7.6	24.9 ± 6.5	77.7 ± 3.7	81.8 ± 1.2
Hindgut [colon (except appendix), rectum]	84.7 ± 1.1	50.8 ± 2.9	23.7 ± 2.3	73.1 ± 3.0	68.4 ± 1.0

Source: Ref. 44.

tastases should be analogous to that for other neoplasms with similar metastases. Local excision to prevent bleeding, tenesmus, and obstruction is reasonable if surgical therapy is directed in a palliative fashion. The role of various chemotherapeutic agents is limited, but streptozotocin, 5-fluorouracil, doxorubicin, ß-interferon, and cyclosphosphamide have all been utilized with at best modest benefit (86).

7.10 Liver

Hepatic carcinoids are commonly found in association with metastatic spread of neoplasms originating at distant sites such as the appendix, small intestine, or rectum (18). In contrast, primary carcinoid tumors of the liver are exceptionally rare clinical entities, with only 43 cases described in the literature (20,93–95), comprising only 0.41% of all carcinoid lesions (44). Carcinoids of the liver present in a characteristically young population (42.2 ± 16.6 years) (17); the reason for this age distribution is unclear. No specific gender predominance for primary hepatic carcinoids is noted.

The signs and clinical symptoms of hepatic carcinoids—either primary or metastatic—are related to the destruction of viable hepatic parenchyma by the tumor mass, such as pain, a palpable mass, gastric outlet obstruction, and weight loss. Interestingly, the carcinoid syndrome occurs in only 22% of these patients (16).

Histologically, carcinoids of the liver resemble well-differentiated hepatocellular carcinomas, which may complicate an initial diagnosis. Hepatic carcinoids are usually characterized by the presence of biogenic amines, which may be visualized by formaldehyde-induced fluorescence. In addition, electron microscopy may be performed to confirm the diagnosis (96). Carcinoids can be distinguished from hepatocellular carcinomas by the existence of membrane-bound secretory granules within tumor cells (dense core granules 100—200 nm in diameter), nuclear monomorphism, and Grimelius-positive cytoplasmic granules. It has been suggested that neuroendocrine cells within bile ducts may migrate into intrahepatic ducts and give rise to the neuroendocrine tumor; other theories propose that neuroendocrine differentiation occurs in malignant stem cells.

The diagnosis of hepatic carcinoid tumors is often challenging by diagnostic imaging alone, as a variety of other hepatic lesions may resemble carcinoid disease. The typical ultrasonographic finding is that of a hyperechoic mass with multiple cystic lesions. Computed tomography often reveals low-density, moderately enhancing areas, which demonstrate a cystic pattern. Angiography, now only rarely employed in the detection of carcinoid lesions, can demonstrate multiple hypervascular and centrally located radiolucent areas within the liver. In the past, percutaneous fine needle aspiration (FNA) or needle biopsy followed by immunological and electron microscopic (EM) assessments were recommended for diagnosis. However, transhepatic access is a potentially dangerous procedure for neoplasms such as biliary cystadenocarcinoma (97), and these maneuvers have fallen out of favor. Since secondary hepatic carcinoids exceed primary lesions by far, a careful search for primary disease must be undertaken. Abdominal and chest CT imaging, bronchoscopy, and hepatic venous sampling may be appropriate procedures prior to a careful intraoperative exploration.

Most patients undergoing surgery exhibit a favorable outcome (5-year survival of 53%). The survival rate for patients receiving multimodal therapy is similar to that of those patients treated by surgery alone, although the number of such patients is low (98).

gamma camera, uptake is recorded at 4 hours postadministration, and further studies may be undertaken at 24 and (rarely) 48 hours, by which time renal and hepatic background activity has significantly dissipated. The associated use of single positron emission computed tomography (SPECT) imaging provides further enhancement of the sensitivity of this study and precise identification of lesions that are either occult or unsuspected. That the entire body can be imaged at one time is of considerable advantage since it enables the detection of covert lesions, which might otherwise be either undetectable (outside of an evaluated area) or require multiple (expensive and time consuming) different imaging studies for identification.

In the identification of extrahepatic tumors, the sensitivity of SRS alone is equal to that of conventional imaging methods (CT and MRI) combined (112). The combination of the use of conventional imaging methods in addition to SRS results in the identification of over 95% of hepatic metastases (Fig. 4); it has been reported that undertaking an Octreoscan leads to an alteration in therapeutic plan for up to 20% of patients.

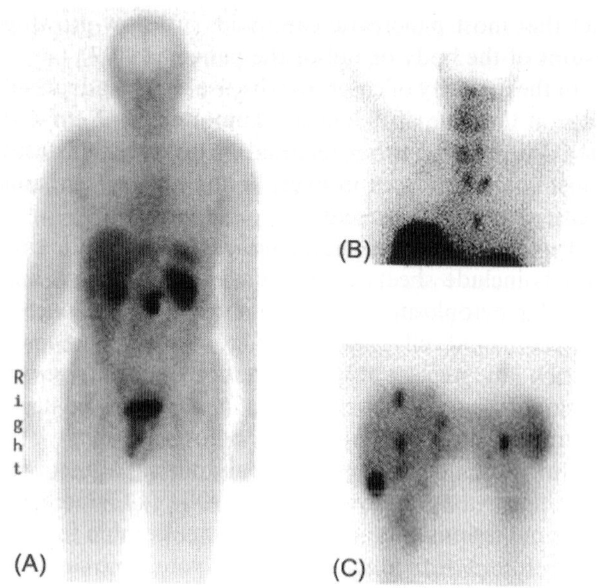

Figure 4 Octreoscan scintigraphy is advantageous in that one scan is capable of providing a whole-body image. Thus, localization of primary disease and metastases can be undertaken in a single study. (A) Anterior view of ^{111}In-pentetreotide scintigram demonstrates a solitary gastrinoma just to the left of midline at the level of the inferior pole of the left kidney. The presence of tracer in the liver, spleen, kidneys, and urinary bladder is normal. (B) Multiple chest metastases expressing SST_R2; the primary was an ileal carcinoid. (C) Diffuse hepatic gastrinoma metastases in a planar SPECT image.

8.2 Invasive Studies

8.2.1 Endoscopic Ultrasonography

EUS, in experienced hands, is of particular utility in determining the extent of carcinoid tumors of the duodenum and stomach; it is also especially useful in the identification of small tumors in the pancreatic head and the localization of duodenal microcarcinoids (usually <1 cm), since these are often submucosal and cannot be visualized with endoscopy alone. EUS has an overall sensitivity of 80–85% and specificity of approximately 95%, although the technique is substantially user dependent (117).

8.2.2 Intraoperative Ultrasonography

IOUS is performed by the operating surgeon, often with the assistance of an ultrasonographer. It has become a technique of considerable utility, allowing the surgeon not only to confirm the site of very small pancreatic or hepatic lesions but to identify multicentricity and otherwise occult lesions that may be too small to palpate.

8.2.3 Portal Venous Sampling

In the majority of cases this time-consuming, expensive, and technically difficult procedure does not specifically localize the tumor but provides only evidence of a region of interest. In patients who have had previous surgery and in whom a recurrence is suspected, the development of post-surgical collateral vessels may complicate the interpretation of such a study. This procedure is rarely recommended and is indicated only in unusual circumstances.

8.2.4 Selective and Provocative Angiography

Selective angiography can provide a reasonable degree of localization of lesions within the pancreas or liver. Provocative angiography involves the injection of calcium or pentagastrin into the hepatic, gastroduodenal, superior mesenteric, and splenic arteries, while serial blood samples from the hepatic and peripheral veins are assayed for hormone levels (118). The invasive nature of these procedures is not without risk, but in situations which are otherwise difficult to resolve angiography may be warranted.

9 THERAPY OVERVIEW

9.1 Pharmacological Management

9.1.1 Cytotoxic Drugs

Medical management of the carcinoid tumor has focused on cytotoxic drugs and pharmacological control of the bioactive products of the tumor. Several cytostatic regimens have been utilized to treat patients with carcinoid syndrome, and response rates of 20–40% have been reported with the combination of streptozotocin and doxorubicin in selected small groups of patients. Used individually, these agents, as well as 5-fluorouracil and cyclophosphamide, have been disappointing (119). Etoposide may be more effective, either alone or in combination with cisplatin (120). Overall, chemotherapeutic responses have not proven durable. In addition, the side effects of cytotoxic therapy often outweigh its transient benefits. The low efficacy of these chemotherapeutic drugs may be secondary to the low proliferative rate of carcinoid tumors.

9.1.2 Recombinant Drug Therapy

Recombinant leukocyte α-interferon may be of some use in the treatment of disseminated carcinoid tumors and carcinoid syndrome (121), although it is associated with significant toxic side effects in some individuals. It can ameliorate flushing and diarrhea and may even induce a degree of tumor regression in some patients (122).

Initial trials with human leukocyte interferon appeared promising (123). Nearly half of all patients demonstrated a biochemical response, whereas an additive effect was observed in patients who also underwent hepatic arterial embolization (124). More recently, however, other investigators have reported that the effects of α-interferon on midgut carcinoid tumors are transient and accompanied by substantial side effects (125). The loss of durability in the interferon response may relate to the development of neutralizing antibodies (126). Preliminary reports suggest that the combination of interferon with octreotide is more advantageous than monotherapy.

9.1.3 Somatostatin Analogues

The somatostatin analogue octreotide has enabled control of many of the symptoms of carcinoid syndrome. Given its minimal side effects, the improvement in quality of life has been highly significant and there is evidence that a degree of arrest of tumor growth also occurs in some patients (127). Octreotide has also been found to be effective in the management of carcinoid crisis, which is characterized by profound hypotension and tachycardia often associated with mortality (128).

Carcinoid Syndrome. Although its potential chemotherapeutic value has not yet been defined, octreotide is clearly the most effective means of ameliorating carcinoid syndrome. Its pharmacological activities are diverse. Octreotide inhibits the release and synthesis of bioactive agents from the carcinoid tumor (129) and induces inhibitory G-proteins with action on the intracellular signaling of amines and peptides. Octreotide also possesses potent preabsorptive actions in the gastrointestinal tract, which may diminish the secretory diarrhea of the carcinoid syndrome. Although Dharmsathaphorn et al. (130) reported as early as 1980 that somatostatin inhibited carcinoid flushing and diarrhea, the clinical application of this observation was limited by the 1- to 2-minute biological half-life of native somatostatin. The long-acting stable synthetic somatostatin analogues octreotide (previously identified as SMS 201-995) and RC-160 have eliminated this shortcoming. The octapeptide octreotide shares with native somatostatin the Phe-Trp-Lys-Thr amino acid sequence that confers biological activity but resists proteolysis because the first and fourth of these amino acids have been replaced by D-stereoisomeric forms. Octreotide has a 90- to 120-minute half-life and may therefore be used clinically by subcutaneous injection on a twice or three times-daily schedule.

Carcinoid Crisis. Octreotide is also currently the agent of choice for prophylaxis of the carcinoid crisis (24). Patients with carcinoid tumors may exhibit profound hypotension or bronchospasm on induction of general anesthesia or manipulation of the tumor due to release of bioactive agents from the lesion (33). Carcinoid crisis may also occur during the initiation of chemotherapy, during arterial embolization, or during fine needle biopsy of a liver metastasis (131). The carcinoid crisis is probably elicited by stress-associated endogenous catecholamines, which, in turn, stimulate secretion of carcinoid tumor products (33). Pretreatment with octreotide prevents these reactions and antagonizes the effects of such products in established crisis situations. Octreotide should be administered in doses of 100–400 μg subcutaneously before, during, and after embolization, surgery, or other tumor manipulation. Prior evaluation by pentagastrin provocation tests may be used to document adequate protection against provoked release of hormones (33). If somatostatin blockade has not been employed and a carcinoid crisis occurs during tumor manipulation, 100 μg of octreotide should be injected intravenously.

Antitumor Activity. Laboratory observations have stimulated interest in the use of somatostatin analogues as antineoplastic agents. Somatostatin has been reported to inhibit centromere separation stimulated by epidermal growth factor, as well as DNA replication and cell division (132). Octreotide has been shown to inhibit the growth of human pancreatic cancer cells implanted into nude mice (133). Such laboratory observations have paralleled occasional reports of tumor arrest or shrinkage in patients with somatostatin receptor–bearing pancreatic islet cell tumors and metastatic carcinoids treated with somatostatin analogues (134). However, antineoplastic clinical use of somatostatin analogues must await larger clinical trials.

Dosing and Administration. Octreotide may be administered initially at 100–200 μg subcutaneously twice daily and then increased as needed up to 1500 μg/d in divided doses with minimal side effects. This treatment regimen has been reported to decrease urinary 5-HIAA concentrations and control diarrhea in 85% of patients (135). The carcinoid flush is also usually moderated by this therapy, although bronchospasm may be a more persistent problem. Delineation of the effects of octreotide on the cardiac aspects of the carcinoid syndrome must await longer follow-up. More recently, depot or long-acting repeatable (LAR) analogues (136) have proven to be as clinically efficacious as octreotide with the advantage of requiring only monthly injection.

9.1.4 Receptor-Mediated Isotope Therapy

^{111}Indium Pentetreotide. Radiolabeled somatostatin analogues target neuroendocrine and other tumors, such as carcinoid, which express high levels of type 2 somatostatin receptor (SST_R2). We have previously reported ^{111}In-pentetreotide scintigraphy to have a sensitivity and specificity of 75% and 100%, respectively, for the localization of gastroenteropancreatic tumors (137).

Modlin et al. (137) have conducted a phase I/II trial to evaluate the therapeutic safety of ^{111}In-DTPA-octreotide (^{111}In-pentetreotide) in the treatment of gastroenteropancreatic tumors (GÉPT). Patients with unresectable advanced malignancy, at least one tumor bearing site documented by ^{111}In-pentetreotide uptake, and no further conventional therapeutic options were included. Four cycles of ^{111}In-labeled pentetreotide at one of three radiation dose levels were administered to 39 patients, who were scrupulously monitored for changes in hematological and renal function profile as well as evidence of disease progression. Follow-up included frequent phlebotomy, follow-up octreotide scintigraphy, and biannual computed tomography.

A majority of the 39 patients enrolled in this therapeutic safety trial experienced only mild or moderate side effects, including transient myelosuspression. One patient developed transient acute renal tubular necrosis but successfully underwent six cycles of radiotherapy without developing renal failure. Of evaluable patients with gastroenteropancreatic disease, 77% demonstrated radiographic stability or modest improvement of disease, 80% had stable or improved symptoms, and 56% experienced stability or a notable decrease in at least one measured tumor hormone marker over the course of therapy. The hematological and renal safety as well as the therapeutic efficacy of radiolabeled pentetreotide at divided doses of only 300 mCi suggest that higher doses of this agent, or perhaps other higher-energy emitters, could be used safely for the treatment of otherwise untreatable neuroendocrine tumors.

Alternative Isotopes. A further consideration is the development of alternative isotopes with different radioemission profiles which may confer improved tumoricidal effect. The use of isotopes with potentially superior therapeutic properties such as yttrium (138) or lutetium (139) is currently under study, and preliminary results are promising. It is likely that intravenous isotopic therapy may become a major therapeutic strategy in dealing with metastatic carcinoid disease. The use of pentetreotide labeled with ^{90}yttrium, which emits higher-energy β-particles and has greater tissue penetration than that of ^{111}indium (140,141), may potentially lead to a higher delivery of radiation to a larger part of a tumor expressing SST_R2. Trials with this agent have been conducted in xenografts (142) and have recently have been initiated in humans. Similarly, it may also be possible to link more than one isotope to the receptor ligand and thus target the tumor with a cocktail of isotopes with varying tissue penetrations.

9.2 Surgery

Although the introduction of octreotide has proven to be a major advance in the clinical management of the carcinoid syndrome, surgery remains the most effective treatment for both local tumor effects and symptoms caused by the secretory agents. The precise surgical management depends on the localization and size of the lesion.

Site-specific guidelines for surgical therapy of carcinoid tumors throughout the gut are outlined above. In general, treatment consists of radical surgical excision of the tumor, although gastric (type I and II) and rectal carcinoids (and possibly duodenal carcinoids) may be managed with local excision. Overall 5-year survival is excellent for carcinoids of the appendix (81%) and rectum (82%), whereas small intestinal (55%), gastric (58%), and colonic carcinoids (60%) exhibit a far worse prognosis (Fig. 5). Five-year survival for gallbladder (41%) and pancreatic (36%) carcinoids is even more dismal (14).

9.2.1 Nonmetastatic Disease

The management of nonmetastatic carcinoid tumors is reasonably well accepted. Lesions in the ileum or right colon should be resected en bloc with regional mesenteric lymph node drainage. Tumors in the appendix < 1 cm in diameter are unlikely to be metastatic and may be treated by simple appendectomy. Tumors ≥2 cm are associated with a high incidence of regional spread and should be resected by formal right hemicolectomy (67). Patients with nonmetastatic carcinoid tumors in the second part of the duodenum have a better prognosis than those with similarly located duodenal adenocarcinomas and are therefore excellent candidates for pancreaticoduodenal resection if the patient's medical status is not a contraindication.

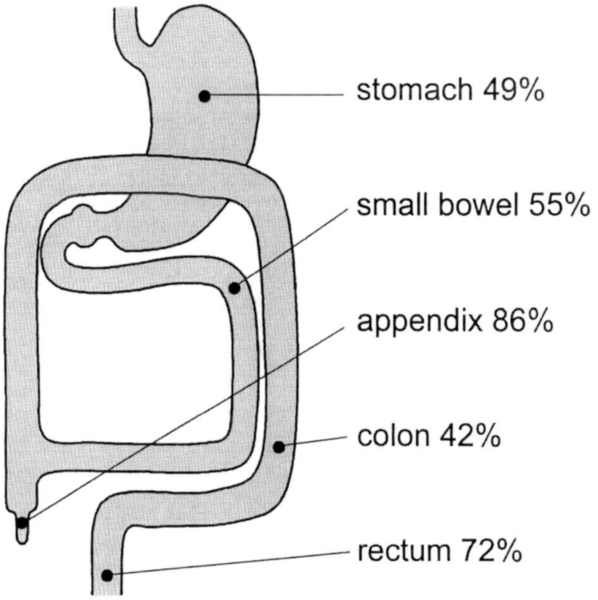

Figure 5 Overall 5-year survival rates of 10,878 carcinoid tumors by site. (From Ref. 44.)

9.2.2 Metastatic Disease

Palliative (Cytoreductive) Surgery. As a result of broader biochemical testing and improved diagnosis of the syndrome, substantial numbers of metastatic carcinoid tumors are identified without evidence of a primary tumor. Although a thorough search should be made for the primary tumor in patients with hepatic metastases, the course of the disease is generally dominated by the hepatic tumor burden. An undiscovered primary tumor is not likely to later become clinically significant, although occasionally lesions in the ileum may bleed, obstruct, or perforate (143).

Patients with carcinoid syndrome from hepatic metastases have a particularly poor quality of life, and surgical resection of tumor foci may reduce associated symptoms and improve survival. Aggressive interventional cytoreduction by hepatic resection or induced hepatic ischemia has therefore been proposed to decrease the hepatic tumor burden and palliate carcinoid symptoms (144). Cryosurgical debulking of hepatic carcinoid metastases has been described for palliation of carcinoid syndrome, but its efficacy awaits rigorous evaluation. Similarly, the use of high-energy radiofrequency probes has achieved some popularity. Both modalities require formal evaluation, and each has limitations in terms of damage to bile ducts and vessels.

Although as few as 10–25% of patients with hepatic metastases from carcinoid may be curable by conventional hepatic resection (145), anecdotal experience has suggested that debulking hepatic metastases may substantially palliate systemic symptoms of carcinoid or other endocrine tumors (146). Palliative resection may be considered when 90% of the tumor can be safely extirpated. McEntee et al. (147) reviewed their experience with aggressive cytoreductive hepatic resection in 37 patients, 24 of whom had carcinoid tumors with the remainder having islet cell tumors. Although significant palliation was achieved in most patients, the duration of palliation was short and a relatively high morbidity was encountered. Thus, although effective palliation may be achieved by aggressive cytoreductive partial hepatectomy, the benefits may be brief and the morbidity substantial.

Transplantation. Hepatic transplantation is currently undertaken in some centers provided that the patients are good surgical risks and have carcinoid metastases that appear curable only by total hepatectomy (148). This management option is potentially attractive since it offers cure rather than palliation to patients with these slowly growing tumors. However, although early results are promising, more data are needed before total hepatectomy can be advocated on a general basis (149).

9.2.3 Emergent Surgery

Carcinoid tumors may infrequently present with massive gastrointestinal bleeding, intussusception, and bowel obstruction from tumor or fibrosis (150). Mesenteric ischemia caused by fibrotic obstruction of the mesenteric vasculature (151) or retroperitoneal fibrosis (152) is sometimes identified. In each case, the primary intervention should be directed to the emergency that has required celiotomy. Since such patients are often acutely ill and unstable, it may be wise in emergency settings to defer definitive or extensive carcinoid tumor surgery until a second procedure. Arterial embolization may serve a role in patients for whom an open procedure may be too dangerous (153).

9.3 Minimally Invasive Intervention

Induced hepatic ischemia may achieve the palliative benefits of hepatic cytoreduction without its shortcomings. Ischemic treatment of carcinoid tumors of the liver is possible because these tumors are primarily supplied by the hepatic artery. Hepatic parenchyma can remain viable via portal vein perfusion despite hepatic arterial occlusion (154). Ischemia may be achieved by hepatic artery ligation, temporary occlusion, or embolization (Fig. 6). These methods differ in completeness, distribution, and duration of ischemia. In addition, surgical ligation has the disadvantage of preventing future angiographic access to the hepatic arterial tree for repeated induction of hepatic ischemia. Selective embolizations of hepatic artery branches cause complete but temporary ischemia by filling the distal arterial tree with embolization material.

Several centers have achieved satisfactory palliation of the midgut carcinoid syndrome by embolization and have reported parallel biochemical evidence of tumor necrosis (145,155,156). For instance, induced ischemia of hepatic lesions leads to a marked decrease in urinary excretion of 5-HIAA for at least 72 hours after embolization (145). Embolization has a high success rate in properly prepared and selected patients in centers that have accrued substantial experience with this procedure. In a Swedish series (145), one third of the patients who underwent bilateral embolizations showed biochemical normalization of tumor markers accompanied by a marked regression of the tumor. During a 5-year follow-up period, less than 10% of patients required repeat embolizations due to recurrence of symptoms. The use of embolization with associated cytotoxic agents (chemoembolization) has been studied but has yet to yield any significant advantages. However, hepatic artery embolization combined with sequential chemotherapy has been slightly more encouraging, with one trial documenting a reduction of tumor size in 78% of patients (157).

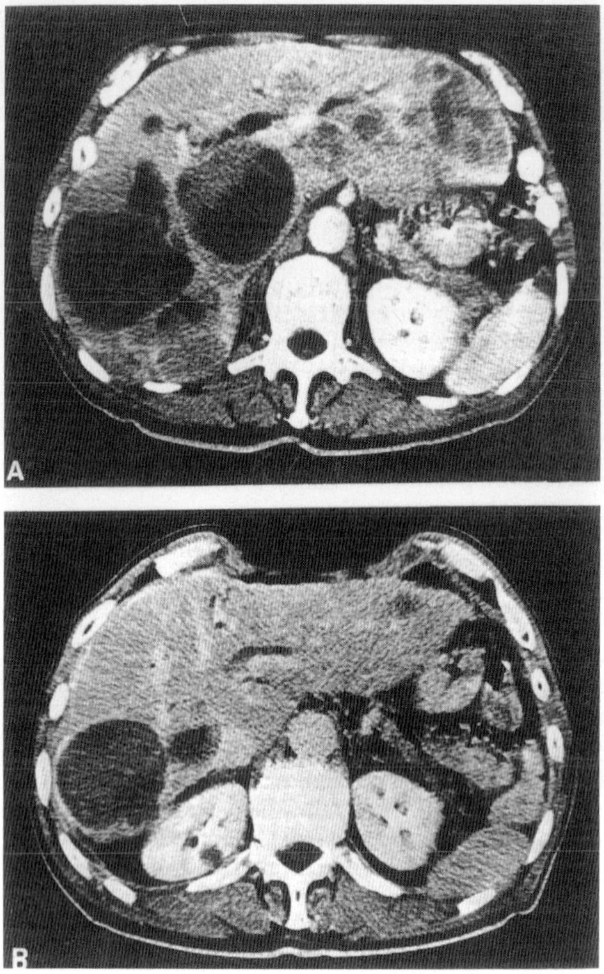

Figure 6 (A) Abdominal CT images of a 68-year-old patient with diffuse hepatic carcinoid metastases evident on preoperative scan. (B) Significant tumor regression is seen 3 years following open cytoreductive therapy, hepatic arterial embolization, and octreotide therapy. Note the dramatic reduction in hepatic left lateral segment size. (From Ref. 13.)

Side effects of embolization may include transient nausea, emesis, fever, and abdominal pain. Occasional paroxysmal episodes or major fluid shifts and alterations in cardiopulmonary function can be safely controlled by administration of octreotide. Although collateralization of the tumor arterial supply may cause recurrence of symptoms after either embolization or operative ligation, embolization may be repeated even in patients who are unable to tolerate a surgical procedure. Appropriate pharmacological preparation is essential to maximize the safety of such maneuvers.

It should be emphasized that hepatic embolization performed after carcinoid metastasis is already well established may result in little improvement in actual patient survival despite symptomatic palliation, although Mitty et al. (156) reported a 2-year increase in survival in 18 patients compared with historical controls. Earlier and repeated embolization with improved techniques that allow more distal and selective permanent embolization will probably result in better survival figures in the future (145). However, in patients in whom a curative resection is potentially achievable by unilobar hepatectomy, this should be attempted rather than a palliative embolization provided the medical condition of the patient permits.

10 TREATMENT ALGORITHM

A logical plan of management is likely to optimize the outcome for most patients. The choice among various treatment modalities for carcinoid disease must be individualized for each patient and reflect the experience of the team of physicians involved.

On initial suspicion of the carcinoid syndrome, patients should undergo a biochemical, radiological, and endoscopic workup designed to characterize the humoral output of the tumor and define its anatomical location(s) (Fig. 7). Although usually serotonin and 5-HIAA output are conventionally measured at this time, in clinical practice it is apparent that plasma chromogranin is currently the most effective screening tool. Assessment of the production of other bioactive peptides and amines is likely to become important as antagonists for other bioactive substances such as tachykinins and growth factors are developed.

The next step is delineation of the tumor site and identification of metastases. The best overall study is the octreotide scan, although other modalities such as CAT scan may be useful adjuncts in more complex circumstances.

After detailed evaluation and tumor localization, celiotomy should be performed under octreotide blockade. The entire primary tumor is resected, if possible. If this is not feasible, then biopsy is performed for diagnosis and as much of the tumor as possible is debulked. Intestinal tumors are generally extirpated by anatomical en bloc resection unless they are <1 cm in size. Mesenteric nodes are excised en bloc, and aortic lymph nodes in the area of drainage are removed. Cholecystectomy prevents gallbladder ischemia after future hepatic embolization and protects against the possible sequelae of sludging and cholecystitis if long-term octreotide therapy is employed. Superficial liver lesions should be removed by wedge excision if feasible. Major anatomical hepatic resections should ideally not be undertaken at the time of intestinal surgery.

One month after surgery, repeat clinical, biochemical, and topographic staging should be undertaken. If evidence of residual disease remains, the patient's tumor should be restaged. Patients demonstrated to have unilobar hepatic disease who represent good surgical risks should be considered for hepatic resection 3–6 months after the original procedure. Patients with bilobar hepatic disease and patients who cannot tolerate hepatic resection should undergo hepatic embolization. In either case, the invasive procedure should be performed during somatostatin blockade, as outlined above.

All patients are followed closely, with serial plasma chromogranin or urinary 5-HIAA levels (if the chromogranin assay is not available) at 3-month intervals. Octreotide scintigraphy and abdominal CT should be obtained every 6 months for the first 2 years. Patients who develop new clinical, biochemical, or anatomical evidence of tumor recurrence or renewed hormonal symptoms should be restaged and managed accordingly. Typically, this includes re-embolization and continued or escalating the octreotide therapy. Patients with anatomical evidence of recurrence should, in addition, undergo biochemical testing to verify that the recurrent tumor is truly a carcinoid and not a second primary adenocarcinoma. Trophic factors secreted by the carcinoid may predispose such patients to a second neoplasm (158).

Patients with any evidence of residual disease or symptomatology should be placed on high-dose LAR octreotide; such therapy will remove or ameliorate any symptoms. There is also reasonable evidence to indicate that high-dose octreotide is capable of stabilizing tumor growth in up to 50% of patients with neuroendocrine tumor disease (159). Given its relatively low adverse effect profile, depot injection of this agent appears to be a reasonable stategy.

31. Feldman JM. Carcinoid tumors and syndrome. Semin Oncol 1987; 14:237–246.
32. Sjoerdsma A, Weissbach H, Udenfriend S. Simple test for diagnosis of metastatic carcinoid (argentaffmoma). JAMA 1955; 159:397.
33. Ahlman H, Ahlund L, Dahlstrom A, Martner J, Stenqvist O, Tylen U. SMS 201–995 and provocation tests in carcinoid patients in preparation for surgery and hepatic arterial embolization. Anesth Analg 1988; 67(12): 1142–1148.
34. Modlin IM, Tang LH. Approaches to the diagnosis of gut neuroendocrine tumors: the last word (today). Gastroenterology 1997; 112:583–590.
35. de Herder WW, Lamberts SW. Somatostatin and somatostatin analogues: diagnostic and therapeutic uses. Curr Opin Oncol 2002; 14(1):53–57.
36. Majcher SJ, Lee ER, Reingold IM, Boyle J, Haverbach BJ. Carcinoid syndrome in bronchogenic carcinoma. Arch Intern Med 1966; 117:57–63.
37. Hayashi H, Nakagawa M, Kitagawa S, Yamada T, Ishida K, Kurumaya H. Immunohistochemical analysis of gastrointestinal carcinoids. Gastroenterol Japon 1993; 28(4):483–490.
38. Cheek RC, Wilson H. Carcinoid tumors. Curr Probl Surg 1970; 7:4–31.
39. Brenner S, Heimlich H, Widman M. Carcinoid of esophagus. NY State J Med 1969; 69:1337–1339.
40. Lindberg GM, et al. Atypical carcinoid of the esophagus: a case report and review of the literature. Cancer 1997; 79:1476–1481.
41. Brown RS, et al. Carcinoid tumor of the esophagus. J Clin Gastroenterol 1994; 19:338–339.
42. Siegal A, Swartz A. Malignant carcinoid of the esophagus. Histopathology 1986; 10:761–765.
43. Cadiot G, Laurent-Puig V, Thuille B, Lehy T, Mignon M, Olschwang S. Is the multiple endocrine neoplasia type 1 gene a suppressor for fundic argyrophil tumors in the Zollinger-Ellison syndrome? Gastroenterology 1993; 105:579–582.
44. Surveillance, Epidemiology, and End Results (SEER) Program Public-Use Data (1973–1999), National Cancer Institute, DCCPS, Surveillance Research Program, Cancer Statistics Branch, released April 2002, based on the November 2001 submission.
45. Kulke MH, Mayer RJ. Carcinoid tumors. N Engl J Med 1999; 340(11):858–868.
46. Moesta KT, Schlag P. Proposal for a new carcinoid tumour staging system based on tumour tissue infiltration and primary metastasis: a prospective multicentre carcinoid tumour evaluation study (West German Surgical Oncologists' Group). Eur J Surg Oncol 1990; 16: 280–288.
47. Rindi G, Luinetti O, Cornaggia M, Capella C, Solcia E. Three subtypes of gastric argyrophil carcinoid and the gastric neuroendocrine carcinoma: a clinicopathologic study. Gastroenterology 1993; 104(4):994–1006.
48. Annibale B, Azzoni C, Corleto VD, di Giulio E, Caruana P, D'Ambra G, Bordi C, Delle Fave G. Atrophic body gastritis patients with enterochromaffin-like cell dysplasia are at increased risk for the development of type I gastric carcinoid. Eur J Gastroenterol Hepatol 2001; 13(12): 1449–1456.
49. Lehy T, Mignon M, Cadiot G, Elouaer-Blanc L, Ruszniewski P, Lewin MJ, Bonfils S. Gastric endocrine cell behavior in Zollinger-Ellison patients upon long-term potent antisecretory treatment. Gastroenterology 1989; 96(4):1029–1040.
50. Thomas RM, Baybick JH, Elsayed AM, Sobin LH. Gastric carcinoids: an immunohistochemical and clinicopathologic study of 104 patients. Cancer 1994; 73: 2053–2058.
51. Nakamura S, Linda M, Yao T, Fujishima M. Endoscopy features of gastric carcinoids. Gastrointest Endosc 1991; 37:535–538.
52. Box JC, Watne AL, Lucas GW. Small bowel carcinoid: review of a single institution experience and review of the literature. Am Surg 1996; 62:280–286.
53. Davies MG, O'Dowd G, McEntee GP, Hennessy TP. Primary gastric carcinoids: a view on management. Br J Surg 1990; 77:1013–1014.
54. Berge T, Linell F. Carcinoid tumours: frequency in a defined population during a 12-year period. Acta Pathol Microbiol Scand 1976; 84:322–330.
55. Burke AP, Thomas RM, Elsayed AM, Sobin LH. Carcinoids of the jejunum and ileum: an immunohistochemical and clinicopathologic study of 167 cases. Cancer 1997; 79:1086–1093.
56. Kotsis T, Voros D, Paphiti A, Frangou M, Mallas E. Duodenal gangliocytic paraganglioma as a radiological moving defect. Dig Surg 2000; 17(6):636–640.
57. Stamm B, Hedinger CE, Saremaslani P. Duodenal and ampullary carcinoid tumors: report of 12 cases with pathological characteristics, polypeptide content and relation to the MEN-I syndrome and von Recklinghausen's disease (neurofibromatosis). Virchow Arch A 1986; 408:475–489.
58. Burke AP, Federspiel BH, Sobin LH, Shekitka KM, Helwig EB. Carcinoids of the duodenum: a histologic and immunohistochemical study of 65 tumors. Am J Surg Pathol 1989; 13(10):828–837.
59. Yamamoto C, Aoyagi K, Suekane H, et al. Carcinoid tumors of the duodenum: report of three cases treated by endoscopic resection. Endoscopy 1997; 29:218–221.
60. Marshall JB, Bodnarchuk G. Carcinoid tumors of the gut: our experience over three decades and review of the literature. J Clin Gastroenterol 1993; 16:123–129.
61. Peck JJ, Shields AB, Boyden AM, Dworkin LA, Nadal JW. Carcinoid tumors of the ileum. Am J Surg 1983; 146:124–132.
62. Lundqvist M, Wilander E. A study of the histopathogenesis of carcinoid tumors of the small intestine and appendix. Cancer 1987; 60:201–206.
63. Johnson LA, Lavin P, Moertel CG, Weiland L, Dayal

Y. Carcinoids: the association of histologic growth pattern and survival. Cancer 1983; 51:882–889.
64. Assadi M, Kubiak R, Kaiser G. Appendiceal carcinoid tumors in children: does size matter? Med Pediatr Oncol 2002; 38(1):65–66.
65. Masson P. Carcinoid tumors (argentaffin tumors) and nerve hyperplasia of the appendicular mucosa. Am J Pathol 1928; 4:181–212.
66. Shaw PA. The topographical and age distributions of neuroendocrine cells in the normal human appendix. J Pathol 1991; 164:235–239.
67. Moertel CG, Weiland LH, Nagorney DM, Dockerty MB. Carcinoid tumor of the appendix: treatment and prognosis. N Engl J Med 1987; 317:1699–1701.
68. Glasser CM, Bhagavan BS. Carcinoid tumors of the appendix. Arch Pathol Lab Med 1980; 104:272–275.
69. Anderson JR, Wilson BG. Carcinoid tumours of the appendix. Br J Surg 1985; 72:545–546.
70. Rothmund M, Kisker O. Surgical treatment of carcinoid tumors of the small bowel, appendix, colon and rectum. Digestion 1994; 55(3):86–91.
71. Roggo A, Wood WC, Ottinger LW. Carcinoid tumors of the appendix. Ann Surg 1993; 217:385–390.
72. Bowman GA, Rosenthal D. Carcinoid tumors of the appendix. Am J Surg 1983; 146:700–703.
73. Ponka JL. Carcinoid tumors of the appendix: report of thirty-five cases. Am J Surg 1973; 126:77 83.
74. Meckel JF. Ueber die Divertikel am Darmkanal. Arch Physiol 1809; 9:421.
75. Fabricius Hildanus W. Selectae observationes chirurgicae quinque & viginti. Item, de gangraena et sphacelo tractatus methodicus. Geneva: G. Cartier, 1598.
76. Thorek P. Meckel's diverticulum. In: Thorek P, ed. Anatomy in Surgery. Philadelphia: JB Lippincott, 1962: 394.
77. Weinstein EC, Dockerty MB, Waugh JM. Neoplasm of Meckel's diverticulum. Int J Surg 1963; 116:103.
78. Weber JD, McFadden DW. Carcinoid tumor in Meckel's diverticula. J Clin Gastroenterol 1989; 11(6):682–686.
79. Soltero MJ, Bill AH. The natural history of Meckel's diverticulum and its relation to incidental removal: a study of 202 cases of diseased Meckel's diverticulum found in King County, Washington, over a fifteen year period. Am J Surg 1976; 132(2):168–173.
80. McFadden D, Jaffe BM. Surgical approaches to endocrine producing tumors of the gastrointestenal tract. In: Cohen S, Soloway RD, eds. Hormone-Producing Tumors of the Gastrointestinal Tract. New York: Churchill Livingstone, 1985:139–157.
81. Ratanarapee S, Manonukul J, Parichatikarond P. Carcinoid tumor of Meckel's diverticulum. J Med Assoc Thailand 1982; 65:556–561.
82. Ballantyne GH, Savoca PE, Flannery JT, Ahlman MH, Modlin IM. Incidence and mortality of carcinoids of the colon: data from the Connecticut tumor registry. Cancer 1992; 69:2400–2405.
83. McDonald RA. A study of 356 carcinoids of the gastrointestinal tract. Am J Med 1956; 21:867–872.
84. Spread C, Berkel H, Jewell L, Jenkins H, Yakimets W. Colon carcinoid tumors: a population-based study. Dis Colon Rectum 1994; 37:482–491.
85. O'Brian DS, Dayal Y, DeLellis RA, Tischler AS, Bendon R, Wolfe HJ. Rectal carcinoids as tumors of the hindgut endocrine cells: a morphological and immunohistochemical analysis. Am J Surg Pathol 1982; 6:131–141.
86. Mani S, Modlin IM, Ballantyne G, Ahlman H, West B. Carcinoids of the rectum. J Am Coll Surg 1994; 179: 231–248.
87. Davidson ED, McDougal WS. Elevated serum acid phosphatase levels with rectal carcinoid tumor. Gastroenterology 1976; 70(1):114–116.
88. El-Salhy M, Wilander E, Lundqvist M, et al. Glucagon and glucagon-like immunoreactive cells in mid- and hindgut carcinoids. Acta Pathol Microbiol Immunol Scand 1988; 96:537–542.
89. Enblad P, Wilander E, Busch C, Glimelius B. The expression of carcinoma associated antigens and blood group related antigens in rectal carcinoids. Dis Colon Rectum 1988; 31:450–453.
90. Soga J. Carcinoids of the rectum: an evaluation of 1271 reported cases. Surg Today 1997; 27(2):112–119.
91. Tsioulias G, Muto T, Kubota Y, et al. DNA ploidy pattern in rectal carcinoid tumors. Dis Colon Rectum 1991; 34:31–36.
92. Demartines N, von Flue MO, Harder FH. Transanal endoscopic microsurgical excision of rectal tumors: indications and results. World J Surg 2001; 25(7):870–875.
93. Kehagias D, et al. Imaging findings in primary carcinoid of the liver with gastrin production. Br Inst Radiol 1999; 72:207–209.
94. Krishnamurthy SC, et al. Primary carcinoid tumor of the liver: report of four resected cases including one with gastrin production. J Surg Oncol 1996; 62:218–221.
95. Smith AL, Auldist AW. Successful surgical resection of an hepatic gastrinoma in a child. J Pediatr Gastroenterol Nutr 1984; 3:801–804.
96. Nicholas S. Primary hepatic carcinoid tumor: an electron microscopic and immunohistochemical study. Anat Path 1991; 95(2):172–175.
97. Läuffer JM, Baer HU, Maurer CA, Stoupis C, Zimmerman A, Buchler MW. Biliary cystadenocarcinoma of the liver: the need for complete resection. Eur J Cancer 1998; 34:1845–1851.
98. Porter A, Ostrowski M. Successful treatment of malignant carcinoid tumor with intravenous cisplatinum. Eur J Surg Oncol 1988; 14:703–704.
99. Läuffer JM, Zimmermann A, Krahenbuhl L, Triller J, Baer HU. Epithelioid hemangioendothelioma: a rare hepatic tumor. Cancer 1996; 78:2227–2318.
100. Joel W. Karzinoidtumor der Gallenblase. Zentralbl Allg Pathol 1929; 46:1–4.

52

Endocrine Tumors of the Gastrointestinal Tract

Maha T. Barakat, John A. Lynn, and Stephen R. Bloom

Imperial College London, London, England

1 INTRODUCTION

Second to the brain, the gastroenteropancreatic system provides the richest source of regulatory peptides originating from the cells of the diffuse neuroendocrine system (1). Tumors of these cells result in varied conditions such as gastric carcinoid, islet cell tumors, and duodenal paragangliomas. We refer the reader to Chs. 47 and 51 for a more detailed exposition of pancreatic neuroendocrine tumors and for gastrointestinal carcinoids.

2 WORLDWIDE INCIDENCE

The clinical incidence of gastrointestinal neuroendocrine tumors is between 0.3–0.7/100,000, although the incidence at postmortem is 2/100,000 (2,3). More than 50% of neuroendocrine tumors in clinical practice are of the "carcinoid" type occurring mostly in the extrapancreatic gastrointestinal tract and lung. The remaining neuroendocrine tumors are mostly pancreatic and include insulinomas, gastrinomas, VIPomas, and glucagonomas. These pancreatic neuroendocrine tumors have been detected at a rate of 0.3–1.6% of unselected autopsies in which only a few sections of pancreas were examined and in up to 10% of autopsies in which the whole pancreas was systematically investigated (4).

3 RISK FACTORS—ENVIRONMENTAL AND GENETIC

Gastroenteropancreatic endocrine tumors occur both sporadically and as part of the autosomal dominant multiple endocrine neoplasia type 1 (MEN1) syndrome. The *MEN1* gene, which encodes a protein of 610 amino acids (menin), is located on chromosome 11q13 and is believed to function as a tumor suppressor (5). In a series of 34 sporadic pancreatic endocrine tumors, mutations in the *MEN1* gene were found in 12 (34%) (6). Native menin has been shown to bind to JunD, an activator protein-1 (AP-1) transcription factor, inhibiting JunD's activation of transcription (7). Furthermore, menin represses p65-mediated transcriptional activation on NF-κB sites (8). These observations suggest that menin's ability to interact with NF-κB proteins and its modulation of NF-κB transactivation contribute to menin's tumor suppressor function.

4 DEMOGRAPHICS—GENDER, AGE, RACE, OR ETHNIC ORIGIN

Male-to-female ratio varies with the different series, but in a large American series of patients with carcinoid, the male-to-female ratio varied from 0.47 to 0.66, depending on the primary site (9). When carcinoid tumor occurs as part of the MEN1 syndrome, it occurs in the thymus in more than two thirds of men, whereas in more than 75% of women it occurs in the lung. The median age of patients with carcinoid is 55 in those with symptoms and 52 in those without. There seems to be a higher age-adjusted incidence rate in the African American male population (2.12/100,000 population per year) (9).

5 PHYSIOLOGY

The myriad of regulatory peptides originating from cells in the gastroenteropancreatic system are involved in endocrine, paracrine, and autocrine communication as well as neurocrine, where the peptides act as neurotransmitters and neuromodulators (1,10–12). Indeed, there may be many more peptides we have not yet discovered. Figure 1 illustrates the complexity of the cell-to-cell communication in the gastrointestinal tract, and Table 1 demonstrates the plethora of gut hormones and peptides (13,14).

6 CLINICAL FEATURES—CLASSIC AND SUBTLE PHENOTYPIC EXPRESSIONS

Gastroenteropancreatic neuroendocrine tumors can be divided into functioning and non-functioning tumors. The "functioning" tumors release detectable peptide hormones into the circulation and are usually associated with defined syndromes. These tumors may release several peptides, only some of which may produce symptoms. Similarly it is not uncommon for a tumor that originally secreted one peptide to undergo dedifferentiation and subsequently co-secrete other peptides. The tumors are slow growing, and, in the case of functioning tumors, the symptoms are usually due to the secreted peptides rather than tumor bulk. Moreover, there may be several years (average 7.5) between the onset of symptoms and final diagnosis with neuroendocrine tumors of the small intestine (15). With the exception of carcinoid tumors, which occur more frequently outside the pancreas, gastroenteropancreatic neuroendocrine tumors occur mostly in the pancreas (see Table 2) (13, 16–19).

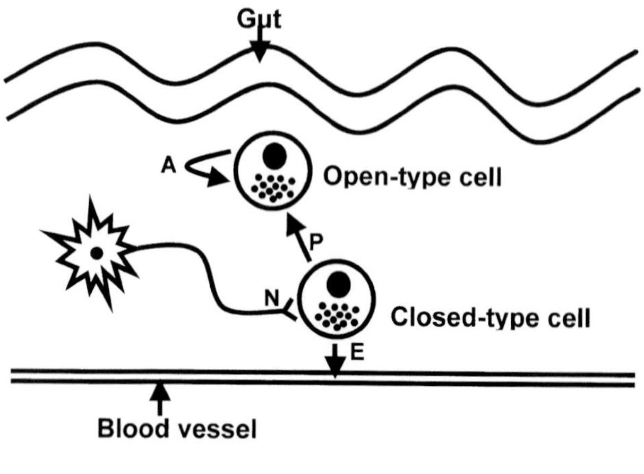

Figure 1 Cell-to-cell communication in the gastrointestinal tract. Open-type endocrine cells are sensitive to luminal contents, while closed-type cells mostly respond to stretch. Cells may secrete hormones into the blood to influence distant targets (endocrine, **E**), to stimulate neighboring cells (paracrine, **P**), or to control their own secretions (autocrine, **A**). They may also modulate or be stimulated by local neurons (neurocrine, **N**). (Adapted from Ref. 13.)

Carcinoid is the term used to describe tumors derived from serotonin-producing enterochromaffin (EC, or Kulchitsky's) cells, but there is a spectrum of different syndromes depending on which cell and which hormone or hormones are produced. Some authors feel the term carcinoid to be archaic because of this wide spectrum (20). The classical carcinoid syndrome of flushing, hypotension, diarrhea, wheezing, and heart disease occurs in fewer than 10% of patients with carcinoid. Of more than 600 patients reported with carcinoid syndrome, 93–94% had raised serotonin levels, whereas only 25–30% of the more than 7000 patients without the syndrome had raised levels (21). High serotonin levels seem to predict the development of carcinoid heart disease. Tumors deriving from the gastric histamine-secreting enterochromaffin-like (ECL) cells produce an "atypical" carcinoid syndrome. These ECL cells contain low serotonin but often secrete the serotonin precursor 5-hydroxytryptophan (5-HTP). The flushing produced by these foregut carcinoids is often more intense, with a purplish hue and protracted duration; it is also more extensive, involving the limbs as well as the upper trunk, and frequently followed by telangiectasia (21).

Carcinoid most frequently occurs in the gut (73.7%) followed by lung (25.1%); within the gut, the frequencies are small bowel (28.9%), appendix (18.9%), and rectum (12.6%) (9). Fewer than 1% of all carcinoids occur in the ovary, pancreas, liver, and gallbladder. Predisposition to metastatic spread depends on location and size (9,14). Table 3 summarizes the relationship between site, metastatic potential, and 5-year survival (9).

It is accepted that the tumors termed "nonfunctioning" may actually produce a hormone or peptide that we cannot detect given current techniques. These nonfunctioning tumors tend to be more aggressive and present with symptoms of tumor bulk (22).

Table 1 Gastrointestinal Regulatory Hormones

Hormone	Location in gut	Cell of origin
Gastrin-cholecystokinin family		
Gastrin	Gastric antrum	G-cell
Cholecystokinin (CCK)	Duodenum	I-cell
Growth factors		
Transforming growth factor-α (TGF-α)	Gastric fundus	Enterochromaffin-like cell (ECL)
Insulin-like growth factor-α (IGF-1)	Gastric fundus	Enterochromaffin-like cell (ECL)
Insulin	Pancreas	β-cell
Pancreatic polypeptide family		
Pancreatic polypeptide (PP)	Pancreas, colon	F-cell
Peptide YY (PYY)	Ileum, colon, pancreas	L-cell
Neuropeptide Y (NPY)	Throughout gut	Myenteric and submucosal neurons
Secretin-glucagon family		
Secretin	Duodenum, jejunum	S-cell
Proglucagon-derived peptides, Pancreas	Pancreas	α-cell
Glucagon		
Glucagon-like peptide-1 (GLP-1)		
Glucagon-like peptide-2 (GLP-2)	Ileum	L-cell
Proglucagon-derived peptides, intestine		
GLP-1(7-36)amide		
GLP-2		
Oxyntomodulin	Duodenum, jejunum (ileum, colon)	K-cell
Glicentin		Intrinsic neural elements
Gastric inhibitory peptide (GIP)	Throughout gut and pancreas	
Vasoactive intestinal polypeptide and related peptides		
Vasoactive intestinal polypeptide (VIP)		
Peptide histidine isoleucine (PHI)		
Peptide histidine methionine (PHM)		
Pituitary adenylate cyclase-activating peptide (PACAP)		
Growth hormone-releasing factor (GRF)		
Tachykinin family		
Neurokinin A	Throughout gut	Intrinsic and extrinsic afferent nerves
Neurokinin B	Throughout gut	Intrinsic and extrinsic afferent nerves
Substance P	Throughout gut	Intrinsic and extrinsic afferent nerves Enterochromaffin-I cell
Neurotensin and related peptides		
Neurotensin (NT)	Ileum, jejunum, duodenum	N-cells, enteric neurones
Neuromedin N		
Xenopsin		
Xenin		
Bombesin and related peptides		
Bombesin	Throughout gut	Enteric nerves
Gastrin-releasing peptide (GRP)	Throughout gut	Enteric nerves
Neuromedin B	Throughout gut	Enteric nerves
Neuromedin C	Throughout gut	Enteric nerves

(*continued on next page*)

Table 1 Continued.

Hormone	Location in gut	Cell of origin
Calcitonin gene–related peptides		
Calcitonin gene–related peptide (CGRP)	Throughout gut	
Calcitonin		
Adrenomedullin		
Amylin		Enteric nerves
Somatostatin	Gastric and duodenal epithelia	D-cell
	Throughout gut and pancreas	Extrinsic and intrinsic neurons of intestinal myenteric and submucosal plexuses
Motilin	Small intestine	Open-type M-cell
Galanin	Throughout gut and pancreas	Enteric neurones
Chromogranins and secretogranins	Throughout gut and pancreas	Dense vesicles of secretory granules
Chromogranin A (CgA)		
Chromogranin B (CgB)		
GAWK (CgB 420–493)		
Secretogranin II (SgII)		
Opioid peptides	Colon	Enterochromaffin-I cell
Cocaine and amphetamine-regulated transcript (CART)	Throughout the gut	Enteric neurons
Neuromedin U	Throughout the gut	Enteric neurons
Nonpeptides		
Histamine	Gastric fundus	Enterochromaffin-like cell (ECL)
Serotonin	Duodenum	Enterochromaffin cell
	Colon	Enterochromaffin-I cell, Enterochromaffin-N cell

Other gut hormones include PTHrP, ghrelin, endothelin-1, trefoil peptides, guanylin, and uroguanylin.
Source: Adapted from Refs. 13, 14.

7 BIOCHEMICAL MARKERS FOR FUNCTIONING TUMORS

As discussed above, neuroendocrine tumors secrete many peptide hormones and amines (see Table 1). Biochemical markers for neuroendocrine tumors can be divided into general and specific markers. General neuroendocrine tumor markers include chromogranins, pancreatic polypeptide, and HCG subunits. Chromogranin A (CgA) derives its name from its original discovery in the catecholamine-containing chromaffin granules of the adrenal medulla (23) and is located alongside specific hormones in large dense-core vesicles of neuronal and neuroendocrine cells. Chromogranin B (CgB), another secretory granule protein, is also widely distributed in neuroendocrine cells, although CgA seems to be present in some cells that do not express CgB (24). CgA-positive tumors by immunocytochemistry include anterior pituitary, parathyroid, medullary thyroid, gastroenteropancreatic, ectopic ACTH, ganglioneuromas, neuroblastomas, pheochromocytoma, small-cell lung, and prostate tumors. The exceptions are the prolactin-producing cells of the pituitary and some pancreatic β-cell tumors, which show positive staining for CgB. Other general stains for neuroendocrine tumors include neuron-specific enolase (NSE), pancreatic polypeptide, and peptide histidine-methionine (25–27).

Plasma CgA is elevated in 94% and pancreatic polypeptide in 74% of endocrine pancreatic tumors (28). In a study with patients with malignant carcinoid and gastroenteropancreatic tumors, CgA was elevated in 99%, CgB in 88%, CgC (secretogranin II) in 6%, and pancreastatin in 46% (29). The highest levels of plasma CgA are seen in metastatic carcinoid (particularly midgut), whereas plasma CgB is usually a better marker for benign insulin-producing tumors. A fragment of CgB termed GAWK (CgB-420-493) is a 74-amino-acid peptide originally isolated from human pituitaries, and high plasma concentrations are found in various neuroendocrine tumors including pancreatic, pheochromocytoma, medullary carcinoma of the thyroid, and

Table 2 Tumor Syndromes of Gastrointestinal Neuroendocrine Tumors

Tumor type	Frequency of pancreatic NET tumors (%)	Malignancy (%)	Tumor location	% with MEN1	Syndrome
Insulinoma	70–75	< 10	Pancreas > 99%	4–5	Hypoglycemia Weight gain
Gastrinoma	20–25	> 50	Duodenum 70% Pancreas 25%	20–25	Abdominal pain Diarrhea Peptic ulceration
VIPoma	3–5	> 50	Pancreas 90%	6	Secretory diarrhea Hypokalemia Achlorhydria Metabolic acidosis Flushing
Glucagonoma	1–2	> 70	Pancreas 100%	1–20	Necrolytic migratory erythema Diabetes Cachexia Thromboembolic disease
PPoma	< 1	> 60	Pancreas 100%	18–44	Pain Weight loss Diarrhea
Somatostatinoma	< 1	> 50	Pancreas 55% Duodenum Jejunum 44%	45	Steatorrhea Diabetes Gallstones Weight loss
Carcinoid	< 1 mostly extrapancreatic	90	Midgut 75–87% Foregut 2–33% Hindgut 1–8% Unknown 2–15%	Rare	Classical carcinoid: Flushing Diarrhea Wheeze Cardiac fibrosis Pellagra dermatosis
ACTHoma CRFoma	< 1	> 99	Pancreas 4–14% (of all ectopic ACTH)	Rare	Cushing's syndrome Pigmentation
PTHrPoma	< 1	> 99	Pancreas	Rare	Hypercalcemia Nephrolithiasis Nephrocalcinosis Osteoporosis
Calcitoninoma	< 1	> 80	Pancreas	16	Diarrhea, flushing
GRFoma	< 1	50	Pancreas 30% Lung 54% Jejunum 7%	16	Acromegaly
Nonfunctioning	< 1	> 80	Pancreas + gastrointestinal tract	18–44	Symptoms of tumor bulk Weight loss

Source: Adapted from Refs. 13, 16, 19.

Table 3 Carcinoid Tumors—Relation Between Site, Metastatic Potential, and 5-Year Survival

Site	% of all carcinoids	Regional metastases	Distant metastases	5-year survival with no metastases	5-year survival with regional metastases	5-year survival with distant metastases
Small intestine	28	39%	31%	65%	66%	36%
Appendix	19	27%	9%	94%	85%	34%
Colon	8	33%	38%	71%	44%	21%
Rectum	13	7%	7%	81%	47%	18%
Stomach	3	10%	21%	64%	40%	10%

Source: Data from Ref. 9.

ACTH-producing lung tumors. High levels are seen with pancreatic endocrine tumors, making GAWK a useful tumor marker (30). In another study, elevated pancreastatin was found in 33%, whereas GAWK was elevated in 50% of patients with pancreatic neuroendocrine tumors (31).

Some tumors secrete multiple hormones (32), and as many as 62% have elevated gastrin despite only 30% presenting with peptic ulceration. Specific markers for carcinoid include urinary 5HIAA, neuropeptide K, substance P, or other tachykinins. Urinary 5HIAA and neuropeptide K show high sensitivity in midgut carcinoid, with lower sensitivity in foregut and hindgut carcinoid (33). For other neuroendocrine tumors, specific fasting hormones such as gastrin, glucagon, pancreatic polypeptide, somatostatin, neurotensin, and VIP (vasoactive intestinal polypeptide) can be measured. An elevated gastrin after withdrawal of proton pump inhibitors for at least 2 weeks and of H2-blockers for at least 3 days is not specific to gastrinoma, and other causes need to be excluded such as atrophic gastritis, hypercalcemia, and renal impairment. Basal gastric acid output studies are often required to distinguish primary from secondary hypergastrinemia, where spontaneous basal acid (proton) outputs of 20–25 mmol/hr are almost diagnostic and >10 mmol/hr suspicious. Should there be equivocal results of basal acid output and fasting gastrin or difficulty stopping pharmacological treatment for the gastrin assay, for example, in case of occurrence of severe symptoms or strong risk of perforation, then the intravenous secretin test is indicated. Whereas a normal response to intravenous secretin is a fall in serum gastrin, a rise of more than 200 pg/mL (100 pmol/L) offers a sensitivity of 85% for the presence of gastrinoma (34).

With regards to the diagnosis of insulinoma, insulin and C-peptide levels need to be interpreted in the presence of hypoglycemia, and a 3-day fast may be required to achieve this (see below). Other hormones such as PTHrP for the diagnosis of a PTHrPoma can be measured in the non-fasting state.

8 BIOCHEMICAL ASSAYS—BASAL, PROVOCATIVE, SUPPRESSIVE

If a diagnosis of carcinoid is suspected and urinary baseline fasting hormones are normal, the pentagastrin test with measurements of plasma tachykinins is quite sensitive (35). In the case of gastrinoma, the secretin test with gastrin measurements has a sensitivity of 80–85% (34,36). The diagnosis of insulinoma requires the measurement of insulin and C-peptide in the presence of hypoglycemia (glucose at or below 2.2 mmol/L). A 3-day fast may be required to achieve this allowing free access to noncaloric fluids. By 24 hours, 66% of insulinomas develop hypoglycemia and by 48 hours, >95% of insulinomas can be diagnosed (37). If hypoglycemia is achieved, simultaneous plasma and urine samples need to be taken for sulfhonylurea analysis to exclude drug-induced hypoglycemia.

9 LOCALIZATION BY IMAGING—NONINVASIVE, INVASIVE, SELECTIVE SAMPLING

In 1998 and 1999 a Delphi consensus was performed to establish guidelines for standardized diagnostic imaging of neuroendocrine tumors (38). With the exception of insulinomas, functional and nonfunctional tumors of the pancreas are detectable with somatostatin-receptor scintigraphy (SRS) with a sensitivity of up to 90% and specificity of 80% (39–41). Insulinomas rarely express somatostatin receptors, thereby limiting the sensitivity of SRS to 10–50% (42). However, there is increasing agreement that malignant insulinomas express somatostatin receptors, and SRS is recommended for staging of confirmed or suspected malignant disease.

In the case of noncarcinoid neuroendocrine tumors, the pancreas is the main source of the primary lesion. Pancreatic surgery is difficult, and the surgeon needs as much information about location of the lesion as possible. The pancreas is best visualized with a dedicated pancreatic and abdominal CT and, more recently, endoscopic ultrasonography (EUS). Several studies have shown that EUS has a sensitivity of 80–90% for imaging pancreatic neuroendocrine tumors (43–47), whereas extrapancreatic tumors could be detected with lower sensitivities (48–50). In one series, EUS showed the highest sensitivity in localizing insulinomas (94%) compared with SRS (12%), transabdominal ultrasound (12%), CT (29%), and MRI (13%) (47). Furthermore, EUS showed the highest accuracy in detecting pancreatic gastrinomas, but failed to detect 50% of extrapancreatic gastrinomas. In nonfunctioning neuroendocrine pancreatic tumors, EUS provided the best information regarding local invasion and regional lymph node involvement. The smallest lesion visualized was a 5 mm tumor in the pancreatic head.

As one can appreciate, the localization of very small pancreatic gastrinomas and insulinomas is often difficult even with endoscopic ultrasound, and at this institution we find that selective angiography with secretagogue injection into the main pancreatic arteries invaluable. The main pancreatic arteries, gastroduodenal, superior mesenteric, inferior pancreaticoduodenal, and splenic, are cannulated separately, and the images are analyzed carefully for the presence of a vascular blush. Gastrinomas can be stimulated with intra-arterial secretin or calcium, and insulinomas with intra-arterial calcium. The chosen secretagogue (secretin or calcium) is then injected into each of the arteries individually and venous samples are collected from the hepatic vein. Normally there should be a fall in gastrin and insulin levels with the secretagogue. In the presence of a gastrinoma or insulinoma, gastrin and insulin levels (respectively) at least double after 30 seconds of the injection (51–55). This offers the surgeon important information on which artery supplies the tumor and if more than one lesion is present. With MEN1 there may coexist an insulinoma and a gastrinoma in the same patient, and this technique can differentiate between the two when both insulin and gastrin levels are checked. Tumors smaller than 0.5 cm have been localized by this technique. Finally, it is crucial to know if hepatic metastases are present prior to resection of the pancreatic primary, since this would alter management. A key strength of selective angiography with intra-arterial injection is that the hepatic artery can also be cannulated and injected with secretagogue. Small liver metastases can be confidently excluded if there is no rise in gastrin or insulin after injection into the hepatic artery. Indeed, calcium stimulation can be used to detect most neuroendocrine tumors of the pancreas, since in the presence of a tumor the calcium acts as a secretagogue and different hormone levels can be checked.

If a diagnosis of carcinoid has been made (e.g., with carcinoid syndrome symptoms or incidental tumor found on chest x-ray– and histology-confirmed carcinoid), SRS imaging is often helpful as the first imaging modality in localization. A fine-cut CT scan can then be performed in the region of uptake in the scintigraphy. If the SRS suggests bowel as the source of the carcinoid, then endoscopy (upper or lower depending on the site) is indicated. In the presence of a negative SRS, CT thorax and abdomen are recommended.

Another imaging modality available with carcinoid is positron emission tomography (PET) where the serotonin precursor 5-hydroxytryptophan (5-HTP) labeled with ^{11}C is used instead of ^{18}F-labeled deoxyglucose (FDG) (56). This showed increased uptake and irreversible trapping of tracer in carcinoid tumors. The uptake was selective and the resolution so high that more liver and lymph node metastases could be detected with PET than with CT, MRI, or SRS. During follow-up, there was a >95% correlation between changes in urinary 5HIAA and changes in the transport rate constant for 5-HTP tracer in PET. Several other tracers have been investigated, such as the monoamine oxidase inhibitor harmine, with promising results in nonfunctioning neuroendocrine tumors.

Other localization procedures for pancreatic tumors include the use of intraoperative ultrasound, and this seems to provide additional valuable information to the surgeon. More recently, radioguided surgery has been applied to the field of gastroenteropancreatic tumors. Intraoperative gamma probes are able to detect accumulation of the tracer (^{111}In DTPA-D-Phe1)-pentetreotide more efficiently (>90%) than somatostatin receptor scintigraphy (68–77%), including lesions <5 mm in size. Furthermore, radio-guided surgery identified 57% more lesions than the "palpating finger (57)."

Very few gastroenteropancreatic tumors are positive on MIBG scanning. This is because they derive from an endodermal origin, not neuroectoderm, and catecholamine-synthesizing machinery is rarely found. For this reason MIBG is not useful in the gastroenteropancreatic group of neuroendocrine tumors either in diagnostic scanning or in therapeutics (58).

10 STAGING—CLINICOPATHOLOGICAL CLASSIFICATION

Gut neuroendocrine tumors were first classified by William and Sandler in 1963. Since then numerous nomenclature systems have been developed. Over the last decade, an experienced group of pathologists have devised a new classification of neuroendocrine gastroenteropancreatic tumors based on clinicopathological patterns (59–61). Tumors are termed functioning neuroendocrine tumors according to their leading clinical and endocrine profile. Those tumors without plasma hormone elevation and lacking endocrine symptoms are labeled nonfunctioning neuroendocrine tumors. The presence of a specific endocrine hyperfunction syndrome seems to be as important as purely pathological features for predicting biological behavior of the tumor (62,63) (see Tables 1 and 2). Table 4 summarizes the proposed classification into benign, uncertain and malignant gastroenteropancreatic tumors (61).

11 TREATMENT

11.1 Curative Surgery

11.1.1 Resection of the Primary Lesion

In principle, a primary lesion that has not metastasized should be resected if surgically possible. This is certainly true with regards to insulinoma, where a subcentimeter lesion may cause sudden death as a result of endocrine hyperfunction rather than tumor bulk or metastases. Futhermore, 90% of insulinomas can be resected by enucleation and local pancreatic resection is rarely necessary.

11.1.2 Resection of Liver Metastases

The presence of liver metastases may not necessary exclude attempted curative surgery. Curative hepatic surgery may be considered if the primary had been previously resected or is potentially resectable, if the metastatic disease is confined to the liver and resectable, and if there is sufficient hepatic reserve to withstand the resection. Surgical techniques have improved considerably since the initial studies a few years ago. In recent series, survival values are similar with 4 to 5-year survival of 70–85% with curative surgery (64–68). Prognostic factors favoring prolonged survival (>1 yr) included previous resection of the primary tumor (42 months median disease-free survival) and 4 or fewer metastases resected (46 months median disease-free survival) (68).

Table 4 Proposed Classification Into Benign, Uncertain, and Malignant Gastroenteropancreatic Tumors

Risk factor	Benign	Uncertain	Malignant
Size (mm)	≤20	>20	>20
Local infiltration	No	Yes	Yes
Angioinvasion	No	Yes	Yes
Atypia	No	Yes	Yes
Gross invasion	No	No	Yes
Metastases	No	No	Yes

Source: Ref. 61.

11.1.3 Liver Transplantation

In rare situations, where there are too many or unresectable liver metastases, a liver transplant in addition to resection of the primary may be performed. This depends on the nature of the tumor and may offer significantly prolonged survival, although the mortality associated with the procedure is high. Experience with liver transplantation for metastases confined to the liver is limited. There has been a meta-analysis of liver transplantation for neuroendocrine tumors with 30 cases (13 foregut and 15 pancreatic primaries) (69). Survival was 52% after 1 year. Of the 12 patients who died within the first year, 6 died as a consequence of the transplant procedure itself and 6 died from tumor recurrence. Transplantation clearly has to be considered only in highly selected cases. At our institution a patient who was diagnosed with pancreatic PTHrPoma underwent resection of the primary 17 years ago. She subsequently developed liver metastases and underwent a liver transplant 10 years ago. She remains alive, and recently discovered pleural and peritoneal recurrences are being treated with radiolabeled octreotide.

11.2 Medical

Medical treatment should be initiated until the time of curative resection of the tumor or continued long term if surgery is not feasible. The precise medical treatment depends on the endocrine syndrome produced by the neuroendocrine tumor. The treatments are summarized in Table 5.

11.2.1 Somatostatin Analogues

As evident from Table 5, somatostatin analogues seem to be an effective symptomatic treatment in a number of the neuroendocrine tumors. This effect of somatostatin has been known for some time (70,71). Somatostatin is expressed throughout the body, and somatostatin

Table 5 Specific Medical Treatments for Some Neuroendocrine Tumor Syndromes

Endocrine syndrome	Treatment options
Carcinoid syndrome	Antihistamines (H1 and H2 antagonists)
	Cyproheptadine, nicotinamide
	Somatostatin analogue if SRS scan positive
	Interferon-α
Insulinoma	Dietary modifications
	Diazoxide
	Guar gum
	Intravenous dextrose if period of fasting
	Somatostatin analogue if SRS scan positive (malignant)
Gastrinoma	High-dose proton pump inhibitor
Glucagonoma	Somatostatin analogue (high dose)
	Anticoagulation
	Insulin if diabetes mellitus
VIPoma	Rehydration + potassium supplements
	Somatostatin analogue (high dose)
	May need bicarbonate in acute attacks
Somatostatinoma	Pancreatic enzyme replacement
	Insulin if diabetes mellitus
PTHrPoma	Rehydration
	Bisphosphonates
	Somatostatin analogue
Nonfunctioning	Somatostatin analogue if SRS scan positive and progressive disease

immunoreactivity is found frequently in neuroendocrine tumors (72). There are five somatostatin receptors (sstr1-5), and the two longer-acting analogues (see Fig. 2) of somatostatin (lanreotide and octreotide) bind preferentially to sstr2 and to a lesser degree to sstr5 (73,74).

It has been demonstrated that octreotide and lanreotide exert their effects on hormone secretion and antiproliferative effects predominantly via sstr2 (73–76). In fact, most gastroenteropancreatic neuroendocrine tumors express all five sstrs, but those lacking sstr2 do not respond to long-acting somatostatin analogues. Only 50% of insulinomas express sstr2 (76). Therefore, long-acting somatostatin analogues benefit only those with sstr2-positive tumors.

It is known from both in vitro and in vivo experiments that somatostatin and its analogues exert antiproliferative effects. Acting mainly via sstr2 and sstr5 to induce cell growth arrest at the G1 phase of the cell cycle, somatostatin exerts both a cytostatic and a cytotoxic effect (77). There were also early case reports of tumor regression (78–81). This prompted several phase II trials to study the effects of octreotide and lanreotide in patients with metastatic neuroendocrine tumors where there was CT-documented evidence of tumor progression (i.e., a 25% increase in tumor size over 1 year) (82–85). These trials showed that partial tumor regression is a rare event, occurring in 3–5% of patients treated with high-dose analogues, and stabilization of tumor growth is the most favorable event, occurring in 36–70% of patients.

Where the tumor is termed "nonfunctioning," the use of somatostatin analogues is agreed upon in cases where the SRS scan is positive and there is tumor progression (>25% tumor growth in one year) or evidence of high mitotic rate from histology (using the

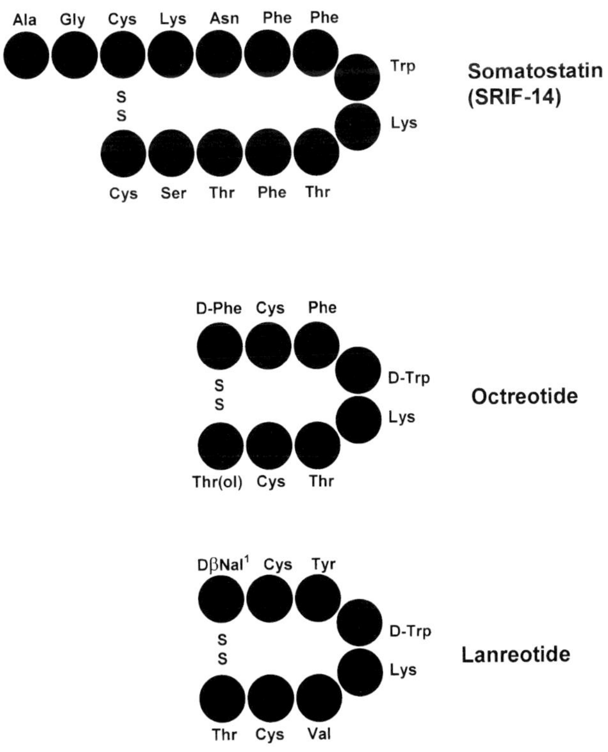

Figure 2 Secondary structure of somatostatin and its analogues. *DβNal = β-(2-naphthyl)alanine.

Ki67 value, CD44 expression, or somatostatin receptor content) (58). Should the tumor be a progressive nonfunctioning carcinoid with a negative SRS scan, the consensus opinion is that interferon-α should be the first-line medical therapy.

11.2.2 Interferon-α

The antitumor effects of interferon-α include direct and indirect mechanisms. The direct effects include antiproliferation (blocks G1-S phase), apoptosis, differentiation, and antiangiogenesis. Indirectly, it also increases class I antigens on tumor cells and thereby induces autoimmunity. Its use was first introduced for the treatment of carcinoid in 1982 because of its ability to stimulate natural killer cells and control hormone secretion, symptoms, and tumor growth (86).

The largest studies using interferon-α in malignant neuroendocrine tumors (mostly carcinoid) show a 42% biochemical and 14% tumor response in carcinoid and a 51% biochemical and 12% tumor response in neuroendocrine pancreatic tumors (87,88). Most therapeutic protocols for malignant carcinoid today use recombinant α-interferons, particularly IFN-α-2b. The recommended doses are 3–9 MU every day or every other day subcutaneously. However, the dose should be titrated individually according to the patient's weight, sex, and age. Oberg has suggested that the leukocyte count should be used for titrating the interferon dose aiming at reducing the number of leukocytes to below 3.0×10^9/L (89). However, side effects of interferon-α are frequent and include most commonly flu-like symptoms in 89%, weight loss in 59%, fatigue in 51%, and depression in 50%. Other side effects include hepatotoxicity, autoimmune disorders, and the development of neutralizing antibodies.

11.2.3 Combination of Octreotide and Interferon-α

The combination of octreotide and interferon-α has shown to be beneficial in some studies as compared with either agent alone (90,91). However, in a recent study 80 therapy-naïve patients (apart from surgery) were treated in a prospective randomized trial with either the somatostatin analogue, interferon-α, or the combination. No difference in antiproliferative response was found between the monotherapies and the combination of the two (58,89).

11.2.4 Chemotherapy

The place of chemotherapy in malignant gastroenteropancreatic neuroendocrine tumors always has to be discussed in a multidisciplinary fashion. Surgical excision, hepatic arterial (chemo)embolization, somatostatin analogues, and interferons need prior consideration, particularly in slowly growing tumors (where the growth in tumor size is < 25% in 1 year). Chemotherapy has different efficacies depending on the tumor type and differentiation and seems to be superior in the treatment of pancreatic neuroendocrine tumors (response rates 40–69%) than in metastatic carcinoid (response rates ~ 20%) (92).

In well-differentiated pancreatic neuroendocrine tumors, streptozotocin and adriamycin appear to offer the best results (93) with a 69% response rate, survival prolongation (median 2.2 years), tumor progression inhibition, and tumor shrinkage in two thirds of patients. In undifferentiated neuroendocrine tumors, the chemosensitivity is similar to that of small-cell carcinoma of the lung. A 67% response rate with a median survival of 1.75 years has been reported using a combination of etoposide (VP16) and cisplatin (CDDP) (94). This combination was not effective in differentiated neuroendocrine tumors. More recently, etoposide and cisplatin have also been effective in the treatment of heavily pretreated patients with poorly differentiated and highly aggressive neuroendocrine tumors (95). Objective response rates of 50–56% were seen with a median response duration of 9 months. Patients with endocrine pancreatic tumors and foregut carcinoids seemed to benefit most from this combination. Midgut carcinoid responded poorly, and there was a significant toxicity rate with nephrotoxicity (53%) and neutropenia (64%). Eriksson's group in Sweden is currently studying the beneficial effect of adding the organic thiophosphate compound amifostine to their etoposide/cisplatin regimen. This compound has been recently introduced to protect against chemotherapy-induced hematological and nonhematological toxicity. If successful in lowering toxicity, amifostine will prove an exciting development in this field. There is clearly a need for new and more active chemotherapeutic agents and regimens, including combinations with other treatment modalities such as hepatic arterial occlusion.

11.3 Interventional Radiology

11.3.1 Hepatic Artery Embolization

The majority of metastases from gastrointestinal neuroendocrine tumors will be in the liver. The liver derives dual blood supply, receiving 20–25% of blood from the hepatic artery and 75–80% from the hepatic portal vein. Metastases in the liver will derive their blood supply through new vessels arising from the hepatic artery and not the portal vein. This therefore provides the therapeutic option of occluding branches of the hepatic artery supplying the metastases without infarcting the liver, assuming that the portal vein is patent. Indeed, it is imperative to confirm this before the procedure. Various particulate materials have been used for the occlusion, including gel foam powder and polyvinyl alcohol microspheres of 150–500 μm diameter. Several reports have indicated that selective hepatic arterial embolization can reduce both hormonal symptoms and tumor burden in patients with both carcinoid and pancreatic neuroendocrine tumors (96–98). The objective response varies between 50 and 90%, and the median duration of response between 10 and 15 months. Symptomatic and biochemical responses (40–90%), often occurring within hours to days, are more frequent than radiological responses (15–40%). The procedure has a high rate of postembolic syndrome, including pain, fever, nausea, leukocytosis, and derangements in liver enzymes (in 50–90%). More severe complications with renal failure, hepatic abscess, liver necrosis, intestinal and cholecystic necrosis occur in 10% of patients, with a mortality of 3–7%.

The complications can be minimized by operator expertise and a formal hospital protocol with preembolization intravenous methylprednisolone, meticulous fluid balance pre- and postembolization requiring central venous pressure monitoring, intravenous octreotide, aprotinin, broad-spectrum antibiotics, and oral allopurinol. With carcinoid, the patient requires additional oral cyproheptadine and nicotinamide, while with insulinoma the blood glucose needs careful monitoring. If there has been a significant response to embolization in an individual patient, then it should be offered again when symptoms recur. There is no consensus as to the optimal timing and frequency of hepatic embolizations between different centers.

11.3.2 Chemotherapy Combined with Hepatic Arterial Occlusion

Several reports have indicated that hepatic arterial occlusion for liver metastases from carcinoid has an immediate effect, which lasts up to one year. In a large retrospective analysis, it has been shown that treatment with a combination of arterial occlusion and systemic chemotherapy with 5FU-streptozotocin alternated with adriamycin-dacarbazin had a 20% higher response rate and a longer tumor growth control time from 4 to 22 months for pancreatic neuroendocrine tumors and from 10 to 24 months for the carcinoid tumors (99). However, conclusions from this study must be guarded since the patients were not randomized and the patient groups were different.

11.3.3 Chemoembolization

Chemoembolization is a combination of hepatic artery embolization with local cytotoxic chemotherapy. Approximately 87% of patients respond to this therapy for an average of 11 months. The response is observed as tumor reduction in 50% of cases and diminution of symptoms of hormonal hypersecretion in 63%. The mean survival is 2 years (100). The mean survival from the onset of symptoms is 57 months, 47 months from the diagnosis of metastases and 24 months from the first treatment (101). More recently, chemoembolization was compared with curative hepatic resections and provided a median survival after treatment of 32 months (range 7–63 months) and an actuarial 5-year survival of 40% (68). Prognostic factors in achieving a sustained response (>1 year improvement in symptoms or radiology) included prior resection of the primary tumor, more than 4 chemoembolization procedures, and liver metastases 5 cm or smaller. Chemoembolization is only palliative but has great functional benefits for patients with hypersecreting tumors. The relative merits of chemoembolization in comparison with hepatic artery occlusion alone or hepatic artery occlusion followed by systemic chemotherapy are not yet clear.

11.3.4 Hepatic Radioembolization

Radioembolization is an experimental technique currently being applied to palliative treatment of hepatic metastases (102). Microspheres are labeled with a radioisotope (such as yttrium 90) and injected into branches of the hepatic arteries supplying liver metastases. There is therefore simultaneous hepatic embolization and local irradiation (brachyradiotherapy). There is still limited experience with this method, and we await further refinements to the technique.

11.4 Hepatic Cryosurgery

Hepatic cryosurgery for metastases involves placing a cryoprobe into each metastasis resulting in cellular damage and subsequent tumor destruction. It can be used for palliation of bilobar liver metastases, but is contraindicated when the tumor occupies >40% of the liver. In a small series of eight patients, the treatment resulted in symptom-free survival of 12 months (median) and overall survival with disease of 25 months (median) (103). Further studies and comparisons with other treatment options are needed to elucidate the effectiveness of cryosurgery and its impact on long-term survival.

11.5 Palliative (Cytoreduction) Surgery

Many of the published studies on hepatic resections include both potentially curative and palliative surgery. In earlier studies, palliative cytoreductive surgery alone did not prolong survival in patients with hepatic metastases from gastroenteropancreatic neuroendocrine tumors and provided an average of 6 months symptom relief if $>90\%$ of the tumor volume was removed (104). Furthermore, since the liver metastases are so often diffusely distributed throughout the liver, surgical resection of these is only possible in 5–8% of patients and was associated with a high complication rate (33%) and mortality rate (9%) (105). More recent series have shown better outcomes with improved surgical techniques. Among 34 patients who underwent hepatic resections, 15 had potentially curative and 19 palliative resections (66). The median survival had not been reached, but the estimated 5-year survival was 85% in the patients with complete resections and 63% with palliative resections.

11.6 Radiolabeled Somatostatin Analogues

Trials are currently underway with the use of radiolabeled somatostatin analogues as an alternative form of therapy targeted against tumor cells expressing the somatostatin receptor sstr2. Initially the diagnostic radiolabeled compound ^{111}In-DTPA-octreotide was used. However, the better higher-energy compound ^{90}yttrium-DOTA-DPhe1-Tyr3-octreotide has a high sstr2 specificity. When used in 10 patients with malignant neuroendocrine tumors and positive SRS scans, this resulted in tumor volume reduction in two patients and partial remission or stable disease in two patients (106). There is one report with the use of ^{90}yttrium-lanreotide in a patient with gastrinoma (107). This form of targeted radioactive therapy is currently a very exciting therapeutic option, and we await results of further trials, particularly on survival.

12 PROGNOSIS

If the primary gastroenteropancreatic neuroendocrine tumor is nonmalignant and resectable at diagnosis, the patient has a high cure rate. The survival of patients with malignant neuroendocrine tumors largely depends on the resectability at diagnosis and the rate of growth of the tumor. In series where the majority of patients have undergone curative surgery, the 5- and 10-year survival rates exceed 50%. In unresectable tumors, the presence or development of liver metastases and the degree of differentiation determine survival. The reader is referred to the sections on survival with various combinations of medical and interventional therapies.

REFERENCES

1. Polak JM, Bloom SR. Regulatory peptides of the gastrointestinal and respiratory tracts. Arch Int Pharmacodyn Ther 1986; 280(suppl 2):16–49.
2. Bax ND, Woods HF, Batchelor A, Jennings M. Clinical manifestations of carcinoid disease. World J Surg 1996; 20(2):142–146.
3. Caplin ME, Buscombe JR, Hilson AJ, Jones AL, Watkinson AF, Burroughs AK. Carcinoid tumour. Lancet 1998; 352(9130):799–805.
4. Kimura W, Kuroda A, Morioka Y. Clinical pathology of endocrine tumors of the pancreas. Analysis of autopsy cases. Dig Dis Sci 1991; 36(7):933–942.
5. Marx SJ, Agarwal SK, Kester MB, Heppner C, Kim YS, Skarulis MC, et al. Multiple endocrine neoplasia type 1: clinical and genetic features of the hereditary endocrine neoplasias. Recent Prog Horm Res 1999; 54:397–438.
6. Wang EH, Ebrahimi SA, Wu AY, Kashefi C, Passaro E Jr, Sawicki MP. Mutation of the MENIN gene in sporadic pancreatic endocrine tumors. Cancer Res 1998; 58(19): 4417–4420.
7. Agarwal SK, Guru SC, Heppner C, Erdos MR, Collins RM, Park SY, et al. Menin interacts with the AP1 transcription factor JunD and represses JunD-activated transcription. Cell 1999; 96(1):143–152.
8. Heppner C, Bilimoria KY, Agarwal SK, Kester M, Whitty LJ, Guru SC, et al. The tumor suppressor protein menin interacts with NF-kappaB proteins and inhibits NF-kappaB-mediated transactivation. Oncogene 2001; 20(36):4917–4925.
9. Modlin IM, Sandor A. An analysis of 8305 cases of carcinoid tumors. Cancer 1997; 79(4):813–829.
10. Polak JM, Bloom SR. The diffuse neuroendocrine system in gastroenterology. Biochem Soc Trans 1980; 8(1):19–22.
11. Bloom SR, Polak JM. Gut hormones in disease. Scand J Gastroenterol Suppl 1983; 82:1–5.
12. Polak JM, Bloom SR. Some aspects of neuroendocrine pathology. J Clin Pathol 1987; 40(9):1024–1041.
13. Taheri S, Ghatei MA, Bloom SR. Gastrointestinal hormones and tumor syndromes. In: De Groot LJ, Jameson JL, eds. Endocrinology. Philadelphia: WB Saunders, 2001:2547–2558.
14. Lauffer JM, Zhang T, Modlin IM. Review article:

current status of gastrointestinal carcinoids. Aliment Pharmacol Ther 1999; 13(3):271–287.
15. Makridis C, Rastad J, Oberg K, Akerstrom G. Progression of metastases and symptom improvement from laparotomy in midgut carcinoid tumors. World J Surg 1996; 20(7):900–906.
16. Aldridge MC, Williamson RCN. Surgery of endocrine tumours of the pancreas. In: Lynn J, Bloom SR, eds. Surgical Endocrinology. Oxford: Butterworth-Heinemann Ltd, 1993:530–520.
17. Arnold R, Simon B, Wied M. Treatment of neuroendocrine GEP tumours with somatostatin analogues: a review. Digestion 2000; 62(suppl 1):84–91.
18. Schindl M, Kaczirek K, Kaserer K, Niederle B. Is the new classification of neuroendocrine pancreatic tumors of clinical help? World J Surg 2000; 24(11): 1312–1318.
19. Jensen RT. Endocrine tumors of the gastrointestinal tract and pancreas. In: Braunwald E, Fauci AS, Kasper DL, Hauser SL, Longo DL, Jameson JL, eds. Harrison's Principles of Internal Medicine. New York: McGraw-Hill, 2001:593–603.
20. Gilligan CJ, Lawton GP, Tang LH, West AB, Modlin IM. Gastric carcinoid tumors: the biology and therapy of an enigmatic and controversial lesion. Am J Gastroenterol 1995; 90(3):338–352.
21. Vinik AI. Carcinoid tumors. In: De Groot LJ, Jameson JL, eds. Endocrinology. Philadelphia: WB Saunders, 2001:2533–2546.
22. Legaspi A, Brennan MF. Management of islet cell carcinoma. Surgery 1988; 104(6):1018–1023.
23. Blaschko H, Comline RS, Schneider FH, Silver M, Smith AD. Secretion of a chromaffin granule protein, chromogranin, from the adrenal gland after splanchnic stimulation. Nature 1967; 215(96):58–59.
24. Winkler H, Fischer-Colbrie R. The chromogranins A and B: the first 25 years and future perspectives. Neuroscience 1992; 49(3):497–528.
25. Tapia FJ, Polak JM, Barbosa AJ, Bloom SR, Marangos PJ, Dermody C, et al. Neuron-specific enolase is produced by neuroendocrine tumours. Lancet 1981; 1(8224):808–811.
26. Hamid QA, Bishop AE, Sikri KL, Varndell IM, Bloom SR, Polak JM. Immunocytochemical characterization of 10 pan-creatic tumours, associated with the glucagonoma syndrome, using antibodies to separate regions of the pro-glucagon molecule and other neuroendocrine markers. Histopathology 1986; 10(2):119–133.
27. Yiangou Y, Williams SJ, Bishop AE, Polak JM, Bloom SR. Peptide histidine-methionine immunoreactivity in plasma and tissue from patients with vasoactive intestinal peptide-secreting tumors and watery diarrhea syndrome. J Clin Endocrinol Metab 1987; 64(1):131–139.
28. Eriksson B, Arnberg H, Lindgren PG, Lorelius LE, Magnusson A, Lundqvist G, et al. Neuroendocrine pancreatic tumours: clinical presentation, biochemical and histopathological findings in 84 patients. J Intern Med 1990; 228(2):103–113.
29. Stridsberg M, Oberg K, Li Q, Engstrom U, Lundqvist G. Measurements of chromogranin A, chromogranin B (secretogranin I), chromogranin C (secretogranin II) and pancreastatin in plasma and urine from patients with carcinoid tumours and endocrine pancreatic tumours. J Endocrinol 1995; 144(1):49–59.
30. Sekiya K, Ghatei MA, Salahuddin MJ, Bishop AE, Hamid QA, Ibayashi H, et al. Production of GAWK (chromogranin-B 420-493)-like immunoreactivity by endocrine tumors and its possible diagnostic value. J Clin Invest 1989; 83(6):1834–1842.
31. Yasuda D, Iguchi H, Funakoshi A, Wakasugi H, Sekiya K, Misawa T, et al. Comparison of plasma pancreastatin and GAWK concentrations, presumed processing products of chromogranin A and B, in plasma of patients with pancreatic islet cell tumors. Horm Metab Res 1993; 25(11):593–595.
32. Wood SM, Polak JM, Bloom SR. Gut hormone secreting tumours. Scand J Gastroenterol Suppl 1983; 82:165–179.
33. Janson ET, Holmberg L, Stridsberg M, Eriksson B, Theodorsson E, Wilander E, et al. Carcinoid tumors: analysis of prognostic factors and survival in 301 patients from a referral center. Ann Oncol 1997; 8(7):685–690.
34. Frucht H, Howard JM, Slaff JI, Wank SA, McCarthy DM, Maton PN, et al. Secretin and calcium provocative tests in the Zollinger-Ellison syndrome. A prospective study. Ann Intern Med 1989; 111(9):713–722.
35. Norheim I, Theodorsson-Norheim E, Brodin E, Oberg K. Tachykinins in carcinoid tumors: their use as a tumor marker and possible role in the carcinoid flush. J Clin Endocrinol Metab 1986; 63(3):605–612.
36. McGuigan JE, Wolfe MM. Secretin injection test in the diagnosis of gastrinoma. Gastroenterology 1980; 79(6): 1324–1331.
37. Friesen SR. Update on the diagnosis and treatment of rare neuroendocrine tumors. Surg Clin North Am 1987; 67(2):379–393.
38. Ricke J, Klose KJ, Mignon M, Oberg K, Wiedenmann B. Standardisation of imaging in neuroendocrine tumours: results of a European delphi process. Eur J Radiol 2001; 37(1):8–17.
39. Krenning EP, Kwekkeboom DJ, Bakker WH, Breeman WA, Kooij PP, Oei HY, et al. Somatostatin receptor scintigraphy with [111In-DTPA-D-Phe1]-and [123I-Tyr3]-octreotide: the Rotterdam experience with more than 1000 patients. Eur J Nucl Med 1993; 20(8):716–731.
40. Termanini B, Gibril F, Reynolds JC, Doppman JL, Chen CC, Stewart CA, et al. Value of somatostatin receptor scintigraphy: a prospective study in gastrinoma of its effect on clinical management. Gastroenterology 1997; 112(2):335–347.

41. Lebtahi R, Cadiot G, Sarda L, Daou D, Faraggi M, Petegnief Y, et al. Clinical impact of somatostatin receptor scintigraphy in the management of patients with neuroendocrine gastroenteropancreatic tumors. J Nucl Med 1997; 38(6):853–858.
42. Modlin IM, Tang LH. Approaches to the diagnosis of gut neuroendocrine tumors: the last word (today). Gastroenterology 1997; 112(2):583–590.
43. Glover JR, Shorvon PJ, Lees WR. Endoscopic ultrasound for localisation of islet cell tumours. Gut 1992; 33(1):108–110.
44. Lightdale CJ, Botet JF, Woodruff JM, Brennan MF. Localization of endocrine tumors of the pancreas with endoscopic ultrasonography. Cancer 1991; 68(8):1815–1820.
45. Palazzo L, Roseau G, Salmeron M. Endoscopic ultrasonography in the preoperative localization of pancreatic endocrine tumors. Endoscopy 1992; 24(suppl 1): 350–353.
46. Rosch T, Lightdale CJ, Botet JF, Boyce GA, Sivak MV Jr, Yasuda K, et al. Localization of pancreatic endocrine tumors by endoscopic ultrasonography. N Engl J Med 1992; 326(26):1721–1726.
47. Zimmer T, Scherubl H, Faiss S, Stolzel U, Riecken EO, Wiedenmann B. Endoscopic ultrasonography of neuroendocrine tumours. Digestion 2000; 62(suppl 1):45–50.
48. Thompson NW, Czako PF, Fritts LL, Bude R, Bansal R, Nostrant TT, et al. Role of endoscopic ultrasonography in the localization of insulinomas and gastrinomas. Surgery 1994; 116(6):1131–1138.
49. Ruszniewski P, Amouyal P, Amouyal G, Grange JD, Mignon M, Bouche O, et al. Localization of gastrinomas by endoscopic ultrasonography in patients with Zollinger-Ellison syndrome. Surgery 1995; 117(6):629–635.
50. de Kerviler E, Cadiot G, Lebtahi R, Faraggi M, Le Guludec D, Mignon M. Somatostatin receptor scintigraphy in forty-eight patients with the Zollinger-Ellison syndrome. GRESZE: Groupe d'Etude du Syndrome de Zollinger-Ellison. Eur J Nucl Med 1994; 21(11):1191–1197.
51. Doppman JL, Miller DL, Chang R, Maton PN, London JF, Gardner JD, et al. Gastrinomas: localization by means of selective intraarterial injection of secretin. Radiology 1990; 174(1):25–29.
52. Doppman JL, Miller DL, Chang R, Shawker TH, Gorden P, Norton JA. Insulinomas: localization with selective intraarterial injection of calcium. Radiology 1991; 178(1):237–241.
53. Fedorak IJ, Ko TC, Gordon D, Flisak M, Prinz RA. Localization of islet cell tumors of the pancreas: a review of current techniques. Surgery 1993; 113(3):242–249.
54. O'Shea D, Rohrer-Theurs AW, Lynn JA, Jackson JE, Bloom SR. Localization of insulinomas by selective intraarterial calcium injection. J Clin Endocrinol Metab 1996; 81(4):1623–1627.
55. Goldstone AP, Scott-Coombes DM, Lynn JA. Surgical management of gastrointestinal endocrine tumours. Baillieres Clin Gastroenterol 1996; 10(4):707–736.
56. Eriksson B, Bergstrom M, Orlefors H, Sundin A, Oberg K, Langstrom B. Use of PET in neuroendocrine tumors. In vivo applications and in vitro studies. Q J Nucl Med 2000; 44(1):68–76.
57. Adams S, Baum RP. Intraoperative use of gamma-detecting probes to localize neuroendocrine tumors. Q J Nucl Med 2000; 44(1):59–67.
58. Role of Somatostatin Analogues in Oncology. European Neuroendocrine Tumor Network (ENET). February 24–27, 2000, Innsbruck, Austria. Round Table Discussion. Digestion 2000; 62(suppl 1):98–107.
59. Kloppel G, Heitz PU. Classification of normal and neoplastic neuroendocrine cells. Ann NY Acad Sci 1994; 733:19–23.
60. Capella C, Heitz PU, Hofler H, Solcia E, Kloppel G. Revised classification of neuroendocrine tumors of the lung, pancreas and gut. Digestion 1994; 55(suppl 3):11–23.
61. Rindi G, Capella C, Solcia E. Cell biology, clinicopathological profile, and classification of gastro-enteropancreatic endocrine tumors. J Mol Med 1998; 76(6):413–420.
62. Kloppel G, Heitz PU. Pancreatic endocrine tumors. Pathol Res Pract 1988; 183(2):155–168.
63. Solcia E, Sessa F, Rindi G, Villani L, Riva C, Buffa R, et al. Classification and histogenesis of gastroenteropancreatic endocrine tumours. Eur J Clin Invest 1990; 20(suppl 1): S72–S81.
64. Que FG, Nagorney DM, Batts KP, Linz LJ, Kvols LK. Hepatic resection for metastatic neuroendocrine carcinomas. Am J Surg 1995; 169(1):36–42.
65. Chen H, Hardacre JM, Uzar A, Cameron JL, Choti MA. Isolated liver metastases from neuroendocrine tumors: does resection prolong survival? J Am Coll Surg 1998; 187(1):88–92.
66. Chamberlain RS, Canes D, Brown KT, Saltz L, Jarnagin W, Fong Y, et al. Hepatic neuroendocrine metastases: does intervention alter outcomes? J Am Coll Surg 2000; 190(4):432–445.
67. Jaeck D, Oussoultzoglou E, Bachellier P, Lemarque P, Weber JC, Nakano H, et al. Hepatic metastases of gastroenteropancreatic neuroendocrine tumors: safe hepatic surgery. World J Surg 2001; 25(6):689–692.
68. Yao KA, Talamonti MS, Nemcek A, Angelos P, Chrisman H, Skarda J, et al. Indications and results of liver resection and hepatic chemoembolization for metastatic gastrointestinal neuroendocrine tumors. Surgery 2001; 130(4):677–682.
69. Bechstein WO, Neuhaus P. Liver transplantation for hepatic metastases of neuroendocrine tumors. Ann NY Acad Sci 1994; 733:507–514.
70. Anderson JV, Bloom SR. Neuroendocrine tumours of the gut: long-term therapy with the somatostatin

analogue SMS 201–995. Scand J Gastroenterol Suppl 1986; 119:115–128.
71. Wynick D, Bloom SR. Clinical review 23: the use of the long-acting somatostatin analog octreotide in the treatment of gut neuroendocrine tumors. J Clin Endocrinol Metab 1991; 73(1):1–3.
72. Polak JM, Bloom SR. Somatostatin localization in tissues. Scand J Gastroenterol Suppl 1986; 119:11–21.
73. Reisine T, Bell GI. Molecular biology of somatostatin receptors. Endocr Rev 1995; 16(4):427–442.
74. Patel YC, Srikant CB. Subtype selectivity of peptide analogs for all five cloned human somatostatin receptors (hsstr 1–5). Endocrinology 1994; 135(6):2814–2817.
75. Buscail L, Esteve JP, Saint-Laurent N, Bertrand V, Reisine T, O'Carroll AM, et al. Inhibition of cell proliferation by the somatostatin analogue RC-160 is mediated by somatostatin receptor subtypes SSTR2 and SSTR5 through different mechanisms. Proc Natl Acad Sci USA 1995; 92(5):1580–1584.
76. Wulbrand U, Wied M, Zofel P, Goke B, Arnold R, Fehmann H. Growth factor receptor expression in human gastroenteropancreatic neuroendocrine tumours. Eur J Clin Invest 1998; 28(12):1038–1049.
77. Sharma K, Srikant CB. Induction of wild-type p53, Bax, and acidic endonuclease during somatostatin-signaled apoptosis in MCF-7 human breast cancer cells. Int J Cancer 1998; 76(2):259–266.
78. Kraenzlin ME, Ch'ng JC, Wood SM, Bloom SR. Can inhibition of hormone secretion be associated with endocrine tumour shrinkage? Lancet 1983; 2(8365–66): 1501.
79. Clements D, Elias E. Regression of metastatic vipoma with somatostatin analogue SMS 201-995. Lancet 1985; 1(8433):874–875.
80. Shepherd JJ, Senator GB. Regression of liver metastases in patient with gastrin-secreting tumour treated with SMS 201–995. Lancet 1986; 2(8506):574.
81. Wiedenmann B, Rath U, Radsch R, Becker F, Kommerell B. Tumor regression of an ileal carcinoid under the treatment with the somatostatin analogue SMS 201–995. Klin Wochenschr 1988; 66(2):75–77.
82. Arnold R, Trautmann ME, Creutzfeldt W, Benning R, Benning M, Neuhaus C, et al. Somatostatin analogue octreotide and inhibition of tumour growth in metastatic endocrine gastroenteropancreatic tumours. Gut 1996; 38(3):430–438.
83. di Bartolomeo M, Bajetta E, Buzzoni R, Mariani L, Carnaghi C, Somma L, et al. Clinical efficacy of octreotide in the treatment of metastatic neuroendocrine tumors. A study by the Italian Trials in Medical Oncology Group. Cancer 1996; 77(2):402–408.
84. Eriksson B, Renstrup J, Imam H, Oberg K. High-dose treatment with lanreotide of patients with advanced neuroendocrine gastrointestinal tumors: clinical and biological effects. Ann Oncol 1997; 8(10):1041–1044.
85. Faiss S, Rath U, Mansmann U, Caird D, Clemens N, Riecken EO, et al. Ultra-high-dose lanreotide treatment in patients with metastatic neuroendocrine gastroenteropancreatic tumors. Digestion 1999; 60(5):469–476.
86. Oberg K, Funa K, Alm G. Effects of leukocyte interferon on clinical symptoms and hormone levels in patients with mid-gut carcinoid tumors and carcinoid syndrome. N Engl J Med 1983; 309(3):129–133.
87. Oberg K, Eriksson B. The role of interferons in the management of carcinoid tumors. Acta Oncol 1991; 30(4):519–522.
88. Eriksson B, Oberg K. An update of the medical treatment of malignant endocrine pancreatic tumors. Acta Oncol 1993; 32(2):203–208.
89. Oberg K. Interferon in the management of neuroendocrine GEP-tumors: a review. Digestion 2000; 62(suppl 1):92–97.
90. Janson ET, Oberg K. Long-term management of the carcinoid syndrome. Treatment with octreotide alone and in combination with alpha-interferon. Acta Oncol 1993; 32(2):225–229.
91. Frank M, Klose KJ, Wied M, Ishaque N, Schade-Brittinger C, Arnold R. Combination therapy with octreotide and alpha-interferon: effect on tumor growth in metastatic endocrine gastroenteropancreatic tumors. Am J Gastro-enterol 1999; 94(5):1381–1387.
92. Rougier P, Mitry E. Chemotherapy in the treatment of neuroendocrine malignant tumors. Digestion 2000; 62(suppl 1):73–78.
93. Moertel CG, Lefkopoulo M, Lipsitz S, Hahn RG, Klaassen D. Streptozocin-doxorubicin, streptozocin-fluorouracil or chlorozotocin in the treatment of advanced islet-cell carcinoma. N Engl J Med 1992; 326(8):519–523.
94. Moertel CG, Kvols LK, O'Connell MJ, Rubin J. Treatment of neuroendocrine carcinomas with combined etoposide and cisplatin. Evidence of major therapeutic activity in the anaplastic variants of these neoplasms. Cancer 1991; 68(2):227–232.
95. Fjallskog ML, Granberg DP, Welin SL, Eriksson C, Oberg KE, Janson ET, et al. Treatment with cisplatin and etoposide in patients with neuroendocrine tumors. Cancer 2001; 92(5):1101–1107.
96. Ajani JA, Carrasco CH, Charnsangavej C, Samaan NA, Levin B, Wallace S. Islet cell tumors metastatic to the liver: effective palliation by sequential hepatic artery embolization. Ann Intern Med 1988; 108(3):340–344.
97. Carrasco CH, Chuang VP, Wallace S. Apudomas metastatic to the liver: treatment by hepatic artery embolization. Radiology 1983; 149(1):79–83.
98. Eriksson BK, Larsson EG, Skogseid BM, Lofberg AM, Lorelius LE, Oberg KE. Liver embolizations of patients with malignant neuroendocrine gastrointestinal tumors. Cancer 1998; 83(11):2293–2301.
99. Moertel CG, Johnson CM, McKusick MA, Martin JK Jr, Nagorney DM, Kvols LK, et al. The management of

patients with advanced carcinoid tumors and islet cell carcinomas. Ann Intern Med 1994; 120(4):302–309.
100. Wallace S, Ajani JA, Charnsangavej C, DuBrow R, Yang DJ, Chuang VP, et al. Carcinoid tumors: imaging procedures and interventional radiology. World J Surg 1996; 20(2):147–156.
101. Stokes KR, Stuart K, Clouse ME. Hepatic arterial chemoembolization for metastatic endocrine tumors. J Vasc Interv Radiol 1993; 4(3):341–345.
102. Andrews JC, Walker SC, Ackermann RJ, Cotton LA, Ensminger WD, Shapiro B. Hepatic radioembolization with yttrium-90 containing glass microspheres: preliminary results and clinical follow-up. J Nucl Med 1994; 35(10):1637–1644.
103. Bilchik AJ, Sarantou T, Foshag LJ, Giuliano AE, Ramming KP. Cryosurgical palliation of metastatic neuroendocrine tumors resistant to conventional therapy. Surgery 1997; 122(6):1040–1047.
104. McEntee GP, Nagorney DM, Kvols LK, Moertel CG, Grant CS. Cytoreductive hepatic surgery for neuroendocrine tumors. Surgery 1990; 108(6):1091–1096.
105. Soreide O, Berstad T, Bakka A, Schrumpf E, Hanssen LE, Engh V, et al. Surgical treatment as a principle in patients with advanced abdominal carcinoid tumors. Surgery 1992; 111(1):48–54.
106. de Jong M, Bakker WH, Krenning EP, Breeman WA, van der Pluijm ME, Bernard BF, et al. Yttrium-90 and indium-111 labelling, receptor binding and biodistribution of [DOTA0,d-Phe1,Tyr3]octreotide, a promising somatostatin analogue for radionuclide therapy. Eur J Nucl Med 1997; 24(4):368–371.
107. Leimer M, Kurtaran A, Smith-Jones P, Raderer M, Havlik E, Angelberger P, et al. Response to treatment with yttrium 90-DOTA-lanreotide of a patient with metastatic gastrinoma. J Nucl Med 1998; 39(12):2090–2094.

53

Liver Transplantation for Neuroendocrine Tumors

Myron E. Schwartz and Sander S. Florman

Mount Sinai School of Medicine, New York University, New York, New York, U.S.A.

1 OVERVIEW

Liver metastases from neuroendocrine tumors (NET) are often slow growing compared to other common solid tumors. Their successful treatment with a variety of modalities, including transplantation, has been reported widely. Approaches include observation, medical therapy with somatostatin analogues, embolization with or without chemotherapy, resection, and liver transplantation. Each of these options has been advocated, and good short- and medium-term results have been reported. This is more a reflection of the favorable biology of these tumors than of the merits of any particular therapy. Because the likelihood of permanent cure by any treatment is remote, the challenge in this disease is to outline a rational basis for choosing among the various options to provide patients with the best and longest-lasting palliation possible.

Liver transplantation is the accepted therapy for end-stage cirrhosis, with excellent long-term patient survival achievable in most cases. Transplantation has also come to be recognized as the best treatment for early but unresectable primary hepatocellular carcinoma, with results equaling those obtained in benign disease (1). The role of liver transplantation in treatment of tumors metastatic to the liver, on the other hand, is far less clear, and the results have historically been poor (2,3).

Liver metastasis is generally the result of hematogenous dissemination of tumor from the primary site. For tumors arising in the gut, where venous drainage is via the portal system, the liver is commonly the first place where metastases appear. Lymphatic metastasis typically occurs concurrently with hematogenous spread, but resection of the primary site can encompass the regional lymphatic bed.

Surgical cure in some patients with liver metastases does appear to be possible. A long-term follow-up study performed in 1997 examined survival in 456 patients who underwent liver resection between 1985 and 1991 for metastatic colonic carcinoma (the most frequent tumor type for which resection of metastases is performed). There were 96 actual 5-year survivors (21%), 52 (11% of the original population) of whom experienced no tumor recurrence and may well have been cured by the liver resection (4).

Not surprisingly, factors that predict survival after resection of liver metastases (fewer than 4 lesions, unilobar disease, and ability to achieve tumor-free margins) also predict ease of resectability; patients with large, multiple, bilobar metastases for whom transplantation might be proposed are highly likely to recur (5). While transplantation may reduce (though not eliminate) the likelihood of hepatic recurrence compared to resection, the majority of patients in whom recurrence develops after liver resection present with extrahepatic disease. As the available limited literature on the subject bears out, transplantation for unresectable metastatic colon cancer is very unlikely to be curative (2,3). While it is not easy to glean from the literature, the same appears true for unresectable metastatic NET.

2 CLASSIFICATION OF NEUROENDOCRINE TUMORS

2.1 Clinical Relevance

NETs of gastrointestinal or pancreatic origin comprise a diverse group of tumors with varying biology and natural history. The clinical consequences of these tumors may be the result of either their physical presence as space-occupying lesions or of the production of hormones or hormone-like substances that cause remote effects. When liver metastasis occurs it is almost always multifocal in both lobes, although this may not be immediately evident. Not uncommonly, symptoms related to bulky liver metastases are the initial presentation; in some cases a careful search reveals the site of the primary tumor, while in others the location of the primary remains obscure despite thorough investigation.

NETs have been classified according to anatomical site of origin, hormonal production, and rate of proliferation (6,7). There is no universally accepted unifying nomenclature, but each basis of classification has relevance to treatment decisions, including the decision to transplant.

2.2 Site of Origin

Based on the embryonic derivation of the site of origin, NETs may be classified as being of foregut, midgut, or hindgut origin. Foregut NETs most commonly arise in the pancreas. Often referred to as pancreatic endocrine tumors (PETs), these neoplasms may produce a wide array of peptide hormones with associated clinical syndromes. About 35% of PETs are considered nonfunctioning; while these produce no active substances, they often produce measurable peptides such as chromogranin A (8). The likelihood of clinically malignant behavior correlates to a significant degree with patterns of hormone production: insulin-producing tumors, for example, are rarely malignant, but gastrin-producing tumors and nonfunctioning PETs commonly are. From an anatomical standpoint, the lymphatic drainage of the pancreatic bed is such that tumors that metastasize widely to the liver invariably invade regional nodes as well in a way that generally precludes surgical cure (9).

Tumors of midgut origin, arising in the small bowel or proximal colon, are more uniform in their pattern of hormone production, producing the array of substances that, when released in sufficient amounts, give rise to the carcinoid syndrome. The term carcinoid tumor, at one time applied to the entire spectrum of NETs, is now more properly applied specifically to tumors of mid-and hindgut origin (7). The likelihood of metastasis correlates with the location of the primary tumor: tumors arising in the rectum, for example, are less likely to metastasize than those arising in the small bowel. The regional lymphatic bed of the small bowel and colon is more readily resected en bloc with a primary tumor than that of the pancreas, a factor that has been mentioned as being of relevance to the decision for transplantation (10). From the authors' perspective, however, since cure is not the chief aim of transplantation, the distinction between midgut and foregut origin is not a major factor in deciding whether transplantation is indicated.

2.3 Hormone Production

NETs are commonly classified according to patterns of hormone production (Table 1). As mentioned above, there is fairly consistent correlation between the hormones produced and both the location of the primary tumor and the histological (and biological) grade of the tumor. From the standpoint of treatment decisions, including the decision to transplant, hormone secretion can be a very important factor. Despite the advent of pharmacological agents that are able to counter hormone-related symptoms (e.g., proton pump inhibitors for gastrinoma, somatostatin analogues for VIPoma, H1 and H2 blockers for carcinoid tumors), patients may develop disabling or life-threatening complications due to hormones released from NET liver metastases. The best palliation is achieved in such cases by resection of the metastases; if their number and distribution pre-

Table 1 Hormones Produced by Neuroendocrine Tumors

Gastrin
Kallikrein
Glucagon
Calcitonin
Histamine
Substance P
Somatostatin
HCG subunits
Prostaglandins
Neurokinin A, B
Neuropeptide K
Chromogranin A, B, C
Pancreatic peptide (PP)
Insulin, proinsulin, C-peptide
Vasoactive intestinal peptide (VIP)
Serotonin and metabolites (5-HIAA, MeImAA)

clude partial hepatectomy, transplantation may be the best solution.

2.4 Rate of Proliferation

Most current literature dealing with classification of NETs focuses considerable attention on the degree of differentiation of the tumor. Based on cytological characteristics and markers of proliferative rate such as Ki 67 staining on immunohistochemistry, NETs may be graded as adenoma, well-differentiated, or poorly differentiated carcinoma. Grading of NETs in this way has proven clinically useful in estimating prognosis (6, 11,12). Because the decision to transplant is not based on intent to cure but rather on the likelihood of a reasonably long period of palliation, transplantation becomes a relatively less rational choice in patients with rapidly proliferating, poorly differentiated carcinomas (13,14).

3 ASSESSMENT OF THE PATIENT WITH NEUROENDOCRINE LIVER METASTASES

Evaluation of patients with NET liver metastases must encompass complete characterization of the tumor with regard to proliferative rate and hormone production, excellent liver imaging to accurately define the extent of liver involvement, an assessment of the adequacy of control of the primary tumor, delineation of the extent and location of extrahepatic metastases, and the physiological state of the patient.

3.1 Characterization of the Tumor

A complete discussion of the biochemical assessment of patients with NETs is beyond the scope of this chapter. In order to counter possible hormone-related symptoms, to help estimate prognosis, and to establish useful markers of tumor activity, a complete profile of tumor-related hormonal products should be checked. Even patients with so-called "nonfunctioning" tumors typically have elevated levels of substances such as chromogranin A, which may be useful as markers of tumor activity after treatment (8).

A recent study by Rosenau et al. suggests that patients with tumor immunohistochemistry demonstrating rapid proliferation as evidenced by a high proportion of cells staining positive for Ki 67 or demonstrating increased metastatic potential as evidenced by regular staining for the adhesion molecule E-cadherin have diminished survival after transplantation (14). At the University of Göteborg, Sweden (a center with a large experience in this disease), patients with tumors exhibiting >10% Ki 67 positivity on immunohistochemistry are excluded from consideration for transplantation (13). These studies can be performed on paraffin-embedded tissue from a prior biopsy and should be obtained as part of transplant evaluation.

3.2 Assessment of Liver Involvement

Either computed tomography (CT) or magnetic resonance imaging (MRI) may be employed to assess the extent of liver involvement. Scans must be performed after the administration of intravenous iodinated contrast material (CT) or gadolinium (MRI). Unlike most other metastatic liver tumors, NET metastases are commonly hypervascular; dual-phase CT or MRI should thus be performed to provide maximal information.

The quality of imaging studies with which patients present for evaluation varies widely; the import of the decisions riding on imaging studies is such that referral centers must insist on top-quality images, even if studies of inferior quality have only recently been obtained elsewhere. Scans should be reviewed with the intent of resection. Particularly in patients with symptoms related to hormone production, liver resection employing the technique of tumor enucleation without regard for the classically desired 1 cm tumor-free margin may offer long-term benefit (15,16).

3.3 Assessment of the Primary Site

In patients with NET liver metastases, the primary tumor may be discovered before, at the time of, or after the recognition of liver involvement, or, in a small minority of patients, not at all (there is some debate over whether the liver may represent the primary site for such tumors). Certainly, the liver is a "fertile field" for these tumors, and the common observation that liver metastases typically grow faster and larger than their primary progenitors is supported by experimental evidence (17,18). In cases where the primary tumor has been resected, the pathology report should be reviewed to determine the adequacy of the resection and the extent of nodal involvement. Imaging with CT and octreotide scan are used to search for residual regional disease.

It is not unusual for the primary tumor to be discovered by careful assessment of imaging studies including CT and octreotide scan when a patient presents with symptoms related to liver metastases. The body and tail of the pancreas have proven the most common site of origin in such cases. While there may be room for debate as to the proper course (19), it has been our practice to consider resection of the primary tumor early in the course of treatment of such patients, in recent years via laparoscopic distal pancreatectomy (20). The aim of this approach is to remove the source of ongoing metastasis, since there is no effective regional therapy such as chemoembolization for the pancreas. In patients with impaired liver function from extensive tumor load, who are not good candidates for preliminary resection of the primary, combined liver transplantation and resection of the primary tumor may be the most rational approach.

There is, as mentioned, a minority of patients who present with extensive NET liver metastases in the absence of a detectable primary tumor. In such cases, it is our practice to proceed with treatment of the liver and to continue surveillance in anticipation of the discovery of the primary site. While it is comforting to have dealt with the primary before considering such a radical treatment for the liver as transplantation, ultimately, since the aim is palliation and not cure, identification of the primary is not, in our opinion, a strict prerequisite to proceeding with liver transplantation. Thus far in our experience, we have taken two patients for transplant without prior identification of the primary site, and in both cases the primary was discovered on intraoperative assessment to lie within the pancreas.

3.4 Evaluation of Extrahepatic Disease

The presence of extrahepatic disease does not logically preclude liver transplantation for NET metastases; as has been discussed, the likelihood of cure is remote regardless of their presence or absence. Nevertheless, a complete picture of the extent of disease is valuable both in planning treatment and in properly informing the patient. Common sites of extrahepatic metastasis include abdominal lymph nodes, lung, and bone; CT of the chest and abdomen and bone scan are thus routinely performed. As the majority of NETs demonstrate avidity for octreotide, nuclear scanning with labeled octreotide is often useful in the detection of disease in unlikely locations as well as to confirm the nature of questionable disease seen on imaging studies (21). More recently, radiolabeled metaiodobenzylguanidine (MIBG) and positron emission tomography (PET) scans have proven similarly useful, particularly in patients with less well-differentiated tumors, in identifying occult sites of disease (22).

3.5 Physiological Assessment of the Patient

Among all the treatments that have been advocated for NET liver metastases, liver transplantation is surely the most radical, with the greatest morbidity and mortality; its value as a tumor treatment diminishes in direct proportion to the likelihood of treatment-related death. Careful assessment of cardiac, pulmonary, and renal function is part of every transplant evaluation. Diverse factors such as obesity, smoking, diabetes, psychiatric issues, and advancing age must all be figured into the complex decision for transplant.

4 THE TRANSPLANT OPERATION

Liver transplantation techniques have been well described elsewhere (23); the technical aspects of transplantation in patients with NET metastases are essentially the same as for other indications. Transplantation in these cases is typically facilitated by the fact that the patients do not generally have underlying liver disease with associated portal hypertension and coagulopathy. On the other hand, bulky disease may complicate the hepatectomy. If the primary tumor has not been resected, or if additional extrahepatic tumor is present at the time of transplant, concomitant procedures such as lymphadenectomy, distal pancreatectomy, pancreaticoduodenectomy, or gastrointestinal resection may be performed.

Anesthesia management in patients with hormonally active NETs is potentially complicated. Administration of H1- and H2-histamine receptor antagonists and corticosteroids and continuous infusion of the somatostatin analogue octreotide are useful in preventing the release of hormonal mediators that can cause wide fluctuations in blood pressure and may result from intraoperative tumor manipulation (24).

In selected cases, some centers have advocated multivisceral, or "cluster," procedures wherein radical excision of the pancreas, duodenum ($\pm$ stomach), bile duct, and liver is performed en bloc in an attempt to completely remove the primary tumor with its lymphatic bed and any locoregional metastases (13,25,26). Transplantation is then performed, either with a multivisceral graft or with a liver alone.

Results of these operations have generally been disappointing, with high early morbidity and mortality; patients who receive multivisceral grafts require increased immunosuppression and have had a high incidence of Epstein-Barr virus–related posttransplant lymphoproliferative disorder. Too few procedures have been performed and followed long term to allow for a good estimate of any increased likelihood of cure from multivisceral resection. In the absence of such data, our approach has been to perform separate resection of the primary and of the liver, rather than embark on the more extensive en bloc procedures (27).

4.1 Tumors and Immunosuppression

Immunosuppression is required for transplantation to be successful, except in the case of identical twins. The mainstay of liver transplant immunosuppression has been the calcineurin inhibitors cyclosporine and tacrolimus. There is now considerable evidence that these medications are associated with an increased incidence of skin malignancies and lymphomas (28). On the other hand, there is no clear association between immunosuppression and the incidence or rate of growth of nonlymphoid solid organ tumors (29). Despite this lack of evidence, there remains a level of concern about administering immunosuppressive drugs to patients with cancer. There is conflicting data as to whether cyclosporine and tacrolimus, which are known to augment liver regeneration, may influence the course of recurrence of primary hepatocellular carcinoma after transplantation (30–32). Even if such were the case, the relevance to recurrence of metastatic tumors would be unclear. The recent introduction of sirolimus, an immunosuppressive drug with demonstrated anticancer activity, may offer help in preventing both liver rejection and tumor recurrence (33).

5 A RATIONAL APPROACH TO THE PATIENT WITH NEUROENDOCRINE LIVER METASTASES

As alluded to in the overview at the beginning of this chapter, it is the generally slow-growing nature of neuroendocrine tumors rather than the benefit of any particular therapy that explains the relatively long survival of patients with neuroendocrine liver metastases as compared to those with metastases from other sources. Nevertheless, most patients with this disease ultimately develop significant symptoms and die as a result. The challenge for those who care for them is to choose wisely among the available modalities in order to maximize both the quality and the length of life. Bearing in mind that cure by any means is ultimately unlikely, it seems most reasonable to withhold the most radical treatment (i.e., liver transplantation) until it is clear that the patient is in imminent trouble and that treatment options less likely to result in serious complication or death have been exhausted. Thus, while the focus of this chapter is liver transplantation, a limited discussion of the array of treatment options seems appropriate to provide adequate context within which to place the transplant option.

5.1 Observation/Medical Therapy

After obtaining blood and tissue sufficient to fully characterize the tumor, consideration should be given to a period of observation in the patient newly diagnosed with neuroendocrine liver metastases. When possible, this allows the physician and the patient to gain some perspective on the nature of the particular tumor with which they are faced; for it must be admitted that, despite the various tests and classification schemes that have been developed, the clinical behavior of the tumor cannot be predicted with complete accuracy. In considering the merits of active intervention, it should always be kept in mind that patients with liver metastases from NETs have a 30% overall 5-year survival and a median survival of 3–4 years *without* treatment (15,34,35).

For those patients with minimal or no symptoms or with hormone-related symptoms that are readily controlled medically (e.g., proton pump inhibitors in gastrinoma), such observation, with periodic imaging and biochemistry to monitor progression, may provide a significant period of good quality life with no risk of treatment-related morbidity. Upon evidence of tumor progression, the somatostatin analogue octreotide may be added; its demonstrated tumoristatic properties come at low physiological (but not monetary) cost (36,37).

5.2 Liver Resection

There is a considerable body of literature advocating resection as the preferred treatment for neuroendocrine liver metastases when technically possible (16,38–41). While these many studies quote respectable medium-term survival figures, close review reveals that reports of cure as evidenced by disease-free survival beyond 5 years are few and far between; in the Mount Sinai series of 16 resections, there are none. Resection should be viewed, then, not as qualitatively different than treatments such as radiofrequency ablation or chemoembolization, but rather as an alternative means to tumor reduction with its unique advantages and disadvantages. In the authors' practice, resection is the least commonly employed of these alternatives in the treatment of patients with NET metastases.

The clearest indication for resection is in the patient with a single or limited number of large, symptomatic tumors that are technically amenable to complete resection. In competent hands, resection can be carried out with low (0–2%) mortality, and after the limited period of surgery-related morbidity the patient may experience prolonged symptom relief without need for repeated interventions. By contrast, large tumors (>4 cm) are not technically suitable for percutaneous ablation techniques, and control in such cases with chemoembolization is both less certain and considerably more drawn out.

The role of subtotal resection is, in the authors' view, limited to cases with documented slow progression of tumors that are producing hormone-related symptoms. As the degree of symptoms is related to the bulk of tumor, significant surgical reduction in tumor volume can result in significant periods of symptom relief quicker and more certainly than can other modalities.

5.3 Ablative Techniques

These technologies extend the ability of the surgeon to physically eliminate tumor tissue and should be viewed as complementary rather than as competing with surgery (42). Because the majority of patients present with multifocal involvement of the liver, these techniques that, like resection, focus on particular tumors are not likely ever to become the mainstay of therapy.

5.3.1 Radiofrequency Ablation

Radiofrequency ablation (RFA) may be performed percutaneously and with the latest available technology is effective in destroying tumors up to 4–5 cm in diameter. Because it is uncommon for patients to present with a limited number of tumors all of which are amenable to RFA, this will rarely be the primary treatment. More commonly, RFA finds application intraoperatively as an adjunct to surgery to treat small lesions that are present deep within the liver of a patient undergoing resection, or percutaneously in treating new tumors that develop during follow-up after resection.

5.3.2 Cryosurgery

Cryosurgery, performed as an open procedure in all but a few centers, is capable of destroying larger tumors and is similarly employed as an adjunct to resection; the indications for cryosurgery are those for resection. The readiness with which cryosurgery is employed is, in general, inversely related to the skill of the operator in performing hepatectomy; the morbidity is no less than that of resection, and patients undergoing cryoablation of large tumors may in fact suffer serious consequences related to the release of substances by the necrotic tumor following treatment.

5.4 Chemoembolization

The typically highly vascular nature of neuroendocrine metastases renders them good targets for chemoembolization (43,44). A catheter is inserted via the femoral artery and advanced into the hepatic artery, followed by injection of contrast. Tumors light up as a blush of contrast; the catheter is then advanced into the branches of the artery supplying the tumor, and injection is made first of chemotherapeutic agents followed by particles to occlude small branches of the artery. As the liver has a dual blood supply, nourished by both the hepatic artery and the portal vein, whereas liver metastases derive their blood supply virtually entirely from the artery, this treatment disproportionately kills tumor relative to surrounding liver. The arterial occlusion produced by chemoembolization is transitory, allowing for repeated treatment. Because it is delivered via the hepatic artery, which supplies (albeit with a number of anatomical variations) the entire liver, chemoembolization may be employed perfectly well in cases of diffuse metastasis.

In order to minimize side effects resulting from the destruction of large amounts of tumor, patients with extensive metastases are generally treated in multiple sessions, treating only a portion of the liver at any one sitting. In patients deemed by virtue of symptoms, extent of liver involvement, or rate of progression to require treatment, chemoembolization is the most commonly employed approach at Mount Sinai. With repeated chemoembolizations it is often possible to maintain patients with diffuse liver involvement who get to the point of requiring therapy, over a period of years, with an acceptable quality of life.

5.5 Liver Transplantation

Considering all of the foregoing discussion, the role of liver transplantation is clear: for patients who are physiologically capable of withstanding the transplant surgery, have slowly progressive disease, extensive, life-threatening liver involvement, and no overwhelming extrahepatic disease, a liver transplant may provide a number of years of good-quality life when no other options remain.

Is it possible that this strategy of withholding the one treatment that definitively removes all liver metastases until other options have been exhausted deprives some patients of an opportunity for cure? While such possibility exists, from all that is known of this disease the likelihood is small, and treatment of subsequent recurrence will be complicated by the need to consider the transplanted liver and associated immunosuppression. Furthermore, the up-front 15% 1-year mortality associated with the transplant procedure independent of tumor-related issues in all likelihood more than cancels out any such benefit (45).

A decision to transplant is of little practical import if a donor organ is not available. An increasing demand for liver transplantation over recent years has not been accompanied by a commensurate rise in the number of available cadaveric donor organs. As a result, donor livers are in short supply. The system for prioritizing recipients of cadaveric donor livers in the United States is based on a score [Model for End-Stage Liver Disease (MELD) score], ranging from 6 to 40, that reflects the degree of medical urgency of the candidates. The score is calculated based on levels of serum bilirubin and creatinine and the standardized prothrombin time (INR) (46).

While there are certain conditions, including early hepatocellular carcinoma, that have been singled out as being exceptional and warranting special priority despite low calculated scores, metastatic NET is not among them. Thus, unless patients receive special case dispensations from a panel comprising representatives of all liver transplant centers in the region, it is in effect impossible to obtain cadaveric donor livers with which to transplant patients with metastatic NET until their liver function is severely affected. The limited Mount Sinai experience with waiting until liver function has been impaired to the point of gaining waiting list priority has been dismal. Since 1998, adult living donor liver transplantation has provided an alternative source of donor organs, offering the potential for more timely transplantation and improved results (47).

6 REPORTED EXPERIENCE WITH LIVER TRANSPLANTATION FOR NEUROENDOCRINE TUMORS

There are a number of small single-center series reporting results of liver transplantation for NET metastases (Table 2) (13,14,25,48 49–56). In a 1998 meta-analysis of 103 patients from 23 centers for whom follow-up data had been reported, Lehnert found the 1-year and 5-year survival rates to be 68% and 47%, respectively, with a 5-year disease-free survival rate of 24% (data on 18 patients regarding recurrence was not available). Age > 50 years and transplantation combined with upper abdominal exenteration or Whipple's operation were identified as adverse prognostic factors on multivariate analysis (57).

In 1997, Le Treut published the collected French experience with liver transplantation for NET comprising 31 patients from 11 centers. With a median follow-up of 57 months, 1-year and 5-year survival rates were 58% and 36%, respectively (10). The most significant factor correlating with outcome was whether the pri-

Table 2 Single Center Series of Liver Transplant for Neuroendocrine Metastases

Author (Ref.)	Year	No. of patients	Median follow-up (months)	1-yr survival (%)	5-yr survival (%)	Actual 5-yr disease-free survivors
Mt. Sinai[a]	2002	11	62	73	36	1
Olausson et al. (13)	2002	9	22	89	—	0
Rosenau et al. (14)	2002	19	38	89	80	3
Ringe et al. (48)	2001	5	22	80	—	0
Coppa et al. (49)	2001	9	39	100	70	—
Pascher et al. (50)	2000	4	42	100	50	1
Frilling et al. (51)	1998	4	54	50	50	0
Dousset et al. (52)	1996	9	29	33	33	0
Anthuber et al. (53)	1996	4	11	25	0	0
Alessiani et al. (25)	1995	14	—	—	—	—
Routley et al. (54)	1995	11	—	82	57	—
Arnold et al. (55)	1989	4	30	50	—	0
Makowka et al. (56)	1989	5	32	60	—	0

[a] Unpublished data; see Table 3 for case details.

Table 3 Transplantation

Patient no.	Age	Sex	Type	1° resection	Alive	Disease free	Survival (months)	Comments
1	40	F	N/F	Distal pancreas[a]	N	N	79	
2	52	M	VIP	Distal pancreas	Y	Y	119	Prior hepatectomy
3	56	M	N/F	Distal pancreas	N	N	41	
4	51	M	N/F	Distal pancreas[a]	N	N	76	
5	56	F	N/F	Whipple[a]	N	N	0	Pulmonary embolus POD#4
6	57	F	Carcinoid	Appendix	N	N	0	Intraoperative death
7	24	F	N/F	Distal pancreas[a]	N	N	16	Living donor
8	56	F	N/F	Not identified	N	N	19	NET unrecognized pretransplant
9	59	M	VIP	Distal pancreas	N	N	0	Prior hepatectomy; intraoperative death
10	56	F	Carcinoid	Ileum	Y	N	13	Living donor
11	56	F	Carcinoid	Rectum	Y	N	11	Living donor

[a] Performed at the time of transplant.
N/F, nonfunctioning; VIP, vasoactive intestinal peptide.

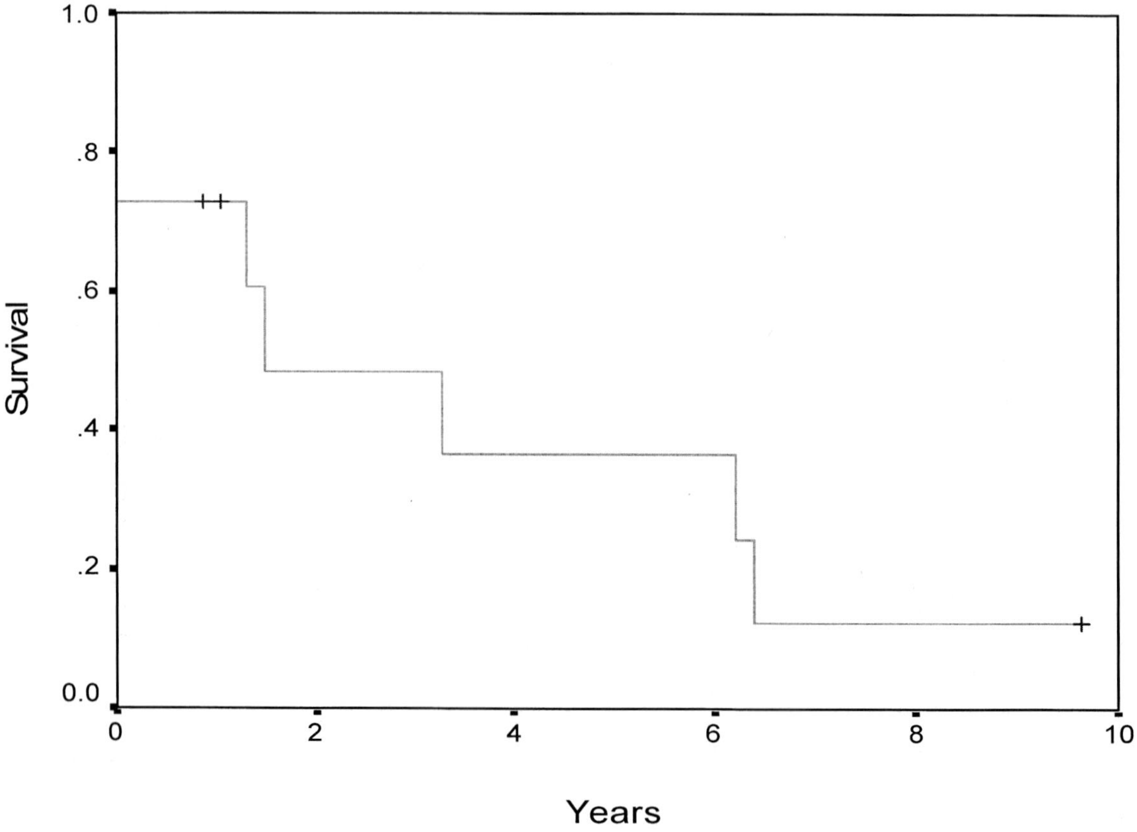

Figure 1 Mt. Sinai patient survival after liver transplant for neuroendocrine metastases.

mary tumor was a carcinoid (69% survival at 5 years) versus PET (8% survival at 4 years).

In reviewing the literature, one is struck by the relatively short period of follow-up in most studies. While most report 5-year survival rates, none has a median follow-up of 5 years. Among the studies that report disease-free survival in an unambiguous way, only 5 patients who were disease-free at 5 years can be identified out of 83 transplant recipients, thus confirming the impression that cure of this disease by transplantation is a very unusual occurrence.

7 THE MOUNT SINAI EXPERIENCE

Since April 1992, 43 patients with NET liver metastases have been evaluated at The Mount Sinai Hospital. Of this group, 15 received only medical therapy. Sixteen patients underwent hepatic resection, either for localized tumor in hopes of cure or for debulking of symptomatic metastases. Fourteen patients were evaluated and listed for transplantation; of these, 11 were transplanted (Table 3). Of the 3 patients listed but not transplanted, one was lost to follow-up, one died 14 months after listing from progressive disease, and one remains waiting more than 4 years after being placed on the waiting list. With a median follow-up of 62 months, our 1-year posttransplant survival is 73%; 5-year survival is 36% (Fig. 1).

Since 1998, we have considered patients with NET metastases in whom transplant is indicated for living donor liver transplantation. Availability of a living donor frees the patient from the need to compete with other transplant candidates on the waiting list and enables the transplant team, in consultation with the patient and treating physicians, to optimize the timing of the procedure. Three of the last five transplants performed at Mount Sinai for NET metastases were performed using living donors, including one case where the donor and recipient were identical twins, thus obviating the need for immunosuppression.

8 CONCLUSION

Liver transplantation for the treatment of metastatic neuroendocrine tumors is radical. While cure is not impossible, it is certainly not probable. The world's experience with transplantation for this indication is limited to fewer than 150 cases with widely varying results and few 5-year disease-free survivors. Nevertheless, there is a role for liver transplantation in carefully selected patients with favorable tumors (i.e., biologically less aggressive). Transplantation is indicated in physically fit patients with unresectable neuroendocrine tumor metastases that, despite optimal medical management, are causing uncontrollable symptoms due to tumor bulk and/or hormone production. Liver replacement should be considered a complementary part of the armamentarium of potential therapies for these patients.

REFERENCES

1. Mazzaferro V, Regalia E, Doci R, Andreola S, Pulvirenti A, Bozzetti F, Montalto F, Ammatuna M, Morabito A, Gennari L. Liver transplantation for the treatment of small hepatocellular carcinomas in patients with cirrhosis. N Engl J Med 1996; 334:693–699.
2. Pichlmayr R. Is there a place for liver grafting for malignancy? Transplant Proc 1988; 20:478–482.
3. Penn I. Hepatic transplantation for primary and metastatic cancers of the liver. Surgery 1991; 110:726–734.
4. D'Angelica M, Brennan MF, Fortner JG, Cohen AM, Blumgart LH, Fong Y. Ninety-six five-year survivors after liver resection for metastatic colorectal cancer. J Am Coll Surg 1997; 185:554–559.
5. Fong Y, Cohen AM, Fortner JG, Enker WE, Turnbull AD, Coit DG, Marrero AM, Prasad M, Blumgart LH, Brennan MF. Liver resection for colorectal metastases. J Clin Oncol 1997; 15:938–946.
6. Capella C, Heitz PU, Höfler H, Solcia E, Klöppel G. Revised classification of neuroendocrine tumours of the lung, pancreas and gut. Digestion 1994; 55:11–23.
7. Creutzfeldt W. Carcinoid tumor: development of our knowledge. World J Surg 1996; 20:126–131.
8. Stridsberg M, Öberg K, Li Q, Engstrom U, Lundqvist G. Measurements of chromogranin A, chromogranin B (secretogranin I), chromogranin C (secretogranin II) and pancreostatin in plasma and urine from patients with carcinoid tumours and endocrine pancreatic tumours. J Endocrinol 1995; 144:49–59.
9. Johanson V, Tisell LE, Olbe L, Wangberg B, Nilsson O, Ahlman H. Comparison of survival between malignant neuroendocrine tumours of midgut and pancreatic origin. Br J Cancer 1999; 80:1259–1261.
10. Le Truet YP, Delpero JR, Dousset B, Cherqui D, Segol P, Mantion G, Hannoun L, Benhamou G, Launois B, Boillot O, Domergue J, Bismuth H. Results of liver transplantation in the treatment of metastatic neuroendocrine tumors. Ann Surg 1997; 225:355–364.
11. Pelosi G, Bresaola E, Bogina G, Pasini F, Rodella S, Castelli P, Iacono C, Serio G, Zamboni G. Endocrine tumors of the pancreas: Ki-67 immunoreactivity on paraffin sections is an independent predictor for malignancy. A comparative study with proliferating-cell nuclear

antigen and progesterone receptor protein immunostaining, mitotic index, and other clinicopathologic variables. Hum Pathol 1996; 27:1124–1134.
12. Gould VE, Gould KA. E-cadherin as tumor differentiation marker and as architectural determinant. Hum Pathol 1999; 30:1273–1275.
13. Olausson M, Friman S, Cahlin C, Nilsson O, Jansson S, Wangberg B, Ahlman H. Indications and results of liver transplantation in patients with neuroendocrine tumours. World J Surg 2002; 26:998–1004.
14. Rosenau J, Bahr MJ, von Wasielewski R, Mengel M, Schmidt HHJ, Nashan B, Lang H, Klempnauer J, Manns M, Boeker KHW. Ki67, E-cadherin, and p53 as prognostic indicators of long-term outcome after liver transplantation for metastatic neuroendocrine tumors. Transplantation 2002; 73:386–394.
15. Soreide O, Berstad T, Bakka A, Schrumpf E, Hanssen LE, Engh V, Bergan A, Flatmark A. Surgical treatment as a principle in patients with advanced abdominal carcinoid tumors. Surgery 1992; 111:48–54.
16. Chamberlain RS, Canes D, Brown KT, Saltz L, Jarnagin W, Fong Y, Blumgart LH. Hepatic neuroendocrine metastases: does intervention alter outcomes? J Am Coll Surg 2000; 190:432–445.
17. Havelaar IJ, Sugarbaker PH, Vermess M, Miller DL. Rate of growth of intraabdominal metastases from colorectal cancer. Cancer 1984; 54:163–171.
18. Hara Y, Ogata Y, Shirouzu K. Early tumor growth in metastatic organs influenced by the microenvironment is an important factor which provides organ specificity of colon cancer metastasis. J Exp Clin Cancer Res 2000; 19:497–504.
19. Akerstrom G, Hessman O, Skogseid B. Timing and extent of surgery in symptomatic and asymptomatic neuroendocrine tumors of the pancreas in MEN 1. Langenbecks Arch Surg 2002; 386:558–569.
20. Patterson EJ, Gagner M, Salky B, Inabnet WB, Brower S, Edye M, Gurland B, Reiner M, Pertsemlides D. Laparoscopic pancreatic resection: single-institution experience of 19 patients. J Am Coll Surg 2001; 193: 281–287.
21. Ahlman H, Wängberg B, Tisell LE, Nilsson O, Fjalling M, Forssell-Aronsson E. Clinical efficacy of octreotide scintigraphy in patients with midgut carcinoid tumours and evaluation of intraoperative scintillation detection. Br J Surg 1994; 81:1144–1149.
22. Bombardieri E, Maccauro M, De Deckere E, Savelli G, Chiti A. Nuclear medicine imaging of neuroendocrine tumours. Ann Oncol 2001; 12(suppl 2):S51–S61.
23. Busuttil RW, Klintmalm GB, eds. Transplantation of the Liver. Philadelphia: WB Saunders Co, 1996.
24. Claure RE, Drover DD, Haddow GR, Esquivel CO, Angst MS. Orthotopic liver transplantation for carcinoid tumour metastatic to the liver: anesthetic management. Can J Anesth 2000; 47:334–337.
25. Alessiani M, Tzakis A, Todo S, Demetris AJ, Fung JJ, Starzl TE. Assessment of five-year experience with abdominal organ cluster transplantation. J Am Coll Surg 1995; 180:88–89.
26. Starzl TE, Todo S, Tzakis A, Podesta L, Mieles L, Demetris A, Tepperman L, Selby R, Stevenson W, Stieber A, Gordon R, Iwatsuki S. Abdominal organ cluster transplantation for the treatment of upper abdominal malignancies. Ann Surg 1989; 210:374–385.
27. Curtiss SI, Mor E, Schwartz ME, Sung MW, Hytiroglou P, Thung SN, Sheiner PA, Emre S, Miller CM. A rational approach to the use of hepatic transplantation in the treatment of metastatic neuroendocrine tumors. J Am Coll Surg 1995; 180:184–187.
28. Otley CC, Pittelkow MR. Skin cancer in liver transplant recipients. Liver Transpl 2000; 6:253–262.
29. Kelly DM, Emre S, Guy SR, Miller CM, Schwartz ME, Sheiner PA. Liver transplant recipients are not at increased risk for nonlymphoid solid organ tumors. Cancer 1998; 83:1237–1243.
30. Freise CE, Ferrell L, Liu T, Ascher NL, Roberts JP. Effect of systemic cyclosporine on tumor recurrence after liver transplantation in a model of hepatocellular carcinoma. Transplantation 1999; 67:510–513.
31. Ceriello A, Mezza F, Cozzolino S, Pettinato G, Mancini A, Santaniello W, Calise F, Cuomo O. Role of immunosuppression in recurrence after liver transplantation for diethylnitrosamine-induced tumors in rats. Transpl Int 1994; 7(suppl 1):S204–S207.
32. Steininger R, Herbst F, Fugger R, Muhlbacher F, Fritsch A. Immunosuppression does not enhance tumor growth after orthotopic liver transplantation for hepatoma. Transpl Int 1992; 24:2690–2692.
33. Luan FL, Hojo M, Maluccio M, Yamaji K, Suthanthiran M. Rapamycin blocks tumor progression: unlinking immunosuppression from antitumor efficacy. Transplantation 2002; 73:1565–1572.
34. Moertel CG. Karnofsky memorial lecture: an odyssey in the land of small tumors. J Clin Oncol 1987; 5:1502–1503.
35. Thompson GB, van Heerden JA, Grant CS, Carney JA, Ilstrup DM. Islet cell carcinomas of the pancreas: a twenty year experience. Surgery 1988; 104:1011–1017.
36. Arnold R, Trautmann ME, Creutzfeldt W, Benning R, Benning M, Neuhaus C. Somatostatin analogue octreotide and inhibition of tumour growth in metastatic endocrine gastroenteropancreatic tumours. Gut 1996; 38: 430–438.
37. Skogseid B. Nonsurgical treatment of advanced malignant neuroendocrine pancreatic tumors and midgut carcinoids. World J Surg 2001; 25:700–703.
38. Wängberg B, Westberg G, Tylén U, Tisell L, Jansson S, Nilsson O, Johansson V, Schersten T, Ahlman H. Survival of patients with disseminated midgut carcinoid tumours after aggressive tumour reduction. World J Surg 1996; 20:892–899.
39. Que FG, Nagorney DM, Batts KP, Linz LJ, Kvols LK.

Hepatic resection for metastatic neuroendocrine carcinomas. Am J Surg 1995; 169:36–42.
40. Azimuddin K, Chamberlain RS. The surgical management of pancreatic neuroendocrine tumors. Surg Clin North Am 2001; 81:511–525.
41. Grazi GL, Cescon M, Pierangeli F, Ercolani G, Gardini A, Cavallari A, Mazziotti A. Highly aggressive policy of hepatic resections for neuroendocrine liver metastases. Hepatogastroenterology 2000; 47:481–486.
42. Siperstein AE, Berber E. Cryoablation, percutaneous alcohol injection, and radiofrequency ablation for treatment of neuroendocrine liver metastases. World J Surg 2001; 25:693–696.
43. Moertel CG, Johnson CM, McKusick MA, Martin JK Jr, Nagorney DM, Kvols LK, Rubin J, Kunselman S. The management of patients with advanced carcinoid tumours and islet cell carcinomas. Ann Intern Med 1994; 120:302–309.
44. Drougas JG, Anthony LB, Blair TK, Lopez RR, Wright JK Jr, Chapman WC, Webb L, Mazer M, Meranze S, Pinson CW. Hepatic artery chemoembolization for management of patients with advanced metastatic carcinoid tumors. Am J Surg 1998; 175: 408–412.
45. United Network for Organ Sharing. <*http://www.unos.org*> Accessed August, 2002
46. Kamath PS, Wiesner RH, Malinchoc M, Kremers W, Thierneau TM, Kosberg CL, D'Amico G, Dickson ER, Kim WR. A model to predict survival in patients with end-stage liver disease. Hepatology 2001; 33:464–470.
47. Miller CM, Gondolesi GE, Florman S, Matsumoto C, Munoz L, Yoshizumi T, Artis T, Fishbein TM, Sheiner PA, Kim-Schluger L, Schiano T, Shneider BL, Emre S, Schwartz ME. One hundred nine living donor liver transplants in adults and children: a single-center experience. Ann Surg 2001; 234:301–311.
48. Ringe B, Lorf T, Dopkens K, Canelo R. Treatment of hepatic metastases from gastroenteropancreatic neuroendocrine tumors: role of liver transplantation. World J Surg 2001; 25:697–699.
49. Coppa J, Pulvirenti A, Schiavo M, Romito R, Collini P, Di Bartolomeo M, Fabbri A, Regalia E, Mazzaferro V. Resection versus transplantation for liver metastases from neuroendocrine tumors. Transplant Proc 2001; 33: 1537–1539.
50. Pascher A, Steinmullr T, Radke C, Hosten N, Wiedenmann B, Neuhaus P, Bechstein WO. Primary and secondary hepatic manifestation of neuroendocrine tumors. Langenbecks Arch Surg 2000; 385:265–270.
51. Frilling A, Rogiers X, Malago M, Liedke O, Kaun M, Broelsch CE. Liver transplantation in patients with liver metastases of neuroendocrine tumors. Transplant Proc 1998; 30:3298–3300.
52. Dousset B, Saint-Marc O, Pitre J, Soubrane O, Houssin D, Chapuis Y. Metastatic endocrine tumors: medical treatment, surgical resection, or liver transplantation. World J Surg 1996; 20:908–915.
53. Anthuber M, Jauch K-W, Briegel J, Groh J, Schildberg FW. Results of liver transplantation for gastroenteropancreatic tumor metastases. World J Surg 1996; 20: 73–76.
54. Routley D, Ramage JK, McPeake J, Tan KC, Williams R. Orthotopic liver transplantation in the treatment of metastatic neuroendocrine tumors of the liver. Liver Transpl Surg 1995; 1:118–121.
55. Arnold JC, O'Grady JG, Bird GL, Calne RY, Williams R. Liver transplantation for primary and secondary hepatic apudomas. Br J Surg 1989; 76:248–249.
56. Makowka L, Tzakis AG, Mazzaferro V, Teperman L, Demetris AJ, Iwatsuki S, Starzl TE. Transplantation of the liver for metastatic endocrine tumors of the intestine and pancreas. Surg Gynecol Obstet 1989; 168:107–111.
57. Lehnert T. Liver transplantation for metastatic neuroendocrine carcinoma. Transplantation 1998; 66:1307–1312.

54

Cytoreduction of Neuroendocrine Tumors

Håkan Ahlman and Michael Olausson

Sahlgrenska University Hospital, Göteborg, Sweden

1 INTRODUCTION

The term carcinoid tumors originally covered gastroenteropancreatic endocrine tumors, which were divided according to their embryological origin into foregut carcinoids (broncho-pulmonary, thymic, stomach, duodenum, upper jejunum, pancreas), midgut carcinoids (lower jejunum, ileum, appendix, and cecum), and hindgut carcinoids (colon, rectum) (1). This classification does not relate to the natural history and clinical behavior of these tumors, so a revised classification was proposed taking into account tumor location, tumor size, angioinvasion, hormone production, histological grade, and proliferative index (2). Using this classification the digestive neuroendocrine (NE) tumors are divided into well-differentiated tumors (WDEC) comprising carcinoid tumors of the gastrointestinal tract and endocrine pancreatic tumors (EPT) and poorly differentiated endocrine carcinomas (PDEC). NE tumors are usually diagnosed at a late stage, when the patients has disseminated disease and hormonal symptoms. The work-up of these patients includes CT/MRT, octreotide scintigraphy, hormonal screening, and analysis of tumor biopsies. The histopathological examination aims at classifying the tumor with respect to origin and biological behavior. Immunohistochemical staining for amine and peptide hormones and synaptic vesicle proteins can be helpful in defining the origin of the tumor (3). Analysis of growth pattern, degree of NE differentiation, and proliferative capacity may provide prognostic information (4). Such analysis includes evaluation of tumor cell growth, degree of cellular/nuclear atypia as well as presence, or absence, of necrosis; these factors are then weighed into a histological grade (G1–G3) scale. The NE differentiation is evaluated by antibodies against proteins of the neurosecretory granules (chromogranin A, synaptophysin) or cytosolic markers (neuron specific enolase, PGP 9.5). WDEC are immunopositive for all markers in the majority of tumor cells, while PDEC often lack the granular markers with cytosolic markers retained. The proliferative capacity can be assessed by counting of mitoses, but is more reliably estimated by analyzing the fraction of tumor cells that express the Ki67 antigen (4). Following the histopathological analysis, NE tumors can be broadly divided into WDEC with good, or intermediate, prognosis and PDEC with sinister prognosis. Other factors, e.g., angiogenic capacity, expression of adhesion molecules, and specific genetic changes, may prove to be prognostic tools in the future and also indicators of responsiveness to medical treatment.

Bronchial and thymus carcinoids are derived from the embryological foregut. Bronchial carcinoids can be typical (carcinoid morphology, few mitoses, and absence of necrosis), with good prognosis, or atypical (nuclear atypia and deranged architecture, increased mitotic activity, or presence of necrosis), with intermediate prognosis (5) in contrast to large-cell neuroendocrine carcinomas and small-cell lung carcinomas with poor prognosis (6,7). Thymic carcinoids were recognized as a separate entity by Rosai and Higa (8). Asymptomatic tumors may be incidentally detected, while symptomatic patients may present with ectopic production of ACTH and GHRH, usually at an advanced stage. Thymic carcinoids often have slow progression, but are invariably malignant.

Cytoreductive surgery is sometimes required for other NE tumor types, e.g., the rare cases of malignant pheochromocytoma/paraganglioma with excessive catecholamine (CA) secretion or medullary thyroid carcinoma (MTC) with diarrhgenic syndromes or ectopic ACTH production.

2 PREOPERATIVE CONSIDERATIONS

Prior to all interventional treatment of NE tumors, the tumor type and hormone production must be assessed. Patients with midgut carcinoids are pretreated with long-acting somatostatin analogues, e.g., octreotide ($100\ \mu g \times 4$ s.c.), to prevent carcinoid crises during intervention. In case of a crisis reaction (severe facial flushing, bronchoconstriction, and hypotension), adrenergic drugs should be avoided, since carcinoid tumor cells may express adrenoceptors and a vicious circle with excessive release of serotonin and tachykinins can be initiated. Instead, the surgical manipulation should be interrupted, volume substituted according to hemodynamic parameters and titrated doses of octreotide and cortisone given. Spinal anesthesia with markedly reduced arterial blood pressure may elicit carcinoid crises due to compensatory release of CA from the adrenals, in turn activating serotonin release from the tumor. For postoperative pain epidural analgesia is preferred (9). Foregut carcinoids with excess production of histamine may cause an "atypical carcinoid syndrome" (generalized flushing, bronchoconstriction, hypotension, lacrimation, and cutaneous edema). Hepatic arterial embolization of liver metastases in these patients may be contraindicated due to uncontrollable release reactions. Correct diagnosis relies on analysis of the main histamine metabolite methylimidazole acetic acid (MelmAA) in urine. Patients with histamine-producing tumors are optimally pretreated with a combination of somatostatin analogues, blockade of histamine (H_1 and H_2) receptors and cortisone. Histamine-liberating agents, e.g., morphine and tubocurarine, should be avoided (10). For patients with glucagonoma or VIPoma, preoperative treatment with octreotide is usually sufficient. Skin lesions (necrolytic migrating erythema), sometimes associated with glucagonomas, can heal rapidly with octreotide, antibiotics, and amino acid supplementation prior to surgery. During this period, low-dose heparin is recommended due to increased risk of thrombosis. Patients with gastrinoma maintain their medication with omeprazol for a period after removal of the tumor, since they have elevated gastric acid secretion due to hypertrophy of the gastric mucosa. Patients with large insulinomas may require hypertonic glucose after tumor removal, and close glucose monitoring is necessary.

Surgical treatment of patients with advanced pheochromocytomas/paragangliomas present specific problems due to cardiovascular effects caused by excessive release of CA, which may activate α-adrenoceptors, leading to vasoconstriction and reduced plasma volume (not compensated for by vasodilatation via β_2-adrenoceptors), and β-adrenoceptors, resulting in tachycardia. The combination of enhanced afterload and tachycardia can damage the myocardium. With successively increased dosage of the α-adrenoceptor blocker phenoxybenzamine, vasoconstriction is reduced and plasma volume normalized. During medical treatment tachycardia may appear as a consequence of vasodilatation or presynaptic blockade of α-adrenoceptors. First at the stage with normalized plasma volume the tachycardia can be corrected by the use of β-adrenoceptor antagonists. Attention should be paid to tumors with preferential secretion of epinephrine, i.e., predominant activation of β-adrenoceptors. Too rapid institution of treatment with phenoxybenzamine may lead to vasodilatation and circulatory collapse. Intraoperative control of vascular tone can also be obtained by nitroprusside or adenosine; the latter drug has an antiarrhythmic effect on the sensitized myocardium. Certain drugs should be avoided, e.g., sympathomimetics (ketamine), stimulants of autonomic ganglia (succinylcholine), CA-uptake inhibitors (droperidol), vagolytics (atropine), and halothane, which may induce arrythmias (see Ref. 11). In case major debulking is planned, a first step of noninterventional cytoreduction, e.g., radiotherapy with ^{131}I-MIBG or chemotherapy (cyclophosphamide, dacarbazine, and vincristine), can be tried in order to reduce tumor burden and secretion of CA (12,13). For palliation, α-methyltyrosine may have additional effects, since this drug reduces the synthesis of CA.

3 SURGICAL TREATMENT OF LOCOREGIONAL DISEASE

Adequate treatment of locoregional disease is a prerequisite for subsequent tumor resection with curative intent. There is an evident correlation between the size of the primary NE tumor and presence of metastatic disease for lesions in certain regions, e.g., appendix and rectum (14). Tumors less than 1 cm are cured by simple excision/appendectomy, while larger or locally invasive tumors require more extensive surgery (15). In case of small intestinal midgut carcinoids, tumor size does not seem to influence prognosis (16). Two thirds of small midgut carcinoids (< 1 cm) have microscopic spread to lymph nodes, and almost half of the patients have liver metastases (17). Midgut carcinoids may be multiple and require resection of involved intestine and mesentery. The tumors are often accompanied by retroperitoneal fibrosis or desmoplastic mesenteric reaction, which may lead to constriction and kinking of the bowel and intestinal ischemia. The primary surgical treatment should therefore include dissection and removal/reduction of the central mesenteric lymph nodes mobilizing the small intestine for adequate resection and preventing vascular compression (18).

Gastric carcinoids are divided into four subtypes: hypergastrinemia induces hyperplasia of enterochromaffin-like cells with subsequent progression into small multiple carcinoids in the corpus-fundus region. This condition can be associated with chronic atrophic gastritis (type I) or be part of a setting with MEN-1 gastrinoma (type II). Type III tumors are larger solitary lesions, not associated with hypergastrinemia, and type IV tumors comprise very rare tumor types including PDEC. Type I lesions are usually benign and are probably best managed by endoscopic excision and follow-up. The role of antrectomy to reduce gastrin levels in order to reverse hyperplasia/neoplasia of enterochromaffin-like cells has not been strictly evaluated. Type II lesions may require wider excision, or gastric resection. Type III tumors and PDEC require cancer surgery, when resectable (19).

The surgical management of EPT also varies with tumor type, e.g., enucleation of small benign insulinomas or pancreatic resection of larger, more aggressive tumors of both functional or nonfunctional types. The MEN-1 pancreas is a surgical enigma, which may lead to repeat surgical procedures of successively diagnosed tumors, eventually ending up with subtotal, or completion pancreatectomy (Fig. 1) (20). For patients with nonfunctonal EPT and bilateral liver metastases, most authors advise pancreatic resection only in patients with symptoms like pain or bleeding. In one series of nonfunctional EPT, palliative pancreatic resections were performed in 12 patients and compared with 22 nonresected patients without evident survival advantage (4.5 versus 3.2 yr). The small difference may be explained by smaller tumors in the resected group (21). In case of biliary or gastric outlet obstruction, by-passes are performed. Operative biliary by-pass is usually preferred, since individual patients with EPT may have long survival (22).

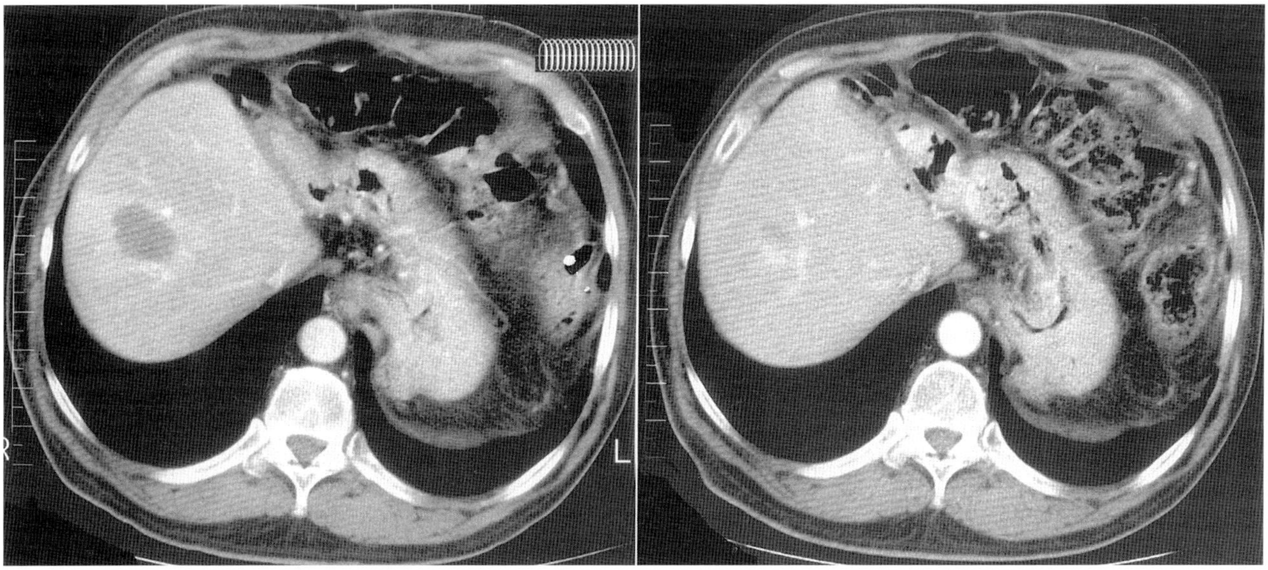

Figure 1 CT in a patient with the MEN-1 syndrome subjected to completion pancreatectomy and left hepatectomy due to metastatic EPT. One centrally located metastasis in the residual right liver was treated with radiofrequency ablation. The dark area represents the coagulation necrosis (left). Three months later marked shrinkage of the necrotic area (right). After completion of treatment the patient had normal tumor markers and negative octreotide scintigraphy.

For successful primary surgery of bronchial carcinoids, not only complete removal of tumor and careful lymph node dissection is required, but also optimal sparing of lung parenchyma. In contrast to lung cancer, wide resection margins are not required. Peripherally located tumors are managed by wedge resection or resections of segments or lobes; centrally located tumors by bronchotomy, excision, and bronchoplasty, sleeve resections of bronchi, and more rarely pneumonectomy. Endoscopic treatment of bronchial carcinoids by YAG laser can be used to palliate airway obstruction in patients with advanced disease (23). Large-cell neuroendocrine carcinomas and small-cell lung carcinomas are best treated by chemotherapy. In the former tumor type resection may be attempted, if distant metastases are not present (6,7).

The surgical treatment of primary NE tumors and locoregional disease is not controversial. Treatment of patients with liver metastases is more demanding and may involve several interventional modalities. For future randomized studies on the role of medical treatment in advanced disease, primary surgery by an experienced surgeon is of importance to prevent local complications by the tumor and correctly stage the tumor disease. In case liver transplantation is planned as a second step, it is import to resect all extrahepatic tumor. There is no general agreement when to start the palliative surgical treatment, e.g., gastrinomas metastatic to the liver can show most variable growth rates in different patients, which influences the decision making (24).

4 INTERVENTIONAL TREATMENT OF LIVER METASTASES

The surgical/interventional treatment for liver metastases can be divided into four modalities: liver resection, vascular interventions, other peroperative procedures, and liver transplantation.

4.1 Liver Resection

Anatomical liver resection can be performed for lesions located within any of the eight liver segments, each supplied by branches of the hepatic arteries and portal vein and each drained by one hepatic duct (Fig. 2A). For curative resections good clearance margins are required, but for WDEC resected for palliation, the margins can be narrowed and local tumors can be removed by atypical resections. The extension of tumor is assessed by inspection, palpation, and intraoperative ultrasound. The latter technique allows good definition of liver anatomy and reveals the relationship between the tumor and the portal/hepatic venous pedicles. This is of special importance if techniques like cryo- or laser therapy are used.

In the sagital projection the liver is divided by the three principal hepatic veins, which delineate the major liver resections: left hepatectomy (removal of segment no. II–III), right hepatectomy (removal of segment no. V–VIII), and trisegmentectomy, which also includes removal of segment no. IV and sometimes the caudate lobe (segment no. I). Resection of individual segments requires identification and subsequent ligation of its portal pedicle. This can be difficult for segments no. VII–VIII and may cause impaired venous drainage from the residual lower segments. Superficial liver metastases along the edges of the liver are safely removed by wedge excisions and plugging with absorbable fibrin to secure hemostasis.

4.1.1 Left Hepatectomy

The left middle hepatic veins have their junctions at variable levels and can usually be controlled separately outside the liver (Fig. 2D). Division of the liver parenchyma can be performed by several techniques, e.g., the finger fracture technique with subsequent ligation of blood vessels and bile ducts.

4.1.2 Right Hepatectomy

The most common variant in arterial anatomy is replacement of the right hepatic artery by a branch of the superior mesenteric artery. For right-sided liver tumors, preoperative angiography or MR angiography is therefore valuable. For right hepatectomy, the right hepatic vein can be controlled outside the liver (Fig. 2B). It is important to obtain control of the free edge of the lesser omentum by clamping in order to prevent bleeding. Inflow occlusion is established by the so-called Pringle's maneuver. The safe duration of total ischemia of the liver at normothermia may exceed 1 hour but can be lower with hepatic dysfunction. Therefore, the shortest possible clamping should be used, since the procedure is associated with intestinal congestion and accumulation of metabolites. Intermittent clamping in 15-minute periods is usually advised (see Ref. 25).

4.1.3 Extended Right Lobe Resection

In some cases extended right lobe resections, leaving only the two left liver segments, can be performed (Fig.

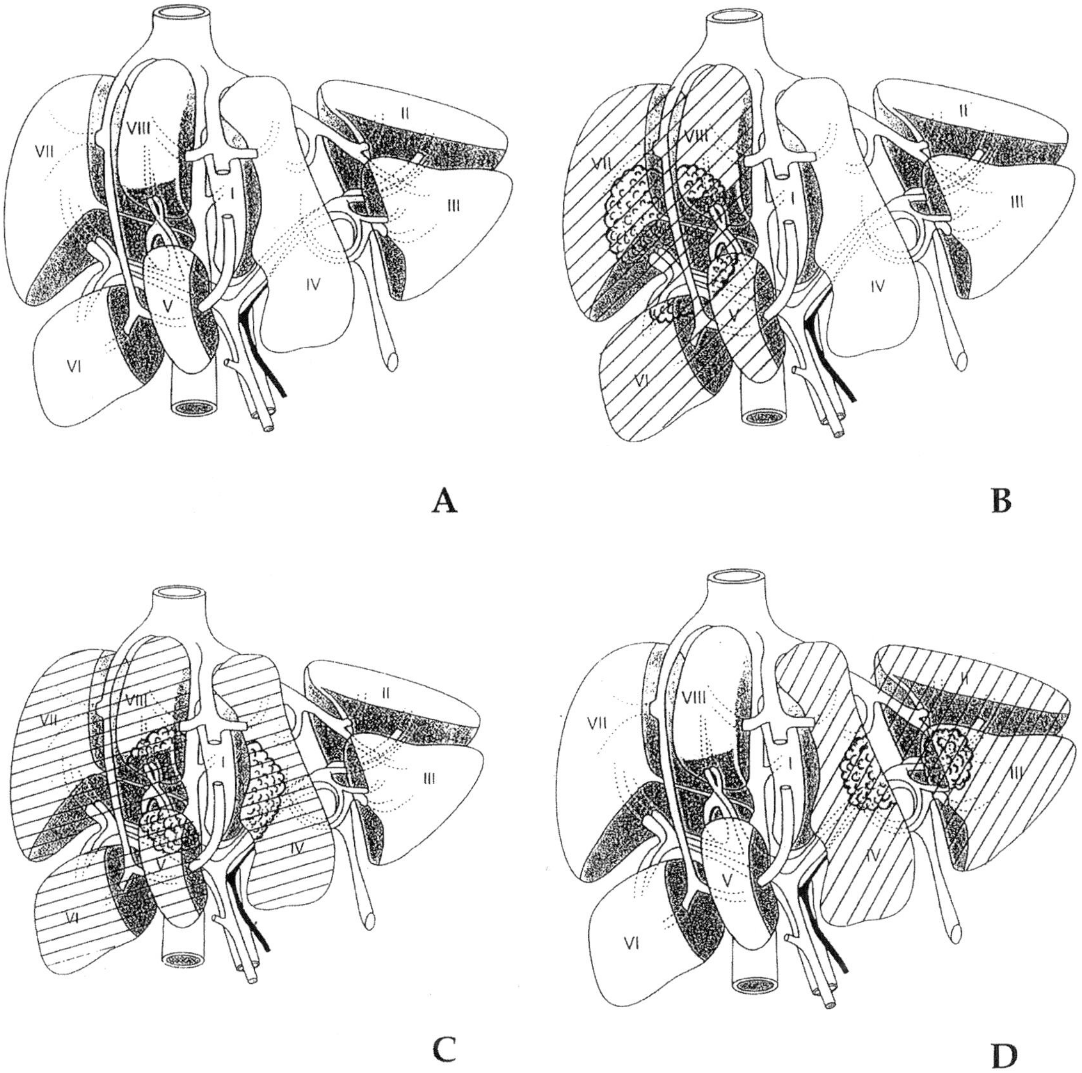

Figure 2 (A) Segmental anatomy of the liver: (B) right hepatectomy; (C) extended right lobe resection; (D) left hepatectomy.

2C). A residual liver less than 20–25% of the original volume may lead to hepatic failure. One way to reduce morbidity and mortality in these cases is to use preoperative portal embolization of the right liver lobes carrying the lesions. This procedure induces hypertrophy of the intact left liver during a 4- to 6-week period, so the planned resection can be safely performed (26).

4.1.4 Metastasectomy

Metastasectomy of multiple lesions usually requires intermittent clamping of inflow vessels, incision by diathermy, and blunt dissection. To obtain good cytoreduction the principles of anatomical resection, wedge resection, and metastasectomy are often combined. Division of the liver parenchyma often includes the use of an ultrasonic surgical aspirator, which destroys the parenchyma without damaging the biliary and vascular structures and allows accurate placement of ligatures/clips. Also, the harmonic scalpel, or hydrojet devices, can be used. All of these techniques facilitate bloodless resections. To minimize oozing from the cut surface, techniques to assist hemostasis can be used, e.g., rapid-setting fibrin glue or an argon beam coagulator. The operative mortality for elective liver surgery must be kept low. In most series figures of $< 5\%$ are reported (25). Prophylactic use of antibiotics has reduced infectious complications. The morbidity is more frequently associated with sepsis than with bleeding.

4.2 Results of Liver Surgery

Over the last decade very active surgery has become increasingly more common as primary treatment of low-grade NE tumors (WDEC) and their metastases. Curative liver surgery (i.e., no gross residual tumor) should be considered for all patients with resectable disease, since this is the only long-term effective strategy (27). Palliative liver surgery can be considered for some patients with slow tumor growth and severe hormonal symptoms. Palliative liver resections are generally performed in patients in whom more than 90% of the tumor volume can be safely excised (28,29). In clinical series of patients with NE tumors some 10 years ago, the liver resection rate with curative intent was low, about 10% (30,31). This was partly ascribed to the fact that the tumors had diffuse spread in the liver at clinical presentation (30). In our own consecutive series of 64 patients with the midgut carcinoid syndrome and liver metastases (Fig. 3), 14 patients (22%) with lesions limited to the right or left liver lobes underwent intentionally curative liver surgery and normalized their tumor markers, i.e., chromogranin A in plasma and urinary 5-HIAA (18). In more recent American and French series (33–35) curative, or palliative, liver resections could be performed in as many as 40–50% of patients with NE tumors. In all the reported series at centers of expertise, the mortality was low (< 5%) and the complication rate below 30%.

One evident problem with an active liver surgery program is that many resections are considered curative at the time of surgery but later proven not to be. With access to sensitive diagnostic tools (tumor-secreting hormones, general NE tumor markers, octreotide scintigraphy and SPECT, spiral CT and MRT) and careful follow-up, subclinical disease can be discovered and limited lesions re-resected (36). This strategy has been successful in patients with NE tumors treated by liver transplantation; in our own experience octreotide scin-

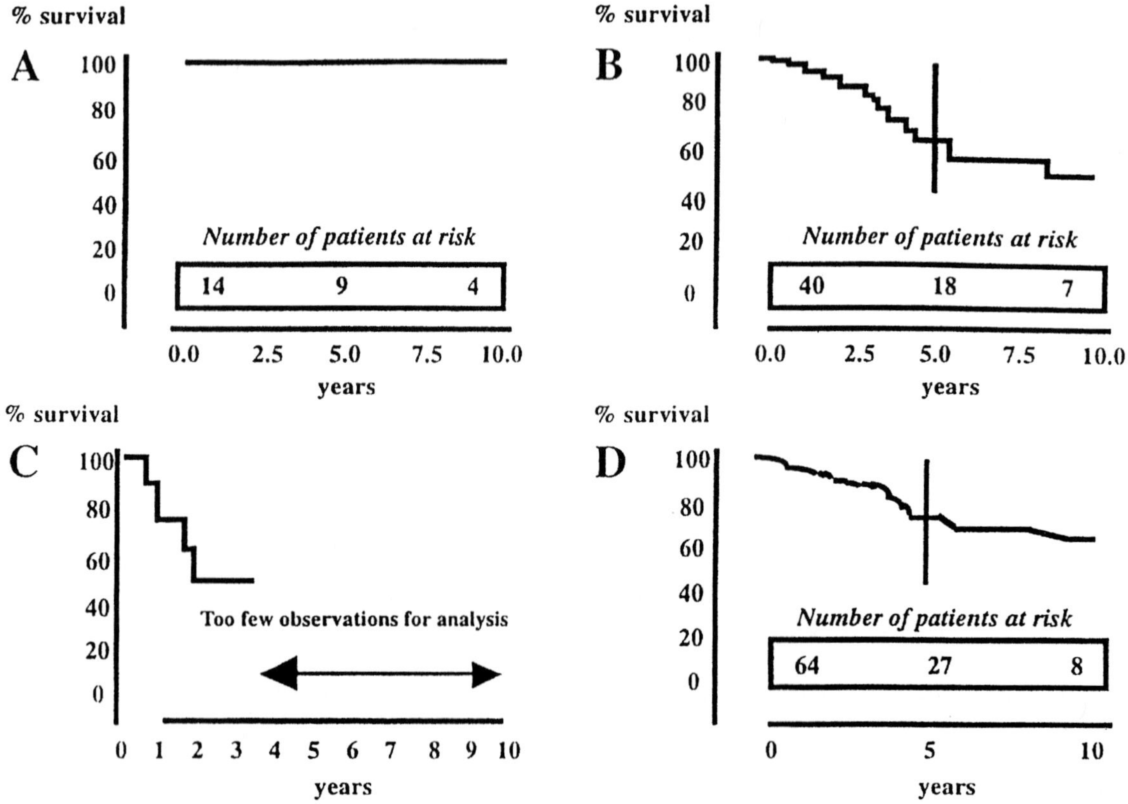

Figure 3 Kaplan-Meier survival analysis of 64 consecutive patients with the midgut carcinoid syndrome: (A) patients with sole surgical treatment (primary surgery + liver surgery) ($n = 14$); (B) patients with bilateral liver tumors treated by primary surgery, embolization and octreotide ($n = 40$); (C) patients with sole medical treatment (octreotide combined with chemotherapy/interferon) after primary surgery due to complicating diseases ($n = 10$); (D) panel represents survival in the entire series.

tigraphy and SPECT were superior to biochemical markers from the recurrent tumor (37). If multiple liver metastases recur, vascular interventions or ablative treatments are at hand. In case there is no extrahepatic disease, patients with nonresectable recurrent liver tumors may be candidates for transplantation.

More than 10 years ago Norton et al. (38) reported the outcome of very aggressive surgery in selected patients with advanced gastrinoma. They all underwent major liver resections combined with other debulking procedures at tumor progression, followed by chemotherapy. On a short-term basis good symptomatic relief and markedly reduced tumor markers were seen with this strategy. Out of 42 consecutive patients with EPT treated over a 10-year period at the NIH, 17 were resected and 25 deemed inoperable and medically treated (33). There seemed to be a 5-year survival advantage in the surgically treated group (79%) versus the medically treated group (28%) in this selected series. There was no operative mortality, but the tumor recurred in all surgically treated patients within 8 years. On the other hand, such delay of the tumor growth with a long medication-free interval, also observed for midgut carcinoids (18), is a major therapeutic advantage in itself. Mc Entee et al. (29) from the Mayo Clinic reported encouraging results in 1990 in 37 patients (carcinoids or EPT) treated with liver resection. The early series included 17 curative resections (9 patients had hormonal symptoms); 8 were completely relieved of symptoms and 5 of these were alive after 2 years without evidence of disease. Twenty patients underwent palliative resections (16 patients had hormonal symptoms); 8 experienced symptom relief and 5 were alive after one year. In a later review from the Mayo Clinic (34) 74 patients with metastatic NE tumors had undergone liver resection (41 patients had midgut carcinoids). The 4-year survival was 73%, even though nearly two thirds of the procedures were palliative. There were no differences in survival between patients with curative or palliative procedures. Symptomatic response to liver resection was seen in 90% with a mean duration of response of almost 20 months. Resection of large (>10 cm) dominant lesions was clearly related to symptom relief and reduction of tumor markers. The role of resection for enhanced survival has still not been proven in randomized studies.

4.3 Vascular Interventions

Markowitz in 1952 (39)] first proposed hepatic vascular interventions as therapeutic procedures. The rationale for ischemic treatment of NE tumors of the liver is their main blood and oxygen supply from the hepatic artery (40–42) with maintained portal perfusion of the normal liver parenchyma. Ischemia can be achieved by several techniques directed against the hepatic artery: ligation, selective embolization, or temporary occlusion. The methods differ in completeness, distribution, and duration of ischemia (43).

4.3.1 Ligation

Ligation of the hepatic artery was clinically introduced more than 30 years ago (41). It has been largely abandoned due to difficulties in obtaining adequate ischemia (due to the rich collateral blood supply to the liver) and consequently short-term palliation (<6 m), significant mortality in patients with advanced disease, and restricted possibilities for repeat vascular interventions (42).

4.3.2 Selective Embolization

Selective embolization of the hepatic arteries causes a temporary but complete ischemia, since the arterial tree distal to the point of injection is filled with embolization material (45). Contraindications are tumor burden exceeding 50% of the liver volume, occlusion of the portal vein, hyperbilirubinemia, and persistently elevated liver enzymes. Relative contraindications are contrast allergy, coagulopathies, extrahepatic tumor dominance, or poor performance status of the patient (46). In our experience patients with tumor volumes exceeding 50% can safely undergo this type of treatment using titrated superselective embolizations well separated in time (intervals of 2–4 weeks). A similar strategy can be followed for patients with previous hemihepatectomy and recurrent tumors in the residual liver. Immediately before embolization an arteriogram is performed to demonstrate the arterial anatomy, tumor blood flow, and patency of the portal vein (Fig. 4) (47,48). Both absorbable and nonabsorbable embolization materials have been used, e.g., gelfoam powder and alcohol-Ivalon particles (46, 49). The need to maintain an open route for repeat procedures excludes the choice of steel coils in the proximal arterial segment. Aiming at complete ischemia of long duration efforts have been directed toward smaller permanent emboli to obtain a good peripheral ischemia without passage into the liver sinusoids (45,50).

4.3.3 Chemoembolization

Chemoembolization is embolization combined with liver-targeted intra-arterial administration of chemotherapy. Hajarizadeh et al. (51) found symptomatic improvement to 5-FU in carcinoid patients with a mean duration of 2 years associated with significant tumor

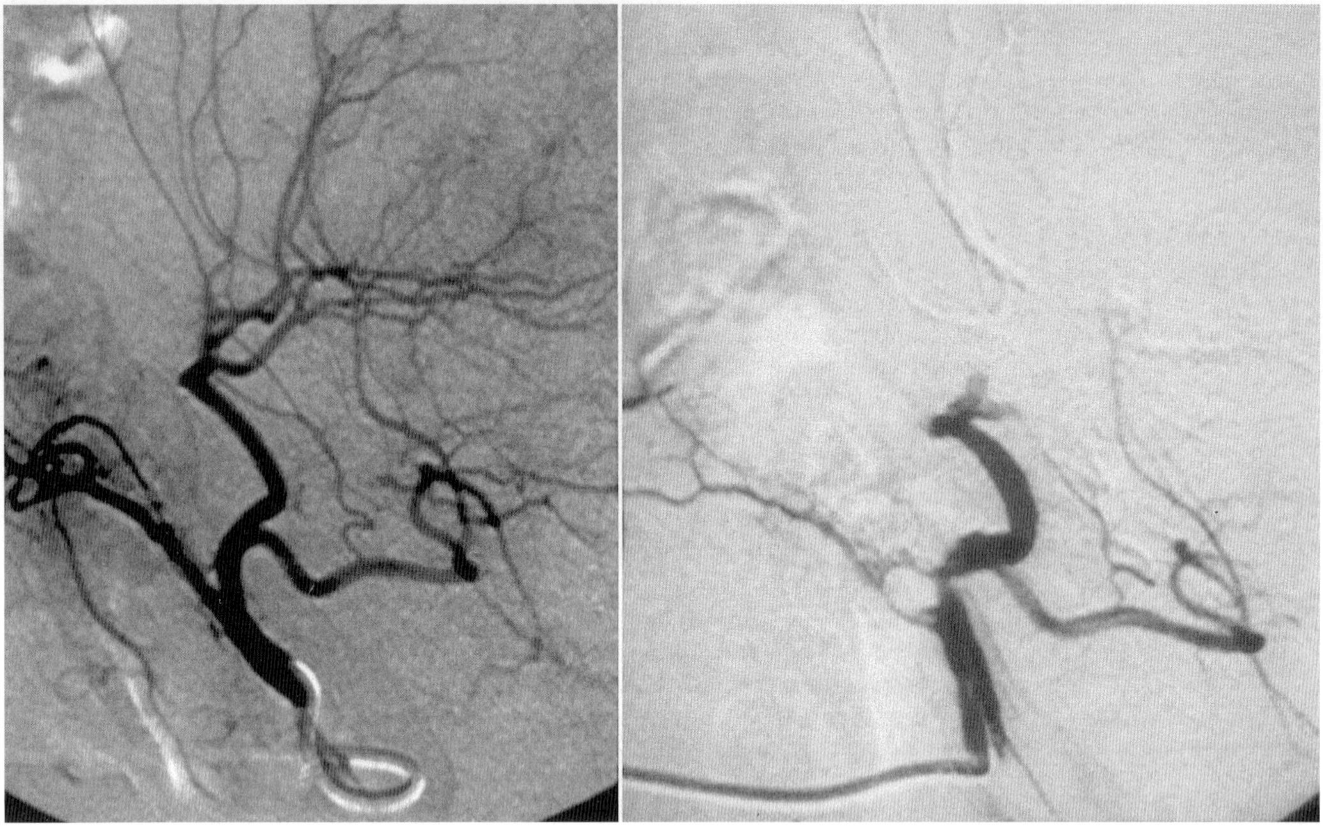

Figure 4 Arteriogram in a patient with midgut carcinoid and liver metastases before (left) and 10 minutes after embolization (right).

regression in half of the patients. Up to 72% sustained tumor control has been reported for advanced NE tumors using repeat treatment and other cytotoxic drugs (doxorubicin, mitomycin C, and cisplatinum) (52–54). Pronounced tumor regression has been reported with a modified embolization procedure using iodized oil, doxorubicin, and gelfoam particles (54). The relative merits of chemoembolization versus selective embolization await further studies.

4.3.4 Radioembolization

Pilot series have been performed using so-called radioembolization; i.e., microspheres labeled with the β-emitter ^{90}Y were used as embolization material. Since tumor arterioles are much wider than those supplying the normal parenchyma, deposition of labeled microspheres resulted in threefold higher radiation exposure in tumor than in normal liver tissue (55). A minor part ($<5\%$) of the activity delivered reached the lungs due to AV shunting in the liver. Unresolved problems are exact dosimetry, which requires good estimates of tumor volume, and nonhomogeneous distribution of microspheres. Furthermore, radiation-induced damage may lead to necrotic areas with redistribution of microspheres.

4.3.5 Temporary Occlusion

Some centers have reported good symptom palliation related to biochemical and clinical tumor responses in patients with the midgut carcinoid syndrome using temporary occlusion of the hepatic artery via external vessel loops (positioned during surgery) and repeat periods of applied ischemia (56). For long-term treatment, temporary occlusion can be applied via a port-operated tourniquet around the hepatic artery. A combination of peripheral embolization and temporary proximal occlusion can have additive effects in therapy-resistant cases.

4.3.6 Clinical Response to Liver Ischemia

Hepatic arterial embolization is accompanied by liver pain, transient elevation of liver enzymes, nausea, and usually a late fever reaction (24–48 hr). Embolization may lead to serious complications in individual patients (gallbladder ischemia, pancreatitis, liver abscess, vascular damage and aneurysm formation, hepatorenal syndrome, and hormonal crises). The mortality in the major series is < 5%, which should serve as a quality standard (46). To minimize adverse reactions, several precautions can be undertaken, which include first of all an experienced interventional radiologist, but also the use of co-axial catheter systems for superselective catheterization with low risk of vascular damage, prophylactic use of octreotide, cholecystectomy at time of primary surgery (to eliminate the risk for gallbladder perforation), intravenous hydration, and hemodynamic monitoring to reduce the risk for development of the hepatorenal syndrome (9,43).

To monitor the outcome of ischemic therapy, CT and biochemical tumor markers are used. According to our follow-up schedule these investigations are compared with preoperative results in the outpatient clinic 1 month after completion of embolization therapy (18). It would be a therapeutic advantage if the response to ischemia could be followed closer to embolization. For this purpose we have tried to develop better monitoring systems. We observed general tumor regression in individual patients subjected to unilateral embolization indicating activation of systemic antitumor effects, e.g., activation of natural killer (NK) cells (57). In one series responsive patients developed rapid lymphocytosis with predominance of NK cells; in vitro the cytotoxic activity of isolated lymphocytes from these patients increased shortly after embolization. The observed early immunological responses closely correlated with late monitoring of therapeutic effects (58). MR-spectroscopy of liver tumors before and shortly after embolization with regard to energy-rich phosphates may give information on the degree of ischemia and is under investigation.

4.4 Results of Ischemic Treatment

The result of ischemic treatment of liver metastases is obviously dependent on stage of the disease. Coupe et al. (59) reported a series of 63 consecutive carcinoid patients with advanced stage, of whom 30 were embolized for palliation. The survival after angiography, or angiography and embolization, was similar in both groups. Mitty et al. (60) reported long-term follow-up of 18 patients treated with embolization with prolongation of the expected survival by 2 years. Carrasco et al. (50) treated 25 patients with the carcinoid syndrome. The vast majority of patients showed both biochemical responses and tumor regression with an average duration of one year. Marlink et al. (61) introducd a different protocol for embolization in patients with severe symptoms; two successive embolizations were performed within one week leading to rapid symptom palliation. In our own study patients with midgut carcinoids were embolized in two settings one month apart after primary surgery (resection of primary tumor, optimal surgical reduction of extrahepatic disease, and prophylactic cholecystectomy) (18). Our 40 patients could be divided into two equally large groups: responders with more than 50% tumor reduction and pronounced reduction of 5-HIAA excretion (80%) and nonresponders with less than 50% tumor reduction and a moderate 5-HIAA reduction (30%) with clear survival advantage in the former group. The overall long-term results of embolization showed 60% survival at 5 years (Fig. 3). In a Norwegian study of patients with the midgut carcinoid syndrome, the response rate to interferon (IFN) was twice as high in patients subjected to prior embolization indicating additive effects. It should be noted that IFN is a potent enhancer of NK cell cytotoxicity (62). In a recent multicenter study of the midgut carcinoid syndrome, the patients were stratified according to 5-HIAA levels (more or less than 500 μmol/24 hr) and presence, or not, of valvular heart disease. After primary surgery, the tumors of the liver were treated by embolization and thereafter the patients were randomized to treatment with octreotide alone, or in combination with IFN. There was no survival advantage for combined medical treatment versus octreotide alone, but the time to tumor progression was significantly prolonged for patients treated with the combination of drugs (63). Moertel et al. (42) treated 111 patients with liver metastases of NE tumors ischemically and continued with systemic chemotherapy (doxorubicin, dacarbazine, streptozotocin, and 5-FU sequentially) in 71 patients. The study was not randomized, but still indicated additive effect between ischemic and medical treatment with enhanced median survival time (from 27 to 49 months).

Reviewing our first 94 embolizations in patients with the midgut carcinoid syndrome, we met with the following complications: three patients occluded the main hepatic artery (one hepatic abscess), but all had excellent symptom relief. One patient developed an aneurysm of the hepatic artery after the first embolization and a fatal hepatorenal syndrome after the second procedure. These complications together with one case of pancreatitis were all seen among the first 11 embolizations before the introduction of a coaxial catheter system. At the subsequent 83 embolizations only two minor complications were seen (transient renal insufficiency and cardiac arrythmia).

4.5 Intraoperative Procedures

4.5.1 Radioguided Surgery

Taking advantage of the high expression of somatostatin receptors (SSTR) by several NE tumors, attempts to develop radioguided surgery using a hand-held scintillation detector after preoperative injection of radiolabeled somatostatin analogues have been evaluated. The indications for radioguided surgery would be recurrent tumors in regions not easily investigated by other methods (e.g., neck metastases of MTC, carcinoids, and EPT), small EPT (e.g., the MEN-1 syndrome), and as control of adequate tumor removal (e.g., residual carcinoid metastases in the mesenteric root after lymph node dissection). Promising results have been reported, but scintillation detection is clearly not sensitive enough to detect microscopic tumor growth or microadenomas (64).

4.5.2 Regional Hyperthermia

At advanced stage of histamine- or CA-producing tumors, ischemic liver treatment is potentially dangerous due to uncontrollable release of tumor products. In individual patients with the foregut carcinoid syndrome we have used cytotoxic drugs (melphalan and cisplatinum) delivered by regional hyperthermic liver perfusion. During perfusion the venous effluent from the liver with vasoactive substances was shunted from the systemic circulation, thus avoiding vasomotor effects. Cytostatic perfusion of the isolated liver with simultaneous filtration of portal vein blood and a maintained systemic circulation were made possible by a special perfusion catheter inserted in the cava. The surgical technique involves isolation of the hepatic artery, portal vein, and cava inferior and superior to the liver together with a temporary portocaval shunt that allows blood flow rates to be maintained in both the hepatic artery and portal vessels (65). Repeat hyperthermic perfusion can be difficult to perform due to intense fibrotic reaction of the vessels used for perfusion.

4.5.3 Local Ablation

In elderly patients or patients with progressive tumors after previous treatment, percutaneous alcohol injections into isolated liver lesions can be performed (66). The volume of individual metastases is estimated ultrasonographically and the lesions are injected with equal volumes of absolute alcohol. During injection the lesions develop high echogenicity. With repeat injections marked symptom palliation related to reduced tumor markers and proven tumor necrosis can be achieved. Alternatively, the tumor can be destroyed by cryosurgical techniques, which also have the advantage that multiple lesions can be treated at a single session. The cellular damage is caused by intra- and extracellular crystal formation, dehydration, and vascular damage (67). Cryosurgery is less effective close to large vessels ("heatsink") and should not be used for large tumors due to risk for coagulopathies, respiratory distress syndrome, and acute renal failure. Cryoprobes can be equipped with intraoperative ultrasound for tumor localization. Modern cryoprobes can destroy tumors deep in the liver without damaging the normal overlying parenchyma. In short series good symptomatic relief has been reported (68,69). Metastatic liver tumors can also be treated by interstitial laser or most recently by radiofrequency ablation (70–72), causing selective thermocoagulation. Lesions close to large vessels can usually be treated, since the vessels are protected by cooling due to blood stream effects. These techniques can be used intraoperatively or percutaneously. Ultrasound is usually the imaging guidance, but open thermosensitive MR systems for monitoring of coagulative effects are being developed (73). These local ablative techniques can be used as complement to liver resection (Fig. 1) or for recurrent tumors in the residual liver after resection.

5 FUTURE TECHNIQUES

5.1 SSTR-Targeted Radiotherapy

This is a recent approach to deliver localized radiotherapy. Since NE tumors frequently express high numbers of SSTR (mainly SSTR2 and 5 with high affinity for octreotide, which is the basis for octreotide scintigraphy) and internalize these receptors after ligand binding, the radiopharmaceutical will accumulate in the tumor cells (74). The first attempts were made by i.v. injections of therapeutic amounts of the diagnostic substance DTPA-D-Phe^1-octreotide (75). ^{111}Indium is a low-energy β-emitter with Auger electrons and the observed therapeutic effects were modest. Therefore, the high-energy β-emitter ^{90}Y was complex bound to ^{90}Y-DOTA-D-Phe^1, Tyr^3-octreotide in order to reach tumoricidal radiation. In preliminary series individual patients have been reported with significant tumor regression, or stable disease, after multiple treatments (76). Adverse effects can be seen mainly from the bone marrow and kidneys. We have used this type of therapy (^{177}Lu-DOTA-Tyr^{3}-octreotate) as complement to a carcinoid patient with liver transplant and extrahepatic nonresectable recurrent tumors, which led to stable disease and markedly reduced tumor markers 6 months after completion of radiotherapy.

5.2 Imatinib (ST1571)

Inhibition of intracellular signaling from tyrosine kinases associated with certain proteins/receptors by this drug is a novel therapeutic principle of great promise in certain diseases as chronic myeloid leukemia (chimeric BCR-ABL protein with tyrosin kinase activity) and gastrointestinal stroma cell (GIST) tumors (constitutive activation of tyrosine kinase from the *c-kit* receptor) (77). Similar tyrosine kinases are also associated with platelet-derived growth factor (PDGF) receptors. Digestive NE tumors may express PDGF subtypes and their receptors on both tumor cells and surrounding stroma (78). In preliminary studies such patients have been treated with imatinib, leading to antitumor effects. If the treatment is proven effective as in GIST tumors, the surgical treatment should be timed with optimal tumor regression in order to avoid too aggressive cytoreduction.

ACKNOWLEDGMENTS

This work was supported by grants from the Swedish MRC (5220) and the Swedish Cancer Society (3911).

REFERENCES

1. Williams E, Sandler M. The classification of carcinoid tumours. Lancet 1963; 1:238.
2. Capella C, Heitz P, Höfler H, Solcia E, Klöppel G. Revised classification of neuroendocrine tumors of the lung, pancreas and gut. Digestion 1994; 55:11–23.
3. Jakobsen AM, Andersson P, Saglik G, Andersson E, Kölby L, Erickson JD, Forssell-Aronsson E, Wängberg B, Ahlman H. Differential expression of vesicular monoamine transporter (VMAT)1 and 2 in gastrointestinal endocrine tumours. J Pathol 2001; 195:463–472.
4. Rindi G, Azzoni C, La Rosa S, Klersy S, Paolotti D, Rappel S, Stolte M, Capella C, Bordi C, Solcia E. ECL cell tumor and poorly differentiated endocrine carcinoma of the stomach: prognostic evaluation by pathological analysis. Gastroenterology 1999; 116:532–542.
5. Travis WD, Rush W, Flieder DB, Falk R, Fleming MV, Gal AA, Koss MN. Survival analysis of 200 pulmonary neuroendocrine tumors with clarification of criteria for atypical carcinoid and its separation from typical carcinoid. Am J Surg Pathol 1998; 22:934–944.
6. Jiang SX, Kameya T, Shoji M, Dobashi Y, Shinada J, Yoshimura H. Large cell neuroendocrine carcinoma of the lung: a histologic and immunohistochemical study of 22 cases. Am J Surg Pathol 1998; 22:526–537.
7. Clark R, Ihde DC. Small-cell lung cancer: treatment progress and prospects. Oncology 1998; 12:647–658.
8. Rosai J, Higa E. Mediastinal endocrine neoplasm of probable thymic origin, related to a carcinoid tumor Clinicopathologic study of 8 cases. Cancer 1972; 29: 1061–1074.
9. Ahlman H, Åhlund L, Dahlström A, Martner J, Stenqvist O, Tylén U. The use of SMS 201-995 and provocation tests in carcinoid patients in preparation for surgery and hepatic arterial embolisation. Anesth Analg 1988; 67:1142–1148.
10. Ahlman H, Wängberg B, Nilsson O, Grimelius L, Granérus G, Modlin IM, Stenqvist O, Scherstén T. Aspects of diagnosis and treatment of the foregut carcinoid syndrome. Scand J Gastroent 1992; 27:459–471.
11. Owen R. Anesthetic consideration in endocrine surgery. Anesthesia 1986; 41:71.
12. Kimmig B, Adolph J. Eisenhut selektive nuklearmedizinische Therapie mit MIBG. In: Zum Winkel K, ed. Wirkungssteigerung der Strahlentherapie maligner Tumoren. Berlin: Springer-Verlag, 1987:116–123.
13. Averbuch SD, Steakley CS, Young RC, Gelmann EP, Goldstein DS, Stull R, Keiser HR. Malignant pheochromocytoma: effective treatment with a combination of cyclophosphamide, vincristine, and dacarbazine. Ann Intern Med 1988; 109:267–273.
14. Moertel CG. An odyssey in the land of small intestinal tumours. J Clin Oncol 1987; 5:1502–1522.
15. Rothmund M, Kisker O. Surgical treatment of carcinoid tumours of the small bowel appendix colon and rectum. Digestion 1994; 55(suppl 3):86–91.
16. Norton JA. Surgical management of carcinoid tumors: role of debulking and surgery for patients with advanced disease. Digestion 1994; 55(suppl 3):98–103.
17. Makridis C, Öberg K, Juhlin C, Rastad J, Johansson H, Lörelius LE, Åkerström G. Surgical treatment of midgut carcinoid tumors. World J Surg 1990; 14:377–385.
18. Wängberg B, Westberg G, Tylén U, Tisell LE, Jansson S, Nilsson O, Johanson V, Scherstén T, Ahlman H. Survival of patients with disseminated midgut carcinoid tumours after aggressive tumour reduction. World J Surg 1996; 20:892–899.
19. Ahlman H, Kölby L, Lundell L, Olbe L, Wängberg B, Granérus G, Grimelius L, Nilsson O. Clinical management of gastric carcinoid tumors. Digestion 1994; 55 (suppl 3): 77–85.
20. Tisell LE, Ahlman H, Jansson S, Grimelius L. Total pancreatectomy in the MEN-1 syndrome. Br J Surg 1988; 75:154–157.
21. Evans DB, Skibber JM, Lee JE, Cleary KR, Ajani JA,

Gagel RF, Sellin RV, Fenoglio CJ, Merrell RC, Hickey RC. Nonfunctioning islet cell carcinoma of the pancreas. Surgery 1993; 114:1175–1182.
22. Prinz RA, Badrinath K, Chejfec G, Freeark RJ, Greenlee HB. "Nonfunctioning" islet cell carcinoma of the pancreas. Am J Surg 1983; 49:345–349.
23. Chughtai TS, Morin JE, Sheiner NM, Wilson JA, Mulder DS. Bronchial carcinoid—twenty years experience defines a selective surgical approach. Surgery 1997; 122:801–808.
24. Sutliff VE, Doppman JL, Gibril LF. Growh of newly diagnosed untreated metastatic gastrinomas and predictors of growth pattern. J Clin Oncol 1997; 15:2420–2431.
25. Benjamin IS. Management of secondary endocrine tumours of the liver. In: Lynn J, Bloom SR, eds. Surgical Endocrinology. Oxford: Butterworth-Heinemann, 1993: 538–547.
26. Farges O, Belghiti J. Options in the resection of endocrine liver metastases. In: Mignon M, Colombel JF, eds. Recent Advances in the Pathophysiology and Management of Inflammatory Bowel Diseases and Digestive Endocrine Tumours. Paris: John Libbey Eurotext, 1999: 335–337.
27. Miller CA, Ellison EC. Therapeutic alternatives in metastatic neuroendocrine tumors. Surg Oncol Clin North Am 1998; 7:863–879.
28. Foster JH, Lundy J. Liver metastases. Curr Probl Surg 1981; 18:157–202.
29. Mc Entee GP, Nagorney DM, Kvols LK, Moertel CG, Grant CS. Cytoreductive hepatic surgery for neuroendocrine tumours. Surgery 1990; 108:1091–1096.
30. Galland RB, Blumgart LH. Carcinoid syndrome: surgical management. Br J Hosp Med 1986; 35(166):168–170.
31. Hughes KS, Sugarbaker PH. Resection of the liver for metastatic solid tumors. In: Rosenberg SA, ed. Surgical Treatment of Metastatic Cancer. Philadelphia: Lippincott, 1987:125–164.
32. Söreide O, Berstad T, Bakka A, Schrumpf E, Hanssen LE, Engh V, Bergan A, Flatmark A. Surgical treatment as a principle in patients with advanced abdominal carcinoid tumors. Surgery 1992; 111:48–54.
33. Carty SE, Jensen RT, Norton JA. Prospective study of aggressive resection of metastatic pancreatic endocrine tumours. Surgery 1992; 112:1024–1032.
34. Que FG, Nagorney DM, Batts KP, Linzl J, Kvols LK. Hepatic resection for metastatic neuroendocrine carcinomas. Am J Surg 1995; 169:36–43.
35. Dousset B, Saint-Marc O, Pitre J, Soubrane O, Houssin D, Chapuis Y. Metastastic endocrine tumors: medical treatment, surgical resection, or liver transplantation. World J Surg 1996; 20:908–915.
36. Ahlman H, Wängberg B, Tisell LE, Nilsson O, Fjäling M, Forssell-Aronsson E. Clinical efficacy of octreotide scintigraphy in patients with midgut carcinoid tumours and evaluation of intraoperative scintillation detection. Br J Surg 1994; 81:1144–1149.
37. Olausson M, Friman S, Cahlin C, Nilsson O, Jansson S, Wängberg B, Ahlman H. Indications and results of liver transplantation in patients with neuroendocrine tumors. World J Surg 2002; 26:998-1004.
38. Norton JA, Sugarbaker PH, Doppman JL, Wesley RA, Maton PN, Gardner JD, Jensen RT. Aggressive resection of metastatic disease in selected patients with malignant gastrinoma. Ann Surg 1986; 203:352–359.
39. Markowitz JC. The hepatic artery. Surg Gynecol Obstet 1952; 95:644–646.
40. Gelin LE, Lewis D, Nilsson L. Liver blood flow in man during abdominal surgery II. The effect of hepatic artery occlusion on the blood flow through metastatic tumor nodules. Acta Hepatosplenol 1968; 15:21–24.
41. Cho KJ, Reuter SR, Schmidt R. Effects of experimental hepatic artery embolization on hepatic function. Am J Roentgenol 1976; 127:563–567.
42. Moertel CG, Johnson CM, McKusick MA, Martin JK Jr, Nagorney DM, Kvols LK, Rubin J, Kunselman S. The management of patients with advanced carcinoid tumors and islet cell carcinomas. Ann Intern Med 1994; 120:302–309.
43. Geterud K, Tylén U, Jansson S, Stenqvist O, Tisell LE, Ahlman H. Hepatic arterial embolization in the treatment of the midgut carcinoid syndrome and other advanced endocrine tumours metastatic to the liver. J Intervent Radiol 1990; 5:69–76.
44. Almersjö O, Bengmark S, Engevik L, Hafström LO, Nilsson LA. Hepatic artery ligation as pretreatment for liver resection of metastatic cancer. Rev Surg 1966; 23: 377–380.
45. Chuang VP, Wallace S. Hepatic artery embolization in the treatment of hepatic neoplasms. Radiology 1981; 140:51–58.
46. Ajani JA, Carrasco CH, Wallace S. Neuroendocrine tumors metastatic to the liver vascular occlusion therapy. Ann NY Acad Sci 1994; 733:479–487.
47. Allison DJ, Modlin IM, Jenkins WJ. Treatment of carcinoid liver metastases by hepatic-artery embolisation. Lancet 1977; 2:1323–1325.
48. Pueyo I, Jimenez JR, Hernández J, Brugarolas A, Garcia-Moran M, Garcia-Muniz JI, Arroyo F. Carcinoid syndrome treated by hepatic embolization. Am J Roentgenol 1978; 131:511–513.
49. Lunderquist A, Ericsson M, Nobin A, Sandin G. Gelfoam powder embolization of the hepatic artery in liver metastases of carcinoid tumor. Radiologie 1982; 22:65–70.
50. Carrasco CH, Charnsangavej C, Ajani J, Samaan NA, Richli W, Wallace S. The carcinoid syndrome: palliation by hepatic artery embolisation. Am J Roentgenol 1986; 147:149–154.
51. Hajarizadeh H, Ivancev K, Mueller CR, Fletcher WS, Woltering EA. Effective palliative treatment of meta-

static carcinoid tumors with intra-arterial chemotherapy/chemoembolization combined with octreotide acetate. Am J Surg 1992; 163:479–483.
52. Venook AP, Stagg RJ, Lewis BJ, Chase JL, Ring EJ, Maroney TP, Hohn DC. Chemoembolization for hepatocellular carcinoma. J Clin Oncol 1990; 8:1108–1114.
53. Perry LJ, Stuart K, Stokes KR, Clouse ME. Hepatic arterial chemoembolization for metastatic neuroendocrine tumours. Surgery 1994; 116:1111–1116.
54. Ruszniewski P, Rougier P, Roche A, Legmann P, Sibert A, Hochlaf S, Ychou M, Mignon M. Hepatic arterial chemoembolisation in patients with liver metastases of endocrine tumors. Cancer 1993; 71:2624–2630.
55. Andrews JC, Walker SC, Ackermann RJ, Cotton LA, Ensminger WD, Shapiro B. Hepatic radioembolization with yttrium-90 containing glass microspheres: preliminary results and clinical follow-up. J Nucl Med 1994; 35:1637–1644.
56. Nobin A, Månsson H, Lunderquist A. Evaluation of temporary liver dearterialization and embolization in patients with metastatic carcinoid tumor. Acta Oncol 1989; 28:419–424.
57. Wängberg B, Geterud K, Nilsson O, Jansson S, Dahlström A, Tylén U, Ahlman H. Embolisation therapy in the midgut carcinoid syndrome—just tumour ischemia? Acta Oncol 1993; 32:251–256.
58. Wängberg B, Ahlman H, Tylén U, Nilsson O, Hermodsson S, Hellstrand K. Accumulation of natural killer cells after hepatic artery embolisation in the midgut carcinoid syndrome. Br J Cancer 1995; 71:617–618.
59. Coupe MO, Hodgson HJF, Hemingway A, Allison DJ. The effect of hepatic artery embolization on survival in the carcinoid syndrome. J Intervent Radiol 1989; 4: 179.
60. Mitty HA, Warner RRP, Neuman LH, Train JS, Parnes IH. Control of carcinoid syndrome with hepatic artery embolization. Radiology 1985; 155:1623–1626.
61. Marlink RG, Lokich T, Robins SR, Clouse ME. Hepatic arterial embolization for metastatic hormone-secreting tumors: technique, effectiveness and complications. Cancer 1990; 64:2227–2232.
62. Hanssen LE, Schrumpf E, Kolbenstvedt AN, Tausjö J, Dolva LO. Treatment of malignant metastatic midgut carcinoid tumours with recombinent human α-2b-interferon with or without prior hepatic artery embolization. Scand J Gastroenterol 1989; 24:787–795.
63. Kölby L, Persson G, Franzén S, Ahrén B, for the Swedish MRC Group on Endocrine Abdominal Tumours. Effect of interferon-alpha on survival in patients with disseminated midgut carcinoid tumours—a prospective randomised study. In press.
64. Wängberg B, Forssell-Aronsson E, Tisell LE, Nilsson O, Fjälling M, Ahlman H. Intraoperative detection of somatostatin-receptor-positive neuroendocrine tumours using indium-111-labelled-DTPA-D-Phe^1-octreotide. Br J Cancer 1996; 73:770–775.
65. Schersten T, Ahlman H, Wängberg B, Granérus G, Grimelius L. Hyperthermic liver perfusion chemotherapy in the treatment of the foregut carcinoid syndrome. Lancet 1991; 338:568–569.
66. Kölby L, Wängberg B, Ahlman H, Jansson S, Forssell-Aronsson E, Erickson JD, Nilsson O. Gastric carcinoid with histamine production, histamine transporter and expression of somatostatin receptors. Digestion 1998; 59:160–166.
67. Charnley RM, Doran J, Morris DL. Cryotherapy for liver metastases; a new approach. Br J Surg 1989; 76: 1040–1041.
68. Bilchik AJ, Sarantou T, Foshag LJ, Giuliano AE, Ramming KP. Cryosurgical palliation of metastatic neuroendocrine tumors resistant to conventional therapy. Surgery 1997; 122:1040–1048.
69. Cozzi PJ, Englund R, Morris DL. Cryotherapy treatment of patients with hepatic metastases from neuroendocrine tumors. Cancer 1995; 76:501–509.
70. Dowlatshahi K, Bhattacharya AK, Silver B, Motalen T, Williams JW. Percutaneous interstitial laser therapy of a patient with recurrent hepatoma in a transplanted liver. Surgery 1992; 112:303–606.
71. Bilchik AJ, Rose DM, Allegra DP, Bostick PJ, Hsueh E, Morton DL. Radio frequency ablation: a normally invasive technique with multiple applications. Cancer J Sci Am 1999; 6:356–361.
72. Matsui Y, Nakagawa A, Kamiyama Y, Yamamoto K, Kubo N, Nakase Y. Selective thermocoagulation of unresectable pancreatic cancers by using radiofrequency capacitive heating. Pankreas 2000; 1:14–20.
73. Kettenbach J, Silverman SG, Hata N, Kuroda K, Saiviroonpurn P, Zientara GP, Morrison PR, Hushek SG, Black PM, Kikinis R, Jolesz FA. Monitoring and visualization techniques for MR-guided laser ablations in an open MR system. J Magn Reson Imaging 1998; 8: 933–943.
74. Andersson P, Forssell-Aronsson E, Johanson V, Wängberg B, Nilsson O, Fjälling M, Ahlman H. Internalization of ^{111}In-DTPA-D-Phe^1-octreotide. J Nucl Med 1996; 37:2002–2006.
75. Krenning EP, Kooij PP, Pauwels S, Breeman WA, Postema PT, De Herder WW, Valkema R, Kwekkeboom DJ. Somatostatin receptor: scintigraphy and radionuclide threapy. Digestion 1996; 57(suppl 1):57–61.
76. Smith MC, Liu J, Chen T, Schrau H, Yeh CM, Jamav F, Valkema R, Bakker W, Kvols L, Krenning E, Pauwels S. OctreoTher: ongoing early clinical development of a somatostatin receptor—targeted radionuclide for antineoplastic therapy. Digestion 2000; 62(suppl 1):69–72.
77. Goldman JM, Melo JV. Targeting the BCR-ABL tyrosine kinase in chronic myeloid leukemia. N Engl J Med 2001; 344:1084–1086.
78. Chaudhry A, Papanicolaou V, Öberg K, Heldin CH, Funa K. Expression of platelet-derived growth factor and its receptors in neuroendorine tumors of the digestive system. Cancer Res 1992; 52:1006–1012.

55

Medical Management of Neuroendocrine Gastrointestinal Tumors

Kjell Öberg

Uppsala, University Hospital, Uppsala, Sweden

Håkan Ahlman

Sahlgrenska University Hospital, Göteborg, Sweden

1 INTRODUCTION

The clinical management of metastatic neuroendocrine tumors necessitates a multimodal approach, including surgery and other means of cytoreductive treatment, radiotherapy, and medical treatment. Surgery and other forms of cytoreduction have been dealt with in previous chapter, therefore this chapter will concentrate on radiotherapy and medical treatment of neuroendocrine gastroentero-pancreatic (GEP) tumors (1,2). The long-term natural history of neuroendocrine GEP tumors is not known because until recently an effective treatment for patients with functional syndromes did not exist and therefore patients often died of complications of hormonal excess rather than from the tumor per se (3,4). In a study of 212 patients with Zollinger-Ellison syndrome (ZES), 31% had died at a mean follow-up of almost 14 years. Only half of these deaths were due to tumor progression, particularly in bone and liver, and to ectopic ACTH production (4). In a recent large study involving 185 patients with ZES, the 10-year survival rate was not significantly different among patients in whom no tumor was found and patients with tumors that were completely resected, and patients in whom tumors were resected without biochemical cure (84%, 96%, and 93%, respectively) (5). However, in patients with unresectable disease, the 10-year survival rate was only 30% (5). This study demonstrates that development of metastatic liver disease is the primary determinant of survival in patients with ZES. In patients with malignant carcinoid disease and the classical carcinoid syndrome, the 5-year survival rate was 20% and the median survival from time of diagnosis was only 2 years two decades ago (6,7). However, today, when a more aggressive cytoreduction is performed combined with medical treatment such as somatostatin analogues and α-interferons, the median survival has significantly increased more than 5 years from start of treatment (8). Nevertheless, a majority of patients with neuroendocrine GEP tumors present with metastatic disease at the time of diagnosis; therefore, surgery and other means of cytoreductive treatment is seldom curative, indicating a need for medical treatment in a significant number of patients (9–11). The evaluation of medical treatment has been difficult because a large number of studies of medical therapy include small numbers of patients, mixing together endocrine pancreatic tumors, bronchial carcinoids, and intestinal carcinoids. Many studies do not take into account differences in biological behavior between classical midgut carcinoids, bronchial carcinoids, and endocrine pancreatic tumors. Very few randomized trials of medical therapy have been published to date. In addition, many clinicians are still reluctant to treat patients with neuroendocrine GEP tumors with no or limited clinical symptoms, because they have been assumed to have a good prognosis. Today there is no medical treatment for bulky metastatic disease that cures the patient. However, the quality of life for patients with functioning tumors has been significantly improved by the introduction of biological treatment, particularly somatostatin analogues and interferon-α (IFN-α).

2 RADIOTHERAPY

External radiotherapy has limited value in the treatment of patients with malignant neuroendocrine GEP tumors. Today, this kind of therapy is mainly used for treatment of brain metastases and pain related to bone metastases. In these two situations, long-lasting palliation can be obtained by using this technique (12).

Tumor-targeted radioactive treatment has been performed over recent years initially using ^{131}I-MIBG (meta-iodo-benzylguanidine). The objective response rates of MIBG therapy have been limited with symptomatic improvement in 30–40% of patients and biochemical responses in 7–10% (13). This kind of treatment has been recently updated by a group from the Netherlands with long experience of MIBG therapy in carcinoids. The authors showed that predosing with nonradiolabeled MIBG resulted in improved targeting of ^{131}I-MIBG with a prolonged palliation and biochemical response in the patients (14). This finding was further supported by preclinical data in BON-1, neuroendocrine cells xenografted to nude mice that predosing with cold MIBG increased tumor to nontumor radioactivity rates by two-, to threefold. Targeted radiotherapy is not an option in patients with negative or weakly positive MIBG scintigraphy. However, nonradiolabeled MIBG might enhance uptake in patients with low initial uptake (14).

A majority of neuroendocrine GEP tumors, both intestinal carcinoids and endocrine pancreatic tumors, express high-affinity somatostatin receptors. A majority of endocrine pancreatic tumors, with the exception of insulinomas, express receptor subtypes 2 and 5 (sst_2 and sst_5) in high numbers and with high affinity. Classical midgut carcinoids also express the same subset of somatostatin receptors. Tumor-targeted treatment with radioactive somatostatin analogues (^{111}In-DTPA-octreotide, ^{90}Y-DOTA-octreotide) has been developed during recent years (15–17). In a recent study, 41 patients with neuroendocrine tumors were subjected to treatment with ^{90}Y-DOTA-TOC, a β-emitting radionuclide based on octreotide. It binds to somatostatin receptors 2 and 5, and the radioactivity is then internalized into the tumor cell and transported to the cell nucleus. The treatment consisted of four intraveneous injections of a total of 6,000 MBq/m^2 of ^{90}Y-DOTA-TOC, administered at 6-week intervals (18). The overall response rate was 24%. For endocrine pancreatic tumors, the response rate was 36%. Complete remissions were found in 2%, partial remission in 22%, and minor responses in 12%. The median follow-up was 15 months. The median duration of response was not reached at 26 months, and the 2-year survival rate was 76% for all neuroendocrine tumors and 83% for endocrine pancreatic tumors. Patients suffering from the carcinoid syndrome achieved a significant reduction of symptoms, and the treatment was well tolerated. Side effects included grade III cytopenia in 5% and vomiting shortly after injection in 23%. No grade III or IV renal toxicity was observed. The first attempts with somatostatin analogue–based tumor-targeted treatment were made by injection of therapeutic amounts of the diagnostic substance ^{111}In-DTPA-D-Phe-octreotide (15,16). ^{111}Indium is a low-energy β-emittor with Auger electrons, and the observed therapeutic effects were modest. It did not include significant tumor reductions but merely reduction of clinical symptoms. Therefore, the high-energy β-emittor ^{90}ytrium, which is complex bound to DOTA-D-Phe-Tyr^3-octreotide, is a step forward. This compound is now evaluated in several phase II studies in different neuroendocrine tumors. One dose-limiting problem with this kind of treatment is kidney toxicity, but infusion of amino acids is now used to reduce the renal peptide reabsorption. Patients receiving cytotoxic treatment prior to radioactive treatment and with low bone marrow reserve are also a therapeutic challenge (19). Early clinical trials with other isotopes, such as ^{177}lutetium, has started, where this compound is bound to DOTA-octreotate. This compound is both γ- and β-emitting and demonstrates similar side effects as ^{90}Y-DOTA-octreotide treatment. No results have so far been published. It has also been suggested that a combination of ^{90}Y-DOTA-octreotide and ^{177}lutetium-DOTA-octreotate might be of value in the treatment of patients with multiple metastases of different size because of different capacity for these isotopes to penetrate into the tumor. The benefit of this combination has to be demonstrated in forthcoming clinical trials. The precise role of tumor-targeted radioactive somatostatin analogue treatment should be defined in randomized clinical trials.

3 MEDICAL TREATMENT

The management of clinical symptoms related to malignant neuroendocrine GEP tumors has improved significantly over the last decades. The introduction of proton pump inhibitors has facilitated the management of patients with neuroendocrine pancreatic tumors secreting gastrin and presenting with ZES. Today most patients with ZES and hypersecretion of acid are clinically controlled by these kinds of medication. There are very few patients dying of bleeding gastric ulcers today (20). The management of the carcinoid syndrome has been a therapeutic challenge over the years. In earlier days, serotonin inhibitors such as methysergide, cyproheptadin, and ketanserin were used to reduce the symptoms of flushing and diarrhea (21,22). Today, all these substances are replaced by treatment with somatostatin analogues (23). If the patient only presents with diarrhea related to a carcinoid tumor, loperamide or ondansetron can control these symptoms. A combination of histamine H1 and H2 receptor antagonist is effective in patients with a carcinoid syndrome that is caused by gastric or bronchial carcinoids secreting histamine (24). Prednisone in doses of 20 mg/day gives occasional relief in some cases with severe flushing.

Somatostatin analogues (octreotide, lanreotide) are effective at relieving symptoms and decreasing hormone levels when self-administered every 6–12 hours subcutaneously in patients with the carcinoid syndrome (23,25). Today, long-acting formulations of both compounds are available, which have significantly improved quality of life for patients with symptomatic neuroendocrine GEP tumors (see below). In a significant number of patients with malignant neuroendocrine GEP tumors, medical treatment can control the clinical symptoms for many years but is not curative. The antitumor medical therapy includes combinations of different agents, such as cytotoxic agents, α-interferons, and somatostatin analogues. Such combinations can be used from the start of treatment in patients with significant clinical symptoms but can be added consecutively during the course of disease when one type of treatment is failing.

3.1 Chemotherapy

Chemotherapy has been considered the gold standard for treatment of most neuroendocrine GEP tumors. However, it has usually been reported with variable criteria for assessing antitumor responses and in a limited number of patients. Cytotoxic treatment is today used predominantly in patients with tumors that show high proliferative capacity and large tumor burden. That means that the proliferation index analyzed by the antibody Ki-67 (MIB-1) should be above 5%. Chemotherapy has shown the most benefit in high proliferating tumors such as malignant endocrine pancreatic tumors and bronchial carcinoids. Classical midgut carcinoid with low proliferating capacity (Ki-67 usually < 2%) has not demonstrated any advantage of regular cytotoxic treatment (1, 2, 8, 26–29). Streptozotocin-based therapy in combination with fluorouracil and doxorubicin is the most widely applied cytotoxic treatment for neuroendocrine tumors. However, a large variety of different cytotoxic agents has been tried in endocrine pancreatic tumors as well as in classical carcinoids (Tables 1,2) (26–42). It has been suggested that functioning tumors, such as gastrin, insulin, and VIP-secreting tumors, respond better to cytotoxic treatment than non-functioning tumors, but that has not been found in larger studies (41–43). It has also been suggested that dacarbazine (DTIC) might be more effective in patients with glucagon-producing tumors than other types of tumors. That has not been confirmed when compiling data from different studies. It is difficult to predict the therapeutic outcome only from tumor type and hormone secretion. The therapeutic decisions should be based on tumor biology parameters such as proliferation capacity, angio-invasion, and metastatic spread. Streptozotocin (STZ), a glucose-nitrosourea compound, originally derived from a *Streptomyces* species, has been in clinical use since 1967 (44). In preclinical studies it was found to have cytotoxic effect on rat pancreatic islet cells and has been used in combination with other agents. The current first-line regimens for most types of endocrine pancreatic tumors is a combination of streptozotocin + 5-fluorouracil (5-FU) or doxorubicin. In one study where streptozotocin + doxorubicin was compared with streptozotocin + 5-fluorouracil and chlorozotocin alone, the response rates were 69%, 65%, and 30%, respectively, and the median duration of response was 18 months for doxorubicin combination and 14 months for the 5-FU combination and 17 months for the chlorozotocin group (42). Survival for patients treated with the doxorubicin combination was significantly longer. Streptozotocin alone generated response rates of 20–40%. There is still a debate as to whether the combination of streptozotocin with doxorubicin is better than with 5-FU. At our center we usually start with 5-FU, because a combination of streptozotocin and 5-FU can be used for long-term treatment as there are no upper limit in terms of total

40. Ruszniewski PH, Rougier P, Andre-David F. Prospective multicentric study:chemotherapy with streptozotocin (STZ) and 5-fluorouracil (5-FU) for liver metastases in Zollinger-Ellison syndrome (ZES). Gastroenterology 1989; 96:A431.
41. Moertel CG, Hanley JA, Johnson LA. Streptozotocin alone compared with Streptozotocin plus fluorouracil in the treatment of advanced islet-cell carcinoma. N Engl J Med 1980; 303(21):1189–1194.
42. Moertel CG, Lefkopoulo M, Lipsitz S, Hahn RG. Streptozotocin-doxorubicin, streptozotocin-fluorouracil, or chlorozotocin in the treatment of advanced islet cell carcinoma. N Engl J Med 1992; 326(8):519–523.
43. Eriksson B, Arnberg H, Lindgren PG, Lorelius LE, Magnusson A, Lundqvist G, Skogseid B, Wide L, Wilander E, Oberg K. Neuroendocrine pancreatic tumours: clinical presentation, biochemical and histopathological findings in 84 patients. J Intern Med 1990; 228(2):103–113.
44. Weiss RB. Streptozotocin: a review of its pharmacology, efficacy and toxicity. Cancer Treat Rep 1982; 66(3):427–438.
45. Moertel CG, Kvols LK, O'Connell MJ, Rubin J. Treatment of neuroendocrine carcinomas with combined etoposide and cisplatin. Evidence of major therapeutic activity in the anaplastic variants of these neoplasms. Cancer 1991; 68(2):227–232.
46. Ansell SM, Pitot HC, Burch PA. A phase II study of high dose paclitaxel in patients with advanced neuroendocrine tumors. Cancer 2001; 91:1543–1548.
47. Moertel CG, Johnson CM, McKusick MA. The management of patients with advanced carcinoid tumors and islet cell carcinomas. Ann Intern Med 1994; 120: 302.
48. Drougas JC, Anthony LB, Blair TK. Hepatic artery chemoembolization for management of patients with advanced metastatic carcinoid tumors. Am J Surg 1998; 175:408.
49. Kim KYH, Ajani JA, Carrasco CH. Selective hepatic arterial chemo-embolization for liver metastases in patients with carcinoid tumor or islet cell carcinoma. Cancer Invest 1999; 17:474.
50. Eriksson BK, Larsson EG, Skogseid BM. Liver embolizations of patients with malignant neuroendocrine gastrointestinal tumors. Cancer 1998; 83:2293.
51. Diaco DS, Hajarizadeh H, Mueller CR. Treatment of metastatic carcinoid tumors using multimodality therapy of octreotide acetate, intra-arterial chemo-therapy and hepatic arterial chemoembolization. Am J Surg 1995; 169:523.
52. Diamandidou E, Ajani JA, Yang DJ. Two-phase study of hepatic artery vascular occlusion? with microencapsulated cisplatin in patients with liver metastases from neuroendocrine tumors. AJR Am J Roentgenol 1998; 170:339.
53. Marlink RG, Lokich JJ, Robins JR, Clouse ME. Hepatic arterial embolization for metastatic hormone-secreting tumors. Technique, effectiveness, and complications. Cancer 1990; 65:2227.
54. Stokes KR, Stuart K, Clouse ME. Hepatic arterial chemoembolization for metastatic endocrine tumors. J Vasc Intervent Radiol 1993; 4:341.
55. Jacobsen MB, Hanssen LE, Kolmannskog F. Interferon-α2β, with or without prior? hepatic artery embolization: clinical response and survival in midgut carcinoid patients. Scand J Gastroenterol 1995; 30: 789–796.
56. Guillemin R. Somatostatin: the early days. Metabolism 1993; 41(suppl 2):1–4.
57. Ho LT, Chen RL, Chou TY, Fong JC, Wong PS, Chou CK. Pharmacokinetics and effects of intravenous infusion of somatostatin in normal subjects—a two-compartment open model. Clin Physiol Biochem 1986; 4:257–267.
58. Pless J, Bauer W, Briner U, Doepner W, Marbach P, Maurer R, Petcher TJ, Reubi JC, Vonderscher J. Chemistry and pharmacology of SMS 201-995, a long-acting octapeptide analogue of somatostatin. Scan J Gastroenterol 1986; 21(suppl 119):54–64
59. Pless J. Chemical structure—pharmacological profile of Sandostatin®. In: O'Dorisio TM, ed. Sandostatin in the Treatment of GEP Endocrine Tumors. Berlin: Springer, 1989:3–13.
60. Eriksson B, Tiensuu Janson E, Bax NDS, Mignon M, Morant R, Opolon P, Rougier P, Öberg KE. The use of new somatostatin analogs, lanreotide and octastatin, in neuroendocrine gastro-intestinal tumors. Digestion 1996; 57(suppl 1):77–80.
61. Eriksson B, Renstrup J, Imam H, Öberg K. High-dose treatment with lanreotide of patients with advanced neuroendocrine gastrointestinal tumours: clinical and biological effects. Ann Oncol 1997; 8:1–4.
62. Kvols LK, Moertel CG, O'Connell MJ. Treatment of the malignant carcinoid syndrome. Evaluation of a long-acting somatostatin analogue. N Engl J Med 1986; 315:663–666.
63. Gorden P, Comi RJ, Maton PN, Go VLW. Somatostatin and somatostatin analogue (SMS 201-995) in treatment of hormone-secreting tumors of the pituitary and gastrointestinal tract and non-neoplastic diseases of the gut. Ann Intern Med 1989; 110:35–50.
64. Öberg K, Norheim I, Lundqvist G, Wide L. Treatment of the carcinoid syndrome with SMS 201-995, a somatostatin analogue. Scand J Gastroenterol 1986; 119: 191–192.
65. Maton PN, Gardner JD, Jensen RT. Use of long-acting somatostatin analogue SMS 201-995 in patients with pancreatic islet cell tumors. Dig Dis Sci 1989; 34:285–291.
66. Scarpignato C. Somatostatin analogues in the management of endocrine tumors of the pancreas. In: Mignon M, Jensen RT, eds. Endocrine Tumors of the Pancreas. Basel: Karger, 1995:385–414.

67. Lamberts SW, van der Lely AJ, De Herder WW, Hofland LJ. Octreotide. N Engl J Med 1996; 334:246–254.
68. Wood SM, Kraenzlin ME, Adrian TE, Bloom SR. Treatment of patients with pancreatic endocrine tumours using a new long-acting somatostatin analogue: Symptomatic and peptide response. Gut 1985; 26:438–444.
69. Jockenhovel S, Lederbogen s, Olbricht T. The long-acting somatostatin analogue octreotide alleviates symptoms by reducing post-translational conversion of prepro-glucagon to glucagon in a patient with malignant glucagonoma, but does not prevent tumor growth. Clin Invest 1994; 72:127–133.
70. Harris A, Redfern JS. Octreotide treatment of carcinoid syndrome: analysis of published dose-titration data. Aliment Pharmacol Ther 1995; 9:387–394.
71. Buscail L, Estève JP, Saint-Laurent N. Inhibition of cell proliferation by the somatostatin analogue RC-160 is mediated by somatostatin receptor subtypes SSTR2 and SSTR5 through different mechanisms. Proc Natl Acad Sci USA 1995; 92:1580–1584.
72. Imam H, Eriksson B, Lukiniius A. Induction of apoptosis in neuroendocrine tumors of the digestive system during treatment with somatostatin analogs. Acta Oncol 1997; 36:607–614.
73. Fassler JE, Hughes JH, Cataland S. Somatostatin analogue: an inhibitor of angiogenesis? Biomed Res 1988; (suppl):181–185.
74. Yamada Y, Reisine T, Law SF. Cloning and functional characterization of a family of human and mouse somatostatin receptors expressed in brain, gastro-intestinal tract and kidney. Proc natl Acad Sci USA 1992; 89:251–255.
75. Schaer JC, Wser B, Mengod G, Reubi JC. Somatostatin receptor subtypes, SSTR-1, SSTR-2, SSTR-3 and SSTR-5 expression in human pituitary, gastroenteropancreatic and mammary tumors: Comparison of mRNA analysis with receptor autoradiography. Int J Cancer 1997; 70:530–537.
76. Janson ET, Stridsberg M, Gobl A. Determination of somatostatin receptor subtype 2 in carcinoid tumours by immunohistochemical investigation with somatostatin receptor subtype 2 antibodies. Cancer Res 1998; 58:2375–2378.
77. Reubi JC, Koppeler A, Waser B. Immunohistochemical localization of somatostatin receptors, SSTR-2A in human tumors. Am J Pathol 1998; 153:233–245.
78. Rocheville M, Lange DC, Kumar K, Sasi R, Patel RC, Patel Y. Subtype of the Somatostatin receptor assemble as functional homo- and heterodimers. J Biol Chem 2000; 275:7862–7869.
79. Lancranjan I, Bruns C, Grass P. Sandostatin-LAR: Pharmaco-kinetics, pharmaco-dynamics, efficacy, and tolerability in acromegalic patients. Metabolism 1995; 44:18–26.
80. Ruszniewski P, Ducreux M, Chayvialle JA. Treatment of the carcinoid syndrome with the long-acting somatostatin analogue lanreotide: a prospective study in 39 patients. Gut 1996; 39:279–283.
81. Trendle MC, Moertel CG, Kvols LK. Incidence and morbidity of cholelithiasis in patients receiving chronic octreotide for metastatic carcinoid and malignant islet cell tumours. Cancer 1997; 79:830–834.
82. Bartholomeo M, Bajetta E, Buzzoni R. Clinical efficacy of octreotide in the treatment of metastatic neuroendocrine tumors. A study by the Italian Trials in Medical Oncology Group. Cancer 1996; 77:402–408.
83. Arnold R, Trautmann ME, Creutzfeldt W. Somatostatin analogue and inhibition of tumor growth in metastatic endocrine gastroentero-pancreatic tumors. Gut 1996; 38:430–438.
84. Ricci S, Antonuzzo A, Galli L. Octreotide acetate long-acting release in patients with metastatic neuroendocrine tumors pretreated with lanreotide. Ann Oncol 2000; 11:1127–1130.
85. Öberg K, funa K, Alm G. Effects of leukocyte interferon on clinical symptoms and hormone levels in patients with midgut carcinoid tumors and carcinoid syndrome. N Engl J Med 1983; 309:129–133.
86. Öberg K, Norheim I, Lind E. Treatment of malignant carcinoid tumors with human leukocyte interferon: long-term results. Cancer Treat Rep 1986; 70:1297–1304.
87. Smith DB, Scarffe JH, Wagstaff J. Phase II trial of rDNA alfa 2b interferon in patients with malignant carcinoid tumor. Cancer Treat Rep 1987; 71:1265–1266.
88. Doberauer C, mengelkoch B, Kloke O. Treatment of metastatic carcinoid tumors and the carcinoid syndrome with recombinant interferon alpha. Acta Oncol 1991; 30:603–605.
89. Moertel CG, Rubin J, Kvols LK. Therapy of metastatic carcinoid tumor and the malignant carcinoid syndrome with recombinant leukocyte A interferon. J Clin Oncol 1989; 7:865–868.
90. Välimäki M, Järvinen H, Salmela P. Is the treatment of metastatic carcinoid tumor with interferon not as successful as suggested? Cancer 1991; 67:547–549.
91. Creutzfeldt W, Bartsch HH, Jacubaschke U. Treatment of gastrointestinal endocrine tumours with interferon-α and octreotide. Acta Oncol 1991; 30:529–535.
92. Öberg K, Eriksson B, Tiensuu Janson E. The clinical use of interferons in the management of neuroendocrine gastroenterpancreatic tumors. Ann NY Acad Sci 1994; 733:471–478.
93. Veenhof CHN, de Wit R, Taal BG. A dose-escalation study of recombinant interferon-alpha in patients with a metastatic carcinoid tumour. Eur J Cancer 1992; 28:75–78.
94. Biesma B, Willemse PHB, Mulder NH. Recombinant interferon alpha-2b in patients with metastatic apudomas: effect on tumours and tumour markers. Br J Cancer 1992; 66:880–885.

95. Nobin A, Lindblom A, Mansson B. Interferon treatment in patients with malignant carcinoids. Acta Oncol 1989; 28:445–449.
96. Öberg K, Eriksson B, Tiensuu Janson E. Interferons alone or in combination with chemotherapy or other biologicals in the treatment of neuroendocrine gut and pancreatic tumors. Digestion 1994; 55(suppl 3):64–69.
97. Grandér D, Öberg K, Lundquist M-L. Interferon-induced enhancement of 2́5́- oligoadenlyate synthetase in midgut carcinoid tumours. Lancet 1990; 336:337–340.
98. Dirix LY, Vermeulen PB, Fierens H. Long-term results of continuous treatment with recombinant interferon-α in patients with metastatic carcinoid tumors—an antigiogenic effect? Anticancer Drugs 1996; 7:175–181.
99. Andersson T, Wilander E, Eriksson B. Effects of interferon on tumor tissue content in liver metastases of human carcinoid tumors. Cancer Res 1990; 50:3413–3415.
100. Detjen KM, Welzel M, Brembeck FH. Molecular mechanisms of interferon-α- mediated growth inhibition in human neuroendocrine tumor cells. Gastroenterology 1999; 118:735–748.
101. Imam H, Gobl A, Eriksson B, Öberg K. Interferon-alpha induces bcl-2-proto-oncogene in patients with neuroendocrine gut tumor responding to its antitumor action. Anticancer Res 1997; 17:4659.
102. Zhou Y, Gobl A, Wang S, Jacobsen MB, Janson ET, Hains GK III, Radosevich JA, Öberg K. Expression of p68 protein kinase and its prognostic significance during IFN-α therapy in patients with carcinoid tumors. European Journal of Cancer 1998; 34:2046–2052.
103. Zhou Y, Wang S, Gobl A, Öberg K. The IFN-α regulation of interferon regulatory factor-1 (IRF-1) and IRF-2 has therapeutic implication in carcinoid tumors. Ann Oncol 2000; 11(6):707–714.
104. Janson ET, Rönnblom L, Ahlström H. Treatment with alpha-interferon versus alpha-interferon in combination with streptozocin and doxorubicin in patients with malignant carcinoid tumors: a randomized trial. Ann Oncol 1992; 3:635.
105. Tiensuu Janson EM, Ahlström H, Andersson T. Octreotide and interferon alfa: a new combination for the treatment of malignant carcinoid tumours. Eur J Cancer 1992; 28A:1647–1650.
106. Arnold R. Antiproliferative treatment of metastatic neuroendocrine gastro-enteropancreatic tumors: effect of combination therapy with octreotide and α-interferon. In: Mignon M, Colombel JF, eds. Recent Advances in the Pathophysiology of Inflammatory Bowel Diseases and Digestive Endocrine Tumors. Paris: John Libbey, 1999:292–295.
107. Rönnblom LE, Alm GV, Öberg K. Autoimmune phenomena in patients with malignant carcinoid tumors during interferon-α treatment. 1991; 30:537–540.
108. Goldman JM, Melo JV. Targeting the BCR-ABL tyrosine kinase in chronic myeloid leukemia. N Engl J Med 2001; 344:1084–1086.
109. Chaudry A, Papanicolaou V, Öberg K, Heldin CH, Funa K. Expression of platelet-derived growth factor and its receptors in neuroendocrine tumors of the digestive system. Cancer Res 1992; 52:1006–1012.
110. Dennis PB, Fumagalli s, Thomas G. Target of rapamycin (TOR): balancing the opposing forces of protein synthesis and degradation. Curr Opin Genet Dev 1999; 9:49–54.

Index